CONTENTS

Maternal-Infant Nursing Care

THIRD EDITION

Maternal-Infant Nursing Care

ELIZABETH JEAN DICKASON RN, MA, MED

Professor Emeritus,
Queensborough Community College,
Bayside, New York;
Nurse Consultant,
East Chatham, New York

BONNIE LANG SILVERMAN RNC, MS, NNP,
PHD CANDIDATE

School of Public Health and Health Sciences,
Department of Epidemiology and Biostatistics,
University of Massachusetts at Amherst,
Amherst, Massachusetts

JUDITH A. KAPLAN RN, ACCE, PHD

Assistant Professor, Nursing,
Nassau Community College,
Garden City, New York

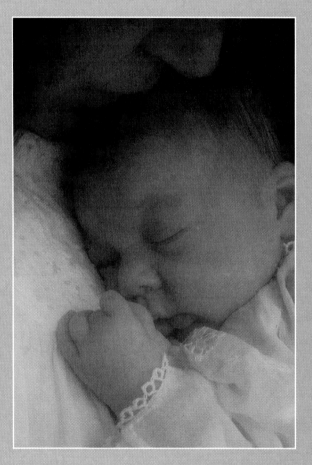

with 668 illustrations

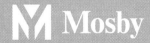

St. Louis Baltimore Boston Carlsbad Chicago Naples New York Philadelphia Portland
London Madrid Mexico City Singapore Sydney Tokyo Toronto Wiesbaden

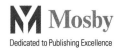

Mosby
Dedicated to Publishing Excellence

A Times Mirror
Company

Vice President and Publisher: Nancy L. Coon
Editor: Michael S. Ledbetter
Developmental Editor: Nancy L. O'Brien
Project Manager: Dana Peick
Production Editor: Dottie Martin
Manuscript Editors: Dan Begley, Dottie Martin
Designer: Amy Buxton
Manufacturing Manager: Betty Mueller
Cover Art: SuperStock, Inc.

A NOTE TO THE READER:
The author and publisher have made every attempt to check dosages and nursing content for accuracy. Because the science of pharmacology is continually advancing, our knowledge base continues to expand. Therefore we recommend that the reader always check product information for changes in dosage or administration before administering any medication. This is particularly important with new or rarely used drugs.

Printed in the United States of America
Composition by Accu-color, Inc.
Printing/binding by Von Hoffmann Press

Mosby–Year Book, Inc.
11830 Westline Industrial Drive
St. Louis, Missouri 63146

Library of Congress Cataloging-in-Publication Data

Dickason, Elizabeth J.
    Maternal-infant nursing care / Elizabeth Jean Dickason, Bonnie
Lang Silverman, Judith Kaplan. — 3rd ed.
      p. cm.
    Includes bibliographical references and index.
    ISBN 0-8151-2517-8
    1. Maternity nursing. 2. Pediatric nursing. 3. Family nursing.
I. Silverman, Bonnie Lang. II. Kaplan, Judith, RN, PhD.
III. Title.
    [DNLM: 1. Maternal-Child Nursing. WY 157.3 D547m 1997]
RG951.D53 1997
610.73'678–dc21
DNLM/DLC   97-10756
for Library of Congress   CIP

97 98 99 00 01 / 9 8 7 6 5 4 3 2 1

Contributors

Camille Bodden, MS, RN
Assistant Professor,
Department of Nursing,
Queensborough Community College,
Bayside, New York
Chapters 13 and 15

Carolyn D'Avanzo, DNSc, RN
Assistant Professor,
Women's Health, Health Promotion
  Unit,
School of Nursing,
University of Connecticut,
Storrs, Connecticut
Chapter 2

Darlene M. Del Prato, MS, RNC
Faculty, Maternal-Child Nursing,
School of Nursing,
St. Joseph's Hospital Health Center,
Syracuse, New York
Chapter 26

Madeline Hogan, MS, RN
Instructor,
Maternal and Child Nursing,
Nassau Community College,
Garden City, New York
Chapters 3, 4, 17

Beth A. Iovanne, MSN, RNC, NNP
Neonatal Nurse Practitioner,
Lawrence & Memorial Hospital,
New London, Connecticut
Chapter 29

Nancy V. Jackson, EdD, RN
Clinical Associate Professor,
Division of Nursing,
New York University,
New York, New York
Chapters 18, 19, 20

Suwersh Khanna, EdD, RNC
Assistant Professor,
School of Nursing,
Pace University,
Pleasantville, New York
Chapter 23

Ann Marie Menendez, MSN, RNCS
Assistant Professor,
Department of Nursing,
Queensborough Community College,
Bayside, New York
Chapter 8

Barbara A. Redding, MS, EdD, RN
Associate Professor,
College of Nursing,
University of South Florida,
Tampa, Florida
Chapter 27

Toni Ross, PhD, PNP, RN
HIV Clinical Scholar,
Mount Sinai Medical Center,
New York, New York
Chapter 25

Mary Ann Shea, JD, RN
Attorney at Law,
Midwest Medical/Legal Services,
St. Louis, Missouri
Chapter 30

Kathleen Rice Simpson, MSN, RNC
Perinatal Clinical Nurse Specialist,
St. John's Mercy Medical Center,
St. Louis, Missouri
Chapter 14

Francine Stier, MA, RN
Childbirth Educator,
Mount Sinai Hospital,
Hartford, Connecticut
Chapters 5 and 6

Consultants

Carol M. Arnold, MS, RN, ACCE
Assistant Clinical Professor,
Texas Woman's University,
Dallas, Texas

Eugenia Sawyer Barrington, BS, BSN, MPH, RN
Associate Professor,
Texarkana College,
Texarkana, Texas

Joea E. Bierchen, RN, BSN, MSN, EdD, FNP
Professor Emeritus,
St. Petersburg Junior College,
St. Petersburg, Florida

Alice Day, BS, MS, RN
Assistant Professor,
South Georgia College,
Douglas, Georgia

Sylvia Delaney, MS, RN, IBCLC
Clinical Nurse Specialist,
Lactation Consultant,
Long Island Jewish Medical Center,
New Hyde Park, New York

Kathleen Didominicis, BSN, MSN, RN
Professor of Nursing,
Moraine Valley Community College,
Palos Hills, Illinois

Dustine N. Dix, MS, RN
Clinical Instructor,
University of North Carolina-Chapel Hill,
Chapel Hill, North Carolina

Denise D. Estridge, BSN, MPH, RN
Nursing Instructor,
Guilford Technical Community College,
Jamestown, North Carolina

Polly D. Fehler, AS, BSN, MSN, RN
Instructor of Nursing,
Tri-County Technical College,
Pendleton, South Carolina

Lynn R. Grommet, MNSc, RNC
Faculty,
East Arkansas Community College,
Forrest City, Arkansas

Linda Hildenbrand, RN, BSN, MS
Hagerstown Junior College,
Hagerstown, Maryland

Judith J. Hilton, MSN, RNC
Assistant Professor of Nursing,
Lenoir-Rhyne College,
Hickory, North Carolina

Marilyn Hurt, MSN, RN
Garland Community Hospital,
Garland, Texas

Patricia M. Jacobson, BSN, MSN, RN
Nursing Instructor,
Bullard Havens Regional Vocational-Technical School,
Bridgeport, Connecticut

Jill Janke, ANP, DNSc, RN
Associate Professor,
School of Nursing and Health Sciences,
University of Alaska-Anchorage,
Anchorage, Alaska

Karyn London, PA
HIV Clinical Scholar,
Adult AIDS Clinic,
Mount Sinai Medical Center,
New York, New York

Diane B. Longobucco, MSN, RNC, APRN
Clinical Nurse Specialist,
Women and Children Services,
St. Francis Hospital and Medical Center,
Hartford, Connecticut

Valerie Scott Massimo, MSW, DOCTORAL CANDIDATE
SUNY-Rockefeller College of Social Welfare;
Adoption Training Specialist,
New York State Department of Social Services,
Albany, New York

Carol F. Metcalf, MPH, RN
Truckee Meadows Community College,
Reno, Nevada

Patricia L. Nash, RNC, MSN, NNP
NNP Manager,
Cardinal Glennon Children's Hospital,
St. Louis, Missouri

Patti Fern Nicks, MSN, RN
Nursing Faculty,
Angelina College,
Lufkin, Texas

Linda D. O'Boyle, BS, MS, RNC, EdD
Associate Professor,
Barton College,
Wilson, North Carolina

Winifred A. Olmstead, MSN, RN
Faculty, School of Nursing,
Saint Joseph's Hospital Health Center,
Syracuse, New York

Linda L. Putsché, MS, RNC
Assistant Professor,
The Union Memorial Hospital School of Nursing,
Baltimore, Maryland

Rosemary Scarangella, MEd, RNC, OGNP
Nurse Practitioner,
Planned Parenthood;
Assistant Professor,
Nassau Community College,
Garden City, New York

Sharleen H. Simpson, MSN, MA, PhD, ARNP
Associate Professor,
University of Florida,
Gainesville, Florida

Cheryl A. Smith, MSN, RNC
Lead Nurse, Perinatal Clinician,
Women's Health Services,
DeKalb County Board of Health,
Lithonia, Georgia

Jean E. Staffeld, BSN, MEd, RN
Instructor,
Providence Hospital School of Nursing,
Sandusky, Ohio

Sue A. Tedford, MNSc, RN
Level III Coordinator,
Jefferson School of Nursing,
Pine Bluff, Arkansas

Sue G. Thacker, AS, BSN, MS
Associate Professor,
Wytheville Community College,
Wytheville, Virginia

Colleen E. Tracy, MS, RN
Nursing Instructor,
Anoka Ramsey Community College;
Staff Nurse,
Fairview-Riverside Medical Center,
Minneapolis, Minnesota

Mary Starkey Wallace, MSN, RN
Chairperson, ADN Program,
Wallace State College,
Hanceville, Alabama

Celesta L. Warner, BSN, MS, RN
Instructor,
Wright State University-Miami Valley College of Nursing
  and Health,
Dayton, Ohio

Donna Wilsker, BSN, MSN, RN
Assistant Professor of Nursing,
Lamar University-Beaumont,
Beaumont, Texas

Preface

Nursing care today must be focused on assessment of body systems in order to plan interventions and on education for self-care by the mother for both herself and her infant. Short hospital stays have become the dominant influence in how maternal and infant nursing care is delivered. Home care before and after birth is still unstandardized. Women have to manage all their care, often stumbling along. Because of managed care policies, it appears that care for women has taken steps backward. Additional alternatives need to be created, and the most viable of these is increased client education for self-care.

Therefore a nursing text for a changing environment must prepare a nursing practitioner for new roles, emphasizing assessment, client education, and home care. The nurse must thoroughly understand the normal progression of pregnancy and childbirth to identify, plan, and intervene for the health care requirements of pregnant clients. To promote this understanding and to emphasize that childbearing is a normal and natural process, the complete normal cycle of pregnancy, labor, and birth is first presented. The student who comprehends the normal processes and patterns is best prepared to identify the complications that may occur and thus implement the appropriate nursing interventions.

Of particular importance in maternity nursing is the impact of the client's cultural background and family. The nurse must be aware of the cultural influence and family dynamics to identify specific needs and to develop an individualized plan of care. Cultural considerations and family interactions are woven throughout the text beginning in Chapter 2, in which three ethnic groups are discussed in detail.

The client must be considered as the *person-in-environment* before any planning takes place. Unless the students can learn to listen attentively—separating their own needs and biases from those of the clients—their planning will be superficial.

STRUCTURE

This text is clinically oriented. Care plans and reality-based nursing planning engage the student in interaction with "the way things are." Frank discussion of the socioeconomic risk factors of sexually transmitted diseases (STDs), substance abuse, spouse abuse, poverty, and powerlessness will find echoes in real life situations. The stu-

dent is challenged to become involved in seeking changes in routine health care, which often misses the real needs of the high-risk client.

In spite of the universality of the childbearing and parenting experience and the health needs of families in our society, maternal and infant nursing often has been taught in brief courses. The sequence of this text is structured so that it can be used in a short course. The text proceeds from women's health care through the normal, usual experiences of pregnancy, birth, and recovery. Once this foundation has been established, the student can quickly grasp the physiologic basis of complications. Thus, in an *integrated* curriculum, this structure facilitates the use of pregnancy complications in discussion of body system alterations within medical-surgical nursing courses.

Traditionally, maternity texts have been locked into the time sequence of trimesters, divisions derived from an outdated way of viewing care. The sequence that is based on body system adaptation to pregnancy or complications has more validity because most problems of pregnancy begin before or early in the pregnancy. For each complication of pregnancy, the physiology of the body system is reviewed and rationales for alterations are explained.

Several main threads are woven throughout the text. Physical assessment is stressed consistently as the basis of data collection before planning. The nursing process serves as a structural framework.

The collaborative role of nursing is recognized, and delineation of nursing and medical functions is noted. **Clinical Management** in each area delineates the overlapping role of medicine, midwifery, and nursing, and **Nursing Responsiblities** separate the nursing role. Pharmacologic factors that change during both pregnancy and lactation are discussed in detail in Chapter 16 and in the **Drug Profiles** throughout the text that contain the most current information on drugs commonly used in pregnancy and childbirth. Infection is now a major concern, and the most up-to-date information on STDs and other perinatal infections is discussed in Chapter 25, while universal precautions are emphazied in each area of care.

Finally, legal aspects are covered in specific detail, especially the accountability for documentation. The high rate of litigation in perinatal care requires that students understand the responsiblity for ensuring both maternal and fetal health. Chapter 14 emphasizes accountability in monitoring labor progress, and Chapter 30 reviews the legal and ethical aspects of nursing in this area.

FEATURES

Our goal has been to make this text a tool for which both teaching and learning are made easy. The text is interactive, that is, the student is engaged in responding to the material and in developing decision-making capabilities, rather than just memorizing data. This is a user-friendly learning guide for students. For example, features start with easy readability. **Learning Objectives** are listed at the beginning of each chapter to provide the reader with a basic guide to the major points in the chapter. **Key Terms** are defined on first use, highlighted to reinforce student learning, and tested at the end of each chapter. Definitions to most of the key terms are included in the glossary. **Key Points** end each chapter, reviewing major points and guiding students to make connections and synthesize information. Finally, more than 600 full-color illustrations enhance understanding of anatomy and physiology, assessment, nursing skills, and procedures and birth sequences.

Additional learning tools include these features:

Research boxes remind the student that nursing must contribute to the development of criterion-based research and base its practice on valid findings.

Procedures important for specific areas of nursing care are outlined in many chapters.

Nursing Care Plans are based on real cases and are guides for the student, not to copy but to refer to in making their own plans.

Decision Trees are created when nursing decisions must be rapid and complex. These are created for nonreassuring fetal heart rate patterns, preterm labor, gestational diabetes, infant resuscitation, and accidental injury during pregnancy.

Care Paths sometimes replace care plans in hospital settings, therefore three Care Paths are given as guidelines in labor, recovery from cesarean birth, and care of the newborn.

Cultural Awareness boxes contain brief discussions of cultural variations the student might encounter in maternity nursing.

Self-Discovery boxes are included in many chapters when content personally affects a student who may be learning for the first time "the way things work" in sexuality, family planning, pregnancy, childbirth, and parenting. Self-Discovery boxes highlight personal questions to consider and perhaps record in a journal.

Student Resource Shelf follows each chapter reference list to guide the student toward further reading. References are annotated.

Test Yourself feedback questions are found throughout each chapter. Students who cannot answer the questions should reread the material immediately preceding each box. Selected answers are provided in the Appendix.

Study Questions are located at the end of each chapter, and answers immediately follow.

Clinical Decisions are found throughout the text to help the student think about decision making in novel situations. These can be used in classes or conferences as open-ended discussion topics. When possible, suggested answers are in the Appendix.

TEACHING-LEARNING PACKAGE

A number of ancillary products for both instructors and students are offered with this text.

An **Instructor's Resource Manual** is designed to help faculty develop lectures, reinforce teaching through classroom and clinical activites, and evaluate student comprehension. This valuable resource includes lecture outlines, chapter overviews, core learning activities, and enrichment activities for a better student. Each unit includes a short-answer quiz.

A **Test Bank** contains more than 500 test questions with an answer key, correlated with page numbers and degree of difficulty. This test bank is included in the Instructor's Manual and is also available electronically in Microtest III, using Computest for the PC format. The disk is accompanied by a users' guide. Computest allows intructors to edit, add, delete, or select questions on the computer before printing out the test.

A **Student Learning Guide** contains suggestions for journal entries, learning activities, case studies, crossword puzzles, and quizzes to reinforce student learning. The material in this guide is also included in the Instructor's Resource Manual.

Overhead Transparencies are provided for 40 of the full-color illustrations from the text, helping instructors to assist classroom learning.

The authors of this text seek to enhance the nursing student's grasp of the field of maternal and infant nursing care. Remembering that pregnancy and birth affect all members of the family, the student is encouraged to gain an understanding of care for each person in her context and her environment.

TO THE STUDENT

You will enjoy reading this text because it is user-friendly. Your maternity course will be short and filled with new experiences. You will interact with these experiences and often be tempted to personalize what is happening. To sort out feelings and reactions, this is a good time to start a personal journal. Record your ideas, experiences, and feelings. Some students keep the last pages of their lecture notebook as personal record; others keep a diary. To help you get started, reflection questions called **Self-Discovery** are

marked with the symbol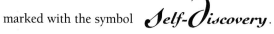

Clinical Decisions help you develop skills to make decisions. A short client situation is given for which there may be several answers. Discuss these together with classmates or in conference. Some of these have suggested answers in the Appendix.

Test Yourself questions are found throughout each chapter. The questions check if you understood the preceding paragraphs. Try to answer them before checking the answers supplied in the Appendix.

Study Questions end each chapter. The first question tests your knowledge of the key terms in the chapter. Answers are immediately following the study questions.

Key Points **Key Points** can be used to summarize the chapter. Turn these into questions, and see if you are clear about the answers.

Student Resource Shelf contains annotated references especially relevant to a student who wishes to learn more about a subject that has been discussed in the chapter.

There are also **Drug Profiles**, marked with the symbol

, that summarize the major drugs you will use in maternity and infant care.

Research Boxes, indicated with the symbol ,

describe current research in specific areas. Remember that nursing must base its practice on valid research findings.

We live in a multicultural society and must learn how pregnancy and parenting are viewed by each cultural group with which we work. Look for **Cultural Awareness** boxes marked with the symbol . In your journal, record clinical situations in which, to allow good nursing care, cultural differences required specific knowledge.

The nursing process always guides our planning. Assessment must come first. This text emphasizes assessment of physical status and psychosocial needs. Only after learning the normal parameters can you learn to detect when things are going wrong. For this reason, too, the text begins with normal pregnancy and birth and then discusses how complications occur and are treated. The nursing process guides care planning and evaluation. Suggested diagnoses and outcomes are given for major care needs. You may use these, but the **Nursing Care Plan** is specific for the case that precedes it. Thus you may use these for a guide, but you need to individualize your own plans. Evaluation cannot be done unless answers to certain questions are sought. Therefore evaluation in this text always is in the form of questions to be answered. Learn to ask the *right* questions. You will also find **Care Paths** and **Decision Trees**—methods used in hospital settings to guide care.

Nursing accountability is emphasized because childbirth places two clients at risk. Legal issues and documentation of nursing activity are major emphases in the material you will be learning. For instance, fetal monitoring and assessment are involved in two thirds of the litigation in this area; failure to monitor correctly or to document or report changes often is the basis of a legal charge against a nurse. For this reason, even while a student, you must learn the patterns that signal nonreassuring fetal responses.

Finally, ethical issues and care of socially high-risk women will involve you in debate about "what is right" in maternity care. Our care depends on recognition of discrimination in quality of care for the affluent and for those in poverty. Nurses are learning to be advocates for their clients and to produce models of care for high-risk women that include creative problem solving.

Sometimes you may feel overwhelmed by the mass of material a textbook must include. Concentrate on learning basic anatomy and physiology of the pregnant woman and the newborn. Then, subsequent variations leading to complications will be easier to understand. Our goal is to assist you in building the basis for competence in caregiving, which is your goal.

Acknowledgments

A collaborative work depends on the efforts of many people: the authors of each section, the editors, and the production and art and design personnel. This text is indeed a result of the creative process for which there were many ideas and discussions.

First, we particularly want to thank our nursing students who shaped our teaching methods because they freely interacted with the content and with their clients. Readers of the manuscript helped clarify content by asking the question, "What does the student of maternity and infant nursing care need to know?"

Illustrations were generously shared by Fredda Diamond; St. John's Mercy Medical Center, St. Louis; Baby-Think-It-Over, Eau Claire, Wisconsin; Corometrics, Wallingford, Connecticut; PPG Medical Systems, Pleasantville, New York; March of Dimes Birth Defects Foundation, White Plains, New York; Ross Laboratories, Columbus, Ohio; Mead Johnson Company, Evansville,

Indiana; Oxford Instruments, Oxon, England; American Cancer Society, Atlanta; American Heart Association, Dallas; and Community Health and Family Planning Council, New York.

Many illustrations are modified from classics in the field. Derivative work is seen today, but the forefathers and foremothers shaped our thinking, and we have chosen to reproduce their work. Photographers include Camille Bodden, Brian Hopewell, James Suddath, Mark Sick, John Young, R.O. Roberson, Richard Silverman, Rollie Trapp, Martha Schult, Victoria Langer, Marjorie Pyle, RNC, of *Lifecircle,* Costa Mesa, California, and Michael S. Clement, MD, of Mesa, Arizona.

The creation of a text of this complexity would not be possible without the full support of the editorial, production, and art and design staff. Thanks go to Michael Ledbetter, our editor; Nancy O'Brien, our developmental editor; Dana Peick, our project manager; Dottie Martin, our production editor; and Amy Buxton, our designer.

Finally, many families participated by sharing experiences and photographs. Special thanks to the Suddath, Livingstone, Hopewell, Bodden, Schult, Roberson, Trapp, and Silverman families.

We are indeed indebted to our computers and to our families who supported this endeavor to its fullest.

Elizabeth Jean Dickason
Bonnie Lang Silverman
Judith A. Kaplan
with Martha Olson Schult

Contents

UNIT *Two*

PREGNANCY

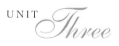

UNIT *Three*

LABOR, BIRTH & RECOVERY

UNIT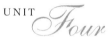

NEWBORN CARE

UNIT *Five*

PREGNANCY AT RISK

UNIT *Six*

NEWBORN AT RISK

UNIT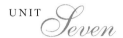

MATERNAL-INFANT NURSING ISSUES

One

Foundations *of* Maternal-Infant Nursing

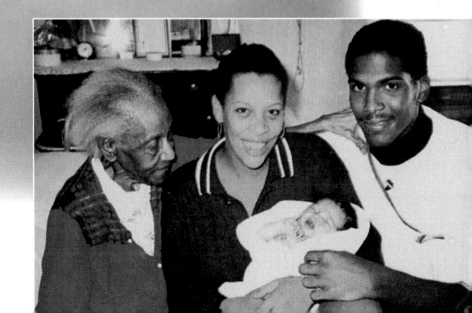

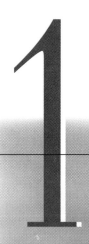

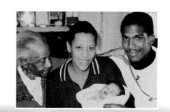

1. Contemporary Maternal-Infant Nursing Care

Learning Objectives

- Describe four trends in delivery of maternity and infant care.
- Identify examples of community and professional standards of care.
- Identify sources of resistance to full participation in family-centered maternity care.
- Differentiate between independent and collaborative nursing functions.
- Define steps used in the formation of a nursing diagnosis.
- Discuss socioeconomic and educational factors that result in better provision of prenatal care.
- Discuss problems contributing to maternal and infant morbidity and mortality.
- List four components of informed consent, comparing the nurse's and physician's roles in obtaining consent.

Key Terms

Assault
Battery
Clinical Nurse Specialist
Community Standards of Care
Emancipated Minor
Informed Consent
Malpractice
Morbidity
Mortality
Negligence
Neonatal
Nurse Entrepreneur
Nurse Practitioner
Perinatal
Prenatal Abuse
Professional Standards of Care

GOAL OF CARE

The goal of maternal and infant nursing care is the birth of a healthy infant into a family able to parent appropriately. This text assumes that childbearing is a developmental challenge for the woman and her family. The birth of an infant always changes things. Life will be different for the parents because the patterns of their relationship will change. These changes are especially felt when the first child is born.

With the birth of an infant, some parents feel more in touch with a spiritual dimension, brought about by the wonder at new life. When things go well, there is awe and a sense of joy. Because the spiritual dimension is tapped, if technologic or physiologic problems occur, fear and anxiety may seem more intense for the parents.

Family Coping

Family coping will always be tested in pregnancy and parenting. There is the potential for growth in family relationships or the possibility of distancing from the perceived problem. Usually only the woman is seen during health care visits. Often it is not until problems arise that health care personnel inquire about the father's adaptation.

No one should assume that parenting is a natural skill developed through instinct. Children learn to parent by

2

watching their own parents. When role models are inadequate, however, conflict may exist among the new parents' societal expectations, their own needs, and their memories of "how to do it." The nurse must recognize that parents may have feelings of low self-esteem and guilt because of their own ideas of what a good parent is. Regardless of the situation, these parents need support in their efforts to raise children.

Individual Coping

An individual is expected to accomplish specific tasks associated with the developmental age. If these tasks are achieved, the individual can progress to the next growth task and mature with some degree of competence and self-esteem. Application of this concept to parenthood can help the nurse understand the ways in which parenthood conflicts with other circumstances in a person's life. Pregnancy and parenting can be considered a maturational crisis, presenting a challenge in learning how to cope. For example, an adolescent mother trying to establish her own identity may have difficulty focusing on the needs of her infant, or woman in the midst of a career challenge may feel a conflict between self-actualization through her work and through parenting.

Every effort must be made to support the parent. It is said that the new mother needs to be mothered so she can mother. This statement can be extended to include both parents. Smoyak (1977) states:

> Children do not become normal adults unless nurtured in some type of close continuing social unit, where norms are clearly set, where self-esteem is fostered, and where separateness/connectedness issues are worked on openly and directly. The most important work of parents as socializing agents is to get each succeeding generation to want to go on. Parents, in one way or another, have to accomplish getting their children "hooked" on the idea of continuity. Simply put, they have to make it pleasant to be alive, and further, to suggest that one's "debt" for such pleasure is to pass it on to the next person or generation.

It is important for nurses not to personalize their own family history while working with childbearing families. The nursing student may find that much of the content of this course is personally meaningful. However, each childbearing family is unique. Culture and structure of the family need to be considered before plans are made by health care personnel. While learning the support role of the nurse, remember to focus on discovering the environmental and psychosocial forces affecting families. These forces may contribute to parents' ways of reacting to stress. In addition, some parents do not respond in positive ways to pregnancy or to their children. The increasing incidence of elective abortion, child abuse, and child neglect must be a concern of all health professionals. Chapter 2 introduces the family in its context.

As a maternity nurse, it is important to communicate and interact with families during the stressful time of pregnancy. Differences in developmental level, culture, value systems, socioeconomic status, and education all influence the way in which people react to the process of childbearing and childrearing. Nursing interactions may help parents identify special characteristics of their infant, form a parent-child bond, and facilitate acceptance of their child and their role as a parent. Because nurses often have limited time to spend with the childbearing family, it is essential to involve other members of the health team to maximize the benefits associated with these interactions.

Klaus and Kennell (1982) identified specific behaviors that parents demonstrate in early attachment with their newborn. These bonding or attachment behaviors include skin-to-skin contact and eye contact. It is important for the nurse to observe these interactions and intervene when the parent appears to be hesitant or frightened. Chapter 8 explains the process of bonding in detail, and Chapter 20 discusses ways of working with parents as they learn to understand their child's patterns of growth and development.

Factors Influencing Goal Achievement

To achieve the goal of supporting healthy childbearing, the following information is useful in determining if any problems interfere with a positive outcome for the pregnancy or birth:

1. Know the positive or harmful environmental factors influencing family functioning.
2. Assess the state of the family's emotional and physical health.
3. Know if there are genetic or environmental factors that may harm the infant.
4. Assess whether the family has reasonable access to adequate health care during and after pregnancy.
5. Assess whether the parents have access to childbirth preparation classes.
6. Identify if there are any complications during pregnancy that will affect maternal or fetal condition or the newborn infant.
7. Determine what the mother has experienced during labor and birth and how she is recovering.
8. Have an idea of how much informed common sense about childrearing the parents bring to the process.
9. Know if there are unusual financial, social, psychologic, or physical constraints that prevent caring for the infant.

TRENDS IN MATERNAL-INFANT CARE

Recent trends in maternal-infant care include regionalization, managed care, critical pathways, community standards of care, rising cesarean birth rates, cost containment, early discharge, and effects of diagnosis-related groups.

Regionalization

Complications that may occur after birth may result in transferring the neonate to a tertiary care hospital. Separation of the neonate from the family creates a more stressful situation in which parents may demonstrate a grief response or inadequate coping mechanisms. Therefore before the birth, a mother at risk may be transferred to a tertiary (large, centrally located) medical center. At these facilities, high-risk infants are born in an area adjacent to a neonatal intensive care unit (NICU), thus eliminating the need to transport the infants after birth. This trend is called *regionalization* and has lowered infant death rates. It includes the trend of some small hospitals closing their maternity services because their back-up care for high-risk infants and mothers was not adequate.

Managed Care

To ensure the health of clients and avoid the high costs of specialists and hospitalizations, there is a trend toward *managed care*. Managed care provides a structure for continuous delivery of health services that includes services such as case management, health and nutrition education, and transportation. For example, a managed care prenatal program may include a preconception program that provides risk assessment, contraception counseling, immunizations, and health promotion education. Client education is tailored to meet the diversity of age, culture, and education levels. Case management promotes improved health outcomes thereby decreasing health costs (McKnight and Burns, 1994).

Critical Pathways

Nurses are the health care providers who are most consistently at the client's bedside. To enhance client-centered care, nurses have developed guidelines known as critical pathways. These "health care maps" guide nurses and clients through the most direct course of treatment. Specific tasks or outcomes are marked at certain timed points. Areas for data collection and documentation can also be included. By helping clients and staff identify necessary goals, client satisfaction increases and staff frustration decreases. Critical pathways have been proved cost efficient by decreasing length of hospitalization and increasing quality of care. Critical pathways include interventions from other disciplines and departments such as social work, home care, pharmacy, and dietary (Grayson, 1993; McGregor, 1994). In this text such pathways are called "Care Maps."

Community Standards of Care

Transport of known high-risk mothers before birth and all at-risk infants when stabilized after birth is standard care for almost all community hospitals now. **Community standards of care** are criteria expected from practitioners working in a particular setting or geographic area. These standards develop through time and are subject to improvement.

Use of technologies such as fetal monitoring and ultrasound is now a community standard of care. Community standards of care always are considered in legal action; therefore physicians are hesitant to omit any step in treatment of the pregnant woman. As a result, sometimes the client may be made to feel that she must comply with multiple examinations when she would prefer not to do so.

Rising Cesarean Birth Rates

With the use of fetal monitoring and ultrasound for prenatal evaluation of fetal condition has come an increased rate of cesarean births, which has the following positive aspects: (1) distressed infants are rescued before potential injury occurs, and (2) maternal mortality and morbidity may be prevented. Negative aspects include: (1) potential complications of surgery and anesthesia, (2) high cost, (3) maternal discomfort from a potentially unnecessary operation, and (4) grief related to the loss of the "natural" delivery experience. Federal health planners have called for a serious attempt to reduce the numbers of repeat cesarean births. Today a trial of vaginal birth after cesarean (VBAC) is recommended if conditions permit.

Increased Cost of High-Technologic Care

As the medical profession has developed increasingly sophisticated technology, costs have escalated. For example, the minimum cost for an ultrasound screening is more than $300. This examination may be repeatedly ordered, along with fetal monitoring, for a woman who is in the last weeks of her pregnancy if there is question of a problem. In fact, today maternity care is a lucrative business, and several hospitals in the same location may compete to attract clients. Hospitals will advertise, provide tours, and seek client evaluation of services (Box 1-1).

At the same time, cost containment is an important trend in health care. Early discharge with home care is becoming more common. Cost containment changes the way nurses plan the care for the mother. Home care has been included in the text for this reason (see Chapters 17 and 20).

Early Discharge

Just 40 years ago, a woman was hospitalized for 7 days after birth. Bed rest was maintained for 3 days, and physical activity was increased gradually, throughout a long period. Recovery was called *confinement*. Through the years, however, health care personnel have realized that early return to normal activities is the best course for uncomplicated births. In the 1980s most mothers were

▌ *Box* 1-1   **Sample Advertising Descriptions of Hospital Birth Settings in One City**

SETTING 1: PRIVATE HOSPITAL
Labor-delivery-recovery and postrecovery (LDRP) rooms. All rooms have TV, VCR, stereo, CD player, refrigerator, sofa bed, and private bathroom with whirlpool tub for use during labor.

SETTING 2: HEALTH MAINTENANCE ORGANIZATION (HMO)-RUN HOSPITAL
Users of HMO (only) can have normal birth in labor, delivery, and recovery rooms. Pastel decorated space with

TV, sofa bed, maple furniture, and view of the river. After 1 day, transfer to semiprivate family-centered unit.

SETTING 3: UNIVERSITY HOSPITAL CENTER
Spare surroundings but the place for high-risk pregnancies and births. Labor in shared rooms with TV and chair. Move to delivery room, then to mother-baby unit for recovery. Praised for expert nursing care and best neonatal intensive care (one of only two units in the city).

---

hospitalized for 3 to 4 days for normal vaginal delivery and 5 to 7 days for cesarean births. Currently, many mothers are discharged after 12 to 24 hours for normal vaginal delivery and by the fourth postpartum day following an uncomplicated cesarean birth (McGregor, 1994).

Effects of Diagnosis-Related Groups

Some women request early discharge because they are well prepared for self-care or because of financial constraints. Others may be discharged early because of the rules of *diagnosis-related groups* (DRGs). These groups assign a predetermined number of days deemed, first by federal government guidelines and now by many private insurance companies, as essential for hospital treatment of a particular condition and for which the hospital will receive payment. However, not all clients fit into these established categories, and therefore some persons may be slated for discharge before they are ready. Others are discharged early because they do not qualify for assistance and have no insurance. Several states are reconsidering such early discharge and have passed legislation requiring insurance companies to pay for a full 48 hours of care after vaginal delivery.

Implications for nursing care

Although DRG guidelines allow 2.7 days for an uncomplicated vaginal birth and 4.3 days for a cesarean birth, many insurance companies are urging doctors toward earlier client discharge. Before, nurses had at least 2 to 3 days to evaluate recovery and to prepare parents as primary care givers. If women go home during critical recovery time, they must express needs, learn lessons, assimilate information, and prove comprehension by return demonstrations in a brief time. Therefore it is essential that nurses act as advocates for women and children, participate in the development of health care policies, and develop new approaches to physical assessment, psychosocial evaluation, and teaching (Wood and Ransem,

1994). Prenatal education is essential in reducing the need for formal postpartum classes. Prenatal and postdelivery inclusion of the father in this teaching is essential in preventing the mother from being overloaded with information and responsibilities and ensuring that he is not left out of the planning process.

Home care

Early discharge with home care is common and is an effective way to follow through on immediate postbirth care. Some health care centers have developed comprehensive follow-up care; others provide visits only to adolescent mothers or those with psychosocial or medical problems. In situations when women are not supported by extended families, if they are sent home before they are fully recovered or before they understand how to care for the infant, the first few weeks at home can be difficult. Home care is an area where **nurse entrepreneurs** are developing independent practice because some area institutions have not yet developed good home monitoring or follow-up care.

T E S T *Yourself* 1-1 _____

a. Explain how managed care influences the outcomes for the pregnant client.
b. List three disadvantages to early (24 hour) discharge of the maternity client.

FAMILY-CENTERED MATERNITY CARE

The postpartum unit and newborn nursery were once separate areas. Infants stayed in the nursery, except during feeding, and were cared for by neonatal nurses. Because of greater emphasis on parents' rights and their need to learn primary care of the infant, the concept of *rooming-in* was introduced. Rooming-in allows the mother-infant dyad to stay in the same room for an extended period. Benefits include feeding the infant on demand and facilitating the attachment process. Nurses have a greater opportunity to observe the parent caring for their newborn thus promoting childcare teaching and providing assistance as necessary (Weiss and Armstrong, 1991).

The rooming-in concept has been revised in the philosophy of *family-centered maternity care* (FCMC). In this framework, the mother and child are considered a unit, a *dyad,* with one nurse assigned to their primary care. Within FCMC, infant assessments are performed at the bedside with maternal checks. Parents are encouraged to record feeding times and amounts and voiding and stooling patterns. In this way, although the nurse is still responsible for determining the stability of the newborn, the parents begin to see the factors involved in their child's care. They become aware of sleep patterns and are more comfortable with the newborn's behavior. Because parents have fewer nurses with whom to relate, they may be freer to ask for and obtain assistance, reassurance, and instruction. Care of the mother-infant dyad has been demonstrated to be efficient and effective. Breastfeeding is enhanced in this setting (Figure 1-1). Wide surveys have proven FCMC to be the most effective means of postbirth care for mother and infant (Enkin et al, 1995).

Box 1-1

CLINICAL DECISION

Observe the policies of the institution with which you are familiar. If FCMC is not used, why? Is the rationale client or administration centered?

Many hospitals have rebuilt or constructed new family-centered units where the partner and sometimes siblings may join the mother during all or part of the birth process. In a *labor-delivery-recovery* (LDR) *room,* the woman is not moved from place to place during the labor process, but once settled in her room, she completes the birth there (when all is normal) and spends a few hours of recovery in the same room with the infant at her side. Where the census of births is not too high, some units have LDRP rooms, labor-delivery-recovery and postrecovery (or postpartum) rooms in which the woman stays for the entire hospital period. This LDRP plan usually is not feasible in a unit with a high census.

Homelike Birth Settings

In some states, clients may choose a more homelike birth setting outside of the hospital. Certified nurse- and lay-midwives actually may monitor the birth in the woman's home. Or, with her partner, siblings, and friends, she may come to a birthing center to be assisted by a nurse-

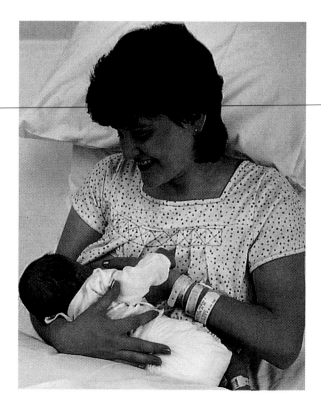

Figure 1-1 Breastfeeding is enhanced in facilities using family-centered maternity care. (Courtesy Ross Laboratories, Columbus, Ohio.)

midwife. These freestanding centers have back-up assistance available from an adjacent hospital if problems occur during the birth process. The client in such a center usually will go home within 12 to 24 hours. In addition, women who elect home or birthing center births are screened for potential problems before the decision is made. High-risk pregnancies need the more extensive resources of a hospital.

Fathers

Traditionally, the father was an observer during the intrapartum period. Not only was he an inactive participant in the birth event but also he was not permitted in the delivery area. Today, the picture is different. Most fathers choose to participate in childbirth preparation classes, which allows them to be a vital part of the process, supporting the mother during birth. With increased societal emphasis on shared parenting and the recognition of paternal bonding, many fathers are active in care giving and enjoy the closeness it brings. Almost universally, hospitals have an open visiting policy for fathers. Fathers are involved in infant care classes and are instructed with the mothers.

Although many cultures encourage the father's participation in the entire birth event, many do not. For example,

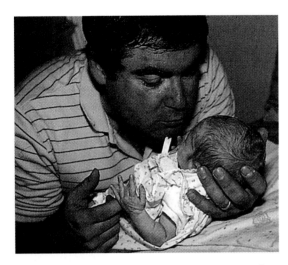

Figure 1-2 Father involvement is to be encouraged in family-centered maternity care. (Courtesy Marjorie Pyle, RNC, *Lifecircle.*)

traditionally, it was considered improper and unacceptable for Asian men to be with their wives during childbirth. Other societies see it as unmasculine to be involved in "women's business." Care must be taken to respect each person's feelings and not impose one's own values while giving encouragement and support.

The nurse who has developed rapport with a father reluctant to be in the labor or birthing area may effect significant change by being supportive. The FCMC setting encourages the father to share the birth experience, introduces the grandchild to the grandparents, and welcomes siblings to meet the new infant (Figure 1-2).

These changes promise a richer birth experience for the family, but they also create a challenge for nurses in maternity care. Because of the focus on promoting independence for the family, the nurse has a new role.

Directions for Maternity and Infant Care

The role of nursing is changing. Wood and Ransem (1994) described major trends in society, which include significant changes in health care. Nursing can grow as society shifts from an industrial to an information base. There is also a move toward self-help and networking in health care. Many options are presented when a care issue arises; a person no longer passively allows the first opinion to prevail. The search for alternative care options has become important. The nurse now functions as an integral member of the health care team working in a collaborative relationship with the physician and client.

Health information is available to almost everyone. The distribution of information about human immunodeficiency virus (HIV) infection, for example, has reached every household in the United States. The dis-tribution of complete health information still is uneven, yet clients are more knowledgeable than ever before. You will work with couples who have some knowledge but who always need additional knowledge so that they may care for their own needs.

The role of nursing in maternal and infant care is increasingly "high tech" yet needs to remain "high touch," illustrated by the nurse's role during the birth process. As a primary care provider, the nurse must determine what the family needs, participate in intensive technical monitoring, and give support. Coordination of care demands an ability to look beyond technical tasks to see the family. It is more important to be *holistic* in maternity nursing care and to not isolate the mother or infant from the rest of the family.

The nurse must promote self-monitoring, self-care, and infant care and nurturing. It is no longer enough to get the mother through recovery; she must also be helped in her new role as nurturer of the infant. It is essential for the nurse to integrate multicultural family theory into care during the childbearing cycle and find a personal balance between technical and educative-supportive care.

PUTTING THEORY INTO PRACTICE

Maternity nursing benefits from increased application of theory to practice. Nurses have a more consistent rationale for interventions than in the past. Nursing actions no longer come only from physicians' orders, although collaborative functions often are written on the order page.

A number of theoretic conceptual models are used to achieve a framework for nursing practice. Fawcett (1988) stated that "Conceptual models are ways of approaching a problem, a framework or context in which events may be viewed." You will recognize these models throughout the text. Research findings also are clarifying ways of practice. For example, the work of Klaus and Kennell on bonding theory has been one of the important changes directing maternal-infant care in the last decade. In addition, use of the nursing process has become a standard of care.

Nursing Research

Nursing research is concerned with the study and assessment of nursing problems or phenomena. Creative research studies enable nurses to find ways to improve nursing practice and client care. Nursing research can be qualitative, quantitative, or a combination of both methods. Qualitative research is concerned with describing phenomena through observation, historical documents, and content from interviews. Data are coded and analyzed to determine categories and major themes that may be used to develop nursing theory. Quantitative research involves controlled research methods that develop and test theories by examining relationships among variables. Data are analyzed through statistical means with acceptance or rejection of hypotheses. Both types of research are important and necessary to improve clinical practice, client care, and outcomes.

Research in parent-child health tends to focus on current priorities in the delivery of health care to childbearing families. For many years, there have been practices unsupported by careful research studies; practices ensured by custom and habit rather than a sound scientific basis. Now many of these practices are being questioned and research studies will determine whether actions are beneficial, ineffective, or actually harmful to the pregnant woman and her infant.

Abstracts and discussion of research studies concerned with childbearing are included throughout the text because nurses have a responsibility to stay current with what is being confirmed through research studies.

Professional Standards of Care

Many groups interested in maternal and child health have proposed standards of care. The American Nurses' Association (ANA) has developed standards of care for nursing in each specialty area. The Association of Women's Health, Obstetric, and Neonatal Nurses (AWHONN), formerly the Nurses Association of the American College of Obstetrics and Gynecology (NAACOG), has also detailed standards for each area. These standards are used when policies and procedures are formulated for an area of health care. Standards may be referred to as a guide for care and as a reference if a question of negligence arises. **Professional standards of care** are also changing, with greater demands on and accountability of the maternity nurse than ever before. (See Appendix 1B for perinatal standards).

As care becomes more technologically sophisticated, nurses are required to continue updating their knowledge and skills. For example, it is unacceptable for a nurse who is hired to work with women during labor to say, "I couldn't provide the care she needed because I didn't know how to do it." If a nurse is assigned to work in a specialized area, the hospital must provide orientation, and the nurse must study how to manage care and must insist on a supervised apprentice orientation period.

Obstetric nurses are *advocates for women*, often seeing that necessary referrals are done and that other personnel communicate clearly. Nurses may help smooth roadblocks in care services and ensure that treatments are fully understood while the client's rights are respected.

Physicians, Midwives, and Nurses

In maternity care, a special emphasis must be placed on collaborative relationships among physicians, midwives, and nurses. In many settings collegial relationships have developed during the last decade. As nursing theory is developed and nursing roles are clarified, there is hope that nurses will be assertive and professional in relationships with physicians and midwives so that quality care is made available to maternity clients.

Legal Obligations

A nurse caring for mothers and infants has a special need to give safe and competent care. The legal obligations of maternal-infant care have assumed a greater importance than in earlier decades because people are more knowledgeable and because there are two clients for whom suit may be brought. There also are many kinds of technology in use and options for care. Decisions may be made rapidly in changing situations. As a result, documentation has become increasingly important. The idea that *it was not done if it was not written* is the current belief in the courts. For example, the nurse who is a primary nurse in the labor area may become involved in situations in which legal and ethical decisions will be made with little time to consider alternatives. This nurse must document actions and client responses as soon as possible.

Some important legal issues in maternity and infant nursing include emancipated minors, informed consent, assault and battery, prenatal abuse (see Chapter 27), the obligation to report child abuse, negligence and malpractice (see Chapter 30), and the Pregnant Patient's Bill of Rights.

Emancipated minor

An **emancipated minor** is a person less than the legal age who is a parent, is in the military, lives away from home, or is self-supporting and thus has all the legal rights of an adult.

Informed consent

To protect autonomy and to avoid duress, the client must freely give **informed consent** before any invasive treatment or procedure is performed. Each client has the right to refuse consent. She must receive a full explanation (in her primary language) of the benefits and risks to herself or the unborn child (*fetus*). She must be given, in language she understands, the alternative choices of treatment or nontreatment with the goals of care. Then she must sign a consent form. The consent should be obtained by the physician or nurse practitioner, and the conference and signature or merely the signature must be witnessed by another person (usually the nurse). If the *signature alone* is witnessed, a note to that effect should be added to the consent form. The nurse should provide time for the client to ask any questions that occur later and be aware that a client may change her mind.

Assault and battery

To threaten to do harm to an individual is **assault**. To harm or touch a person without consent (except in an emergency) is **battery**.

Any nursing procedure should be fully explained *before* the client is *touched*. Even though a formal consent is not required, to preserve a trusting nurse-client relationship, it is important to educate the client about the reasons for and results of care before initiating the procedure. Nurses must advocate for their clients, especially in clinical situations where the woman may be seen by a number of physicians and students. Remember, *touching someone without consent constitutes battery.*

Prenatal abuse

Because it is more evident that prenatal care reduces the incidence of infant morbidity and mortality, **prenatal abuse** is becoming a legal issue. If the woman does not protect the fetus by maintaining her own health or seeking prenatal care or continues to abuse substances that may injure the fetus, she may be held liable for damages to the fetus (Rhodes, 1990). This is a controversial issue discussed further in Chapter 27.

Obligation to report child abuse

It is mandatory for health care professionals to report suspected child abuse. These professionals know about signs and symptoms of child abuse and therefore are responsible for informing the appropriate agency so the matter may be investigated. Failure to report may result in a fine or liability for damages. Permissive reporting is allowed for community persons who believe the child has been abused. These individuals are protected by legislation from suit when a good-faith report is given (Rhodes, 1987). Chapter 30 reviews sample cases for which legal aspects in the **perinatal** period must be considered.

Self-Discovery

What do you think are the issues with prenatal abuse when it includes maternal exposure to smoking, alcohol, or drugs? ∼

Negligence and malpractice

Negligence is failing to make sure a client understands a treatment or procedure, to inform the client fully regarding consequences of interventions, or to follow set protocols in a situation that could result in harm. **Malpractice** is failing to do the reasonable or prudent practice expected by a professional in the specific situation or performing actions outside of one's area of competence that result in injury. Negligence may apply to any person. Malpractice is narrowed to the professional; it is

professional negligent conduct. Such negligence may be further defined in the following way:

In a health care agency, a nurse has the duty to provide care for clients. This duty may be interpreted as malpractice when a *breach of duty* occurs by *omission* (e.g., forgetting to check a monitor, give medication, instruct in home self-care, or notify a physician of a change in client status). The breach also may occur by *commission* (e.g., giving the wrong medication or identifying the infant incorrectly). In some way the breach of duty must cause physical or mental injury to the client. It must be shown that the commission or omission of an act by the nurse resulted in physical injury or unnecessary pain and suffering. A busy health care unit is not an excuse for failure to act correctly. Nurses must follow hospital policies and procedures, acting within their job descriptions and scope of practice as written in the state license.

When there are legal or ethical issues with a case, staff members may consult the hospital risk-management team. No delay should occur before advice is sought from the risk manager. Chapter 30 details legal and ethical aspects of maternity care and discusses actual cases that have arisen in suits and in risk-management decisions.

Box 1-2

CLINICAL DECISION

Describe a situation that occurred during your maternity nursing rotation that might have become a basis for a legal suit. What were the nursing implications?

Pregnant Patient's Bill of Rights

The Pregnant Patient's Bill of Rights develops some aspects of what is the right thing to do when a woman is receiving care during pregnancy, labor, birth, and recovery (see Appendix 1A). This document does not have the force of a rule or regulation, but it can guide the nurse's thinking in upgrading care to be as "right" as possible in a setting.

EXPANDED CARE ROLES FOR NURSES

The roles of nursing in maternity care have been expanded, and further education may offer nurses the opportunity to participate in more independent practice. Several choices are available today. A nurse may become a clinician, such as a lactation consultant, through continuing education and concentration in an area that brings additional responsibility in the hospital. The nurse also may become certified in a specialty area, such as neonatal intensive care. In the same way, women's health practitioners offer a wider range of health care services than nurses with only a basic background. Today a number of programs offer specialization. Almost all clinical programs require a baccalaureate degree in nursing and basic experience in the chosen specialty area for a nurse to proceed to a master's degree program or take a qualifying examination in a specialty.

Nurse Practitioner

A **nurse practitioner** is a professional licensed nurse who, with additional study, develops a specialization in maternity, neonatal, or perinatal nursing or in women's health care. This practitioner may manage care of well clients or stabilized ill clients.

Clinical Nurse Specialist

A **clinical nurse specialist** is a professional licensed nurse who has completed a master's degree in a specialty area and will usually be in a role to upgrade nursing practice in client care areas.

Certified Nurse-Midwife

A certified nurse-midwife (CNM) is a professional midwife who is certified according to the requirements of the National Certifying Board of the American College of Nurse-Midwives. This person is educated in nursing and midwifery. A nurse-midwife also may have a baccalaureate, master's, or doctoral degree in public health administration, nursing, or a health-related science.

International definition of midwife

A *midwife* is a person who, having been regularly admitted to a midwifery educational program fully recognized in the country in which it is located, has successfully completed the prescribed course of studies in midwifery and has the qualifications to be registered and legally licensed to practice midwifery.

Midwives must be able to give the necessary supervision, care, and advice to women during pregnancy, labor, and the postpartum period; to conduct deliveries on their own responsibility; and to care for the newborn and infant. This care includes preventive measures, detection of abnormal conditions in mother and child, procurement of medical assistance, and execution of emergency measures in the absence of medical help.

The midwife has an important task in counseling and education for clients and the family and community. The work should involve antenatal education and preparation for parenthood and extends to certain areas of gynecology, family planning, and child care (Richmond and Wise, 1986).

The CNM may practice in hospitals, clinics, health units, domiciliary wards, or any other service.

Since the 1930s, nurses have been entering nurse-midwifery. Before then, the majority of midwives had no nursing education. There is pressure on the American College of Nurse-Midwives to admit lay-midwives into professional training programs. However, few states have practicing lay-midwives.

Lay-midwife

Throughout the world, most births are attended by lay-midwives who have received some training or who, by experience, are accorded the responsibility of normal births. Several states in the United States do license lay-midwives. The Midwives Alliance of North America (MANA) is the group with which they are encouraged to affiliate.

Birth attendant

The birth attendant is internationally recognized as a health care worker who fulfills a useful role in areas where health services are not sufficiently developed. In most countries, on-the-job orientation and working experience enable the birth attendant to assist women during childbirth and the immediate postpartum period, including newborn home care.

NURSING EDUCATION

Currently the trend in nursing education is to prepare a general practitioner. This has resulted in a decrease in specialty areas, such as maternity nursing, for the nursing student. Although different rationales are used, none take into account that this area of health care affects more families than any other. Maternal and infant care can seem simple at first. It may be assumed that the nurse is dealing with primarily healthy people. However, with advances in medicine, many clients with chronic diseases or even organ transplants are having children. Although gaining rapport, teaching, guiding, and assessing require a certain level of nursing interaction, the nurse must use the nursing process to assess, plan, diagnose, and implement and evaluate safe care for the childbearing family. Close monitoring and preventive health care during the childbearing cycle assures better outcomes for the expectant woman and fetus. No matter what area of specialization is chosen by the nurse, every nurse should have a basic knowledge of the way a family functions during the childbirth cycle (Box 1-2).

What is the focus of maternity nursing? Nursing students already have studied sociology, psychology, human growth and development, and anatomy and physiology. Using this knowledge, the nursing student may best learn the following functions in this area of nursing:

1. Assessment of the impact of family structures on parenting
2. Preventive health teaching regarding risk factors in the environment
3. Teaching regarding child-spacing or infertility
4. Preventive health care during the childbearing cycle
5. Monitoring of pregnancy, labor, and recovery
6. Assessment of maternal adjustment to the pregnancy

▌ *Box* 1-2 **Maternal-Infant Practice Competencies for Graduates of Nursing Programs**

1. The graduate of a program in nursing will practice maternal-infant nursing based on theoretic and empiric knowledge of normal and selected abnormal patterns of biophysic and psychosocial growth and development of the pregnant woman, fetus, newborn, and family.

2. The graduate of a program in nursing uses the nursing process to assess, diagnose, plan, implement, evaluate, and revise a safe plan of nursing care based on standards of practice to achieve mutually agreed on priorities and goals with the healthy childbearing family.

3. The graduate of a program in nursing assists families in understanding and coping with normal developmental and common situational crises during childbearing.

4. The graduate of a program in nursing promotes the maintenance and restoration of the reproductive health of individuals and families during the preconceptional and interconceptional phase and of individuals who decide not to bear or cannot bear children.

5. The graduate of a program in nursing is expected to maintain and upgrade his or her knowledge, develop proficiency in psychomotor skills, and reevaluate appropriateness of affective behaviors required for maternal-infant nursing practice.

6. The graduate of a program in nursing collaborates with nurses and others in using community resources to provide care to childbearing families.

7. The graduate of a program in nursing improves maternal-infant nursing practice through use of research findings and evaluation of current practice.

From Sherwen LN: *MICC: The Maternal-Infant Core Competency Project,* White Plains, NY, 1987, March of Dimes Birth Defects Foundation.

7. Education about self-monitoring techniques during pregnancy, labor, and recovery
8. Screening of risk factors for mother and infant
9. Assessment of levels at risk
10. Support of body systems if mother or baby is stressed or ill
11. Assessment of newborn status and gestational age
12. Promotion of attachment and parent-infant bonding
13. Promotion of parents' total care of the infant
14. Education for support of positive nurturing

In addition, you should master the descriptions of normal anatomy and physiology for childbearing. This knowledge will benefit your understanding of body systems and their function during the childbearing cycle of a family's life.

Use of the Nursing Process

Implementation of the nursing process as a way of approaching nursing problems (health care problems for which a nurse can intervene) has developed rapidly in the last decade. The nursing process is derived from a scientific method and in its current form is similar to the methods used by other professional groups such as social workers. Although terminology may change slightly, the process has been integrated into the nursing approach. Nursing process played an important part in the development of critical pathways. Clarification of nursing and client care expectations fosters a client's compliance with care, thus diminishing frequency of readmissions. In the nursing process, the client is a partner who agrees to the goals, which are detailed in the category known as *expected outcomes.*

Collaborative approach

The beginning nursing student may have difficulty determining the relationships among independent, interdependent, and dependent actions in the health care field. The nursing process allows you to determine independent nursing actions, actions you may initiate under the professional nursing license defined by the nurse practice act in each state. Generally, this definition includes diagnosing and treating human responses to health problems.

Much of hospital-based nursing practice includes *collaborative* or *interdependent* actions based on medical regimens and suggestions or orders from other disciplines (e.g., respiratory, dietary, or physical therapy departments) that may be involved in the client's care. Others have called this role "dependent," but that term is too restrictive because a great deal of input is required by the nurse, who coordinates care 24 hours of the day. When the problem is primarily medical, some have called it a "clinical problem" to distinguish it from nursing problems. The goals for these clinical problems are set primarily by the physician, and interventions are prescribed on the order sheet.

Nurses need to develop and use management skills when coordinating client services to provide holistic care.

Management skills involve anticipating needs and planning interventions to meet these needs before problems arise.

Ideally, when collaborative problems occur, medical *and* nursing professionals should identify the goals of care because both are involved in analyzing, monitoring, recording, and evaluating the client's progress. In this text when there is overlap, the situation is discussed under the heading of *Clinical Management.*

Assessment phase: data collection

When a nurse is assigned to a client with a potential health problem, nothing should be done until data is collected from a variety of sources. First, obtain the client's health history, statements about current signs and symptoms, and family situations affecting care needs. Next, perform a physical assessment to detect other problems and confirm subjective statements. The physician or midwife will order diagnostic tests to determine the medical problem. From these sources, the nurse identifies client care problems requiring nursing intervention.

Analysis phase: nursing diagnosis

Problems that can be managed through nursing interventions are selected, categorized, and put in order of priority. Problems that need resolution by other health care professionals are referred to the appropriate departments. The most difficult task is to analyze the data and identify the nursing diagnostic statement that applies to the problem. It is important to understand the defining characteristics of the problem because some diagnoses appear to overlap.

A steady effort has been made to clarify diagnoses. Since 1973 the conference on classification of nursing diagnoses meets biannually to study and tighten classifications. This group is the North American Nursing Diagnosis Association (NANDA). This text uses the NANDA diagnostic listing released in 1996. In maternity care, problem-oriented nursing diagnoses do not always apply. Positive health behaviors, adequate coping, and knowledgeable clients do not fit the framework. It is therefore important to be aware of a new approach based on developmental tasks. Starn and Neiderhauser (1990) used Roy's adaptation model to undergird nursing diagnoses and planning. Other health-related diagnoses are in the process of development.

Each statement must be individualized by adding an etiologic component, or factors that influenced or precipitated the health problem. The second part of the diagnostic statement, "related to," are factors that can be affected by nursing activity. The diagnoses will not direct nursing care as intended if they contain causes that need medical, economic, or social services intervention. The statement should not be related to unchangeable factors. (e.g., "dysfunctional grieving related to death of the infant"). The death is a fact; no one can intervene. Instead, this nursing diagnosis might be stated in several ways, depending on the situation of the client: "dysfunctional grieving related to unsupportive significant others in family, unrealistic expectations of self, or unresolved anger." You should not reword medical etiologies, nor be too vague in the etiologic statement of the nursing diagnosis.

Although each client and family is unique in its needs, there are often commonalities during pregnancy. Uncomplicated gestations necessitate changes or adaptations that we recognize as expected (Box 1-3). Women experiencing complicated pregnancies have additional needs specific to each situation but may share many of these additional diagnoses (Box 1-4). In this text there are suggestions for nursing diagnoses. Because every client has different sets of data, these are only a guide for your planning. The following are some common choices.

Ambivalence. When a woman becomes pregnant, ambivalence is a major feeling during the first trimester. Depending on her delight in or anxiety about being pregnant, she will react to the discovery of potential problems in fairly consistent ways. For many women, bearing a child continues to be considered a way of expressing the feminine role.

Lowered self-esteem. A woman who does not feel successful because of losing the pregnancy or having complications may suffer from lowered self-esteem. Depending on her support system, her situation may confirm old feelings of insecurity and low self-worth. Lowered self-esteem is seen especially in teen pregnancies and in women who have suffered spouse abuse. It may be too complex to determine the source of the unsuccessful feelings; however, referral for additional help can be important for this person.

Health-seeking behaviors. Health-seeking behaviors always will need to be considered. Because self-monitoring is essential during pregnancy, information giving is a major nursing role in prenatal care. Absolutely basic to any cooperation in self-care is the understanding of what to do and why.

Family processes, altered. Family coping always will be tested by pregnancy. The childbearing process may foster growth in relationships or result in distancing. Changes in relationships have the ability to alter parenting and coping skills. Alteration in family coping or individual coping may become one of the highest priorities in care. Referrals for support services, information, and empathetic conversation are an important part of nursing care.

Fear or anxiety for self or infant. A degree of fear and anxiety for self and for the infant always will be present. In many cases, fear is well founded. Many women have read about their conditions and may have many questions. The nurse should encourage the woman to express how she copes with difficult problems. If desired, the nurse can help find a chaplain or counselor to talk with her further. Enlist the support of the extended family.

▌ *Box* 1-3	**Nursing Diagnostic Statements for Uncomplicated Pregnancies**

Activity intolerance, risk for	Injury, risk for
Anxiety	Knowledge deficit
Body image disturbance	Management of therapeutic regimen, individual: effective
Caregiver role strain, risk for	Nutrition, altered: less than body requirements
Constipation	Nutrition, altered: more than body requirements
Coping, ineffective individual	Oral mucous membrane, altered
Family processes, altered	Parent/infant attachment, altered: risk for
Fatigue	Personal identity disturbance
Growth and development, altered	Role performance, altered
Health maintenance, altered	Sexuality patterns, altered
Health-seeking behaviors	Sleep pattern disturbance
Infection, risk for	Urinary elimination, altered

▌ *Box* 1-4	**Nursing Diagnoses for More Complicated Pregnancies**

Fear	Pain
Fluid volume excess	Parental role conflict
Fluid volume deficit	Powerlessness
Gas exchange, impaired	Self-esteem, situational low
Grieving, anticipatory	Social isolation
Grieving, dysfunctional	Tissue perfusion, altered: risk for
Management of therapeutic regimen, individual: ineffective	Urinary retention
Mobility, impaired	

Grieving. Pregnancy and childbirth may involve some measure of *grieving.* Parents may experience grief when they have a cesarean birth instead of the anticipated vaginal delivery, when the neonate is not the "perfect" child because of a physical defect, or even because of the birth of a child of an undesired gender. Intense grief is usually experienced after intrauterine death, abortion, or neonatal death. Chapter 26 suggests ways of interacting to support the grieving couple.

Planning phase: expected outcomes

The nursing process statement must provide a focus for the goals of care, which are specified in the *expected outcomes* or evaluative criteria. Planning includes setting outcomes with the client and listing summaries of interventions. Planning precedes nursing actions. These objectives should be specific, individualized, and measurable and should list a specified amount of time for achievement. The care paths used in many settings are part of the planning phase. It is important to date and sign the plan and update, revise, reevaluate, and reanalyze it as necessary. In this text, there are suggested outcomes. Reword these to individualize the nursing plan of care.

Implementation phase: nursing interventions

Implementation is nursing intervention. The information written on the care plan or Kardex should be formulated with the client's entire hospital stay in mind. However, the client's condition usually changes, and these plans are updated, revised, or discontinued regularly as needed. If the nurse selects a nursing diagnosis with a formulated plan and does not intervene so that the client makes progress toward the expected outcomes, or if the client does not learn the needed self-care skills before discharge, it may be thought of as negligence by the nurse.

Nursing intervention should be related to the etiologic statement, and it is within your *independent function* to modify the environment to prevent hazards; to assist with activities of daily living (ADL), rest, sleep, and maintaining body functions; to guide and teach self-care and medication activities; and to support, socialize with, and be an advocate for the client. These actions do not require direction from others.

In addition, nursing actions also can be collaborative, such as when you monitor progress, maintain supportive technologic equipment, carry out physicians' orders to

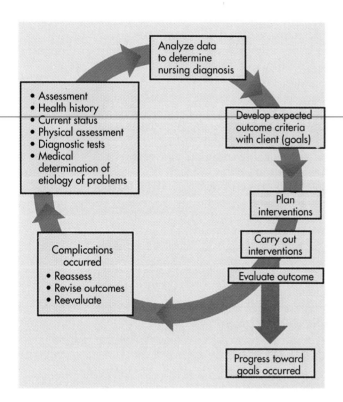

Figure 1-3   The circular nature of the nursing process.

medicate and perform treatments, or prepare the client for surgery.

Evaluation phase

If the client has been involved with formulation of expected outcomes of care, the nurse, together with the client, should be able to determine whether there has been progress toward resolution of the problem. Otherwise, you may only hope that the client understands and is motivated to perform self-care activities. It is important to validate hopes with proof. During discharge planning, special efforts must be made to ensure that the client understands self-care and infant care. If she shows that she does, documentation must reflect that fact. If she still has questions or difficulty, documentation should reflect that also. Figure 1-3 shows the nursing process in sequence but in a continuous, circular manner.

In this text there are questions related to the outcomes. Always ask questions first as you seek to evaluate. These questions need to be answered before documenting evaluation statements.

HOW MAY MATERNAL AND INFANT CARE BE EVALUATED?

The results of health care are reflected in **morbidity** (illness) and **mortality** (death) statistics. These statistics

are important in determining whether there has been progress in achieving the overall goals of health planning and care. Throughout this text, you will see statistics of risk. These risk statements will assist you in focusing on the frequency with which complications occur. You should be aware of the complications that carry the highest risk of morbidity and mortality and those that should be preventable with good prenatal care. This country, with its abundance of physicians and hospitals, should have much lower maternal and infant mortality and morbidity rates. Nurses must work together with other health professionals to identify causes of and solutions for these problems and work toward change in the delivery of adequate care.

Although maternal mortality has been reduced, as seen in Table 1-1, the United States continues to have a high infant mortality rate. This country now ranks seventeenth in relation to infant mortality statistics from other industrialized nations. A few years ago, the ranking was twelfth (Atrash, Alexander, Berg, 1995). The major causes of infant mortality in the perinatal period are related to socioeconomic factors affecting lifestyle, drug abuse, poor nutrition, and access to health care. Premature birth especially contributes to infant death and illness (MMWR, 1996).

Prenatal care is an important vehicle for providing needed services to pregnant women. It is a major reason for the significant decrease in maternal mortality seen during the last few decades. The decreased mortality also is related to the use of antibiotics and increased understanding of the processes of the maternal-fetal physiology and intervention when problems occur. The success of prenatal care is reflected in the statistics. The point in her pregnancy at which the mother seeks prenatal care is directly related to the amount of schooling she has had. Those with less schooling begin care much later (Fiscella, 1995).

Even though the rates of death have dropped significantly in the last 50 years, black women and immigrants from Central and South America have 2.8 to 3 times the rate of death as white women (see Table 1-1). These statistics show a continuing discrepancy in the quality and availability of health care. Women in certain ethnic groups are more likely to seek care later in pregnancy or only when things go wrong. Illegal immigrants especially may not seek care at all, coming to the hospital or clinic during labor without having obtained previous care. Puerto Rican mothers are least likely to seek early care. Women with lower incomes who come from Central and South America also are less likely to seek early care (Ventura et al, 1995). This is due to several factors including inability to pay, distance from care providers, and lack of money for transport or child care. Most women seek care when it is available, low cost, "user-friendly," and perceived to be sympathetic.

The way a woman is treated in the office or clinic setting influences her compliance, self-esteem, and ability to pre-

Table 1-1	**Maternal Death Rates**

MATERNAL MORTALITY TERMINOLOGY

Maternal Death

Arises from any cause while pregnant or within 42 days of the end of pregnancy (even if abortion or ectopic pregnancy). For international comparisons, the World Health Organization (WHO) divides the postbirth period into two periods: 1 to 7 days and 8 to 42 days.

Direct maternal death

Results from obstetric complications or from interventions, omissions, or incorrect treatment during these days

Indirect maternal death

Results from a previously existing disease or one that developed during pregnancy that was aggravated by the effects of pregnancy

Nonmaternal death

Results from accidental or incidental causes unrelated to pregnancy or its management

Maternal death rate

Number of all maternal deaths per 100,000 live births.

Race	1950	1960	1970	1990	1994
All races	83.3	37.1	24.7	7.9	7.8
White	61.1	26.0	14.4	5.6	5.0
Nonwhite	221.6	97.9	55.9	16.5	18.2

Compiled from National Center for Health Statistics: Annual summaries of births, marriages, divorces, and deaths, United States Vital Statistics Reports.

Table 1-2	**Infant Death Rates**[*]

INFANT DEATH RATE
Number of deaths in first year of life, including first 28 days

Neonatal mortality

Number of deaths from birth through first 28 days of life, regardless of prematurity

Fetal mortality

Number of deaths of infants after twentieth week of development but before day of birth

Perinatal mortality

Combination of fetal and neonatal mortality figures

Rate	1950	1960	1970	1990	1994
Infant death rate	29.2	26.0	19.9	9.0	7.99

Compiled from *Morbidity and Mortality Weekly Reports* and National Center for Health Statistics.
*Per 1000 live births.

pare for the birth. For example, one clinic makes a special effort to see each woman within 1 hour of her appointment time. The same clinic also provides a social worker, nutritionist, and physician or midwife located in the same facility. At another clinic in the same city, women come early to take numbers before being seen by a health care professional. They sit all day waiting to be called at intervals to be weighed, to provide urine samples, and finally to see the midwife or physician. Often, they are tired and hungry when they leave. The wasted time is not used to educate these women about prenatal and infant care.

There is national interest in preventing pregnancy complications and premature births. The Surgeon General set goals for the year 2000 that include a special emphasis on reducing mortality for infants of poor families (Table 1-2). To reach these goals health care professionals must analyze deficiencies. The following statement by Richmond and Wise (1986) still holds true:

> We raise these issues because we are deeply distressed, both by these numbers and by the tone of our national debate regarding our commitment to the less advantaged in our society, and particularly to the children of the less advantaged in our society. We often hear the rationalization that we can no longer afford to assure a healthier beginning for these children. We often hear that we are entering a period of "scarce resources."
>
> Our national budget is over 1 trillion dollars, . . . 11% spent on health care. Resources are hardly scarce; they are merely competitive. Unfortunately, children are not competing very well for their just share of our national resources. Let it be stated clearly that our inability to reach the Surgeon General's goals for better infant health is a reflection of our inaction and our lack of national commitment, not our lack of capability.

More than 15 years ago, the Carnegie report on the status of the nation's families suggested the following four ways that families could receive supportive help (Kenniston and The Carnegie Council on Children, 1978):

1. Perhaps the simplest way is to encourage and provide better education for future parents, including the opportunity for adolescent parents to have experience with children, learning growth and development and methods of child care.
2. Day care facilities need to encourage the participation of parents and other family members so they can continue to be primary care givers in the upbringing of their children.
3. A wider recognition by society of the important role of parenting must underlie any regulatory changes in institutions supporting the family. It is hoped that this recognition would bring more support to ease the child-care problems of working parents by allowing tax breaks, child allowances, and more flexible working hours. It would also allow a parent to stay at home to be a full-time parent if he or she chose to do so.
4. New family income and health care programs need to replace welfare payments. The stability of the poor family is in jeopardy, and such families may need dramatic supports to allow survival.

It is interesting and discouraging to consider progress since that report. In many ways, the poor family has not benefitted; however, some advances in child care and flexible working hours have been made. In 1988 the National Commission to Prevent Infant Mortality repeated some of the following concerns from reports it had issued 20 years before:

1. Broaden private and public health insurance coverage for childbearing women and for infants.
2. Extend Medicaid coverage for infants and for pregnant women with incomes up to 200% of federal poverty levels.
3. Coordinate and fund public programs of family planning.
4. Simplify applicant procedures for Medicaid.
5. Increase providers of maternity care for low-income women.
6. Increase public awareness of the problems of morbidity and mortality.

Since 1988 Medicaid has been extended for pregnant women. Other services are available but accessible only if someone contacts the woman. Recent challenges to Medicaid coverage and food programs may alter services.

Causes of Problems

Maternal chronic disease

For a few women, chronic disease has been recognized and treated before pregnancy. For example, the woman with preexisting diabetes will know that pregnancy places additional stress on her system and on the balance of glucose that has been achieved. She may be managing her condition skillfully, and yet her system may be thrown out of balance by the changes induced by pregnancy. However, because of her experience, she may need less care than the woman whose diabetes is first diagnosed during pregnancy. The new diabetic client will need teaching and support to master self-monitoring (see Chapter 24).

Hypertension and cardiovascular disease are major health problems in this country. Depending on genetic inheritance, health status, and stress, a pregnant woman already may have chronic hypertension or cardiac dysfunction. Although more common in the older population, hypertension also is found in younger people. If a pregnant woman has a previously elevated diastolic blood pressure, she can become increasingly hypertensive and may need hospitalization. Pregnancy-induced hypertension (PIH) occurs exclusively during the second part of pregnancy and may occur in those without a history of hypertension (see Chapter 22).

Cardiac dysfunction in young adults usually is a result of rheumatic fever, congenital defects, or hypertensive disease. Pregnancy places stress on the cardiovascular system and can increase cardiac problems in some women. However, today fewer cases of rheumatic fever are seen, and the incidence of cardiac disease during pregnancy has diminished (See Chapter 23).

Pregnancy-related problems

A high-risk pregnancy may be lost by spontaneous abortion before the fetus is viable. Approximately 20% of all pregnancies are lost in this way, many for reasons that are not traceable to any pathologic problem. Known maternal factors include poor nutrition, anemia, borderline fertility, and chronic disease. In addition, approximately 30% of aborted conceptions are lost because of poor implantation or because of a malformed, poorly developing embryo.

After the age of viability, an abnormal outcome may result when a pregnancy ends in a stillbirth or neonatal death or results in a compromised infant with a less than optimal chance for a healthy life.

Prenatal period. Problems related to the site of implantation or to the structure of the placenta make up a large group of the complications of pregnancy. The uterine structure normally accommodates itself to the growth and development of the infant, the amniotic fluid, and the placenta. If the placenta is poorly situated, early hemorrhage may result. If the placenta separates from the uterine wall, fetal hypoxia or death may result. Much of prenatal care involves assessment and diagnosis of potential problems with placental or fetal growth. Chapters 11 and 14 describe these means of evaluation. Chapters 8, 9, and 10 describe the care given to the pregnant woman.

Labor and birth. A few women have difficulty with the birth process either because of problems with the forces of labor or the mechanisms of labor. The nurse participates in monitoring and assessment and assists the physician or midwife during operative interventions. When a woman needs assisted birth, it is important to identify the requirements for information and support for both the woman and her partner. The experience may be frightening, and there always is much concern for the infant (see Chapters 13 and 15).

Recovery. Recovery problems may include hemorrhage, depression, and infection. Types of infection that alter maternal and fetal health are described in Chapter 25. Infection is a focus of maternal care today. The prevalence of sexually transmitted diseases (STDs) and the ease with which the fetus may become infected have directed attention to the important issues of prevention. The importance of asepsis, universal precautions, and education cannot be overemphasized.

The incidence of women with drug dependencies also has increased. Depending on geographic location or urban or rural settings, you may encounter women who use addictive drugs during pregnancy. Most nurses encounter women who smoke excessively or abuse alcohol. Because of the adverse effects of these substances on the fetus, every effort must be made to encourage the pregnant woman to avoid drug use during pregnancy. In some states a woman may be sued for child abuse if she continues intake of these adverse chemicals. When a newborn's test results are positive on a toxicology screen, the case is referred to a child welfare agency, and the woman may not be able to care for her child until she receives treatment. Chapter 29 reviews care of these infants, and Chapter 27 describes the care of women at high risk because of social problems.

High-Risk Infant

Birth-associated problems

If an infant is born before its development is completed, immaturity in every body system will handicap normal growth. Immaturity and low birth weight are no longer considered the same thing; however, approximately two thirds of low-birth-weight infants also are born prematurely. One third of these small infants are fully developed but have poor fetal weight gain because of intrauterine stress or malnourishment. If all premature and low-birth-weight infants are included in a single group, they account for approximately 65% of all deaths in the first year of life.

The handicaps and long-term effects produced by intrauterine stress or malnourishment should not be underestimated. If the infant is subjected to a reduced nutritional or oxygen supply, optimal development is prevented. Active and passive smoking is linked clearly with low birth weight and prematurity (see Chapter 10).

The problems of preterm and postterm infants differ in degree and cause, but the same interventions often are used for both (see Chapter 29). The beginning practitioner will not do primary care in the NICU for these infants, yet the signs of developing problems, the risk factors, and the ways of supporting body systems should be recognized. The nurse in the NICU will need additional clinical education to function in a collaborative role in the care of these ill infants. However, the beginning practitioner who understands the signs of and the risk factors for neonatal problems can provide preventive care and support for parents.

Environmental chemicals

A number of teratogens may disturb body function or growth, and their effects on the development of the fetus have been identified. Chapter 28 identifies environmental agents that are toxic to sperm or ova before conception and those that alter structure, biochemistry, or growth of the fetus.

Many occupational health rules are circumvented in the workplace. Regulations must be enforced to prevent workplace pollution. In addition, environmental protection must be a major issue for health in the 1990s. Chemical effluents are entering the environment every day, and the list of offending chemicals is long. Not only can there be an immediate effect from these chemicals but also genetic defects may result from mutations and may be passed to the next generation. Nurses can be in the forefront of those who defend health by seeking changes in and compliance with environmental laws.

Genetic problems

Approximately 3% to 4% of birth defects are from traceable genetic causes. The study of genetics is rapidly developing, and many diseases of unknown etiology are now linked to a chromosomal or single gene defect (see Chapter 28).

CONFIDENTIAL MEDICAL REPORT   (Each question MUST be answered)

Only for scientific purposes approved by the Board of Health; not open to inspection or subject to subpoena

NAME OF CHILD _____   BIRTH NO. _____

	10. Race: White, African-American, American Indian, Other (specify)	11. Ancestry (e.g., African-American, Chinese, Cuban, German, Italian Puerto Rican, etc.)	12. Education (Record highest yr. completed) Elm./High School 0-12 / College 1-4 5+		13. Occupation: Mother Father	14. Kind of business or industry	15. Employed during this pregnancy
Mother	10a.	11a.	12a.		13a.	14a.	15a. 1☐Yes 0☐No
Father	10b.	11b.	12b.		13b.	14b.	

16. Previous pregnancies (complete all sections)

Total number of previous pregnancies	Born alive			Spontaneous terminations				Induced terminations			
	Now living	Now dead		Less than 13 weeks	13 to 19 weeks	20 weeks or more		Less than 13 weeks	13 to 19 weeks	20 weeks or more	
a. Number____ None ☐	b. Number____ None ☐	c. Number____ None ☐	d. Number____ None ☐	e. Number____ None ☐	f. Number____ None ☐	g. Number____ None ☐	h. Number____ None ☐	i. Number____ None ☐

17. Prior terminations Type	Date Month Year	18. Date last normal menses began Month Day Year	19. Prenatal care			20. Mother's blood group and Rh
a. First live birth			a. Date first visit to any provider Month Day Year	b. Providers (check all that apply) 1.☐ Hosp. 4.☐ SHF 2.☐ MIC 5.☐ Pvt Phy 6.☐ Other 3.☐ Other Clinic	c. Total number of visits to all providers _____ 0☐ None	
b. Last live birth						
c. Last other termination						

21. Primary financial coverage this birth 1.☐ Medicaid 2.☐ HMO 3.☐ Other 3rd Party 4.☐ Self	22. During this pregnancy, did Mother participate in: 1.☐ WIC 4.☐ AFDC 2.☐ SNAP 5.☐ Other 3.☐ PCNP Specify_____ 0 ☐ None	23. Check if Mother was 1.☐ Private physician's client 2.☐ General services client	24. Was hospital of this delivery a: 1.☐ Prelabor referral for high risk 2.☐ Emergency transfer before delivery Specify transfer from _____ 0 ☐ Neither

Figure 1-4 Worksheet for preparing the birth certificate.

Vital Statistics

Birth statistics

A birth worksheet is made out by the parents 1 or 2 days after birth and completed and signed by the physician. A copy is sent to the Bureau of Health or the city registrar to be recorded, and an official certificate is sent to the parents several weeks later. Copies of statistics from all birth certificates are sent to the National Center for Health Statistics.

The birth worksheet shown in Figure 1-4 shows the categories to be filled in by the parents. The certificate should give the full name of the infant and the father's surname as last name if the couple is married, or the infant's surname may also include the mother's maiden name if the couple desires. If the mother is single, the child receives her surname unless official *paternity papers* are attached to the form and submitted with the initial certificate. Changing names later may require an appearance in court.

Race needs interpretation. "White" includes most Hispanic people such as Mexican, Mexican-American, Cuban, and Puerto Rican. "Other" includes all who are not grouped into the white or black categories, such as Asians, Native Americans, Eskimos, and Asian Indians. The country or ethnic group of parental origin (e.g., Korean, Japanese, German, Italian) should be listed. Since 1989 the infant has been assigned the race of the mother. Because these worksheets were revised in 1989, more information

will be available through this national data collection required for all birth certificates. The second part of the certificate is a confidential medical report not open to inspection or subpoena (see Chapter 21, Figure 21-1).

Maternal mortality and morbidity

Statistics are collected from 10% of the hospitals throughout the United States, and statistical projections are made on the basis of data from these reporting hospitals. Table 1-1 gives definitions and rates of maternal death and lists statistics that indicate the improvement in health care (see also Box 1-5). In recent years the morbidity and mortality rates for the major pregnancy problems of hemorrhage, hypertension, and infection have been reduced through more comprehensive health care. However, as can be seen by the numbers, health care is unevenly applied to women in this society.

Although fewer women die from infection, the number of cases of infection during pregnancy is increasing. The rate of spontaneous and elective abortion is relatively unchanged. The incidence of pregnancy in adolescents remains high (see Chapter 8), and the incidence of pregnancy in older women is increasing. A woman older than 35 is considered at higher risk because she may have concurrent chronic disease and lowered fertility.

A study of maternal mortality in the United States from 1979 to 1986 (Atrash et al, 1990) has shown that maternal

Box 1-5	Categories of Maternal Mortality

Complications of pregnancy, childbirth, and the puerperium
Ectopic pregnancy
Toxemias of pregnancy and the puerperium, except abortion
  with toxemia
Hemorrhage of pregnancy and childbirth
Abortions
  Abortions induced for legal indications

Abortions induced for other reasons
Spontaneous abortions
Other and unspecified abortions
Sepsis of childbirth and the puerperium
All other complications of pregnancy, childbirth, and the
  puerperium
Delivery without mention of complication

Maternal deaths are those assigned to complications of pregnancy, childbirth, and the puerperium, category numbers 630-676 of the *Ninth Revision International Classification of Diseases,* 1975. Rates per 100,000 live births in specified group.

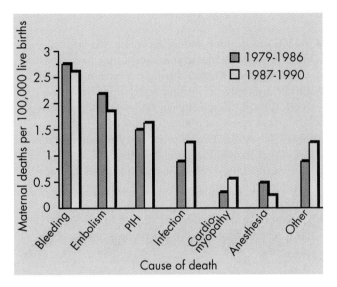
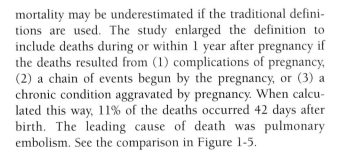

Figure 1-5   Pregnancy-related mortality from 1979 to 1986 compared with 1987 to 1990. (From Berg et al: Pregnancy-related mortality in the United States, 1987-1990, *Obstet Gynecol* 88[2]:161, 1996.)

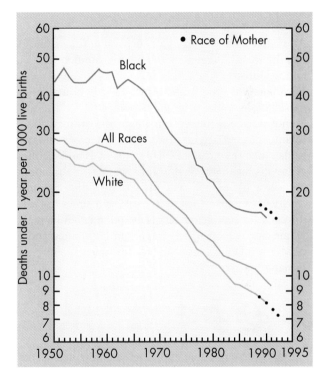

Figure 1-6   Infant mortality by race in the United States from 1950 to 1992. Beginning in 1989, race for live births is tabulated according to race of the mother instead of the father. (From *Monthly Vital Statistics Report,* 43[6S]:1 1995.)

mortality may be underestimated if the traditional definitions are used. The study enlarged the definition to include deaths during or within 1 year after pregnancy if the deaths resulted from (1) complications of pregnancy, (2) a chain of events begun by the pregnancy, or (3) a chronic condition aggravated by pregnancy. When calculated this way, 11% of the deaths occurred 42 days after birth. The leading cause of death was pulmonary embolism. See the comparison in Figure 1-5.

Infant mortality and morbidity

Mortality figures must account for deaths from the age of viability, which is a gestational age of 20 weeks (Figure 1-6). Few of the small infants 20 to 28 weeks old survive,

but the potential is there. Therefore the terms identified for infant mortality in Table 1-2 are necessary. An infant that is more developed than 20 weeks, weighs 1 lb or more, or is 16.5 cm crown-to-rump who dies in utero is called an *intrauterine fetal death,* meaning one who is stillborn. Loss of a younger fetus is called an *abortion.* If there is no heartbeat or respiratory effort at birth, the infant is listed as a death in utero and becomes part of the fetal and **perinatal** death rate. Of the infants who survive birth, the **neonatal** period—from day 1 to 28—is crucial. Premature infants or those with birth defects especially may die within these 28 days and are listed in the neonatal mortality statistics. The infant death rate includes all deaths of liveborn infants from birth through the first birthday. Box 1-6 lists the categories of causes of infant death. Parental responses to infant death are discussed in Chapter 26.

Maternity and infant care continues to need nursing interventions. Along with changes in policies supporting health of mothers and infants, perhaps community education, parenting classes in school, and emphasis on prenatal care will all contribute to a reduction in morbidity and mortality for mothers and children.

Box 1-6	Categories of Causes of Deaths of Infants less than 1 Year Old

All causes
Congenital anomalies
Hyaline membrane disease and respiratory distress syndrome
Asphyxia, anoxia, and other hypoxic conditions
Immaturity, unqualified
Complications of pregnancy
Difficult labor, with and without birth injury
Conditions of placenta and umbilical cord

Key points

- All maternity and family care focuses on the birth of a healthy infant. Pregnancy is a time to promote parenting skills.
- Each family is unique and brings varied cultural expectations to the perinatal period.
- Trends in care include putting high-risk women and infants into tertiary hospitals. Thus much of the day-to-day maternity care of smaller hospitals and birthing centers is for the normal healthy woman and infant.
- Increasing use of high-tech care has raised the costs of care. Early discharge to reduce costs sometimes has been too early for complete assessment and interventions.
- Home care is increasingly important for women and newborn infants. This is an area for independent nursing practice.

- FCMC has become widely accepted, and fathers, friends, siblings, and grandparents may have a part in supporting the woman during the birthing process.
- Physician, midwife, and nurse relationships must work toward being collegial rather than competitive.
- The nurse has legal obligations for care in the obstetric setting. Lawsuits are not unusual, and it is important to avoid nursing liability.
- Community and professional standards of care are considered when negligent actions are being questioned.
- Collaborative and independent care functions can be clear when using the nursing process to focus care planning.

Study Questions

1-1. Select the terms that apply to the following statements:
   a. Rates of death for mothers or infants _____
   b. A person less than legal age living independently of her or his family _____
   c. The most important factor in the successful outcome of a pregnancy _____
   d. The chief consideration about whether a lawsuit is possible _____
   e. Numbers of persons who become ill because of conditions related to pregnancy _____
   f. Actions that a nurse may initiate under professional license _____

1-2. Name four factors influencing a healthy pregnancy outcome.

1-3. Match the terms with their definitions.
   a. Nurse practitioner
   b. Birth attendant
   c. Midwife

   1. Assists women during childbirth and postpartum period
   2. Certified in nursing and midwifery
   3. Professional, licensed specialized nurse
   4. Licensed nurse with a master's degree in a specialty area

1-4. Match the terms with their definitions.
   a. Death in utero before 20 weeks
   b. Death of a live born infant at 2 days
   c. Death of fetus at 32 weeks

   1. Neonatal mortality
   2. Perinatal mortality
   3. Abortion
   4. Fetal mortality

Answer Key

References

*Arnold LS et al: Lessons from the past, *Matern Child Nurs J* 14(2):79, 1989.

Atrash HK et al: Maternal Mortality in the United States, 1979-1986, *Obstet Gynecol* 76(6):1055, 1990.

Atrash HK, Alexander S, Berg CJ: Maternal mortality in developed countries: not just a concern of the past, *Obstet Gynecol* 86(4 Pt 2):700, l995.

Enkin M et al: *A guide to effective care in pregnancy and childbirth,* ed 2, Oxford, 1995, Oxford University Press.

*Fawcett J: Conceptual models and theory development, *J Obstet Gynecol Neonatal Nurs* 15(6):400, 1988.

Fiscella K: Does prenatal care improve birth outcomes? A critical review, *Obstet Gynecol* 85(3):468, 1995.

Fleischer R, Sala J: Pregnancy after organ transplantation, *J Obstet Gynecol Neonatal Nurs* 24(5):413, 1995.

Grayson M: Next steps for nursing, *Hosp and Health Netw* 67(16):26, 1993.

*Hughes D et al: *The health of America's children: maternal and child health data book,* Washington, DC, 1987, Children's Defense Fund.

*Kenniston K, The Carnegie Council on Children: *All our children: the American family under pressure,* New York, 1978, Harcourt Brace Jovanovich.

*Klaus M, Kennell J: *Parent-infant bonding,* ed 2, St Louis, 1982, Mosby.

McGregor, LA: Short, shorter, shortest: improving the hospital stay for mothers and newborns, *MCN Am J Matern Child Nurs* 19(2): l, 1994.

McKnight M, Burns J: Four ways to improve your prenatal program, *Business and Health* 12(5):47, 1994.

National Centers for Health Statistics: Advance report on final mortality statistics, 1994, *MMWR* 45(ss-3):1, 1996.

Price C: Associate degree nursing education: challenging premonitions and resourcefulness, *Nursing Forum* 30(4):26, 1995.

*Rhodes AM: The nurse's legal obligations for reporting child abuse, *Matern Child Nurs J* 12(5):313, 1987.

Rhodes AM: Maternal liability for fetal injury, *MCN Am J Matern Child Nurs* 15(1):41, 1990.

*Classic reference.

*Richmond JB, Wise PH: Midwifery and medicine in America, *J Nurse Midwifery* 31(5):219, 1986.

*Smoyak SA, ed: Symposium on parenting, *Nurs Clin North Am* 12(3):4, 1977.

Starn J, Neiderhauser V: A MCN model for nursing diagnosis to focus intervention, *MCN Am J Matern Child Nurs* 15(3):180, 1990.

Ventura SJ et al: Advance report of final natality statistics 1993, *Monthly Vital Statistics Report* 44(3S):2, 1995.

*US National Commission to Prevent Infant Mortality: *Death before life: the tragedy of infant mortality,* Washington, DC, 1988, The Commission.

Weiss ME, Armstrong M: Postpartum's mothers' preferences for nighttime care of the neonate, *J Obstet Gynecol Neonatal Nurs* 20:290, 1991.

Wood S, Ransem V: The 1990s: a decade for change in women's health care policy, *J Obstet Gynecol Neonat Nurs* 23(2):139, 1994.

Student Resource Shelf

Enkin M et al: *A guide to effective care in pregnancy and childbirth,* ed 2, Oxford, 1995, Oxford University Press.
Complete review of worldwide research databases and standards of care with analysis of degrees of effectiveness. Shows that many common practices in care are useless.

Gennaro S: Research utilization: an overview, *J Obstet Gynecol Neonatal Nurs* 23(4):313, l994.
Introductory article to an issue directed at research in maternity care.

Scoggin J: How nurse-midwives define themselves in relation to nursing, medicine and midwifery, *Nurs Midwife* 41(1):36, 1996.
Describes a study of how midwives define their occupational identity.

York R: Maternal factors that influence inadequate prenatal care, *Public Health Nurs* 10(4):241, 1993.
Identifies factors that influence the woman's decision to seek prenatal care.

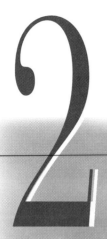

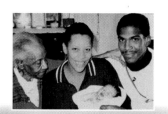

The Family *in a* Multicultural Society

The word *family* has a variety of meanings and applies to different groupings. Families can be defined by the nature of the bonds that tie their members together. A *biologic family* is defined by blood relationships, the relationships of parent to child and sibling to sibling. The biologic family is the fundamental, historical way in which people view a family. The *legal family* is defined by the civil or religious bonds of marriage and adoption. The *functional family* is distinguished by shared household living, responsibilities, and activities. The *ethical family* is determined by basic expectations of trust, reliability, loyalty, and long-term commitment.

Of course, all of these bonds overlap in a family. However, families are not uniform. Each is as unique as its individual members. How one interacts and communicates and the values and attitudes held are influenced by one's ethnic background and social class, the cultural environment in which one lives, and the parents' child-rearing practices. Individuality is shaped by the family context; actions are governed by characteristics of the family. One family might find a specific behavior acceptable and normal, whereas another family might find it unfamiliar. Family life is therefore rich and varied.

While the "typical" family of a generation ago included a homemaker mother, working father, and children, only approximately 10% of today's families fit that description. In addition, only 26% of all households in the United States are composed of a married couple residing with their own children. Approximately 40% of all marriages are remarriages, so that in approximately 20% of all households with children, one parent is a biologic parent and the other is a stepparent (Andersen and Sabatelli, 1995). One out of every four children lives in a single-parent family; for African-American children it increases to one out of every two (National Center for Children in Poverty, 1990).

Beginning with the abstract term "family," generalizations about basic or core features that apply to all families can be made. From this point, you can understand the diverse dynamics and structures that will be found within families with whom you will interact.

FAMILY AS A SYSTEM

Another word for family is *system*, the totality of objects with their mutual interactions. The **family system** is the primary and most powerful system to which you belong (Murray and Zentner, 1993). The family is changed even before the arrival of a new member. Family attachment to the fetus begins in utero, and subsequent interactions continue throughout the new member's life span. The new family member will be imprinted by the family's history, structure, and style. This process of imprinting and being imprinted by the family and carrying the pattern for interaction into other areas of life is the "output" of a family system.

Goals and Purposes

All systems are goal-directed (Whitchurch and Constantine, 1993), and the primary goal of the family system is its own survival. Secondary goals are physical survival and personal development. Terkelsen (1980) suggests that family members interact with intense **attachment behavior** (e.g., love, caring, affection, loyalty). These interactions continue throughout life. Membership in the family, through birth, adoption, or marriage, is virtually permanent. The purposes of these interactions are physical survival and personal development for all members. Personal development can occur only when there is security about physical survival. These goals are achieved when the family achieves the following four objectives:

1. Reproduction, recruitment, and release of family members: Families give birth to or adopt children, rear them to maturity, and release them as self-sufficient adults to start families of their own. They also incorporate new members by marriage and establish policies by which other persons become family members.
2. Physical maintenance: The family meets the needs of each member for food, clothing, and shelter. These material resources are acquired and allocated by family members responsible for procuring income, managing the household, and caring for members.
3. Socialization of children: The family guides the indi-

vidual's internalization of increasingly mature and acceptable patterns in areas such as controlling elimination, food intake, sexual drives, and aggression. Through the establishment of types and intensity of interactions, patterns of affection, and administration of sanctions, conformity to family norms is encouraged.

4. Emotional maintenance: Individual emotional development depends on the satisfaction of emotional needs. The family unit is committed to creating and sustaining the senses of being valued, cared about, accepted, and the sense of permanence of ties of affection. As members are rewarded for achievements, encouraged to succeed, and helped to overcome crises, a sense of satisfaction and purpose is provided. These family objectives are summarized by Terkelsen (1980) in his following definition of "the good enough family:"

> A family is sufficient or good enough to the extent that it is matching specific elements of structure to specific needs . . . . The idea is this: If you give a living thing what it needs, it *grows itself up*. That is, *under conditions of need attainment*, growing up is something that the organism does for itself. The heart of the matter is that *need attainment* is the mainspring of development. And despite our complexity, we human beings share this property with the rest of the living world. The implication for our notion of sufficiency is simply this: the task of the family is to create a resource, in the form of interpersonal enactments, that matches or meets a need. When the family performs this task, each member "grows itself up."

You will deal with families that are not "good enough," families that cannot meet the needs of their members because of financial, physical, or emotional handicaps. Part of your responsibility may be to assess the sufficiency of families to carry out their purpose.

Stages of Development

Although there is currently a trend toward later marriage and childbearing, most people in our culture marry in their twenties and thirties and have children who start first grade at age 6, throw the household into a turmoil in their teens, and move out as young adults. Their parents are then left to deal with each other, their own aging parents, retirement, and eventually death (Carter and McGoldrick, 1989). This pattern suggests different stages in the family's history. At each stage certain developmental tasks must be accomplished to successfully navigate subsequent stages. When families are remarried or blended, or when there is single parenthood, the stages are even more complex, requiring considerable adjustments and compromise. By carefully examining these stages, one can learn the **stage-appropriate tasks** of the family system. In addition to understanding a model of the successful family, one can identify the family's developmental stage. It is also possible to recognize how well the family accomplishes its tasks.

Each individual moves through these stages of development: fetus, infant, toddler, child, adolescent, and adult. Each term label denotes a stage of development at which different processes or tasks take place. Erikson (1950) outlined the maturational tasks of the individual in psychosocial terms. Growth means movement through stages of development; attainment of the ensuing stage depends on accomplishment of the tasks of the previous stage. There is a predictability about family development that helps nurses know what to expect of a given family at any given stage. Much as each individual who grows, develops, matures, and ages undergoes the same successive changes and readjustments from conception to senescence as every other individual, the life cycle of individual families follows a *universal sequence* of family development.

A number of models based on stages in the family's history have been useful for describing the life cycle of families. While stage models are less applicable to more complex family situations such as blended or single-parent families, models still provide a useful way to view family life cycles. The Carter and McGoldrick (1989) model includes six stages: (1) single young adults, (2) the couple, (3) families with young children, (4) families with adolescents, (5) families launching their adolescents, and (6) families later in life. The first three stages concern learning in this text and aid in conceptualizing how effectively couples will negotiate the new responsibilities of the childbearing period.

The single young adult

In this stage of the family life cycle the young adult separates from the family of origin, hopefully without fleeing reactively to a substitute emotional refuge. This phase is a cornerstone that will influence all succeeding stages in the family life cycle. It is a time for individuals to develop personal life goals, keeping what is useful from the family of origin while defining new goals that are theirs alone. This newly-formed independence results in new ways of relating to parents that are less hierarchic.

Forming of families through marriage: the couple

In the second stage of the family life cycle, the couple establishes themselves as a unit separate emotionally and financially from their families of origin. Traditionally the marriage ceremony is the rite that signals the beginning of a new family. Despite the way in which a couple validates their union, all couples must form a durable relationship capable of carrying out the tasks of the later stages. The couple's investment in their relationship is crucial. This beginning is connected to the couple's completion of tasks in their own families of origin (i.e., achieving a sufficient degree of solid personal identity and emotional independence). It is the successful completion of the *individuation–separation process* of growing up in the family that makes the successful founding of a new family possible. A marriage is not so much a beginning as a stage in a multigenerational process.

Becoming parents: families with young children

Whether the second stage is successfully negotiated or not, all couples face decisions about children: to have or not to have them, how many to have, and when to have them. From conception, the newcomer affects the relationship. The arrival of the child transforms a *dyadic* (two-person) system into a *triadic* (three-person) system, and the structure (patterns of interaction) changes profoundly. The previously childless couple must make space in their relationship for another person. The child deprives the new parents of privacy and time for each other. Without care, a triangle in which two members are close and the third is an outsider can develop. In young families the father may feel left out because the mother forms an intense alliance with "her" child. The outsider may become more involved in work and leave most of the responsibility for running the household and parenting to the mother. In the modern two-paycheck and often two-career marriage, the division of childcare responsibilities and household chores may become a source of conflict for the couple. The challenging task of the childbearing family is to establish an interactional structure in which there is time and space for the needs of the couple as a couple, while the needs of the children are met.

A child's extremely rapid development from a suckling infant requiring frequent feedings to a toddler capable of crawling and climbing requires an almost constant process of readjustment on the part of the parents. With each new child, family structure and function goes through a process of reorganization. Readiness for parenthood, personality traits, life experiences, and positive or negative interactions among family members will determine how successfully the family negotiates this process (May and Perrin, 1985). Responses of siblings generally depend upon age, developmental level, and their perceptions relative to security within the family system.

As the nurse addressing the needs of the childbearing family, one should be sensitive to these tasks of system realignment. The nurse should be alert to the constant readjustment to the changing needs of growing children through the years that causes energy depletion and a lack of privacy. The single parent is at even greater risk for not having personal needs met. This may cause resentment, leading to the potential for abusive behaviors.

FAMILY PATTERNS

Repetitive patterns of interactions in the family determine who, when, and to whom members relate. There can be many patterns of interaction: (1) the *pattern of communication* describes who says what to whom and in what way, (2) the *pattern of power* describes who influences whom and how, and (3) the *pattern of role performance* describes who does what. Knowledge of internal family dynamics may appear to be outside the scope of the nurse's responsibility. It is true that contact with the client does not allow a comprehensive view of the inner workings of the family. However, the individual is *embedded* in the family system and cannot truly be understood without attention to it. The family focus allows you to see that an individual's self-understanding, role expectations, value orientation, and motivation are not simply within the individual; these develop in interaction with the other members of the family system.

Boundaries

Boundaries refer to the invisible lines around individuals and groups that protect the separateness and autonomy of family members and define who participates and in what ways. The boundaries may be visible; for example, the closed door that separates the parents' bedroom from the children's room is a boundary between marital and sibling subgroups. Of course, a boundary may not be obvious. Parents may decide not to discuss certain matters in front of children. That decision becomes a family rule regulating information shared. It also identifies a boundary. Family rules that regulate information shared, the access members have to one another, and the activities in which members are permitted to participate create boundaries.

These boundaries are not fixed, like those dividing a map into political territories. Boundary-making in the family is a dynamic process that balances the comfort of members with their interaction with the outside. The usual purpose is to protect members from intrusive threats and to permit interchange. Thus boundaries should be flexible.

An individual's boundary preserves the right to be a separate person. However, this boundary must be flexible enough to promote interaction so the individual feels and is recognized as a family member. The person needs to be emotionally connected to other family members and able to give and receive support and affection. Sometimes a boundary goes around a troublesome child, labeled a "black sheep." Audible comments align others together, leaving out the one who does not seem to conform. Such negative boundaries may be difficult to alter. Similarly, the boundary around a couple provides an area for the satisfaction of their needs without the intrusion of in-laws, children, and others. At the same time, this boundary must be flexible enough to permit contact between them and their children, their families of origin, and the external environment. The achievement of clear, firm, and flexible boundaries is a constant challenge as the family develops.

Disengagement patterns

Minuchin and Fishman (1981) characterize the failures of adequate boundary-making as **disengagement**. When boundaries are overly rigid, they restrict contact among individuals, the family system, and outside systems. Rigid boundaries result in disengaged families, and members of these families are *underresponsive* to one another. The individual feels distant and isolated. The behavior of the individual seems to be of no concern to the others. In a disengaged family, distance may permit autonomy, but it may also minimize affection and deprive the individual of support. You may detect disengagement when parents display a surprising ignorance of important information about their children, for example. Or you may notice that a mother is tearful as she talks to you about her fears, but her husband sits beside her, seemingly unmoved by her distress. An absence of conflict and a lack of concern for one another's interests are signs of the disengaged family and may suggest that it may be difficult for you to connect with its members.

Enmeshed patterns

The opposite of rigid boundaries is diffuse boundaries. Whereas the rigid boundary is impermeable, the diffuse boundary is overly permeable. In the nuclear family with diffuse boundaries, the parents and siblings are overly close; individuals are dependent on one another. Minuchin and Fishman (1981) call these **enmeshed families**. Any action by one member triggers strong and immediate reactions from the others. In contrast to disengaged parents, enmeshed parents may spend too much time with their children and do things for them that the children could do for themselves. You can recognize the enmeshed family when its members interrupt each other, speak for each other, and argue with each other. You won't be able to finish your conversation with the mother-to-be without intrusions from other members, and you may find yourself included in a family argument.

It is important to recognize that boundaries may vary according to cultural group. Disengagement may characterize families in certain cultural groups where the paternal authority is unquestioned. Conversely, in many groups, diffuse boundaries are the norm. For example, the boundaries of an African-American family may function well as diffuse and more flexible. Aunts, uncles, and cousins may be involved in primary support of the mother. Kinship networks may not follow genograms of first-degree relatives as in other families. This is true also of extended families from cultures where many relatives may be involved in caring for the child. The nurse should ask who will be taking a direct care role for the newborn and who will be providing a supporting role for the mother (Figure 2-1).

Tracing a Genogram

An understanding of family structure helps you to understand what happens when a child is born. The birth of a

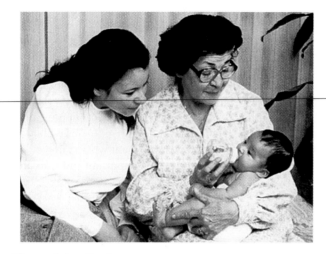

Figure 2-1 The family support system extends beyond parents.

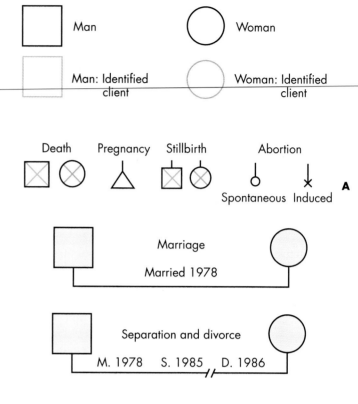

child calls for a radical restructuring of the family. The stages of this restructuring can be diagramed by the use of a **genogram** (Figure 2-2, *A* and *B*), a format for drawing at least a three-generation diagram of a family tree to record information about family members and relationships.

Self-Discovery

Are you able to follow your family line for more than three generations? Note your family origins. Which cultural or ethnic patterns have entered the family? Which have remained strong influences? Draw your family genogram. ~

TRANSITIONS: CHILDLESSNESS TO PARENTHOOD

Whether it is a nuclear, single parent, remarried, or blended family, the establishment of stable and affectionate relationships between parents and child is essential for healthy growth. In nuclear or blended families, in addition to bonding to their child, parents must bond to one another. They must establish firm, clear, and flexible boundaries between themselves and their children. As parents, they have responsibility for nurturance and guidance, but as a couple, they must meet each other's needs. If overinvolvement as parents results in underinvolvement as spouses, either or both parents can feel isolated or unsupported.

As a nurse, you are a privileged participant during the first days of a couple's transition from childlessness to parenthood. This transition is not easily navigated, as Nichols (1984) reminds us in the following:

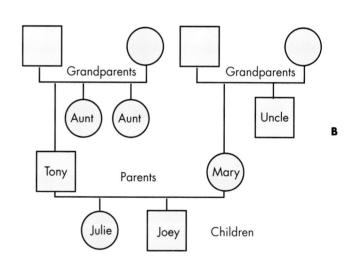

Figure 2-2 A, The standardized symbols for a genogram developed by McGoldrick. **B,** Family genogram.

All too often, husband and wife give up the space they need for supporting each other when the children are born. Husband and wife are sustained as a loving couple and enhanced as parents if they have time to be alone together—alone to talk, alone to go out to dinner occasionally, alone to fight, and alone to make love. Unhappily the demands of small children often make parents lose sight of their need to maintain a boundary.

STRESSES ON THE FAMILY SYSTEM

Families do not exist by themselves; they exist in the real order, with other families and people. Our beliefs and laws spell out the way things should be, but we live and practice the way things are. For example, we say in general that marriage ought to be monogamous, that premarital sex and marital infidelity are taboo, that marriage should last until death, that children belong to parents, and that the state interferes with their socialization only under extreme circumstances, but reality is much different. The family is considered to be the economic unit for consumption, mutual property, and inheritance, and it is the residential unit until the child achieves majority. Our laws support these ideas about marriage and the family.

The actual behavior of many American families is often in direct conflict with these assumptions. The family reacts to tensions from within and social stressors from without.

Social Factors

Marriage rate

The marriage rate is the number of marriages per 1000 population, not just those eligible to marry (persons older than 15 and unmarried). The rate was 9.1 in 1994, a low rate in comparison with prior years (Figure 2-3). In the 1950s the estimated median age of a woman at first marriage was 20 years; one half of the women who married were younger than 20. Most women married before having children. In contrast, 31% of all the births in 1993 were to unmarried women, which is 1% more than in 1992 (MVSR, 1995).

These figures reflect the divorce trends and the change in cultural insistence on marriage before childbearing. In the 1990s the overall birth rate has declined approximately 1% per year and in 1994 was at the lowest point in 15 years (MVSR, 1995).

Today women are postponing marriage longer than their mothers did. More women are enrolled in higher education programs, and preparation for a career has assumed a greater importance for the future. When both partners in a marriage expect to work, preparation allows the potential for a higher income. In addition, the possibility of remaining unmarried, being childless, or being divorced raises the need to be prepared for an income-producing occupation.

Fertility rate

The fertility rate is the number of live births per 1000 of the women aged 15 to 44. Figure 2-4 shows the general trends in fertility. Beginning in the early 1990s the rate has been falling approximately 2% a year. (The rate was 67.6 in 1993). The declining birth rate reflects the aging of the baby-boom generation, who are reaching their middle to late forties; there are fewer women in the population of

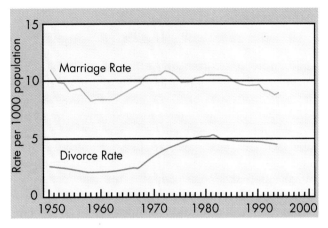

Figure 2-3 Marriage and divorce rates: United States, 1950-1994. (From Monthly Vital Statistics Report 43[13]:4, 1995.)

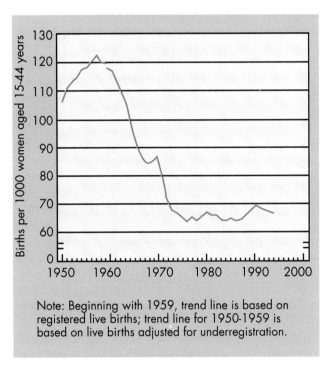

Note: Beginning with 1959, trend line is based on registered live births; trend line for 1950-1959 is based on live births adjusted for underregistration.

Figure 2-4 Fertility rates: United States, 1950-1994. (From Monthly Vital Statistics Report 43[13]:4, 1995.)

younger age groups. It also reflects the concern parents have to afford the costs of caring for and educating their children. Of the population of women in the childbearing years, 20% are childless; one third of these women have impaired fertility (MMWR, 1995).

Today a growing number of men and women are voluntarily sterilized after having their desired number of children (see Chapter 5). Therefore women are having fewer children and reaching the end of childbearing earlier than their mothers.

Divorce rate

The Census Bureau defines a family as two or more persons related to each other by blood, marriage, or adoption who live together. The divorce rate has remained stable in the past few years and now accounts for more than 40% of single-parent families (MVSR, 1995). Half of the states have adopted some form of no-fault divorce laws, which allows a marriage to be terminated without any expectations of punitive consequences—after the negotiation of joint property settlements and arrangements for the maintenance of children and the spouse (see Figure 2-3).

The highest incidence of divorce occurs in families with preschool children and school-age children. Two thirds of women who divorce do so before age 30, and seven eighths of all women who divorce do so before middle age. Most children are less than 7 years of age when their parents separate or divorce. As a result, many families are single-parent or remarried families.

Contraception

The basic tension within marriage is between the desire to provide a stable family structure for rearing children and the desire to achieve a satisfying and meaningful relationship with the opposite sex. Effective contraception essentially separates reproduction and the sexual relationship. Mate selection on the basis of sexual compatibility may not coincide with mate selection on the basis of suitability for establishing and maintaining a family. Perhaps too much has been expected of the institution of marriage if men and women expect to find their only sexual relationship, their only partners-in-dialogue, their primary valuation and appreciation as persons, and the fulfillment of their romantic longings within one person. Perhaps the family established by marriage has always suffered from this inner tension of romance versus reproduction, but until the turn of the century, family behavior was more rigidly controlled by social mores, public opinion, and ecclesiastic and civil law. As we enter the twenty-first century, great changes in American society have removed much of the framework of external social control. The result is more and more families with alternative structures or lifestyles that differ from the traditional idea. The nurse should be aware that in most societies of the world, mate selection is not primarily the choice of the two partners but is affected by extended family wishes.

Self-Discovery

List benefits young couples may receive if their families select the marriage partner. ~

Mobility

One of the most potent forces that changed the family was the shift from a primarily rural and agricultural society to an urban and industrial society. This relocation of work from farm to city disrupted extended family structures. Only the nuclear family tended to migrate, which left the extended family behind. The average American household consisted of five persons from 1890 to 1910 but shrank to four persons from 1920 to 1950; the last census showed that it has shrunk even further—to three persons.

High residential mobility is still a mark of American society. Forty million Americans, 18% of the population, move every year. There is a debate about the extent of this separation from the extended family, and it is probably rare for a nuclear family to be completely isolated from the family network. However, although contact may be maintained and help obtained in extended crises, contacts are usually short and limited. Telephone calls and visits on holidays are no substitute for living in the same house or on the same street.

Therefore the parents become the sole child rearers in the geographically and socially isolated nuclear family. However, when the mother and the father become the only effective models that the children can emulate, other influences become value determiners, including schools, adolescent subculture, and the popular media. This turning away from parental values and expectations has been a source of intergenerational conflict in modern American families.

Consequences

Single-parent families

The demography of single-parent families is difficult to express accurately. A single mother may live with her parents, or with a boyfriend. In these cases the child has other adults in its social environment. To have the following descriptions of a single-parent household be accurate, the definition must be based on living arrangements of only one adult in the household (Bumpass and Raley, 1995) (Figure 2-5). Being a single parent will make more difficult the objectives of the family system: establish an income, maintain a household, develop social relationships in the community, and teach children to become productive members of that community. The challenges of the childbearing years of development are coping with energy depletion and lack of privacy. The danger of task overload can be great for the single mother or father with young children.

When a mother or father divorces, the children experience the loss of the other parent. The majority of the time the children stay primarily with the mother, however, increasingly, the father will gain primary custody. In the case of the mother, if she had not been employed outside of the home before the divorce, the children also experience loss of the mother's time through her employment.

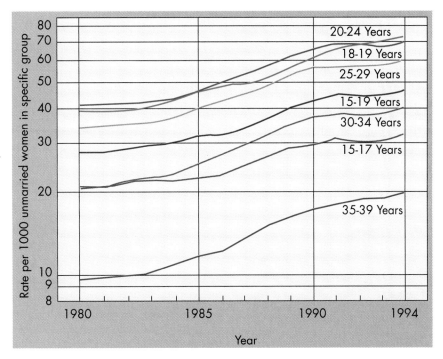

Figure 2-5 Birth rates for unmarried women, by age of mother: United States, 1980-1994. (From Monthly Vital Statistics Report 44(suppl 11):9, 1996.)

The divorced mother or father also may be cut off emotionally from the extended family system of in-laws. Divorced men and women tend to have fewer friends and belong to fewer organizations than married couples. The social isolation experienced by these parents tends to intensify the parent-child relationship.

Although the percentage of single-parent families has doubled since 1970, it may be a temporary arrangement. Because many divorced persons remarry, the single-parent family may serve as a transition for the parent from one marital partner to another and between parenthood and stepparenthood.

Remarried families

Remarried families, **blended families**, or **reconstituted families** are complex family systems that result from the remarriage of persons who have lost their first spouses through death or divorce. If these persons are already parents, the remarriage creates family relationships involving stepparents, stepchildren, stepsiblings, and stepgrandparents. If the spouses have children between them, there are also half-siblings. A child in a stepfamily can have two "mothers," three or four sets of grandparents, full siblings, half-siblings, and stepsiblings. In this case it can be difficult to answer questions about family and the nature of family relationships.

The stepfamily is becoming more common. Carter and McGoldrick (1989) provide the following important reminder to all who have to deal with stepfamilies:

Unfortunately, the "instant intimacy" that remarried families expect of themselves is impossible to achieve and the new relationships are all the harder to negotiate because they do not develop slowly, as intact families do, but must begin midstream, after another family's life cycle has been dislocated. Naturally, second families carry the scars of first families. Neither parents, nor children, nor grandparents can forget the relationships that went before. Children *never give up their attachment* to their first parent, no matter how negative the relationship with that parent was or is. Having the patience to tolerate the ambiguity of the situation and allowing each other the space and the time for feelings about past relationships is crucial to the process of forming a remarried family.

The challenge of forming a remarried family will increase in difficulty, depending on whether the spouses have no children from previous marriages (difficult), have grown children (more difficult), or have young or adolescent children who still require parenting (most difficult). Both parents and children will need time to adjust to their new relationships (Table 2-1).

The birth of a child to a remarried couple has many possible ramifications for the stepfamily. The couple's decision to have a child may come from a loving commitment or more problematic motivations—to assure spousal commitment, to demonstrate family solidarity, to satisfy cultural expectations, or to surpass the parenting results of the former marriage. Despite the motivations of the parents, other factors play a part in how the birth of a child affects family structure. If both spouses are parents from

Table 2-1	Selected Differences Between Traditional Nuclear Family and Stepfamily

Nuclear Family	Stepfamily
This family originates with marriage of never-married persons who are childless; thus the family is born of individuals coming together in step-by-step progression from courtship to marriage through parenthood.	This family originates with remarriage of divorced or widowed persons who may or may not be childless; thus the new family is born of separation and loss (usually an unfinished process) preceding rapid entry into instant multiple roles.
First marriage joins the two families of origin of each partner.	Remarriage involves interweaving three, four, or more families whose previous life cycles had been disrupted by death or divorce (and may join spouses of differing life-cycle stages [e.g., father of adolescent children and never-married wife]).
Both biologic parents are included.	One biologic parent who exists as a memory (in the case of death) or as a noncustodial parent outside the family circle may be excluded.
Relationship between spouses predates the relationship between parent and child.	Relationship between natural parent and child predates the relationship of the new couple.
Biologic mother has 9 months to prepare for her role as mother.	Stepmother (whether or not she has a child or children of her own) has indeterminate period of acquaintance with children to assume role of primary mother, other mother, comanager, or friend.
Natural parents have important postnatal period of bonding to develop psychologic attachment with child.	Stepparent has postmarriage period of adjustment to develop familial affection for spouse's children.
Natural parents begin parenting an infant who knows no other parent.	Stepparent begins parenting children of various ages who have lost a parent through divorce or death.
Couple bond of the natural parents (normally) takes priority over all other family relationships and provides a solid foundation for a unified household.	Natural bond between biologic parent and child can take priority over the new marital bond and can create a competitive or conflicting environment of divided loyalties. This is not an inevitable consequence but a possibility.

previous marriages or if one of the spouses has not previously had children, the birth of the new child has a different impact. The ages of stepchildren also make a difference. Young stepchildren may fear that they will be loved less than the newcomer. Conversely, the new half-brother or half-sister can serve as a link between stepsiblings and the couple and thus bring **cohesiveness** to the stepfamily. A nurse can bring a special service to the new mother by being sensitive to and allowing her to talk about the emotional issues involved in such a birth.

Adolescent parents

One segment of single-parent families that presents special needs is the teenage parent. The United States leads nearly all other developed nations in its incidence of pregnancy among teenage women (see Figure 2-5). Teenage childbearing varies by race of the mother. Childbirths to women less than age 20 are uncommon for Chinese (1%), Japanese (3%), and Filipino and other Asian mothers (6%). White American teenage mothers had a rate of 11%. Hawaiian teenage mothers (17%) and Native American mothers (20%) approached the 23% rate for African-American mothers (MVSR, 1995).

Even within a racial group outcomes vary depending on socioeconomic class and most recent country of origin. Of teenage Hispanic mothers of Cuban and South and Central American background, 7% to 9% were younger than 20 years old compared with 17% to 22% of mothers of Mexican and Puerto Rican background (MVSR, 1995). These statistics are general statements that point to areas where health care providers should address improved delivery of services.

With the stigma of illegitimacy largely removed, less than 5% of teenage mothers surrender their infants for adoption. However, only one in five of 30,000 girls younger than 15 who become pregnant each year receive any prenatal care during the first 3 months of pregnancy. The medical consequences of pregnancy in adolescence and care for adolescent mothers and fathers are discussed in Chapter 8.

Economics and the Family

Every family exists within a socioeconomic context, and there are great differences in financial security. Those who exist in an impoverished physical context (i.e., those who live in substandard housing and have inadequate clothing and insufficient food) and those families who enjoy an abundance of food, clothing, and housing face different issues. The key to material abundance is regular employment that rewards the worker with an income. Many parents do not have such employment and cannot provide for their children.

Poverty

Poverty is statistically defined in the United States by the government **poverty level**, which changes from year to year. Approximately 20% of all children less than age 18 live in families whose income is below the poverty level. Half of these children live in households headed by women (i.e., single-parent families maintained by the mother). This development is being called the "feminization of poverty." Thus an American child has one chance in 10 of being poor if the father is the provider and has one chance in two of being poor if the mother is the provider. Without a legitimate, stable job role the poor adult man or woman has great difficulty functioning as a parent. The chronic stress of surviving puts the stability of the poor family at risk.

The life cycle of poor families was clearly drawn by Colon (1980). The young adult, thrown out of or tearing away from the family of origin, ill-equipped with the skills necessary to do well in a technologically complex society, enters an unmarried or married state. Because of limited job options, the adolescent boy frequently cannot form a supporting relationship, and the young childbearing girl emerges as the organizing force within the family. After childbirth, as the father becomes peripheral to the family or disengaged, the mother, who is chronically overburdened and often depressed, may be unable to respond to her children on an individual basis. The children, without attention from their mother or absent father, fail to develop the cognitive, affective, and communication skills that will enable them to benefit from a middle–class-oriented school system. These children are usually absorbed by peer culture.

Poverty can frustrate the goals of the family. Not every family living below the poverty level can be described by this "worst possible" scenario. On the other hand, to function properly as parents, people need the support of the larger economic system. The initiatives taken by government health services need better implementation so that the children and families may develop in healthy directions.

IMPORTANCE OF CULTURE

Families do not exist in isolation. They are connected to the extended family and the families of origin (Figure 2-6). The new couple's understanding of what it means to be a husband, wife, or parent is derived from their respective families. Their parents learned these understandings from their parents.

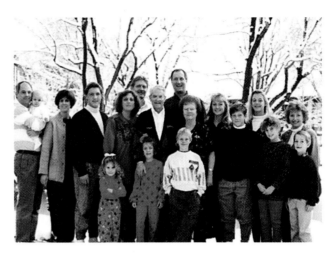

Figure 2-6　An extended family including grandparents, parents, and grandchildren.

Every social or human system has a belief system, a set of beliefs, values, and rules regarding what is true and desirable. These beliefs create a sense of cohesiveness and belonging among members and thus promote the goals of the family system and the development of individual members in harmony with societal expectations. Each family does not start from scratch to create its beliefs. Families do not exist in a vacuum. Each family is connected to other families by race, religion, and national or geographic origins that create a sense of commonality, which, transmitted through generations, is called **ethnicity**. "Ethnicity patterns our thinking, feeling, and behavior in obvious and subtle ways. It plays a major role in determining what we eat, how we work, how we relax, how we celebrate holidays and rituals, and how we feel about life, death, and illness" (Giordano, McGoldrick, and Pearce, 1982). You must understand the client's family culture and beliefs about pregnancy, parenthood, infant care, and contraception to provide personal care.

Culture is the sum of the beliefs and values about the world and human existence, the language, foods, habits, skills, arts, architecture, and institutions of a people in a given time. Ethnicity is the particular social and cultural heritage shared by a group. This ethnicity is a common ancestry that is a biologic descent from common ancestors intertwined with culture and transmitted through time by the biologic descendants of people. Inherited culture makes Jews Jewish, Italians Italian, and Africans African, for example, by providing a sense of identity. With the rapid social changes of the current period, culture and ethnicity are becoming "diluted," and the disparity between grandparents and grandchildren often centers on how differently from the "old ways" the younger generation acts and lives.

In the United States cultural groups from all over the world have coexisted for more than 200 years. This coexistence has not been smooth and has not produced a "melting pot" of national homogeneity in which ethnic differences have disappeared. Rather, it has produced a "salad bowl" effect in which the uniqueness of cultural groups has often been retained.

Although there is a mainstream of values that we can attribute to the middle class, not every ethnic group has been *acculturated* (i.e., absorbed and transformed by the cultural mainstream). How affected a person may be by ethnic background may not be simple to determine. It depends on the length of time the family has lived in the country, the number of generations born after immigration, the number of intermarriages (cross-cultural marriages) that have occurred, the strength with which family tradition has maintained ethnic identity, and the degree that the family has chosen to assimilate into the larger society.

Ethnic Values

People live and are usually governed by *values*—rules that shape their attitudes, beliefs, and behaviors. Cultural groups generally have dominant ethnic value orientations that they share with other members of the group (Box 2-1). Such ethnic value orientations provide a starting point for becoming acquainted with the cultural views of other ethnic groups.

All human beings experience life on the basis of their particular cultural values and assumptions. Most of these assumptions are outside their awareness. You will also see clients through your own "cultural filter." If you have mainstream American values, you may expect the client to keep appointments punctually and to follow schedules for health care (Time: Future). You may pay more attention to what the client is doing to help herself rather than how she is doing (Activity: Doing). You may resent the "intrusiveness" of the client's family (Relational: Individual). You will expect her to be confident of improvement (Man-Nature: Mastery-over-Nature). Finally, you may not understand if she feels that something she did wrong was the source of her illness (Basic Nature of Man). When misunderstanding happens, you may be judging the client by the standards of your cultural system and be guilty of **ethnocentrism**, believing that your cultural values are the "correct" ones. You must be aware of your client's values and recognize the differences from yours. You can do this if you become aware of your own values and develop a sensitivity to clients' values.

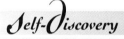

Consider the ethnic value orientations from each of the five categories in Box 2-1. Which ones best describe your family? Which ones best describe your own values? ~

| Box 2-1   Ethnic Value Orientations

TIME
Attitudes about the temporal focus of human life
Past: Values tradition
Present: Values "now" with no sense of urgency
Future: Values planning for the future, being on time, saving time, and places importance on novelty and youth

ACTIVITY
Attitudes about patterns of action in interpersonal relations
Doing: Values personal accomplishments and emphasizes getting the job done
Being: Values self-expression and spontaneous emotion
Being-becoming: Values the development of different aspects of the person in a rounded, integrated fashion

RELATIONAL ORIENTATION
Attitudes about relating in groups
Individual: Values autonomy vs responsibility and emphasizes pursuit of self-interest
Collateral: Values consensus and equal distribution of power
Lineal: Values hierarchic organization, including authority from above and obedience from below

MAN-NATURE ORIENTATION
Attitudes about one's relationship to the natural (and/or supernatural) environment
Mastery-over-Nature: Values one's power and technology to solve all problems
Harmony-with-Nature: Values a balance between human actions and the forces and influences in the heavens and on earth
Subjugation-to-Nature: Values human passivity and endurance in the face of uncontrollable forces

BASIC NATURE OF MAN
Attitudes about the innate good or evil in human behavior
Neutral-Mixed: One is born neither good nor evil but is a clean slate upon which parents, school, community, and nation leave their imprint
Evil: One is born evil but is perfectible and is thus in need of discipline, rules, and regulations
Good: One is born good but is corruptible and must avoid temptation

Modified from Spiegel J: An ecological model of ethnic families. In Giordano J, McGoldrick M, Pearce JK, eds: *Ethnicity and family therapy*, New York, 1982, The Guilford Press.

Nurses can be informed about ethnic patterns in several ways. Literature that describes ethnicity is available, but perhaps the best way to learn about ethnic beliefs is to learn from clients or from family members themselves. The maternity nurse must consider cultural influences on the client, some of which are identified in Box 2-2. In following chapters cultural variations are discussed in relation to practices during pregnancy, labor, and birth. Various patterns of family interaction will become evident. Stereotyping and assuming values and motivations to be true will interfere with your assessment and planning of nursing care. Therefore it is wise to learn to listen to the differences people have. Table 2-2 lists selected birth practices for different cultural groups.

Culture is not the only factor to be considered when assessing and understanding your client as a member of a family system. Gender, social class, and economic status are also important. As further study, choose additional reading from the Student Resource Shelf at the end of this chapter.

NURSING RESPONSIBILITY FOR CULTURALLY AWARE CARE

In the 1960s nursing educators began to recognize the need for including multicultural or **transcultural nursing** concepts in the curricula of schools of nursing and to determine what constitutes "culturally appropriate" care. This process can be fostered by first gaining an understanding of factors that influence health and illness behaviors in various cultural groups (Tripp-Reimer, Brink, and Saunders, 1988). Another framework for assessment of such factors (Giger and Davidhizar, 1995) uses six categories evidenced by all cultural groups: communication, space, social organization, time, environmental control, and biologic variations. This framework in client assessment can help to clarify similarities and differences among ethnic groups. It is used as a unifying principle for the following discussion of three of the many cultural groups in

the United States. When studying other groups, using the same six categories will organize learning.

Providers need to give greater consideration to the interaction of culture with the health care environment and how that influences client actions and behavior (Box 2-3). Discomfort with providers in an antepartal clinic, for example, may cause women either to not accept services or to be noncompliant. The nurse should not dismiss cultural health beliefs or practices as unscientific or primitive without further evaluation. By defining whether such practices are efficacious (helpful), neutral (may be helpful and are not harmful), dysfunctional (harmful), or uncertain (possibly harmful), the nurse can support practices that promote health and discourage those that may be damaging (Giger and Davidhizar, 1995). If a health practice is efficacious, it provides health benefits, even though the scientific reason may be nebulous. Home remedies such as spices, herbal teas or massage, or the use of prayer are examples of practices that may be efficacious, or that may be neutral—doing neither good nor harm.

Self-Discovery

If you have origins outside of the mainstream American culture, consider what different relatives have said about pregnancy and birth practices. Note their comments to share with your classmates. Together decide which practices are efficacious, which are neutral, and which are dysfunctional or uncertain. ~

Southeast Asian-Americans

Communication

Perhaps nothing is more essential to the nurse-client interaction than effective communication. It is through both verbal and nonverbal communication that the client

---

▌ *Box* **2-2**   **Cultural Beliefs Relevant to Maternal Nursing Care**

Fertility: Man's virility demonstrated in having a child; woman blamed for infertility

Family planning: Contraception contradicts desire for large families or religious tenets

Pregnancy: Norms for activity and rest, sexual intercourse, social relations, emotional climate, touching

Labor and delivery: Position assumed during delivery; management of pain

Postpartal care: Reestablishing body balances, restoring bodily purity

Food: Food restrictions and preferences

Cause of disease: Attribution of symptoms to social and interpersonal conflict or supernatural activity

Pain: Denial or exaggeration of pain, fatalistic acceptance of pain as punishment

Treatment: Reliance on folk practitioners (e.g., spiritual advisors, lay midwives, herbalists)

Maleness and femaleness: Attitudes and behaviors toward sex of child

Parenting: Roles of mother and father; involvement of the extended family

Table 2-2	**Cultural Birth Practices**
Pregnancy/Birth	**Recovery/Newborn**
CAMBODIA Childbirth is a "cold" condition. Mother must stay warm; covers head with towel.	Woman refuses to bathe after delivery or drink iced drinks. Lying-in for 1 week. Might not hold infant right after delivery. No compliments about infant to avoid evil spirits.
DOMINICAN REPUBLIC Satisfy cravings during pregnancy.	Traditional women do not bathe, wash hair, or have intercourse for 40 days. Protect child from evil spirits by wearing red. May save umbilical cord.
ETHIOPIA Mother may turn away from newborn as symbol of rejection of pain caused by infant. Some women may have ritual circumcision.	Mother may be confined for 2 to 4 weeks. Colostrum perceived as not good for infant. Sugar water given until milk produced.
HAITI Birth in squatting or semiseated position, supported by husband or close relative.	Placenta may be buried beneath doorway or burned. Postpartum is a "hot" state; avoid hot foods.
INDIA Must satisfy cravings because these are fetal desires. Husband should not be present. Female relatives assist.	Family members care for infant for first 10 days. Mother rests. Naming rites only after 10 days or when astrologically beneficial. Boys valued more than girls, especially as firstborn.
JAPAN Natural childbirth without anesthesia often preferred. Labor silently and eat during labor for strength.	Long recovery period (as long as 3 months). Remain indoors. May not wash for 1 week. Children highly prized, number limited.
PHILIPPINES During pregnancy wash often to have a clean infant. Avoid sexual intercourse during pregnancy. Western technology in use for deliveries.	Mother keeps warm and rests for 10 days, without bathing. Special bath at 2 weeks.
SOUTH KOREA Stoic response to labor pain. Father not allowed at birth.	Thanks offerings immediately after birth. Avoid cold, no iced drinks. Warm special postpartum foods. Only sons' births celebrated.
SWEDEN Any position to deliver, even underwater. Father/siblings may stay in unit overnight and witness birth.	As long as 12 months of paid leave for newborn care. Wide range of choices for newborn care.
THAILAND Home birth with father holding mother's head and shoulders between his knees.	Father buries placenta. Many rituals during postpartum month. Mother keeps warm during recovery.

From Geissler E: *Pocket guide to cultural assessment,* St Louis, 1994, Mosby.

| Box 2-3 | Characteristics of the Culturally Competent Practitioner |

- Moves from cultural unawareness to an awareness and sensitivity of her/his own cultural heritage
- Recognizes her/his own values and biases and is aware of how they may affect clients from other cultures
- Demonstrates comfort with cultural differences that exist between her/himself and clients
- Knows specifics about the particular cultural group(s) with which he/she is working
- Understands the historical events that may have caused harm to particular cultural groups
- Respects and is aware of the unique needs of clients from diverse communities
- Understands the importance of diversity within and between cultures
- Endeavors to learn more about cultural communities through interactions with clients, participation in cultural diversity workshops and community events, readings on cultural dynamics, and consultations with community experts
- Makes a continuous effort to understand the other's point of view
- Demonstrates flexibility and tolerance of ambiguity and is nonjudgmental
- Maintains a sense of humor and an open mind
- Demonstrates a willingness to relinquish control in clinical encounters, to risk failure, and to look within for the source of frustration, anger, and resistance
- Acknowledges that the process is as important as the product

From Randall D: *Culturally competent HIV care*, Rockville, Md, 1994, Public Health and Human Services, Maternal Child Bureau.

expresses her needs and desires to the nurse, and the nurse responds. Yet because communication is "culture bound," misunderstandings may arise when the nurse and client are from different cultures. The frank speech and direct gaze of the American nurse may be considered rude by an Asian client. Alternately, the nurse may perceive the passive attitude and averted gaze of the client as evidence of evasion and inability to confront problems.

When a Southeast Asian woman enters a maternity service, her unspoken goal may be to be a "good" patient and cause her to yield outwardly to the wishes of authority figures such as health providers. She may smile, nod, and answer "yes" to requests of care givers. But the smile may mask confusion, and the nod and affirmative answer may mean only that she hears, not that she understands or agrees (D'Avanzo, 1992). If English fluency is a problem, the use of translators or family members may help. Keep in mind, however, that the client may be reluctant to share intimate or confidential information in the presence of others. Because family elders often play a key role in deci-

sion making, the nurse also must be careful not to act in ways that may be interpreted as disrespectful to them, or the nurse-client relationship will be jeopardized.

The cultural norm for Cambodian and Laotian women tends to be subservience to male authority, such as their husbands or eldest sons, but Vietnamese women are usually the prime movers in making health care decisions for their families. Subjects such as childbearing, sex, or contraception, however, may not be considered appropriate topics to discuss when men are present. It may also be considered shameful to cry out during birth in the presence of a man.

Nurses often communicate through touch, yet an action such as stroking the hair of a laboring Southeast Asian woman may be distressing to her. The head is considered the most sacred and honorable part of the body and should not be touched except by close intimates. The nurse's hands on the infant's head and the removal of vernix after delivery also may be interpreted adversely.

Space

The culture in which we live, and even our geographic locations within cultures, determine our views of personal space. One's "comfort zone" relative to personal space varies within cultures and from culture to culture (Haber et al, 1992). The loss of control over personal boundaries is frequently mentioned by Southeast Asian women as a negative aspect of U.S. maternity care. Vietnamese women often prefer a female friend to be present during delivery. Laotian women may prefer the husband to be present. Hospital policies that allow "fathers only" in delivery rooms may therefore be distressing to some Southeast Asian groups.

Squatting also is common for delivery in Southeast Asia, and although it may be less traumatic for both mother and infant (Paciornik, 1990), it is often viewed as primitive by U.S. care givers and may not be allowed. Many women state that they feel embarrassed because of the loss of privacy and control over their personal space during the process of labor and delivery, but this may be particularly acute for the Southeast Asian woman. The nurse should maintain a sense of acceptance regarding her client's need for modesty, such as allowing her to tie a draw sheet around her in sarong-fashion during the laboring process. The presence of female midwives, if available, also will help mitigate some of this discomfort.

Social organization

In all cultures, children learn social behavior such as basic beliefs and common ties from their parents and others with whom they have contact (Figure 2-7). These interactions have long-standing effects regarding their attitudes and beliefs about important life events or milestones such as the childbearing process. Individuals within cultures generally embrace to some degree the con-

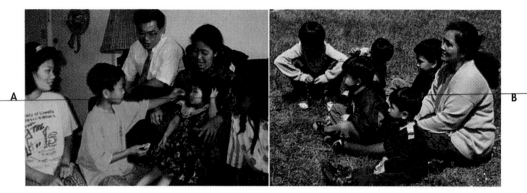

Figure 2-7 A, B Southeast Asian families may be large and closely spaced. They are often a tightly knit group.

cept of ethnocentrism, which maintains that one's own culture is best (and often implies that others are inferior). Variations occur within ethnic groups, but individuals within cultural groups share certain common traits, such as religious beliefs and food preferences. These necessarily affect health behaviors and relationships with care givers during the maternity cycle.

Religious beliefs, such as Buddhism, often influence how Southeast Asians react to life events and health practices. Pain or other suffering may be seen as punishment for transgressions in this or previous lives; thus help-seeking behaviors are considered inappropriate. Adherents to this teaching often appear stoic. They may smile and say they are "okay" even when they are experiencing postpartum pain, which makes assessment of nonverbal behavior even more important. The nurse should also be aware that because of the small body size of many Asians, average medication doses for pain may be too large.

Animism, especially prominent in Laotian hill tribe people, is rooted in the idea that gods, demons, and spirits control one's life. Help from a shaman may be sought to purge the person of maladies. Strings may be tied on the infant's wrists or ankles, or amulets may be worn to prevent "soul loss" and later illness. Removal of such items by health care professionals should be done with extreme caution and thoroughly explained to the family.

Heat and cold

Closely tied to religious beliefs, Chinese medical tradition rests on principles of universal balance and harmony between the equal and opposite forces of yin (hot) and yang (cold). Childbirth is seen as a critical time when women are in a "cold" state that may lead to future illness. To balance this state, Southeast Asian women may wish to eat "hot" foods in the postpartum period to "strengthen the blood:" meats and soups with chili and black peppers, sweets, and wine steeped with herbs. Cold drinks such as ice water and juices may be avoided. Steamed rice is a dietary staple and is preferred with all meals.

Time

Cultural groups often differ in their perception of time, which influences their perceptions relative to past, present, or future orientations. The future orientation of most North Americans allows for greater appreciation of the benefits of preventive health care and the need to be on time for appointments. Most Southeast Asians, however, come from a system where health care is *crisis oriented,* with symptom relief in the *present* as the goal. In addition to herbal medicines from the Chinese tradition, many Asians are used to taking facsimiles of Western drugs that are sold over the counter in Southeast Asia. On occasion this causes problems during childbirth such as resistance to certain antibiotics. It is important therefore to determine whether herbal or other medicines are being taken during pregnancy in addition to any prescribed medications. The *present orientation* of Southeast Asians also presents problems relative to the American appointment system. Whatever is occurring at any given moment may take precedence over the future, including prenatal or postpartum appointments. Such time orientation, perfectly reasonable to the Southeast Asian, is usually annoying to an American nurse, who may believe the client is being irresponsible and "noncompliant."

Environmental control

Most individuals prefer to maintain some control over their general surroundings or environment. Hospital settings, however, are notorious for making clients of all cultures feel they are in an alien environment where health care providers control their actions. The biomedical approach of most health care settings in the United States and Canada is often in conflict with traditional health care practices. For example, food preferences of Southeast Asian women after delivery would be considered *neutral,* provided the needs for optimal nutrition are met (Figure 2-8).

Ritual disposal of the placenta by Laotian clients is another neutral practice. However, some Southeast Asian women believe they should discard colostrum as "old"

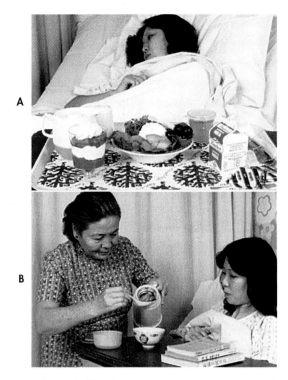

Figure 2-8 **A,** The first postpartum meal may be refused by some Asian women because, **B,** special foods are considered essential for recovery in the Asian culture. (Courtesy Concept Media, Irvine, Calif.)

milk and feed the infant rice paste or boiled sugar water for several days after delivery. This practice would constitute a *dysfunctional* traditional practice because of the benefits of colostrum in bolstering newborn immunity. The taking of potentially harmful herbs or over-the-counter medicines also constitutes a dysfunctional traditional practice. Nurses should seek to accept and support traditional health practices that are neutral or efficacious, while discouraging those that are dysfunctional or uncertain.

Biologic variations

Most nurses are educated to standardized norms that do not include cultural variations among racial groups. Therefore significant deviations from the norm, such as short stature in Asians, may be seen as unusual, even though they are within the norms of that cultural group.

As a group, Asians born abroad are generally shorter in stature and weigh less at birth than their American counterparts. Infants also differ in appearance by the epicanthic folds of the eyelids; smaller, flatter noses; larger teeth; and skin color. Mongolian spots—bluish spots that resemble bruises in the lumbosacral region—are commonly found in Asians (see Chapter 18). It is also rare to find an Rh-negative blood type in Asians.

Asians may metabolize drugs differently. If a cesarean birth is required, care givers should be aware that analgesics and muscle relaxants may produce different reactions in Asians. The muscle relaxant succinylcholine, for example, may cause prolonged muscle paralysis in an Asian client (Giger and Davidhizar, 1995). It is apparent that knowledge of biologic variations among cultural groups is an essential and integral part of the process of client assessment.

African-Americans
Communication

Variations in the way standard English is spoken become evident as one travels across the United States. In African-Americans, many of these variations in grammar, syntax, and pronunciation have been traced to several West African languages and are called black English. White nurses may have difficulty understanding words or phrases or may perceive these cultural variations as inferior or uneducated speech, which serves only to decrease communication and widen the gap between provider and client.

The importance of effective nurse-client communication in improving the health of African-American women and their children cannot be overestimated. The white nurse must move beyond any limitations of language that may occur and convey a willingness to communicate.

As is true with clients who speak languages other than English, clarification of meanings of words or phrases is essential. Familiarity with health-related terms that may be used by African-Americans, such as "miseries" for pain, helps nurses substitute more understandable phrases. As is true for Asian clients, nonverbal behaviors such as smiling or nodding may not indicate agreement or that the client is attentive to what the nurse is saying. Naming children takes on special significance for African-Americans. There is a current trend to give infants traditional African names that convey special meanings. In addition, "power names" may be given; it is felt that such names may provide opportunity for the child to identify with that powerful person or thing in the future.

Space

African-Americans, not unlike other ethnic groups such as Central Americans, may have a greater tolerance for physical closeness. What may seem to the nurse like too many people and too much confusion in the room may be perfectly comfortable for an African-American. If the nurse's discomfort shows, the client may misinterpret the source of the nurse's discomfort to mean he or she is uncomfortable with African-Americans, especially if the client has had prior experiences with health providers that made her feel inferior. The African-American woman may prefer a female attendant during childbirth. She may request that a sister or her mother pray with her.

Social organization

The description of the United States as a "melting pot" is recognized as out-of-date. The United States today more closely resembles a "salad bowl," where cultures intermingle and assimilate but retain their own cultural characteristics. As an ongoing consequence of segregation, many African-Americans have not been fully assimilated into mainstream America, and their lifestyles often are unequal in addition to being separate (Cherry and Giger, 1995).

The morals, beliefs, and attitudes of African-American culture were shaped by the destructive process of slavery that virtually obliterated family security and structure. Many traits shared within the group, however, such as food preferences and religion, serve to strengthen cultural ties and bring self-esteem and a sense of community. Most cultures have "food taboos" during pregnancy, often learned from mothers or other female family members. In the southern United States African-Americans have reported that they believe they should avoid fresh fruits, vegetables, and acidic foods during pregnancy (Cooksey, 1995). The incidence of pica, where substances such as clay or laundry starch are eaten, has been reported and may be greater in African-American women than in white women (Cooksey, 1995).

Religion is important in the lives of many African-Americans. Through the years it has been a source of hope and exuberant expression. Churches within black communities also serve an important social function because the advice of the minister is sought for both social and health-related situations. Health professionals may find it helpful to enlist the support of the minister to bridge gaps between themselves and clients (Cherry and Giger, 1995).

The high incidence of single female-headed African-American families accompanied by a lack of educational opportunities and low income is a major concern (Wilson, 1987). African-American adolescents, as compared with European-American adolescents, are three times as likely to give birth and five times as likely to be single parents (Frager, 1991). By comparison, while European-Americans are reported to have the highest rates for early sexual experiences, they also have the highest rates of induced abortions (Aneshensul et al, 1990).

When the African-American woman enters the maternal-child unit at the hospital, she may be the prime decision maker with regard to her health, or she may look to the family matriarch for advice (Figure 2-9). The matriarch is often a strong survivor of multiple social problems, and the "glue" that binds and strengthens her family.

Time

Because the majority of health professionals in the United States are from the Anglo culture, their perception of time is future-oriented. Many African-Americans also share this perception of the importance of time and being on time. They may, however, hold the view that time is more flexible and that lateness of as long as an hour is acceptable (Cherry and Giger, 1995). Time also may not be valued because of a history of poverty, discouragement,

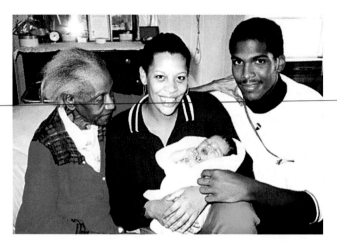

Figure 2-9   The extended family is important in an African-American family. Here, the new infant is brought to greet the great, great-grandmother. (Courtesy Camille Bodden.)

and the belief that things will not change for the better regardless of one's actions.

Present happenings may be more important than future events to African-Americans. This present time orientation may negate the need to be on time for appointments, take medicines on time, or practice preventive health care. Health care may become crisis-oriented, particularly when compounded by a lack of financial resources. An example of how present orientation, expressed as a lack of concern for illness prevention, may correlate with poor pregnancy outcome in African-American women was given by Burks (1992). The most common reason given for late prenatal care in her study was lack of awareness of the pregnancy. The second most common response was denial or ambivalence. The greatest influence on African-Americans seeking services was illness or undesirable physical symptoms (i.e., crisis care). It is clear that health care providers must be flexible regarding time when clients are present oriented, yet convey the importance of seeking prenatal care before problems arise.

Lack of future orientation is common among most teenagers. There also may be other time-related impediments to care, such as the distance to the provider and the difficulties inherent in getting there. Because of rising malpractice costs, rural obstetric services are harder to obtain (Bushy, 1990). McClanahan (1992) suggests that home health care nurses could provide much-needed antenatal services to this population.

It is common for individuals in all cultures to practice some degree of self-treatment such as the use of aspirin, vitamins, or heat before seeking the aid of practitioners. When assessing African-American clients it is important to determine what specific remedies have been used, for how long, and how successful they have been in alleviating symptoms without putting value judgments on such practices.

Biologic variations

Compared with white infants, African-American infants at birth weigh approximately 240 g less, have head circumferences 0.7 cm smaller, and are 2 cm shorter in length. This seems to be true only after the thirty-fifth week of pregnancy, when gestational growth slows for African-American infants (Cherry and Giger, 1995). Because lactose intolerance is present in a large percentage of African-Americans, cow's milk formula may not be tolerated (see Chapter 10).

Skin pigmentation is determined by the amount of melanin in the skin. Mongolian spots, melanocytes deep within the skin layers, are commonly found in African-American infants. These are blue-gray in color and are frequently seen in the lumbosacral region. These bluish-gray markings also may be present in other areas and may appear to be bruises.

Some of the most difficult health and social problems confronting African-Americans today relate to substance abuse. Cocaine use has been cited as the cause of 10% of the cases of low birth weight (LBW) in African-American newborns in certain communities. It is known that cocaine use is associated with increased risk of abruptio placentae, intrauterine growth retardation, and preterm delivery. Currently, acquired immunodeficiency syndrome (AIDS) is the leading cause of death for African-American women between the ages of 14 and 44 in New York and New Jersey. African-American and Hispanic women constitute 17% of the female population in the United States but represent 73% of the women with AIDS (Kazanjian and Eisenstat, 1995). Given the woman's role within the African-American family unit, these figures are catastrophic (see Chapter 25).

Mexican-Americans

Communication

As a result of high fertility rates and increased immigration, the Mexican-American (alternatively Mexicano or Chicano) population in the United States is steadily increasing. They are a heterogeneous group, ranging from acculturated second- or third-generation individuals to illegal immigrants in search of better economic conditions. Many live in the Southwestern United States and travel freely back and forth across the border, thereby retaining more of their language and cultural customs than some other Hispanic groups. Many Mexican-Americans are employed in farm work or other low-paying jobs where there is little opportunity to learn English. Although Spanish is the dominant language, they may speak one of more than 50 dialects or may blend Spanish and English in a way that is incomprehensible to speakers of either language.

When communicating with health care providers, children are frequently relied on to complete paper-work and to translate. Communications are guided by cultural concepts. "Platica" mandates a low-keyed approach to conversation, whereas "simpatia" encourages respectful outward agreement that may mask either a lack of understanding or agreement. Small talk by the provider before interviewing is considered to be polite and necessary to acquiring desired information, whereas joking or direct confrontation may be perceived as rude or disrespectful.

Large families are valued, and fertility rates of Mexican-American women are markedly higher than other Hispanic groups such as Puerto Ricans and Cubans. They have the lowest rates of early sexual activity but the highest rates of teenage births. They use contraception to prevent pregnancy less often and infrequently have abortions if pregnancy results (Aneshensul, 1990).

Publicly supported health services are available to persons without citizenship in the United States provided that proof of identification such as income, residence, or number of dependents can be provided. Undocumented aliens without the legal right to be in the United States are therefore ineligible for public assistance such as Medicaid or Medicare. In some communities, however, free clinics exist for such individuals, supported by private funding such as grants and donations. These clinics frequently are staffed by health care professionals who volunteer time and expertise. Illegal Mexican immigrant women who are pregnant frequently avoid medical facilities, which might reveal their illegal status to the authorities. A U.S. Department of Health and Human Services survey reported that 32% of persons of Hispanic origin are not covered either by private or public health insurance, compared with 12% of white Americans and 22% of African-Americans (Urrutia-Rojas and Aday, 1991).

The prevalence of premature births is relatively higher (Mendoza et al, 1991), and the miscarriage-stillborn rate for Mexican women who are farm workers is more than double that of other population groups (reflecting concern about pesticides). Despite poverty and the lack of prenatal care, it has been observed that LBW is infrequent in infants of Mexican-born women.

Women of Mexican-origin born in the United States have higher incomes, educational status, and more health care access than native Mexicans, yet their infants have a 60% higher risk for LBW than Mexican-born women. This phenomenon is attributed to an increase in smoking and drinking and a decrease in weight gain during pregnancy in American born women.

The roles of Mexican-American women are changing as they interact with American women and encounter the multiple stressors of low education, poverty, and prejudice. Divorce rates are increasing, and the number of Hispanic female heads of households is approximately twice that of non-Hispanic households (U.S. Bureau of the Census, 1990). When a husband is present in the household, he is more likely to be dominant in health care decision making. Recognition of this factor by the nurse will help to ensure that prenatal appointments are kept and that the family experiences greater satisfaction with the care received.

Space

Mexican-Americans usually enjoy physical closeness and are more comfortable with smaller interpersonal distances within their family and social groups than many white Americans. As is true of many new immigrants, it is common for several related families to live together; therefore the client is used to the presence of many people. Because giving birth is a joyous event for Mexican-Americans, the client may be overwhelmed by well-wishers. Nurses who are unaccustomed to this cultural pattern should exercise patience and understanding toward visitors while ensuring that the client also receives adequate care, including rest.

Modesty is highly valued in the Mexican-American culture, and exposure of intimate body parts and touching of genitalia during labor and delivery is frequently a source of intense embarrassment. This may be expressed by the woman as "feeling hot." Female nurses and physicians who avoid undue exposure of the client are usually well accepted, whereas treatment by men may be refused for modesty's sake. The client may be wearing a *muneco*, a cord that is placed under the breasts with a knot over the umbilicus. Because this is believed to ensure a safe delivery, the nurse should not attempt to remove it.

There is generally a strong bond of affection between Mexican-American women and their female relatives, and the cultural norm is to have one or several present during childbirth. The nurse should be aware that abnormalities, should they occur, may be ascribed to cosmic or environmental events. For example "pujos," umbilical protrusion in the infant, is thought to be due to contact by the infant with a menstruating woman; "mal puesto" refers to abnormalities caused by magic; and earthquakes may cause breech deliveries. "Susto," or loss of the soul is thought to be related to a fright during pregnancy. The spirit may be returned by sweeping the mother with herbs as she lies outstretched on the floor.

Social organization

The processes of adaptation and integration into mainstream American life by Mexican-Americans depend primarily on whether their presence is sanctioned and they are given the privileges of legal status (Salgado de Snyder, 1986). Families that have been in the United States for generations are part of the mainstream and enjoy levels of economic success similar to other Americans. Cultural identity remains strong, with many immigrants consistently helping to maintain their economically less fortunate relatives in Mexico.

For undocumented immigrants, there is constant fear of arrest and deportation by authorities. In addition, they may be exploited at will by employers because they have no legal rights. Such immigrants, at risk for multiple stress-related physical and emotional problems, are the least likely to seek health services. Mexican-Americans underutilize health and social services and are substantially less likely to begin prenatal care early. They frequently obtain late or no prenatal care at all.

The concept of "compadrazgo" or coparenthood helps to maintain and protect the child. Godparents are chosen who usually have greater socioeconomic status than the parents and are agreeable to taking coresponsibility for the child's welfare. This is considered both an honor and a responsibility, and the godparents and child usually maintain a close relationship throughout their lives.

Although family ties are generally strong, language and other educational skills propel Mexican-American children into the mainstream faster than the parents, often causing disruption of traditional roles and relationships. The integration of women into the work force has also necessitated changes in traditional gender roles. However, the tendency to solve problems within the family and to give mutual aid generally remains. Group needs are superior to individual needs, and the dishonor or shame of an individual affects the whole family. In some families, intense emotional attachment to the family (called familism) and to places and things is believed to retard both individual and collective progress (Kulpers, 1991).

Time

Most Mexican-Americans who are of the second or third generation have the future-oriented perception of time that is common to most Americans. Studies of students, for example, indicate that time perceptions of Mexican-American students are similar to their white American counterparts, even though they maintain strong cultural ties to the Mexican community. These acculturated Mexican-Americans can be depended on to keep prenatal appointments, take medications appropriately, and to value prevention strategies that are likely to ensure good pregnancy outcomes. They usually have the resources to obtain prenatal and postpartum care, either through private or public means.

The Mexican-American who is a newer arrival may have a present time orientation more similar to Southeast Asian clients. Such an orientation gives little credence to future possibilities and may cause families to spend years of savings on events such as weddings or religious festivals. This lack of future orientation, combined with a sense that they are controlled by external supernatural forces, often delays upward mobility and cultural integration (Kulpers, 1995). Because they perceive time as elastic, these Mexican-Americans may be late or not appear for scheduled prenatal or postpartum appointments unless they are not feeling well. They may not follow medication schedules and may devalue activities that focus on long-term planning or prevention. Health teaching that emphasizes the present or short-term may be best accepted. Some Mexican-Americans cannot look beyond the day-to-day struggle to survive.

Environmental control

The nurse should make every effort to provide cultural comfort when the Mexican-American client enters a health care setting. The client's beliefs and use of health practices that are culturally appropriate for her should be assessed, so that support can be given to those that appear to be efficacious or neutral and can be an adjunct to scientific health care. If the nurse does not reject these nonharmful cultural practices, the client is more likely to be receptive to health teaching relative to those practices that appear either dysfunctional or uncertain. Health is frequently seen as either good luck or as a reward from God for a sinless life.

Although some cultural practices, such as ensuring a good weight gain during pregnancy are efficacious, certain practices most often held by new immigrants, can be dangerous. A child with symptoms of crying, diarrhea, loss of weight, and high fever may be thought to be the victim of *"mal ojo,"* the evil eye, caused by being looked at by a person with supernatural powers. Touching the infant is believed to prevent or help cure this condition. Eggs and water may be mixed and put under the infant's bed to drive out the evil influence, rather than seeking health care. Symptoms of severe dehydration, such as a depressed anterior fontanelle, may be ascribed to an imbalance between the fontanelle and hard palate. The mother may pull hairs, apply eggs to the infant's head, or hold it in a head-down position to attempt to alleviate the depression (Ruiz, 1985) (Figure 2-10).

Mexican-American women are less likely to breast-feed than white American women and may wean the infant earlier. They generally believe that a fat infant is a healthy infant and observe that formula-fed babies are fatter. One concern is that some women use whole milk rather than formula to feed the infant. Mexican-American women also may believe colostrum to be "dirty" and may delay breast-feeding for a day or two. In addition, a period of quarantine for as long as 40 days, called *"la cuarentina,"* which includes abstention from various activities, including sexual relations, may be observed by the mother (Coreil and Mull, 1990).

Folk healers. Before seeking health care, or concurrently, the client may consult one or more folk healers within her community. Family members pass down knowledge of treating illness just as mothers and grandmothers do in the white American culture. Self-medication is also common in Mexico. Alternatively, a "yerbero" who specializes in spices and herbs may be sought. For serious physical or emotional complaints, the client may seek help from a male "curandero" or female "curandera" whose gift of healing derives from both Native American and Roman Catholic traditions and who usually provides care in his or her home. This traditional practitioner may pray, give herbs, massage, counsel, or use white or black magic as part of the cure. Imbalances between the person and God, and hot and cold elements, are believed to contribute to illness (Ruiz, 1985). In some ethnic communities in the United States curanderos and curanderas have successfully worked with health practitioners for the mutual benefit of the client. The primary goal of treatment is to free the client of the sin that has made her sick, while restoring the balance of heat and cold.

Heat and cold. Mexican-Americans share some of the beliefs held by Southeast Asians in relation to cold and wind. Cold is to be avoided after delivery. Because water and wind are considered "cold" regardless of the temperature, the Mexican-American mother may prefer not to shower and may insist that doors and windows be kept closed. Inability to become pregnant is believed to be related to a "cold" womb and is treated with heat. A decrease in the mother's milk supply after birth is considered to be a result of "coldness," and heat, such as hot herbs, may be used to increase lactation.

Some Mexican-Americans believe that pregnancy is a "hot" state, and that they should dissipate the heat by bathing and by not ingesting "hot" foods. Acidic foods and fresh fruits and vegetables also may be avoided, and the prevalence of pica in the form of eating clay has been

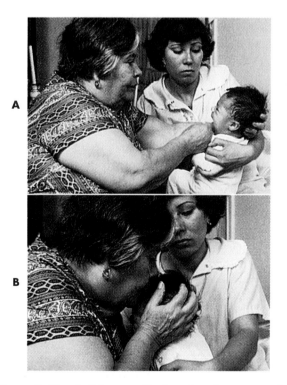

Figure 2-10 A, B In some Mexican-American groups the grandmother has special rituals to perform for the infant.
(Courtesy Concept Media, Irvine, Calif.)

reported (see Chapter 10). Conversely, after birth they are considered to be in a cold state, and cold foods such as dairy products and chicken may be avoided.

Biologic variations

Depending on their ethnic heritage, Mexican-Americans range from being pure Mongoloid (Native American) to pure Caucasian of Spanish descent (Salgado de Snyder, 1986) with corresponding darker to lighter skin coloring.

Mexican-Americans are at greatest risk for health problems related to communicable disease: diarrhea resulting from gastroenteritis and parasitic infestations and skin disorders. Tuberculosis is common in Mexico and is frequently found in newly arrived immigrants and migrant workers. Hispanics are also overrepresented (21%) in the number of AIDS cases in the U.S. population (Kazanjian and Eisenstat,

1995). Nurses should use both prenatal and postpartum contacts as an opportunity to educate clients about this disease and encourage behavioral change in persons at high risk. Finally, higher death rates from pneumonia, and traumatic injuries resulting from violence, accidents, alcohol and drug use have been documented (Magar, 1990).

When a Mexican-American woman seeks health care for her pregnancy, the nurse should ensure that an accurate and complete assessment, including laboratory work, is done for the woman, particularly if she is a new arrival to the United States. Because there is high incidence of diabetes and hypertension, repeated assessments should be done throughout the pregnancy. As with all ethnic variations, the nurse needs to develop cultural competence for the groups that are seen in the clinic and hospital or home care setting (Rorie, Paine, Burger, 1996).

Key Points

- A family may be defined as biologic, legal, functional, and ethical. Each family is unique in its emphasis on and configurations of these aspects.
- The overall goal of a family is physical survival and the personal development needed to mature and pass on a secure life to the next generation.
- A "good enough" family provides basic needs for its members and provides an environment wherein each member "grows itself up."
- Individuals and families move through predictable stages of growth and development. Stressors may inhibit development from one stage to the next.
- Patterns of communication, power, and role performance demonstrate family dynamics and influence family health.
- Cultural factors influence client actions and behavior relative to childbearing.

- Ethnicity patterns our thinking, feeling, and behavior in obvious and subtle ways. Nurses with mainstream American ethnicity patterns must give sensitive multicultural care to those with differing ethnic backgrounds.
- The divorce rate greatly affects the family by increasing complexity of relationships and often results in single parents, who may easily become depleted of the energy needed for parenting.
- Remarried or blended families may adjust easily or with difficulty depending on the new spouses' previous marriages and number of children who still require parenting.
- Adolescent parenting rates vary from group to group and carry psychosocial and economic problems into attempts to build a family.

Study Questions

2-1. Select the terms that apply to the following statements:
   a. America is facing a new, divorce-related social problem called the "feminization of poverty." Often, single mothers live on lower incomes that are below the _____.
   b. At every stage of human development, intimacy, love, and commitment are important. These three words describe _____.
   c. If the statement is made "Italians and Polish place great emphasis on family weddings," this statement describes _____.
   d. A child is cast into the role of a parent and is required to care for younger children because a single parent goes to work. This is a change in _____ tasks.
   e. When one looks at the interactions of a family causing one member to be labeled a "black sheep," one is looking at family _____.
   f. The primary goals of the family are _____ and _____.

2-2. The highest incidence of divorce in the 1990s occurs between:
   a. Couples with college-age children.
   b. Middle-aged men and women.
   c. Couples with preschool and schoolchildren.
   d. Retired men and women.

2-3. Match the terms with their descriptions.
   a. Family members do not share much time or feeling   1. Boundaries
   b. Brothers and sisters help each other and are loyal   2. Enmeshment
   c. Defines who is in or out of the inner family circle   3. Cohesiveness
   d. Parent and one sibling seem overly dependent on each other   4. Disengagement

2-4. A Vietnamese woman refuses the presence of her husband in labor, despite the urging of the nurse. This cultural difference illustrates her preference to:
   a. Be alone during childbearing.
   b. Avoid her husband.
   c. Be accompanied by a female friend.
   d. Have her mother-in-law with her.

2-5. If a Hispanic woman is not punctual for clinic appointments, she may be indicating a cultural value of:
   a. Activity:Being
   b. Time:Present
   c. Man-Nature:Passivity
   d. Time:Future

Answer Key

2-1. *a,* Poverty level; *b,* attachment behaviors; *c,* ethnicity; *d,* stage-appropriate behavior; *e,* boundaries; *f,* physical survival; personal development. 2-2: c. 2-3: *a,* 4; *b,* 3; *c,* 1; *d,* 2. 2-4: c. 2-5: b.

References

Andersen S, Sabatelli R: *Family interaction: a multigenerational developmental perspective,* Boston, 1995, Allyn and Bacon.

Aneshensul C et al: Onset of fertility-related events during adolescence: a prospective comparison of Mexican-American and non-Hispanic white females, *Am J Public Health* 80:959, 1990.

*Arrendondo R et al: Alcoholism in Mexican-Americans: intervention and treatment, *Hosp Community Psychiatry* 38:180, 1987.

*Beal W: Separation, divorce and single parent families. In Carter EA, McGoldrick M, eds: *The family life cycle: a framework for family therapy,* New York, 1980, Gardner Press.

Becker TM et al: Mortality from infectious diseases among Mexico's American Indians, Hispanic whites, and other whites, *Am J Public Health* 80:320, 1990.

Bumpass LL, Raley RK: Redefining single-parent families: cohabitation and changing family reality, *Demography* 32(2):97, 1995.

Burks J: Factors in utilization of prenatal services by low income Black women, *Nurse Pract* 17:34, 1992.

Bushy A: Rural determinants in family health: considerations for community health, *Fam Comm Health* 12:29, 1990.

*Carter B, McGoldrick M: *The changing family life cycle: a framework for family therapy,* Boston, 1989, Allyn and Bacon.

Centers for Disease Control: US AIDS cases reported through February 1992, *HIV/AIDS Surveillance* March 1992.

Cherry B, Giger J: Black Americans. In Giger J, Davidhizar R, eds: *Transcultural nursing,* St Louis, 1995, Mosby.

*Colon F: The family life cycle of the multiproblem poor family. In Carter EA, McGoldrick M, eds: *The family life cycle: a framework for family therapy,* New York, 1980, Gardner Press.

Cooksey NR: Pica and olfactory cravings of pregnancy: how deep are the secrets? *Birth* 22(3):129, 1995.

Coreil J, Mull J: *Anthropology and primary health care,* Boulder, Colo, 1990, Westview Press.

D'Avanzo C: Bridging the cultural gap with Southeast Asians, *MCN Am J Matern Child Nurs* 17:204, 1992.

*Duvall EM: *Marriage and family development,* ed 5, Philadelphia, 1977, Lippincott.

*Erikson E: *Childhood and society,* New York, 1950, W W Norton & Co.

Frager B: Teenage childbearing part I: the problem has not gone away, *J Pediatr Nurs* 6:131, 1991.

Geronimus A, Andersen H, Bound J: Differences in hypertension among US black and white women of childbearing age, *Public Health Rep,* 1990.

Giger J, Davidhizar R: *Transcultural nursing,* ed 2, St Louis, 1995, Mosby.

*Giordano J, McGoldrick M, Pearce J, eds: *Ethnicity and family therapy,* New York, 1982, Guilford Press.

Haber J et al: *Comprehensive psychiatric nursing,* ed 4, St Louis, 1992, Mosby.

*Kay M, ed: *Anthropology of human birth,* Philadelphia, 1982, F A Davis.

Kazanjian PH, Eisenstat SA: Human immunodeficiency virus. In Carlson K, Eisenstat SA, eds: *Primary Care of Women,* St Louis, 1995, Mosby.

Kulpers J: Mexican-Americans. In Giger J, Davidhizar R, eds: *Transcultural nursing,* St Louis, 1995, Mosby.

*Levitan S, Belous R, Gallo F: *What's happening to the American family?* ed 2, Baltimore, 1988, Johns Hopkins University Press.

Magar V: Health care needs of Central American refugees, *Nurs Outlook* 38:239, 1990.

* Classic reference.

*May K, Perrin S: The father in pregnancy and birth. In Hanson S, Bozett F, eds: *Dimensions of fatherhood,* Beverly Hills, 1985, Sage Publ.

McClanahan P: Improving access to prenatal care, *J Obstet Gynecol Neonatal Nurs* 21:280, 1992.

Mendoza F et al: Selected measures of health status for Mexican-American, mainland Puerto Rican and Cuban-American children, *JAMA* 265:227, 1991.

*Minuchin S, Fishman H: *Family therapy techniques,* Cambridge, 1981, Harvard University Press.

Murray R, Zentner J: *Nursing assessment and health promotion strategies throughout the life span,* ed 5, Norwalk, Conn, 1993, Appleton & Lange.

National Center for Children in Poverty: *Five million children: a statistical profile of our poorest children,* New York, 1990, Columbia University School of Public Health.

National Center for Health Statistics: Advance report on final mortality statistics, 1989, *Monthly Vital Statistics Report* 40(suppl 2): 1992.

National Center for Health Statistics: Fertility rates: United States 1950-1994, *Monthly Vital Statistics Report* 43(13):4, 1995.

National Center for Health Statistics: Marriage and divorce rates: United States 1950-1994, *Monthly Vital Statistics Report* 43(13):4, 1995.

National Center for Health Statistics: Birthrates for unmarried women, by age of mother: United States 1980-1994, *Monthly Vital Statistics Report* 44(suppl 11):9, 1996.

*Nichols MP: *Family therapy: concepts and methods,* New York, 1984, Gardner Press.

Paciornik M: Commentary: arguments against episiotomy and in favor of squatting for birth, *Birth* 17:104, 1990.

*Randolph L, Gesche M: Black adolescent pregnancy: preventions and management, *J Community Health* 11:10, 1986.

Rorie JL, Paine LL, Burger MK: Primary care for women: cultural competence in primary care services, *J Nurs Midwifery* 1(2):92, 1996.

*Ruiz P: Cultural barriers to effective medical care among Hispanic-American patients, *Ann Rev Med* 36:63, 1985.

*Salgado de Snyder V: Factors associated with acculturative stress and depressive symptomatology among married Mexican immigrant women, *Psych Women Quart* 11:475, 1986.

* Classic reference.

*Terkelson KG: Toward a theory of the family life cycle. In Carter EA, McGoldrick M, eds: *The family life cycle: a framework for family therapy,* New York, 1980, Gardner Press.

*Tripp-Reimer T, Brink P, Saunders J: Cultural assessment: content and process, *Nurs Outlook* 32:78, 1988.

Urrutia-Rojas C, Aday L: A framework for community assessment: designing and conducting a survey in a Hispanic immigrant and refugee community, *Public Health Nurs* 8:20, 1991.

US Bureau of the Census: The Hispanic population in the United States: March 1989, *Current Pop Reports Series* P-20, No 444, Washington, DC, 1990.

*US Bureau of the Census: *Statistical abstracts of the United States,* 1988 annualed 108, Washington, DC, 1988.

Whitchurch GG, Constantine LL: Systems theory. In Boss P et al, eds: *Sourcebook of family theories and methods: a conceptual approach,* New York, 1993, Plenum.

*Wilson J: *The truly disadvantaged: the inner city, the underclass and public policy,* Chicago, 1987, University of Chicago Press.

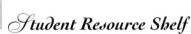

Student Resource Shelf

Geissler E: *Pocket guide to cultural assessment,* St Louis, 1994, Mosby.
Comprehensive guide to various ethnic groups worldwide, including customs and childbearing issues.

Giger J, Davidhizar R: *Transcultural nursing,* St Louis, 1995, Mosby.
Framework for cultural assessment and intervention techniques applied to specific cultural groups in the United States.

Ramer L: *Culturally sensitive caregiving and childbearing families,* White Plains, NY, 1992, March of Dimes Birth Defects Foundation.
A self-study module for study of transcultural nursing. Includes cultural profiles of major groups in the United States.

Spector R: *Cultural diversity in health and illness,* ed 4, Stamford, Conn, 1996, Appleton & Lange.
Comprehensive guide to major ethnic groups in United States with emphasis on delivery and acceptance of health care.

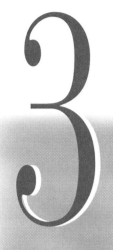

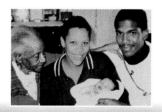

Human Reproduction & Sexuality

Learning Objectives

- Identify major reproductive structures of men and women.
- Describe the physiologic changes initiating puberty, menstruation, and fertility.
- Explain feedback mechanisms of the menstrual cycle and describe hormone action in each phase.
- Compare and contrast the decline in fertility in men and women.
- Identify the phases of the sexual excitement cycle for men and women.
- Differentiate between the concepts of gender and sexuality.
- Describe the expression of sexuality across the lifecycle.

Key Terms

Ampulla	Oocytes
Areola	Oogenesis
Cervix	Ova
Corpus Luteum	Ovaries
Ejaculation	Ovulation
Endometrium	Pelvic Floor
Epididymis	Penis
Estrogen	Perimetrium
Fallopian Tubes	Progesterone
Fimbriae	Proliferative Phase
Follicle-Stimulating	Prostaglandins
Hormone (FSH)	Prostate
Follicular Phase	Puberty
Fundus	Pubescence
Gametes	Scrotum
Gender Identity	Secretory Phase
Gonads	Semen
Graafian Follicle	Seminiferous Tubules
Ischemic Phase	Sexuality
Leydig's Cells	Spermatozoa
Luteal Phase	Spermatogenesis
Luteinizing Hormone	Spinnbarkeit
(LH)	Testes
Menarche	Testosterone
Menopause	Uterus
Menstrual Phase	Vagina
Menstruation	Vas Deferens
Myometrium	Vulva

The human reproductive system is highly complex and the internal development and maturation of this system involve a precise harmony between several systems of the body. To understand the process of childbirth, the reproductive structures must first be understood.

A review of the male and female reproductive systems will help to better understand what is necessary for successful conception, pregnancy, and birth. The intricate interworking of the human reproductive cycle underlies the remainder of this text. When a clear picture of the

45

reproductive structures and "how they work," is understood, it becomes easier to assess and plan nursing care more readily.

Although clearly different, male and female reproductive anatomies are initially identical or *undifferentiated*. There is no cellular difference until about the fifth week after conception. At that time primordial sex cells, originating in the walls of the yolk sac, begin to develop and migrate into the embryo to form the **gonads,** the major sex organs. At this point the sex of the embryo can be determined only microscopically. External genitalia begin differentiation by the end of the eighth week, with completion by the twelfth week. Because of the common beginning of both male and female reproductive systems, there are apparent parallels in several structures and in the function of the sexual hormones as development continues.

MALE REPRODUCTIVE ANATOMY

Although it may appear that male sexual structures are more external than internal, only the penis and the supportive scrotum are external. The testes, the storage and transport ducts, the accessory structures of the seminal vesicles, the prostate, and the bulbourethral glands are all internal structures (Figure 3-1).

External Structures

The **penis** is a long, flexible structure located in front of the scrotum and below the symphysis pubis. The penis contains the urethra, which is used as a passageway for urine and semen. The penis is divided into the body, or shaft, and a rounded end known as the glans. The glans is smooth and, like its female counterpart (the clitoris), is extremely sensitive to stimuli. At birth, the penis is covered by the prepuce, or foreskin, which may be circumcised for religious, cultural, or hygienic reasons, leaving the glans exposed.

The shaft of the penis consists of three urethral layers surrounded by three longitudinal layers of tissue: two *corporae cavernosae* and one *corpus spongiosum*. Although the penis is normally flaccid, with sexual excitation blood flow increases in the penis, and venous exit is impaired. The tissue becomes engorged and the organ stiffens, becoming erect to penetrate the female vagina.

The **scrotum,** a baglike structure, is suspended behind the penis. It is a supportive structure that holds the testes. The scrotum is divided by a septum (partition) of connective tissue so each testis has its own compartment. The scrotum acts to protect the internal structures by means of sensitivity to touch, pain, and temperature, as it constricts to pull the testes closer to the body. To continue spermatogenesis, the temperature of the testes must remain cooler than core body temperature. The scrotum automatically tightens close to the body when environmental temperature is cold and becomes looser when the temperature is warm. (Jeans that fit too tightly may inhibit spermatogenesis.)

Internal Structures

The **testes** are two white, oval glands about 2 inches in size and weighing about 12 g each. These develop within the peritoneal cavity until about the twenty-eighth week of fetal development, then begin descent through the inguinal canal into the scrotal sac. The testes will remain outside the abdominal cavity, suspended in the external scrotum to maintain the lower-than-core body temperature necessary to produce and maintain **spermatozoa** (mature sperm). Failure of the testes to descend results in *cryptorchidism,* or undescended or ectopic testes.

Each testis is protected by a fibrous tissue layer called the *tunica albuginea.* This membrane covers the testis and then extends inward as septa (dividers) that create hundreds of individual lobes. The effect is similar to that found in orange or grapefruit sections. The "fruit" of each lobe is a long mass of threadlike fibers, tightly coiled to fit in this small space. These fibers are the **seminiferous tubules,** the site of **spermatogenesis** (sperm production). Surrounding these tubules are Sertoli's cells, which secrete nourishment for the developing spermatozoa (Figures 3-2 and 3-3).

Other specialized cells are contained in the interstitial tissue. Clusters of **Leydig's cells,** stimulated by hormones from the anterior pituitary gland, produce the male hormone **testosterone,** responsible for male sexual characteristics and functioning.

The ends of all the seminiferous tubules join to form a common collection area known as the *rete testis,* which

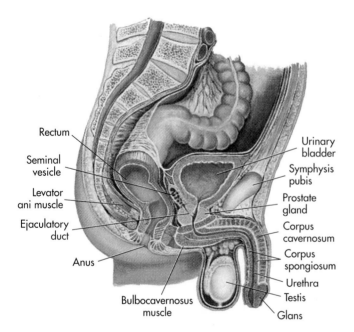

Figure 3-1 Male reproductive organs. Sagittal section of pelvis showing placement of male reproductive organs.

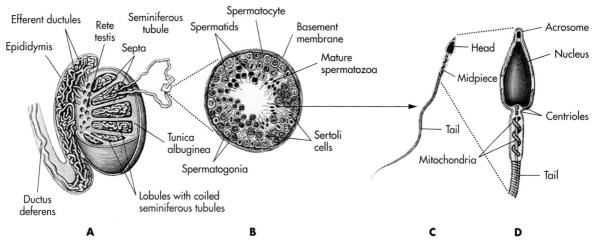

Figure 3-2 Histology of the testis. **A,** Gross anatomy of the testis with a section cut away to reveal internal structures. **B,** Cross-section of a seminiferous tubule. Spermatogonia are near the periphery, and mature sperm cells are near the lumen of the seminiferous tubule. **C,** Mature sperm cell. **D,** Head of a mature sperm cell. (Courtesy Bill Ober.)

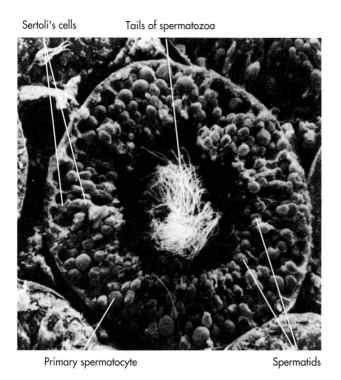

Figure 3-3 Scanning electron micrograph of cross-section of seminiferous tubule. Primary spermatocytes, spermatids, and Sertoli's cells can be seen in wall of tubule, and tails of spermatids undergoing transition into mature spermatozoa can be seen extending into tubule lumen. (From Kessel RG, Kardon RH: *Tissues and organs: a text-atlas of scanning electron microscopy,* New York, 1979, WH Freeman & Co.)

leads to ducts that enter the **epididymis**, the storage structure located on the lateral and posterior sides of each testis. Here the sperm mature, nourished by secretions within the coiled tube, and remain until ejaculation.

Sperm exit each epididymis via a **vas deferens**, a tube about 40 cm long that connects to the prostatic urethra.

The vas deferens joins the spermatic cord and passes through the inguinal canal into the pelvis, where it meets with the vas deferens from the other side. These two vas deferens then join with the seminal vesicles (located posterior to the bladder) at the ejaculatory ducts to receive alkaline fluid that is rich in nutrition and contains prostaglandins. Although the function of these fluids is not fully understood, they may enhance fertilization and aid the zygote in reaching the uterus.

The ejaculatory ducts enter the **prostate**, a gland below the bladder that surrounds the urethra, in the same way that a balloon on a Foley catheter surrounds the catheter. Composed of numerous glands embedded in fibromuscular tissue, the prostate is pierced by the ejaculatory ducts. It is here that the majority of the ejaculatory fluid is formed. This fluid facilitates sperm motility and protects sperm from the acidic vaginal environment. Additional fluid is added by the bulbourethral (Cowper's) glands. The combination of these ejaculatory fluids plus sperm is called **semen**, which is emptied into the prostatic urethra and expelled by **ejaculation** (Figure 3-4).

Spermatogenesis

The primitive germ cells enter the gonads at the fifth week of life and later become part of the seminiferous tubules. In contrast to the woman, there are no partially developed sex cells in the male gonads at birth. Instead production of sex cells starts at puberty under the influence of gonadotropic hormones. Testosterone stimulates sperm maturation or spermatogenesis. The spermatogonia develop into primary spermatocytes and then undergo the first meiotic division to become secondary spermatocytes. Unlike the female cells, however, there is no delay in further maturation, and these cells immediately begin the final change into mature spermatozoa. Although mature sperm may remain in the epididymis for

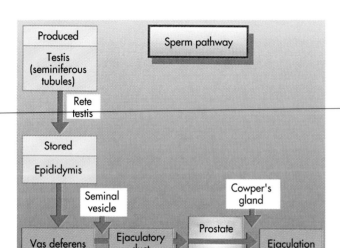

Figure 3-4   Sperm pathway.

FEMALE REPRODUCTIVE ANATOMY

Female sexual anatomy is also divided into internal and external portions (Figure 3-5). Internal structures are the ovaries, fallopian tubes, uterus, and vagina. The vulva is the main external female structure. Although not directly involved in reproduction, the breasts are considered accessory sexual structures.

Internal Structures

Ovaries

The primary controlling organs of female reproduction are the two **ovaries**. These two small organs, similar to almonds in shape and size, are located beside (but not attached to) the uterus and are suspended by the ovarian ligament. The ovaries serve both to develop **ova**, the female sex cells or gametes, and to produce hormones (**estrogen** and **progesterone**).

Oogenesis. Production of ova, **oogenesis**, begins in the third to fifth week of embryonic life, when primitive germ cells begin to form, migrate to the gonads, or ovaries, and turn into oogonia (early ova). These undergo rapid mitosis (cell division), develop into primary **oocytes**, and enter the first meiotic (sex cell) division, but they *do not complete this division until puberty*. By the seventh month of fetal life, the oocytes are surrounded by tissue that later becomes follicles. Although there are 700,000 to 2 million primary oocytes at birth, the number is reduced to about 40,000 by puberty. At this time, hormones from the anterior pituitary gland stimulate ripening of one ovum and its release from the ovary. This process, called **ovulation**, leaves the once smooth ovarian surface scarred and gives it its characteristic bumpy appearance.

Fallopian tubes

The **fallopian tubes**, also known as oviducts, lie adjacent to the ovaries at one end and are attached to the uterus at the other end. The tubes are approximately 4 inches (10 cm) in length and have a rich blood supply. Cells line the tubes and secrete proteins to nourish the ovum as it travels to the uterus.

Each fallopian tube is divided into three segments: the infundibulum, the ampulla, and the isthmus. The straight, narrow tubal isthmus attaches the tubes to the uterus just below the fundus. The wide, funnel-shaped infundibulum

up to 6 weeks, depending on the frequency of ejaculation, most sperm live only 2 to 3 days once deposited in the female vagina.

Characteristics of sperm

At any time, one portion of the seminiferous tubule may contain primary spermatocytes in meiotic division while another portion contains secondary spermatocytes becoming spermatids (see Figure 3-3). Millions of sperm are produced at the same time; in one ejaculation of semen there may be as many as 20 to 60 million. Only one will fertilize the ovum; the others die en route or are altered in the uterus or fallopian tubes.

Each spermatozoon is made up of a head and a tail (see Figure 3-2, *C* and *D*). The acrosome, nucleus, and centrioles make up the head, which carries half the number of chromosomes (the haploid number) needed for the new cell that will become the fetus. The head is the portion of the sperm that penetrates the ovum wall. The tail or flagellum is long and flexible to propel the sperm through the female genital tract, then it drops off as the head enters the ovum. See Chapter 6 for a discussion of sperm and infertility.

Hormonal Control

The hypothalamus is responsible for hormonal control in men and women. It produces hormone-releasing factors that cause the anterior pituitary gland to secrete the actual gonad-stimulating hormones, including **follicle-stimulating hormone** (FSH) and **luteinizing hormone** (LH). These hormones initiate production of **gametes** (sex cells) and sex hormones. Hormonal changes governing fertilization and pregnancy are described in Chapters 7 and 9.

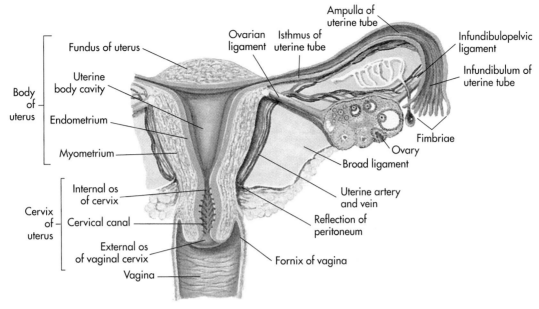

Figure 3-5   Female pelvic organs in a frontal section. The entire uterus is shown, with the upper portion of the vagina and the left uterine tube and ovary.

is fringed and wrapped around the ovaries but is not attached to them. The fingerlike projections of the infundibulum, the **fimbriae,** swell at ovulation, and these, the cilia that line them, and the entire tube reach out to capture the ovum, sweeping it up into the tube. This action captures the ovum as it is released from its follicle, preventing it from being absorbed in the abdominal cavity. The ovum is propelled through the tube by the cilia, hairlike projections that move rhythmically. Fertilization usually takes place in the middle portion of the tube, the **ampulla.**

Uterus

Commonly known as the "womb," the **uterus** lies behind the pubic bones and between the rectum and bladder (see Figure 3-11). It has the shape of an inverted pear and is about the size of a fist. It is normally hollow and flat and its walls almost touch. The uterus provides a nourishing and protective environment for the developing embryo and fetus.

Segments of the uterus. The uterus is divided into the corpus and cervix. The corpus, the upper two thirds of the uterus, is further divided into the fundus, cornua, body, and uterine isthmus.

The **fundus** is the rounded, top portion of the uterus, easiest to palpate through the abdominal wall. It extends above the cornua, the wide segments where the tubal isthmus enters the uterus. The body is the center part, and the uterine isthmus, which contains the uterine canal, is the narrower, bottom segment leading to the cervix.

Uterine layers. The walls of the uterus are made up of two distinct tissue layers and a third covering layer. The **perimetrium,** an outer, serosal covering, is an exten-

sion of the parietal peritoneum. The inner layer, the **endometrium,** is composed of three sublayers. The first and second layers slough off when menstrual blood and tissue are shed and then rebuild during the first part of the cycle. Mucous cells of the endometrium temporarily produce nutrients for the fertilized ovum.

The middle layer, the **myometrium,** is composed of layers of smooth muscle fibers that extend in three directions. These fibers intertwine with and connect to elastic tissues and blood vessels throughout the uterine wall, and they also connect to the dense, inner layer of the endometrium (see Figure 3-5). Like the endometrium, the myometrium has three sublayers:

1. The outer myometrial layer is found mostly in the fundus. The longitudinal fibers are needed to push the fetus downward at birth.
2. The middle muscle fibers are interlaced in a figure 8 pattern, encircling large blood vessels. The middle layer contracts strongly during labor. These muscles are important for hemostasis (cessation of bleeding) and control of blood loss after birth.
3. The inner layer is most concentrated where the fallopian tubes join the fundus and around the internal os. These muscles act as sphincters to prevent menstrual blood from ascending into the tubes, as well as to hold the contents of the uterus during pregnancy.

Cervix

The **cervix** is composed of elastic smooth muscle and connective tissue and is approximately 2.5 cm in length and diameter. The cervical canal has two openings: the *internal os,* connected to uterine tissue, and the *external os,* which is the portion seen at the end of the vagina. The color of the endocervical lining is pink in a nonpregnant state but turns bluish with pregnancy (see Chapter 9).

The cervix feels pressure but has few nerve endings. From cells in the lining, it produces mucus that lubricates and cleanses the vagina. Mucus production is altered by the menstrual cycle and pregnancy.

TEST *Yourself* 3-2 _____

Fill in the blanks.
a. Secretions that nourish the ovum are _____.
b. Structure that traps the ovum at ovulation is _____.
c. Mechanisms that provide for ovum transport down the tube are _____.
d. Usual site of fertilization is _____.
e. Layer of uterus that contracts during labor is _____.
f. Site where vaginal lubrication produced is _____.

Circulation. The major blood supply to the uterus and cervix comes from the aorta as it divides at the umbilical level into the two iliac arteries. Each of the iliac arteries then divides into a hypogastric artery and then into a uterine artery. The ovarian artery also joins the uterine artery after supplying the ovary. During pregnancy the blood vessels further proliferate and enter at every level of the myometrium.

Innervation. Parasympathetic fibers from sacral nerves stimulate vasodilation and inhibit muscle contraction. Efferent sympathetic motor nerves (T5 through T10) reach the uterus through the uterosacral ligament ganglia, affecting vasoconstriction and the ability to contract (see Chapter 13). Although the autonomic system regulates action of the uterus, the uterus can also relax and contract on its own. Radiating pain sensations from the uterus connect in the paracervical areas and proceed upward to levels T11 and T12 of the spinal cord.

Ligaments. To bear the weight of a pregnant uterus, a strong and well-developed support system within the pelvis is required. This system is provided by the following ligaments attached to the ovaries and uterus:

1. *Broad ligaments* are two ligaments that are double folds of the parietal peritoneum. These cover the uterus like sheets hanging on a line (Beischer and MacKay, 1993). Suspended within them are the fallopian tubes, ovaries, blood vessels, and round and ovarian ligaments. The broad ligaments are made of loose connective tissue and help keep the uterus in place.
2. *Cardinal ligaments* are the chief support for the uterus. Actually the base of the broad ligament, these ligaments extend from the cervix to the pelvic walls and wrap the ureter and uterine vessels.
3. *Round ligaments* are parallel with the broad ligament. These two pieces of smooth muscle and connective tissue attach to the uterus at the cornua and pass through the inguinal canal, ending in the labia majora.

4. *Uterosacral ligaments* are two cordlike folds of peritoneum extending from the lower cervix to the fascia over the second and third sacral vertebrae, attaching on either side of the rectum. These encircle the rectum posterior to the uterus, forming Douglas' cul-de-sac behind the cervix.
5. *Ovarian ligaments* attach the ovaries to the cornua.

Vagina

Commonly called the "birth canal," the **vagina** serves as the passageway from the internal reproductive organs to the external genitalia. It is a long, tubular structure, about 10.5 cm in length, between the vaginal *introitus* (opening) and the uterine cervix. It slants upward and slightly posterior when the woman is standing. Because it meets at a *right angle* with the cervix, its anterior wall is shorter than its posterior wall by about 1.5 cm. The distal vagina terminates in a cul-de-sac known as a *fornix,* a space surrounding the cervix. Seminal fluid after coitus collects in the fornix, keeping sperm near the cervix.

The inner walls of the vagina, called the *rugae,* are smooth, folded gland-containing mucous membranes. These foldings allow for the pronounced stretching of the vagina during childbirth. Vaginal membranes range from wet to dry, influenced by hormones and sexual excitation, and generally maintain an acidic environment hostile to invading bacteria.

Pelvic floor

The **pelvic floor,** a muscular diaphragm, supports the structures within the pelvic cavity. Its most important segments are the circumvaginal muscles, the levator ani, and the fascia that covers it. Areas not completely covered by this muscle are filled with the coccygeal and piriformal muscles. The perineal body—the muscular tissue between the lower vaginal introitus and the anus—serves as an anchor for genital muscles and ligaments. Changes during pregnancy and labor and after birth are discussed in Chapters 9, 13, and 17.

External Structures

Vulva

The **vulva** is the female external genitalia. The *mons,* made up of soft, fatty tissue, lies directly over the symphysis pubis and becomes covered with hair just before puberty (Figure 3-6). The mons divides into two folds of skin or "lips," called the *labia majora,* which are covered with hair on the outside but smooth inside. When these outer labia are spread, the thin, pink inner *labia minora* can be seen; these inner labia are smooth, hairless, and extremely sensitive to pressure, touch, and temperature. Both sets of labia cover and protect the *vestibule,* which contains the urethral meatus, vaginal introitus, and clitoris.

Urethral meatus and vaginal introitus. The urethral meatus (the entrance of the urethra) opens approximately

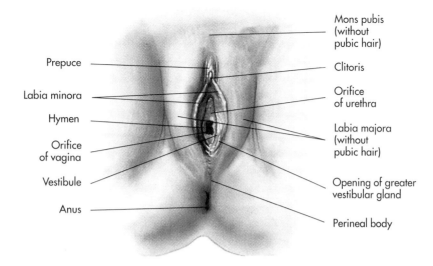

Prepuce

Labia minora

Hymen

Orifice of vagina

Vestibule

Anus

Mons pubis (without pubic hair)

Clitoris

Orifice of urethra

Labia majora (without pubic hair)

Opening of greater vestibular gland

Perineal body

Figure 3-6 External genitals of the female. (Courtesy David J Mascaro & Associates.)

1 cm below the clitoris. The vaginal introitus is surrounded by and sometimes partially covered by a thin membrane called the *hymen.* Perivaginal glands (also called Bartholin's glands)—small round buds thought to produce fluid for lubrication during intercourse—are on either side of the introitus. The fourchette, a thin membranous ridge at the back of the vestibule, is formed by the juncture of the labia majora and minora.

Clitoris. On the anterior of the vulva, the labia minora join to form a soft fold of skin or hood called the *prepuce,* which partially covers the clitoris. Like the penis, the clitoris is also composed of a glans and a shaft. The glans is small and round and is filled with many nerve endings and a rich blood supply. The shaft is a cord connecting the glans to the pubic bone; within it is the major blood supply of the clitoris. The vestibular bulbs are erectile tissue along the sides of the vestibule; these blood and nerve supplies account for engorgement, swelling, and sensitivity during sexual stimulation. Sebaceous glands secrete *smegma,* a fatty substance with a distinct odor similar to that of the smegma from the penis.

Breasts

The mammary glands begin to develop during the sixth week of fetal life, but only the main lactiferous ducts are formed before birth. The glands remain undeveloped until puberty, when growth occurs in response to circulating hormones. During pregnancy the glands complete development in preparation for lactation (see Chapter 17). Breasts are called secondary sex organs because they are not directly involved with reproduction.

Structure. The breasts consist of two mammary glands located on each side of the chest wall, attached by connective tissue and covered with and given shape by fatty tissue. The breasts extend from the second to the sixth or seventh rib and lie between the sternum and the axillary border with an axillary tail extending upward and laterally. Although size and

shape vary a great deal from woman to woman, a breast is generally dome-shaped and weighs between 100 and 200 g. Symmetry between both breasts is rarely perfect, but contours should be smooth with no dimpling, lumps, or retracted areas (Figure 3-7). The breasts are highly vascular structures, and blood vessels enlarge during pregnancy.

In each breast there are 15 to 20 lobes, each containing clusters of alveoli, which resemble tiny bunches of grapes. These are richly lined with capillaries to absorb nutrients from the blood for milk production (lactation). The smallest parts of alveoli are the *acini,* the saclike end of the glandular system. The acini are lined both with epithelial cells that secrete colostrum and milk and with muscles that contract to expel milk.

Little canals, or *ductules,* exit the alveoli and join to form larger canals, the lactiferous ducts. During lactation, milk flows from the alveoli, through the duct system, and into balloonlike storage sacs called *lactiferous sinuses.* The sinuses merge into openings on the nipple. The nipple is a round, pigmented portion of fibromuscular tissue and may be firm and elevated, flat, or even inverted. It is sensitive to temperature and tactile stimuli. Surrounding the nipple is the **areola,** the smooth, pigmented circle of skin containing tiny sebaceous glands (Montgomery's tubercles) that secrete the fatty substances needed to lubricate and protect the nipple. Muscle fibers that tighten to create nipple erectness are also within the areola.

TEST *Yourself* 3-3 _____

Fill in the blanks.
a. Cells that secrete colostrum are _____.
b. Canals that carry milk are _____.
c. Storage site of milk is _____.
d. Glands that lubricate the nipple are _____.

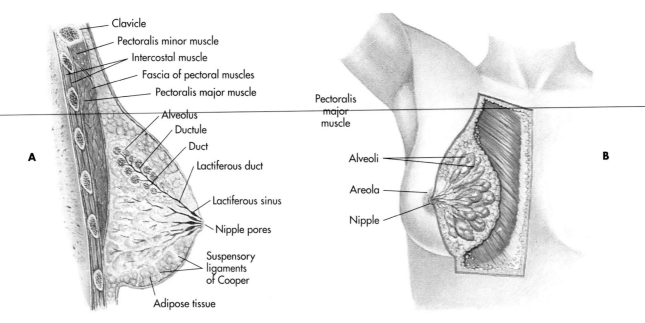

Figure 3-7   The female breast. **A,** Sagittal section of a lactating breast. Notice how the glandular structures are anchored to the overlying skin and to the pectoral muscles by the suspensory Cooper's ligaments. Each lobule of glandular tissue is drained by a lactiferous duct that eventually opens through the nipple. **B,** Anterior view of a lactating breast. Overlying skin and connective tissue have been removed from the medial side to show the internal structure of the breast and underlying skeletal muscle. In nonlactating breasts the glandular tissue is much less prominent, with adipose tissue composing most of each breast.

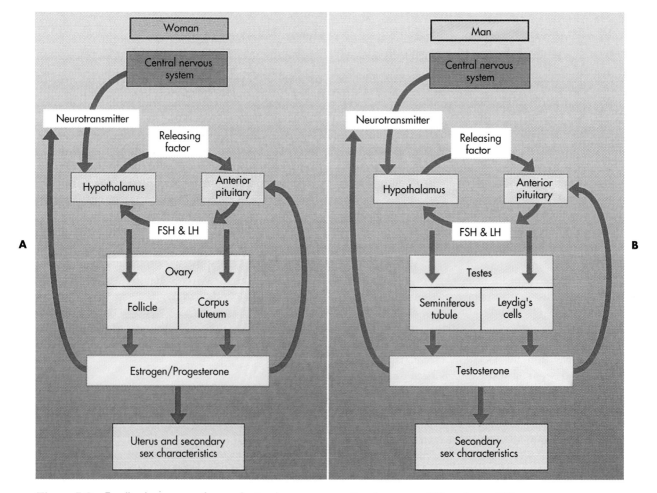

Figure 3-8   Feedback process of reproductive hormone secretion in woman **(A)** and man **(B).**

Hormonal influences. Estrogen and progesterone increase vascularity in the breasts and stimulate acini and duct growth. Water and fatty secretions are increased, resulting in fullness, heaviness, and discomfort during the premenstrual period. During pregnancy the breasts respond to estrogen and progesterone, human placental lactogen (HPL), and prolactin (PRL) to prepare and develop a fully functioning lactating system (see Chapter 17).

PUBESCENCE AND PUBERTY

Both males and females reach sexual maturity through a system of growth and change known as **pubescence.** One to 2 years before puberty, secondary sex characteristics begin to appear with the development of pubic and axillary hair, breast budding, and gradual breast enlargement. Males experience characteristic deepening of the voice, development of body hair, and enlargement of the genitalia. Secondary sex characteristics continue to develop slowly for the next few years after the onset of puberty.

A marked growth spurt precedes puberty by about 1 year. During this period of pubescence, 20% to 25% of linear growth occurs, as males add 8 to 12 inches to their height and females add 2 to 8 inches to theirs. Body weight increases by 20 or 30 pounds during this period. Hands and feet grow first, then long bones; this explains why the young grower often seems so awkward. In girls, linear growth is considered almost complete once menstruation starts, since there is epiphyseal closure under estrogen influence. The age at which the growth spurt associated with puberty begins varies from person to person. Puberty occurs *as growth slows.*

Puberty begins for girls with the first menstrual period, called **menarche.** For boys the first nocturnal emission (ejaculation of semen) begins puberty. In the United States the average age of menarche is 12.3 years; boys mature 6 to 12 months later. However, puberty can occur at any time between the ages of 9 and 15 for girls and between 10 and 17 for boys.

At puberty children move into adolescence, the time of preparation for adulthood; adolescence generally includes the ages from 13 to 19. It is often called the "period of transition" because the teenager's emotions and mind attempt to keep up with rapid physical changes.

Ovulation and therefore pregnancy can occur even before menarche occurs or a menstrual pattern is established. During this time, adolescents can find themselves as parents, "children having children," before being emotionally or developmentally ready. Teenage pregnancy is discussed in detail in Chapter 8.

Onset of Puberty

Hormonal factors

The onset of puberty is controlled by a complex process beginning when the gonads are differentiated in the

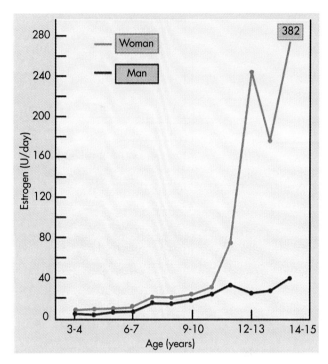

Figure 3-9   Excretion of estrogen in urine of children. Sudden change occurs in girls just before puberty.

embryo. The hormone feedback process is similar in both the male and female (Figure 3-8).

There is a sudden surge of estrogen in girls (Figure 3-9). LH and FSH are active in the first part of the menstrual cycle. FSH stimulates the **graafian follicle,** causing it to mature and resulting in rising estrogen levels. LH plays a role when the follicle is ripe and mature; it triggers follicular rupture and release of the ovum. For the boy, FSH and LH produce androgens necessary for spermatogenesis and testosterone production.

Other hormones also participate in the rapid maturation that occurs during puberty, including the somatotropic (growth) hormone (STH), adrenocorticotropic hormone (ACTH), and thyroid hormone. Hormonal interplay functions on a feedback mechanism; that is, hormonal levels and glandular activities are interdependent and reciprocal.

In females, hormonal levels change with the menstrual cycle. FSH activates several ovarian follicles to grow and mature each cycle. As the follicles mature, they produce estrogens that initially stimulate additional FSH secretion. At the same time, the LH level rises, reaching its peak about 16 to 18 hours before ovulation. This peak is frequently used to study the menstrual cycle of a woman experiencing fertility problems (Figure 3-10). LH and estrogens peak immediately before ovulation. When one follicle becomes the "ripest," it ruptures and releases the mature ovum.

There is only a slight drop in estrogen levels after ovulation, and then as progesterone levels rise, FSH and LH production decreases, suppressing the maturation of another follicle while the body prepares to receive a fertilized ovum.

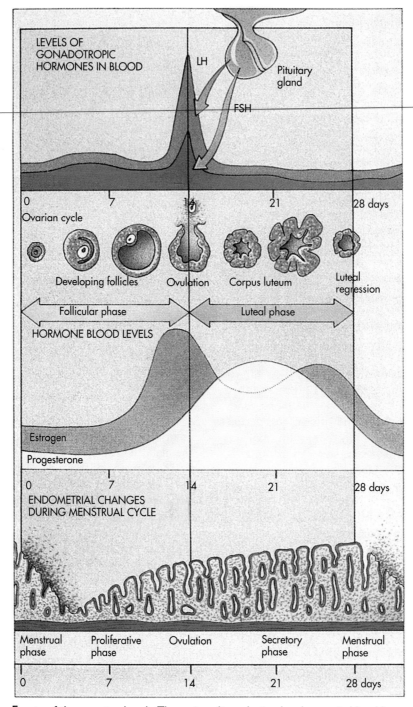

LEVELS OF
GONADOTROPIC
HORMONES IN BLOOD

LH

Pituitary
gland

FSH

0   7   14   21   28 days

Ovarian cycle

Developing follicles   Ovulation   Corpus luteum   Luteal
regression

Follicular phase   Luteal phase

HORMONE BLOOD LEVELS

Estrogen

Progesterone

0   7   14   21   28 days

ENDOMETRIAL CHANGES
DURING MENSTRUAL CYCLE

| Menstrual phase | Proliferative phase | Ovulation | Secretory phase | Menstrual phase |

0   7   14   21   28 days

Figure 3-10   Events of the menstrual cycle. The various lines depict the changes in blood hormonal levels, the development of the follicles, and the changes in the endometrium during the cycle. (Courtesy Kevin A Sommerville.)

(During pregnancy, higher levels of estrogen and progesterone also suppress follicle growth and ovulation.)

After ovulation, LH induces changes in the ruptured follicle. The empty follicle, now known as the **corpus luteum**, because of its yellow color, continues to function under the influence of LH by releasing progesterone. Progesterone, estrogen, and LTH prepare the uterine lining for implantation of the fertilized ovum by thickening its mucous membrane and increasing its blood supply. If the ovum is not fertilized, the levels of estrogen and progesterone begin to fall.

Then the hypothalamus is no longer inhibited by estrogens and begins again to secrete the follicle-stimulating hormone-releasing factor (FSHRF)—a gonadotropin-releasing factor—to the anterior pituitary, which in turn releases FSH and restarts the cycle.

Hormones called **prostaglandins** (PGs), produced in most organs of the body, both affect smooth muscle contractility and hormonal activity during menstruation and ovulation and influence fertility, cervical mucous properties, motility of the fallopian tubes, and contractility of the uterus. In addition PGs contribute to spontaneous abortion and influence the onset of labor.

Menarche

The first menstrual period, called the menarche, usually occurs between 11 and 13 years of age. Although the precise mechanism for menarche is unknown, it is thought to be related to maturation of the hypothalamus. Menarche appears to also be triggered by attainment of a specific percentage of body fat (17%) and body weight (approximately 48 kg or 105 lb). Although follicle secretion of estrogen has begun in a cyclical pattern 2 to 3 years before puberty, the sufficient level of estrogen necessary to establish a consistent hormonal cycle does not occur until puberty begins.

Menstrual Cycle

It takes approximately 1 month for the female to complete her reproductive cycle, from the start of the ripening follicle to the shedding of the uterine lining. The monthly discharge of blood, cellular material, and mucus is called **menstruation** and lasts 3 to 6 days on the average. The length of the cycle varies from woman to woman and may even vary during the course of a year for the same woman. Although the average cycle occurs every 28 to 30 days, the length may vary by as much as 5 to 10 days. Some women have 21-day cycles, whereas others only menstruate every 32 to 35 days. Many factors influence the length of the cycle, including illness, stress, fatigue, environmental conditions, and hormonal differences. Periodic changes may be described by phases or cycles: the *ovarian cycle* is divided according to hormonal activity, and the *uterine* or *endometrial cycle* is described by the varying thickness of the endometrium. Both phases occur simultaneously (see Figure 3-10).

Uterine cycle

The first day of menstrual flow is the first day in the endometrial or uterine cycle and marks the beginning of the **menstrual phase.** By the time this cycle ends, the endometrial lining is thin, estrogen levels are low, and the uterus is dormant. The time from cessation of menses until the beginning of ovulation is the **proliferative phase**, marked by enlargement of the endometrial glands in response to new estrogen stimulation. The endometrial layers become very thick and filled with blood. The cervical mucus becomes abundant, thin, and clear, and its pH changes to a more alkaline state to allow for and to encourage (to "welcome") the entry of sperm. The mucus becomes very stretchable during ovulation, a condition known as **spinnbarkeit** (see Chapter 5).

After ovulation the **secretory phase** begins. Under the influence of progesterone, the endometrial cells swell and dilate in preparation for the fertilized ovum. If fertilization and implantation do not occur, the levels of estrogen and progesterone fall. Vasoconstriction occurs, causing a decreased blood supply to the endometrium; this in turn results in tissue breakdown, beginning the **ischemic phase.** As endometrial tissue sloughs off, capillaries break, and blood begins to escape with the tissue and mucus as the menstrual phase begins again.

Ovarian cycle

The ovaries also go through rhythmic, cyclical changes. Each primary oocyte within the ovary is surrounded by several layers of cells that will become a follicle. Estrogen-producing cells surround the follicle as it matures. In each cycle, only one follicle from approximately 40,000 matures into a graafian follicle, which ruptures to liberate the ovum. Although other follicles develop simultaneously, once one ripens and ruptures the others decrease in size. The exception to this rule occurs with fraternal twins, when two follicles mature and rupture and are fertilized by two different sperm (see Chapter 21).

There are two ovarian phases. The **follicular phase** begins immediately after menses and ends about midway through the uterine cycle. During this phase the follicle matures, with final maturation and release of the ovum influenced by a surge of LH from the anterior pituitary gland (see Figure 3-10). Note especially in Figure 3-10 the developing follicle in relation to the growth of the endometrial tissue.

The **luteal phase** begins when the graafian follicle ruptures and the ovum is released. After rupture, follicle walls collapse to form the corpus luteum, which has a life span of 10 to 12 days unless the ovum is fertilized. During that span the corpus luteum produces progesterone, a thermogenic hormone. As a result, there is a change in body temperature, a sign used to aid in contraception (see Chapter 5). In most cycles the ovum is not fertilized and the corpus luteum degenerates, becoming a dry, scarred area called the *corpus albicans,* which produces no hormones. Estrogen and progesterone levels drop, body temperature returns to the preovulatory range, and the spongy, edematous layer of the endometrium sloughs off.

Menstruation begins for most women 14 days (± 2 days) after ovulation, regardless of the length of the menstrual phase. Variation in the length of the cycle is a result of a slower or more rapid buildup of the endometrium and follicle during the follicular or proliferative phase. See Chapter 4 for discussion of altered menstrual patterns.

Self-Discovery

During the time you are studying maternity nursing, record the signs and symptoms of each menstrual cycle in yourself, a partner, or an adolescent in your family. Note whether stress changes menstrual timing. ~

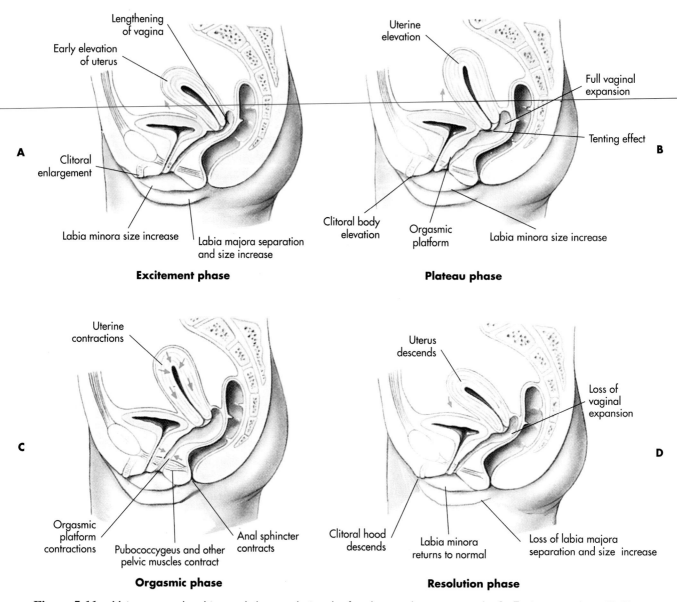

Figure 3-11   Major external and internal changes during the female sexual response cycle. **A,** Excitement phase. **B,** Plateau phase. **C,** Orgasmic phase. **D,** Resolution phase. (Courtesy Medical and Scientific Illustration, Crozet, Va.)

HUMAN SEXUALITY

Sexual Response

Both men and women respond to sexual stimulation by experiencing a cycle of events. Masters and Johnson (1966) characterize the cycle by describing four phases: *excitement, plateau, orgasm,* and *resolution.* In both sexes these phases are characterized by vasocongestion (increased blood supply) and myotonia (muscle tension with increased contractility). Both sympathetic and parasympathetic neural pathways are involved, and hormones play a part; testosterone and serotonin and dopamine release influence both male and female responses.

Both sexes are stimulated by physical, psychologic, and emotional factors. Although the genitals and breasts are the most sensitive erogenous areas, any part of the body can cause sexual arousal, initiating the physical response cycle (Figure 3-11).

The excitement phase

Physical or mental stimuli trigger this initial phase. Heart rate, respirations, and blood pressure rise, and skin sensitivity is heightened. Parasympathetic stimulus increases blood flow to the genitals and breasts.

Female. For the woman the pooling of blood (vasocongestion) causes the clitoris to swell and increases vaginal lubrication from the vestibular glands. The inner two thirds of the vagina expands, and the labia majora and minora enlarge and open.

Male. Response in the male is also initially caused by parasympathetic vasodilation. Blood flow increases into

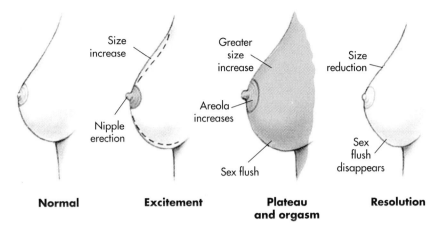

Size increase

Nipple erection

Greater size increase

Areola increases

Sex flush

Size reduction

Sex flush disappears

Normal   **Excitement**   **Plateau and orgasm**   **Resolution**

Figure 3-12   Changes in the breast during the female sexual response cycle. (Courtesy Medical and Scientific Illustration, Crozet, Va.)

the corpora cavernosa, causing engorgement that constricts veins and prevents venous drainage. The penis becomes enlarged and erect (tumescent), and the testicles draw closer to the body.

Plateau phase

As arousal continues, sexual and muscle tension heighten. A "sex flush" occurs, and there may be a red rash or blotches over the chest, neck, or other parts of the body (Figure 3-12).

Female. As the woman experiences the plateau phase, vasocongestion causes the vagina to swell, narrowing the canal and introitus to increase penile friction. The inner labia thicken, the highly sensitive clitoris is pulled up to the pubic bone for protection, and the uterus and cervix are drawn away from the vagina.

Male. This phase is characterized by an increase in the length and diameter of the head and shaft of the penis. The testicles enlarge and press closer to the body. There is deepening of the color of the penile head, and the preejaculatory fluid appears as a prelude to the orgasmic phase.

Orgasmic phase

Orgasm is the shortest of the phases and is brought about by rhythmic muscular contractions, ranging from mild genital throbbing to intense spasms or sometimes involuntary rigidity or thrashing movements of the entire body. Brain wave changes occur, and as the person focuses on pleasurable sensations, "black out" or altered level of consciousness may occur.

Female. Female orgasm is felt in the clitoris and throughout the genital and pelvic areas. Three to ten contractions less than one second apart occur in the outer one third of the vagina, the uterus, fallopian tubes, and the perirectal area. These rhythmic pulsations are thought to aid the sperm in entering the cervix and in moving upward through the reproductive tract (see Figure 3-11).

Male. The male orgasm consists of two stages. At the peak of excitement, sympathetic fibers trigger the release of sperm from the epididymis to travel through the duct system. The prostate, seminal vesicles, and bulbourethral glands secrete fluids to nourish and transport the sperm. Extra blood is forced to the base of the urethra to close it during orgasm, preventing sperm from being pushed up into the bladder. This is called "emission," and once this occurs ejaculation is inevitable. Seconds later, impulses from sympathetic fibers cause muscle contractions of the penis and urethra that force semen out the urethra in spurts. These contractions are less than one second apart and can be felt in the testicles and rectal area (Figure 3-13).

Resolution

After orgasm, resolution allows the body to return to the prearousal state. As engorgement decreases, pressure that has trapped blood in the genitals begins to decrease. Organs return to normal size, color, and position. Vital signs return to normal levels.

Female. Because more blood may remain trapped, the woman's erectile tissue remains engorged and sensitive, and she may be able to respond to stimulus by reentering the plateau phase and quickly experiencing another orgasm.

Male. Men experience "refractory" periods during which there cannot be another orgasm, even if the penis remains erect. The time of this refractory period varies among individuals.

Gender and Sexuality

Sexuality encompasses far more than just the gender of a person or sexual activity. It involves physical, emotional, and cultural factors and is an intrinsic part of each human being. Sexuality begins at conception with sex determina-

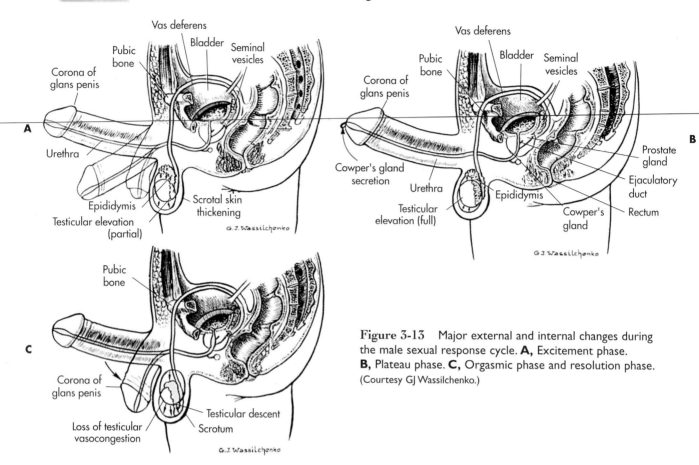

Figure 3-13 Major external and internal changes during the male sexual response cycle. **A,** Excitement phase. **B,** Plateau phase. **C,** Orgasmic phase and resolution phase. (Courtesy GJ Wassilchenko.)

tion, grows in infancy and childhood as the child learns to relate to the people and the world around him or her, and continues until death.

Though the term **sexuality** is often linked only with physical attraction and genital activity, sexuality is intrinsic to and influences every aspect of a person's life. The product of many factors, sexuality impinges on a person's choices of career, sexual partner(s), friends, and interests. It influences self-perception and how one is viewed by others. Sexuality enervates, motivates, and defines the individual and also grows and changes as the person does. Establishing gender identity and sexual roles and choosing a sex partner are all parts of that ongoing process.

Gender Identity

Though sex is established at conception and sexuality is influenced from birth, awareness and one's views of self as male or female develops more slowly. At age 2 or 3 the child can state "I'm a boy" or "I'm a girl"; by age 6 there is realization that gender is permanent.

This **gender identity** is related to how a child is treated and the reaction of the child to others. Enactment of *gender role* occurs when the child starts to behave as either a girl or a boy by copying actions of others of the same sex and, by the age of 6, scrupulously avoiding actions associated with the opposite sex. Play in later childhood allows

the child to practice gender roles as he or she perceives them by doing what is established as appropriate for men or women. Gender identity governs behavior and helps define actions within the sex role, but it may also limit role performance if it includes rigid ideas.

Sexual orientation

A person's sexual orientation refers to the romantic attraction to and sexual desire for another person or persons. A person who is heterosexual seeks relationships and sexual interaction with persons of the opposite sex. A male homosexual or female lesbian is attracted to a person of the same sex. The term "orientation" rather than sexual "preference" is used more often since attraction to a particular sex is thought to be an intrinsic quality rather than a choice (Reinisch and Beasley, 1990).

Homosexuality and lesbianism, considered by some as the result of abnormal development, have long carried a stigma. Blame for both orientations was placed on numerous factors such as a domineering mother, a weak father, or same-sex childhood play. Though the reason for being homosexual instead of heterosexual is still not understood, labeling homosexuality as a disorder or abnormality is known to be inappropriate. A man or woman's sexual orientation is simply a part of the whole person. A person cannot be "cured" of attraction to the same sex, nor does a person have mental or sexual problems simply because of his or her expression of sexuality. Neither childhood nor adolescent periods of same-sex activity is known to determine adult attraction and behavior (Thorne, 1994).

OVERVIEW OF SEXUALITY ACROSS THE LIFE CYCLE

Sexuality involves physical, emotional, and cultural factors and is an intrinsic part of each human being. Sexuality is experienced in different ways across the life cycle, from birth until death, and is a basic component in achievement of developmental tasks (Berger, 1988).

Before Birth and During Infancy

Physical sexual response occurs in the developing fetus; penile erections have been observed during ultrasound examinations during pregnancy. After birth, changes in hormonal levels and reaction to pleasurable feelings may trigger involuntary genital responses in the newborn.

According to Erikson (1978), the infant's developmental task during the first year of life is achievement of "trust vs mistrust." Consistent response to physical and emotional needs is essential to provide the infant with security, gratification, and pleasure and also to set the stage for future sexual experience. When parents touch, hold, and cuddle an infant, they teach the infant that physical stimulation is necessary and good. They are also responding to the infant's communication. Though parents expect a smiling response from a contented infant, they may be surprised that there is also a genital response to pleasurable feelings.

With growth comes exploration, and this often begins with the infant's exploration of his or her own body; finding fingers to suck and genitals to touch is a way of discovering self and learning to obtain comfort and happiness independently. At this early age, seeking sexual pleasure does not have an interactional component, but instead the activity is repeated simply because it "feels good."

Childhood

By the time a child is 3 years old, his or her curiosity runs rampant. Self-stimulation is common in the toddler, as is developing interest in other children's and the parents' bodies. For the toddler the next task of "autonomy vs shame and doubt" will include exploring abilities, testing limits, and checking for parents' approval.

As toddlers seek the ability to rule their own bodies, toilet training begins. Perception of genitalia expands to include elimination and the pleasure gained by controlling elimination. The child realizes that a high value is placed on being private and keeping clean.

By the age of 4 or 5, the child has an increased interest in sex and sexual differences, with more frequent masturbation, investigation of adult bathroom practices, and instances of playing "doctor" with other children. As the child works on the task of establishing "initiative vs guilt" he or she takes on new tasks with great excitement. Children want to please parents or caregivers and are vulnerable to their responses. Disapproving or punitive reactions to behavior causes guilt feelings to be associated with expressing sexuality. Since same-sex groups are more common at this stage, there is a developmental "homosexual centered" period, but this type of behavior is not predictive of specific adult sexual orientation.

During the period between ages 5 and 12, the child strives to achieve the school-age developmental task of "industry vs inferiority." The child seeks to identify with and have the approval of admired others and begins to take pleasure in them. Sexual exploration may be a way of trying out the gender roles with which the child has identified. Comfort with these roles and satisfaction in their performance is part of a child's completion of this middle-school task.

Though the child of this age needs physical contact with the parents, many parents are uncomfortable with this; they believe that cuddling, touching, and holding are only appropriate for young children, or they may fear that the child will respond in a sexual manner to physical signs of affection. As a result the child may be physically isolated from the time of preschool through adolescence, a time when reassurance during the many changes of this period is important.

Adolescence

During puberty, sexual feelings intensify and physical reactions occur, such as more frequent erections and nocturnal emissions ("wet dreams") in boys and increased vaginal secretions in girls. Fantasies are heightened and masturbation activity is increased. Because pubertal changes occur at different rates, those who are still prepubescent may be envious, anxious, or embarrassed, whereas those going through these changes may have decreased self-esteem and may try to fit in with peers by looking and acting as much alike as possible. As teens work to complete the task of "identity vs role confusion," sexual activity may be the tool used to feel accepted, popular, and "adult." Needs and care for adolescents are discussed in Chapter 8.

Adulthood

Men and women begin to view sexual activity as a way to establish relationships or to strengthen closeness with a partner. They risk sharing themselves in an effort to achieve "intimacy vs isolation." This is the period of establishing careers and starting families, and young adults learn to use their sexuality to help define themselves.

At this stage the interest in, frequency of, and response to sexual activity differ between men and women. The term "sexual peak" is used to describe frequency of orgasms experienced. For men the peak occurs in adolescence and the early twenties, whereas for women the peak generally occurs from the mid-twenties to the mid-forties.

Parenthood may be a sexual stressor in early adulthood. New roles add unexpected physical and emotional demands to the parents and challenge them to maintain intimacy while giving increased attention to the growing child. Pregnancy and any complications may limit intercourse or any orgasm-stimulating activity (see Chapter 8).

After childbirth, women may be reluctant to resume sexual activity because of fatigue, changes in body image, or fear of a closely spaced pregnancy. The combination of being a mother and a lover may cause the woman to feel conflict. Fathers also experience conflicting feelings and often feel "left out" of physical affection and attention, now directed primarily at the infant (see Chapter 17).

Middle Adulthood

Parenthood is still a reality for many at this stage, but others have moved on to relating to grown children and grandchildren. These adults are settled into career tracks and seek new areas of interest as they pass through the developmental phase of "generativity vs stagnation." Part of the task of achieving generativity includes sharing with members of the next generation and acting as role models for them. Sexuality may not change radically, but some adaptation for physical changes may be needed. The woman goes through **menopause** between her late forties and early fifties. Changes in ovarian function, menstruation, and hormonal levels result in vaginal changes, including decreased elasticity, dryness of tissue, and decreased lubrication during arousal. Lower estrogen levels result in breast tissue loss, the potential for osteoporosis, and cardiovascular complications. Sexual activity may decline in frequency, and arousal may take longer. Body image may cause a woman to feel less desirable. See Chapter 4 for more discussion of this period.

Men experience fewer reproductive changes than women and a more gradual decrease in hormonal levels. They may, however, notice slower arousal, fewer spontaneous erections, decreased intensity of orgasm, and less ejaculate. Because men continue to produce sperm into later years, the term "male menopause" actually refers to the man's emotional responses to the effects of normal aging processes rather than to a cessation of fertility.

Because arousal may take longer in both men and women, these changes may have a positive effect on sexual activity by increasing the time spent in the period of foreplay or stimulation. Feelings of intimacy may be enhanced by this need. Men and women in this age group may be more emotionally secure and more able to express romantic feelings, even though adult children are often surprised that parents are still sexually active.

Late Adulthood

Normal physical changes and acute or chronic medical problems may interfere with regular patterns of sexual activity in the older adult. Expressions of sexuality do not cease as frequency of intercourse decreases. Those who have had satisfying relationships throughout the years are generally able to continue sexual activity with some adjustments.

The last of Erikson's developmental tasks is "integrity vs despair," indicating that older persons must come to terms with all the changes in their lives. Being comfortable with sexuality and seeing it as an invigorating force makes this transition easier.

Key Points

- Male and female anatomy is initially identical until about the fifth week of development.
- Because of the common beginning of both male and female reproductive systems, there are parallels in the structures and the function of sexual hormones.
- The spermatozoa live 2 to 3 days after ejaculation, whereas the ovum survives only 24 hours.
- Pubescence precedes puberty by about 2 years. Gradual development of secondary sex characteristics signals the approach of puberty.
- Most girls and women are not well educated about the menstrual cycle, despite monthly experiences.

- Estrogen and progesterone levels counteract several of each other's effects but also work together to achieve others.
- Human sexuality is an integral part of a person's life regardless of whether intercourse is practiced.
- Surrounded with cultural values and restrictions, adolescents may try to break parental restrictions through sexual experimentation. For this reason clear, cause-and-effect education about sexual activity is important early in adolescence.

Study Questions

3-1. Select the terms that apply to the following statements:
   a. The mobile end of the fallopian tube is the ———————.
   b. The uterine layer responsible for contractions during birth is ———————.
   c. Except for the days around ovulation, the vaginal environment is usually ——————— because of its pH.
   d. ———————, a hormone found in many body tissues, is involved in uterine cramping during menstruation.
   e. The continuous process of forming the male reproductive cell is ———————.
   f. Sperm are formed first in the ———————.

3-2. Which is true of spermatogenesis?
   a. Immature sperm begin to develop in Leydig's cells.
   b. Sperm do not develop until testicular descent into the scrotum.
   c. Spermatozoa develop at puberty under the influence of hormones.
   d. Sexual excitation triggers formation of spermatozoa.

3-3. The portion of the uterus that extends above the insertion of the fallopian tubes is the:
   a. Cervix.
   b. Body.
   c. Isthmus.
   d. Fundus.

3-4. Which hormone raises body temperature at ovulation?
   a. Estrogen
   b. Progesterone
   c. FSH
   d. HCG

3-5. Fertilization usually occurs in the:
   a. Fimbriae.
   b. Ampulla.
   c. Cornua.
   d. Uterus.

3-6. Menarche is defined as the first:
   a. Cycle of ovulation.
   b. Menstrual period.
   c. Development of sex characteristics.
   d. Complete hormonal cycle.

3-7. Match the length of the menstrual cycle with what you know of its phases.
   a. If Marie ovulates on day 20 of her cycle, when would her next menstrual period likely begin?
   b. If Jane ovulates on day 12 of her cycle, when would her next menstrual period likely begin?
   1. Day 34
   2. Day 32
   3. Day 28
   4. Day 26

Answer Key

3-1: *a,* Fimbria; *b,* myometrium; *c,* acidic; *d,* prostaglandin; *e,* spermatogenesis; *f,* seminiferous tubule. 3-2: *c.* 3-3: *d.* 3-4: *b.* 3-5: *b.* 3-6: *b.* 3-7: *a,* 1; *b,* 4.

References

Beischer NA, MacKay EU: *Obstetrics and the newborn,* ed 3, Philadelphia, 1993, Harcourt Brace Jovanovich.
*Berger KS: *The developing person through the life span,* ed 2, New York, 1988, Worth.
Cunningham G et al: *Williams obstetrics,* ed 19, Norwalk Town, Conn, 1993, Appleton & Lange.
*Erikson EH, ed: *Adulthood,* New York, 1978, WW Norton & Co.
*Gray H: *Anatomy of the human body,* Philadelphia, 1985, Lea & Febiger.
Hite S. *The Hite report on the family,* New York, 1994, Grove Press.
*Masters WH, Johnson VE: *Human sexual response,* Boston, 1966, Little Brown and Co.

* Classic reference.

*Moore K: *Essentials of human embryology,* Philadelphia, 1988, BC Decker.
Reinisch J, Beasley R: *The Kinsey Institute new report on sex,* New York, 1990, St Martins Press.
Thorne B: *Gender play,* New Jersey, 1994, Rutgers.

Student Resource Shelf

Blackburn ST, Loper DL: *Maternal, fetal, and neonatal physiology,* Philadelphia, 1992, WB Saunders.
A standard text for nurses and nurse midwives on the physiology of pregnancy and birth.

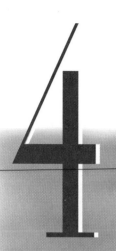

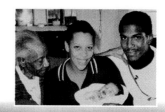

4

Women's Health Care

The birth of today's approach to women's health care is the result of a long and complicated gestation. As women become more aware of their needs and more assertive in seeking solutions, traditional approaches are rapidly changing. Previously, only reproductive issues were recognized as needing management by physicians; general health issues were often ignored, misdiagnosed, or mis-understood. As clients, women perceived that the physician held the power, determined what needed to be done to treat a particular problem, and chose the course of therapy. Unsuccessful treatment often left the woman with the realization that her complaints were seen as vague and psychogenic and that she would "just have to live with it."

Difficult menstruation, body changes after menopause, and even nongynecologic symptoms such as chest pain or abdominal discomfort were all too frequently given inappropriate attention or inadequate follow-up care. The woman's acceptance of a passive and cooperative role left her with little choice but to simply accept and follow instructions, whether these were helpful or not.

CHANGES IN WOMEN'S HEALTH CARE

Current approaches to women's health care are the result of societal trends in feminism and consumerism. Women are no longer satisfied with having limited input concerning their diagnoses and treatments. The focus now is on providing holistic health care that values the woman's participation and cooperation, demystifies the health care experience, and creates a more collegial environment in which the woman is the true owner and caretaker of her body. At the same time the role of the physician is evolving from authoritative and hierarchic to consultative and supportive.

As the philosophy toward woman's health care has changed, so have the settings and the providers of care. Although care is still based primarily in obstetric-gynecologic settings, centers that manage women's comprehensive health needs are being developed.

In this changing environment, nursing has developed more fully the role it has always played in health care. Nurses, long known as advocates, teachers, and counselors, now play expanded roles as primary care givers and serve as clinical nurse specialists, nurse practitioners, and certified nurse-midwives. Women can now receive comprehensive assessment, planning, treatment, education, counseling, and support from nurses who either work in collaborative practices with physicians or who operate their own private practices. Although some women find it difficult to accept diagnoses and prescriptions from someone other than a physician, many appreciate the new approach.

Goals of Care

Goals for women's health, once focused on the treatment of problems, now emphasize maintenance of wellness; these goals promote self-care through education and support. The primary objective of this care is to **empower** each woman—to give back to her control over her body and its health by treating her as an informed and independent learner, by respecting her decisions about how she will be treated, and by encouraging her to share information with other women. Along with her practitioner, each woman is seen as a partner in health care, and she is encouraged to contribute the expertise that only she has—knowledge of her own body and mind. Complete physical, psychologic, and sexual wholeness is the expected outcome of this challenging new approach.

These goals are set to meet the needs of the ever-changing population of women: the young and the old, the physically challenged and the chronically ill, the sexually active heterosexual and the lesbian, the corporate executive and the homeless mother. Wellness for all women is the ultimate goal.

THE HEALTH VISIT

A woman's first impression of the health care setting will influence her decision of whether to continue seeking care there. The surroundings of the place, the level of respect and privacy shown, and the attitudes of all staff members combine to make the experience a positive and valuable one. If the woman is shown respect and courtesy in an unhurried atmosphere and believes the staff is sensitive to her feelings, her anxiety will be relieved and she will be more at ease.

Health History

After initial introductions are made and explanations of personnel and their roles are given, the woman's health history is carefully taken by interview, in writing, or a combination of the two (Figure 4-1). Questions should be clear, nonthreatening, and specific. When the history is taken verbally, adequate privacy must be provided to encourage the woman to answer honestly without fear of embarrassment or of being overheard while disclosing relevant information. The history should include any areas that might affect the woman's health or the maintenance of her health. Many components of her life, including her medical, surgical, reproductive, nutritional, sexual, psychologic, social, occupational, economic, cultural, and religious status are reviewed, as is any history of substance use or abuse.

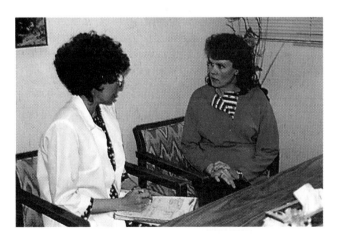

Figure 4-1 Each client is interviewed to identify individual concerns. (Courtesy Marjorie Pyle, RNC, *Lifecircle*.)

The woman's educational level is evaluated so that teaching is personalized to meet her level of understanding. When the health history is complete, it should be reviewed so that both the woman and the interviewer can ask questions or clarify information.

Physical Assessment

General examination

The woman often perceives the physical examination as an unpleasant event. Being inspected while undressed; having her body touched, probed and palpated; and assuming uncomfortable and embarrassing positions make her feel a loss of privacy, dignity, and control. Many women avoid health care because of these reasons. Offering explanations to the woman, providing her with a private and secure area to change into a patient gown, and not exposing her body parts unnecessarily can alleviate some anxiety. Even encouraging the woman to keep socks or a shirt on can make her feel less exposed. In addition, allowing the woman to sit at a 30- to 45-degree angle instead of lying flat allows eye contact and communication during the genital and pelvic examination. Provision should be made to allow someone of the woman's choosing to stay with her at all times. If the examiner is a man, a female staff member should be present to guard against any misunderstanding or misinterpretation of conduct.

Examination of the woman may range from a simple reproductive assessment to a complete physical review of systems if her care is not being followed by another practitioner. Vital signs, height, and weight always are obtained, and cardiopulmonary wellness should also be ascertained.

Laboratory work may include complete blood count and electrolytes, glucose, cholesterol, and triglyceride values. For a woman at risk for **sexually transmitted diseases** (STDs), testing for hepatitis B, syphilis, gonorrhea, and, with the woman's consent, human immunodeficiency viral (HIV) infection will be included. Urine is analyzed for blood, glucose, acetone, and protein, and, if indicated, a Tine or purified protein derivative (PPD) test may be used to detect tuberculosis exposure. During the gynecologic examination, specimens may be obtained for culture or cytologic analysis of vaginal mucus and cells.

Gynecologic examination

The gynecologic assessment includes examination of the breasts, vulva, vagina, cervix, and uterus. The rectum should also be included in the evaluation.

Breasts. Breast examination is an essential part of any woman's physical examination, with a clear explanation of the procedure and findings given. The procedure should be performed in both upright and supine positions, allowing for visual inspection and palpation. The woman should be encouraged to perform **breast self-examination** before, along with, or after the practitioner.

Self-Discovery

Teach yourself or a relative to do a breast self-examination (see Procedure 4-1).

Genitalia. The genital and pelvic examination may cause anxiety and discomfort for the woman experiencing it for the first time. The procedure should be explained before the woman lies on the examining table, and she should be asked if she wishes to have a partner, family member, or friend stay with her during the examination. She is then assisted to a supine position, with her head and shoulders elevated and supported comfortably. This relaxes the rectus muscles, allowing easier examination of the vagina. Stirrups support her feet, and she is instructed to move her buttocks to the bottom end of the table. The areas not being visualized are draped, and she is warned to expect touch before it is done. To encourage her role as an active participant, the woman may be given a mirror so that she is able to observe what the examiner is doing and learn about her own normal anatomy for self-examination.

For many women the experience of looking at, touching, and becoming thoroughly familiar with their genitalia may be a natural and comfortable one. Others, however, because of personal, cultural, or religious influences, consider this experience difficult, embarrassing, or even distasteful. By teaching this aspect of self-care as part of total health maintenance, the nurse may alleviate anxiety and foster within the woman a sense of self-mastery and control. If the woman does not wish to participate in the examination, she is still informed of the results of each step.

The external genitalia are first inspected for infection, lesions, and trauma. A speculum that is warmed and lubricated with water is then inserted into the vagina to visualize the vaginal vault, walls, and cervix (Figure 4-2). Secretions or drainage are noted, and specimens for the Papanicolaou smear or culture may be obtained. Once the speculum is removed, a bimanual pelvic examination is performed, with two fingers of one hand inserted into the vagina while the examiner's other hand palpates the uterus and adnexae for size, position, shape, tenderness, and masses (see Chapter 9, Figure 9-11).

There should be little or no discomfort during the vaginal, pelvic, and rectal examinations. Most women tend to tense before digital or speculum insertion; some grab the table or someone's hand. Although this may seem reassuring, it actually increases the resistance the examiner encounters and causes discomfort for the woman. Preparing the woman for the sensations of pressure and assisting her with techniques such as slow, rhythmic breathing and visualization will relax vaginal and pelvic floor muscles, allowing easier access for examination.

PROCEDURE 4-1

Teaching Breast Self-Examination

The procedure for manual self-examination is recommended by the American Cancer Society and may be performed either while standing or lying down. The best time to do breast self-examination is right after your period, when breasts are not tender or swollen. If you do not have regular periods or sometimes skip a month, do it on the same day every month.

1. Lie down and put a pillow under your right shoulder. Place your right arm behind your head.

2. Use the finger pads (the top third of each finger) of your three middle fingers on your left hand to feel for lumps or thickening.

3. Press firmly enough to know how your breast feels. If you are not sure how hard to press, ask your health care provider or try to imitate the way your health care provider uses the finger pads during a breast examination. Learn what your breast feels like most of the time. A firm ridge in the lower curve of each breast is normal.

4. Move around the breast in a set pattern. You can choose either (A) the circle, (B) the up and down line, or (C) the wedge. Use the same pattern every time. Doing this will help you to make sure that you have gone over the entire breast area and to remember how your breast feels.

5. Now examine your left breast using right-hand finger pads.

6. If you find any changes, see your physician right away.

The nurse should also teach the woman to palpate up into the axilla to examine the tail of the breast. In front of a mirror, the woman should inspect for skin dimpling or pulling, redness or swelling, and nipple changes.

The examiner may also ask the woman to stand with both arms above her head and press the palms of both hands together. This contracts the chest muscles and makes some tumors more obvious.

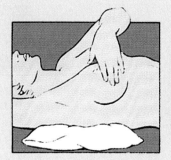
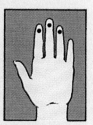

Finger Pads

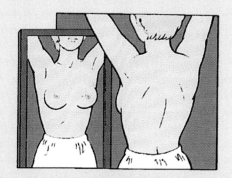

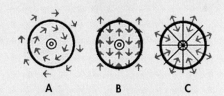

A   B   C

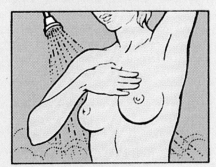

(Courtesy American Cancer Society)

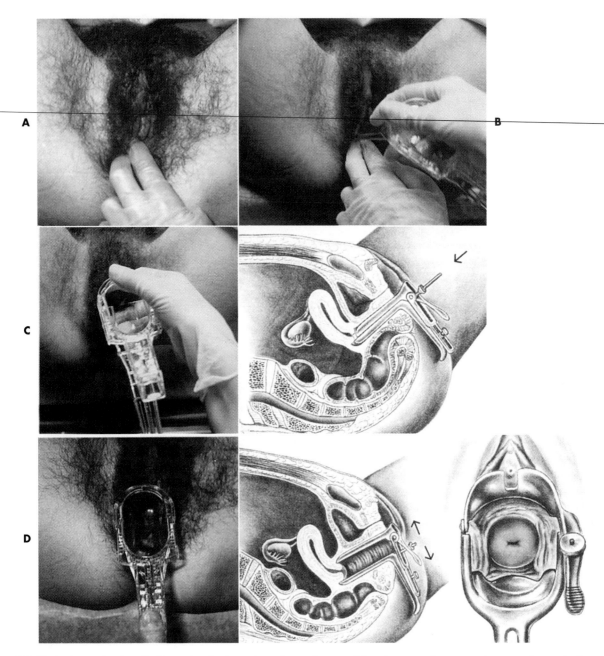

Figure 4-2 Vaginal examination. **A,** Preparing for insertion of speculum: applying downward pressure in posterior vaginal opening with two fingers. **B,** Inserting closed speculum over fingers. **C,** Directing speculum downward at 45-degree angle. **D,** Speculum in place, locked and stabilized. Note cervix in full view. (From Seidel HM et al: *Mosby's guide to physical examination,* ed 3, St Louis, 1995, Mosby.)

After changing gloves, the examiner assesses the rectum by palpation with a lubricated gloved finger. A specimen may be obtained at this time for a *guaiac* test (blood in the stool). Tissues should be provided to remove the lubricant.

Safety is important when the woman returns to a sitting position. As the examiner supports her back, she is instructed to move up on the table and lower both legs together.

Postexamination discussion. Explanation and discussion of results, goal setting, and planning should take place outside the examining room when the woman is fully clothed and comfortable. This is a time for clarification, collaboration, explanation, teaching, support, and counseling (Figure 4-3). Before the woman leaves the office, she should know both how to obtain the results of any tests she had and the person with whom she can discuss the tests. If she needs a second visit, one should be scheduled at this time.

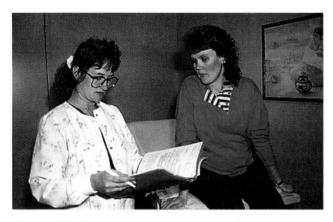

Figure 4-3 After the physical examination, findings should be discussed and self-care taught. (Courtesy Marjorie Pyle, RNC, *Lifecircle*.)

WOMEN'S HEALTH EDUCATION

Gynecologic Hygiene

General hygiene is an important part of any person's total health maintenance. In our society, cleanliness is considered extremely important, and emphasis is placed on eliminating, preventing, or disguising natural body secretions and odors. Perineal hygiene in particular is a major concern for most women, and products abound that promise "freshness" to their users. Although cleansing is necessary, frequent use of soap and water usually is sufficient to maintain hygiene. Over-the-counter (OTC) feminine hygiene products often contain chemicals that can alter normal flora, irritate tissues, predispose the woman to infection, and disguise conditions that should be assessed and treated by a professional. Towelettes, deodorants, and sprays are unnecessary for most women and should be avoided.

Though many women consider douching useful or even essential to ensure cleanliness, douches should be employed only if ordered as a specific treatment. Even then, they should be used with caution. Douches are administered by gravity, with the bag held less than 24 inches above hip level, and never with the force of a bulb syringe. The nurse instructs the woman to use warm water (not hot) to prevent tissue trauma and to avoid instilling the solution under pressure, which could force the fluid or air into the uterus and out into the abdominal cavity. Douching may be associated with ascending infection into the fallopian tubes (see Chapter 25).

Menstrual Hygiene

Menstruation is perceived as a particular hygiene problem for women. Because of its normal musky odor, menstrual flow is a source of embarrassment for Western women. Most often, bleeding is absorbed by disposable

sanitary pads or napkins made of natural or synthetic absorbent materials. Culture or finances may necessitate the use of homemade fabrics such as cloth rags. Whatever the woman's choice, care must be taken to protect others from exposure to her blood by careful disposal or washing of the pads.

Many women prefer the use of internal vaginal tampons, either alone or with a sanitary pad. Made of a combination of cotton and synthetic fibers, tampons are small and compact for insertion with or without an applicator, and they expand as they absorb vaginal drainage. If inserted without trauma, positioned properly, and changed once every 4 hours (sooner if saturated), tampons are a safe, comfortable, and effective way to eliminate the bulkiness of a pad and the chance of bleeding through or around it. Some women are unable to use tampons because of physical limitations or sensitivity to the products. Others may feel uncomfortable with genital manipulation or with handling the soiled tampon. For those who wish to use tampons, correct use does not damage the hymen or affect virginity. Teenagers as well as adult women may use them.

Careful hand washing is essential with the use of tampons, both before and after insertion. Proper disposal to prevent contamination from blood is also an important consideration. Most tampons may be flushed in toilets that are connected to a sewer system, but to prevent bacterial buildup, they should not be flushed if a septic tank is used. Applicators may or may not be flushable. Tampons may also be wrapped and disposed of appropriately in the garbage.

Tampons come in different absorbencies to accommodate various menstrual flow patterns. The least absorbent size should be used to ensure that it will be changed often enough. This is important for the prevention of toxic shock syndrome, a condition arising from the growth of bacteria in the warm, moist, and nutritive medium that a saturated tampon provides.

Toxic Shock Syndrome

Toxic shock syndrome (TSS) is a multisystem, bacterial infection that is severe, acute, and potentially fatal. TSS was first described as a syndrome affecting children and adolescents in 1978 (Todd et al, 1978). After this report, TSS was noted among menstruating women and in 1980 was linked with the use of superabsorbent tampons.

Although the exact pathogenesis of TSS is unknown, it is generally accepted that the syndrome is a response to a toxin (TSST-1) produced by the *Staphylococcus aureus* bacterium. Other organisms associated with TSS-like syndromes are group A and specific group B streptococci (Schlievert, Gocke, Deringer, 1993), but these are not usually associated with tampon use and are seen in skin and tissue infections (Wood, Potter, Jonasson, 1993).

Nonmenstrual TSS may occur in association with puerperal (postpartum) sepsis, postcesarean delivery infection, mastitis, staphylococcal wound, or skin infection that includes boils, infected abrasions, burns, or insect bites. Whereas menstrual-associated TSS is declining, nonmenstrual TSS appears to have remained constant (Reingold, 1991).

Risk

Though TSS may affect women, men, and children of any age, it occurs most frequently among young menstruating women. Cases among women are largely associated with the use of tampons. TSS has also been observed with use of contraceptive diaphragms and sponges, though not in significant numbers. The incidence of menstrual-associated TSS has declined from 1 to 16 cases per 100,000 people in 1980 to the current rate of 1 to 3 cases per 100,000 women (Reingold, 1991). This decrease in the rate of TSS may be the result of intense media warnings about safe use of tampons.

Reasons for increased susceptibility to TSS during menstruation or after birth are unclear. *S. aureus* is more often isolated from the vagina during these times, suggesting some changes in the normal flora related to the increased presence of menstrual fluid or lochia. Unused tampons have not been shown to carry pathogens, but research on the composition of tampons suggests a connection with the production of TSST-1.

Tampons, especially superabsorbent ones, contain significant amounts of menstrual flow and provide a medium for the growth of *S. aureus,* thus supporting toxin production. Tampons may also transport organisms from the external genitals or unwashed hands. Additionally, consistent tampon use may cause local irritation or trauma, creating a portal of entry for organisms.

Signs

The characteristic symptoms of TSS reflect multiple system involvement. Onset may be sudden, with flulike symptoms present, such as high fever, chills, sore throat, headache, muscle pain (myalgia), vomiting, diarrhea, and hypotension. Within 1 to 2 days a characteristic macular sunburnlike rash appears. Mucous membranes of the vagina and oropharynx may appear beefy red; ulcerations of mucous membranes may develop later. Generalized desquamation or sloughing and peeling of the skin, including skin on the end of fingers and toes and on palms and soles, occur 1 to 2 weeks after onset of TSS (see Box 4-1).

TSS leads to vasodilation from toxins and increased capillary permeability, resulting in the loss of significant amounts of fluid from the central circulation. This leads to hypotension and decreased tissue perfusion. All major organs can be affected, with cardiac, renal, pulmonary, and nervous system manifestations of this septic shock. When death occurs, it is from cardiac arrhythmias, res-

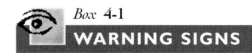

Box 4-1
WARNING SIGNS

Toxic Shock Syndrome

The Centers for Disease Control considers toxic shock syndrome to be present when desquamation of the skin occurs in conjunction with five additional symptoms:
- Sudden fever higher than 101° F
- Diarrhea
- Vomiting
- Muscle aching (myalgia)
- Rash similar to sunburn

piratory failure, and disseminated intravascular coagulation. Survivors may suffer prolonged sequelae, including renal failure, gangrene of fingers and toes, peripheral neuropathies, memory impairment, and the inability to concentrate.

Clinical management

Because no specific diagnostic tests exist to identify TSS, the diagnosis is based on the recognition of clinical signs associated with the syndrome. Treatment depends on early recognition and requires integrated care for and support of cardiac, respiratory, renal, hepatic, metabolic, and central nervous system functions. For this reason the woman is usually placed in an intensive care setting. Vigorous and persistent fluid resuscitation is uniformly required, with monitoring of blood pressure, renal function, and central venous pressure. After cultures are obtained, aggressive antibiotic therapy is begun to decrease both the severity of the infection and the chance of recurrence.

Nursing responsibilities

The nurse plays a significant role in the prevention and detection of TSS. Ongoing teaching is essential, and the nurse must anticipate the learning needs of the individual woman involved. Women should be advised of basic hygiene practices such as washing hands before and after tampon insertion. Labia should be held open with one hand while the tampon is inserted with the other hand. Tampons should be changed frequently (every 1 to 4 hrs) or according to the manufacturer's guidelines, and a woman should use the least absorbent tampon that will meet her needs. It is also suggested that tampons should not be used overnight or in the first 8 weeks after childbirth (Creehan, 1995).

Vaginal contraceptive devices should also not be worn for a prolonged period of time and should not be used to control menstrual flow. Tampons and vaginal contraceptives should be avoided if possible when infections (e.g., boils) occur on other parts of the body (see Chapter 5).

Women should be advised that if they "lose" tampons or contraceptive devices, they should see a health care provider immediately.

VAGINAL INFECTIONS

Vulvovaginitis

Women commonly seek treatment for inflammation and infections of the vulva and vagina when the discharge, pain, or pruritis generally associated with these conditions interferes with comfort, self-esteem, or usual activities.

Bacterial Vaginosis

Bacterial vaginosis (BV) is caused by *Gardnerella vaginalis,* formerly called *Haemophilus vaginalis* or nonspecific vaginitis, and is associated with a change in normal vaginal flora. Predisposing factors appear to be sexual intercourse (especially with multiple partners), the use of an intrauterine device (IUD), vaginal tissue damage, and the presence of a sexually transmitted disease.

Signs

A woman may often be asymptomatic, thus delaying diagnosis and treatment. However, many women (up to 50%) do experience characteristic symptoms: copious amounts of thin, watery or milky grayish white to yellow secretions that have a distinctive "fishy" odor. Odor may be more noticeable after intercourse, when semen and vaginal secretions alter pH and release chemicals that produce the odor. Vaginal pH will be lower than 4.5, and microscopic examination of vaginal mucus shows presence of "clue" cells—epithelial cells covered with bacteria.

Clinical management

The most common treatment for the *nonpregnant* woman is metronidazole, 500 mg orally bid for 7 days. Alternate therapy is a single oral dose of metronidazole, 2 g, or metronidazole gel, 0.7% administered intravaginally bid for 5 days. More severe side effects of nausea, heartburn, and a metallic taste may be present with the single dosage regimen. Those taking metronidazole should be taught to avoid alcohol consumption during treatment and for 48 hours after treatment because of the drug's Antabuselike effects, causing facial flushing, headache, abdominal cramps, nausea and vomiting, fever, tachycardia, palpitations, hypotension, and the feeling of chest constriction (Wilson, 1996).

To avoid the potential teratogenic effects of metronidazole, the pregnant woman may take ampicillin, 500 mg every 6 hours for 7 days. Alternate treatment may include clindamycin, 300 mg po, bid for 7 days, and clindamycin cream, 2% intravaginally at bedtime for 7 days.

Local treatment with povidone iodine suppositories or chlorhexidine is also effective when applied directly on the affected area and does not produce unpleasant side effects.

Treatment of sexual partners is not indicated, unless there are recurrent or persistent infections, but the couple should use a condom until treatment is complete and symptoms are no longer present.

Vaginal Candidiasis (Moniliasis)

Candidiasis is the second most common vaginal infection, with about 75% of all women reporting an infection at least once during their reproductive years. Like bacterial vaginosis, infections with *Candida albicans* are related to changes in the balance of vaginal flora. Other factors include recent antibiotic therapy, diabetes mellitus, or excessive intake of carbohydrates or dairy products. Hormonal changes such as those associated with pregnancy or the use of oral contraceptives seem to have an effect. In addition, using feminine hygiene products or wearing tight-fitting pants and noncotton underwear may alter the vaginal environment enough to allow Candida to thrive. The newborn may be infected during birth. (See Table 4-1 for more information and Chapter 19 for treatment of the newborn.)

Signs

The most common symptoms of vaginal candidiasis are mild to severe vulvovaginal pruritis, burning, soreness, dyspareunia, and external dysuria. The thick vaginal discharge is white and "cheesy" in texture and often appears as white, curdlike plaques adherent to vaginal walls and the cervix. Physical and speculum examinations frequently reveal reddened vulval and vaginal tissue. Marked leukocytosis on the slide may indicate the presence of a second infection, such as trichomoniasis.

Clinical management

Recommended treatments for acute vaginal candidiasis include a number of "-azole" vaginal creams, ointments, suppositories, and tablets. Commonly used medications are butoconazole nitrate cream, clotrimazole cream or tablets, miconazole cream or suppositories and terconazole cream or suppositories. For mild to moderate cases, single dosage regimens may be recommended, such as tioconazole 6.5% ointment, 5 g intravaginally, or 1 clotrimazole 500 mg, vaginal tablet. Oral agents have not as yet been approved by the FDA for use in acute vaginal candidiasis, but they may be used to treat recurrent infections. Ketoconazole, 200 mg twice a day for 5 to 14 days, fluconazole, 100 to 150 mg in a single dose, or itraconazole, 200 mg daily for 3 days may be ordered. The woman may also be treated prophylactically with oral ketoconazole, 100 mg daily for 6 months, oral fluconazole, 150 mg once a month, clotrimazole, 500 mg tablet each month, or terconazole, one application at bedtime for 7 days. It is

Table 4-1   Commonalities of Sexually Transmitted Diseases

Risk Factors	Symptoms	Diagnosis	Patient Teaching	Fetal/Newborn Effects
Unprotected sexual contact or use of oral contraceptives, IUD, or diaphragm	Discharge from urethra or vagina	Culture prepared: oropharyngeal cervical vaginal rectal urethral	Genital hygiene Principles of asepsis	Intrauterine death Congenital anomalies Newborn infection
Multiple sexual partners	Dysuria	Serologic testing	Safer sex	Conjunctivitis
Smoking or drug or alcohol use	Dyspareunia	Visualization	Treatment of partner(s)	Oral infection
Age 16-24	Discomfort, such as pain or pruritis		Use of medications	Respiratory tract infection
High stress levels	Many STDs asymptomatic		Follow-up care	
	Symptoms more common in women		No conferred immunity	

Courtesy Carol A. Mottola, PhD, RN.

important to watch for adverse reactions to these medications; hepatotoxicity is a major side effect of ketoconazole, and fluconazole and itraconazole may cause nausea and diarrhea.

Other treatment options may include the use of intravaginal boric acid suppositories. Women with recurrent candidal infections may find oral ingestion of yogurt with live lactobacillus or even douching with plain yogurt to be helpful. The woman's treatment of this infection should be monitored in a clinic.

Male sexual partners are not routinely treated, unless recurrence is frequent. If both partners are using miconazole cream, sexual intercourse may actually help spread the medication into the vagina; otherwise, abstinence or intercourse with a condom is encouraged.

Trichomonas Vaginalis

Trichomonas vaginalis is a sexually transmitted disease responsible for approximately 25% of symptomatic vaginal infections. It is estimated that 2.5 to 3.0 million women contract trichomonal infections annually in the United States. In addition to the female vagina, *T. vaginalis* inhabits the urethra of both men and women. The infection has an incubation period of 4 to 28 days. Hot tubs and whirlpool baths have been suggested as means of transmission for the infection, but this is unproven. The likelihood of acquiring trichomonal infections is greater for those with multiple sexual partners.

Signs

Approximately 50% of women with trichomoniasis may be symptom free. Symptoms when present include discharge that is gray to yellow-green (occasionally malodorous), vaginal pruritus, dyspareunia, and dysuria. Examination reveals labia that may be pallid or erythematous. Discharge may be present on the vulva, and speculum examination frequently reveals excessive discharge and a "strawberry-like" friable cervix. Vaginal walls may be erythematous. Gonorrhea cultures should be obtained for women with trichomoniasis because as many as 50% of affected women may have concomitant infection with *Neisseria gonorrhoeae*.

Clinical management

Treatment is recommended both for symptom-free persons and those with symptomatic trichomonal infection. Treatments of choice are a single dose of oral metronidazole, 2 g, or metronidazole, 500 mg twice a day for 7 days. Clotrimazole antifungal cream provides symptomatic relief and has produced cure among some women, but often creams are not curative. Teaching must also include the Antabuse effect that occurs when alcohol is taken with metronidazole.

Since metronidazole is contraindicated during early pregnancy because of the potential for teratogenic effects on the fetus, first trimester symptomatic relief may be achieved by using a *gentle*, dilute vinegar douche: place 2 tablespoons of vinegar in 1 L of water or a saline douche and use daily for 1 week, then twice weekly until the first trimester is over.

Referral of the woman's sexual partner(s) for evaluation and treatment is recommended to prevent reinfection. A woman should be advised to abstain from intercourse or to use condoms until she and her sexual partner(s) complete therapy and cure is documented.

Nursing responsibilities

With any vulval or vaginal irritation, planning focuses on relief of symptoms and prevention of recurrence, and women should be encouraged to do the following:

- To relieve some discomfort, maintain hygiene by frequent gentle cleansing of the vulva, wiping from front to back after elimination, and avoid chemical sprays or powders.
- Carefully follow proper application instructions and dosage regimens if analgesic creams or ointments are used.
- Avoid tight clothing, and use underwear and pantyhose with at least cotton crotches to allow better air flow to the genital area and to prevent increased temperature.
- Use latex condoms for "safe sex" to prevent the spread of infection or exposure to other infections.

If vaginitis is recurrent or frequent, the woman should receive follow-up attention from a nurse practitioner or medical practitioner to rule out underlying causes, such as diabetes or a secondary STD.

Other Sexually Transmitted Diseases

Women must be assessed for other STDs. The incidence of syphilis, once considered under control, is now on the rise, as is the incidence of gonorrhea. Chlamydia is the most frequently reported female STD today. Human papillomavirus (HPV), which causes genital warts, affects not only the woman's total health but predisposes her to other infections and increases her risk for cervical cancer. If the woman becomes pregnant, most STDs can be transmitted to the infant in utero or at birth (see Chapter 25 for full discussion).

Pelvic inflammatory disease

A consequence of an STD, **pelvic inflammatory disease (PID)** or salpingitis (inflammation of the fallopian tubes) may be asymptomatic or present with sharp or chronic lower pelvic pain, chills, malaise, gastrointestinal disturbances, a purulent discharge, or irregular bleeding.

Risk factors for PID include nulliparity, multiple sexual partners, repeated STDs, and IUD use. Definitive diagnosis is made by laparoscopy.

Acute PID may require hospitalization, treatment with intravenous (IV) antibiotics, and removal of an IUD, if present. Surgery may be needed to repair damaged tubes or remove scar tissue (see Chapter 6 for more discussion of PID).

Human immunodeficiency virus and hepatitis B

Today two viruses threaten women as potentially lethal infections. Hepatitis B (HBV) and human immunodeficiency virus (HIV), the virus responsible for acquired immunodeficiency syndrome (AIDS), can be acquired through sexual relations with an infected partner, and the rate of both is increasing in the female population. In 1991, 11% of new hepatitis B cases and about 10% of reported HIV infections occurred in women (Horton, 1992).

The health threat that AIDS poses to women is increasing in severity. Women are contracting the disease from sex partners infected through drug use, previous sexual activity, or exposure to contaminated blood. Education is essential for control and treatment of HIV in women. Women who have been exposed to the HIV infection should be taught to recognize early gender-specific indicators:

- Chronic candidal (yeast) infections, especially if they are not relieved by local antifungal treatments
- Recurrent episodes of PID or genital warts
- Menstrual irregularities or amenorrhea

The full effect of HIV on the families of the affected women and on society in general is yet to be seen, but as the number of persons with HIV increases, so must services, teaching, and support systems.

PSYCHOSOCIAL CONCERNS

Women are at risk for more than reproductive problems. They experience a higher proportion of emotional problems than men do, particularly with eating disorders, substance abuse, and depression. Alcohol and drug use has risen; smoking, however, is reported to be on the decrease (American Cancer Society, 1996).

Potential for Abuse

Women are at risk for becoming victims of physical and sexual abuse. Traditional and cultural views of the woman, particularly the view of wife as property, devalue a woman and render her powerless. Though traditions are changing, domestic violence and instances of rape appear to be more frequent, although this trend may be because more cases than before are now being reported. It has been estimated that 21% to 30% of women have been beaten by a partner at least once and that 1 in 600 women are rape victims (Horton, 1992). (See Chapter 27 for a discussion of abuse during pregnancy).

Symptoms of abuse are often hidden by the woman or overlooked by caregivers. Physical examination must include careful attention to warning signs of repeated unexplained injuries, frequent emergency department visits, and bruises or scars. Studies show that practitioners do not screen routinely for abuse; further, if they do find evidence, they may not report it or make referrals. They may fear invading privacy or feel inadequate or frustrated when they cannot "cure" the situation (Parsons et al, 1995). Building a relationship of trust, respect, and confidentiality with the woman may encourage her to admit to the trauma. Collaboration with counselors trained in helping rape or abuse victims may also aid these victimized women.

Age does not protect a woman from abuse, and an increasing number of older women are being treated and counseled as victims of abuse from spouse and children. Fear, guilt, and shame often prevent them from reporting their situations, and the health practitioner must be sensitive to all physical signs and verbal and nonverbal clues.

PHYSICAL CONCERNS

Chronic Diseases

Many women live with chronic physical conditions. Hypertension, hypercholesterolemia, hyperlipidemia, and diabetes mellitus are common, and the rate of autoimmune disorders such as lupus erythematosus and rheumatoid arthritis is significant (see Chapters 22, 23, and 24). Menopausal women are also at risk for osteoporosis and coronary artery disease.

ALTERED MENSTRUAL PATTERNS

For most women, the menses occurs on a 28- to 30-day schedule and lasts 3 to 7 days. For some women, more debilitating symptoms may need treatment. Primary **dysmenorrhea** begins about a year after menarche and can include nausea, vomiting, diarrhea, headache, pelvic abdominal pain, lower back pain, and an increased menstrual flow. Prostaglandins are implicated in dysmenorrhea; the levels rise threefold in the time from the follicular phase to the luteal phase of the cycle (Speroff, 1994). Secondary dysmenorrhea occurs after normal cycles have been established for some time and may usually be related to pelvic pathology, especially to endometriosis. Secondary dysmenorrhea may be related to the use of an IUD, to PID, to uterine fibroids, or to endometrial polyps.

There may be severe cramping on the first day of the cycle or for several days after. Pain may be relieved by nonpharmocologic methods: rest, local heat, massage of abdomen or back, exercise as tolerated, and relaxation techniques. Some women require medication to alleviate pain. Current therapy includes antiprostaglandins such as ibuprofen (Motrin), naproxen (Naprosyn, Anaprox), and ketoprofen. Some studies suggest beginning the dosages 2 to 3 days before menstruation. Women accustomed to taking antiprostaglandins should be cautioned that these nonsteroidal antiinflammatory drugs (NSAIDs) are not recommended during pregnancy or lactation. In addition, some women use transcutaneous electrical nerve stimulation (TENS) (see Chapter 16), or hormones such as birth control pills may be used to interrupt menses for a time in certain women.

Amenorrhea

Amenorrhea is primary if menarche has never occurred. Small or poorly nourished girls and athletes may have a delay in reaching the level of adequate body fat needed to trigger menstruation. Family history may indicate a potential for problems. In general, primary amenorrhea is not considered a problem until age 16.

Secondary Amenorrhea

Secondary amenorrhea occurs as a woman approaches menopause. Anatomic conditions may cause secondary amenorrhea if the outflow tract is affected or if there are problems with the ovary, endometrium, or anterior pituitary or hypothalamus glands. Anorexia and strenuous exercise can also cause cessation of menses or irregular pauses. Body fat must be maintained at 22% of total body weight to maintain menstruation, or hypothalamic function will be depressed (Hernandez and Atkinson, 1996). Athletes often have amenorrhea after intense training.

Dysfunctional Uterine Bleeding

Dysfunctional uterine bleeding refers to abnormal uterine bleeding when the pelvic examination is otherwise within normal limits. Common causes are estrogen withdrawal, estrogen breakthrough during the cycle, and progestin breakthrough. Terms used to define specific problems include the following:

- *Oligomenorrhea*—intervals greater than 35 days
- *Polymenorrhea*—intervals less than 21 days
- *Menorrhagia*—regular intervals but excessive flow and duration
- *Metrorrhagia*—irregular intervals and excessive flow and duration

The goal of treatment is to replace the hormone that is missing. Medroxyprogesterone acetate (MPA) may be given to treat both oligomenorrhea and metrorrhagia by changing the endometrium and then allowing it to slough off when the medication is stopped, like a "medical curettage" (Speroff, 1996). Oral contraceptives may be helpful, or progestin may be given via an IUD to deliver it directly to the endometrium if the bleeding is chronic and not helped with other treatments. Gonadotropin-releasing hormone (Gn-RH) agonists may also be used to thwart coagulation defects. Last resorts are surgical endometrial ablation or hysterectomy in an older woman (Hernandez and Atkinson, 1996).

Premenstrual Syndrome

Premenstrual syndrome (PMS) describes a wide variety of symptoms as listed in Box 4-2. Symptoms are present only in the luteal phase of the cycle in the 5 to 11 days before menstruation. These changes must be noted in at least two consecutive cycles to be considered PMS. The precise cause of PMS is not known, but theories suggest hormone imbalance with changes in endorphin levels, abnormal

> ▌ *Box* **4-2**   **Common Changes (Symptoms) Experienced with Premenstrual Syndrome***
>
> **PHYSICAL**
>
> Water retention   Change in eating patterns
> Weight gain   Fatigue
> Muscle and joint   Changes in sleep patterns
>   discomfort
> Breast tenderness
>
> **EMOTIONAL**
>
> Radical mood and
>   temperament swings
> Heightened irritability
>   and anger
> Depression
> Loss of interest in usual
>   activities
>
> **COGNITIVE**
>
> Decreased ability to
>   concentrate
>
> *These changes are noted in the late luteal phase of the menstrual cycle and usually resolve with the onset of menses.

prostaglandin metabolism, thyroid function, and aldosterone secretion as possibilities (Speroff, 1996). Other reports cite lower levels of magnesium, zinc, and vitamins B_6, E, and A (Hsia and Ling, 1990). External stresses may also play a part in the woman's perception of PMS and its severity.

Risk

It is estimated that at least 40% of women in the United States experience PMS routinely; about two thirds of these are incapacitated for a period of time by the symptoms. Epidemiology elsewhere is difficult to calculate; cultural norms influence a woman's awareness or willingness to speak of such difficulties.

Clinical management

Nonpharmacologic approaches are successful in treating some PMS symptoms. Avoidance of caffeine, salt, fat, sugar, and refined and processed foods is suggested, as is increased exercise that may raise endorphin levels. Recommended foods include nuts, seeds, whole grains, legumes, vegetables and fruits, and vegetable oils. Holistic practitioners often prescribe vitamins, such as B_6, E, and A, and minerals, such as zinc, magnesium, and calcium. Herbs such as *dong quai*, the "woman's ginseng" (Stein, 1995) and evening primrose oil may also be beneficial, though care must be taken to avoid overdosing with these substances.

Certain medications may also be helpful in alleviating discomfort: spironolactone for bloating; mefenamic acid in the luteal phase; aspirin and acetaminophen, danazol, naltrexone, bromocriptine, clonidine, or D-fenfluramine for pain. Gn-RH agonists that inhibit ovarian activity or progestins such as MPA may decrease uterine irritability (Chuong, 1995).

CLIMACTERIC

The reproductive capabilities of a man and a woman vary as both age. A man does not experience as dramatic a reduction in hormonal production as does a woman; thus a man's reproductive function changes more gradually. In the man, psychologic changes produce a sense of the loss of youth and vigor and perhaps a realization that life goals may not have been met. Some subtle physical changes take place in the man such as the gradual diminution of the testosterone level, which causes loss of skin elasticity and loss of muscle mass, but unless the man experiences a pathologic change in his reproductive anatomy, sperm production and fertility do not decrease.

For the woman, however, a definite and dramatic change in reproductive functioning occurs. She experiences a period of transition known as the **climacteric**, during which gonadal activity slows and ultimately ceases completely, resulting in physical and psychologic changes.

The climacteric is divided into phases:

1. *Premenopausal*—reproductive years before menopause
2. *Menopausal*—first 12 months after permanent cessation of menses
3. *Postmenopausal*—period beginning 1 year after last menses and referring to the rest of woman's life
4. *Perimenopause*—period lasting from the onset of signs of approaching menopause to approximately 1 year after last menses

Although menstruation may not cease until around the age of 50, it may begin earlier in women who smoke or have received chemotherapy, who are thinner, or who live at high altitudes. Premenopause may start as early as 36 to 42 years of age, with alteration in hormonal production. As the number of healthy ovarian follicles declines and sensitivity to gonadotropins decreases, estrogen levels fluctuate, with resultant changes in the menstrual cycle. Irregularities in menstruation and differences in character and duration of menstrual flow are often noted.

Physiologic Components

Menopause is defined by the occurrence of the last menses. At this point ovulatory function ceases. In response to the drop of estrogen levels, changes in estrogen-dependent tissues occur and menopausal symptoms appear.

Hot flushes and flashes

Low estrogen levels affect stability between the hypothalamus and the autonomic nervous system and contribute to triggering the classic hot flushes or flashes experienced by 85% of menopausal women. Flushes also coincide with surges of luteinizing hormone (LH). The characteristic sign of flush is visible reddening of the skin on the face, neck, and chest; the characteristic sign of flash is a feeling of intense heat. Diaphoresis may occur. These flush and flash episodes take place most frequently at night and in times of stress, and surprisingly hyperthermia does not occur. In fact, core body temperature *drops* during these flashes.

Genitourinary changes. In response to decreased estrogen levels, the tissues of the vagina, vulva, urethra, and bladder begin to atrophy. The vagina becomes thin and flattened. Secretions decrease and so does lubrication in response to sexual stimulation. The urethra shifts closer to the vaginal introitus, increasing the risk of infection and discomfort. **Dyspareunia** (pain during vaginal intercourse) may decrease the woman's interest in coitus.

Because the sphincter has less tone, stress incontinence resulting from coughing or sneezing may cause leakage of urine. An increase in the frequency of urinary tract infections is also related to decreased estrogen levels.

Osteoporosis. Much attention has been paid recently to **osteoporosis** as a sequela of menopause. Bone mass peaks at about 30 years of age and is sustained by adequate calcium intake, regular exercise, and circulating estrogen levels. Loss of ovarian function at menopause increases bone resorption dramatically for 3 to 4 years (Baran, 1994; Lindsay, 1996). Bone mass loss is related to the effect of low estrogen on calcitonin levels, allowing calcium loss from the bone and resulting in increased bone fragility and postural changes from curvature of the spine.

Cardiovascular changes. Lower levels of estrogen affect the cardiovascular system. During the premenopausal period, estrogen may lower low-density lipoprotein (LDL) serum levels and raise high-density lipoprotein (HDL) serum levels, decrease plaque formation, and possibly improve coronary blood flow by dilating coronary vessels (Moore and Dunham-Noonan, 1996). With lower estrogen levels, these protective mechanisms are withdrawn, increasing the risk of myocardial infarction (MI) and cerebrovascular accidents.

General symptoms of menopause commonly include those less well-defined causes, such as fatigue, joint pain, dizziness, and palpitations.

Neurologic and emotional changes. The inability to concentrate and the loss of memory are frequent occurrences in perimenopausal women. This happens because estrogen affects the availability of neurotransmitters such as tryptophan and serotonin and because estrogen receptors are found in the hippocampus (the learning center of the brain) (Sherwin, 1996; Pearlstein, 1995). Emotional symptoms such as insomnia, nervousness, irritability, depression, and abrupt mood swings are equally as common and frequently more disturbing than the physical symptoms. Often in the past, only somatic discomforts were treated, and women were advised either to simply accept the emotional symptoms or to seek psychiatric help to deal with them. Today's emphasis on more holistic care makes it easier for women to adjust to menopause and postmenopause.

Surgical menopause. Surgery to remove all or part of the reproductive organs may be indicated by an otherwise untreatable condition such as cancer. In these cases the woman has to deal not only with the implications of a serious medical condition and the stress of undergoing surgical procedures, but she must also adjust to the physical and psychologic effects of oophorectomy (removal of the ovaries) or hysterectomy (removal of the uterus). The menopausal symptoms caused by sudden cessation of ovarian function may be severe, especially the hot flushes and flashes. Change in body image of self-esteem resulting from the loss of reproductive ability may be worsened by the neurologic and emotional results of decreased estrogen. Therefore in addition to teaching hormonal therapy, the nurse must include in the plan of care actions designed to meet the woman's total needs.

Care During the Climacteric

If the average age for menopause is 52 years, women today will live approximately one third of their lives as postmenopausal persons. Many women have no difficulties adjusting to this new phase, whereas others need help to deal with problems related to hormonal changes. Nurses can help women accept menopause as a natural and nonpathologic process and realize that measures are available to ease the transition.

Nonpharmacologic interventions

Common unpleasant but non-critical menopausal adaptations may be treated or prevented simply, without the need for medical interventions.

Interventions for hot flushes and flashes. Wearing layered, porous clothing, avoiding hot areas, and drinking cool liquids help lessen flash sensations. Relaxation techniques, especially slow, rhythmic breathing and avoidance of stress, have been shown to increase vasomotor control, alleviating the embarrassment and discomfort that this sensation usually involves. Pharmacologic interventions may include belladonna or ergotamine tartrate (Hammond, 1996).

Interventions for genitourinary changes. Kegel exercises help decrease stress incontinence (see Chapter 9). Lubrication with water-soluble jelly or oils and application of estrogen creams can compensate for vaginal dryness and tightness, making intercourse easier.

Interventions to improve general health. Eliminating smoking is a healthy response to menopause. Adherence to a diet low in refined sugars, alcohol, caffeine, and sodium helps control body weight. These actions, along with an exercise and relaxation regimen and stress reduction in general, promote total wellness and relieve individual symptoms.

Interventions for emotional lability. Emotional and psychologic symptoms can be affected by diet and exercise. Physical activity increases dopamine and circulating endorphin levels. Individual or group support and counseling are of major help to the menopausal woman, offering her the opportunity to share her experiences with a professional and with other women. Often the ability to talk freely to an interested person or persons who can validate perceptions and offer practical advice may determine how easily a woman manages to cope during this time.

Alternative therapies. The perimenopausal woman may also be offered information on alternative therapies prescribed by holistic health practitioners, such as the use of vitamins, minerals, herbs, aromatherapy, acupressure and acupuncture, or gemstones and gem essences (Stein, 1995; Ito, 1994).

Prevention of coronary artery disease. Decreased estrogen levels contribute to the major health problems of coronary artery disease, the leading cause of death in women. Diet modifications significantly reduce the risk of developing this disease. Cholesterol and triglyceride levels can be lowered by limiting daily fat intake to 30% of the total calories, with no more than 10% of fat intake from saturated fats. The diet is then balanced by obtaining 20% of the total daily calories from protein and by obtaining 50% to 60% from complex carbohydrates, especially those high in fiber.

Elimination of other risk factors such as smoking can make a critical difference in the severity of cardiovascular changes.

Prevention of osteoporosis. The postmenopausal decrease in estrogen levels can cause osteoporosis, which predisposes the woman to fractures and their disabling sequelae. Exercises that put stress on the bones, such as brisk walking, jogging, and weight lifting can slow bone resorption and increase bone mass, but these exercises are most effective when done consistently in the premenopausal years. As estrogen levels drop, calcium, fluoride, and vitamin supplements (especially vitamin A) may slow bone loss. A daily calcium intake of 800 to 1500 mg is recommended, taken with vitamin D to aid in absorption. Newer therapies include calcitonin (usually synthesized in the thyroid), which decreases bone turnover and resorption. Since it affects only the skeleton, calcitonin has few side effects but does have the drawback of being given by a subcutaneous route daily. An intranasal form of calcitonin is being developed to make it easier to use. Biphosphonates such as Didronel have proven helpful by slowing bone metabolism but are awaiting approval by the FDA. These drugs should be taken in the morning with breakfast but for optimum absorption, not with caffeine or calcium (Baran, 1994; Lindsay, 1996).

These preventive measures can spare the woman not only from the general discomforts related to osteoporosis—lessening of height, kyphosis, and backache—but also from serious complications—fractures related to increased bone fragility and poor healing potential and respiratory compromise stemming from thoracic anatomic changes.

TEST *Yourself* 4-1 _____

List two signs in each of the following phases of the climacteric and also list the nonpharmacologic interventions for each sign.
a. Premenopause
b. Menopause
c. Postmenopause
d. Perimenopause

Hormone replacement therapy

Although women can "learn to live" with some results of menopause, the trend is to prescribe **hormone replacement therapy** (HRT). Some women are more at risk for serious cardiovascular problems and osteoporosis because of heredity, physical status, or lifestyle. Other women find that alternate therapies are unsuccessful. For both sets of women, HRT will usually be prescribed (Lichtman, 1996).

Much is written about both the benefits and risks of taking estrogen or estrogen with progesterone to simulate premenopausal levels. Estrogen has been proven to dramatically reduce the incidence of cardiovascular crises such as MI in postmenopausal women (Philosophe and Seibel, 1991). It has been estimated that the number of women that suffer an MI is halved when estrogen replacement is given. By affecting liver metabolism, estrogen maintains the level of HDL and prevents hypercholesterolemia, a known component of coronary heart disease. Estrogen also acts as a vasodilator and affects platelet aggregation.

Concern exists about the possible connection between estrogen and breast and endometrial cancers, raising the question of whether **estrogen replacement therapy** (ERT) increases a woman's risk for malignancy. Many breast tumors are estrogen-receptor positive, meaning that they require and thrive on estrogen. Women with a strong family history of breast cancer or those who have had cancer themselves generally are not considered candidates for ERT, although this is no longer viewed as an inviolable rule. Some researchers question whether ERT does in fact increase the risk of breast cancer, citing studies that the estrogen levels of pregnancy do not increase mortality rates if all other variables are equal, and that pregnancy after breast cancer seems not to have a negative effect on prognosis (Archer, 1991). It has also been stated that routine low doses taken to prevent osteoporosis and cardiovascular disease have not been clearly proven to increase the risk of breast cancer (Speroff, 1994). Questioning risks and benefits may help the woman decide whether to use ERT.

In addition to its effects on circulation and bones, ERT treats vaginal atrophic changes, loss of bladder control, vasomotor instability, insomnia, decreased libido, mood swings, depression, and memory loss related to menopause. Its benefits cannot be disputed, although its risks must be considered.

Because estrogen is conjugated in the liver, ERT should be withheld if the woman has an active liver disease or chronic impaired liver function. Acute thrombophlebitis, a history of gallbladder disease in pregnancy, or a current pregnancy all are contraindications to ERT.

Estrogen and cancer. Estrogen is implicated in endometrial cancer because of its hyperproliferative effect on the tissue lining, causing cellular dysplasia that can become cancerous. Women who have had unexplained vaginal bleeding should consider having an endometrial biopsy before deciding on ERT.

The risk of endometrial cancer can be decreased by adding progesterone to the HRT regimen. Progesterone has a protective effect related to decreasing estrogen-receptor activity and breaking down estradiol. Unfortunately, progesterone does not have as positive an effect on the cardiovascular system and actually can lower HDL levels. Giving natural nonandrogenic progesterone and limiting the dose seem to alleviate this problem.

The dose amount and duration of treatment appear to be factors in the connection between HRT and cancer. It is generally accepted that the smallest dose should be given for the briefest length of time. HRT may be given as short-term therapy to alleviate symptoms during menopause, tapering off after cessation of menses, or it may be given as a long-term prophylactic measure. To achieve the desired effect on the cardiovascular, genitourinary, and skeletal systems, it may be necessary to take HRT for life. This may pose a significant problem since some studies suggest that although there is no significant increase in breast cancer when HRT is used for up to 5 years, there may be a 30% increase in the cancer rate when HRT is continued for more than 15 years (Sitruk-Ware and Utian, 1991).

Choices of treatment. Replacement regimens should be individualized and based on the woman's needs and tolerance. Doses should be adjusted to obtain the most favorable effects from the smallest amount of medication. Other risk factors may actually play a larger role in cancer formation than do the hormones. Obesity, for example, is strongly linked to both breast and endometrial cancers because estrogen is metabolized in fat cells, and levels of estrogen will be higher as fat cell mass rises. Controlling these factors may allow the hormones to be used with less risk.

Natural estrogens are used most often and are less potent than synthetic preparations. Estrogens can be taken orally, parenterally, transdermally, by subcutaneous implant, or in the form of a gel, cream, suppository, or vaginal ring. The oral route affects liver metabolism, aiding in maintenance of the HDL level but possibly overloading the liver and causing gastrointestinal upset. Vaginal rings, which deliver medication more directly but may be irritating and cause inflammation and infection, are not as commonly used.

The easiest and most constant route is the *transdermal patch*, which is changed only twice a week and allows slow absorption, keeping levels constant. The Estraderm patch (estradiol) can irritate the skin but is usually well tolerated.

Dosage routines. Oral estrogen may be taken according to either a sequential or continuous regimen. In the sequential regimen, 0.65 mg of conjugated estrogen or 1.0 mg of micronized estradiol is taken either daily or from the first to the twenty-fifth day of the month. Progesterone is added as MPA, 10 mg daily for the first 14 days of the month or the last 10 days of estrogen administration. Progesterone is available in natural or synthetic form, and the nonandrogenic type is usually chosen to eliminate the hormone's effect on HDL levels. MPA (Provera) is commonly used, and oral dosages vary according to form and route. For women experiencing surgically induced menopause, unopposed estrogen therapy is given only if the uterus has been removed. If there is an intact uterus, progesterone should be added.

The continuous regimen involves taking both estrogen and progesterone daily, with the progesterone decreased to MPA 2.5 mg (Speroff, 1994).

If HRT is sequential, withdrawal bleeding occurs in the week that nothing is taken; if it is continuous, breakthrough menses can occur on an irregular basis. Most women find this difficult once the menses have ceased.

The decision to use HRT ultimately rests with each woman. She should be helped in assessing her greatest risks and the options available to controlling them. Asymptomatic women may chose to avoid pharmacologic interventions because of fear of cancer, dislike of taking medication daily, or discomfort with resumed menstruation (Scalley and Heinrich, 1993; Johnson, Lilford, Mayers, 1995). Women who choose HRT should continue to be monitored carefully and should be screened meticulously according to guidelines.

CANCER IN WOMEN

According to the American Cancer Society (ACS), the mortality rate for women from cancer of all sites has risen 50% in 30 years, increasing from 128,553 deaths in 1962 to 245,740 in 1992. It is estimated that currently 262,440 women a year die from cancer.

Lung Cancer

Though the number of deaths from lung cancer has declined in men between 1962 and 1992, there has been a 438% increase in the number of deaths for women. It is estimated that as many as 158,700 deaths occurred from lung cancer in 1996. Since 1987, more women have died from lung cancer than from breast cancer, making it the leading cause of cancer death in women.

Risk

Smoking and exposure to secondary smoke are the major causes of lung cancer, with industrial and environmental pollutants, tuberculosis, and radiation also considered risk factors. In planning to teach about preventing lung cancer, the nurse should be aware of the following:
- Smoking has decreased in women over age 18 since 1974.
- Over 70% of adults started smoking daily before the age of 18.
- Of women with incomes below the poverty level, 28% are smokers.
- Each year, about 3000 nonsmoking adults die because of exposure to secondary cigarette smoke (ACS, 1995).

Although noncarcinogenic lung tissue may return to normal if smoking is stopped, some tumors may continue to grow for years *even after cessation of smoking*. Consequently the overall 5-year survival rate after treatment is only 13% regardless of the stage of diagnosis.

Signs

Persistent cough, blood-tinged sputum, chest pain, and recurring bronchitis or pneumonia may be presenting signs. Chest radiograph, bronchoscopy, and sputum cytologic examinations aid in the diagnosis of lung carcinoma, but early detection is difficult because symptoms are often evident only after the growth is well established, large enough for detection by radiograph. Depending on staging and tumor type, options include surgical removal, radiation, and chemotherapy.

Clinical Management

The type and stage of the cancer determine the course of treatment. Although surgery may remove localized tumors, chemotherapy and radiation therapy are often added because metastasis usually occurs by the time of diagnosis. Small cell carcinoma may be treated successfully with only radiation and chemotherapy.

Breast Cancer

Breast cancer continues to be a major threat to women, with the ACS estimating occurrence rates of 1 in every 9 women by age 85. It is estimated that in 1996, 184,300 new cases of invasive breast cancer were diagnosed, with 44,300 deaths occurring. For European-American and Hispanic women, cancer mortality has declined in the past 5 years, but for African-American women there is actually an increase. This disparity is attributed to the difference in awareness of both the need for and the availability of cancer screening and treatment.

Risk

Increased risk of breast cancer exists for women who are older than 40 years of age, have a personal or family history of the disease, have a history of benign breast disease, have never had children (nulliparity), or whose first pregnancy occurred after 30 years of age. Because current studies show an increased connection between estrogen and breast cancer, early menarche and late menopause are now being added as risk factors. High doses of ERT or prolonged treatment with ERT may increase the chances of breast cancer in women already at risk.

Other possible links with breast cancer are high intakes of both fat and caffeine and smoking. Obesity may also increase chances of breast cancer because estrogen metabolism occurs partly in fat cells. Studies are now being conducted on the possible connection between breast cancer and pesticides, chemical exposure, physical activity, alcohol consumption, and induced abortion, although no definitive links have been confirmed.

Screening

The simplest and probably most important screening method women can use is manual breast self-examination. Every woman should know how to examine her breasts and should practice breast self-examination monthly. A clinical physical examination by a professional is recommended every 3 years for 20- to 40-year-old women and every year for women over 40 (see Procedure 4-1).

Mammography is an important part of early detection. Although there is some controversy about its safety and efficacy, it still is endorsed by the ACS as a necessary part of screening. Guidelines include a baseline mammogram by age 40, repeated every 1 to 2 years between ages 40 and 49, and once a year for women older than 50. Suspicious lumps or areas on a mammogram should always be followed up with biopsy for definitive diagnosis.

For younger women and those with denser breast tissue, examination by ultrasound (sonogram), computerized axial tomography (CAT), positron emission tomography (PET), and magnetic resonance imaging (MRI) may prove more beneficial. Although universal agreement on the timing of specific procedures does not exist, it is known that consistency in screening affects success in diagnosis and treatment. Until mammography is readily available to all women regardless of their economic status, diagnosis will be denied to many in need and mortality will increase among the poor.

New research on breast cancer is promising. In 1994 two breast cancer genes were isolated, BRCA-1 and BRCA-2, which may allow better screening for women with high family cancer rates. In 1996 the FDA approved CA 15-3, a blood test that detects cancer antigens. This blood test is successful in detecting recurring tumors and is thought to be able to identify abnormal cell growth 5 months earlier than other detection methods. At present this test is considered more effective at ruling out primary cancers than diagnosing the occurrence of the cancer.

Early detection is the key to successful treatment of breast cancer. In an effort to project a prognosis, a system was developed on the basis of **cancer staging:** factors considered are primary tumor location and size (T), degree of nodal involvement (N), and presence of metastasis (M) (spread of cancer to other body sites). In general the lower the staging number, the better the prognosis. Treatment regimens are also based on the staging at diagnosis. (See Box 4-3 for an explanation of the various stages.)

Signs

The most common sign of breast cancer is a painless mass in the breast, although this may be absent in some women. Other significant changes include thickening, swelling, or dimpling of the skin of the breast, other skin irritations such as bumpiness or color change (orange skin), or a change in configuration of the breast. Changes in the nipple—inversion, erosion, or tenderness—or the presence of discharge may also indicate the presence of a tumor.

Clinical Management

Early detection and treatment by surgery, hormonal manipulation, chemotherapy, radiation therapy (radiotherapy), or a combination of these treatments can increase the survival rate to around 90%, depending on staging at diagnosis.

It is essential that each woman understands the available treatment options and is given adequate time to choose. Since the shock of learning that she has cancer often prevents the woman from absorbing facts and details initially, she may need to have repeated explanations and opportunities to seek the information necessary to make an informed decision.

Depending on the staging of the cancer, the woman's other risk factors, and her personal preference, surgery can remove only the tumor (lumpectomy) with a circle of tissue around it, or it can remove the entire breast (mastectomy). The "simple" mastectomy takes only breast tissue, leaving muscle and the chest wall intact. This procedure is usually accompanied by a regional node dissection to detect the presence of malignant cells in the lymph system. Studies have shown that long-term survival rates after lumpectomy with subsequent radiotherapy are as high as for those women who undergo mastectomy or mastectomy with radiotherapy (Henderson, 1995; Harris, 1991). A mastectomy and node dissection may be recommended if there has been any invasive spread of the tumor.

If a mastectomy is necessary, various techniques for reconstructive surgery can make it easier for the woman to retain a good body image and adjust to this major procedure. In addition, emotional support and practical assistance are available from self-help groups such as the ACS's "Reach to Recovery."

Hormonal manipulation. After the tumor is removed, it is tested for estrogen-receptor sensitivity. Tumors that are sensitive to estrogen receptors rely on the presence of estrogen for growth. This growth can be inhibited or prevented by binding the receptor sites and blocking estrogen uptake with a drug such as tamoxifen (Nolvadex). Researchers are investigating the prophylactic use of this method in women with high-risk profiles. Tamoxifen and other hormones such as progestins, estrogens, and androgens are generally considered more effective in post- rather than premenopausal women.

Chemotherapy. Aggressive systemic treatment with a variety of chemotherapeutic agents is employed with or without surgical intervention. Chemotherapeutic treatment has produced encouraging results, although many women find it difficult to cope with the side effects of this therapy. However, advances in the management of side effects such as severe nausea have eased treatment considerably. Autologous bone marrow transplantation is also suggested to treat the devastating bone marrow suppression that may be caused by the chemotherapy regimen.

Radiation therapy. Whether the tumor or the entire breast is removed, the tumor may be treated locally by a course of radiotherapy for 5 to 6 weeks. Preoperative radiation is often used to shrink larger tumors and to reduce the extent of surgery.

Most women are treated by multiple modalities, depending on staging, tumor type, estrogen assay, and general condition. Each treatment plan should be individualized and thoroughly explained so that the woman is able to make a well-informed decision.

▌ *Box* 4-3	**Staging for Breast Cancer**

Stage I	Tumor is 2 cm or less
Stage II	Tumor more than 2 cm, less than 5 cm
Stage III	Tumor more than 5 cm in greatest dimension
Stage IV	Tumor of any size with extension to chest/or skin

From American Cancer Society: *Cancer facts and figures*, New York, 1996, The Society.

Cervical Cancer

The rate of cervical cancer has decreased about 2% per year since 1988, but an estimated 15,700 new cases will occur annually resulting in 4900 deaths. Women at greater risk for cervical cancer are those whose first intercourse occurred before the age of 18, who have multiple or promiscuous partners, and who smoke. History of infection with herpes simplex virus type 2 or human papillomavirus (genital warts) may predispose cervical cells to cancerous changes. Cervical cancer is most prevalent in African-American women, whose mortality rate is twice that of white women, and among women in lower socioeconomic groups. This may be the case because some women lack access to health teaching and the financial means to obtain screening services. As with breast cancer, cervical cancer is described by staging (Box 4-4).

Signs

Signs of cervical cancer may include abnormal uterine bleeding or spotting and abnormal vaginal discharge. Pain and systemic symptoms are late manifestations. *Papanicolaou's stain test*, or the Pap smear, is considered the main test for early detection and thus is an important factor in the treatment of cervical cancer. The ACS recommends that the first Pap smear be performed when the woman becomes sexually active or by the time she is 18 and that it be repeated every year with a pelvic examination. After three or more consecutive negative smear results, testing may be performed every 1 to 3 years, depending on the woman's risk status. Some experts believe that the test should be repeated once after the initial smear, and if both results are negative, the woman should have routine Pap smears every 3 years until age 35 and then every 5 years until age 60 when no further testing is necessary.

Clinical management

Precancerous cervical changes may be treated with *cryosurgery* (destruction of cells by extreme cold) or by *electrocoagulation* (destruction of cells through intense heat or electrical charges). Local surgery may remove the tumor, or more extensive surgery may be needed in later stages. Radiotherapy is also used.

Nursing considerations

For the Pap smear to be as accurate as possible, the woman should be instructed to refrain from douching, from using any vaginal products, and from having intercourse for 24 hours before the test. The examiner must use only water as a lubricant and must follow accepted procedures for obtaining the cervical sample. Cells mistakenly taken from the vaginal walls or vault yield false negative results.

The woman should also be taught genital self-examination to detect changes on the labia and at the vaginal introitus. Changes in color of the vaginal tissue and the presence of lesions or discharge can then be assessed early and treated.

Endometrial Cancer

An estimated 34,000 new cases of endometrial cancer will be diagnosed annually, with 6000 deaths resulting. In general women at the highest risk for endometrial cancer are over 50, have a history of failure to ovulate, are infertile, have heavy or unusual periods, have problems with diabetes or obesity, and prolonged use of tamoxifen or ERT, especially without a progesterone component. Since estrogen exposure has a strong connection to this cancer, menopausal women with a family history of endometrial cancer or other compromising factors should have an endometrial biopsy before beginning ERT.

Other risk factors of endometrial cancer include the history of diabetes, gallbladder disease, hypertension, obesity, and pelvic radiation. Pregnancy seems to decrease the risk of endometrial cancer, as does oral contraceptive use, which actually halves the risk and provides protective effects that last up to 15 years after use is discontinued. If cervical cancer is detected early, survival rates at 5 years can be as high as 89%; for cancer of the endometrium the survival rate at 5 years is as high as 94%.

Signs

Abnormal uterine staining or bleeding outside the menstrual cycle, especially in postmenopausal women, may be an early sign of endometrial cancer. Pain and weight loss occur late in the disease. The Pap smear is only partially effective in detecting endometrial cancer. A pelvic examination by a health professional should be performed annually for women over 40, and an endometrial biopsy should be done at menopause for high-risk women.

Clinical management

Surgery and radiation are the usual therapies for uterine carcinoma. A hysterectomy is avoided as much as possible, especially in premenopausal women, but in later

---

Box 4-4   Staging for Cervical Cancer

Stage 0	In situ, intraepithelial carcinoma
Stage I	Carcinoma confined to cervix
Stage II	Involvement of upper vagina
Stage III	Involvement of lower third of vagina and/or extension to pelvic side wall
Stage IV	Extension beyond the true pelvis

From American Cancer Society: *Cancer facts and figures,* New York, 1996, The Society.

stages of the disease, hysterectomy with salpingo-oophorectomy may be indicated. Later-stage tumors may also require chemotherapy to control metastasis.

TEST *Yourself* **4-2**

Correlate risk factors associated with each type of cancer listed in Box 4-6.

Ovarian Cancer

Ovarian cancer is the third most common reproductive cancer among women and causes death in 61%. An estimated 26,700 new cases will occur annually, leading to 14,800 deaths.

Risk

Ovarian cancer most often occurs in women over age 60. Women who have never been pregnant have twice the risk as those who have given birth. Experiencing a first pregnancy at an early age; an early menopause, and using an oral contraceptive seem to decrease risk. The risk of ovarian cancer doubles for women who have had breast cancer (see Box 4-5 for staging), and there is evidence that a strong family history of ovarian cancer also increases risk.

Signs

Ovarian cancer is often "silent," with vague symptoms that are often not evident until late in the disease. Nausea, vomiting, abdominal bloating, discomfort, or pain commonly occur. In rare instances there is vaginal bleeding. Diagnosis is made by a pelvic examination, transvaginal ultrasound, Doppler imaging, or laparoscopic examination. A new blood test, the Ca-125, may prove helpful for early detection but is believed to produce inconsistent results at the present time. Because diagnosis is often delayed, the overall survival rate is 39% (ACS, 1996).

Clinical management

In addition to surgery, radiotherapy and chemotherapy are the common treatment modalities for women with ovarian cancer. In early stages of the disease, only the involved ovary is removed so that surgical menopause is avoided. In later stages a bilateral oophorectomy is performed, and the fallopian tubes, uterus, and any other intraabdominal lesions may also be removed.

In addition to traditional chemotherapy regimens, a new drug is being used with encouraging results. *Taxol,* derived from the bark of the Pacific yew tree, has been used successfully to treat ovarian cancers that were unresponsive to conventional therapy. This is also being investigated for use with breast and other cancers.

Box 4-5	Staging for Ovarian Cancer
Stage I	Tumor limited to ovaries
Stage II	Tumor involves one or both ovaries with pelvic extension
Stage III	Tumor involves one or both ovaries with peritoneal metastasis outside pelvis
Stage IV	Distant metastasis

From American Cancer Society: *Cancer facts and figures,* New York, 1996, The Society.

Nursing considerations

Women should be encouraged to have consistent physical and gynecologic examinations. Any unexplained symptoms should be followed up promptly and thoroughly, especially in women over the age of 40.

Colorectal Cancer

The rate of colorectal cancer has declined over the last 30 years, in large part a result of more frequent testing of stool for *occult blood,* but there will still be an estimated 133,500 new cases annually, with 54,900 deaths resulting. The rate of survival for colon cancer, if detected at an early, localized stage, is 83%; for rectal cancer the survival rate is 61% (ACS, 1996).

Risks

Personal or family history of colorectal cancer or polyps and inflammatory bowel disease may be risk factors. Other possible risks are physical inactivity and a high fat and low fiber intake. Studies now suggest that ERT and NSAIDs may act protectively.

Signs

Rectal bleeding, blood in the stool, or a change in bowel habits all suggest colorectal cancer. Digital rectal examination, testing stool for blood, and visualization by proctosigmoidoscopy or colonoscopy are recommended to aid in early detection.

Clinical management

Surgery to remove the tumor is the usual therapy, which may then be followed by radiotherapy. Surgery may involve resection (cutting out) of the bowel or the creation of an *ostomy,* bringing a portion of the intestine to the surface of the abdomen for evacuation of stool into an external appliance. Current results for chemotherapy in the treatment of colorectal cancer are encouraging.

Nursing considerations

Teaching should emphasize that a digital rectal examination be performed every year for women over 40 years of age. Available screening procedures should also be taught and encouraged as part of all health teaching (Box 4-6). Analysis of a stool specimen for covert (hidden) blood by use of *guaiac* testing is a simple, effective, and inexpensive tool for spotting tumors; in addition, results can be obtained quickly. Additional teaching should include dietary counseling and should promote the need to increase activity and to report any changes in elimination patterns.

TEST *Yourself 4-3*

  a. What does early detection mean for breast, cervical, and colorectal cancer?
  b. Why is early detection of ovarian cancer so difficult?

Many cancers are preventable; some are treatable or even curable with early detection and intervention. With education and support, women hopefully will be willing and able to make necessary lifestyle changes to avoid developing cancer. Nurses are striving to make cancer testing, services, and treatments available to all so that fewer women will be lost to this deadly disease.

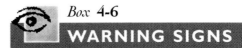

Box 4-6
WARNING SIGNS

Cancer

LUNG
Cough, sputum streaked with blood, chest pain, back pain, recurring lung infections

BREAST
Breast changes that persist throughout the menstrual cycle: a lump, thickening or swelling, skin dimpling or irritation, retraction, distortion, pain, scaliness, nipple tenderness

CERVICAL AND UTERINE
Positive Pap smear, unusual bleeding, pain

OVARIAN
Abdominal enlargement, vague digestive disturbances that persist and cannot otherwise be explained

COLORECTAL
Rectal bleeding, blood in the stool, a change in bowel habits.

Key Points

- Women's health care has changed dramatically in the past 2 decades. It is hoped that the use of traditional settings and the change in practitioner care, which empower women to take control of their health, will improve the total quality of women's health.
- Women who are victims of physical and sexual violence need encouragement and education to admit their situations and to plan for protection.
- Women need teaching and counseling to avoid dangerous STDs and viral diseases such as hepatitis B and HIV, as well as cancers of all sites.

- Women must be made aware of available health resources and be encouraged to take an active part in their own health maintenance.
- Teaching for women should emphasize personal hygiene, with additional specific teaching at appropriate stages about menstruation, dysmenorrhea, premenstrual syndrome, and coping with the climacteric.
- The current role of nursing has been expanded and strengthened by specialists within the profession who are filling the void in women's health care.

Study Questions

4-1. Select the terms that apply to the following statements:
  a. The most important procedure in the detection of breast cancer is _____.
  b. _____ is a potential complication from the use of tampons.
  c. Changes in the frequency, regularity, or quality of the menstrual cycle may signal that the woman in her forties has begun menopause or the _____.
  d. _____ is a common and potentially serious effect of postmenopausal estrogen depletion.
  e. Chlamydial, gonococcal, and trichomonal infections are classified as _____.

4-2. A client states that she is afraid of pain during a pelvic examination. The best nursing normal intervention is to:

   a. Offer her a hand to squeeze during the procedure.

   b. Position her lying flat to relax pelvic muscles.

   c. Encourage her to breathe slowly and rhythmically.

   d. Instruct her to bear down during bimanual palpation.

4-3. Women should be instructed to schedule a mammogram:

   a. When they first become sexually active.

   b. Every 3 years if results of the first one are negative.

   c. Only when a lump is detected by self-examination.

   d. Every year after age 50.

4-4. Preparatory teaching for a woman scheduled for a Pap smear should include:

   a. Refraining from sex for 1 week before the test.

   b. Wearing cotton underwear on the day of the test.

   c. Eliminating douching for 24 hours before the test.

   d. Avoiding the use of aspirin or ibuprofen for 24 hours before the test.

4-5. A decrease in estrogen is related to cardiovascular disease because low estrogen:

   a. Predisposes to obesity.

   b. Precipitates hypertension.

   c. Alters HDL levels.

   d. Causes fluid volume overload.

4-6. Which statement most accurately reflects the connection between the risk of cancer and the use of HRT?

   a. Smoking, obesity, and a poor diet increase the risk when HRT is used.

   b. There is no significant risk with HRT.

   c. HRT should never be continued for more than 2 years.

   d. The cardiovascular benefits of HRT far outweigh the risks.

Answer Key

4-1: *a*, Breast self-examination; *b*, toxic shock syndrome; *c*, climacteric; *d*, osteoporosis; *e*, sexually transmitted diseases. 4-2: c. 4-3: d. 4-4: c. 4-5: c. 4-6: a.

References

*American Academy of Pediatrics: *Report of the committee on infectious diseases,* Elk Grove Village, Ill, 1988, The Academy.

American Cancer Society: *Women and cancer,* Atlanta, 1995, The Society.

American Cancer Society: *Breast cancer facts and figures: 1996,* Atlanta, 1996, The Society.

American Cancer Society: *Cancer facts and figures,* New York, 1996, The Society.

Anderson JR: Early intervention for HIV infection in a gynecologic setting, *J Womens Health* 2(4):343, 1993.

Andrews WC: Continuous combined estrogen/progestin hormone replacement therapy, *Nurse Pract* Part 2, 20(11):1, 1995.

Archer DF et al: Endometrial morphology in asymptomatic postmenopausal women, *Am J Obstet Gynecol* 165(2):317, 1991.

Atkins-Murphy P: Primary care for women: screening tests and preventative services recommendations, *J Nurse Midwife* 40(2):74, 1995.

Baker VL: Alternatives to estrogen replacement: transdermal patches, percutaneous gels, vaginal rings, implants and other methods of delivery, *Obstet Gynecol Clin North Am* 21(1):271, 1994.

Baran DT: Osteoporosis: monitoring techniques and alternative therapies, *Obstetric Clinics* 21(2): 321, 1994.

Chuong CJ et al : A practical guide to relieving PMS, *Contemporary Nurse Practitioner* 1(3):31, 1995.

Clapp JF, Little K: The interaction between regular exercise and selected aspects of women's health, *Am J Obstet Gynecol* 173(1):9, 1995.

Creehan P: Toxic shock syndrome: an opportunity for nursing intervention, *J Obstet Gynecol Neonatal Nurs* 24(6):557, 1995.

Freedman RR, Woodward S: Behavioral treatment of menopausal hot flushes: evaluation by ambulatory monitoring, *Am J Obstet Gynecol* 167(2):436, 1992.

*Classic reference.

Freeman S: Menopause and hormone replacement therapy: complementary therapies, *Contemporary Nurse Practitioner* 1(1):40, 1994.

Geary MA: An analysis of the women's health movement and the impact on the delivery of health care in the United States, *Nurse Pract,* Part 1, 20(11):24, 1995.

Hammond CB: Menopause and hormone replacement therapy: an overview, *Obstet Gynecol* 87(2):2S, 1996.

Harris JR, Recht A: Conservative surgery and radiotherapy. In Harris JR et al, eds: *Breast diseases,* ed 2, Philadelphia, 1991, Lippincott.

Henderson CI: Breast cancer. In Murphy GP, Lawrence WL, Lenhard RE, eds: *Clinical oncology,* Atlanta, 1995, American Cancer Society.

Hernandez E, Atkinson B: *Clinical gynecologic pathology,* Philadelphia, 1996, WB Saunders.

Horton J: *The women's health data book,* New York, 1992, Elsevier.

Hsia LS, Ling MH: Premenstrual syndrome: current concepts in diagnosis and management, *J Nurse Midwifery* 35(6):351, 1990.

Ito D: *Without estrogen: natural remedies for menopause and beyond,* New York, 1994, Random House.

Jensvold MF et al: Menstrual cycle–related depressive symptoms treated with variable antidepressant dosage, *J Women's Health* 1(2):109, 1992.

Johnson N, Lilford RJ, Mayers D: Do healthy asymptomatic postmenopausal women with a uterus want routine cyclical hormone replacement: a utility analysis, *J Obstet Gynecol Neonatal Nurs,* 24(2):35, 1995.

Lauritzen C: Hormone replacement therapy prescribing guidelines: dream or reality? *Int J Gynecol Obstet* 52(suppl 1):S3, 1996.

Lichtman R: Perimenopausal and postmenopausal hormone replacement therapy–part 1: an update of the literature on benefits and risks, *J Nurse Midwife* 41(1):3, 1996.

Lichtman R, Papera S: *Gynecology: well woman care,* Norwalk, Conn, 1990, Appleton & Lange.

Limouzin-Lamouthe MA et al: Childbearing, reproductive control, aging women, and health care: projected ethical debates, *J Obstet Gynecol Neonatal Nurs* 23(2):147, 1994.

Lindsay R: The menopause and osteoporosis, *Obstet Gynecol* 81(2):16S, 1996.

Marty JP: New trends in transdermal technologies: development of the skin patch Menorest, *Int J Gynecol Obstet* 52(suppl 1): S17, 1996.

McGurty MK: Vaginal infections: keys to treatment, *Contemporary Nurse Practitioner* 1(3):18, 1995.

Moore AA, Dunham-Noonan M: A nurse's guide to hormone replacement therapy, *J Obstet Gynecol Neonatal Nurs* 25(1):24, 1996.

Ojeda L: *Menopause without medicine,* Alameda, Calif, 1992, Hunter House.

Parsons L et al: Methods of and attitudes toward screening obstetrical and gynecologic patients for domestic violence, *Am J Obstet Gynecol* 173(2):381, 1995.

Pearlstein T: Hormones and depression: what are the facts about PMS, menopause and hormone replacement therapy? *Am J Obstet Gynecol* 173(2): 646, 1995.

Philosophe R, Seibel M: Menopause and cardiovascular disease: NAACOG's clinical issues in perinatal women's health nursing, 2(4):430, 1991.

Reed BD, Eyler A: Vaginal infections: diagnosis and management, *Am Fam Physician* 47(8):1805, 1993.

Reingold AL: Toxic shock syndrome: an update, *Am J Obstet Gynecol* Part 2, 165(4):1236, 1991.

Scalley EK, Heinrich JB: An overview of estrogen replacement therapy in postmenopausal women, *J Womens Health:* 2(3):189, 1993.

Schlievert PM, Gocke JE, Deringer JR: Group B streptococcal toxic shock-like syndrome: report of a case and purification of an associated pyrogenic toxin, *Clin Infect Dis* 17(1):16, 1993.

Sherwin B: Hormones, mood, and cognitive functioning in postmenopausal women, *Obstet Gynecol* 87(2):20S, 1996.

Sitruck-Ware R, Utian W: *The menopause and hormonal replacement: facts and controversies,* New York, 1991, Marcel Dekker.

Speroff L et al: *Clinical gynecologic endocrinology and infertility,* Philadelphia, 1994, Williams & Wilkins.

Speroff L: Postmenopausal hormone therapy and breast cancer, *Obstet Gynecol* 87(2):44S, 1996.

Stein D: *The natural remedy book for women,* Freedom, Calif, 1995, Crossing Press.

Sullivan JM, Fowlkes LP: The clinical aspects of estrogen and the cardiovascular system, *Obstet Gynecol* 87(suppl 2):41, 1996.

Sweet RL: New approaches for the treatment of bacterial vaginosis, *Am J Obstet Gynecol,* Part 2, 160(2):479, 1993.

Thomas B: Challenges for teachers of women's health, *Nurse Educator* 17(5):10, 1992.

*Todd JK et al: Toxic shock syndrome associated with phage-group-I staphylococci, *Lancet* 36:1116, 1978.

Whitman S et al: patterns of breast and cervical cancer screening at three public health centers in inner city urban areas, *Am J Public Health* 81(12):1651, 1991.

Wilson BA et al: *Nurses drug guide,* Norwalk, Conn, 1996, Appleton & Lange.

Wood TF, Potter MA, Jonasson O: Streptococcal toxic shock-like syndrome: the importance of surgical intervention, *Ann Surg* 217(2):109, 1993.

Zapda J et al: Changes in mammography use: economic need and service factors, *Am J Public Health* 82(10):1345, 1992.

 Student Resource Shelf

Maddox M: Women at midlife: hormone replacement therapy, *Nurs Clin North Am* 27(4):959, 1992.

HRT is the most important menopause-related topic for women to consider. Although the benefits of this treatment do seem to outweigh the risks, each woman needs to make a choice.

Women's health care, *J Nurse Midwife* 36(1): 1991.

Entire issue devoted to various topics in women's health.

Women's health care, *Am J Women's Health* 1(1): 1992.

Contains a number of relevant articles.

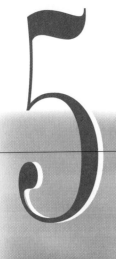

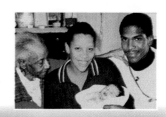

Fertility Care

Learning Objectives

- Describe the advantages and disadvantages of each fertility control method.
- Discuss and explain the application of the nursing process in planning care for clients who seek contraceptive assistance.
- Describe the nursing role in counseling for reproduction and fertility control.

Key Terms

Abstinence
Amenorrhea
Basal Body Temperature (BBT)
Billings Method
Calendar Method
Cervical Cap
Chemical Barriers
Coitus Independent
Coitus Interruptus
Condom
Contraception
Depo-Provera (DMPA)
Diaphragm
Fertility Awareness Method
Intrauterine Device (IUD)
Lactation Amenorrhea Method (LAM)

Mechanical Barriers
Minipill
Natural Family Planning (NFP)
Norplant Subdermal Implant
Oral Contraceptive (OC) ("The Pill")
Pelvic Inflammatory Disease (PID)
"Perfect Use"
Postcoital Contraception
Sexually Transmitted Diseases (STDs)
Spermicide
Surgical Sterilization
Symptothermal Method
Tubal Ligation
"Typical Use"
Vasectomy

FERTILITY ISSUES

Fertility control is not a new concept; in fact, many methods have been used throughout history to prevent pregnancy. Infanticide and abortion were practiced in many primitive civilizations. Withdrawal, douching, and sitting upright to expel the semen were methods common in Biblical times. Women in ancient Egypt used domes formed of hollowed lemon halves to cover the cervix. Other cultures have used tampons or followed elaborate rituals to prevent conception (Schenker and Rabenou, 1993). Today **contraception** refers to the practice of

choosing and using a method to delay, prevent, or space a pregnancy; it affords many fertility alternatives and choices during the reproductive years.

GLOBAL POPULATION CONCERNS

Uncontrolled population growth has been a concern since 1798, the year Thomas Robert Malthus released a treatise detailing the economic and social consequences of unchecked population expansion (Diczfalusy, 1995). World population has doubled since the beginning of this century and is projected to reach 10 billion by the year

2100 (Spira, 1994). Genuine concern exists about having adequate worldwide resources for sustaining such a population. Concern also exists for issues regarding the quality of life, human dignity, access to health and reproductive care, and freedom of choice. The governments of many developing countries have been underwriting family planning programs since the early 1960s, when contraceptive technology improved with the use of oral contraceptives and **intrauterine devices** (IUDs). Thus family planning has become a well-recognized foundation for health care in most developing countries. Since the 1960s there has been recognition that the health care aspect of family planning encompasses, in addition to birth control, the control of **sexually transmitted diseases** (STDs) and maternal, infant, and child well-being.

Access to family planning services, especially in the developing countries of the world, is essential to help limit or slow the exponential growth of population. Child spacing in a noncoercive atmosphere is certainly a goal. In many countries family planning and limitations on the number of children per family are government policy. The Chinese policy of one child per family, for example, includes incentives such as monthly allowances and priorities in housing. Disincentives such as fines for extra births, loss of health coverage, and intense peer pressure characterize some of the official Chinese measures to limit family size (Freedman and Isaacs, 1993). In the 1960s India promoted male sterilization by using payments of food or commodities. Families with numerous births were penalized by being denied their choice of schools, having their free maternity care eliminated, or having limitations placed on their housing choices.

Religious beliefs determine many child spacing efforts. Muslims are allowed by Shari'ah law to space their children (Omran, 1992). Orthodox Jews are limited in their contraceptive choices based on the prohibition of improper destruction of the seed (Gen 38). Thus female contraception is condoned but male contraception is not. The Roman Catholic view prohibits all forms of contraception except the family planning methods and abstinence, since the primary purpose of marriage is procreation. The Protestant Church embraces the philosophy of responsible parenthood, which includes contraception (Schenker and Rabenou, 1993). In the Hindu faith a woman's primary religious duty is fulfilled when she gives birth to a son. The female infant is of less value and not as worthy of the resources (i.e., money, nutrition, education). Buddhist teachings do not stress procreation, but both the Hindu and Buddhist faiths oppose bodily injury, which includes abortion and infanticide.

Cultural factors may influence the type of contraception used in different countries. For instance, female sterilization is used extensively in India, Asia, and Latin America. The IUD is used in China and East Asia. Condom use is popular in Japan. Russia's delivery of contraceptive health care is so lacking that the abortion rate is one of the highest in the world (Djerassi, 1995).

Status of Women

In the Western world the status of women in society has improved since the beginning of the twentieth century. Since the 1960s, the rise of feminist philosophy has resulted in legislation to equalize opportunities for women. Gender equality in many developing nations, however, lags behind in such areas as nutrition, health, income, and personal security. One outcome of the 1994 International Conference on Population and Development in Cairo was the resolution that a prerequisite for reducing poverty, promoting economic growth, and achieving sound population policies is the elimination of social and economic discrimination against women. Whether this ideal will come to fruition depends largely upon the availability of education that empowers women without clashing with existing cultural and religious practices (Diczfalusy, 1995). Legislation enacted on an international level may have little or no effect on women living in certain Muslim countries (Iran, Iraq, and Saudi Arabia), South Asia, or much of sub-Saharan Africa, where religious and customary laws may supersede secular authority (Freedman and Isaacs, 1993). In many northern African countries, practices such as female genital mutilation serve to further subjugate women by compromising their physical and mental health and by increasing the risk of complications during childbirth (Diczfalusy, 1995).

Certain war-ravaged countries in Eastern Europe and Africa have experienced severe repercussions in the health of women and children. The rape and torture of women, the forced continuation of pregnancies resulting from rape, and the escalating levels of STDs further render the surviving women and children at risk for serious health consequences.

Poverty, war, education, religious beliefs, cultural norms, and government policies play an essential role in determining the ability of a couple (the woman in particular) to control reproductive destiny. Contraception is a personal choice; decisions concerning it are as unique as the individual making them. Nursing professionals have a responsibility to those seeking contraception to provide health care with dignity and with respect to the clients' cultural beliefs.

Adolescent Pregnancy

The rising pregnancy rates for adolescents in the United States has caused many health care professionals to be concerned about STDs and unwanted pregnancy. Prevention of adolescent pregnancy is now a high priority in health care delivery in the United States. Innovative programs of sex education with special emphasis on postponing a first sexual encounter can be successful when parents, teachers,

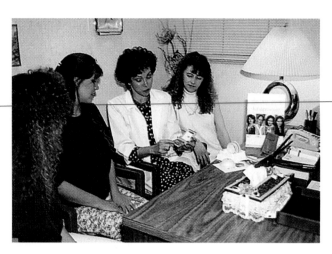

Figure 5-1 Providing personal instruction is the key to gaining the compliance of teenage women. (Courtesy Marjorie Pyle, RNC, *Lifecircle*.)

and the community work together to facilitate change (Creatsas, 1993). Measures such as peer counseling and role playing and mediums such as theater, music, and videos may help young teens develop skills to make informed decisions about sex and resist peer pressures.

Studies have shown that delaying the first sexual experience until the later teen years reduces the number of potential lifetime sexual partners, thus reducing the potential for STDs and unplanned pregnancy (Frost and Forrest, 1995; Oakley, 1995). When school-based health clinics are available, adolescents have access not only to birth control but also to generalized health care. A close, trusting relationship often develops between the teen and the clinic staff, an essential component of successful health care for teens (Beilinson, Miola, Farmer, 1995) (Figure 5-1).

CONTRACEPTION

Accidental or unwanted pregnancies occur when contraception fails or when contraceptive needs remain unmet. Unplanned pregnancies may also be the result of mistiming, a desired pregnancy occurring sooner than planned (Zotti and Siegel, 1995). Meeting contraceptive needs entails focusing interventional efforts on the "user's perspective" (Diczfalusy, 1991), stepping inside the shoes of the client, and understanding the cultural and socioeconomic constraints governing the choice and use of the birth control method. Counseling often is best received when a person is highly motivated to prevent pregnancy, such as after a recent birth.

Contraceptive choices may be limited or enhanced by long-range personal or family goals, the expense of the method, feelings about sexuality, the relationship of the couple, the cultural significance of birth planning in the client's life, and the religious beliefs about and the psy-

chologic importance of pregnancy (Zotti and Siegel, 1995).

An ideal method of birth control follows these criteria:
- Easy to use
- Coitus independent (unrelated to the sexual act)
- Safe
- Inexpensive
- 100% effective
- Produces no side effects
- Acceptable to religious and cultural beliefs and practices of the users

No single method meets all these criteria. The consistency with which a contraceptive method is used is an important factor in the prevention of pregnancy. Contraceptive failure, misuse, and nonuse are especially high among those who are economically disadvantaged, less educated, adolescent, or homeless. Moreover, the less educated and adolescent populations tend to rely on ineffective methods based on hearsay or on methods that are cheaper and more readily available to them. Thus a great deal of work is needed to provide everyone with suitable contraceptive information and follow-up care.

Rates of Effectiveness

Part of the general evaluation of a method's acceptability is its rate of effectiveness. These rates, statistically projected from studies of small samples, use a percentage reading based on the results of the method's use by 100 women for 1 year. The phrase, "per women-years of use" is often used, or a percentage based on the study of 100 women is given. For example, if 100 women use a method for 1 year and 3 became pregnant, the effectiveness rating is 97%, or 3 pregnancies per 100 women per year of use. Without the use of any contraception, approximately 70% of sexually active women would become pregnant within 1 year.

Effectiveness rates can be misleading unless they are placed in careful context. For instance, the package insert statistics included with a contraceptive device (such as oral contraceptives, diaphragms, or condoms) often include "**perfect use**" effectiveness, which refers to the use of the method perfectly and consistently *every time* (e.g., taking the birth control pill every day without fail). Also included in the package insert statistics are the average or "**typical use**" rates, which are the "real world" estimates of typical users. With methods that involve user participation and responsibility (such as with the diaphragm, condom, and spermicide) the gap between the perfect effectiveness and the typical use effectiveness rates may be considerable.

Among the many factors that affect the effectiveness rates, one of the most important is the age of the man or woman using the method. The older a person is, the more skillful, motivated, and diligent he or she usually becomes. Older women may also have more predictable or planned times for intercourse, making contraceptive use easier

(Gladwell, 1993). The rate of effectiveness for contraception increases with other factors as well, such as the income, education, and lifestyle of the person (Mosher, 1990). Some studies have demonstrated that nonsmokers have more consistent contraceptive use and higher effectiveness rates than smokers, perhaps because they take a less risky approach to their lives (Lethbridge, 1991). The most highly motivated contraceptive users seem to be young, single, educated women with careers. This group, perhaps the most successful users of contraception, may approach the "perfect use" statistic for any of the methods they choose. Nurses who counsel contraceptive users must be familiar with the various effectiveness rates so that questions and concerns may be meaningfully addressed.*

Self-Discovery

If you have used a family planning method, how would you describe its ease of use and the side effects for you and your partner? Would you consider an alternate method?

If you have not used a method, imagine a scenario in which you need a method. After reading this chapter, which method appeals to you and why? ∼

Nonhormonal Methods: Fertility Awareness and Natural Family Planning

Natural family planning (NFP) and the **fertility awareness method** are based on the events of the menstrual cycle. The ovum is viable for approximately 1 day after ovulation, and sperm are viable for approximately 2 to 3 days after being deposited in the vagina. Using this knowledge, the couple abstains from unprotected intercourse or uses an additional method of contraception during the woman's "unsafe" time, that is her peak fertile days. A recent study has shown that the unsafe time during each menstrual cycle is during the 6 day period that ends on the day of ovulation (Wilcox, Weinberg, Baird, 1995). Until further research is conducted, the conventional advice given to most couples is that the 10 day fertile or unsafe period is 7 days before ovulation until 2 days after (Hatcher et al, 1994). Because the variation in cycle length occurs before ovulation, many couples use technologic help (i.e., urine testing kits that help detect ovulation).

Natural family planning and fertility awareness methods may include any or all of the following: (1) calendar or rhythm method, (2) basal body temperature method, (3) Billings ovulation method (i.e., cervical mucous changes), and (4) the symptothermal method. Inherent in the use of these methods is a couples' ease in communicating with each other about sexual body functions and their motivation to maintain accurate menstrual cycle records.

Nursing intervention. This involves counseling and teaching about the menstrual cycle, how to maintain and interpret charts of cervical mucous changes, and how to focus on physiologic signs. Situations such as stress, medications, or infection need to be discussed because the usual indicators of fertility may be altered as a result of these. The nurse emphasizes the partners' need for increased communication and flexibility in choosing abstinence or additional birth control when the fertile time occurs.

Rhythm or calendar method

The rhythm or **calendar method** is based on a record of the woman's menstrual cycle during the previous 6 months. The number of days in the shortest and the longest cycles are noted. (Ovulation most often occurs 14 days ±2 days before the next menses). The woman then calculates the first unsafe day (the beginning of the fertile time) by subtracting 20 days from the shortest cycle. The last unsafe day is then determined by subtracting 10 days from the longest cycle. An example of the calculations follows:

Shortest cycle = 25 days   Longest cycle = 32

$$\begin{array}{cc} 25 & 32 \\ -20 & -10 \\ \hline \text{Day 5} & \text{Day 22} \end{array}$$

For the woman in this example the fertile or unsafe period is calculated to be 18 days, from days 5 through 22 of each of her cycles. If the woman in this illustration began her period on May 3, her first fertile day would be May 7 (Day 5), and her last fertile day would be May 24 (Day 22). Using the calendar method alone, this woman must abstain from sexual intercourse (or use another method) for longer than she may desire. To shorten the period of abstinence the couple can add some or all of the following methods.

Basal body temperature

The woman's temperature is taken every day after she awakens and before any physical or emotional activity occurs. She uses a basal thermometer, which measures in 0.1 rather than 0.2 increments so that small changes are easily noted. Before ovulation, the **basal body temperature** (BBT) remains low. Approximately 24 hours before ovulation the temperature dips slightly (0.1° to 0.2°) and then rises sharply within 24 hours. The rise of 0.4° to 0.8°is maintained during the life of the corpus luteum for approximately 12 days. The day before menstruation, the temperature drops again to the previous low levels. (Figure 5-2). This shift is caused by the thermogenic influences of progesterone, which is secreted in higher levels after ovulation. Therefore a temperature elevation lasting 3 days signifies an end to the need for abstinence even if the calendar count has not ended.

*Effectiveness rates used in this chapter are from Hatcher et al, 1994, unless otherwise indicated.

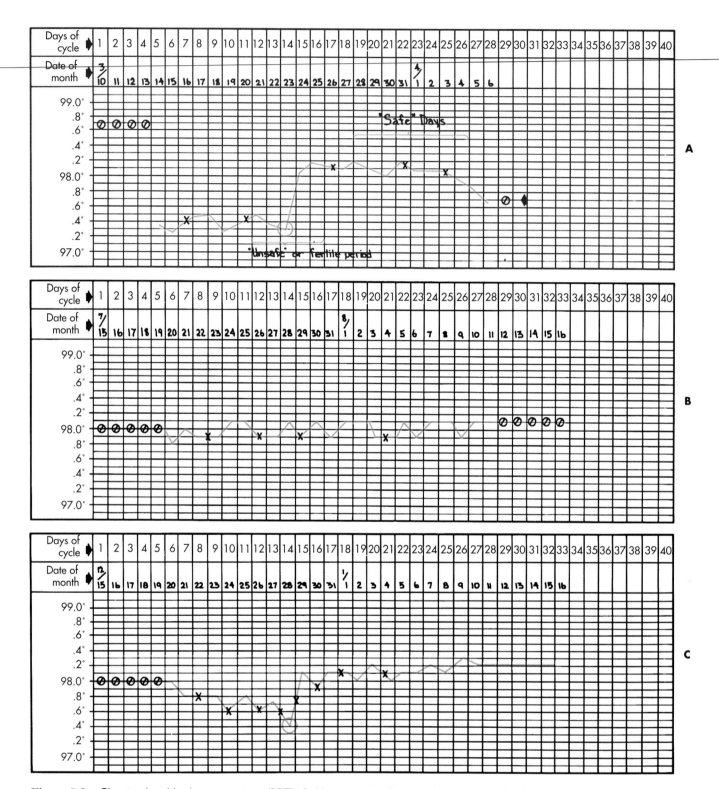

Figure 5-2 Charting basal body temperature (BBT). **A,** Normal cycle. **B,** Anovulatory cycle. **C,** After conception. ∅ , Menstruation; ⊙ , ovulation; **X,** intercourse during previous 24 hours.

Many factors, including infection, stress, fatigue, alcohol use, jet lag, use of electric blankets, or alteration in normal sleep patterns, can alter the expected outcome of the temperature chart. These factors should be noted on the temperature chart.

Methods based on cervical mucous changes

Billings method. The **Billings method** relies on the changes in cervical mucous secretions (see Figure 5-2). After menstruation the discharge appears yellowish and viscid and is impenetrable to sperm. At 2 or 3 days before ovulation, the rising levels of estrogen change the mucus to a clear, colorless liquid similar to an egg white. It now has qualities that "welcome" the sperm, promoting maximum survival. If this mucus were tested, the glucose levels would be increased and the pH would be more alkaline (Figure 5-3). The mucus has a threadability called *spinnbarkeit*. If the mucus is spread on a glass slide (Figure 5-4), a fernlike pattern crystallizes, known as ferning (Billings et al, 1972).The woman is taught to be aware of her vaginal wetness and to recognize the changes that signal ovulation. After ovulation, the mucus again changes under the influence of progesterone to a thick, white, and non-stretchy consistency that is difficult for the sperm to penetrate.

Interference with the natural cycle through the use of contraceptive foams, jellies, or creams, or the through the use of douches, or in the presence of vaginal infections makes any test of the mucus inaccurate. The use of nasal decongestants may also have a drying effect on the mucus.

Symptothermal method. The **symptothermal method** combines the use of the BBT with analysis of cervical mucous changes and makes predictions of ovulation more accurate. In addition to mucous changes, other changes may also be noted and may include increased libido, or midcycle spotting. Mittelschmerz (ovulatory pain) may be indicated in many ways: brief abdominal swelling or pain, rectal pain, lower pelvic pain, or one-sided pelvic pain (Hatcher et al, 1994).

Ovulation testing kits. A urine testing kit that detects hormonal changes during the menstrual cycle may be used at home. Tests now available, such as Q-Test, First Response, and Ovu-Stick, *detect but do not anticipate* ovulation. The Home Ovarian Monitor is being tested as a predictive device and will make testing for contraception or fertility more accurate (Cavero, 1995). Other devices such as the Rabbit, Rite Time, or Ovudate help predict temperature changes during the fertile times. Because the methods are not affected by illness, stress, or activity levels, they are reliable when used in combination with other fertility indicators. If used every month, however, cost is a consideration.

The ovulation detection kits currently available do not give enough advance warning of impending ovulation. A woman who relies solely on external monitoring devices may not become familiar enough with her own bodily changes to determine the unsafe times. Daily observation of cervical mucous changes is a more accurate predictor (Fehring, 1991).

Advantages. No cost is involved in fertility awareness methods, except for a thermometer, charts, or the ovulation detection kits, and there is no need for a prescription. These methods are easy to learn even among disadvantaged populations (Ryder, 1993). Motivated couples are afforded the chance to share in mutual choices. Finally, awareness methods are the only means of controlling pregnancy sanctioned by the Roman Catholic Church.

Effectiveness rates are based on the use of a combination of fertility indicators. According to Hatcher (1994)

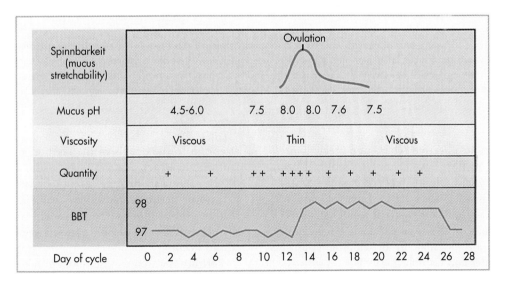

Figure 5-3   Comparison of qualities of cervical mucus during the menstrual cycle. Ovulation occurs when conditions are most favorable. (Redrawn from Moghiss KS. In Wallach EE, Kempers RD, ed: *Modern trends in infertility and conception control,* vol 1, Baltimore, 1979, Williams & Wilkins.)

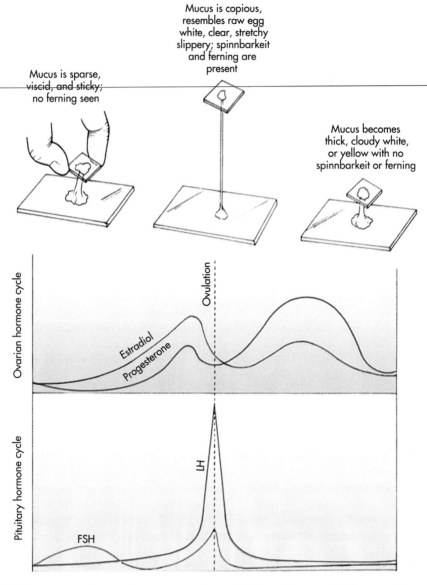

Mucus is sparse, viscid, and sticky; no ferning seen

Mucus is copious, resembles raw egg white, clear, stretchy, slippery; spinnbarkeit and ferning are present

Mucus becomes thick, cloudy white, or yellow with no spinnbarkeit or ferning

Ovulation

Ovarian hormone cycle

Estradiol
Progesterone

Pituitary hormone cycle

LH

FSH

Figure 5-4 Parameters of cervical mucus at ovulation. *Ferning* is the term for the crystalline pattern formed when the mucus is spread on a glass slide, dried, and viewed under a microscope. *Spinnbarkeit* is the term for the egg-white consistency of mucus that is more alkaline, has a higher sodium and glucose content, and is more receptive to sperm. (From Fogel CI, Woods NF: *Health care of women: a nursing perspective*, St Louis, 1981, Mosby.)

the method is more effective when unprotected intercourse is limited to the postovulatory days only. During the first year of typical use the method is approximately 80% effective; meaning that 20% of the women will become pregnant. In stable, long-term relationships, NFP may actually enhance the sexual experience for couples. These methods are popular in developing countries (Ryder, 1993; Ryder and Campbell, 1995).

Disadvantages. The calendar method alone is not reliable because the time of ovulation is difficult to determine and the viability of the sperm or the ovum may vary in some persons. The couple must be motivated to pay attention to the details of the method and must be vigilant about either abstaining or using another method during the unsafe period. Recent menarche with irregular periods or perimenopause may make fertility awareness methods difficult to use. Some women are unable to identify cervical mucus or BBT patterns even with persistent record keeping.

Fertility awareness methods provide no protection against STDs. In fact the use of alternative methods of sexual expression used by some couples during the fertile time, such as oral or anal sex, may increase the transmission of the human immunodeficiency viral (HIV) infection (Hatcher et al, 1994). Fertility awareness methods are not recommended in the early postpartum period because factors such as lack of sleep, breast-feeding, or fatigue may affect the expected signs of fertility.

Lactation amenorrhea method

Hoping to capitalize on the well-known phenomenon that breast-feeding women who do not menstruate rarely become pregnant, researchers are trying to establish guidelines for greater effectiveness of the **lactation amenorrhea method** (LAM). The key to the suppression of fertility is frequent breast-feeding throughout the day, every day, as long as amenorrhea continues. Once spotting or menses begins, other methods of contraception must be implemented.

Women who follow these guidelines have a 2% chance of accidental pregnancy (Rojnik et al, 1995). There is a high probability that the woman who is amenorrheal while breast-feeding will be able to regulate her fertility in the *first* 32 weeks postpartum even if she introduces some supplementation to the infant's feedings. Hatcher et al (1994) recommend relying on the LAM for a maximum of 6 months after birth. After this the pregnancy rate rises to about 6%.

Nursing intervention. This involves not only teaching effective breast-feeding techniques but also counseling about ovulation, spotting, and the return of menses during the recovery period. Counseling should include alternative methods of birth control during the time most postpartal women return to ovulation, approximately 2 months after birth.

Advantages. The woman who uses the LAM must begin with birth control when she experiences her first menses or spotting. Neither cost nor a physician's visit is involved.

Disadvantages. The woman must be extremely confident in her abilities to breast-feed and nourish the infant without reliance on supplementary feedings. Should the woman need to return to work after the birth of the infant or use supplemental bottle milk, the levels of breast milk will diminish and menses may return.

TEST *Yourself* 5-1 ━━━━━━━━━━━

Describe the differences among the following birth control methods: rhythm, Billings, symptothermal, and BBT alone. Which method has the best "perfect use" rating? Compare these rating with the "failure rate" when no contraception is used.

Coitus interruptus

Coitus interruptus (withdrawal) is an ancient method that requires the male to withdraw his penis from the vagina immediately before ejaculation. As a result, semen is not deposited in or near the vagina.

Advantages. The withdrawal method is useful for those who have no other method available. It involves no cost, devices, or chemicals and is available in any situation.

Disadvantages. This method may be extremely frustrating because both partners must maintain control. Withdrawal may be quite difficult for a sexually inexperienced person. Even though ejaculation may be held back, preejaculatory fluid (which may contain semen stored in the prostate or Cowper's glands) can escape before ejaculation. A small drop of semen may contain millions of sperm. It is possible for sperm deposited near the external genitalia to reach an ovum. Thus this method has a failure rate of about 18%. It provides some protection, however, if no other method is available. Coitus interruptus provides no protection against HIV infection because bodily secretions mix during sexual arousal and penetration (Hatcher et al, 1994).

Abstinence

The advent of acquired immunodeficiency syndrome (AIDS) has made **abstinence** a viable option. Among teenagers, however, peer pressure, a feeling of invulnerability, and a tendency toward risk-taking behavior have made abstinence a difficult choice as a method of birth control (Brown et al, 1992).

Sexual expression can involve a range of intimate activities. Touching, cuddling, dancing, massaging each other, and many other activities besides coitus are capable of meeting the needs to be both nurtured and loved and to give them in return. Although sexual expression without intercourse is an extremely effective contraceptive, it is not easily accomplished. Family planning counselors must therefore be supportive of abstinence and help establish programs for young people that enable them to choose abstinence as a method of preventing pregnancy (Hatcher et al, 1994).

Advantages. Abstinence is free, requiring the couple to learn about the body, sexuality, and control over life experience. Using abstinence for contraception allows the couple to explore many other avenues of sexual expression. In the era of AIDS, abstinence is regaining general approval.

Nonhormonal Methods: Barrier Methods

Chemical barriers

Chemical barriers come in a variety of forms—film, foam, jelly, gel, cream, and suppositories—that can be used alone or with a mechanical barrier such as the condom, diaphragm, or cervical cap. Nonoxynol-9 is the active spermicidal (sperm killing) ingredient in most of the products. The **spermicide** destroys the cell membrane of the sperm. Sperm thrive best at an alkaline pH of 8.5 to 9.0. Because the vagina is normally acidic until ovulation, chemical barriers are designed to keep the vaginal pH near 4.

Chemical barriers are inserted deep in the vagina. Though foams, jellies, and gels are instantly effective, sup-

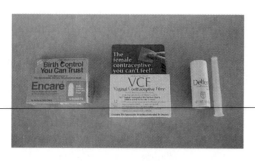

Figure 5-5 Mechanical and chemical barrier birth control devices. Diaphragm, jelly, and foam. (Courtesy Michael Clement, MD.)

positories and films need time to dissolve in the vaginal fluid (5 to 20 minutes). After the chemical barrier is inserted, it is usually effective for about 1 hour. All chemical agents must be used immediately before intercourse (10 to 30 minutes) and therefore cannot be isolated from intercourse. Effects last for about 1 hour; repeated intercourse requires reapplication. The woman should not douche for at least 6 hours after intercourse because it removes the chemical and may allow sperm to enter the uterus. If a chemical barrier is used in the weeks after childbirth, a double application is necessary until the stretched vaginal tissue returns to prepregnant size (Figure 5-5).

Nursing intervention. This involves education about the proper use of the spermicide. Teaching should stress that chemical barriers must be reapplied with every sexual encounter and that there are time limits to their efficacy. It should also emphasize that greater effectiveness is achieved when they are used with other contraceptive measures, such as condoms. Finally the teaching should discuss the precautions to observe.

Advantages. Chemical contraceptives need no prescription, are simpler to use, and may be used more often by adolescents. Products are available in pharmacies and in supermarkets. For the woman who forgets her birth control pill for 2 days or who has infrequent intercourse, a chemical barrier may be especially useful as a temporary measure. When used alone, chemical barriers require no special manipulative skills; insertion is much like that of a tampon. The chemical agents do not alter body physiology but do increase vaginal lubrication. Because of its bacteriostatic effect, spermicide may offer increased protection against STDs, including herpes, gonorrhea, trichomonas, chlamydia, and AIDS. Greater protection, however, occurs when both a chemical barrier and a condom are used.

Current scientific data fail to confirm any risk of birth defects with the use of spermicides at the point of conception or during early pregnancy (Faundes, Elias, Coggins, 1994).

Disadvantages. The failure rate with "typical use" is approximately 21%. A small percentage of women and men experience burning from the agent. Switching from nonoxynol-9 to octoxynol-9 may help with sensitivity. An

additional disadvantage is the amount of liquefied agent discharge. Because the method must be used immediately before intercourse, planning and forethought are involved, making it psychologically more difficult for adolescents, who tend to romanticize spontaneity. Some women dislike the genital manipulation involved.

Mechanical barriers

Mechanical barriers physically prevent sperm from entering the cervix. The condom, diaphragm, and cervical cap are widely used in the United States today. The contraceptive sponge was removed from the market in early 1995 by the manufacturer because of a dispute with the FDA. Since the safety and efficacy of the sponge were not disputed, the manufacturer may one day restore it to production.

Use of a spermicide such as nonoxynol-9 is strongly recommended with the cervical cap, diaphragm, or condom to increase the efficacy of these methods. The woman using a barrier method must learn the proper insertion and care of the diaphragm or cervical cap. Use of oil-based lubricants such as mineral oil, petroleum jelly, butter, or any edictions (Monistat), have a damaging effect on the latex material.

Nursing intervention. This involves teaching the chosen method, stressing signs and symptoms that require immediate attention (e.g., toxic shock syndrome), reviewing the proper placement and removal of the device, and storage techniques. Encourage annual health evaluations, and provide telephone access for any questions.

Diaphragm. The **diaphragm** is a curved rubber dome enclosed by a flexible metal ring that rests in the vagina and covers the cervix. Diaphragms are available in a variety of sizes. A fitting is necessary and the size will need to be changed after pregnancy or weight gain or loss of 10 pounds or more.

Spermicidal cream or jelly (about a teaspoonful) is placed in the cup portion and on the rim of the diaphragm before insertion so that the spermicide contacts the cervix. The contraceptive effect of the diaphragm is attributed partly to its role as a container for the spermicide; any sperm reaching the cervix are incapacitated.

The woman checks for proper placement of the diaphragm by feeling for the cervix, which feels like a rounded knob or the tip of the nose. The anterior rim can be felt resting against the symphysis pubis. Once in place the diaphragm should not be felt by either partner during intercourse. (Note Figure 5-6 for the method of placement).

The diaphragm should remain in place for at least 6 hours after intercourse but no longer than 24 hours because of the risk of toxic shock syndrome. If coitus occurs again within 6 hours and the diaphragm is still in place, an additional application of foam or jelly should be used. The woman should not douche during the next 6-hour period because it may dislodge the diaphragm

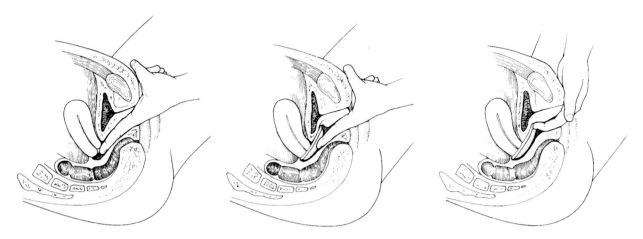

Figure 5-6   Proper placement of diaphragm between posterior fornix and symphysis pubis. (From Fogel CI, Woods NF: *Health care of women: a nursing perspective,* St Louis, 1981, Mosby.)

and force sperm into the cervix. Periodic inspection for holes or tears in the diaphragm and careful cleaning of it are important.

Toxic shock syndrome. Toxic shock syndrome (TSS) occurs occasionally when barrier methods and tampons are used. When a diaphragm is to be used, the nurse should discuss the risk factors and signs of illness (see Box 4-1). The risk of TSS may be significantly reduced if the woman does the following:

- Washes her hands with soap and water before inserting or removing the diaphragm, or cervical cap
- Leaves the device in position for less than 24 hours
- Does not use the device in the immediate postpartum period
- Seeks treatment for any vaginal infection before reusing the device
- Cares for the device with soap and water and lets it dry completely

Advantages. The failure rates for the diaphragm vary depending upon the user's age and the frequency of intercourse. The failure rate is 10% for women who have frequent intercourse and approximately 3% to 4% for women who have less frequent intercourse. Manipulation is required to insert the diaphragm, but the insertion technique is relatively simple to master. For most women the diaphragm neither interferes with physiologic functioning nor alters sexual sensation.

Disadvantages. An accidental pregnancy rate of up to 18% exists among typical first-year diaphragm users. Motivation and preplanning are required to use this method effectively. Expenses include an initial office or clinic visit and the expense of the chemical barrier. Vaginal manipulation may be culturally unacceptable or may be distasteful for some women. The diaphragm may contribute to recurrent cystitis as a result of upward pressure of the rim against the urethra. In unusual coital positions the diaphragm may slip out of place. Sometimes a woman may experience pelvic discomfort, cramps, or

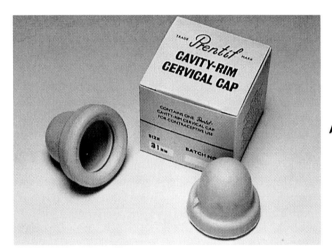

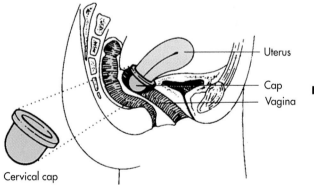

Figure 5-7   **A,** Cervical cap. **B,** Cervical cap placement.

pressure on the bladder or rectum. Allergy to latex or spermicides is a contraindication to its use.

Cervical cap. The Prentif **cervical cap** functions in much the same manner as the diaphragm but is smaller, thicker, and less flexible (Figure 5-7). About ¹/₂ teaspoon of spermicide is placed in the dome before insertion. The rim fits snugly around the base of the cervix and may be left in place for up to 48 hours; it should remain in place for at least 6 hours after intercourse. Repeated intercourse does not require more spermicide. Care for the cap is similar to that of the diaphragm. The cap must be carefully fitted and is obtained through prescription. Failure rates range from 8% to 18%.

Nursing intervention. This involves teaching the woman how to insert and remove the cap, which is slightly more difficult than the diaphragm to place correctly. Precautions about TSS, warnings about using the cap during menstruation, and instructions on care for the device are provided. Handwashing before and after cap insertion is vital.

Advantages. Many similarities exist between the advantages of the cervical cap and the diaphragm. Most cervical cap users express satisfaction with its use. Because the cap is smaller than the diaphragm, it may be less noticeable to both partners. Since there is no pressure on the bladder, fewer urinary tract infections are noted.

Disadvantages. The major drawbacks of the cap are the possible effects of long-term exposure to secretions, spermicides, and bacteria trapped inside it. If the cap is left in place more than 48 hours, vaginal irritation and a foul-smelling odor may result. Trauma to the tissues of the cervix or the vagina during insertion (though rare) and prolonged retention of the cap both contribute to changes in Pap smear results, and the Pap examination should be done before initial use, after three months' use, and then yearly (Hatcher, 1994). Allergy to latex or spermicides, presence of **pelvic inflammatory disease** (PID), or repeated urinary tract infections are contraindications to its use. It is also not recommended for use for 6 to 12 weeks after a full-term birth.

Male condom. The **condom** has been used since the time of the pharoahs in Egypt, though for decorative purposes at that time. The condom was later used to protect against venereal disease and was discovered that it also prevented pregnancy. A condom is basically a sheath that is placed over the erect penis to prevent semen from making contact with the vulva or vagina. A small pouch of airless space should be left at the tip of the condom to catch the ejaculate and to prevent the condom from tearing (Figure 5-8). After ejaculation, the penis must be withdrawn from the vagina while still erect, and care must be taken to prevent the condom from slipping off to prevent semen from entering the vagina. Should the accidental leakage of sperm occur, the insertion of a dose of spermicidal foam or jelly helps but still may not prevent pregnancy.

A spermicidal condom (a condom with a small amount of nonoxynol-9 on its inner and outer surfaces) is highly effective in killing sperm within the condom and in protecting against STDs.

Nursing intervention. This involves teaching the correct placement and removal of the condom, including precautions about the use of oils or petroleum-based products on the latex. Women should be encouraged to choose condoms for their partners. Discuss the differences between condoms for birth control and those for the prevention of STDs. The use of a condom to protect against infection when the woman is using a coitus-independent birth control method (pill, IUD, Norplant) should be emphasized, especially among adolescents.

Advantages. The effectiveness rate of the condom can be as high as 96% if it is used exactly as directed with each coital act. Effectiveness improves with the use of a spermicidal condom or with the use of both a condom and vaginal foam. No prescription is necessary. Condoms are inexpensive and readily available in any pharmacy and even from some vending machines in public restrooms.

Condom use encourages male participation in and responsibility for "safe sex." The condom has been found to be effective in preventing STDs, such as AIDS, trichomoniasis, herpes, chlamydia, gonorrhea, syphilis, and it also protects against reinfection from vaginal infections when one partner is under treatment.

Disadvantages. Typical user failure rates can be as high as 10% to 15%, depending on the study cited. Because the condom covers the glans, some men feel that it curtails some of the pleasurable sensations. To offset this, applying the condom before vaginal penetration can be part of foreplay. A small number of people are allergic to the latex condoms and must use the natural skin type instead, though skin-type condoms *do not* provide protection against STDs. For those who are allergic to latex, clinicians may recommend using the skin sheath underneath a latex condom to maintain protection against STDs.

Female condom. A vaginal pouch or condom for women is a soft polyurethane pouch that is lubricated inside with nonoxynol-9 and has two flexible rings at both ends. One ring surrounds the cervix to keep the pouch stable while the other ring remains outside the vagina to protect the perineum (Figure 5-9). The condom may be inserted up to 8 hours before intercourse, and since it is disposable, it should not be reused. The condom should be removed after intercourse, with care taken not to spill the ejaculate on the perineum. The female condom is approximately as effective as the male condom and theoretically offers excellent protection from STDs.

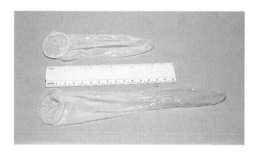

Figure 5-8 Condom. (Courtesy Michael Clement, MD.)

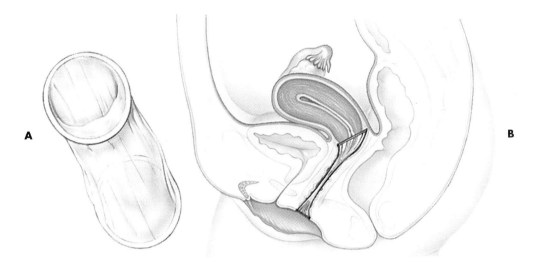

Figure 5-9   A, Female condom or vaginal pouch. **B,** Correctly inserted in vagina. The top ring covers the cervix. (Redrawn from Franklin M: *J Nurse Midwifery* 35(6):371, 1990.)

Nursing intervention. This involves teaching insertion and removal of the device. Provide information about protection against STDs and emphasize handwashing before and after insertion.

Advantages. The female condom is available for use without a prescription. It is less likely to tear than latex and is not affected by oil-based lubricants. The device protects against STDs as effectively as the male condom.

Disadvantages. Some users complain that the condom is difficult to insert and uncomfortable during intercourse for both partners.

Self-Discovery

Visit a drug store and note the cost (per unit) of over-the-counter (OTC) contraceptive methods. What do your findings suggest about compliance in using an OTC method? ~

Intrauterine device

The IUD is a highly effective form of birth control. It is inserted into the uterus and left there for 1 year (Progestasert, shown in Figure 5-10) or up to 10 years (Copper T-380 or ParaGard). The new Levonorgestrel IUD (LNg-20) is coated with a membrane regulating small daily release of levonorgestrel for up to 5 years. The LNg-20 is awaiting FDA approval and is expected to be on the market within the next few years. The GyneFix (CuFix) has a very low expulsion rate because it is anchored to the fundal muscle of the uterus; this device is currently in the testing phase (Van Kets et al, 1995).

In general the IUD is recommended for women who have been pregnant and are in a stable, monogamous relationship—essentially women determined to be at very low

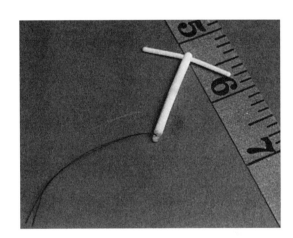

Figure 5-10   Progestasert IUD. (Courtesy Mark 6, New York.)

risk for STDs. Many developing countries have fostered its use because of its low cost and lengthy effectiveness. Most IUDs have been unavailable in the United states in the recent past, however, because of lawsuits involving the Dalkon shield. IUD use in the United States is around 2%; the majority of users are between 30 and 45 years of age.

Mode of action. Although the exact way in which IUDs prevent pregnancy is unclear, it seems that some local effects create a uterine environment hostile to implantation. The addition of metals (copper) and medications (progesterone and levonorgestrel) to the flexible polyethylene provide time-released action in minute amounts. Current theories concerning the mechanism of change within the uterus include the following:

- The IUD acts as a foreign body in the uterus, generating an inflammatory response in the endometrium and keeping it "out of phase" in the menstrual cycle. The inflammatory cells may be spermicidal or may damage the ova so that fertilization is impossible.

- An increase in the local production of prostaglandins inhibits implantation.
- Sperm seem to be immobilized as they pass through the uterine cavity; many fewer sperm are found in the fallopian tubes of IUD users. Ovum seems to move out of the tube more quickly.
- With the progesterone-type IUD, the cervical mucus becomes altered in consistency and the pH slows sperm transport.
- The copper may interfere with the intracellular metabolism within the endometrium.

Despite the presence of an IUD, implantation may occur, though rarely. Women who become pregnant with an IUD in place have an extremely high rate of spontaneous abortion (about 50%). The IUD can be removed early in pregnancy with the result of a lower spontaneous abortion rate. If the pregnancy continues, the IUD tends to become embedded in the maternal side of the placenta and the fetus usually is unharmed by the device. Long-range side effects of the medicated IUDs (copper or progesterone-releasing) on the fetus have not yet been determined. Opponents of the IUD argue that since implantation is prevented, the IUD is essentially an abortifacient (abortion-causing) device. A woman with ethical problems with abortion should be aware of this.

Nursing intervention. This involves obtaining a careful sexual history to determine a good candidate: a woman who is in a monogamous relationship with no history of pelvic infection and is post-birth. The early *danger signs* taught are listed in Box 5-1.

Teach the woman to wash her hands and to always check the position of the IUD string at the cervix. Use a backup method for the first few cycles after insertion. Some women are given prophylactic antibiotics at the time of insertion. Follow-up appointments are scheduled annually.

Advantages. The IUD is coitus independent. The copper-bearing IUD cost is minimal when it is calculated over the 10-year period; expenses include Pap smear, insertion of the IUD, and follow-up office or clinic visits. Failure rates vary in typical use: 0.1% for the LNg-20, 0.8% for Copper T-380, and 2.0% for Progestasert. Expulsion rates are lower and side effects such as cramping and heavy bleeding are less frequent for the progesterone-releasing IUDs. The Progestasert IUD releases 65 µg of the hormone, whereas LNg-20 releases only 20 µg daily, with virtually no systemic absorption for either device.

The ParaGard system is ideal for a woman who has completed her childbearing and desires a coitus-independent method without exposure to the hormonal effects of the birth control pill. The Progestasert method is ideal for the woman who wishes to delay pregnancy for a year or wishes to space a pregnancy. Most women who desire a pregnancy after the IUD is removed are able to conceive as rapidly as non-IUD users.

Disadvantages. The inflammatory process caused by the IUD may increase uterine contractility after insertion and thus result in expulsion of the device. Because the possibility of expulsion may continue for three or four subsequent menstrual cycles, a back-up method of contraception is necessary. A woman may initially experience cramping, heavy bleeding, or pelvic pain during menses. If these symptoms persist, the IUD may have to be removed. After menstruation and for about once a week thereafter, the woman must check with her finger for the nylon threads that protrude into the vagina through the cervix; this action may be distasteful for some women. If there is any doubt about the position or length of the string or if a cycle is missed, the woman should contact her clinician.

The woman with a Progestasert system is six to ten times more likely to have an ectopic pregnancy than the woman with a copper IUD. PID is a complication for all IUD users. The risk is reduced, however, if the woman has only one sexual partner. If an infection develops, the IUD should be removed immediately; vigorous antibiotic therapy will be prescribed.

TEST *Yourself* 5-2

What are three reasons why an IUD would not be recommended for a 25-year-old woman?
Explain why the IUD may be perceived as a device that may cause an abortion and therefore is not used by those who oppose abortion.

Hormonal Control: Oral Contraceptives

The **oral contraceptive (OC)**, also known as **the pill** has been on the market since the early 1960s. A steady decline in the dose of estrogens and progesterones in the pill has reduced serious estrogen-related side effects. Doses of estrogens now range from 20 to 50 µg as compared with the 50 to 150 µg range used in the 1960s. The primary action of the pill is the suppression of ovulation by inhibiting the hypothalamus, the pituitary, and the ovarian release of hormones. Follicle-stimulating hormone (FSH) and luteinizing hormone (LH) are suppressed. Secondary effects are the physiologic responses

Box 5-1

WARNING SIGNS

Intrauterine Device

- **P** Period late (pregnancy suspected), abnormal spotting or bleeding
- **A** Abdominal pain or pain with intercourse
- **I** Infection (abnormal vaginal discharge)
- **N** Not feeling well, fever, chills
- **S** Strings lost (shorter or longer)

of the endometrium, decreased fallopian tube motility, and change in the thickness and pH of cervical mucus. Two types of pills are on the market in the United States: the combined oral contraceptive (the pill) and the progesterone-only contraceptive (the mini-pill).

Combined regimen

Varied combinations of estrogen and progesterone in synthetic form compose the *combined* OC, which is available in three forms:

Monophasic pills contain synthetic estrogen and progesterone in each pill and must be taken for 21 or 28 days. In the 21-day pack the pill is taken for 21 days, then no pill is taken for the next 7 days, during which time menstruation will begin. The 28-day pack has 21 pills with medication and 7 pills with no medication (or with iron only) so that withdrawal bleeding begins during the 7 days.

Biphasic pills contain a certain level of estrogens throughout the cycle. To mimic body patterns in the 21-day pack, there is a small dose of progestins (synthetic progesterones) for 10 days and then a slightly higher dose for 11 days.

Triphasic pills alter the levels of estrogens and progesterones continuously throughout the cycle. The total monthly dose of hormones is less with triphasic pills than with mono- or biphasic pills. The clinician begins by prescribing the lowest possible dose.

Nursing intervention. This focuses on the need for education about oral contraceptive, on information about their method of use, and on the need for an alternate contraceptive method if pills are skipped. A thorough medical history and screening for underlying diabetes, hypertension, or high cholesterol levels will be part of the examination. A telephone follow-up is important. Many family planning providers require informed consent before prescribing oral contraceptives. A list of early danger signals may be included in the consent form (Hatcher et al, 1994) (Box 5-2).

Box 5-2

WARNING SIGNS

Potential Side Effects Associated with Oral Contraceptives

- **A** Abdominal pain (severe): may mean a gallbladder or liver problem
- **C** Chest pain (severe), cough, shortness of breath: may mean a blood clot
- **H** Headache (severe), dizziness, weakness, numbness: may mean hypertension or impending stroke
- **E** Eye problems (vision loss or blurring), speech problems: may mean stroke
- **S** Severe pain in leg, calf, or thigh: may mean blood clot

Failure to take tablets will interrupt the protection. Because of the low dose of the pills, a woman who forgets to take a pill for more than 12 hours must take the missed tablet and use a backup method for that cycle. One study found that missing up to 7 tablets may not be as important as the "timing of the omission in relation to the pill-free interval" (Korver, Goorissen, Guillebaud, 1995).

Advantages. Perfect use of the combined-regimen pill approaches 100% effectiveness. Typical use failure rates of up to 3% may occur because of human error, such as taking an antibiotic, forgetting a pill, having diarrhea or vomiting, and failure to use a backup method.

Coitus independence is achieved for women taking the pill, and many women experience greater satisfaction in the sexual act once the fear of pregnancy has been eliminated. Menses occurs more or less predictably, with a decreased flow.

Possible beneficial side effects of the combined-regimen pill include increased bone mineral density, alleviation of symptoms of premenstrual syndrome, and reduction or elimination of dysmenorrhea, endometriosis, menorrhagia, iron-deficiency anemia (because menstrual blood flow is decreased), benign breast disease, ovarian cysts, and rheumatoid arthritis (ACOG, 1994). Although recent research indicates a lower rate of ovarian and endometrial cancers among combined-regimen pill users (Vessey and Painter, 1995), the risk of cervical adenocarcinomas among long-term users seems to be increased (Ursin et al, 1994; Donovan and Klitsch, 1995). It is unknown whether this finding correlates with the woman's use of the pill or with the likelihood of her having an increased number of sexual partners as a result of "sexual freedom." Careful monitoring is necessary for susceptible women, including those whose mother or sisters have had breast, uterine, or cervical cancer. For healthy, non-smoking women older than 40 years of age, the benefits of preventing pregnancy may outweigh any risks of oral contraceptive use. Thus for most women, the pill has proven very safe.

Disadvantages. The main disadvantages of the combined-regimen pill lie in its side effects. Many of these side effects may be eliminated by careful selection of the ratio of estrogens to progesterone. Comparison of the different chemical formulations of progestins is also essential in choosing the correct pill because each different progestin has an estrogenic effect, an androgenic effect, and an antiestrogenic effect, and all must be tailored to the woman's physical needs. A physician may use an estrogen profile, which provides data on each woman's estrogen levels, to assist in the choice of an acceptable pill.

Side effects related to estrogens tend to mimic the unpleasant symptoms of early pregnancy: nausea, fluid retention, headaches, melasma (chloasma), breast tenderness and fullness, and occasionally blurred vision (Table 5-1). Changing to a lower dose may eliminate these effects.

Table 5-1	Results of Estrogen, Progesterone, and Androgen Excess	
Estrogen	**Progesterone**	**Androgens**
GASTROINTESTINAL SYSTEM		
Nausea, bloated feeling, weight gain	Increased appetite, real weight gain, cholestatic jaundice	Cholestatic jaundice
VASCULAR AND RENAL SYSTEMS		
Fluid retention, venous capillary engorgement	Dilated leg veins	
Occasional occurrence of spider nevi	Depression, nervousness, fatigue	
Headaches (migraine) and perhaps elevation of blood pressure		
A slight chance of thromboembolism in women at high risk		
MUSCULOSKELETAL SYSTEM	Increased muscle mass	Increased muscle mass
UTERUS		
Hypermenorrhea, increased size fibroids	Scanty, short menses, slight endometrial atrophy	
	Dysmenorrhea usually improves; sometimes breakthrough bleeding	
VAGINA		
Leukorrhea, excess secretion	Reduction in lining thickness and secretions; more Candida infection, pruritus	
BREASTS		
Mastaglia, possible enlargement of benign cysts	Regressing of breast tissue	Regression of breast tissue
	Tenderness	Inhibited lactation
SKIN		
Melasma (darkening of skin over nose and cheeks)	Possible occurrence of acne, hair loss, oily scalp	Acne, oily skin, rashes, hirsutism
GLUCOSE METABOLISM		
Increased levels in fasting state	Lowered carbohydrate tolerance	
Decreased glucose tolerance, increased insulin response to glucose		
LIBIDO		
Increased	Decreased	Decreased

Progesterone-related side effects include fatigue, depression, hirsutism, acne, oily skin and scalp, decreased libido, weight gain, headaches, pruritus, low-density lipoproteins (LDL) cholesterol levels, and decreased high-density lipoproteins (HDL) cholesterol levels. Breakthrough bleeding also occurs more often in the first two cycles of use, signifying endometrial adjustment to the new hormone levels. If spotting continues, the woman should see her clinician for reevaluation of the dosage regimen.

Other side effects are hypertension (disappearing when use of the pill is discontinued); acceleration of gallbladder disease in susceptible women; and alteration in certain laboratory data such as liver function tests, sedimentation and coagulation rates, and thyroid and other hormone function tests. Blurring or loss of vision requires immediate discontinuation of the pill. Some women experience a change in the corneal curvature of the eye, requiring a change in contact lenses or glasses.

RESEARCH

PURPOSE OF STUDY
To determine if there is an association between use of oral contraceptives and increasing bone mass density.

LITERATURE REVIEW
Postmenopausal osteoporosis is a health care problem affecting 20 million women in the United States, resulting in more than 1 million bone fractures a year. Total bone mass increases in women in their twenties, peaks in their thirties, then stabilizes or decreases until menopause. By age 50, approximately 10% of vertebral bone mass is lost.

METHOD
The study included 57 premenopausal women. Oral contraceptives were used by 24 of the women for at least 1 year. Bone mass density was measured in both groups.

FINDINGS AND IMPLICATIONS FOR PRACTICE
Bone mass density was significantly higher in the oral contraceptive users than in the nonusers. Bone mass density increased 1% for each year of oral contraceptive use. Oral contraceptives improve bone mass density in both premenopausal and postmenopausal women. It is thought that estrogen combined with progestin may offer the best bone-sparing effects while decreasing the associated risk of thrombosis.

DeCherney A: Bone sparing properties of oral contraceptives, *Am J Obstet Gynecol* 174(1):15, 1996.

During the first 6 weeks of lactation, women are advised against combined OCs because estrogens may diminish milk supply. Furthermore, long-range effects on the infant are unknown.

Postpill **amenorrhea** (abnormal stoppage of the menses) may occur more often in women who begin the pill close to menarche or who had a late menarche. No relationship has been demonstrated between postpill amenorrhea and the length of time the pill has been taken or the type of pill (Hatcher et al, 1994). There may be a delay in the ability to conceive among former pill users. Therefore a woman planning to become pregnant should discontinue the pill 6 to 18 months before she would like to conceive. At least three cycles off the pill are recommended before attempting to conceive. Finally, the pill can affect the proper metabolism of certain vitamins (especially C), and thus supplementation may be required.

Progesterone-only regimen

Progesterone-only oral contraceptives are called "**minipills**" because of the low dose of synthetic progesterone in them. The minipills contain the same progestins available in the combined-regimen oral contraceptive but in smaller doses. If minipills are taken for 21 days, ovulation is not suppressed but fertility is lowered. Pregnancy rates with perfect use are as low as 0.5%, but typical use pregnancy rates may be as high as 13%. Lactating women using the minipill achieve nearly 100% effectiveness.

Progesterone induces physiologic changes that interfere with the endometrial phase and the properties of the cervical mucus. The uterine environment thus becomes hostile to sperm motility and to implantation. Ovulation is inhibited by the alteration of the ovarian-pituitary hormonal interactions.

Nursing intervention. This includes teaching about the mode of action for minipills, the unpredictability of the menstrual cycle, and breakthrough bleeding. Stress that pills not be skipped and that another contraceptive method be used when the pill has been "forgotten." Since the pill is taken every day, it is usually harder to forget.

Advantages. The minipill contains less progesterone than the combined pill so that some of the progesterone-related side effects, including weight gain, candidal vaginitis, and acne, may not occur. Benefits of the minipill include the reduction in or elimination of menses, a decreased incidence of anemia, and a reduction in the presence of menstrual cramps and the pain associated with endometriosis. Its effects are reversed when it is discontinued. When lactating women want hormonal contraception, clinicians prescribe the minipill because it does not diminish the quantity of milk or adversely affect the infant's health. The minipill may be chosen by women older than 35, women unable to take estrogens, and women with a history of headaches or mild hypertension.

Disadvantages. Menstrual cycle disturbance is the most common disadvantage cited by women. Amenorrhea, the lack of cycle control, increased appetite and mild weight gain, and ectopic pregnancies all may occur. Functional ovarian cysts may occur more frequently.

Progesterone subdermal implants
FDA approval of the **Norplant subdermal implant** was given in 1991. This system provides slow release of the synthetic progestin levonorgestrel through six Silastic cylindric capsules placed (using a local anesthetic) under the skin on the inside upper portion of the woman's arm (Figure 5-11). The Norplant device can remain in place for up to 5 years and then must be removed surgically (also under local anesthetic). In 1994, nearly 200 lawsuits were filed against the manufacturer of the Norplant system alleging problems related to the implant: including scarring of tissue and difficulty in removal. (Klitsch, 1995). Problems of scarring and removal are being

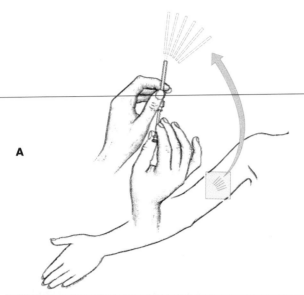

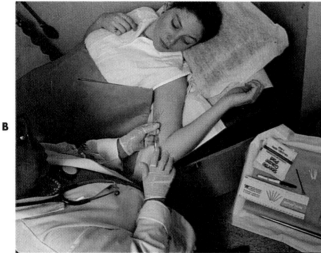

Figure 5-11 **A,** Norplant subdermal implant is one of the newest contraceptive devices. It contains six porous capsules of synthetic progestin. **B,** Capsules are placed just under the skin inside the upper portion of the arm. (**A,** From William C. Andrea; **B,** From Joel Gordon Photography.)

addressed (Shihata et al, 1995). Currently, the product has not been removed from the market.

The Norplant device acts in much the same manner as the progesterone-only minipill and thus has the similar advantages and disadvantages. Accidental pregnancy rates during the 5-year span are similar to surgical sterilization (Thomas and LeMelle, 1995). As a measure to help reduce the rates of adolescent pregnancy, Norplant holds promise because acceptability among teenagers is high (Polaneczky et al, 1994). Efforts to use Norplant in a school-based clinic in Baltimore met with political and social opposition among some groups who consider targeting inner city adolescents to receive Norplant as a

form of "ethnic genocide" (Beilinson, 1995). Clearly, much needs to be done to educate the public about the risks and benefits of Norplant.

Nursing intervention. This includes educating the Norplant user regarding early warning signs and how to care for the site after insertion. Possible complications from Norplant use include the following:

- Abdominal or referred pain (ectopic pregnancy)
- Heavy vaginal bleeding
- Infection and expulsion of a capsule
- Delayed menses after a long period of regular menses
- Migraine headaches or blurred vision

Advantages. The Norplant device has similar advantages as the progesterone-only pill. It seems to have a longer continuation rate than the pill, but this remains to be seen in light of the legal problems mentioned earlier. The Norplant device is coitus independent and desirable because it is immediately reversible when removed.

Disadvantages. The disadvantages are also similar to the progesterone-only pill. Amenorrhea is common in the first year of use, but there may be unpredictable heavy days of bleeding. Removal of the capsules is more difficult than insertion and requires more time. The initial cost is higher than the pill, but throughout a 5-year period it may be less. The pregnancy rate for women weighing more than 70 kg (154 lb) is higher during the 5-year period.

Injectable progestin

Injectable medroxyprogesterone acetate known as **Depo-Provera** (DMPA), was approved for use in the United States in 1992. A dose of 150 mg is given intramuscularly every 12 weeks to inhibit ovulation by suppressing FSH and LH levels. Cervical mucous properties change to make fluids inhospitable to sperm. The first-year failure rate is as low as 0.3%.

Nursing intervention. This includes teaching the effects of DMPA on the menstrual cycle: irregular bleeding patterns, the occurrence of amenorrhea and breakthrough bleeding, and the side effects of progesterone-only pills. Before making a decision about this method, the woman must be informed about the possible risks of breast cancer or osteoporosis with long-term use. Annual health screenings with Pap smear, breast examination and mammog-

CULTURAL AWARENESS

Discuss the implications in the earlier statement that using Norplant subdermal implant contraception for inner city teenagers is a form of ethnic genocide. Is coercion of the teenagers involved?

raphy, and a test of bone density for osteoporosis may be planned by the clinician.

Advantages. The DMPA injections provide contraceptive coverage for longer than 3 months and thus provide protection even if the woman is late for the injection. Amenorrhea may be a welcomed side effect and the incidence of amenorrhea increases the longer a woman uses the DMPA method. The injection is a good choice for a highly effective contraceptive for a short period. Lactating women may safely use this method.

Disadvantages. The common complaint against DMPA is weight gain. Headaches and depression may cause concern. Since there is a slight chance of allergic reaction to the injection, the woman should remain in the facility for a short period after receiving the injection. A decrease in libido sometimes occurs. Finally, a visit every 3 months is difficult for some women.

Postcoital choices

"Morning after" pills are highly effective when used within 72 hours after unprotected midcycle intercourse. **Postcoital contraception** either prevents fertilization or stops the fertilized egg from implanting. Though it is legal and effective, availability is not well advertised. Several postcoital choices exist; a progestogen such as Ovral, an androgen such as Danazol, or an antiprogesterone such as RU 486 may be used (Barnhart and Sondheimer, 1994). Emergency contraception is most effective when used within 24 hours of unprotected intercourse. The risk of contraception is reduced by about 75% with these methods. Considerable resistance to RU 486 still exists because of its controversial abortion-inducing effect when used with prostaglandins. It has been used with considerable success in Europe for postcoital contraception (Baulieu, 1994).

Nursing intervention. This includes guidance about the medication and explanation of side effects. The method is only for *emergency* contraception because of the expected side effects of nausea, vomiting, dizziness, and headache, which subside after the treatment is complete. The subsequent menses usually begins within 3 weeks.

Advantages. The potential for reducing the number of unwanted pregnancies and abortions is good because of its safety and effectiveness. The method is simple and available.

Disadvantages. The lack of general knowledge about the method and the importance of obtaining it within 72 hours is the main disadvantage. For instance, clinics may be closed on weekends.

TEST *Yourself* 5-3 _____

List at least five factors to be considered before choosing a contraceptive method.

Surgical sterilization

Surgical sterilization is usually a permanent measure and should be undertaken only after a great deal of consideration. Though best if both partners sign the informed consent, it is legal in most states when only the client signs. If the person relies on federal or state funding for the procedure, the following regulations apply: the individual must be at least 21 years of age and be mentally competent. Many states require a waiting period of 30 to 90 days between the time that the consent is signed and the procedure is performed. Though surgical sterilization is not considered 100% effective and pregnancies do occur, the failure rate may be lower than 1%, depending upon the surgical technique.

Since psychologic implications accompany the loss of reproductive ability, the person choosing the option of sterilization must explore personal feelings. Reproductive prowess often is equated with the degree of "maleness" or "femaleness" a person feels. Loss of reproductive ability may lower self-esteem. Most men and women who undergo surgical sterilization, however, are not adversely affected. In fact, with fear of unwanted pregnancy gone, many couples report improvement in their sex lives and more frequent intercourse.

Female sterilization. Several surgical techniques exist for sterilization of women. **Tubal ligation** involves tying, clipping, occluding the tubes, and removing the fimbriated ends of the tubes (Figure 5-12). Most approaches make use of a laparoscopy to perform a minilaparotomy, which leaves a small abdominal incision.

The best time for a tubal ligation is within 24 to 48 hours after the woman has given birth, when the tubes have been displaced toward the anterior part of the abdomen and are easily visualized. Local anesthesia can be used. When the procedure is performed on an outpatient basis, the woman may be sent home within a few hours if she is stable. Recovery may be delayed, but there usually are few complications.

The woman may require an analgesic for postoperative pain. She should rest for a few days after the surgery and avoid heavy lifting for a week. Side effects are minimal, and uterine function is not altered. Ovulation still occurs, but the ovum is absorbed into the peritoneal cavity.

Reversal of tubal ligation has become more promising with the use of microsurgical techniques. Pregnancy rates after reversing female surgical sterilization range from 43% to 88%, depending on the technique. Reversal is expensive, requires major surgery, and is not an option for most women (Hatcher et al, 1994).

Advantages and disadvantages. The procedure is safe and recovery is rapid. Coitus independence is achieved, and contraception is permanent and highly effective for the woman whose family is "complete" or who is nearing menopause. Women unsure about their desire to have more children should not use this method. The procedure

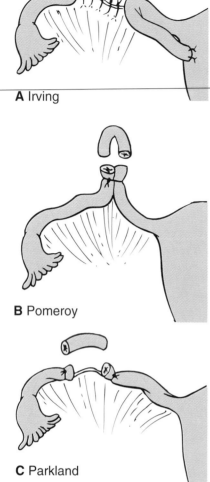

Figure 5-12   Tubal ligation.

A Irving

B Pomeroy

C Parkland

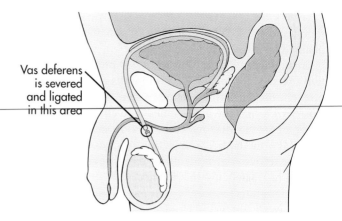

Vas deferens is severed and ligated in this area

Figure 5-13   Vasectomy. Vas deferens has been tied off and severed. Sperm cannot enter ejaculatory duct.

is initially expensive and the method provides no protection against STDs.

Male sterilization. Vas ligation or **vasectomy** is a common form of surgical sterilization and can be performed in the physician's office under local anesthesia. It does not affect the production of male hormones, and sperm, or the ability to have an erection, nor does it alter sexual function. The vas deferens is severed, making passage of the sperm from the testes to the urethra impossible (Figure 5-13). Postoperative care may involve the use of mild analgesics for pain, ice packs on the scrotum intermittently for swelling, and scrotal support. No heavy lifting should be done until the incision has healed. Side effects are rare but can include infection, hematoma, or small spermatic granulomas (ACOG, 1996).

Abstinence from sexual intercourse is required only until the incision heals (approximately 3 days). Sterility is achieved when a minimum of 15 ejaculations have occurred because sperm remain in the area beyond the ligation. The couple is advised to use another method of birth control until analysis confirms that two samples are free of sperm. The man should bring a specimen of the ejaculate for a sperm count 2 to 3 months after surgery and again at 1 year.

Advantages and disadvantages. The cost of a vasectomy is less than the cost of tubal ligation. Responsibility for contraception is shared, and chemicals, barriers, or hormones do not have to be considered any longer. Vasectomized men are not at increased risk for cardiovascular disease. Reversibility is possible with varying results, though surgery for this is expensive. Fifty percent or more of vasectomized men develop antibodies against their own sperm and thus may remain infertile despite a successful reversal. Current studies find no relationship between prostate cancer and vasectomy; protocols for screening vasectomized men remain the same as for the general male population (Hatcher et al, 1994).

Research methods

Many methods currently under investigation in the United States are being used freely in other parts of the world. In this country, stringent FDA guidelines and clinical trials require long-range study of the safety and effectiveness of all new methods. Research funding for innovative methods has dwindled because of fears of litigation by the manufacturers.

Male methods. A nonlatex condom has recently been introduced that has less sensation interference, is nonallergenic, and has more resistance to breakage. Drugs such as testosterone and androgen-related hormones are being tested with progestins to reduce the side effects of solely male hormone injections (Ringheim, 1995). Alexander (1995) reported on research that focuses on changing the sperm's ability to penetrate the ovum. A vaccine to influence the maturation process of sperm is also being investigated (Griffin, 1994).

Female methods. Vaccines that are effective for about a year are currently under study. These substances may provide immunity against sperm or ovum. Since immune responses vary widely, a great deal of work still must be done.

Disposable diaphragms with spermicide included are being studied. Lea's Shield, a silicone dome similar to the diaphragm, is in clinical trials. Lea's Shield has a small loop for easier insertion and removal (Archer et al, 1995). A nonsurgical sterilization technique using quinacrine pellets is being tested but may not be available for many years in this country (Hieu et al, 1993). Finally, there is research on kits that are able to predict ovulation using saliva (Barbato, Pandolfi, Guida, 1993).

There is a chance birth control pills may be sold without prescription within the next decade. Pills taken once a month are being studied. A donut-shaped vaginal ring that releases progesterone may be available within the next few years. This ring would remain in place for 3 weeks and be removed during menses. Norplant developers are working on a double or single-rod system and/or a biodegradable system that dissolves in the body. These new implants would have a shorter life span than the ones currently used. New spermicides that reduce the risk of STDs without changing vaginal flora are being formulated and frameless IUDs that eliminate cramping are also being developed.

Issues to consider

Contraception has been an important issue throughout history. Women who choose to control their own fertility applaud and encourage advances in contraceptive methods. As vehicles for political gain, religious fervor or social change, contraceptive innovations may be used in a way that usurps the woman's control of her own fertility. Attempts by many to deny funding for family planning agencies that also provide elective abortion procedures deny a segment of the population access to reproductive choices.

Proposals to withhold or limit social welfare benefits for families with more than a specified number of children would force these families to prevent pregnancy or else lose the ability to feed and clothe their children. Enforced contraception has surfaced regarding judicial punishment for the crime of child abuse as witnessed by the 1990 *State of California vs. Darlene Johnson* case in which Judge Harold Broadman ordered Darlene Johnson, convicted of child abuse, to obtain a Norplant device or face several years in jail. Similar cases of enforced or coerced contraception appear in certain states that withhold or limit public assistance for women who give birth to a large number of children. The fundamental flaw in the imposition of these policies is the assumption that contraception will somehow cure the child abuser or that the problems of poverty may be alleviated by simply limiting family size (Charo, 1992).

The American Medical Association (AMA) Board of Trustees has taken a strong stand against the political imposition of contraception, pointing out that the freedom to procreate, to refuse medical intervention, and to exercise personal choice in contraception are constitutional rights (Board of Trustees, AMA, 1992).

Box 5-1
CLINICAL DECISION

Mrs. J, 35, is an unemployed single parent of four dependent children. List the advantages and disadvantages of at least three contraceptive choices for her.

Nursing Responsibilities

Contraception has become an integral part of life for many people. Each birth control method available today has risks and benefits associated with its use, and each method carries responsibilities on the part of the user to learn about its side effects, advantages, and disadvantages. All education about fertility control is based on a firm understanding of the anatomy and physiology of reproduction. Using this knowledge, nurses can provide counsel and support to individuals that will enable them to make informed decisions. By becoming truly involved in the broader issues of global concern related to reproductive issues, the nurse makes a further commitment to prevent the subjugation of women and to foster reproductive rights and choices.

ASSESSMENT

To create an accurate picture of the client's needs, the nurse plays a role in acquiring pertinent information, in obtaining a sexual history to identify any dysfunction, in determining whether the couple wishes to delay or prevent pregnancy, and in learning the religious or cultural beliefs that may affect the choice of contraceptive.

Consider the following factors about the contraceptive user when gathering data:

- Educational level
- Socioeconomic level and stress factors
- Age and prior experience with contraception
- Cultural and religious beliefs, myths, and misinformation
- General physical health (careful attention to allergies, e.g., latex and spermicides)
- Motivation levels and career goals
- Menstrual or obstetric history
- Satisfaction with current method

NURSING DIAGNOSES

If a person is experienced with a particular method and is educated and motivated, the nurse may need only to provide new information about the chosen method. In this instance, nursing diagnoses may include the following:

- Health-seeking behavior regarding the chosen method and its use, side effects, and the results it is expected to provide

- Knowledge deficit related to learning about the method and how to apply it
- Altered health maintenance related to the requirements of the method (e.g., the use of the pill or use of other medications while taking the pill)

In a different situation, such as for a young teenager, the nursing diagnoses may need to include more extensive counseling and preparation in the following areas:

- Knowledge deficit regarding availability, advantages, and disadvantages of contraceptive options
- Health-seeking behavior regarding the menstrual cycle, times of peak fertility, and choices of contraceptive method
- Potential for noncompliance in contraceptive use and the degree of protection from STDs the method offers
- Potential for infection that may result from overuse of spermicides, lack of hygiene, or lack of information

EXPECTED OUTCOMES

As part of the process in establishing the appropriate method, the nurse and the client set goals to do the following:

- Select a method appropriate to his or her needs and desires.
- Describe or demonstrate the correct procedure for use.
- List advantages, expected side effects, and precautions to remember.
- Verbalize the need to contact the clinician should harmful side effects or questions arise about the use of the method.
- Report satisfaction or dissatisfaction with the chosen method.

NURSING INTERVENTION

Encouraging open communication between the health care provider and the client is the foundation for nursing intervention. Actions that minimize stress, foster active decision making, and maintain health will maximize the potential for success. For example, when teaching a method that requires manipulation (diaphragm or cervical cap) the nurse explains what to expect and remains available for the

woman's questions or concerns. The nurse's active participation helps lower the woman's anxiety and it also facilitates learning the successful use of contraception, which requires self-monitoring (see the following Clinical Decision).

Box 5-2

CLINICAL DECISION

Teresa is 16 and sexually active, though she is embarrassed to talk about it. She is seeking a contraceptive and you have a chance to counsel her. How would you begin the conversation?

Teaching is an integral part of the nursing care plan for the person desiring birth control. Teaching aids are useful, and the literature available from manufacturers of birth control methods should be given to the client for review at home. Information should include the correct procedure for using a particular method, the advantages and disadvantages of it, risks associated with its use, a demonstration and return demonstration of its correct use, and a discussion concerning unusual circumstances that may arise (such as missed pills or broken condoms) (see Figure 5-13).

EVALUATION

Evaluation entails detecting whether the contraceptive user finds the method satisfactory and also determining whether pregnancy has been prevented. Unacceptable side effects prompt many to seek another method. Determining whether the client has achieved the desired outcomes is not easy. The nurse looks for the following whenever possible:

- Was the client able to describe the use of the chosen method?
- Did the client demonstrate correct use of the method and is the client aware of the problems for which the clinician should be notified?
- Does the client know when to return to the clinic or office for follow-up?

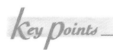

Key points

- Methods based on natural body rhythms are gaining wide acceptance within stable, monogamous relationships because of low cost and increased effectiveness.
- The HIV epidemic has resulted in an increased emphasis on methods that provide an effective disease barrier, such as the correct use of the condom.

- OTC methods are popular but expensive for consistent use. Thus user "forgetfulness" plays a major role in lowered success ratings.
- TSS has occurred with the diaphragm and cervical cap when these devices are left in place longer than recommended.

■ Exposure to STDs must be taken into account when choosing a contraceptive method.

■ The effectiveness of the IUDs depends on the woman's reaction to bleeding, inflammation, and cramping. Those who can tolerate these early effects will find this coitus-independent method quite satisfactory.

■ Hormonal control of fertility seeks to mimic body responses to pregnancy by inhibiting the hypothalamus and the pituitary glands, as well as ovarian hormones.

■ Side effects of the pill mimic early pregnancy. Today low-dose preparations are acceptable to many women.

■ Low-dose progesterone, in pill, implant, or injection form, is an increasingly popular contraceptive method with few side effects.

■ Sterilization is a widely used contraceptive method because of its long-term results. Minisurgery has increased in popularity for both men and women.

Study Questions

5-1. Select the terms that apply to the following statements:
  a. Hormonal methods and sterilization are unrelated to the act of intercourse and thus are _____.
  b. The latex version of the _____ offers protection against HIV infection if used correctly.
  c. The rate of effectiveness that includes reality factors is called _____.
  d. A chemical that stops or kills sperm is called _____.
  e. Women at risk for pelvic inflammatory disease should not use the _____.

5-2. The diaphragm is an effective method of contraception:
  a. When used with spermicide along the rim and inner surface.
  b. Only during the peak fertile time.
  c. When removed within 1 hour of intercourse.
  d. That can be obtained OTC.

5-3. The LAM may be used successfully:
  a. Up to a year after childbirth.
  b. While the mother is supplementing her infant's feedings.
  c. Only if a woman is amenorrheal during lactation.
  d. Instead of a diaphragm.

5-4. Coitus interruptus:
  a. Provides excellent protection from pregnancy.
  b. Provides protection from HIV.
  c. May be used when no other method is available.
  d. May be used successfully by most teenagers.

5-5. The *main* advantage of using Norplant subdermal implant is:
  a. Coitus independence.
  b. Ease of insertion and removal.
  c. Lack of side effects.
  d. The popularity among older women.

5-6. NFP is an effective method of contraception for:
  a. The postpartum mother.
  b. An adolescent having her first sexual experience.
  c. A married woman with one child.
  d. A single mother of three.

References

Alexander CS, Guyer B: Adolescent pregnancy: occurrence and consequences, *Pediatr Ann* 22(2):85, 1993.

Alexander NJ: Future contraceptives, *Sci Am* 136:141, 1995.

American College of Obstetricians and Gynecologists: *Hormonal Contraception,* Technical Bulletin No. 198, 1994, The College.

American College of Obstetricians and Gynecologists: *Sterilization,* Technical Bulletin 222, 1996, The College.

Archer DF et al: Lea's shield: a phase I postcoital study of a new contraceptive barrier device, *Contraception* 52:167, 1995.

Barbato M, Pandolfi A, Guida M: A new diagnostic aid for natural family planning, *Adv Contracep* 9(4):335, 1993.

Barnhart KT, Sondheimer SJ: Emergency contraception, *Curr Opin Obstet Gynecol* 6:559, 1994.

Baulieu EE: RU 486: a compound that gets itself talked about, *Hum Reprod* 9(1):1, 1994.

Beilinson PL, Miola ES, Farmer M: Politics and practice: introducing Norplant into a school-based health center in Baltimore, *Am J Public Health* 85(3):309, 1995.

*Billings EL et al: Symptoms and hormonal changes accompanying ovulation, *Lancet* 282:4, 1972.

Board of Trustees, American Medical Association: Requirements or incentives by government for use of long-acting contraceptives, *JAMA* 267(13):1818, 1992.

Brinton LA et al: Oral contraceptives and breast cancer risk among younger women, *J Natl Cancer Inst* 87:827, 1995.

Brown RT et al: Adolescent sexuality and issues in contraception, *Obstet Gynecol Clin North Am* 19(1):177, 1992.

Cavero C: Using an ovarian monitor as an adjunct to natural family planning, *J Nurse Midwifery* 40(3):269, 1995.

Charo RA: Mandatory contraception, *Lancet* 339:1104, 1992.

Creatsas GK: Sexuality: sexual activity and contraception during adolescence, *Curr Opin Obstet Gynecol* 5:774, 1993.

Diczfalusy E: Contraceptive prevalence, reproductive health, and our common future, *Contraception* 43(3):201, 1991.

Diczfalusy E: Contraceptive prevalence, reproductive health, and international morality, *Am J Obstet Gynecol* 166(4):1037, 1992.

Diczfalusy E: Reproductive health: a rendezvous with human dignity, *Contraception* 52:1, 1995.

Djerassi C: The mother of the pill, *Recent progress in hormone research* 50:1, 1995.

Donovan P: Failure rates for the female condom are moderate; incorrect use is common, *Fam Plann Perspect* 27(3):132, 1995.

Donovan P, Klitsch M: Oral contraceptive users may be at some increased risk of cervical carcinoma, *Fam Plann Perspect* 27(3):134, 1995.

Dugoff L et al: Assessing the acceptability of Norplant contraceptive in four patient populations, *Contraception* 52:45, 1995.

Edwards SR: The role of men in contraceptive decision-making: current knowledge and future implications, *Fam Plann Perspect* 26(2):77, 1994.

Eldridge GD et al: Barriers to condom use and barrier method preferences among low income African-American women, *Women Health* 23(1):73, 1995.

Erwin PC: To use or not use combined hormonal oral contraceptives during lactation, *Fam Plann Perspect* 26(1):26, 1994.

Faundes A, Elias C, Coggins C: Spermicides and barrier contraception, *Curr Opin Obstet Gynecol* 6:552, 1994.

Fehring RD: New technology in natural family planning, *J Obstet Gynecol Neonatal Nurs* 20(3):199, 1991.

Freedman LP, Isaacs SL: Human rights and reproductive choice, *Stud Fam Plan* 24(1):18, 1993.

Frost JJ, Forrest JD: Understanding the impact of effective teenage pregnancy prevention programs, *Fam Plan Perspect* 27(5):188, 1995.

Gladwell M: *Rating contraceptives,* Washington Post, p 37, Jan 4-10 (national weekly edition), 1993.

Grady WR, Tanfer K: Condom breakage and slippage among men in the United States, *Fam Plann Perspect* 26(3):107, 1994.

Griffin PD: Immunization against HCG, *Hum Reprod* 9(2):267, 1994.

Hanna KM: Effect of nurse-client transaction on female adolescents' oral contraceptive adherence, *Image J Nurs Sch* 25(4):285, 1993.

Hatcher RA et al: *Contraceptive technology 1994-1996,* ed 16, New York, 1994, Irvington Publishers.

Hieu DT et al: 31,781 cases of non-surgical female sterilization with quinacrine pellets in Vietnam, *Lancet* 342:213, 1993.

Hillard PJA: Family planning in the teen population, *Curr Opin Obstet Gynecol* 5:798, 1993.

Hinkle LT: Education and counseling for Norplant users, *J Obstet Gynecol Neonatal Nurs* 23(5):387, 1994.

Jimenez SLM: The Hispanic culture, folklore, and perinatal health, *J Perinatal Educ* 4(1):9, 1995.

Klitsch M: Still waiting for the contraceptive revolution, *Fam Plann Perspect* 27(6):246, 1995.

Korver T, Goorissen E, Guillebaud J: The combined oral contraceptive pill: what advice should we give when tablets are missed? *Br J Obstet Gynaecol* 102(8):601, 1995.

Lethbridge DJ: Choosing and using a contraception: toward a theory of women's contraceptive self care, *Nurs Res* 40(5):276, 1991.

Lethbridge DJ: Fertility management in Taiwanese and African-American women, *J Obstet Gynecol Neonatal Nurs* 24(5):459, 1995.

Mastroianni L, Robinson C: Contraception in the 1990s, *Patient Care* 107:118, 1994.

Mellanby A, Phelps F, Tripp JH: Teenagers, sex and risk-taking, *BMJ* 307(3):25, 1993.

Mosher WD: Contraceptive practice in the United States, 1982-1988, *Fam Plann Perspect* 22(5):198, 1990.

Moskowitz EH, Jennings B, Callahan D: *Long-acting contraceptives: ethical guidance for policymakers and health care providers,* Hastings Center Report, Special Supplement S1-S8, Jan/Feb 1995.

Oakley A et al: Sexual health education interventions for young people: a methodological review, *BMJ* 310:158, 1995.

Omran AR: *Family planning in the legacy of Islam,* London, 1992, Routledge.

Parker DA, Harford TC, Rosenstock IM: Alcohol, other drugs, and sexual risk-taking among young adults, *J Subst Abuse* 6(1):87, 1994.

Polaneczky JA: *Norplant and irresponsible reproduction,* Hastings Center Report, Special Supplement S23-S26, Jan/Feb 1995.

Polanecsky M et al: The use of levonorgestrel implants (Norplant) for contraception in adolescent mothers, *N Engl J Med* 331:1201, 1994.

Powderly KE: *Contraceptive policy and ethics: illustrations from American history,* Hastings Center Report, Special Supplement S9-S11, Jan/Feb 1995.

Ringheim K: Evidence for the acceptability of an injectable hormonal method for men, *Fam Plann Perspect* 27(3):123, 1995.

Rojnik B et al: Initiation of contraception postpartum, *Contraception* 51:75, 1995.

Rosenberg MJ et al: Compliance and oral contraceptives: a review, *Contraception* 52:137, 1995.

Rosenthal SL et al: Experience with side effects and health risks associated with Norplant implant use in adolescents, *Contraception* 52:283, 1995.

Ryder B, Campbell H: Natural family planning in the 1990s, *Lancet* 346:233, 1995.

Ryder REJ: Natural family planning: effective birth control supported by the Catholic Church, *BMJ* 307:723, 1993.

Schenker JG, Rabenou V: Family planning: cultural and religious perspectives, *Hum Reprod* 8(6):969, 1993.

Shihata AA et al: Innovative technique for Norplant implants removal, *Contraception* 51:83, 1995.

Spira A: Contraception by the end of the 20th century, *Hum Reprod* 9(3):445, 1994.

Steinbock B: *Coercion and long-term contraceptives,* Hastings Center Report, Special Supplement S19-S22, Jan/Feb, 1995.

Thomas AG, LeMelle SM: The Norplant system: where are we in 1995? *J Fam Pract* 40(2):125, 1995.

Trussell J et al: Contraceptive efficacy of the female condom and other barrier methods, *Fam Plann Perspect* 26(2):66, 1994.

Trussel J et al: The economic value of contraception: a comparison of 15 methods, *Am J Public Health* 85(4):494, 1995.

Tyrer LB: Current controversies and future direction of oral contraceptives, *Curr Opin Obstet Gynecol* 5:833, 1993.

United Nations International Conference on Women (Beijing) Sections C and C2, Articles 91-108, September, 1995.

*Classic reference.

Ursin G et al: Oral contraceptive use and adenocarcinoma of the cervix, *Lancet* 344:1390, 1994.

Van Kets H et al: IUD expulsion solved with implant technology, *Contraception* 51:87, 1995.

Vessey MP, Painter R: Endometrial and ovarian cancer and oral contraceptives—findings in a large cohort study, *British J Cancer* 71(6):1340, 1995.

Visser AP, Bruyniks N, Remennick L: Family planning in Russia: experience and attitudes of gynecologists, *Adv Contracept* 9(2):93, 1993.

Waxman, BK: Up against eugenics: disabled women's challenge to receive reproductive health services, *Sexuality and Disability* 12(2):155, 1994.

Wilcox AJ, Weinberg CR, Baird DD: Timing of sexual intercourse in relation to ovulation: effects on the probability of conception, survival of the pregnancy, and sex of the baby, *N Engl J Med* 333(23):1517, 1995.

Zachariasen RD: Loss of oral contraceptive efficacy by concurrent antibiotic administration, *Women Health* 22(1):17, 1994.

Zotti ME, Siegel E: Preventing unplanned pregnancies among married couples: are services for only the wife sufficient? *Res Nurs Health* 18:133, 1995.

Student Resource Shelf

Monsen RB, Jackson CP, Livingston M: Having a future: sexual decision making in early adolescence, *J Pediatr Nurs* 11(3):183, 1996.
Research that explores the thinking of 12- to 14-year-old adolescents who are becoming sexually active. Discusses ways to enhance the adolescents' sense of having a future unburdened by early pregnancy.

Westoff CL: Current assessment of the use of IUDs, *J Nurse Midwifery* 41(3):218, 1996.
A history of the IUD and a discussion of current IUDs and their potential for safe and effective long-term contraception.

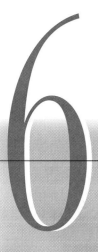

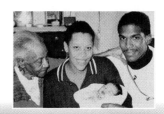

6

Infertility Care

ANALYSIS OF INFERTILITY

For most people, the desire to give birth, to nurture an infant, and to experience parenthood is a basic human need. In the Bible, the story of Abraham and Sarah centers on having a son in their old age (Genesis 17 and 21). For many, the deep longing to procreate is primordial. The "baby boom" generation (those born between 1946 and 1964), many of whom delayed childbearing to pursue educational or career goals, have created demands for reproductive technology as a cure for infertility (Mosher et al, 1991). Delayed childbearing may have an adverse effect on fertility as a progressive decline in fertility is noted after age 35 in the woman and man (Lansac, 1995). A diagnosis of infertility may call into question the self-esteem, goals, aspirations, future plans, and lifestyle of a couple.

Infertility may be perceived as an acute and unanticipated life crisis that may engender grief and guilt (Greil, 1991). Whether the infertile partners choose to pursue the dream of procreation often depends upon the financial abilities, health insurance coverage, emotional support of extended family and friends, and the ability to survive the inevitable emotional turmoil. Caring for the couple with impaired fertility has become a thriving subspecialty of reproductive care. Nurses in this field need to be especially sensitive to the crises that the diagnosis may incur.

Infertility is the inability to achieve conception after 1 year of unprotected intercourse. **Primary infertility** occurs when a couple has never had a child; either the woman has never conceived, or the man has never fathered a child. **Secondary infertility** occurs when a couple has been able to conceive one or more times (regardless of outcome) but has been unable to sustain a current pregnancy. In **unexplained infertility,** no definite cause for the infertility can be found. **Sterility** means that conception is not possible.

Approximately 10% to 15% of couples of childbearing age in the United States are infertile. Factors that cause infertility are almost equally divided between men and women. Unexplained causes may underlie 10% to 15% of infertility cases (Lobo, 1993). In approximately 35% of these couples there are multiple etiologies.

Nursing care usually emphasizes the *couple* as the focus of care. Simultaneous evaluation of both partners is frequently done to ensure an accurate assessment. Nursing care is aimed at the partnership—every intervention has an impact on both people. If one partner receives the diagnosis of infertility or if the infertility remains unexplained, both partners are affected. Once the diagnosis occurs, the partners may undergo a process of grieving for the "lost" procreative identity with its concomitant phases of shock, denial, anger, guilt, depression, and finally resolution (Hirsch and Hirsch, 1995). Male virility and womanliness (or femininity) are frequently intertwined with one's ability to reproduce, therefore infertility may also be inferred as a loss of sexual identity as a man or a woman. Partners may not be in synchrony in terms of the reaction to each aspect of infertility. For instance, the woman may be in the process of denial while the man may be angry or depressed. Nursing care focuses on what the individual may be experiencing but is always mindful of the couple and their relationship. Because the woman in the infertile partnership often carries the greater burden of physical, emotional, and social consequences, it is important to consider the partners as separate and individual as well (Sandelowski, 1994). Frequently the male partner feels excluded from the hub of activities surrounding the woman. Validating his central importance in the process is important. Nursing intervention involves focusing on the most intimate and private aspects of a couples' existence: their sexuality and shared marital intimacy. Sensitivity and respect for the partners' privacy are essential for goal-directed care of infertile partners.

Factors Favoring Fertility

The success or failure of conception depends on many factors, all of which rely on appropriate physiologic function of the reproductive organs (see Chapter 3 for a more detailed description of the menstrual cycle). (See Table 6-1 for elements favoring conception.) The process of conception is possible only during a small number of days in the middle of the menstrual cycle (Wilcox, 1995). Follicle-stimulating hormones (FSH) and luteinizing hormones (LH) trigger ovarian release of estrogens and progesterone that in turn directly affect the cervical, vaginal, and tubal mucosa to respond in ways favoring entry of the sperm. The ovaries respond to FSH stimulation by allowing the follicle to ripen and release a mature ovum. The anatomy of the female reproductive tract must be patent throughout the vagina, cervix, uterus, and fallopian tubes to allow for upward movement of the sperm and for clear passageway of the ova from the ovaries through the fimbriated ends of the fallopian tubes into the uterus. The endometrium must have the appropriate response to hormonal stimulation to be able to nurture and sustain the fertilized ovum (Figure 6-1). Finally, the psychogenic factor, although little understood, needs further study to determine the influence of factors that "allow a baby to come" (Christie, 1994).

The male reproductive organs also respond to the pituitary hormone influences of FSH and LH that affect the testosterone levels and production and motility of sperm in the testes (see Chapter 3 for a more detailed description of the male reproductive physiology). Adequate numbers and effective motility of sperm are essential for the successful travel through the female reproductive tract. Male reproductive anatomy should be patent and anatomically favorable to the deposit of sperm near the woman's cervix. The prostate gland needs to produce the appropriate amount, viscosity, and pH of fluid to aid in the transport of sperm through the female reproductive tract.

CAUSES OF INFERTILITY

When infertility is suspected, investigation of the causes progresses from the simple to the more complex. A detailed health history and physical examination of each partner occurs so the obvious causes of infertility can be ruled out before the couple undergoes further costs in time, money, or emotional and physical stress. For instance, the health history may include assessment of the timing and frequency of sexual intercourse; physical assessment of the reproductive organs; and determination of the presence of chronic disease, nutritional deficiencies, alcohol or drug dependencies, psychologic problems, or recurrent reproductive tract infections.

Table 6-1　Factors Favoring Fertility

Men	Women
REPRODUCTIVE FACTORS	
Unobstructed urethra	Unobstructed tubes
Functioning epididymis, vas deferens, and prostate	Tubal fluids and cilia favoring proper movement of ovum and sperm in tube
Descended testes	
No congenital anomalies	Endometrium adequately prepared to receive fertilized ovum
Normal secretions of genital tract	Cervical mucus receptive to sperm
Ability to penetrate vagina	Cervix competent
Ejaculate deposited at cervix (no retrograde ejaculation or hypospadias)	No congenital anomalies impairing free passage between cervix and tubes
SEX CELL REPRODUCTION	
Normal spermatogenesis producing mature spermatozoa	Normal maturation of graafian follicle and release of ovum
Spermatozoa with adequate numbers and motility	Normal oogenesis producing mature ova
HORMONAL FACTORS	
Hypothalamus-pituitary-gonadal functioning intact	Hypothalamus-pituitary-gonadal functioning intact
Adequate testosterone production	Adequate ovarian hormone production of estrogen and progesterone

Certain occupations or lifestyles pose an increased risk for men and women (e.g., firefighters and workers exposed to hazardous wastes or radiation). In addition, women who have had multiple elective abortions with cervical scarring, abdominal surgery for a ruptured appendix, laparotomies, multiple sexual partners, dramatic alterations in weight, or untreated pelvic inflammatory disease (PID) are at a higher risk for infertility. Use of artificial lubricants, douches, or any agents that alter the pH of the vagina may also affect fertility. Men who have had testicular cancer, surgical repair of hernias, or undescended testicles as children are at a higher risk for infertility as a result of scarring or accidental severing of the epididymis that may have occurred during the surgery.

After obvious causes are ruled out, identifying the source of fertility impairment may require extensive testing (e.g., obtaining blood levels of hormones during the menstrual cycle, male hormone levels, semen analysis, serology, genetic testing). Factors contributing to infertility are outlined in Table 6-2.

Assessment of Female Factors

Ovarian factors

Anovulation, the failure of the ovaries to produce, mature, or release eggs, is the most common ovarian factor leading to infertility. It usually results from an imbalance of hormones at any point in the hypothalamic-pituitary-ovarian interaction. Poor ovulatory function may mean that instead of ovulating with each menstrual cycle, the woman may only ovulate three or four times in a year. This factor may be responsible for 15% to 20% of infertility cases among women. Extensive testing is required to determine the source of any imbalance. In many cases ovulation may be induced by the use of fertility drugs. Polycystic ovarian disease (PCOD), autoimmune ovarian failure, age-related deterioration of the oocytes, and prior treatment with chemotherapy are other factors that cause ovarian-related infertility (Honore, 1994; Jacobs, 1995).

Testing

Detection of ovulation. Daily basal body temperatures (BBTs) are used routinely to determine the approximate time of ovulation (see Chapter 5). Many infertility assessments begin with the use and interpretation of the BBT even though it has been found to be tedious and frequently misinterpreted. Yet, because it is inexpensive and noninvasive and may indicate whether ovulation is occurring, it is often the first assessment tool used. The partners also need to indicate times of sexual intercourse on the BBT chart. Use of an ovulation detection kit may be preferred by some partners. The woman's urine is tested for the surge in LH levels that immediately precedes ovulation. The couple may need to learn how to coordinate the times of sexual intercourse with time of ovulation.

Ultrasonography. To accurately assess the ripening of the graafian follicle and timing of ovulation, vaginal ultrasound testing is frequently used. This testing is usually performed in conjunction with treatments for infertility

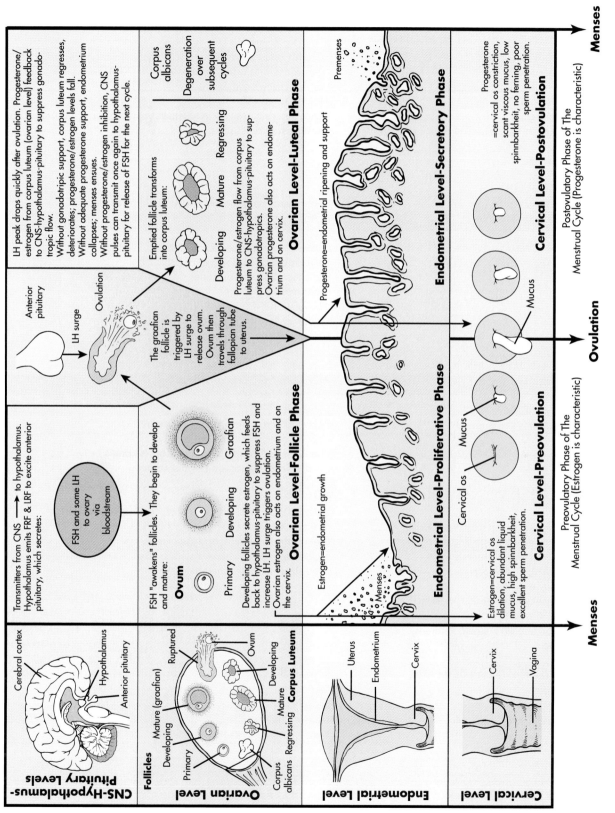

Figure 6-1   Menstrual cycle influences. Note mucus changes (bottom of chart) that correspond to changing hormonal influences. At endometrial and ovarian levels, note development of follicle in relation to growing endometrial tissue. *CNS,* Central nervous system; *FRF,* follicle-releasing factor; *FSH,* follicle-stimulating hormone; *LH,* luteinizing hormone; *LRF,* luteinizing hormone releasing factor.

Table 6-2   **Factors Contributing to Infertility**

Men	Women
GENETIC OR DEVELOPMENTAL FACTORS	
Production of deformed sperm	Chromosomal abnormalities: trisomy or deletions of
Abnormalities of testicles	chromosomes, Turner's syndrome (45 XO), mosaicism
Absence or diminished number of sperm	of sex chromosomes
Abnormal genitalia	Abnormal genitalia
Epispadias or hypospadias	Vaginal, uterine, ovarian abnormalities
Undescended testes (usually repaired during childhood)	Cervical stenosis
Varicocele	
Chromosomal trisomy (XXY)	
HORMONAL FACTORS	
Hyposecretion of pituitary, thyroid, adrenal,	Hypersecretion of hormones released by
or gonadal hormones	pituitary-gonadal activity
	Luteal phase defects
	Excessive production of androgens
	Polycystic ovarian disease (PCOD)
	Hyposecretion of hormones
	Amenorrhea
	Anovulation
	Premenopause or postmenopause
	Congenital adrenal hyperplasia
MECHANICAL OBSTRUCTION	
Retrograde ejaculation	Adhesions from previous surgery
Repair of vasectomy	Endometriosis
Spinal cord injury or disease	Salpingitis
Urethral trauma causing scarring	Repair of ectopic pregnancy surgically
	Uterine polyps or fibroids
	Previous rupture of appendix with peritonitis
	and scar formation on fallopian tubes
CHEMICAL, ENVIRONMENTAL, OR LIFESTYLE FACTORS	
Drug abuse	Drug abuse: tranquilizers, alcohol, cocaine, or nicotine
Alcoholism causing reduced testosterone levels	Strenuous exercise for extended period
Nicotine reducing sperm number and motility	Use of phenothiazines and reserpine
Tight underwear or pants	Exposure to toxic chemicals, pesticides,
Use of phenothiazines and reserpine	radiation, or heavy metals
Excessive hot tub use	Obesity or extremely underweight
Exposure to toxic chemicals, pesticides, radiation,	
or heavy metals	
Agent Orange exposure (in Vietnam veterans)	
Strenuous exercise	
INFLAMMATORY PROCESS AND IMMUNOLOGIC FACTORS	
Mycoplasma infection	Gonorrhea
Prostatitis	Endometriosis
Mumps orchitis	Postabortion sepsis
Epididymitis	Sperm antibodies in vaginal mucus
Other infections with high fevers	
Sperm antibodies—autoimmunity	

Data from Hammond MG, Talbert LM: *Infertility: a practical guide for the physician,* ed 3, Boston, 1992, Blackwell Scientific.

Table **6-2**	**Factors Contributing to Infertility—cont'd**

Men	Women
PSYCHOGENIC FACTORS	
Physical or mental stress resulting in impotence, retrograde ejaculation, or oligospermia	Anorexia nervosa
Poor information regarding sexual techniques	Excessive weight loss
	Amenorrhea
	Poor information regarding sexual techniques and optimal time of the month for conception
CHRONIC ILLNESS OR DEFICIENCIES (MEN AND WOMEN)	
Rare pituitary or adrenal tumor	Renal disease
Cancer of reproductive organs	Cardiac disease
Severe diabetes	Severe nutritional deficiencies
Thyroid disease	Anemia

(i.e., use of fertility drugs to stimulate ovulation or during in vitro fertilization).

Hormonal testing for ovulation includes the following:

- Evaluation of the serum levels of LH at midcycle may be necessary to determine if the LH surge is occurring.
- Evaluation of the progesterone levels will provide a more accurate picture of corpus luteum function. Two samples may be required during the menstrual cycle so that the expected rise in levels of progesterone can be tracked. The progesterone should rise with the LH surge, peak approximately 8 days later, and remain elevated for approximately 2 days until falling in the absence of a pregnancy.
- Midcycle urine testing for estradiol (estrogen) and pregnanediol (progesterone) levels may help determine whether adequate levels exist.
- Routine thyroid function tests may point to hypothyroidism as a cause for anovulation in some women (Shalev et al, 1994).
- 17-ketosteroid testing may determine whether elevated androgens exist that would suppress ovulation. Congenital adrenal hyperplasia or tumors of the adrenals or ovaries may cause elevated levels of these metabolites.

Cervical factors

To be receptive to sperm, the mucus changes to a high spinnbarkheit allowing excellent sperm penetration. Cervical mucous problems may arise from vaginal infections or hormonal deficiencies that prevent the midcycle change and maintain the thick, acidic property of cervical mucus, which inhibit sperm entry. Other cervical mucous problems may be caused by inadequate ovarian function such as (1) luteal phase defects (LPDs), (2) insufficient estrogen or progesterone production, (3) excessive androgen production, and (4) elevated or depressed FSH or LH levels.

Testing

Cervical mucous testing. In fertile women, cervical mucous changes that indicate ovulation begin to occur a few days before ovulation occurs. The mucus changes from a thick, yellowish discharge to the clear, slippery, stretchable substance (the consistency of egg whites). The woman is taught to check for the presence of *spinnbarkheit* (the stretchability of the mucus). When seen under a microscope, the mucus demonstrates a "ferning" pattern (Figure 6-2) that characteristically enables the sperm to travel quickly through it. Women with infertility related to cervical factors may have thick mucus that prevents the sperm from entering the cervix.

Postcoital testing. This is performed after intercourse as close to the time of ovulation as possible. Semen and cervical mucus are retrieved from the woman's cervix within 1 to 24 hours after intercourse (Oei et al, 1995; Wang et al, 1992). Valuable information obtained from this examination includes the adequacy of penile penetration, the quality of the cervical mucus, and whether the sperm have penetrated the mucus. Microscopic examination is performed to determine the presence of infection, spinnbarkheit, ferning, and sperm numbers and motility. The test is relatively simple because the specimen is obtained from the vagina. However, many couples find that having intercourse "on demand" and then being tested is embarrassing and stressful.

Uterine factors

Uterine function is closely aligned with cervical, ovarian, and tubal function. The hormonal influences pre-

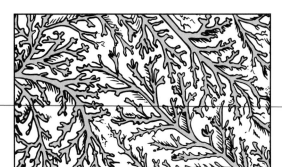

Figure 6-2   Ferning is the term for the crystalline pattern formed when the mucus or amniotic fluid is spread on a glass slide, dried, and viewed under a microscope. (Redrawn from Fogel CI, Woods NF: *Health care of women: a nursing perspective,* St Louis, 1981, Mosby.)

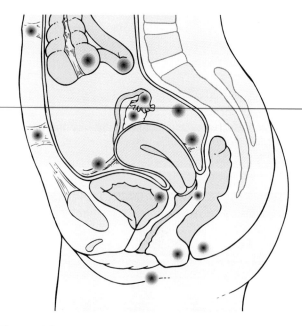

Figure 6-3   Common sites for endometriosis.

pare the uterus for the implantation of the blastocyst when functioning properly. If uterine factors are suspected, the woman may be evaluated for anatomic or structural defects of the uterus that may impede pregnancy (i.e., congenital anomalies). Benign fibroid tumors may cause repeated spontaneous abortion. Uterine infection or inflammation may impede any efforts to become pregnant. Antibiotic therapy may alleviate the infection and restore the endometrial environment.

Endometriosis. Nearly one third of infertile women have **endometriosis,** a condition in which endometrial tissue normally found only in the uterine lining is also found in other body sites. The endometrial tissue that adheres to surrounding organs is known as "implants." The implants are attached most frequently to the ovaries and within the cul-de-sac, the uterosacral ligament, the broad ligament, and even the colon (Perper et al, 1995) (Figure 6-3). These implants within or around the tubes also prevent clear passage of the ovum and sperm. The exact cause is unknown. Newer theories concerning the etiology of endometriosis are focusing on a familial or "genetically preprogrammed condition which occurs as a consequence of immunological malfunction" (Gleicher, 1995). Environmental pollutants (such as dioxins) may weaken the immune system and play a role in the development of endometriosis.

In this misplaced tissue, cyclic bleeding occurs in response to monthly hormonal stimulation, but the tissue cannot be eliminated from the body as menstrual flow. Retention leads to reabsorption, scarring, and adhesions. Some investigators theorize that this endometrial tissue also induces changes in the peritoneal fluid that somehow inhibit oocyte and sperm interaction (Miller et al, 1995). Women with endometriosis may complain of severe dysmenorrhea or may have no signs at all until they are unable to become pregnant. Irregular menses, short cycles

(< 27 days), and heavy bleeding may also characterize the experience of endometriosis.

Testing

Endometrial biopsy. **Endometrial biopsy** involves obtaining a sample of endometrial tissue to be evaluated for the effects of LH. Because endometrial tissue responds to hormonal influence by changes in its thickness, the biopsy is able to confirm appropriate endometrial receptivity to implantation. Luteal phase defects may be detected by this method. The biopsy can be performed in the physician's office within 1 week of expected menstruation. A slender catheter is inserted through the cervix, and endometrial tissue is gently suctioned. A cramping sensation similar to menstrual cramps may be felt while the tissue is being suctioned. The woman may take a mild analgesic (e.g., ibuprofen, Tylenol) before the procedure. Cramping usually stops after the suctioning is completed.

Endoscopy of the endometrium. This allows visualization of the uterus with an endoscope (a flexible tube illuminated with an optical system). Any congenital abnormality of the uterus would be detected (i.e., intrauterine adhesions, polyps, endometritis) (Prevedourakis, 1994). This procedure also takes place in the physician's office. The woman may need a mild analgesic before the procedure.

Ultrasonography. This is frequently used to identify pelvic abnormalities, ovarian cysts, ovarian disease, and masses within the pelvis. Because there is no anesthesia or radiation exposure involved, it is a relatively safe, painless procedure.

Magnetic resonance imaging. Magnetic resonance imaging (MRI) may be used to detect the implants present in endometriosis and uterine fibroids in women with dysmenorrhea or unexplained infertility (de Souza et al, 1995). It is a noninvasive examination that aids in the diagnosis. However, the expense of the procedure may prohibit its widespread use.

Tubal factors

Blockage of the fallopian tubes is often caused by PID, which leaves scar tissue and adhesions as a result of pelvic inflammation or endometriosis. Sometimes the tubes become kinked or twisted. Fibroid growths inside the uterus may block the free passage of the sperm or ovum. Previous pelvic surgery such as appendectomy, ovarian wedge resection, or ectopic pregnancy may have resulted in adhesions or scarring. Tuboplasty or surgical repair of the fallopian tubes may be possible to reduce a tubal ligation; however, fertility rates after surgical repair of the tubes are not encouraging.

Testing

Hysterosalpingogram. **Hysterosalpingogram** is a fluoroscopic examination to assess tubal patency or any distortions in the cervical canal or uterine cavity. It is usually performed immediately after menstruation in the absence of infection and before ovulation or the possibility of pregnancy. The absence of infection is essential because injection of the radiopaque dye through the cervix may cause further spread of infection into the pelvis. When the tubes are normally patent, the dye flows from the cervix, through the uterus, into the tubes, and out into the peritoneum. If the tubes are occluded, the dye does not flow into the peritoneal cavity.

Sometimes, a hysterosalpingogram serves to flush out tubal debris, dislodge adhesions, or induce the normal peristaltic action conducive to fertility by the force of the inward flow of the dye. Sometimes the woman may complain of shoulder pain as the dye enters the peritoneum. This radiographic procedure is performed on an outpatient basis without anesthesia.

Laparoscopy. **Laparoscopy** is a surgical procedure performed in the early follicular phase of the menstrual cycle and requires the use of general anesthesia for the woman. After a small incision is made in the area of the umbilicus, the pelvic area can be viewed with the laparoscope (a thin, flexible illuminated tube with an optical system). Minor surgical repairs such as removal of adhesions on the tubes or lesions from endometriosis may be performed. Because carbon dioxide is used to lift the abdominal wall for a clear view of the pelvic organs, referred shoulder pain may occur after the procedure. The woman may resume normal activities within 1 to 2 days.

Hormonal factors

Hyposecretion or hypersecretion of hormones from the hypothalamic-pituitary-ovarian axis is the most common cause of hormonal infertility. Any imbalance in the delicate interplay of hormones can cause problems such as anovulation, menstrual irregularities, and luteal phase defects. Thyroid disease, diabetes mellitus, and adrenal gland malfunction all have a potentially deleterious effect on fertility. A gradual reduction in the levels of estrogen and progesterone and a reduction in the total number of follicles in the ovaries is noted in most women beginning in their mid-30s (Speroff, 1994). At the same time, FSH levels begin to rise. Rising FSH levels are associated with less competent ovarian follicles and a higher rate of spontaneous abortion as the woman ages (Batista et al, 1995).

Testing. In addition to all the tests mentioned earlier for detection of ovulation problems, serum FSH, serum prolactin, thyroid stimulating hormone (TSH), T3 and T4 levels may be required to assess adequate pituitary or thyroid function. A glucose tolerance test may be needed to assess pancreatic function in light of any other deficiencies that may be found.

Immunologic factors

When a couple is infertile despite normal sperm and hormone levels, assessment of immunologic causes may be the next step of investigation. Many antigens (substances perceived by the body to be "foreign" causing the body to produce antibodies) are present in semen and in the acrosome (head), midpiece, and tail of a sperm. In some cases both men and women produce antibodies against these antigens. The antibodies may be responsible for many cases of unexplained infertility because the sperm may be unable to move freely into the uterus. Some women develop antibodies against their partners' sperm, called *isoimmunization*. When the man develops antibodies against his own sperm, it is called an **autoimmune response.**

Women who develop antiovarian antibodies may have difficulty becoming pregnant even with **assisted reproductive techniques** (ARTs) because they may produce antibodies that destroy the oocyte or the embryo (Shushan, et al, 1995). Serum levels of immunoglobulins are tested in women who are suspected of having antisperm antibodies.

Antibodies against sperm exist in the serum of approximately 12% of infertile women; sperm antibodies are also present in the cervical mucus of some infertile women. Nonvaginal coitus may increase the immune response because the mouth and anus are highly vascular areas that allow for quick entry of the antigen into the body, triggering an antibody response (Moghissi and Wallach, 1985). The new trend among teenagers to avoid loss of virginity through nonvaginal intercourse may have troubling implications for potential loss of fertility.

Environmental and lifestyle factors

The reproductive system is especially vulnerable to the effects of the environment. The use of pesticides, industrial chemicals such as polychlorinated biphenyls (PCBs), and other products used in plastics, detergents, and spermicides are mainly synthetic chemicals that mimic natural hormones like estrogen. The influence of chemicals on human reproductive potential is being given high priority for study. Known environmental factors contributing to infertility are listed on Table 6-2. Cigarettes, alcohol, and marijuana use may lengthen the time needed to conceive (Joesoef et al, 1993). Strenuous exercise (seen in many young people training in gymnastics, ice skating, or ballet) may contribute to amenorrhea and anovulation. Altitude may have an adverse effect on the growth of the follicle. Dry cleaning chemicals, anesthetic gases, textile dyes, noise, lead, mercury, cadmium, and close handling of antibiotics have an effect on the woman's fertility potential (Baranski, 1993). Daughters of women who were given diethylstilbestrol (DES) during pregnancy to prevent miscarriage (during the early 1950s through the late 1960s) are known to have developmentally altered reproductive anatomy and physiology and are frequently infertile as a result.

Identification of occupations or of subgroups of populations at risk for lowered fertility is a first step in heightening awareness of the problem. Obtaining a thorough health history at the beginning of the infertility workup serves to help diagnose the problem.

Genital infection factors

Chlamydia trachomatis, gonorrhea, syphilis, and *Mycoplasma* infections have serious adverse effects on fertility. Sometimes the infections may go undetected in the reproductive tract because of the mild nature of the symptoms. Untreated PID, postabortion sepsis, salpingitis, and endometritis are illnesses that may result. Scar tissue formation may occur after the inflammatory process subsides rendering the woman infertile. (See Chapters 4 and 26 for details on testing for genital infection.) In most cases the organism is highly responsive to antibiotic therapy; culture and sensitivity tests are essential so that therapy may begin before adhesions and irreversible damage occur.

Recurrent pregnancy loss factors

Recurrent pregnancy loss may be considered as part of an infertility workup because spontaneous abortion is a common occurrence within the infertile population. Many causes have been identified: chromosomal abnormalities, uterine anomalies, endocrinologic or immunologic factors, and environmental causes (Daya, 1994). Chronic undetected *Chlamydia trachomatis* infections may add to the risk of spontaneous abortion either from an increase in the antibody production or the inflammatory response to the infection. The risk of recurrent pregnancy loss increases with age (Hakim, 1995). (See Chapter 21 for repeated pregnancy loss.)

Psychogenic factors

Fertility can be influenced by the psyche. Much of the influence of psychologic factors remains unknown or poorly understood. One researcher contends that certain couples unconsciously have lowered fertility in response to situational factors (either psychosocial, interpersonal, or intrapsychic) that create an "unsuitable time to allow a baby to come" (Christie, 1994). The woman's lifelong psychologic task of separating and individuating from her own mother propels her to more mature responsibility toward herself. There is a possibility that a woman with "unexplained" infertility has been unable to resolve internal psychic conflict; an alteration in body functioning may ensue. Unresolved grief or guilt from the death of a parent may also contribute to altered physical abilities, including infertility (Schoener and Krysa, 1996).

Women with "unexplained" infertility may need to have a short period devoted to talking with a therapist to determine whether unresolved feelings of grief or guilt exist (as a possible cause for subfertility) before embarking on the costly and time-consuming process of ARTs. Most infertility centers provide counseling as an integral part of care for the infertile couple.

Assessment of Male Factors

Factors attributable to the man account for approximately 30% to 40% of infertility. Evaluation of the man begins with a complete health history and physical examination to rule out any obvious causes of infertility. Helping the man recall medications used, exposure to toxic chemicals, past or present drug abuse, past febrile illness, steroid use, infections, or sexually transmitted diseases will aid in making the diagnosis. Laboratory analysis of semen and serum determine the adequacy of sperm numbers, shape, and motility and hormonal influences in the process of spermatogenesis. In many cases a specific cause for infertility among subfertile men cannot be found (Sokol, 1996), which may heighten the sense of loss of control for the man (Sherrod, 1992).

Genetic factors

Genetic factors comprise a small percentage of male factor infertility. Cystic fibrosis and XXY chromosome configuration are the most well-known genetic causes of male infertility. Some subfertile men may exhibit a familial component that may be related to an autosomal recessive type of inheritance (Lilford et al, 1994). Further genetic research is necessary in this area.

Hormonal factors

In the man, delayed puberty and congenital or childhood conditions should be recognized long before infertility is suspected (i.e., thyroid disease, adrenogenital syndromes, hypogonadism). Abnormalities in the hypothalamic-pituitary-gonadal axis affect male fertility, and therefore screening is usually warranted. While men who were exposed to prenatal DES before the eleventh gestational week have a higher rate of congenital malformations of the genitalia, no increased incidence of infertility or decreased sexual function is noted (Wilcox et al, 1995).

Serum levels of FSH, LH, testosterone, and prolactin are usually obtained to rule out any form of pituitary or adrenal dysfunction. High levels of FSH may indicate testicular failure (Ross and Nederberger, 1995).

Obstruction of reproductive tract

Varicocele. A **varicocele** is a varicose or swollen vein in the testicle. The swelling elevates the temperature within the testis and thus retards or destroys the process of spermatogenesis. The incidence of varicoceles is as high as 35% in the infertile population. When surgical intervention alleviates the varicosity, 30% to 70% of couples achieve conception (Ross and Nederberger, 1995). Men with varicoceles who also take antihypertensive medications may have impaired ejaculation. Cigarette smoking also has an adverse effect on spermatogenesis among men with varicoceles because of the effects of nicotine on circulation.

Obstructions. Partial obstruction of the epididymis or the vas deferens may sometimes be alleviated with microsurgery. Causes for obstruction range from past genital infections (urethritis, epididymitis, prostatitis) or vasectomy surgery (Hauser, 1995). Diabetes mellitus, spinal injury, or prior pelvic surgery may interrupt sympathetic nervous system flow to the area, which may cause **retrograde ejaculation** (a condition in which the ejaculate flows backward into the bladder rather than out through the urethra).

Testing

Semen analysis. This will examine the most common factors promoting male fertility: sperm production, motility, and basic structure. Adequate numbers of sperm are essential for fertilization. Impairment in the shape or motility (which may be caused by infection, genetic abnormalities, environmental hazards, or antibody production) may prevent the sperm from reaching the fallopian tube. Sperm analysis is usually performed on two separate occasions for increased accuracy. Table 6-3 demonstrates the normal parameters for semen.

Urinalysis. This determines the presence of sperm in the urine, which might indicate retrograde ejaculation. *Pyuria,* a sign of infection in either the urethra or the prostate gland, may be revealed in the urinalysis.

Ultrasonography. Ultrasonography via transrectal ultrasound (TRUS) can be used to view the seminal vesicles, vas deferens, and ejaculatory ducts. It helps to detect obstruction of the system. Doppler ultrasound of the testes can determine the extent of the varicocele if present.

Testis biopsy. This is usually performed on men with a diagnosis of azoospermia. The testis biopsy differentiates between the need for microsurgical repair and disorders of spermatogenesis. In addition, the biopsy provides information for the feasibility of ARTs.

Genitourinary infection

Chlamydia trachomatis, gonorrhea, syphilis, and Mycoplasma infections affect male fertility. These organisms can

---

Table **6-3**	**Normal Values in Semen Analysis**	
Characteristics	**Description**	**Comments**
Color	Opaque	
pH	7.2 - 7.8	Sperm movement inhibited by lower pH levels
Volume	1.5 - 5 ml; mean volume 3.2 ml	Levels above 6 ml cause low concentration of sperm at cervical os
Count	>20 million - 100 million	Count may depend on frequency of ejaculation, fertile men have lower sperm count with more frequent ejaculation
	>30 million normal	Allow 48-72 hours of abstinence before specimen is obtained. More frequent ejaculation in infertile men may increase sperm count
Motility	>50%-60% motile after 2 hours	Graded on scale of 0 to 4 measured 1-2 hours after ejaculation, 2 to 4 is normal
Forward progression	Good forward progression	
Morphology (structure)	>60% normal, oviform	Higher percentage of tapering forms and spermatids associated with varicocele
Viability	>50%	
Leukocytes	<1 million/ml	Increased count indicates infection
Agglutination	None	If persistent, *Escherichia coli* infection or sperm antibodies are present

Data from the World Health Organization Criteria for Normal Sperm Analysis: *WHO laboratory manual for the examination of human serum and semen-cervical mucus interaction,* Cambridge, 1993, Cambridge University Press.

directly affect the quality of semen in many ways. Colonies may attach to the neck of the sperm, causing them to swim in tight circles rather than straight. The bacteria may ingest substances vital for sperm nourishment or may stimulate production of antibodies. Bacteria may cause an inflammation in the prostate gland. In addition, scar tissue may form in the gonads as a consequence of a previous infection and block the sperm from exiting. Bacteria in seminal fluid also play a role in the development of PID with subsequent salpingitis in the woman. Likewise, the woman may harbor bacteria that may spread to the man.

The infections must be diagnosed to be treated. In most cases, bacteria are highly responsive to antibiotic therapy; therefore in addition to the semen analysis and urinalysis, culture and antibiotic sensitivity tests are essential. Certain antibiotics may have adverse effects on spermatogenesis, sperm function, or both. The category of nitrofurans (e.g., Furacin), macrolides (e.g., lincomycin, chloramphenicol), tetracyclines, aminoglycosides (e.g., gentamycin, neomycin), and sulfasalazine in particular may affect these functions (Howards, 1995). Many of these drugs impair fertility during the treatment period only. The benefits and risks of each antibiotic are usually weighed before treatment. Often, both partners are treated even if only one is diagnosed with the infection. In many couples conception may occur after the infection is successfully treated (Shlegel et al, 1991).

Immunologic factors

Men who have undergone vasectomies still produce sperm; however, the sperm are absorbed into the body, not ejaculated into the semen. This reabsorption sometimes promotes antibody production. This autoimmune response is often the cause of continued infertility in a man whose vasectomy is reversed.

Antisperm antibodies. Antibody titers present in the serum of the man may mean that his fertility lowers if the antibodies target his own sperm. If elevated, sperm–bound antibody levels are measured in the semen. If such antibodies exist, the ability of the man's sperm to penetrate and fertilize the human ovum becomes impaired (Howards, 1995).

Cervical mucous penetration. This test allows measurement of sperm migration and penetration through cervical mucus. It differs slightly from **postcoital testing** in that the partner's cervical mucus is not necessary to complete the examination (bovine mucus is used) (Ross and Nederberger, 1995).

Sperm penetration assay. The **sperm penetration assay** (SPA) measures the ability of the sperm to penetrate and fertilize an ovum. A sperm sample is mixed with zona pellucida-free hamster ova in the laboratory. The ability of fertile sperm to penetrate these ova is much greater than among infertile sperm. However, this test may result in a high number of false positive or false negative results. Human sperm that are unable to penetrate hamster eggs may still be able to penetrate human eggs. When used in addition to the postcoital examination, the SPA may provide valuable information about the *potential* for fertilization. In many cases, if the female partner is normal, couples become pregnant despite low sperm counts or the presence of poor motility. Abnormal results of the SPA may be especially unsettling to the man when told he is also unable to fertilize hamster eggs. Information from the test needs to be used as a basis for counseling, psychologic support, and further testing (Seibel and Zilberstein, 1995).

Environmental and lifestyle factors

Factors that may interfere with spermatogenesis include cigarette smoking and drug use including cimetidine (Tagamet) and cocaine. Excessive use of hot tubs or saunas can expose the testes to high temperatures, which have a detrimental effect on sperm production. Wearing tight underpants and trousers may contribute to lowering sperm counts (Parazzini et al, 1995). Chemical warfare may also have a detrimental effect on sperm numbers and motility. The gradual lowering of sperm counts through the past several decades is reported by one researcher (Skakkebaek, Giwercman, and de Kretser, 1994) who postulates an environmental cause (perhaps synthetic chemicals). (See Table 6-2 for known environmental factors contributing to infertility.) Eliminating these factors may be a first step toward fertility.

Psychogenic factors

The infertile man needs to be viewed holistically, that is, physically, psychologically, and socially, to obtain the full picture of the person needing help with an infertility problem. Job or financial stress, family illness, fatigue, or depression may compound the pressures perceived by the person so that fertility may not be possible until the stress is alleviated.

Assessment of Combined Factors

Unexplained infertility

An infertile couple is diagnosed with unexplained infertility when a routine infertility investigation yields normal results and unprotected intercourse has occurred for at least 1 year without a pregnancy. Approximately 10% to 15% of the infertile population is diagnosed with unexplained infertility. Because spontaneous pregnancies do occur among couples with unexplained infertility, a younger couple diagnosed with unexplained infertility after 1 year of unprotected intercourse may not receive as aggressive an approach as an older couple or a couple who has been attempting pregnancy for several years. Many times, subtle defects in the reproductive process may cause the unexplained infertility. More detailed anatomic or physiologic testing may be necessary. Undetected infection in the man or woman may require further culture and sensitivity testing.

TEST *Yourself* 6-1

a. List potential environmental causes of infertility.
b. Which causes of infertility could be eliminated by general education about infertility?

TREATMENT FOR INFERTILITY

The approach for treatment is based on the diagnosis. Planning treatment for the infertile couple involves helping the partners view the diagnosis and intervention realistically. Should the couple find that conceiving or carrying their own biologic child is not possible, the options for parenting are reviewed. With the advanced technologies changing so rapidly, some possible choices might include (but not be limited to) ARTs such as **in vitro fertilization** (IVF), intracytoplasmic sperm injection (ICSI), **gamete intrafallopian tube transfer** (GIFT), **zygote intrafallopian tube transfer** (ZIFT), artificial insemination, surrogate parenting, oocyte donation, and adoption. The nurse remains a strong advocate, providing information about the risks and benefits of each treatment plan. Helping the partners view their chances for a "take home baby" in a realistic framework is essential for decision-making efforts.

Drug or Hormonal Therapy

Replacement therapy may cure infertility in the man or woman diagnosed with hormonal deficiency. For instance, a diagnosis of hypothyroidism or hyperthyroidism might be treated with medications to replace thyroid hormone deficiencies or medication, radioisotopes, or surgery for hyperthyroidism. In many cases when the imbalance is corrected, the restoration of reproductive function may follow.

Restoring ovarian function and ovulation can be accomplished using medications that induce ovulation (see Drug Profile 6-1). Clomiphene citrate (Clomid, Serophene) is the most common ovulation inducer. Clomiphene citrate stimulates FSH and LH secretions by the pituitary. FSH and LH promote growth of the follicle and subsequent ovulation. It is not given in the presence of ovarian or pituitary disease. A complication of clomiphene citrate administration is the possible maturation of multiple follicles which could lead to a multiple pregnancy.

In women resistant to the effects of clomiphene citrate, human menopausal gonadotropin (hMG, Pergonal, menotropin, Metrodin) may be used to induce ovulation. Human chorionic gonadotropin (hCG, Pregnyl) is also given in the cycle to coincide with the LH surge. The administration of hCG at the appropriate time ensures the rupture of the follicle after the hMG or the clomiphene citrate has stimulated the maturation of the follicle (Franks and Gilling-Smith, 1994).

The relationship between the use of ovulation-inducing drugs and the development of systemic lupus erythematosus (SLE) in some susceptible women has been suggested (Ben-Chetrit and Ben-Chetrit, 1994). Further study is necessary in this area.

Luteal phase defects may cause an increase in prolactin levels, which inhibit the secretion of FSH and LH. Ovulation does not occur in women with this disorder. Bromocriptine (Parlodel) may be prescribed to suppress the secretion of prolactin by the anterior pituitary. The drug is discontinued with evidence of ovulation. Prolactin levels and cervical mucous monitoring are done during treatment. Luteal phase defects may also be treated with progesterone (Provera, medroxy-progesterone acetate) suppositories (vaginal or rectal). Using the BBT chart and monitoring the cervical mucus is necessary to assess ovulation.

Additions of low dose gonadotropin agonist (GnRHa, LHRH agonists, Lupron, Buserelin, Zoladex) helps prevent a premature LH surge and multiple release of ova during the induced cycle. Improvement in follicular response and fertilization and implantation rates have been noted with the use of this drug (Tan, 1994a).

Women undergoing treatment with ovulation-inducing drugs are monitored carefully with serum and urine progesterone testing (in some cases on a daily basis) as an indication of impending ovulation. Ultrasound visualization of the follicles may also be required frequently to assess the follicular growth and possible growth of ovarian cysts (in which case the drugs are discontinued for that cycle).

Infertility drugs are expensive. Insurance coverage may be available for some couples, but it is not universal. Once the couple decides to commit to a course of treatment, it is essential to adhere to the schedule of sexual intercourse, laboratory testing, ultrasound testing, BBT charts, and other practices to ensure the optimal outcome. It is important for the couple to completely understand the reality of the time commitment, the prospect of sexual intercourse "on demand," the possibility of lost work time, and meager insurance coverage before making the choice to proceed.

Surgical Intervention

Surgical intervention can provide promising results for eligible couples. The couple is provided with the most recent information on the probable outcomes so that informed decisions may be made. The person undergoing reproductive surgery and the partner must be prepared for the possibility that pregnancy may not be achieved. Among the most common surgical interventions are repairs of congenital anomalies, vasectomies, varicoceles, and removal of tumors affecting reproductive ability. Surgical intervention may also be necessary for many of the ARTs.

Box 6-1

DRUG PROFILE

Drug Therapy for Infertility

Category	Dosage	Usage	Precautions
OVULATION-INDUCING DRUGS			
Clomiphene citrate (Clomid)	Start with 50 mg/day for 5 days beginning on the fifth day of the cycle. May increase dose with subsequent cycles. Doses of >150 mg for 5 days usually not effective. Further infertility evaluation may be necessary.	Nonsteroid estrogen antagonist modifies hypothalamic activity resulting in release of Gn-RH, which causes increase of FSH and LH and development of the graafian follicle. Ovulatory surge should begin 5-10 days after last pill is taken. Couple is advised coitus every or every other day for 1 week beginning 5 days after last day of clomiphene citrate administration. It may be given for as many as 6 cycles. If no pregnancy occurs, a more intensive infertility evaluation is necessary. Couple may want to use ovulation predictor kit. **Pregnancy rates:** ±40%	Evaluate ovulation and plasma progesterone and estrogen levels. Test for pregnancy before administering drug. Endometrial biopsy may be done in third week. **Side effects:** Flushing, hot flashes, abdominal distention, bloating, breast tenderness, nausea, vomiting, visual disturbances, dryness of hair, hair loss. Symptoms cease at the end of treatment. **Adverse effects:** Ovarian enlargement. Medication not continued if visual disturbance (i.e., night blindness) occurs. **Multiple pregnancy risk:** 6%-12% when used alone. High doses may lead to significant antiestrogenic effects and abnormal folliculogenesis.
Bromocriptine mesylate (Parlodel)	1.25 mg/day for 1 week. If tolerated, dosage increased to 1-2 tablets/day (2.5-5 mg/day). Vaginal suppositories available.	Used in women with pituitary adenomas or persistent hyperprolactinemia. Dopamine agonist to reduce serum prolactin levels. Helps restore normal menstrual cycles and inhibits lactation. **Pregnancy rates:** <85%	**Side effects:** Orthostatic hypotension, nausea, vomiting, GI irritation, headache, fatigue, nasal congestion. To avoid symptoms, medication may be taken at bedtime or with meals. Vaginal administration may reduce side effects.
Gonadotropins			
Human menopausal gonadotropin (hMG, Metrodin, Pergonal, menotropin)	Purified gonadotropins contain 75-150 IU of FSH and 75-150 IU of LH given IM. One ampule daily for 7-12 days until a preovulatory follicle develops. Daily dosage varies and is adjusted to individual needs (i.e., response of follicles).	When ultrasound indicates the follicle size is 16-20 mm, hMG is followed by 10,000 IU of hCG to assure rupture of the ripe follicle. Used for women who do not ovulate with clomiphene treatment. hMG is the medication of choice in women with low levels of estrogens and gonadotropins.	Maturation of follicle followed closely to avoid overstimulation. **Side effects:** Not given if FSH or LH is already elevated or if thyroid or adrenal problems or in presence of ovarian cysts. Febrile reaction may indicate possible allergy to drug.

From Bahamondes L et al: The influence of human chorionic gonadotropin administration upon the next ovarian cycle, *Hum Reprod* 10(3):533, 1995.
Harada T et al: Reduced implantation rate associated with a subtle rise in serum progesterone concentration during the follicular phase of cycles stimulated with a combination of gonadotropin-releasing hormone agonist and gonadotropin, *Hum Reprod* 10(5):1060, 1995.
Managing the anovulatory state: medical induction of ovulation, ACOG Technical Bulletin No. 197, September, 1994.
Purvin VA: Visual disturbance secondary to clomiphene citrate, *Arch Ophthalmol* 113(4):482, 1995.
Rossing MA et al: Ovarian tumors in a cohort of infertile women, *N Engl J Med* 331(12):771, Sept 22, 1994.
Whittemore AS: The risk of ovarian cancer after treatment for infertility, *N Engl J Med* 331(12):805, Sept 22, 1994.
BBT, Basal body temperature; *FSH,* follicle-stimulating hormone; *GI,* gastrointestinal; *Gn-RH,* gonadotropin-releasing hormone; *Gn-RHa,* gonadotropin-releasing hormone agonist; *hCG,* human chorionic gonadotropin; *hMG,* human menopausal gonadotropin; *IM,* intramuscularly; *IU,* international unit; *LH,* luteinizing hormone; *PO,* by mouth; *SC,* subcutaneously.

Box **6-1**

DRUG PROFILE—cont'd

Drug Therapy for Infertility

Category	Dosage	Usage	Precautions
Gonadotropins—cont'd			
Human menopausal gonadotropin—cont'd	Ovulation occurs within 36 hours of hCG. Intercourse recommended during the 2 days after hCG administered.	Close monitoring with ultrasound, serum estradiol, LH, and progesterone are essential. **Pregnancy rates:** 20%-90%	**Adverse effects:** After treatment is finished, abdominal distention may indicate ovarian overstimulation. Mild to severe pain may occur. **Multiple pregnancy risk:** ±20%
Human chorionic gonadotropin (hCG)	10,000 IU IM 7-10 days after clomiphene citrate.	hCG is added to clomiphene citrate regimen to ensure rupture of the ripe follicle. **Pregnancy rates:** 20%-90%.	Ultrasonography is used to measure follicle development before administration of hCG. Intercourse is planned for evening of first day after injection and for next 2 days. **Side effects:** Contributes to hyperstimulation syndrome if given with hMG. **Adverse effects:** **Multiple pregnancy risk:** ± 30%
GONADOTROPIN-RELEASING HORMONE THERAPY			
Gonadorelin acetate (Lutrepulse), gonadorelin HCl (Factrel)	A belt is worn around the waist for administration of this drug. Injection administers automatic pulse dose between 10-20 µg pulse. Most women ovulate after 10-20 days of Gn-RH therapy.	For induction of ovulation in women with chronic anovulation and low estrogen and gonadotropin levels who have functioning pituitary and ovary. Stimulates release of FSH and LH leading to folliculogenesis. hCG or progesterone therapy is given after pump is discontinued to support luteal phase. **Pregnancy rates:** 20%-90%	**Side effects:** Headache, lightheadedness. **Adverse effects:** Rare localized phlebitis from pulse injector. **Multiple pregnancy risk:** <12%
SUPPRESSION OF PITUITARY FUNCTION			
Gonadotropin-releasing hormone agonist (Gn-RHa), leuprolide (Lupron), nafarelin (Synarel [inhalant]), Buserelin acetate, goserelin acetate (Zoladex)	Begins on day 3 of menses. Use 1 mg SC daily. Lower dose after estrogen levels checked. hMG may be started.	Alleviates the problem of LH surges associated with sole use of hMG to stimulate ovulation Down-regulates pituitary (depletes LH stores for 2 weeks, followed by hMG) or Gn-RHa and hMG given concurrently. Close monitoring of estrogens and follicles required.	**Contraindications:** Pregnancy, lactation, breast feeding. **Side effects:** Hot flashes, memory and sleep disturbances, irritability, headache, depression, acne. Hypersensitivity, allergy, anaphylaxis may occur. May lose bone density.

Continued.

Box 6-1

DRUG PROFILE—cont'd

Drug Therapy for Infertility

Category	Dosage	Usage	Precautions
SUPPRESSION OF ENDOMETRIOSIS			
Danazol (Danocrine)	Depending upon the severity of the endometriosis, the dosages range from 200-800 mg in 2 or 4 divided doses daily for 4-6 months. Need to begin drug during menses.	Synthetic weak androgen prevents midcycle LH surge so endometriosis is inhibited and tissue regresses and atrophies. Stimulates menopausal effect on endometrial tissue suppressing ectopic implants. It is sometimes used in fibrocystic breast disease to relieve pain and tender nodules.	**Side effects:** Related to reduced gonadotropins: amenorrhea, weight gain, acne, increased skin oils, vasomotor flushing, vasomotor instability, voice changes, fluid retention. Return of ovulation occurs in 60-90 days. Monitor ovulation (either with the kit or BBT charts): drug should not be used during pregnancy
Medroxy progesterone acetate (Provera)	10-30 mg/day PO or 200 mg IM ("Depo") once a month for 6 months. May be given vaginally or rectally.	Sustained progestational effect causes atrophic changes in the endometrial implants. May also be used to sustain corpus luteum after a stimulated cycle in infertility.	**Contraindications:** Thromboembolic disorders, breast or genital carcinoma, undiagnosed vaginal bleeding. **Side effects:** Abdominal bloating. **Adverse effects:** Prolonged anovulation after discontinuing treatment. Not usually recommended for women with primary infertility.

Assisted Reproduction Techniques

The first successful IVF, or test tube conception, was performed in Great Britain in 1978. This accomplishment gave hope to many infertile couples. Since that time, increasingly sophisticated ARTs have evolved to allow many couples to achieve pregnancy. Currently, the research is close to discovering a means for **cryopreserving** (freezing) oocytes. Issues such as cloning and legal rights of the embryo have emerged as potential stumbling blocks in the research of ARTs. With these developments, health care provision, which was once only concerned with the issues of accomplishing a conception and "take home baby," now must face the ethical, moral, and legal issues of postmenopausal pregnancy, "ownership" of extra embryos retrieved during ARTs, and donor oocytes.

In Vitro Fertilization and Embryo Transfer

As stated earlier, IVF and **embryo transfer** (ET) are processes in which the woman's ova are retrieved, transferred to the laboratory, fertilized with the partner's sperm in a petri dish, and the resultant embryo(s) placed within the mother's uterus. In the past the process of retrieving the ovum involved surgical intervention with laparoscopy. Many of the infertility clinics now use a transvaginal ultrasound-directed method of follicle retrieval that does not require anesthesia and may be performed on an outpatient basis (Tan, 1994). The woman is carefully monitored with the use of ultrasound and serum hormone levels to observe the appropriate time to retrieve the ova. The most likely candidates for IVF-ET are women whose fallopian tubes are irreparably damaged. Couples with unexplained infertility may also benefit from this procedure.

To provide a greater opportunity for success, most IVF-ET programs use the technique of **controlled ovarian hyperstimulation** (COH) to encourage the maturation of several ova at once. Medications most often used to accomplish the induction of ovulation include the following:

- Clomiphene citrate alone or in combination with hMG
- hMG alone or in combination with clomiphene citrate
- hCG after a course of clomiphene citrate or hMG to facilitate rupture of the ripe follicles
- Gn-RHa followed by or in combination with hMG to prevent premature LH surge that sometimes occurs. The use of Gn-RHa provides a more controlled stimulated cycle so that the ultrasound and blood testing are not as numerous for the woman (Tan, 1994).

In women who have tubal disease but normal hormonal and ovulatory function, IVF may be attempted without ovarian stimulation. More intensive monitoring is required, but the results are encouraging (Fahy et al, 1995).

Once the ova are retrieved, they are placed in a culture medium with the partner's sperm. If fertilization occurs, the zygote remains in the culture medium until it reaches the 4-8 cell stage of development when the embryo is transferred to the woman's uterine cavity. Frequently, more than one embryo is transferred to increase the chance for success. Embryos unused for a cycle of IVF-ET may be cryopreserved for future IVF attempts. Using the cryopreserved embryos on subsequent attempts may actually improve chances for pregnancy because the woman does not run the risk of ovarian hyperstimulation with possible adverse effects on the endometrium (Frederick et al, 1995).

The success rate of IVF-ET is only approximately 20%. Because most fertility clinics calculate their success rates according to the *number* of pregnancies per IVF-ET, it can be a misleading statistic for many infertile partners. The delivery rate may be substantially lower as a result of spontaneous abortions, preterm deliveries, and stillbirths. The partners need to become educated about the particular clinic they choose. Because IVF-ET is usually a last resort, almost every infertile partner expects success. The financial cost is high because most insurance companies do not provide coverage. Thus the estimated cost for a successful delivery with IVF-ET according to one study is between $67,000 and $114,000. For couples with more difficult problems cost may be as much as $800,000 per delivery. In the same study the authors found that the average charges for a single cycle of IVF ranged from $7,000 to $11,000 (Neumann et al, 1994).

Gamete Intrafallopian Tube Transfer

GIFT was developed in 1984 and closely approximates the IVF-ET process. In GIFT, however, the oocytes are retrieved, combined with the partner's sperm, and placed in the fallopian tube at the normal site of fertilization. There is no waiting period for the ova and sperm to fertilize in the laboratory. The transfer of ova and sperm into the tube may involve laparoscopic surgery with anesthesia for exact placement. GIFT and ZIFT success rates are reported to be 26% to 28%.

Zygote Intrafallopian Tube Transfer

ZIFT is a combination of IVF and GIFT. The ova are retrieved and fertilized in the laboratory with the partner's sperm before being placed in the fallopian tube. Women with at least one functioning fallopian tube are appropriate candidates for GIFT or ZIFT. It is felt that transfer of the ova and sperm or the embryo to the site where fertilization normally occurs provides the fertilized ovum an opportunity to move through the tube in the normal time frame without arriving in the uterus prematurely.

Transvaginal Intratubal Insemination

Many motile sperm are delivered into the fallopian tube using a transvaginal catheter with ultrasound guidance in **transvaginal intratubal insemination** (Toaff et al, 1995). The timing of this procedure is shortly before ovulation to increase the chance for success. COH may be used to promote release of several ova. This new procedure does not involve retrieval of the ova (as in GIFT or ZIFT), so it may be performed in the office without anesthesia. The cost of this procedure is substantially less than GIFT or ZIFT. In transvaginal intratubal insemination, the fimbriated ends of the fallopian tubes must be functioning to pick up the ovum. Timing is crucial—insemination into the tube should occur *before* ovulation. The possibility for ectopic or multiple pregnancy is higher using tubal insemination.

Peritoneal Oocyte and Sperm Transfer

Peritoneal oocyte and sperm transfer (POST) is a procedure that uses ultrasound guidance for retrieval of oocytes to which the partner's sperm is added. The mixture is then placed in the peritoneal cavity near the fimbriae of the fallopian tubes. Luteal support may be necessary in the form of hCG therapy. This procedure has been used successfully for the treatment of unexplained infertility and failed donor insemination. As with GIFT and ZIFT, POST allows accurate control of the number of oocytes transferred; any excess may be inseminated and cryopreserved for future use. POST may be performed with local anesthesia or mild sedation; no surgery is necessary, and the procedure may be done on an outpatient basis (Tan, 1994).

Micromanipulation

Micromanipulation is a new method of approaching the problem of infertility. It involves retrieval of ovum and sperm using techniques in the laboratory that alter the protective coating of the ova (zona pellucida) to allow the sperm to enter (partial zona dissection [PZD]) or directly injecting sperm underneath the zona pellucida (**subzonal insertion** [SUZI]) to "force" fertilization. The newest method to be used is the **intracytoplasmic sperm injection** (ICSI), which can be used even if the man has very few or nonmotile sperm. ICSI may replace the other two methods of micromanipulation because the pregnancy rates are far superior with ICSI (Tarin, 1995). Micromanipulation techniques are usually used in combination with IVF. Pregnancy rates with micromanipulation range from 6% to 49% depending upon the age of the woman (Oehninger, 1995).

Partial zona dissection

In PZD a small slit is made in the zona pellucida that allows the sperm direct access to the oocyte (Figure 6-4, *A*). The low fertilization rate associated with PZD may be

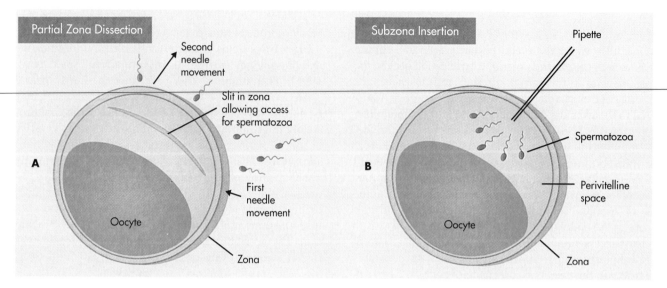

Figure 6-4   Micromanipulation is a new technique for assisting fertilization when sperm quality is poor. **A,** A slit is made in the zona, allowing sperm to enter. **B,** Sperm are inserted through the zona by means of a pipette. (Redrawn from Waterstone J: Investigations in subfertility, *Practitioner* 236:144, 1992.)

caused by the inability of the sperm to enter the slit in the zona pellucida (Van Steirteghem, 1994).

Subzonal insertion

SUZI involves puncturing the zona pellucida with a fine pipette through which a number of spermatozoa are injected (Figure 6-4, *B*). Success rates with SUZI are higher than with PZD.

Intracytoplasmic sperm injection

With ICSI only a single sperm is necessary because it is injected directly into the oocyte (Figure 6-5). Success rates are much higher than PZD or SUZI because this method of "forced" fertilization is effective even in the severest forms of male infertility (Tsirigotis and Craft, 1995).

Oocyte Donation

Oocyte and embryo donation was introduced in 1984. Embryo donation involves retrieval and insemination of ova donated by a woman whose ovulation is induced. The resultant embryos are implanted in the infertile woman whose menstrual cycle is synchronized (using hormone therapy) with the donor. Sperm may be from the recipient's husband or a donor. Pregnancy is quite successful among older recipients whose own oocytes may be faulty. **Oocyte donation** may be done with known or unknown donors. Some fertility clinics ask the recipient to provide a donor who may or may not remain known to the recipient. Oocyte donation between siblings or between daughters and their remarried mothers occurs. One study determined that most

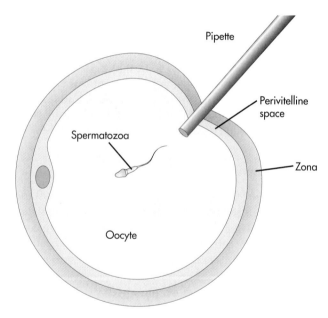

Figure 6-5   Intracytoplasmic sperm injection (ICSI) is a micromanipulation of the sperm and ovum that injects a sperm directly into the oocyte. (Redrawn from Skakkebaek NE, Giwercman A, de Kretser D: Pathogenesis and management of male infertility, *Lancet* 343:1477, June 11, 1994.)

egg donors were able to psychologically give up "ownership" of the egg to provide an opportunity for another woman to be a mother (Snowdon, 1994). Egg donation differs from sperm donation in that retrieval of the oocytes carries a risk for the woman and is more difficult to obtain (Shushan and Schenker, 1994).

Programs involved in oocyte donations establish a registry, similar to a sperm donation registry, where matches based on phenotype likeness are arranged. Because the long-term legal, ethical, and moral ramifications of oocyte donation are still evolving, guidelines set up by the American Fertility Society are used by most centers (Sauer et al, 1993; Ethical Consideration, 1994).

Artificial Insemination

Artificial insemination can be performed using the husband's sperm (**husband insemination** [HI]), a donor's sperm (**artificial insemination by donor** [AID]), or a combination of both. Donated sperm is always frozen or held for at least 6 months to be tested for human immunodeficiency virus (HIV) and then used. The husband's sperm can be freshly inseminated into the partner. Artificial insemination is carefully timed to coincide with ovulation. This method is usually used when the male partner is unable to ejaculate effectively into the vagina (i.e., impotence, hypospadias, retrograde ejaculation, use of antihypertensive medications) or when an immune problem exists (i.e., cervical mucus is hostile to the sperm or antisperm antibodies).

The ejaculate is deposited into the cervical canal or the vaginal vault and kept in place with a diaphragm or cervical cap for 8 hours (see Chapter 5). Two or three inseminations may be required within one monthly cycle; the process may continue for 6 to 12 months until pregnancy occurs. Should a cervical immunologic problem exist, **intrauterine insemination** (IUI) may be performed. Intrauterine insemination means that the ejaculate is injected directly into the uterus through a thin catheter, bypassing the cervical mucus. Sometimes COH is used in conjunction with IUI to synchronize the ripening and rupture of the follicle with the placement of the sperm.

Factors affecting the success rates are the husband's age, duration of the infertility, and regularity of ovulation of the partner (Mathieu et al, 1995). Informed consent is an essential part of the donor insemination process. Before agreeing to undergo donor insemination, the partners need to discuss and agree on whether the offspring is told. Currently, there is a lack of information concerning whether secrecy is best for the child. The dynamics between partners, specifically the degree to which each respects the others' viewpoint, is an important aspect of the process. The fact that the man may be experiencing the infertility, but yet the woman receives the treatment (insemination) may foster feelings of inequality in the man. Another part of the process in donor insemination is that the woman is the biologic parent while the man has no biologic connection to the child. Future events may require knowledge of genetic history and may change the couples' perspective on whether to tell their child. Counseling and careful consideration of these issues are

an integral part of the insemination process (Daniels, Lewis, Gillett, 1995).

ALTERNATIVES TO FERTILITY

Alternatives to fertility are considered when the couple determines that the reality of their situation precludes further attempts to reproduce. For many couples, arbitrary limits are placed before entering the process of pursuing fertility. For others, a monetary, emotional, or physical limit is agreed upon. For instance, many couples will continue to try to become pregnant only by natural means, such as hormone enhancement or diagnostic testing, but will stop short of ARTs (because of their internal discomfort with "test tube" pregnancy). Certain religious opposition to ARTs are factors for many couples. The Vatican opposes any means of ARTs as contrary to the unity of the marriage. Jewish law prohibits insemination of a married woman with sperm other than her husband's. Islamic law condemns artificial insemination by a donor (Mor-Yosef and Schenker, 1995). Financial constraints frequently force couples to decide about alternatives. Many well-meaning relatives of the couple also encourage adoption as a means of "relaxing enough to become pregnant," which may or may not be accurate.

Surrogacy-Host Motherhood

In **surrogacy-host motherhood**, a surrogate or substitute mother accepts an embryo and agrees to carry the pregnancy to term for the infertile couple. The ova and sperm may be donated from the infertile couple or donor ova and sperm may be used. There are cases of the infertile woman's own mother accepting her daughter's fertilized ovum and carrying her own grandchild to term. Hormonal replacement therapy enables even a menopausal woman to support a pregnancy. When the infertile woman produces no ova, donor embryos may be used from cryopreservation units.

The surrogate mother is screened for physical (i.e., general health; infections; habits such as smoking, alcohol, or substance abuse) and psychologic factors before the process begins. The potential for surrogate attachment to the infant is a significant factor. Attachment seems to be greater if the surrogate is a genetic surrogate and a gestational one (i.e., the woman donates the egg and also carries the infant to term for another couple). If the surrogate perceives herself as just the "receptacle" for the genetic parents (i.e., the ova and sperm are from the infertile couple), she may feel that the infant is being made for another. Sometimes, it is not the biologic attachment but rather the "emotional investment the woman has in a pregnancy" (Snowden, 1994). Some grief or mourning about giving up the infant can be expected. Counseling the surrogate mother for a period after the birth may be necessary to help her work through feelings of loss.

Many states lack legislation to protect the rights of all parties involved in a surrogate program. As a result the risk of exploitation on both sides is high. Many safeguards must be provided for the infertile couple and for the surrogate mother. These safeguards include written agreements of assumption of responsibility for the infant, counseling, psychologic screening, screening for genetic diseases or STDs, legal counsel, and tissue typing to determine paternity. Some states protect the surrogate's right to assume some form of parenting role despite a preconception agreement to the contrary (Ethical Consideration, 1994). Legal questions involving injuries suffered by the donor or surrogate in the process of ARTs or the birth of an "imperfect" infant also serve to increase the complexity of the issues. For the most part, legal protection supports the choices made by the infertile partners to meet their reproductive needs.

Adoption

When the infertile couple considers adoption, the solution to their infertility problem may or may not be resolved. They may have undergone years of testing, probing, and questioning about their private lives and habits but are still faced with the inability to conceive. In such cases the couple may need to separate their desire to reproduce themselves from their desire to parent a child. Only the latter need can be met by adoption (Valentine, 1986). Discussions about adoption need to be timed so that the couple has a chance to resolve some of the feelings about their inability to conceive or maintain a pregnancy. Adequate time and opportunity must be afforded the couple to explore their feelings and grieve. Referral to support groups or counseling is frequently necessary. Initial anger and resentment may be expressed toward the nurse who suggests adoption because it may confirm the couple's failure to conceive (Sherrod, 1992). But for many couples, the idea of adoption reaffirms their hope in becoming parents (see Chapter 20).

Childless Lifestyle

As mentioned earlier, childbearing and parenthood are major life events involving goals and plans for the future for most people. When conception does not take place, a deep sense of loss may occur. For the couple to reach the decision to remain childless, the process of mourning for their lost parental role is usually necessary. The couple also needs to reconcile their life choice with that of society. Western society places a high value on parenthood. Subtle messages suggest that the childless couple is not as highly valued as a couple with children. Facing social stigma and ostracism may be a part of the decision to remain childless. Although men and women may differ in their particular adjustment, a sense of shared values, goals, and interests helps the couple adjust to a childless lifestyle. The couple may need much support during this time of transition. Helping the partners refocus the goals for their marriage, review career options, and establish hobbies or outside interests may foster the adjustment to childlessness. Acceptance of a childless lifestyle may be associated with greater marital adjustment through time (Ulbrich et al, 1990).

Nursing Responsibilities

Establishing an ongoing relationship is the start of the nursing process. Care for the partners during the diagnostic phase is collaborative: all health care services (e.g., medical, laboratory, social service) are coordinated to provide a holistic approach. In addition to the detailed health history mentioned previously, the nurse gathers information about the family support system; cultural, ethnic, and religious concerns; and occupational and financial data. Information about the lifestyle of the couple, their educational background, and the pertinent health history of each partner is obtained (including childhood diseases or allergies). It is during the information gathering phase that the nurse forms a basis of trust for the ongoing relationship with the partners. Questions are posed in a neutral tone with sincere interest in the answers given by the individual. Enough time is allowed for the interviewing process to proceed uninterrupted. Documentation of the information gathered is an essential component to nursing responsibility.

Intensely personal discussions about sexual practices and reproductive history are usually difficult for most people. The infertile partners may feel threatened by an invasion of their privacy by a stranger yet feel at the mercy of the health care provider to "solve" their problem. Maintaining a nonthreatening and supportive manner facilitates openness and trust. The process of diagnosing and treating infertility is long and may not provide answers for the partners. Much of the frustration, anger, and disappointment experienced by the couple may be displaced on the nurse during the course of the diagnosis or treatment. Continued support and a nonjudgmental atmosphere are essential for goal-directed care.

Optimally, the nurse who has been a part of the infertility process with the couple throughout the diagnostic phase remains an integral part of the treatment phase. The infertility process may not always proceed in a linear fashion. Treatment may occur during the diagnostic phase but nursing care encompasses the whole continuum. Once the diagnosis is established, the nurse reassesses the individual needs of both partners. The success rates of each possible treatment are stated in terms that the couple can understand (i.e., the "take-home-baby" rates). The nurse provides support to the partners during the process without judging their choices.

ASSESSMENT

When gathering data for the assessment phase, the following factors may be considered:
- Financial needs or constraints that may place undue burdens on the partners to continue the pursuit of fertility
- Education level of the couple
- Stress factors such as work, chronic illness, extended family responsibilities
- Cultural and religious beliefs
- Menstrual, obstetric, and sexual history
- General health (e.g., known allergies, prior abdominal surgeries)
- Level of motivation to follow through with the treatment plan
- Knowledge level of different treatment methods

NURSING DIAGNOSES

Based upon the information gathered during the assessment phase, possible nursing diagnoses may include the following:
- Knowledge deficit(s) regarding diagnostic or treatment procedures, options, financial costs
- Ineffective individual or family coping in relation to adapting to the diagnosis of infertility or decision-making about diagnostic tests or available treatments
- Altered patterns of sexuality related to the invasion of privacy (i.e., providing sperm samples for artificial insemination or IVF) or loss of spontaneity in the sexual relationship
- Potential for infection or injury related to the surgery or treatment regimen
- Self-esteem disturbance in response to the lack or loss of reproductive ability

EXPECTED OUTCOMES

Enabling and encouraging the partners to maintain a sense of control and actively participate in the diagnostic and treatment process may foster the achievement of expected outcomes for the couple. The optimal outcome is that the couple will be able to become pregnant, carry the infant to term, experience a normal delivery of a healthy infant, and successfully adapt to the new family configuration and altered lifestyle. With this optimal result in mind, some expected outcomes are that the couple will be able to do the following:
- Make informed decisions regarding diagnostic and treatment options
- Comply with the diagnostic and treatment regimen by maintaining accurate ovulation-intercourse-menstruation charts
- Adhere to accurate schedules of intercourse and medication should they be prescribed
- Exhibit effective coping behaviors by expressing a sense of self-worth and adequacy and demonstrating the ability to provide mutual emotional support
- Verbalize the need for help in coping and attend counseling sessions when necessary
- Exhibit positive health-seeking behaviors by demonstrating a willingness to alter potentially adverse behaviors (i.e., drug or alcohol consumption or environmental threats to fertility)

NURSING INTERVENTION

Nursing intervention is primarily directed toward assisting the partners to achieve goals. Based upon the nursing diagnoses and expected outcomes, the most common nursing interventions might include the following:
- Providing emotional support before, during, and after diagnostic testing and treatment
- Enabling informed decision-making through teaching of the various diagnostic and treatment options
- Teaching methods of fertility promotion (Box 6-1)
- Informing the partners about what to expect, reasons for the tests, what the results mean, implications for further testing
- Encouraging active participation in the process
- Referrals to outside support systems such as other family members, religious or community resources, and organized support groups such as RESOLVE
- Providing lists of popular books about infertility

EVALUATION

Evaluation of the expected outcomes helps reveal that the partners achieved the goals established previously or altered their expectations. Ask the following questions to evaluate expected outcomes: Did the partners . . .
- Exhibit informed decision-making regarding testing and treatment options?
- Comply with directions for testing and treatment?
- Openly communicate with one another and the members of the health team?
- Use available support systems?
- Select alternatives that met their needs and desires?

Box 6-1

TEACHING PLAN *for* HOME CARE

Fertility Promotion for Couples

- It takes the average couple 6 to 9 months of unprotected intercourse to achieve pregnancy.
- Women who ovulate regularly do so 14 days ±2 days before the next menstrual period. Distinctive changes in cervical mucus indicate that ovulation has probably occurred.
- Use of ovulation predictor tests is helpful.
- The woman may be asked to keep a record of distinctive changes in cervical mucus. This clear, abundant mucus precedes the day of ovulation and provides a transport medium for the sperm. If these changes do not occur, the physician will evaluate hormonal levels.
- The normal fertile man needs 30 to 40 hours to return to his usual sperm production levels after an ejaculation. A man with low sperm count may need as long as 48 hours.
- With a typical menstrual cycle of 28 days (there are many variations in cycle length), intercourse should occur in the following pattern when a woman is trying to conceive:
  > Nights 9 and 12
  > Morning 14
  > Night 15
  > No times in between

  This schedule allows the pituitary gland to stimulate sperm production and provides time for sperm production to return to peak levels. It also maintains active sperm in the female reproductive tract.
- Intercourse should occur three to four times a week during the month to stimulate sperm production.

- Positions are important. The superior (man above) position is best for intercourse with fertility as the goal. The woman's hips should be elevated on a small pillow to facilitate sperm collection in the seminal pool near the opening of the cervix.
- The deepest penetration is advised. The woman may fold her knees on her chest and spread them as far apart as possible.
- At ejaculation, the man should penetrate as deeply as possible and stop thrusting so ejaculation occurs as near the cervix as possible. Withdrawal should occur just after ejaculation.
- When the female orgasm occurs during or after ejaculation, the cervix dips into the seminal pool.
- The woman should remain in bed for 1 hour after ejaculation to hold the seminal pool near the cervix.
- No artificial lubricants should be used. However, saliva, egg white, or olive oil are physiologic and will not hinder sperm mobility.
- No douching should be done before or after intercourse.
- Because intercourse "on demand" or on a "medical schedule" may seem artificial, care should be taken that technique and timing do not destroy an atmosphere of making love. Some men experience temporary impotence. Discussing this with the fertility nurse or physician may lessen tension and promote appropriate function.

From Dickason EJ, McKenzie CA: The infertile family. In Howe J et al, eds: *The handbook of nursing,* New York, 1984, Wiley & Sons.

ISSUES TO CONSIDER

Technologic advances have occurred at such a rapid pace as to outstrip society's ability to establish norms (laws) for application. There are myriad issues pertaining to individual rights, informed consent, family justice, and access to care. The American Fertility Society has attempted to come to grips with this by developing and promulgating a set of guidelines. However, this is only a start, because recommendations are neither mandatory nor legally enforceable. Examples of some issues are as follows:

- Should egg donors be paid? What is a fair price for an egg?
- Should research be allowed on frozen eggs or embryos?
- Should the sale of embryos be legal? Under what circumstances?
- If an embryo was acquired by extralegal means would this constitute kidnapping?
- Under what circumstances might an embryo be legally destroyed? Would it represent manslaughter if an embryo were disposed of by different means?

- In what manner should the cryopreservation of embryos be regulated?
- How is the potential inadvertent incest mitigated?
- Should eggs be harvested from aborted fetuses? If so, how does the process of natural selection proceed?
- What are the social, economic, behavioral, and human ramifications of embryo cloning (when and if this occurs)?
- Does society have a moral obligation to provide access to health services for the treatment of infertility regardless of the ability to pay? Should more urgent community health needs (such as childhood immunizations and well-infant care) take precedence over the needs of the infertile? (Wilder, 1995; Goode and Hahn, 1993; Gabriel, Hoffman, Rosenthal, 1996).

Easy answers to these questions are not possible. Some countries such as Australia, Great Britain, Canada, and Israel mandate state supported coverage for certain types of infertility care, but state funding cannot provide universal access to the most expensive and sophisticated techniques. Human dignity, justice, and equality should be an integral part of the process.

Key Points

- Infertility may be found in as high as 15% of the childbearing population, and 10% to 15% of all cases of infertility are related to unexplained causes.
- Causes of infertility are almost equally divided between men and women.
- The diagnosis of infertility is given if no conception occurs after 1 year of unprotected intercourse.
- Infertility may be primary (no prior conception) or secondary (no current conception after previous pregnancy).
- To determine the cause of infertility, the couple is evaluated for reproductive organ function and sperm and ova adequacy.
- Treatment may be multifaceted and may involve administration of hormones and antibiotics, surgical repair of structural abnormalities, or removal of adhesions or tumors.
- Advanced technologies to assist reproduction include IVF-ET, GIFT, ZIFT, ICSI, and oocyte donation. Other methods of micromanipulation to assist reproduction are being developed.
- Moral, ethical, and legal issues affected by ARTs are in flux. Guidelines and laws to prevent abuse of the system are being developed.
- Nursing care for the infertile couple focuses on assessment and support. Active listening, teaching, counseling, information about referral systems and support groups, and documentation of events are essential components of care.

Study Questions

6-1. Endometriosis is one cause of female infertility. Which of the following statements best describes the cause of endometriosis?
   a. Implants may block the passage of sperm into the cervix.
   b. Dysmenorrhea is always severe and helps in the diagnosis.
   c. Immunologic factors may be the primary cause.
   d. Antibody formation to the partner's sperm causes the implants to form.
6-2. The introduction of semen directly into the uterine cavity is called
   a. Micromanipulation.
   b. Intrauterine insemination.
   c. Autoimmunity.
   d. Transvaginal oocyte retrieval.
6-3. Varicocele is
   a. The formation of antibodies against the man's own sperm.
   b. Usually considered an unexplained factor in infertility.
   c. Cured with improved coital techniques or positions.
   d. A swollen, twisted vein in the testicle.
6-4. The Smiths had one child 5 years ago. They have been trying to conceive for the past 3 years with no success. They are assessed for
   a. Primary infertility.
   b. Secondary infertility.
   c. Age-related infertility.
   d. Enviromental factors.
   e. b, c, and d.
6-5. Low sperm production may be caused by
   a. Environmental factors.
   b. Antibiotic or antihypertensives.
   c. Childhood surgical repair for undescended testicles.
   d. All of the above.
6-6. The "forced" fertilization technique of ICSI is
   a. A method of drilling into the zona pellucida.
   b. Injecting sperm into the zona pellucida.
   c. Injecting sperm into the oocyte.
   d. Allowing the ova and sperm to fertilize in the fallopian tube.

Answer Key

6-1: c. 6-2: b. 6-3: d. 6-4: e. 6-5: d. 6-6: c.

References

American College of Obstetricians and Gynecologists: *Managing the anovulatory state: medical induction of ovulation*, Technical Bulletin No. 197, September 1994.

Baranski B: Effects of the workplace on fertility and related reproductive outcomes, *Environ Health Perspectives Supplements* 101(suppl 2):81, 1993.

Batista MC et al: Effects of aging on menstrual cycle hormones and endometrial maturation, *Fertil Steril* 64(3):492, 1995.

Becker G, Nachtigall RD: Born to be a mother: the cultural construction of risk in infertility treatment in the US, *Soc Sci Med* 39(4):507, 1994.

Ben-Chetrit A, Ben-Chetrit E: Systemic lupus erythematosus induced by ovulation induction treatment, *Arthritis Rheum* 37(11):1614, 1994.

Christie GL: The psychogenic factor in infertility, *Aust N Z J Psychiatry* 28:378, 1994.

Daniels KR, Lewis GM, Gillett W: Telling donor insemination offspring about their conception: the nature of couples' decision-making, *Soc Sci Med* 40(9):1213, 1995.

Daya S: Issues in the etiology of recurrent spontaneous abortion, *Current Opinion Obstet Gynecol* 6:153, 1994.

de Souza NM et al: The potential value of magnetic resonance imaging in infertility, *Clin Radiol* 50:75, 1995.

Ethical consideration of assisted reproductive technologies, *Fertil Steril* 62:5, 1S-125S, 1994.

Fahy UM et al: In-vitro fertilization in completely natural cycles, *Hum Reprod* 10(3):572, 1995.

Flamigni C, Borini A: Counseling post menopausal women for donor in-vitro fertilization and hormone replacement therapy, *Hum Reprod* 10(5):1237, 1995.

Franks S, Gilling-Smith C: Advances in induction of ovulation, *Current Opinion Obstet Gynecol* 6:136, 1994.

Frederick JL et al: Successful pregnancy outcome after cryopreservation of all fresh embryos with subsequent transfer into an unstimulated cycle, *Fertil Steril* 64(5):987, Nov 1995.

Gabriel T, Hoffman J, Rosenthal E: High-tech pregnancies test hope's limit, *NY Times* CXLV(50,299): Jan 7 - Jan 10, 1996.

Gleicher N: Immune dysfunction—a potential target for treatment in endometriosis, *Br J Obstet Gynaecol* 102(suppl 12):4, Oct 1995.

Gomel V: From microsurgery to laparoscopic surgery: a progress, *Fertil Steril* 63(3):464, 1995.

Goode CJ, Hahn SJ: Oocyte donation and in vitro fertilization: the nurse's role with ethical and legal issues, *J Obstet Gynecol Neonatal Nurs* 22:106, 1993.

Greil, AL: Not yet pregnant: infertile couples in contemporary America, New Brunswick, NJ, 1991, Rutgers University Press.

Hakim RB et al: Infertility and early pregnancy loss, *Am J Obstet Gynecol* 172(5):1510, 1995.

Halman LJ et al: Gender differences and perceptions about childbearing among infertile couples, *J Obstet Gynecol Neonatal Nurs* 23(7):593, Sept 1994.

Hauser R et al: Pregnancies after microsurgical correction of partial epididymal and vasal obstruction, *Hum Reprod* 10(5):1152, 1995.

Hirsch AM, Hirsch SM: The long term psychosocial effects of infertility, *J Obstet Gynecol Neonatal Nurs* 2(6):517, July/August 1995.

Honore LH: Pathology of female infertility, *Current Opinion OBGYN* 6:364, 1994.

Howards SS: Treatment of male infertility, *N Eng J Med* 332(5):312, Feb 2, 1995.

Jacobs HS: Polycystic ovary syndrome: aetiology and management, *Current Opinion Obstet Gynecol* 7:203, 1995.

Joesoef MR et al: Fertility and use of cigarettes, alcohol, marijuana and cocaine, *Ann Epidemiol* 3(6):592, 1993.

Kolata G: Chemicals that mimic hormones spark alarm and debate. Sperm counts: some experts see a fall, others poor data, *NY Times* C1:9, March 19, 1996.

Lansac J: Delayed parenting: is delayed childbearing a good thing? *Hum Reprod* 10(5):1033, 1995.

Leke RJI et al: Regional and geographical variations in infertility: effects of environmental, cultural, and socioeconomic factors, *Environ Health Perspectives Supplements* 101(suppl 2):73, 1993.

Lilford R et al: Case-control study of whether subfertility in men is familial, *BMJ* 309(6954):570, Sept 3, 1994.

Lobo RA: Unexplained infertility, *J Reprod Med* 38(4):241, 1993.

Mathieu C et al: Cumulative conception rate following intrauterine artificial insemination with husband's spermatozoa: influence of husband's age, *Hum Reprod* 10(5):1090, May 1995.

Miller KA et al: The effect of serum from infertile women with endometriosis on fertilization and early embryonic development in a murine in vitro fertilization model, *Fertil Steril* 64(3):623, 1995.

*Moghissi KS, Wallach EE: Unexplained infertility, *Fertil Steril* 39(1):5, 1985.

Mor-Yosef S, Schenker JG: Sperm donation in Israel, *Hum Reprod* 10(4):965, 1995.

Morell V: Attacking the causes of "silent" infertility, *Science* 269:775, August 11, 1995.

Mosher WD et al: Fecundity and infertility in the US: incidence and trends, *Fertil Steril* 56(2):192, 1991.

Neumann PJ, Gharib SD, Weinstein MC: The cost of a successful delivery with in vitro fertilization, *N Eng J Med* 331(4):239, July 28, 1994.

Oehninger S et al: Intracytoplasmic sperm injection: achievement of high pregnancy rates in couples with severe male factor infertility is dependent primarily upon female and not male factors, *Fertil Steril* 64(5):977, 1995.

Oei SG et al: European postcoital tests: opinions and practice, *Br J Obstet Gynaecol* 102:621 August, 1995

Parazzini F et al: Tight underpants and trousers and risk of dyspermia, *Int J Androl* 18(3):137, 1995.

Perper MM et al: Dysmenorrhea is related to the number of implants in endometriosis patients, *Fertil Steril* 63(3):500, 1995.

Prevedourakis C et al: Hysterosalpingography and hysteroscopy in female infertility, *Hum Reprod* 9(12):2353, 1994.

Ross LS, Nederberger CS: Male infertility: diagnosis and treatment, *Comp Ther* 21(6):276, 1995.

Sandelowski M: On infertility, *J Obstet Gynecol Neonatal Nurs* 23(9):749, Nov/Dec 1994.

Sauer MV et al (American Fertility Society): Guidelines for oocyte donation, *Fertil Steril* 59:5S, 1993.

Sauer MV, Paulson RJ: Oocyte and embryo donation, *Current Opinion Obstet Gynecol* 7:193, 1995.

Schoener CJ, Krysa LW: The comfort and discomfort of infertility, *J Obstet Gynecol Neonatal Nurs* 25(2):167, Feb 1996.

Seibel M, Zilberstein M: The diagnosis of male infertility by semen quality, *Hum Reprod* 10(2):247, 1995.

Shalev E et al: Routine thyroid function tests in infertile women: are they necessary? *Am J Obstet Gynecol* 171(5):1191, 1994.

Sherrod RA: Helping infertile couples explore the option of adoption, *J Obstet Gynecol Neonatal Nurs* 21(6):465, Nov/Dec 1992.

Shlegel PN et al: Antibiotics: potential hazard to male fertility, *Fertil Steril* 56(2):1235, 1991.

Shushan A, Schenker JG: The use of oocytes obtained from aborted fetuses in egg donation programs, *Fertil Steril* 62(3):449, Sept 1994.

Shushan A et al: Subfertility in the era of assisted reproduction: changes and consequences, *Fertil Steril* 64(3):459, 1995.

Skakkebaek NE, Giwercman A, de Kretser D: Pathogenesis and management of male infertility, *Lancet* 343:1473, June 11, 1994.

Snowden C: What makes a mother? Interviews with women involved in egg donation and surrogacy, *Birth* 21(2):77, June 1994.

Sokol RZ: The diagnosis and treatment of male infertility, *Current Opinion Obstet Gynecol* 7:177, 1995.

Speroff L: The effect of aging on fertility, *Current Opinion Obstet Gynecol* 6:115, 1994.

Tan SL: Luteinizing hormone-releasing hormone agonists for ovarian stimulation in assisted reproduction, *Current Opinion Obstet Gynecol* 6:166, 1994.

Tan SL: Simplifying in vitro fertilization therapy. *Current Opinion Obstet Gynecol* 6:111, 1994.

Tarin JJ: Subzonal insemination, partial zona dissection or intracytoplasmic sperm injection? An easy decision? *Hum Reprod* 10(1):165, 1995.

Toaff ME et al: Controlled ovarian hyperstimulation and transvaginal intratubal insemination as an alternative to gamete intrafallopian transfer, *Fertil Steril* 64(4):777, 1995.

*Classic reference.

Tsirigotis M, Craft I: More experiences with ICSI, *Hum Reprod* 10(4):758, 1995.

Ulbrich et al: Involuntary childlessness and marital adjustment: his and hers, *J Sex Marital Ther* 16(3):147, 1990.

*Valentine D: Psychological impact of infertility: identifying issues and needs, *Soc Work Health Care* 11(4):61, 1986.

Van Steirteghem A: IVF and micromanipulation techniques for male factor infertility, *Current Opinion Obstet Gynecol* 6:173, 1994.

Wang C et al: *The World Health Organization laboratory manual for the examination of human semen and sperm-cervical mucus interaction,* Cambridge, 1992, Cambridge University Press.

Wilcox AJ: Fertility in men exposed prenatally to diethylstilbestrol, *N Eng J Med* 332(21):1411, 1995.

Wilcox AJ, Weinberg CR, Baird DD: Timing of sexual intercourse in relation to ovulation. Effects on the probability of conception, survival of the pregnancy, and sex of the baby, *N Eng J Med* 333(23):1517, Dec 7, 1995.

Wilder BL: Ethical issues related to the new reproductive technologies, *Current Opinion Obstet Gynecol* 7: 199, 1995.

World Health Organization Task Force on the Prevention and Management of Infertility: Tubal infertility: serologic relationship to past chlamydial and gonococcal infection, *Sex Transm Dis* March/April 1995.

Books for Couples

Goldfarb HA: *Overcoming infertility: 12 couples share their success stories,* New York, 1995, Wiley.

Menning BE: *Infertility: a guide for the childless couple,* ed 2, New York: 1988, Prentice Hall.

Simons HF: *Wanting another child: coping with secondary infertility,* New York, 1995, Lexington Books.

Tan SL et al: *Infertility: your questions answered,* Secaucus, NJ, 1995, Carol Publishing Group.

Organizations for Couples

American College of Obstetricians and Gynecologists (ACOG)
ACOG Distribution Center
409 12th Street, SW
Washington, DC 20024-2188

American Fertility Society
2140 Eleventh Avenue South
Suite 200
Birmingham, AL 35205-2800

Fertility Research Foundation
1430 Second Avenue
Suite 103
New York, NY 10021

RESOLVE, Inc.
5 Water Street
Arlington, MA 02174

Adoption Organizations

Adoptive Families of America, Inc.
3333 Highway 100N
Minneapolis, MN 55422

Child Welfare League of America
440 First Street, NW
Washington, DC 20001

 Student Resource Shelf

Holditch-Davis D et al: Fertility status and symptoms in childbearing couples, *Res Nurs Health* 18:417, 1995.
  From the fourth to the ninth month of pregnancy 58 couples (37 of which had a history of infertility) compared common physical and psychologic symptoms.

Sandelowski M: A theory of the transition to parenthood of infertile couples, *Res Nurs Health* 18:123, 1995.
  A theoretic framework of the infertile couples' experiences compared with fertile couples' transition to parenthood. Distinctly different processes were observed.

Schoener CCJ, Krysa LW: The comfort and discomfort of infertility, *J Obstet Gynecol Neonatal Nurs* 25(2):167, 1996.
  Using Kolcaba's framework to provide comfort in infertility, the authors suggest nursing interventions to help couples move along a continuum of ease, relief, and transcendence.

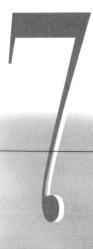

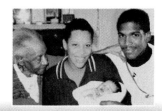

7

Conception &
Fetal Growth

$\mathcal{B}$etween conception and birth, health care begins for the expectant mother and the growing fetus. Many factors are involved in the growth and development of the infant as a separate and unique individual, including the configuration of genes from both parents, the quality of the intrauterine environment, and the external environmental influences.

It is important to distinguish between the concepts of growth and development. *Growth* is an increase in the size and number of cells that causes an organism to gain weight and length. *Development* refers to the changes that occur in primitive cells as they differentiate into tissues that will perform specific functions. This chapter will show how these processes interact during gestation.

When expectant parents inquire about the formation, growth, and development of their infant, the nurse is in an ideal position to encourage the parents' interest and help them understand factors that can affect the health of the fetus.

132

CELLULAR REPRODUCTION

In all body tissue, cells multiply by a process called **mitosis.** To divide, the parent cell duplicates each chromosome so that each new cell is an exact replica (copy) of the parent cell. In mitosis there is first a separation of chromosomes to the opposite sides of the cell before division, then an indentation develops in the center and two identical cells result.

By contrast, a special type of cell division, **meiosis,** must take place in the ovum and sperm to ensure that there will be exactly 23 pairs of chromosomes (46 total) in the new embryo's cells (Figure 7-1). Meiosis causes each oocyte and spermatocyte to contain one member of each pair of chromosomes. This reduction in chromosomes is made possible by a two-step process. The first meiotic division begins much earlier than fertilization. During this step the primary oocyte and primary spermatocyte duplicate their deoxyribonucleic acid (DNA) and double their chromosomes, producing double strands or chromatids.

At the same time, the two members of a chromosome pair often exchange segments of genetic material (Figure 7-2). This "crossing over" between homologous chromosomes causes paternal and maternal genetic material to be randomly recombined so that the genes passed to the infant may be quite different from those in either parent. This is one of the reasons a child may not look or act like either parent.

After the exchange the chromosomes line up near the middle of the cell, and the second meiotic division begins. The cell and chromosomes divide into two new cells, completing the reduction. During oogenesis each of the four cells that results from the two oocyte divisions contains 22 **autosomes** (body cell chromosomes) and one X (sex) chromosome, but only one develops into a mature oocyte. The other three become polar bodies and eventually degenerate and dissolve. By contrast, a spermatocyte divides during spermatogenesis into four types of cells, two containing 22 autosomes and one X chromosome and two containing 22 autosomes and one Y chromosome. *All* these cells become active sperm (Figure 7-3).

Oogenesis

During embryonic life the primary oocytes undergo only a part of the first meiotic division, then these oocytes enter a resting phase until puberty. (This resting phase may vary from 12 to 50 years, providing ample opportunity for damage to the oocytes' genetic material.) When puberty begins, these primary oocytes complete the first meiotic division so ovulation can occur in monthly patterns and the process called **oogenesis** begins. Each month, usually a single primary oocyte begins to increase in size and thickness and develops a protective membrane, the *zona pellucida.* The graafian follicle enlarges, and follicle cells form a thick, fluid-filled layer around the oocyte (see Figure 7-6). As soon as the graafian follicle matures, the oocyte resumes a meiotic division to produce two cells of unequal size: the secondary oocyte and the first polar body. The secondary oocyte receives all the cytoplasm and enters into the second meiotic division. This second division is complete only if the ovum is fertilized. Otherwise the ovum degenerates and is passed out of the body.

Spermatogenesis

Spermatogenesis, which starts as puberty begins and can continue well into the eighth decade of life, is a continuous process, not cyclical, once it begins. It takes about 72 hours for a primary spermatocyte to develop into a mature sperm (see Chapter 3). Primary spermatocytes begin the first meiotic division, which results in two secondary spermatocytes. The secondary spermatocytes then immediately undergo the second meiotic division and the result is four spermatids. These spermatids contain half the number of chromosomes of the primary spermatocyte, as shown in Figure 7-3. (Figure 3-2, *A,* illustrates the anatomic location of the spermatocytes in the seminiferous tubules.) Several stages of the process may occur simultaneously in different parts of the seminiferous tubules.

Because mature sperm have virtually no source of nutrition when separated from the semen, only some survive as long as 72 hours after ejaculation.

FERTILIZATION

Many factors are necessary for effective fertilization of the ovum. Coitus causes an average of 200 to 300 million sperm to be deposited in the vaginal canal close to the cervical os. After ejaculation the life span of sperm is relatively short, and they must quickly move toward the *outer* distal portion of the fallopian tube where fertilization normally occurs. Many factors may impede the journey, a distance of about 21 cm, including incompatible vaginal or cervical fluids, an extremely acidic environment, or a possible narrowing of the cervix, uterus, or tubes (see Chapter 3). However, the estrogenic influences that help change cervical mucous properties to allow for easier sperm penetration are at a peak at ovulation. In addition, the peristaltic actions of the uterine and tubal muscles foster the movement of sperm toward the tube and move the ovum toward the sperm. Prostaglandins found in semen might aid in the rapid transport of sperm toward the tube by affecting the smooth muscle contractions of the uterus. Approximately 2000 sperm reach the fallopian tubes.

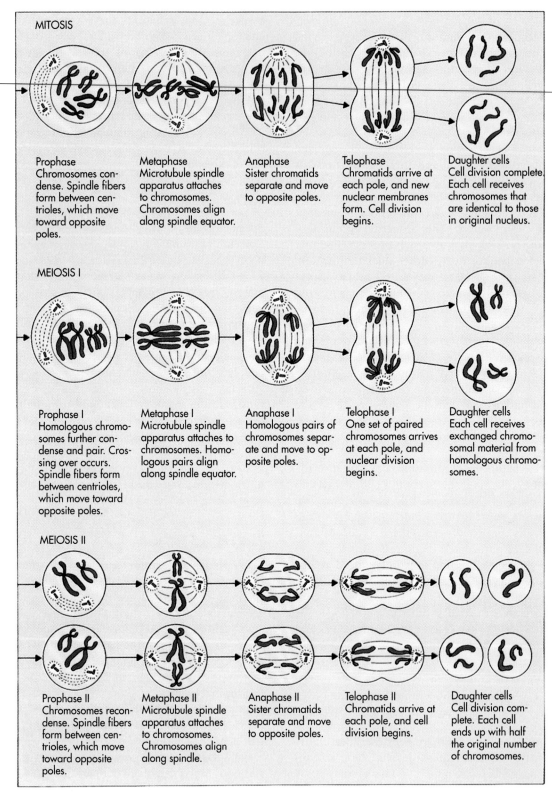

MITOSIS

Prophase
Chromosomes condense. Spindle fibers form between centrioles, which move toward opposite poles.

Metaphase
Microtubule spindle apparatus attaches to chromosomes. Chromosomes align along spindle equator.

Anaphase
Sister chromatids separate and move to opposite poles.

Telophase
Chromatids arrive at each pole, and new nuclear membranes form. Cell division begins.

Daughter cells
Cell division complete. Each cell receives chromosomes that are identical to those in original nucleus.

MEIOSIS I

Prophase I
Homologous chromosomes further condense and pair. Crossing over occurs. Spindle fibers form between centrioles, which move toward opposite poles.

Metaphase I
Microtubule spindle apparatus attaches to chromosomes. Homologous pairs align along spindle equator.

Anaphase I
Homologous pairs of chromosomes separate and move to opposite poles.

Telophase I
One set of paired chromosomes arrives at each pole, and nuclear division begins.

Daughter cells
Each cell receives exchanged chromosomal material from homologous chromosomes.

MEIOSIS II

Prophase II
Chromosomes recondense. Spindle fibers form between centrioles, which move toward opposite poles.

Metaphase II
Microtubule spindle apparatus attaches to chromosomes. Chromosomes align along spindle.

Anaphase II
Sister chromatids separate and move to opposite poles.

Telophase II
Chromatids arrive at each pole, and cell division begins.

Daughter cells
Cell division complete. Each cell ends up with half the original number of chromosomes.

Figure 7-1   A comparison of mitosis with meiosis. During mitosis, chromosomes are duplicated and the cell divides, producing two new cells identical to the first. During meiosis, chromosomes are duplicated only once, but there are two consecutive cellular divisions. This yields four daughter cells, each with half the original number of chromosomes. (Courtesy Raychel Ciemma.)

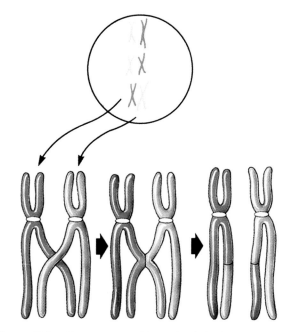

Figure 7-2   Crossing over. Genes (or linked groups of genes) from one chromosome are exchanged with matching genes in the other chromosome of a pair during meiosis. (Courtesy Kevin Somerville.)

Normally, only one of the many sperm reaching the ovum will enter it. The others secrete hyaluronidase, an enzyme found in the acrosome or outer covering of the head of each sperm that helps penetrate the zona pellucida. As fertilization occurs a process called **syngamy** acts to protect the fertilized ovum. During syngamy the ovum completes its second maturational division and extrudes a polar body (Figure 7-4). A reaction in the oocyte cytoplasm occurs just below the cell membrane that causes a barrier to form, preventing other sperm from entering the cell. The tail of the sperm disappears, and the nucleus becomes larger, revealing its chromosomal content. At this point, the structure becomes known as the *male pronucleus,* the sperm nucleus before it fuses with the nucleus of the ovum. The *female pronucleus,* the nucleus of the ovum before it fuses with the nucleus of the sperm, swells. The pronuclei gravitate toward one another and fuse, thus completing fertilization by restoring the full diploid number of chromosomes to the fertilized ovum, which is now the **zygote**. The genetic foundation is now laid for the growth and development of the infant.

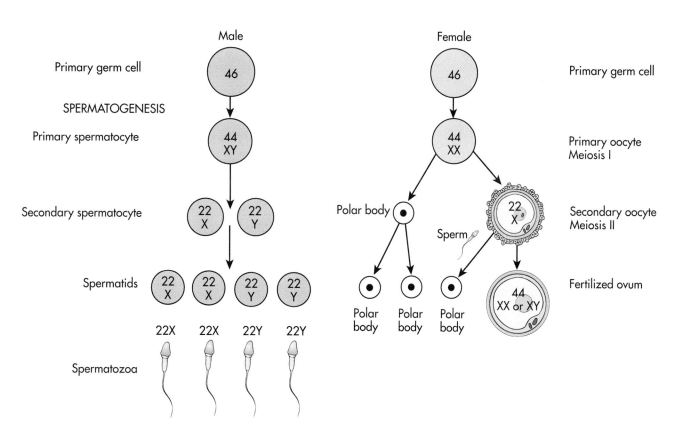

Figure 7-3   Ovum and sperm maturation. Spermatogenesis results in four spermatids, but oogenesis results in only one functional ovum and three polar bodies.

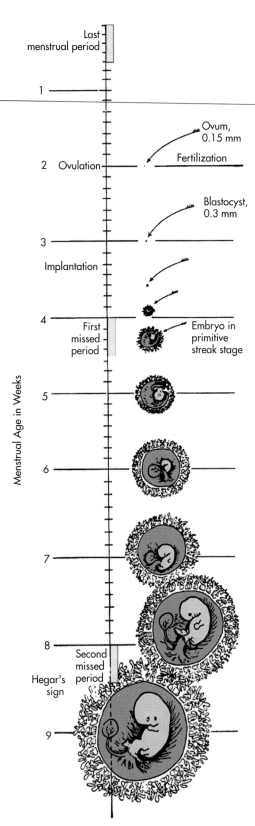

Figure 7-4 Actual size of embryos in relation to mother's menstrual history. Based on 28-day cycle. **Gestational age** is approximately 14 days more than the **fertilization age.** (From Corliss CE: *Patten's human embryology,* ed 4, New York, 1976, McGraw-Hill.)

TEST *Yourself* **7-1** _____

a. After completion of meiosis, each oocyte or spermatozoan will contain only _____ autosome(s) and _____ sex chromosome(s).

b. Exchange of genetic material occurs during _____ of chromatids.

c. Why is the genetic material contained in oocytes at higher risk for damage than that contained in spermatocytes?

d. After the male and female pronuclei fuse, the fertilized ovum is called a(n) _____ .

Determination of Sex

The twenty-third pair of chromosomes are the sex chromosomes (either XX or XY). Females have two X chromosomes; males have an X and a Y chromosome.

The sex of an individual is determined by the presence or absence of the Y chromosome. It was not until 1959 that scientists discovered that embryos carrying the Y chromosome developed as males and those embryos lacking a Y chromosome developed as females.

A **testes determining factor** is thought to be a single gene on the Y chromosome. The male and female genitalia are undifferentiated or in the indifferent stage for the first 6 weeks of the embryo's development. After this, it is thought that the gene on the Y chromosome triggers signals that lead to development of the Leydig's cells that produce testosterone to induce masculinization of the external genitalia. In the absence of this gene (regardless of whether there is a Y chromosome), the embryo becomes a female. Similarly, there may be a single gene on the X chromosome to control a chain of events that triggers feminization of external genitalia.

EMBRYONIC PERIOD

Cleavage

About 24 to 48 hours after fertilization, the zygote divides; the daughter cells resulting from this mitosis are half the size of the fertilized ovum. Continued division results in progressively smaller cells because during this phase the zona pellucida remains intact, keeping the mass of dividing cells at about the same size as the fertilized ovum (Figure 7-5). As cleavage occurs the zygote travels down the fallopian tube toward the uterus. After 3 or 4 days it begins to look like a solid ball of cells, the **morula,** which resembles a mulberry.

Implantation

Approximately 3 to 4 days after fertilization the morula enters the uterus. Cells can be distinguished according to

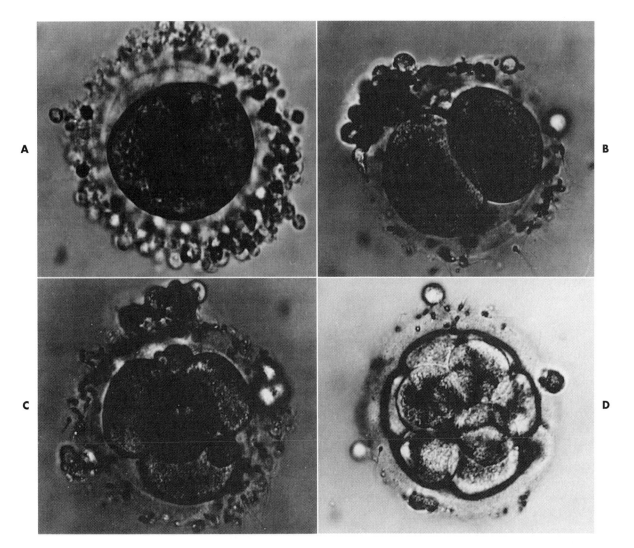

Figure 7-5   Early stages of human development. **A,** Fertilized ovum, or zygote. **B** to **D,** Early cell divisions produce more and more cells. The solid mass of cells shown in **D** forms the morulan early stage in embryonic development. (Courtesy Lucinda L Veeck, Jones Institute for Reproductive Medicine, Norfolk, Va.)

function. Fluid enters the morula and divides the cells into inner and outer cell masses. A cavity (blastocyst cavity) forms and the zona pellucida gradually disappears. The embryo is now called a **blastocyst.** Over the next 2 weeks the inner cell mass differentiates into three layers: ectoderm, endoderm, and mesoderm (Figure 7-6). These primary **fetal germ layers** are the tissues from which all body systems are formed (Box 7-1).

Approximately 7 days after fertilization, a layer of ectodermal tissue on the outside of the blastocyst, the **trophoblast,** begins to burrow into the lining of the uterus; this burrowing is called *implantation* or *nidation.* Trophoblastic cells secrete enzymes that digest or liquefy endometrial tissue. The blastocyst sinks deep into the endometrium, which becomes the *decidua basalis.* Fingerlike projections—villi—of the trophoblast "dig into" and break down uterine tissue and firmly anchor

the blastocyst in the decidua basalis, an area with a rich source of nourishment and oxygen. This activity may be confused with a menstrual period, since some women may experience slight vaginal bleeding at this time. However, by the ninth or tenth day, the epithelium, now called the *decidua capsularis,* has begun to heal over the area in which the blastocyst had become embedded (Figure 7-7).

By the thirteenth day after fertilization the trophoblast has become the chorion, and the villi have become the chorionic villi. By the end of the third month the growth of the embryo causes the decidua capsularis and the decidua parietalis (uterine lining farthest from the implantation site) to compress one another. Only the chorionic villi, also called the *chorion frondosum* now remain in the decidua basalis. These chorionic villi make up the fetal portion of the placenta.

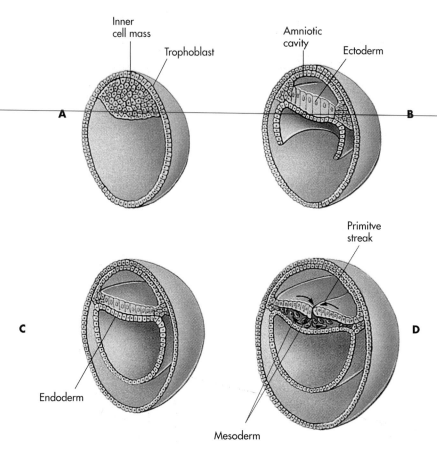

Figure 7-6 Formation of the three primary germ layers. **A,** 3 to 4 days. The amniotic cavity forms within the inner cell mass. **B** and **C,** Second week. Two germ layers are seen—ectoderm and endoderm. The yolk sac is surrounded by endoderm. **D,** During the third week, cells that will become the mesoderm (third germ layer) are sent throughout the embryo by means of the primitive streak. (Courtesy Kevin Somerville.)

Box 7-1	**Organs and Tissues Derived from Germ Layers**

ECTODERM

Central nervous system
Peripheral nervous system
Sensory epithelium of sense organs
Epidermis of hair, nails, subcutaneous glands
Hair follicles
Lens of eye
Enamel of teeth
Hypophysis
Mammary glands

MESODERM

Heart
All connective tissue layers
Bone
Muscles

Cartilage
Blood
Kidneys
Urinary tract
Lymphatic system
Gonadal system
Spleen

ENDODERM

Gastrointestinal tract
Epithelium of respiratory tract, pharynx, tongue, thyroid, parathyroids
Liver
Pancreas
Epithelial lining of bladder and urethra

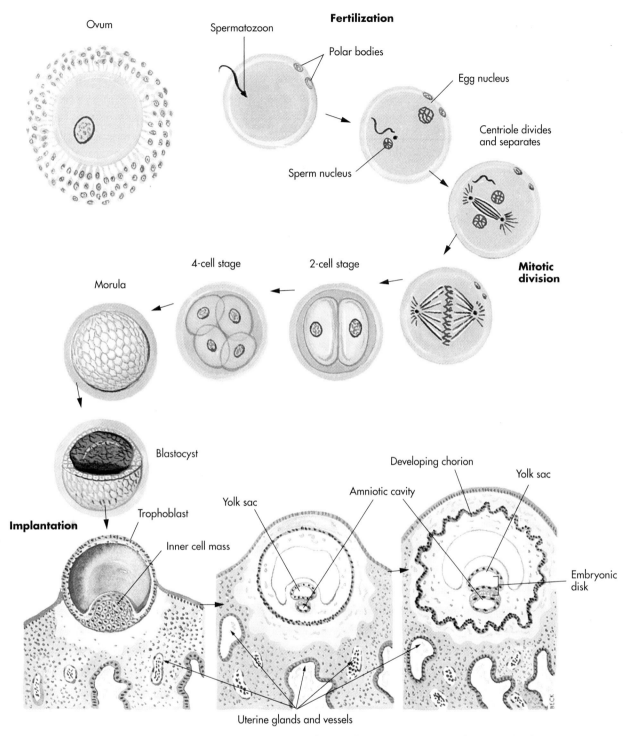

Figure 7-7 Fertilization to implantation and development of the yolk sac. Rapid growth of uterine glands and vessels covers the developing blastocyst at the time of implantation. (Courtesy Ernest W Beck.)

Chorion

The **chorion** develops from the trophoblast and is the outermost membrane and closest to the uterine lining (Figure 7-8). The trophoblast infiltrates maternal tissues with chorionic villi, which are embedded in the decidua basalis. These villi form the fetal side of the placenta. Thus the villi become bathed with maternal blood rich in oxygen and nutrients.

The chorionic villi enlarge by the end of the fourth and fifth months to form 15 to 20 visible placental partitions (cotyledons or "little trees"). In addition, the chorion produces human chorionic gonadotropin (hCG), which helps

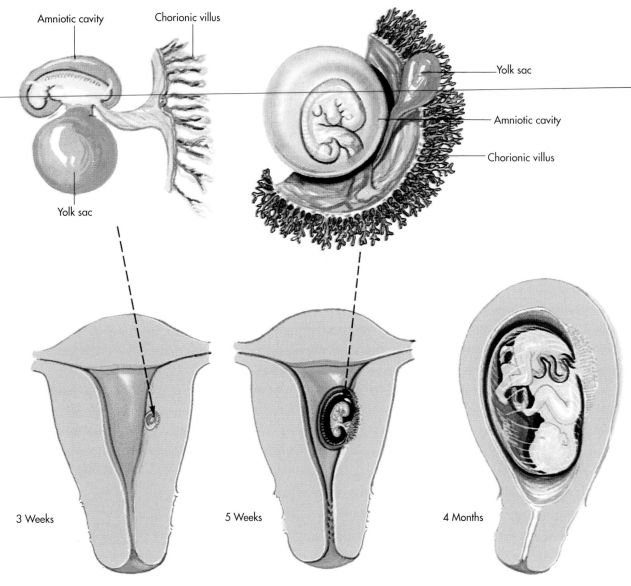

Figure 7-8 Development of the chorion and amnion. Development of the chorion and amniotic cavity to 4 months of gestation. (Courtesy Ernest W Beck.)

sustain pregnancy by preventing the involution of the corpus luteum.

Amnion

The **amnion** appears very early in embryonic life, even before the embryo has taken form. The amnion is small at first, but as it fills with fluid and the embryo grows, it becomes much larger and eventually surrounds the embryo and umbilical cord. Later in pregnancy the amnion expands to fill the entire space of the fetal sac and adheres to the other membrane, the chorion. The amnion and chorion together are known as the fetal membranes (see Figure 7-8).

At term, the amniotic sac contains almost a liter of amniotic fluid, which forms from amniotic cells, urine, and secretions from the lungs and skin of the fetus. This fluid is slightly alkaline and contains albumin, urea, creatinine, lecithin, sphingomyelin, bilirubin, fat, fructose, lanugo hairs, uric acid, and inorganic salts. The amniotic sac cushions the fetus against injury, prevents adhesions of the sticky skin and umbilical cord compression, equalizes pressure, and provides thermal regulation, a medium for fetal movement, and fluid for the fetus to swallow. The fluid is replaced approximately every 3 hours. This secretion and reabsorption is regulated by the amnion cells and fetal swallowing and urinating.

At term, this fluid provides a "wedge" to help soften and dilate the cervix during labor. Amniotic fluid can also provide the physician with valuable diagnostic information when its components are analyzed in high-risk preg-

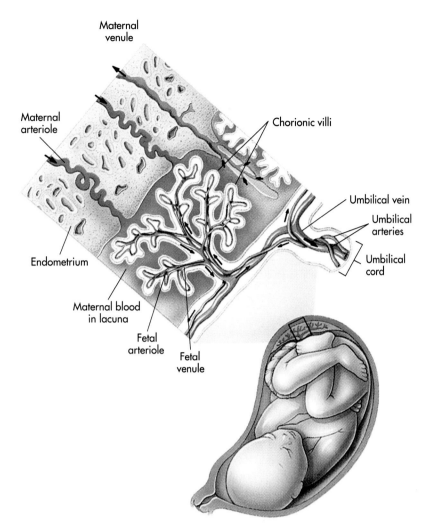

Figure 7-9   Mature placenta. Embryonic blood vessels and maternal blood vessels are in close contact, but there is no mixing of fetal and maternal blood. (Courtesy Christine Oleksyk.)

nancies. Volumes of amniotic fluid greater than average (*hydramnios*) or less than average (*oligohydramnios*) are significant because these variations may be associated with fetal abnormalities (see Chapters 21 and 27).

Placenta

The development and circulation of the **placenta** occur during the third week (Figure 7-9). The placenta is formed at the site of attachment of the chorion to the uterine wall, and both the placenta and its membranes are completely functional by the twelfth week. The placenta expands until it covers about half of the internal surface area of the uterus by the twentieth week.

The placenta secretes hormones essential for maintaining pregnancy. By the third month it takes over production of progesterone from the corpus luteum and it also secretes estriol, an estrogen.

Human placental lactogen (hPL), a hormone similar to prolactin, is also produced by the placenta. This hPL stimulates changes in the mother's metabolic process to ensure that the mother's body is prepared for lactation.

The placenta grows until late in the eighth month. Toward the end of pregnancy it begins to age, secreting hormones in decreasing amounts and gradually becoming less able to effectively exchange nutrients, oxygen, and wastes. Placental aging may be assessed during ultrasound examination (see Chapter 11).

The placental barrier is composed of layers of fetal tissue (trophoblast, connective tissue, basement membrane, and fetal capillary endothelium). It provides some protection to the fetus, but as pregnancy progresses the membrane becomes thinner. The pregnant woman must understand that *virtually everything she puts into her body may cross the placenta*. The placenta acts as the lungs, kidneys, and liver, and the endocrine, digestive, and immune systems until the fetal systems are mature enough to function.

Placental exchange is by *simple diffusion* for oxygen, carbon dioxide, fat-soluble vitamins, and lipids (including narcotics, anesthetics, and barbiturates that are fat soluble). *Facilitated diffusion* and active transport govern glucose, amino acids, calcium, iron, and water-soluble vitamins. *Pinocytosis* controls larger molecules such as globulins, viruses, and antibodies. Other substances pass through by additional means. Large molecules such as immunoglobulin M (IgM), heparin, insulin, or complex cells such as blood cells do not cross the placenta unless there is damage to the placental membrane (Blackburn and Loper, 1992).

There is no direct mingling of fetal and maternal blood, though there may be very isolated exchanges of fetal and maternal blood cells when small leaks occur in the trophoblast, during threatened abortion, or during diagnostic tests such as *chorionic villus sampling* (CVS) and *amniocentesis* (see Chapter 11).

Umbilical cord

While the placenta develops, the *umbilical cord* is also forming. Blood vessels establish a connection between the developing embryo and the placenta via the body stalk. The body stalk and remnants of the yolk sac together form the primitive umbilical cord.

Initially there are four cord vessels. One vein atrophies early in gestation, leaving one larger **umbilical vein** to carry blood from the placenta to the fetus and two small **umbilical arteries** to return deoxygenated blood to the placenta. Approximately 400 ml/min of blood flow through the cord; this flow helps stabilize the soft cord. The cord vessels are also supported by a substance called **Wharton's jelly.** This substance is made up of connective tissue and mucopolysaccharides, and it is covered by amnion that extends up from the fetal side of the placenta and ends at the skin of the abdomen of the fetus. The amount of Wharton's jelly varies widely; it is especially influenced by fetal nutrition, activity, and gestational age. Cord vessels may be constricted in response to stimuli or drugs. The surface of the cord contains no pain receptors; thus cutting the cord is painless.

TEST *Yourself* 7-2 _____

a. The segment of the Y chromosome thought to direct male sexual development is the _____.
b. The embryonic tissue that will become the chorion and placenta is called the _____.
c. Name three functions of amniotic fluid.

Development of the Embryo

The time between fertilization and the fourteenth day of development is called the *preembryonic period*. This is a time of rapid cell division, with differentiation of tissues and the development of the primary germ layers: *ecto-*

derm, endoderm, and *mesoderm.* These three germ layers are the tissues from which all body structures are formed (see Box 7-1).

At the third week the mass of growing cells becomes an **embryo.** The embryonic period is marked by rapid growth and further tissue differentiation, including **organogenesis,** the differentiation and formation of organs. Many organs are developed before the mother realizes she is pregnant. This period is also characterized by extreme susceptibility to adverse environmental influences such as radiation, infection, drugs, or smoking. The shape of the embryo changes dramatically during this stage of development (Figures 7-10 and 7-11).

By the end of the third week, germ layers have begun to form distinct tissues. The ectodermal layer develops into the organs and into the structures that maintain interaction with the outside world, such as the central nervous system (CNS) and brain. The mesodermal layer develops into the supporting tissues of the body (muscle and bone) and the vascular and urinary tract systems so the body can maintain movement and internal function. Finally, the endodermal layer provides for the epithelial linings of most of the systems of the body.

FETAL PERIOD

By the ninth week of gestation the embryo has developed sufficiently to be called a fetus. The fetal period is a time of rapid growth and continues until birth (Box 7-2). Some tissue differentiation still occurs in the genitourinary tract, eyes, and lungs.

By the end of the *first trimester* (conception to week 13), the fetus appears to be a miniature human being. All organ systems have formed and continue to develop the ability to function. However, the fetus is not yet viable outside the uterus because its systems are unable to function independently.

Neurons within the CNS, especially those in the brain, continue to differentiate, proliferate, and grow throughout gestation. Adequate nutrition and the avoidance of **teratogens** (substances that can harm the growing fetus) are vital if development is to proceed normally. Teratogens are discussed fully in Chapter 28. The *second trimester* (week 13 to end of week 26) is characterized by rapid fetal growth, especially in length, and continued cellular differentiation (see Box 7-2). By the end of the second trimester the infant is **viable.**

During the *third trimester* (begins in week 27 and lasts until term [38 weeks]), subcutaneous fat is deposited and the refinement of organ development continues. While reading the following system-by-system descriptions, keep in mind that these amazing processes occur simultaneously and that they are interdependent. Therefore the health of one system often influences the health of others.

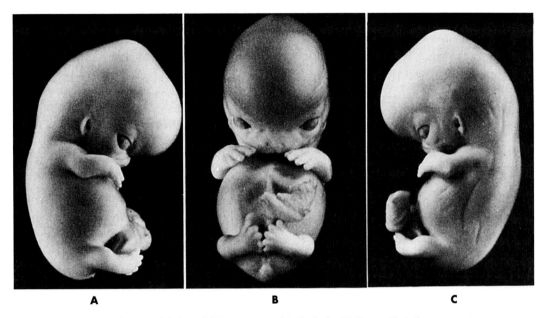

Figure 7-10 Human fetus at 54 days (22.5 mm or inch). **A,** Right. **B,** Front. **C,** Left. (Courtesy R Rugh. Photo by E Ludwig.)

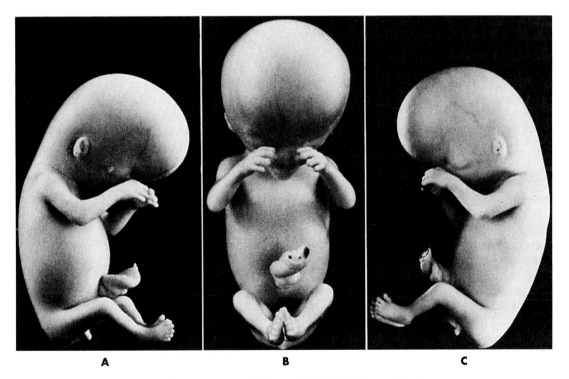

Figure 7-11 Human (male) fetus at 68 days (47 mm). **A,** Right. **B,** Front. **C,** Left. (Courtesy R Rugh. Photo by E Ludwig.)

Box **7-2**   **Embryonic, Fetal, and Placental Milestones at Fertilization Age***

PREEMBRYONIC PERIOD

3 minutes-48 hours

Fertilization, syngamy occur

24-48 hours

First cleavage of zygote occurs

3-4 days

Morula enters uterus

4-5 days

Blastocyst reaches uterus

6 days

Zona pellucida lost
Trophoblast invades decidua basalis, begins to
   become chorion

EMBRYONIC PERIOD

15 days

Implantation complete
Blood vessels form from yolk sac, body stalk, chorion
Primitive streak, mesoderm form
Germ layers begin cell specialization or differentiation
Chorionic villi have circulatory core

18-21 days

Primitive nervous system folding occurs
Heart begins to twitch
Primitive eyes, ears exist
Primitive red blood cells differentiate
Placenta covers approximately one fifteenth of uterus, begins
to function

4 weeks (1 month)

Heart folds, begins asynchronous pulsations; blood pumped
Yolk sac produces blood cells
Brain differentiates into forebrain, midbrain, hindbrain
Head large in proportion to body
Outlines of eyes seen above primitive mouth cavity
Lung buds appear
Gastrointestinal tract, liver, thyroid gland, pancreas, gall-
   bladder can be identified
Somites (future vertebrae) appear on sides of midline
Crown-rump (C-R) length† is 4-5 mm

5 weeks

Limb buds appear
Rapid brain growth occurs
Cranial, spinal nerves develop
Primitive nose, ears, jaws, eyes form

7-8 days

Implantation occurs
Ectoderm, endoderm appear

8-10 days

Clefts in ectoderm form amniotic cavity
Amnion, yolk sac begin to form
Amniotic cells secrete amniotic fluid to protect embryo

13 days

Trophoblast continues to become chorion
hCG appears in urine, serum 10 to 21 days after fertilization
Primary chorionic villi form

Germ cells migrate toward gonads
Umbilical cord forms from body stalk
Heart forms septa
C-R length is 6-8 mm

6 weeks

Trachea, bronchi, lung buds, lips form
Liver produces red blood cells
Central, autonomic nervous systems form
Rudimentary kidney, penis exist
Eyes begin to move to front of face; sensory retinal ends
   form; pigmentation occurs
Cartilage forms; rudimentary bone present
Differentiation of muscles occurs; muscle mass forms over
primitive skeletal shape
C-R length is 10-14 mm

7 weeks

Eyelids form
Gallbladder forms
Liver forms blood cells
Yolk sac declines
Palate, tongue form
Bone cells begin to replace cartilage
Arms, legs move
C-R length is 22-28 mm

8 weeks (2 months)

Hands, feet well formed
Eyes continue to move to front of face; eyelids fuse
Heart has four chambers, beats 40-80 times/min
Major blood vessels form; circulation through umbilical cord
   occurs

*Length of pregnancy is 266 ± 8 days, 38 weeks, or 9 months from fertilization.
†Crown-rump length is the measurement used to determine the fertilization age; it is usually determined by ultrasonography.

▌ *Box* **7-2**   **Embryonic, Fetal, and Placental Milestones at Fertilization Age—cont'd**

Thyroid, adrenal glands, taste buds well formed
External genitalia can be distinguished as male or female

FETAL PERIOD

9 weeks

Fingernails, toenails form
Heartbeat can be heard faintly with ultrasound instruments
Genitalia well developed

10 weeks

Head growth slows; body begins to develop in proportion to it
Limbs reach relative lengths
Bone marrow forms, produces red blood cells
Bladder sac forms; kidneys make urine

11 weeks

Tooth buds appear for temporary teeth
Salivary glands form
Peristalsis begins

SECOND TRIMESTER

16 weeks (4 months)

Fingerprints develop
Arms, legs move frequently
Lips form; facial contours fill out
Skin still loose, wrinkled, pink
Brain forms ridges, cerebrum grows rapidly
Bladder fully formed
Oocytes form in fetal ovaries
Fetus sensitive to light
Meconium (dead cells, mucus, gland secretions) forms, will make up newborn's first stool
C-R length is 14 cm; weight is 180-200 g
200 ml of amniotic fluid present
Amniocentesis possible by 14-16 weeks

20 weeks (5 months)

Anabolic-catabolic exchange begins
Eyelashes, eyebrows, hair on head more abundant
Vernix caseosa (grayish-white, cheeselike substance), lanugo (soft hair) cover, protect fetus
Fetus sucks, swallows, hears sounds

Placenta covers one third of uterine lining
C-R length is 3 cm; weight is 2 g

Thyroid gland secretes hormones
Insulin forms in pancreas.
Liver secretes bile
Urinary tract passages function

12 weeks (3 months)

Lungs take shape; respiratory motion seen
Thumb, forefinger oppose
Vocal cords form
Palate fuses
Swallowing reflex present
Liver begins production of red blood cells
C-R length is 9 cm; weight is 45 g

Brown fat deposits form
Circadian rhythm begins
Respiratory movements occur, become more regular
Myelinization of spinal cord begins
C-R length is 19 cm; weight is 430-480 g
Placenta covers half of uterine lining, weighs 120 g
400 ml amniotic fluid present

24 weeks (6 months)

Eyes complete; eyelids open, close
Alveolar ducts, sacs present; alveolar cells produce pulmonary surfactants (phospholipids that minimize surface tension of respiratory fluids)
Bone ossification begins
Thick vernix covers fetus; head hair very long
Skin layers on hands, feet thicken
Many reflexes appear
C-R length is 23-24 cm; weight is 700-800 g

Continued.

Box 7-2	Embryonic, Fetal, and Placental Milestones at Fertilization Age—cont'd

THIRD TRIMESTER

28 weeks (7 months)

Respiratory, circulatory systems function
Respiratory movements in utero seen by ultrasound
Testes begin to descend
Skin very thin, red, wrinkled, with prominent capillaries underneath
Eyebrows, eyelashes prominent; nails appear
Lanugo begins to disappear
C-R length is 28 cm; weight is 1000-1200 g

32 weeks (8 months)

Subcutaneous fat deposits form to insulate fetus from temperature changes at birth
Skin becomes less wrinkled, red
Fingernails, toenails complete
Alveoli fill; ratio of lecithin, sphingomyelin (L/S) (surfactants) is 1.2:2
More reflexes present
C-R length is 29-32 cm; weight is 1300-2100 g

36 weeks

Brain myelination begins, continues through birth
L/S ratio is 2:1
Sleep-wake cycle more definite
Maternal antibodies transfer to fetus and last for approximately 6 months
C-R length is 32-35 cm; weight is 2500-2800 g
Approximately 1000 ml of amniotic fluid present

38 weeks (term)

Fetus less active because of limited space
Meconium accumulates in intestines
Nails have grown to tips of toes, fingers; creases prominent on soles of feet
Fetus may be able to lift head
Fetal circulation developed
Crown-heel (C-H) length is 46-52 cm C-R length is 35-37 cm; weight is 3000-3600 g
800 ml of amniotic fluid present

Respiratory System: Development and Function

In utero the placenta is a substitute for the nonfunctioning fetal lungs. Oxygenated blood comes to the fetus from the placenta via the umbilical vein. Although fetal lungs are not being used for ventilation and oxygenation, the normal fetus makes respiratory movements in utero. These movements have been demonstrated by real-time ultrasound and are one of the parameters of the biophysical profile (see Chapter 11). These "practice" respiratory movements normally do not draw amniotic fluid into the fetal lungs; they are merely small movements of the chest wall. The respiratory system develops from the endoderm (the same tissue that will give rise to the gastrointestinal system) during day 24 of embryonic life. Bronchi are formed by the sixteenth week of fetal development, and there are primitive lungs by 23 weeks. However, these function only with difficulty because there are not enough alveoli for the necessary exchange of gases. Blood flow to the lungs is also inadequate at this time. Figure 7-12 illustrates the anatomic development of the respiratory system.

Two distinct types of cells are found in the lungs: type I cells, which allow for exchange of gases, and type II cells, which produce **surfactant** at 20 to 24 weeks of gestational age. Surfactant is composed of surface-active compounds that stabilize the alveoli and prevent their collapse with each exhalation. There are two pathways of surfactant production. The first pathway functions from 20 to 24 weeks and continues until birth. However, it is an unstable pathway and is easily inhibited after birth by hypoxia, hypothermia, and acidosis. The second pathway is much more resistant to these stressors but does not fully mature until 35 to 37 weeks of fetal life. Interestingly, stressors on the health of the mother, such as hypertension, preeclampsia, or heroin use, can stimulate the production of surfactant. It is thought that increased amounts of steroids are produced by a mother who is stressed. Pulmonary maturity can be accelerated by giving steroids to a mother before term if enough time is available before delivery of the infant (see Chapter 21).

Respiration is regulated by the respiratory center in the brainstem. Maturation of the CNS progresses as pregnancy continues, with coordination of feeding and respiration occurring at about 34 weeks of gestation. All of these developmental milestones are vital to the discussion of **fetal viability**. The fetus is considered to have reached the age of viability at 20 weeks' gestation, although extrauterine survival at this stage of development is currently almost impossible. When an infant of 20 weeks' gestation seems to be surviving, it is often because there is a discrepancy between the expected date of birth and the real gestational age. The lungs become capable of *borderline* support of extrauterine respiration sometime after 23 weeks of gestation. Adequate respiratory function also depends on maturation of surfactant production and neurologic control of respiration. Since each human being is unique, there is no "magic week" of gestation during which pulmonary maturity is certain.

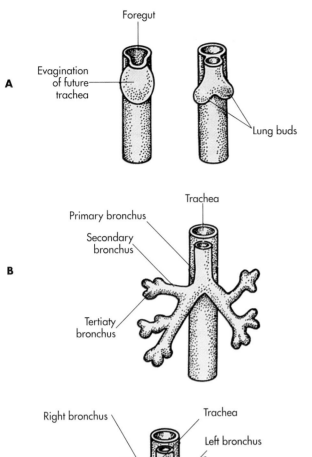

Figure 7-12   Development of the lung. **A,** By 28 days—a single lung bud forms and divides into two buds, forming primary bronchi. **B,** By 35 days—tertiary bronchi branch to form lobules. **C,** After 50 days—continued branching. (Courtesy David J Mascaro & Associates.)

TEST *Yourself* 7-3 _____

a. Which germ layer will form the body's support structures?

b. The second trimester extends from week _____ _____ to week _____; the third trimester extends from week _____ to week _____.

c. If primitive lungs are present by the twenty-third week of gestation, why do you think respiration is so difficult for the infant delivered prematurely?

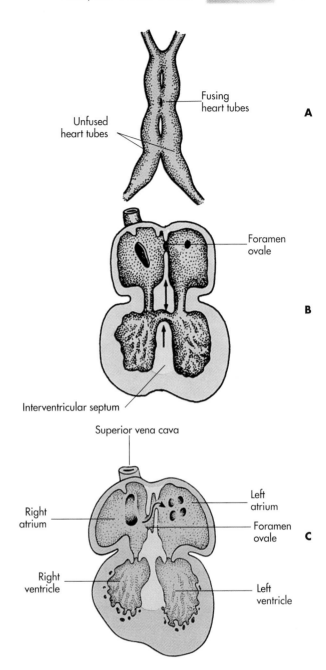

Figure 7-13   Development of the heart. **A,** At 20 days after fertilization—two tubed heart. **B,** At 31 days, note the foramen ovale. The interventricular septum is nearly complete. **C,** At 7 weeks, the flap of the foramen ovale is a one-way door allowing blood to shunt from the right side of the heart to the left. (Courtesy David J Mascaro & Associates.)

Cardiovascular System: Development and Function

With blood circulating by the end of the third week of gestation, the cardiovascular system is the first system to function in the embryo (Figure 7-13). This is necessary because the rapidly growing embryo requires a large quantity of nutrients and produces an equally large amount of waste products. Humans, unlike other animals, have only a small yolk sac for nutritional support during early gestation.

The first indication of cardiac development is seen on day 18 or 19 in the cardiogenic area, where cells cluster to form the cardiogenic cords. These two tubes fuse and then develop strictures and outpouchings that form the primitive heart chambers and vessels. By the end of the fifth week, cells around the heart tubes differentiate into myocardial and pericardial cells. The primitive heart begins beating by day 22, even before the four chambers are well defined. Cardiac muscle develops from tissue that is around the embryonic cardiac tubes. Some of these cells will later form Purkinje's cells, which are the heart's conducting system.

Fetal circulation

The three purposes for fetal circulation are accomplished through the following specialized fetal structures and their functions:

1. Decrease blood flow to the fetal lungs
2. Increase blood flow to the head and the heart
3. Direct blood to the placenta

Fetal circulation differs from adult circulation in several ways. Blood pressure in the adult is lower in the lungs (pulmonary blood pressure) than it is in the rest of the body (systemic blood pressure). In fetal life this condition is *reversed*. Fetal pulmonary blood pressure is higher because fetal pulmonary blood vessels are constricted to divert blood flow away from the nonfunctioning fetal lungs. Fetal systemic blood pressure, however, is lower because blood flow leads to the placenta through blood vessels that are not constricted. Follow Figure 7-14 while reading the following description of fetal circulation.

1. Highly oxygenated blood comes to the fetus from the placenta *via*
2. The **umbilical vein.**
3. This is shunted past the liver *via* the **ductus venosus** and
4. Continues through the inferior vena cava to the right atrium.
5. Poorly oxygenated blood from the lower body flows from the inferior vena cava through the liver and then continues to the right atrium.
6. Most of the highly oxygenated blood from the inferior vena cava is diverted to the left atrium through the **foramen ovale**, a flap that allows blood to flow only from the right to left sides of the heart ("right-to-left shunt").
7. Poorly oxygenated blood from the upper body flows through the tricuspid valve into the right ventricle and *through*
8. The pulmonary artery to the fetal lungs, but
9. Increased pressure caused by fetal pulmonary constriction directs most of this blood away from the pulmonary vessels and to the aorta through the **ductus**

arteriosus; this is another "right-to-left shunt."

10. Simultaneously, highly oxygenated blood in the left atrium, mixed with a small amount of blood from the nonfunctioning fetal lungs, flows through the mitral valve into the aorta. This allows highly oxygenated blood to be directed to the myocardium and the brain.
11. Blood from the ductus arteriosus and the aorta mixes and supplies the rest of the body.
12. The two umbilical arteries (branches of the internal iliac arteries) carry mixed blood back to the placenta for reoxygenation.

TEST *Yourself* 7-4 _____

a. Name three purposes of fetal circulation.
b. Which fetal structure diverts blood from the right atrium to the left atrium?
c. Which fetal structure diverts blood from the pulmonary artery to the aorta?

Metabolic Control

Thermal control

The fetus produces heat in utero, which is dissipated through the placenta to the mother if the mother's temperature is less than that of the fetus (the maternal-fetal thermal gradient). The temperature of the fetus is approximately 0.5° C (0.9° F) above maternal core temperature, which ranges from 37.6° C to 37.8° C (99.8° F to 100.0° F). If the mother becomes febrile, this heat-dissipating mechanism can fail, allowing fetal core temperature to rise. Maternal hyperthermia may not be related to illness. Strenuous exercise or increased environmental temperatures such as those found in hot tubs, saunas, and steam baths can lead to fetal hyperthermia. It has been suggested that fetal or maternal hyperthermia in early development may cause CNS defects such as **anencephaly** (Pleet et al, 1980).

Newborns produce most of their body heat by metabolizing a specialized tissue called **brown fat**, which develops progressively during the last trimester of pregnancy. Sites for brown fat storage in the term infant include the nape of the neck, between the scapulae, in the mediastinum, and surrounding the kidneys.

The control center for heat regulation is located in the hypothalamus and is fully functional in the healthy newborn. Therefore it is the lack of brown fat, and not the lack of temperature control, that places healthy but premature and growth-retarded infants at risk for hypothermia. An insulating layer of fat (white fat) is also deposited during the third trimester. With maturation of the hypothalamus, central control of body temperature is further developed. However, mechanisms for maintaining temperature are still immature at birth; consequently, the neonate does not adapt well to extremes of temperature.

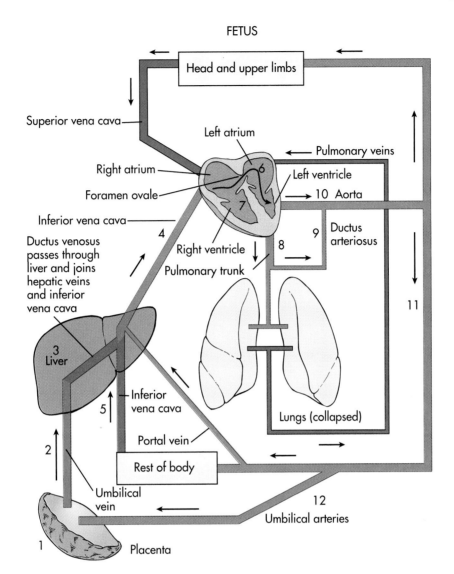

Figure 7-14 The architecture of the fetal circulatory system, showing levels of oxygen saturation in different parts of the system. Blood with the highest oxygen levels is indicated by scarlet color; intermediate values are shown in darker red; purple and the lowest values are shown in blue. (Courtesy G David Brown)

TEST *Yourself 7-5*

a. How is fetal temperature controlled in utero?
b. Why is maternal hyperthermia so serious?

Glucose and calcium

Fetal energy requirements are supplied by maternal metabolism in the form of glucose, lactate, free fatty acids, and amino acids; fetal gluconeogenesis also contributes to energy supplies. This energy is used for both fetal growth and storage of energy for future needs. The rate of energy storage increases toward term as glycogen is stored in the fetal liver and cardiac muscle.

Calcium is supplied to the fetus via active placental transport mechanisms that facilitate transfer from the maternal circulation. Fetal calcium levels are maintained 1 mg/100 ml of blood higher than maternal levels. Maternal calcium levels drop slightly toward term because of fetal needs. Because the growing fetus needs calcium for the development of the bony skeleton, fetal calcium content increases fourfold during the last trimester of pregnancy as bone density progresses. Thus the infant who is delivered prematurely will have decreased calcium stores. If maternal nutritional intake of calcium is inadequate, fetal calcium needs will be satisfied from maternal stores. Chapter 10 discusses maternal nutritional needs.

Integumentary System: Development and Function

Although the *skin* is considered a single organ, it arises from two separate embryologic germ layers. The epidermis, or outermost layer, develops from the surface ectoderm. The dermis is derived from mesenchyme. The skin and its products (mainly vernix caseosa) function mainly in fetal life as protection for underlying structures. Tactile sense is present in utero—a fetus accidentally touched by the needle during amniocentesis will move away from it.

During gestation, cells from the epidermis proliferate and then are shed and replaced. These cells form part of the **vernix caseosa**, a white cheesy substance that protects the skin in utero. The amount of vernix decreases as gestation proceeds, until only a small amount is seen at term in the thigh and axillary creases. Therefore the extent and location of any vernix is observed when assessing the infant's gestational age.

During the eleventh week of gestation, cells proliferate downward and form epidermal ridges in a pattern of grooves and ridges on the soles, fingers, and palms. A unique and permanent genetically determined design forms by 17 weeks of gestation. **Dermatoglyphics**, the study of epidermal ridges and lines, is part of the examination of infants with possible genetic disease, because distinct patterns are sometimes associated with specific syndromes.

Skin color begins to develop prenatally as some cells differentiate into melanoblasts and then melanocytes. The amount of melanin produced in utero varies with race. Infants of African-American parents may vary in skin color from very light to very dark, with darker skin found nearest the nail beds and on the scrotum or labia.

The hair that becomes visible during the twentieth week of fetal life has a fine downy quality and is called *lanugo*. Lanugo is found over the entire fetal body and then recedes with increasing gestational age (see Figure 7-22). By week 36 it can be found only on the fetal shoulders and forehead, and by term most of it is gone.

Sebaceous glands develop along with the hair follicles. Sweat glands are growths that develop from the epidermis downward into the dermis.

Nails begin to appear at the tips of digits during the tenth week of gestation, with fingernails appearing before toenails (Figure 7-15). (Arm development precedes leg development as well.) Nail growth is used to assess gestational age; at week 32 the fingernails are at the fingertips; by week 36 the toenails have reached the ends of the toes.

The *teeth* arise from two embryologic layers. The enamel is derived from the ectoderm; all other tissues have the mesenchyme as their source. Teeth begin to appear in the primitive jaws during the sixth week of gestation. Early proliferations of cells, or tooth buds, will later become the primary or deciduous teeth, which are shed during childhood. Each jaw contains 10 tooth buds that start devel-

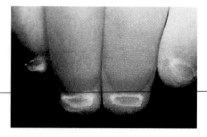

Figure 7-15 Fingernails on a fetus of 15 weeks gestation. (From England MA: *A color atlas of life before birth: normal fetal development,* St Louis, 1990, Mosby.)

oping from the anterior region of the jaw with progression posteriorly. Some precursors to the permanent teeth appear later in gestation, at 10 weeks, whereas others appear even later in the pregnancy. Tooth buds for second and third permanent molars, however, do not appear until after birth, during the fourth month (second molars) and in the fifth year (third molars), respectively.

Mammary glands develop along the mammary ridges, commonly called the milk lines, during the sixth week of gestation. Normally, only those breast buds located in the pectoral region persist. The remaining mammary buds divide and develop the main lactiferous ducts. Further development of lactiferous ducts in the female is postponed until the onset of puberty and continues during pregnancy under the influence of estrogen and progesterone. However, many neonates are born with engorged mammary glands because of the influence of maternal hormones.

Gastrointestinal System: Development and Function

The gastrointestinal tract, or gut, appears during the fourth week of gestation as the embryo folds on itself and incorporates part of its yolk sac. Epithelium, glands, muscles, and fibrous tissues are derived from separate fetal germ layers. Because each of these has a separate arterial supply, the gastrointestinal tract is divided into three anatomic areas: foregut, midgut, and hindgut.

The mouth first appears as a slight depression on the embryo's surface. The lips and palate arise from separate tissue masses of the head and face that grow inward and merge in the midline of the fetus. Clefts in lips or palate occur when either of these masses fails to merge completely. The esophagus grows from the foregut, and a partition, the tracheoesophageal groove, divides it from the beginning trachea. The stomach begins as a dilated area in the foregut as it nears its caudal end. The duodenum forms just past this joint, at the junction between the foregut and midgut. The liver, pancreas, and spleen develop from specialized layers of foregut and midgut. All structures from the common bile duct to the proximal part of the transverse colon are midgut derivatives. The hindgut gives rise to the distal colon, rectum, part of the anal canal, and the urogenital system.

The anus and rectum develop from the *cloaca* (end of the hindgut) as it is divided by the urorectal membrane into the rectum posteriorly and urogenital sinus. The cloaca is covered externally by the cloacal membrane, which must rupture to establish a route for excretion. See Chapter 28 for anomalies of this system.

Development of digestive enzymes continues throughout gestation. Intestinal *disaccharidase* function develops earliest, with mature levels of *maltase* and *sucrase* observed at 6 to 8 months of gestation and mature levels of *lactase* existing only at term. If an infant is born prematurely, however, lactase levels will reach normal levels soon after delivery. Production of some enzymes responsible for protein metabolism does not reach mature levels until term, making vital an external source of some amino acids.

The fetus will "rehearse" later feeding behavior by swallowing amniotic fluid. This does not provide any nutrition to the fetus, but the cellular components of amniotic fluid contribute to the production of meconium. Coordination of suck and swallow reflexes does not occur until about 34 weeks of gestation, but this does not stop the fetus from swallowing amniotic fluid. A fetus will also turn toward his or her fingers if they brush the face (the rooting reflex) and begin to suck on them. Another reflex important for successful feeding without aspiration is the gag reflex. This does not fully mature until the eighth month of gestation.

Meconium, is a tarry black substance that begins to form in the fetal intestine during weeks 13 to 16 of gestation. It consists of secretions from the gastrointestinal tract, including bile pigments, fetal cells and hair contained in swallowed amniotic fluid, and cells sloughed from the intestinal walls.

Although meconium is formed early in fetal life, there should be no passage of it in utero. During a breech position delivery, meconium may be passed as the infant's abdomen is compressed by maternal tissues and perhaps other fetal parts. During times of stress, especially hypoxic stress, the fetal anal sphincter may relax and meconium may be passed, causing the amniotic fluid to become "meconium stained" (see Chapter 14).

TEST *Yourself 7-6*

a. What is meconium?
b. What risk factors can lead to passage of meconium in utero?

Genitourinary System: Development and Function

Renal development and function

Developmental problems of the renal and reproductive systems are relatively common because they develop in close proximity to each other and derive from several common sources of tissues; therefore malformations of the systems may occur together.

Kidneys. The kidneys develop low in the pelvis and seem to move up as they develop, but their location only seems to move because of the growth of the lower part of the body. At about week 12 of gestation the fetal kidneys start to produce hypotonic urine, which contributes to amniotic fluid volume. Absent or malformed kidneys lead to a decrease in amniotic fluid volume, a condition known as oligohydramnios; thus it is important that amniotic fluid be observed during the antepartal period (see biophysical profile in Chapter 11). Although urine production begins in utero, the placental and maternal kidney functions eliminate fetal waste products.

At birth, the term newborn has all the nephrons that will be produced during his or her lifetime. Further growth of the kidney is by hypertrophy not by hyperplasia.

Bladder and urethra. The cloaca is a dilation at the caudal end of the hindgut, divided into the rectal/anal canal and the urogenital sinus by the urorectal septum. The bladder and urethra develop from the urogenital sinus, with additional contributions from surrounding tissues. In the male fetus, production of androgens is vital to the closure of tissues around the urethral tube. If this tube closes abnormally, the urethral meatus will be located on the dorsal (hypospadias) or ventral (epispadias) surface of the penis, rather than at the tip. In very rare instances the abdominal wall fails to close around the bladder, causing exstrophy of the bladder.

Adrenal development and function

The adrenal glands, although in direct contact with the kidneys, have different embryologic origins. Even the cortex and medulla are derived from separate germ layers. The adrenal cortex, which secretes corticosteroids and some androgenic hormones, arises from the mesoderm, whereas the adrenal medulla, which secretes neurohormones (epinephrine and norepinephrine), has the neuroectoderm as its source. The adrenal glands also secrete androgens. Adrenal hyperplasia during gestation can cause masculinization of the female fetus because of the increased amounts of androgens secreted.

During the first half of pregnancy the fetal adrenal glands are large, but they decrease in size as term approaches. Fetal adrenal function may be vital to maintenance of the pregnancy through the active production of steroids. Fetal lung maturity is accelerated by increased fetal steroid production, which occurs during pregnancies complicated by hypertension or preeclampsia and also during labor. Development of the fetal adrenal glands depends on a functioning hypothalamic-pituitary axis. A fetus with major defects in cerebral development, such as anencephaly, also has adrenal hypoplasia.

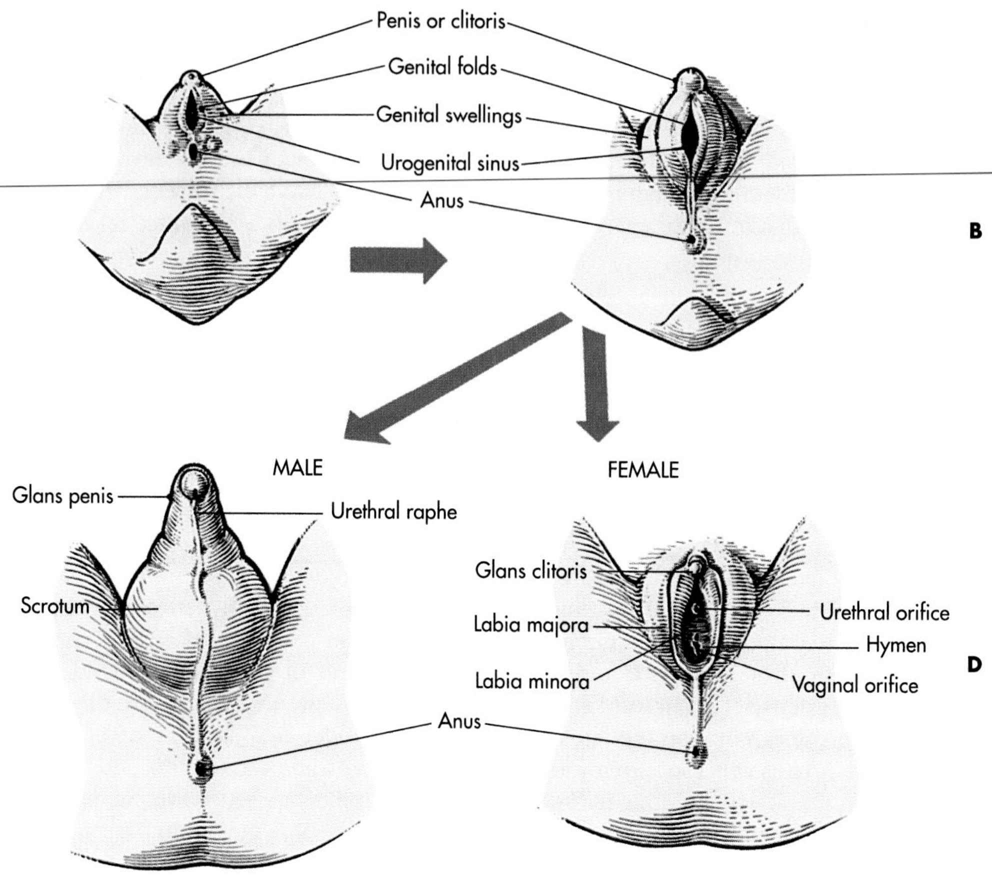

Figure 7-16   Embryonic development of external genitalia. **A** and **B,** Early undifferentiated stages. **C** and **D,** Differentiation into male and female genitalia. (From Langley LL, Telford IR, Christensen JB: *Dynamic anatomy and physiology,* New York, 1980, McGraw-Hill.)

Reproductive System: Development and Function

The reproductive system develops with the urinary system. Testes develop in the fetal abdomen and can be recognized after 7 weeks of gestation. By week 30 of gestation, testes begin to descend through the inguinal canal into the scrotum. Ovaries develop in the abdomen and remain in the pelvic cavity. Figure 7-16 shows development of external genitalia in the male or female fetus (see Chapter 28).

Sexual development continues throughout gestation as the external genitalia change in appearance. These changes are an important part of gestational age assessment. Sexual maturity continues with identification of the infant's somatic sex by both infant and parents and then with the onset of sexual maturity during puberty.

Musculoskeletal System: Development and Function

The musculoskeletal system develops from embryonic mesoderm. Cells from the mesoderm give rise to the embryonic connective tissue, called mesenchyme. Some mesenchymal cells differentiate into myoblasts, the precursors of muscle tissue. Others form fibroblasts (connective tissue), chondroblasts (cartilage), or osteoblasts (bone).

The limbs begin as limb buds that appear on the ventrolateral aspect of the embryo's body near the end of the fourth week. Development proceeds in a proximal-distal manner and is completed by the end of the eighth week of gestation, with completion of the arms preceding completion of the legs by a few days. Limb development is illustrated in Figures 7-17 and 7-18. Bones of the upper and lower extremities that are homologous are the radius, tibia, ulna, and fibula; the thumb and big toe are homologous digits. The growth of the infant's entire skeleton is determined both by genetic endowment and by perinatal environment (see Chapter 28).

Cartilage is seen in the embryo at about 5 weeks of gestation. Bone may develop directly from mesenchymal cells or from cells that first become cartilage and then ossify. Ossification begins in the *diaphysis,* or shaft of long bones, and proceeds in all directions (Figure 7-19). At term, ossification is mostly completed at the diaphyses but has only begun to appear at the *epiphyses,* or ends of the bones. The

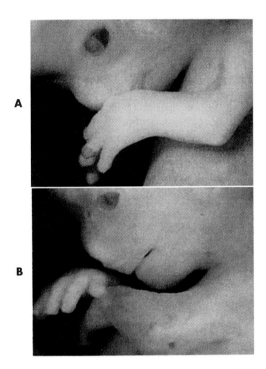

Figure 7-17 Arm development from day 44 to 46. **A,** The arm has bent at the elbow, which points caudally. The arms move in utero from week 7 to 8. **B,** The hands meet and cross in the midline over the thorax. (From England MA: *A color atlas of life before birth: normal fetal development,* St Louis, 1990, Mosby.)

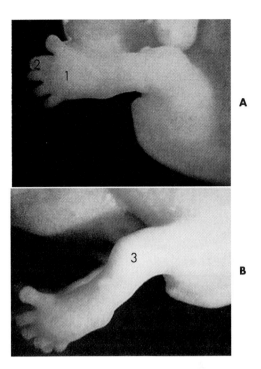

Figure 7-18 Leg development from day 44 to 46. **A,** The soles of the feet (1 and 2) face each other. **B,** The knee (3) points cranially. (From England MA: *A color atlas of life before birth: normal fetal development,* St Louis, 1990, Mosby.)

soft pliability of the skull bones is noticeable at birth. Development of the fetal skeleton depends on maternal supplies of calcium and phosphorus, especially from the end of the embryonic period (8 weeks of gestation) until term, since this is the period of ossification; thus maternal nutrition is important.

Smooth muscles arise from mesenchymal cells located near their associated organs (the digestive tract and elsewhere). *Skeletal muscle* is derived from myoblasts and begins to show its characteristic striations and involuntary movements by the end of the third fetal month. Each skeletal muscle develops near the bone that will be moved by the muscle. It then becomes associated with motor nerves. Adequate development of skeletal muscle depends on adequate amniotic fluid volume. Therefore the fetus crowded into the intrauterine environment because of oligohydramnios will be born with contractures caused by lack of movement.

The normal fetus can perform a wide variety of voluntary and involuntary movements. Both muscle tone and movements change with increasing gestational age, a fact confirmed through ultrasonic examination, by maternal reports of fetal activity, and by direct observations of premature infants. Table 7-1 summarizes characteristics of movements and tone in the development of the infant.

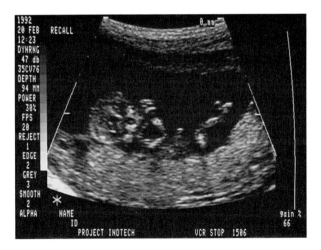

Figure 7-19 Ultrasound print of infant's arms and legs (12 weeks). (Courtesy Advanced Technology Laboratories, Bothell, Wash.)

Neurologic System: Development and Function

Human prenatal and postnatal development proceeds in a cephalocaudal, mass-to-specific, gross-to-fine direction. The nervous system develops from a specialized area of ectoderm called the neural plate about 18 days after conception. The neural plate differentiates into the neural

Table 7-1   **Development of Movements and Tone**

Gestational Age	Muscle Tone (Tonus)	Movements
28 weeks	Absent. Infant lies in extension.	Infant moves spontaneously when awake. Slow and twisting or rapid movements of entire limb occur.
32 weeks	Flexor tone begins in lower extremities. Upper extremities are still extended.	Flexor movements in lower extremities occur in unison. Head turning begins.
36 weeks	Flexor tone increases in lower extremities. Flexion of upper extremities begins.	Vigorous flexion movements of lower extremities now alternate. Neck extension begins.
Term	Flexor tone exists in all extremities.	Alternating movements of all limbs occur. Neck extension continues to improve. Neck flexion begins.

crest and the neural tube. The neural crest becomes the peripheral nervous system, and the neural tube becomes the CNS (brain and spinal cord) (Figure 7-20). The tube is open at the cranial and caudal ends (anterior and posterior neuropores). From day 22 to day 26 after conception, these ends will close by "zipping up" from the thoracic area and proceeding toward the top of the head and "zipping down" from the same area to the base of the spine. Severe developmental defects result from failure of closure in the early days after conception. If the anterior neuropore does not close, the fetus will be *anencephalic*. If the posterior neuropore does not close, the fetus will have some form of *spina bifida*. Prenatal diagnosis is available for many of these major defects (see Chapter 11).

Neural tube growth in the fetus is greater at the cranial end, which will accommodate the brain. The size of the fetal head is related to brain growth and the amount of cerebral spinal fluid.

Development of the brain influences the infant's neurohormonal function and intellectual capacity. The pituitary gland, or hypophysis, is referred to as the "master gland" because of its powerful influence on human function. The two lobes of the pituitary are derived from separate tissues, which explains their separate functions. The anterior pituitary develops from oral ectodermal tissue and is the glandular portion that secretes trophic and growth-stimulating hormones. The posterior pituitary develops from neuroectodermal tissue and secretes antidiuretic hormone and oxytocin. The pituitary gland forms in a specialized area called Rathke's pouch, located in the roof of the fetal mouth. The gland migrates into the base of the brain as development proceeds, but the original site of Rathke's pouch can be felt as a small indentation on the hard palate.

Protection of the brain is an important component of prenatal development. Premature birth threatens neonatal

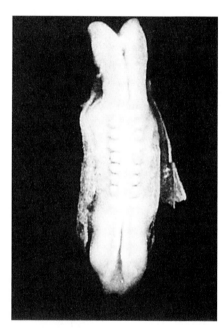

Figure 7-20   The neural tube is fusing, but the anterior and the posterior neuropores are still open (day 22 to 23). (From England MA: *A color atlas of life before birth: normal fetal development*, St Louis, 1990, Mosby.)

neurologic function in several ways. Because the third trimester is the period of increased brain growth, delivery before term forces completion of brain growth in the less than ideal extrauterine environment. The **germinal matrix** is an area of the brain especially vulnerable to damage before 32 weeks of gestation. It is richly supplied with blood vessels that can be easily ruptured, leading to intraventricular hemorrhage (see Chapter 29).

Myelinization

Impulses created by neurons must be transmitted throughout the body. **Myelin** forms an insulating sheath around axons and allows impulses to be conducted in an organized manner. Myelinization begins during the middle of gestation and continues through adolescence. Maturation of sensory and motor functions follows the sequence of myelinization, with mastery of gross motor movements preceding mastery of fine movements.

Fetal responses to external stimuli can be voluntary or involuntary. Motor activity begins early in development with reflex movements occurring at about week 7 of gestation. Spontaneous movements follow at about week 8 of gestation, with swallowing, breathing, and grasping movements (all necessary for postnatal survival) appearing early. By about 16 to 20 weeks of gestation, fetal movements are strong enough to be felt by the mother.

Motor activity

Increased fetal movements and changes in fetal heart rates have been noted when mothers are exposed to a loud noise or if a strong light is directed toward the maternal abdomen. Maternal hunger and anxiety also cause changes in fetal status; the fetus becomes tachycardiac in response to maternal catecholamine secretion during maternal anxiety. The normal fetus alternates periods of rolling and stretching movement with periods of sleep; each part of the cycle lasts about 20 minutes. Heart rate variability decreases during fetal sleep and increases during periods of fetal activity. Reactivity of the cardiac control center to fetal movement is an index of an intact CNS and is examined by the nonstress test (NST) (see Chapter 11).

Special Senses: Development and Function

Fetal sensory systems—touch, smell, vestibular, taste, hearing, vision—develop chronologically (Haith, 1986). The fetus responds to *touch* through the maternal abdominal wall; mothers feel this response. Movement in the uterus provides development of *vestibular function* (the sense of balance and body position). Preterm infants born by 26 to 30 weeks respond to odors. Finally, it is known that newborns discriminate between varying tastes (see Chapter 20).

Vision

Development of vision begins in the fourth week of life. The eyes appear as optic grooves at about 22 days, and all three layers of embryonic tissue are involved in the construction of these complex structures (Figure 7-21). A fetus of about 16 weeks is able to react to light, as evidenced by its startle reflex when a strong beam of light is shone on the mother's abdomen. Later in gestation, at 29 weeks, the same fetus turns toward the light. There is some indication that eye and respiratory movements together can be used to assess prenatal CNS function (Figure 7-22).

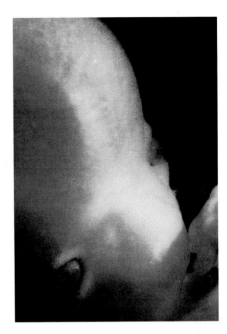

Figure 7-21 At 44 to 46 days of gestation the eyelids have not yet formed. (From England MA: *A color atlas of life before birth: normal fetal development,* St Louis, 1990, Mosby.)

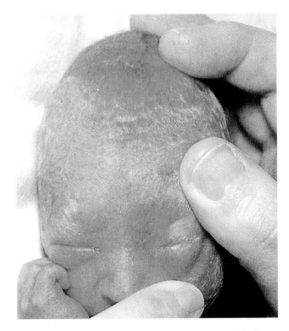

Figure 7-22 Tiny preterm infant whose eyelids do not open (24.6 weeks). (From Beischer MA, MacKay EV: *Obstetrics and the newborn,* ed 3, Philadelphia, 1993, WB Saunders.)

Hearing

The ears develop from several separate structures. The internal ear develops first, beginning with the *otic pit*. Ear structures are mature enough at about 24 to 28 weeks to demonstrate a response to sound and auditory acoustic stimulation is therefore used during prenatal testing to stimulate the fetus. There is debate about the level of decibels to use; only sounds of low frequency seem audible. As gestation progresses, the fetus is able to hear sounds of higher frequency. The fetus is in a "noisy" environment where maternal heartbeat, breathing, and placental and intestinal sounds are heard. Mothers have long reported increased fetal movement in response to loud music and fetal soothing with more placid music.

Hematologic System: Development and Function

Formation of blood, or **hematopoiesis**, parallels cardiovascular development. At about 13 to 15 days of gestation, *angioblasts* organize as "blood islands" in the mesoderm of the yolk sac. Spaces develop within these islands and become lined with the angioblasts, forming the primitive blood vessels and endothelium. Cells of the endothelium then give rise to primitive blood cells. All of this occurs outside the embryo, *in the yolk sac*. Blood is not formed within the embryo until the fifth week of gestation. The primary site for hematopoiesis in the embryo is the liver, which grows larger as this process continues. The liver increases in size and by the ninth week of gestation, it is responsible for about 10% of total fetal weight. Hematopoiesis also gives the liver its red color.

Later in gestation the *reticuloendothelial system,* comprising the liver, spleen, bone marrow, and lymph nodes, becomes the primary site of hematopoiesis. By term, the bone marrow is the main site for production of all red cells and most other cellular blood components, though the liver, spleen, and lymph nodes can be stimulated to produce blood cells during periods of extreme and continued demand.

The *reticulum cell,* the germinal cell for all blood cell production, is found within the reticuloendothelial system. In the lymph nodes, reticulum cells develop into lymphocytes and monocytes. Reticulum cells found elsewhere will yield plasma cells, which provide immune factors. In the bone marrow the reticulum cell will differentiate into either a hemoblast or myeloblast. Hemoblasts undergo several other stages of transformation before emerging as erythrocytes, whereas myeloblasts differentiate into granulocytic leukocytes or megakaryocytes (platelet precursors).

There are many differences in the anatomy and function of fetal blood cells. Fetal erythrocytes are larger in size than adult erythrocytes, though they have a shorter life span (80 to 100 days for fetal cells versus 120 days for adult cells).

Fetal leukocyte function is not always adequate for defense against infection. Implications for the differences between fetal and adult cells are discussed in Chapter 29.

Hemoglobin

Fetal hemoglobin, or Hgb F, is a specialized form of hemoglobin found only during gestation and in early infancy. Hgb F accounts for 70% to 90% of the hemoglobin found in the perinatal period. It has a high affinity or attraction for oxygen, thus ensuring an adequate supply for the rapidly dividing fetal cells.

Blood type

Blood type is determined at conception. As with other genetically transferred traits, blood factors may be dominant or recessive. Incompatibility between maternal and fetal blood may cause fetal and neonatal hemolysis and neonatal jaundice (see Chapter 23).

Coagulation

Fetal ability to synthesize clotting factors is genetically determined. A fetus with inherited defects in the production of clotting factors, such as hemophelia, usually does not show symptoms in utero, even though clotting factors cannot pass from mother to fetus through the placental circulation. In fact, the infant may appear normal for the first few weeks of life.

In the genetically normal fetus and newborn, production of adequate amounts of clotting factors depends on maturation of the liver and the presence of vitamin K. This vitamin is produced in the gastrointestinal tract through the interaction of bacteria, food, and time. Since synthesis of prothrombin and factor VII cannot occur without vitamin K, a parenteral injection of it is given soon after birth (see Chapter 19).

TEST *Yourself* 7-7

a. How does fetal hemoglobin differ from adult hemoglobin?
b. Why is an injection of vitamin K given to newborns?

Immunologic System: Development and Function

The development of immune capability begins in the human fetus between the eighth and fifteenth weeks of gestation. The fetus normally lives in a sterile environment, and the immune system is therefore functioning only in a rudimentary manner. **Passive immunity,** acquired from the mother across the placenta late in pregnancy, offers protection from several pathogens in the early infancy period.

The cells of the immune system, like those of the hematologic system, arise from stem cells, which then become *lymphopoietic* cells (precursors to tissues of the immune system). One type of lymphopoietic cell, called the T cell, is produced first in the thymus and then throughout the body's lymphoid tissues. Another type, the B cell, is produced in an unknown site within the human body. T cells destroy pathogens by phagocytosis; B cells produce antibodies to these pathogens. T-cell function is referred to as *cellular immunity*; B-cell function is called *humoral immunity*. (see Chapter 25 for more on immunity.)

Antibody production

Humans produce five different classes of antibodies: immunoglobulin (Ig) G, M, A, D, and E, each with its own unique chemical structure. IgG, IgA, and IgE are produced by the fetus before the twentieth week of gestation. The *IgG* group is the largest and also the one that provides the most immunity. Only small amounts of IgG are produced by the human fetus, but maternal IgG is actively transported across the placenta. Maternal IgG provides the fetus with passively acquired immunity against many infectious diseases. Blood group antibodies are also in the IgG class and can therefore freely cross the placenta to cause hemolytic disease of the newborn (see Chapter 23).

IgA is the second largest group of immunoglobulins and is produced by lymphoid tissues within the gastrointestinal, urinary, and respiratory tracts. This immunoglobulin protects against local infections, such as those of the respiratory and gastrointestinal tracts. Its presence in human breast milk lowers the incidence of enteric infections in breast-fed infants. IgA can be found in the saliva of neonates after several days of life.

The *IgM* molecule is the largest of all the immunoglobulins and *cannot cross the placenta*. It also is the immunoglobulin that is formed early in the immune response. Therefore any IgM found in the fetus or neonate must be of fetal origin; examination of cord blood for IgM levels can reveal the existence of congenital infection (see Chapter 29).

The exact role of IgD immunoglobulin is not known. IgE is found in elevated amounts in people with atopic allergic disorders. IgE and IgA are produced by the same tissues and are found in external secretions.

TEST *Yourself 7-8*

a. Name the primary differences between fetal and adult red blood cells.
b. How does the fetus acquire passive immunity?

Key points

- Growth and development are distinct but related concepts.
- Fetal growth and development depend on genetic quality and intrauterine and extrauterine environments.
- Mitosis produces cells with the same chromosomal number as the parent cells, whereas meiosis yields cells with one member of each chromosomal pair.
- Meiosis allows for variations in genetic makeup.
- Support structures and circulation arise early in fetal development to supply nutrition for rapid growth.
- Both anatomic (structural) and biochemical (functional) development occur during embryonic and fetal life.
- Although substantial organ system development occurs during the first trimester, the fetus is vulnerable to the effects of teratogens throughout gestation.
- Normal growth and development yield a newborn well equipped to adapt to a supportive extrauterine environment.

Study Questions

7-1. Select the terms that apply to the following statements:
   a. Layer of the embryo from which skin, hair, and nails are created is _____.
   b. Body cell chromosomes are _____.
   c. Double strands of genetic material are _____.
   d. Process by which the size or number of cells increase is _____.
   e. Process by which primitive cells mature is _____.
   f. Process by which the chromosome number is halved is _____.
   g. Structure consisting of two arteries, one vein, Wharton's jelly, and amnion is _____.
   h. Process by which the embryo attaches to the uterine wall is _____.

7-2. The three germ layers are formed and begin differentiation by the end of the second week. The endoderm layer will become:

 a. Linings of the body organs.

 b. Muscle, bone, and cartilage.

 c. The brain and central nervous system.

7-3. Which of the following statements would best describe the 12-week fetus?

 a. It is capable of extrauterine life.

 b. All organs and body systems are completely differentiated.

 c. Although much development has occurred, the fetus is still vulnerable to the action of teratogens.

 d. The placenta forms a complete barrier from the external world.

7-4. What milestone in development occurs around 23 weeks?

 a. The fetal lungs are capable of respiration.

 b. The fetal cardiovascular system is fully formed.

 c. The fetal fingernails have reached the ends of the fingertips.

 d. The fetal brain is completely differentiated.

7-5. Select true or false for the following statements:

 a. Suck and swallow are coordinated by 32 weeks of gestation.

 b. Amniotic fluid cellular components become part of meconium.

 c. The fetus swallows and voids into the amniotic fluid.

 d. There is a time in development when sex appears "neutral."

7-6. The reticulum cell is amazing because it develops in different locations into different cells. Match location with the following cell type:

Cell Type	Location
1. Lymphocyte	a. Bone marrow
2. Hemoblast	b. Lymph node
3. Myeloblast	c. Other reticuloendothelial tissues
4. Monocytes	

Answer Key

7-1: *a,* Ectoderm; *b,* autosomes; *c,* DNA; *d,* growth; *e,* development; *f,* meiosis; *g,* umbilical cord; *h,* implantation. 7-2: *a.* 7-3: *c.* 7-4: *a.* 7-5: *a,* F; *b,* T; *c,* T; *d,* T. 7-6: 1, *b;* 2, *a;* 3, *a;* 4, *b.*

References

Blackburn ST, Loper DL: *Maternal, fetal and neonatal physiology,* Philadelphia, 1992, WB Saunders.

*Haith MM: Sensory and perceptual processes in early infancy, *J Pediatr* 109:158, 1986.

*Pleet HB et al: Patterns of malformations resulting from teratogenic effects of first trimester hyperthermia, *Pediatr Res* 14:587, 1980.

*Classic reference.

Moore KL: *The developing human: clinically oriented embryology,* ed 5, Philadelphia, 1993, WB Saunders.

The classic textbook of human fetal development. Moore extensively illustrates the descriptions and relates the influences of parental health to both normal and abnormal development on the newborn.

Sadler TW: *Langman's medical embryology,* ed 7, Baltimore, 1995, Williams & Wilkins.

Smaller in size than the Moore text but similar in scope. Descriptions of developmental processes are more succinct than those in Moore.

Stine GJ: *The new human genetics,* Dubuque, 1989, Wm C Brown.

An excellent resource for students that clearly illustrates the genetic determinants of human disease. Unfortunately, a more recent revision has not been published.

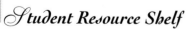

Student Resource Shelf

England MA: *Color atlas of life before birth: normal fetal development,* Chicago, 1990, Mosby.

A fascinating look at the process of fetal development through pictures of fetuses at various stages of gestation. The relationship between the fetus and newborn in terms of anatomy and its function are emphasized.

UNIT

Two

Pregnancy

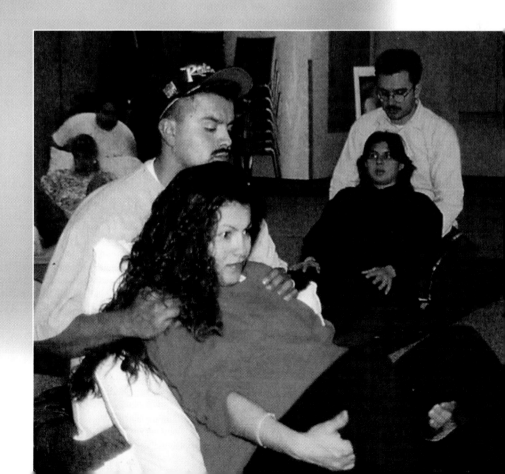

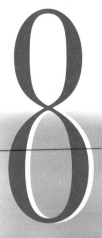

Adaptation *to* Pregnancy

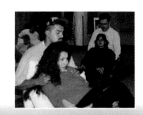

*P*regnancy is a time of major developmental challenges, a time when a woman leaves her identity as a single person and assumes the awesome responsibility of caring for a child. Although some women feel joyful and exhilarated by the challenge, more often a woman may feel ambivalent or even bewildered by it. The changes pregnancy brings will affect all other aspects of the woman's life. To better predict how a pregnant woman will handle this challenge, the nurse must examine the ways in which the woman is nurtured.

Young people learn how to be mothers or fathers from their own parents. Memories of their parents' behavior and attitudes help them develop ideas about what a parent is or should be. Once formed, these ideas are extremely difficult to change. If parent-child relationships were loving, individuals are likely to become loving parents. If relationships were full of distrust and abuse, these patterns are also likely to be repeated in the next generation.

Motivations for pregnancy vary widely. The couple may want to prove their ability to reproduce or to achieve adult status. They may be fulfilling the cultural expectation that "everyone wants children" or may wish to fulfill their parents' wish for a grandchild. A woman may desire to again experience the closeness of the mother-child relationship or to strengthen ties with her partner. More positively, having a child may be viewed as a new beginning, an enriching life experience leading to feelings of creativity and competence. The woman may be reaching the age when she feels that "it's now or never," that she must soon decide to have a baby or risk the inability to conceive or carry a baby to term. However, when the time comes, transition to first-time parenthood is abrupt; the new parents often feel unprepared for the reality of the responsibility.

DEVELOPMENTAL TASKS DURING PREGNANCY

Many **developmental tasks** occur during the psychologic transition from nonparent to parent. This transition parallels and is stimulated by the development of the child within the womb. The overall task of **maternal attainment** is initiated with the diagnosis of pregnancy. The task is completed much later when the mother achieves competence in the mothering role and integrates these mothering behaviors into her other roles (Mercer, 1985; Zabielsky, 1994). A woman who successfully achieves maternal attainment is left with a positive self-image and a healthy relationship with her child.

Pregnancy is influenced by the woman's cultural and social context, and factors such as the woman's age, socioeconomic status, length of marriage, and number of previous pregnancies will affect maternal attainment (Zachariah, 1994). Psychologic factors such as emotional conflict, anxiety, stress, and low self-esteem can have a negative impact on pregnancy outcomes. Conversely, a woman with high self-esteem may be more likely to feel in control of her life and engage in healthful behaviors (Curry, 1994). These behaviors may include getting early prenatal care, exercising, eating healthy foods, and avoiding alcohol, smoking, and caffeine.

The mother's perception that she has support during pregnancy is a key to positive feelings. Zachariah (1994) reported that "a close and intimate attachment with a husband may be one of the more important influences on psychologic well being of women during pregnancy." If the pregnant woman is single or if she is in an unsupportive relationship, there may be added difficulty. Her relationship with her own mother is also significant. The need for an expectant mother to get reacquainted with her own parents is universal. All expectant parents relive past and present relationships with their parents and try to come to terms with unresolved difficulties. If her own mother is available, the expectant mother will need to spend time with her. If her own mother is unavailable, the woman may try to befriend another motherly person to serve as an alternate maternal role model.

There may be unresolved issues of separation and power between mother and daughter. Rivalry between the pregnant woman and her mother may cause friction in every choice, from naming the infant to whether the new grandmother will be invited to help out when the baby comes home. Lederman (1984) reported on the relationship between psychosocial conflicts in pregnancy and progress in labor; those with unresolved conflicts had delayed progress.

First Trimester

Acceptance

During the early weeks of pregnancy the expectant mother tests the reality of her pregnancy. Even after confirmation through tests, she will look for affirmation in other signs and symptoms to reassure herself that the pregnancy is real. First-trimester needs vary, depending on whether the pregnancy is the woman's first. A first pregnancy is like any other first experience, and this expectant mother feels curiosity and concern about the changes ahead. Even the most carefully planned educational program does not fully relieve the anxiety. Although the woman may have chosen to become pregnant, there is always an ambivalence until the idea of being pregnant becomes a reality and an acceptance of the growing fetus, *integration* or **incorporation**, takes place (Tanner, 1969; Rubin, 1984).

The expectant parents' conscious or unconscious motivation and eagerness for pregnancy change the normal degree of **ambivalence** about anticipated life changes. For the first-time mother, pregnancy marks a final break from the girl she once was. She must give up the image of herself as a childless person before she can accept herself as an expectant mother. Some women experience considerable longing for the person they once were, feeling unready for the "mother person" they need to become. This nostalgia is often expressed in dreams and by reviewing images of younger days. Mourning the loss of a previous lifestyle may interfere with acceptance of pregnancy. Inconvenient social circumstances, such as being young and single, may cause the expectant mother to deny the existence of the pregnancy. A disintegrating relationship with the expectant father can cause anger, which may lead to maternal rejection of the fetus.

The following dimensions identified by Lederman (1984) should be considered when assessing the woman's acceptance of the pregnancy:

1. **The desire for the pregnancy and infant.** Some women want an infant but dislike being pregnant. In less healthy cases, some love the warm feelings related to being pregnant but do not look ahead to actually nurturing an infant. However, resolution of negative feelings usually occurs by the third trimester.

2. **Amount of happiness or unhappiness.** For some women, emotional gratification comes from feelings of biologic fulfillment and from their conscious desire for a child despite mood swings and emotional lability. In women with a history of depression, however, pregnancy tends to trigger recurrence of depressed feelings. Low self-esteem greatly increases fears related to labor and the ability to mother the newborn.

3. **Discomfort during pregnancy.** The amount of discomfort experienced during pregnancy varies considerably from woman to woman. When discomfort seems intensified and prolonged, it may indicate a problem with acceptance of the pregnant state.

4. **Acceptance of body changes.** In our society the media have promoted the idea that a thin body is the model for beauty. Many women fear being viewed as "fat" and feel relieved when they look obviously pregnant. Such women look forward to wearing maternity clothing and may choose to begin doing so early in the pregnancy. New views expressed in the media may change perceptions. (See Self-Discovery at right.)

5. **Amount of unresolved ambivalence.** Most women accept pregnancy by the beginning of the third trimester. To assess how well the woman has accomplished this task, discuss her feelings about the infant and help her express how she sees herself as a new mother. Some mothers accept pregnancy but are still unable to imagine themselves as mothers. Women who receive little or no psychologic support may have particular difficulty.

Nurses will need to assess the degree of interference with the woman's acceptance process. For example, ambivalence is natural if a woman must give up a rewarding career or if financial considerations mean that the timing of the pregnancy is poor. These feelings do not mean that the woman has rejected pregnancy; her attitude of happiness or unhappiness is a far more accurate indication of her state of mind. By the end of the first trimester she may begin to look for role models who have had the experience of pregnancy. Rubin (1984) calls this activity **replication.** The woman copies other pregnant women she views as successful mothers by role playing these experts until she can grow into the role of mother.

Concerns

Most pregnant women are concerned during the first trimester with the changes in their own bodies and how these changes will affect their lives. Some of their expressed concerns have to do with the following:

1. Normal symptoms of pregnancy ("Should I worry? Am I normal? What shall I do?")

2. Changes in lifestyle that will result from the pregnancy ("I wonder how pregnancy will make me different.")

3. Changes in relationship with the partner ("How will he accept this pregnancy? How will it change our sexual responses?")

4. Medical care—the sequences and reasons for visits ("How can I get help between visits?")

The pregnant woman may appear to be very self-concerned. She probably will not be able to focus on instructions concerning future events such as labor, delivery, child care, or contraception; thus such topics are best discussed in later visits.

Self-Discovery

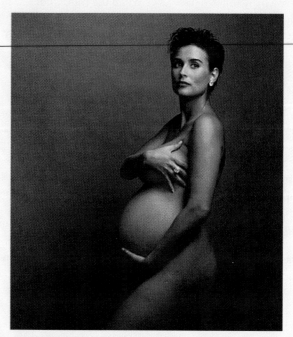

(Copyright Annie Leibovitz/Contact Press Images.)

- *How do you respond to this photograph?*
- *How do the media influence the way women feel about their bodies?*
- *Has this photograph helped women feel that the pregnant body is beautiful? Normal? Natural?*
- *What were women's attitudes about their bodies during pregnancy in your mother's generation? Your grandmothers'? Have they changed?*
- *How would you encourage a woman who feels ugly during pregnancy?* ~

Practical concerns may center around finances, especially if the new infant's arrival will mean curtailment of the family income. There are worries about the expenses of having and raising a child. Women may worry about loss of freedom, increased dependency, or other changes in relationships. Although these concerns are most evident in the first pregnancy, relationships also shift and change with later children.

Signs of Difficulty

Signs of difficulty in first-trimester tasks may be demonstrated as exaggerated discomforts such as severe nausea, sleeplessness, and fatigue, or the woman may complain about discomforts to anyone who will listen. In addition, she may have unresolved anger, feelings of depression, and of hostility toward her partner.

In the first trimester, fatigue-related hormonal effects may lead the woman to take naps and then be wakeful at night. If fatigue is related to night wakefulness, the woman should be asked about feelings of anxiety, dreams, environmental noise, overfatigue during the day, muscle cramping, and nocturia. A woman with a lifestyle that prevents a rest period during the day—a woman who works or has several small children—should be encouraged to discuss with the nurse ways to obtain additional rest.

Although many ambivalent feelings may be expressed about the pregnancy in the first trimester, it is important for the nurse to assess for signs of depression. Mild depression may be related to the many changes brought about by the pregnancy, both physically and psychosocially. Changes in relationships, career plans, or financial matters may be overwhelming for the mother. Encouraging her to talk with significant others and to seek out women who have dealt with these issues may be helpful. Severe depression may hinder the woman in accomplishing her developmental tasks throughout the pregnancy. Symptoms of severe depression include feeling hopeless, apathetic, or worthless; having trouble sleeping, eating (unrelated to normal discomfort of pregnancy), or concentrating; or being plagued by agitation or recurrent thoughts of death. Presence of these symptoms should signal the nurse to refer the woman for further psychiatric evaluation. (See Chapter 26 for complete discussion of interventions for depression.)

Second Trimester

Infant as non-self

By the end of the first trimester, discomforts from physiologic changes have usually disappeared. The expectant mother settles down, and if no physical complications occur, her concerns begin to shift from her own bodily changes to the growing infant. The psychologic task of perceiving the fetus as a growing infant separate from herself, or fetal **differentiation**, is normally complete by the end of the second trimester. This period has also been called *fetal embodiment* (Starn and Niederhauser, 1990).

With the onset of quickening (feeling the fetus move), the parents' thoughts turn inward to the separateness of the child. Though the infant is a part of the parents and familar to them, it is still distinct. Physical sensations, which at first are described as light, fluttering, and exciting, may later seem disruptive. Women complain, "He never leaves me alone! Always giving me a thump when I want to sleep" (Lederman, 1984). Emotional separation between self and the infant is important. Some women report feeling that the infant is a total stranger and are surprised that the infant may have reactions different from their own. For women who have not completed the process of their own task of *individuation* (adolescents, for example), this realization is especially difficult.

Through **visualization** the woman imagines what her child is like and becomes acquainted with it as she notices

what disturbs and what soothes him or her. For instance, a fetus may react to loud rock music with strong movement and be soothed by smooth, lilting melodies. An expectant mother may experiment with and note reactions to rhythmic sensations created when she leans against the spinning dryer or when she rubs firmly in a particular spot. Many "play" with the fetus by pushing against a protruding spot and waiting to be kicked in return. When the expectant mother has a sonogram early in pregnancy, she can actually see her child moving about within her. Women frequently report that this was the first time they understood that another person was really there. Encourage the mother to ask for an ultrasound "photo" of her infant to help her picture the child.

Fears often arise as an expectant mother begins to accept this separateness. This fear does not diminish with later pregnancies, even when the first infant was healthy. A woman may believe that she could not possibly be lucky again after her first infant was "perfect." Often these fears are expressed in dreams about the pregnancy or infant. Some of these dreams are frightening and upsetting to the woman and frequently involve the threat of harm to the infant or to the woman (Blake, 1993).

During the second trimester the process of maternal role attainment includes *internalization,* the mother's use of daydreams using **imagery** to see herself and the infant in various situations. Imagery is especially helpful during times of change. For example, a mother may imagine herself rocking her infant, or an expectant father may picture himself comforting a crying child. This **fantasy** is a normal and valuable part of the process of role attainment (Rubin, 1984) (see Research Box).

Concerns

In general, during the second trimester, the mother is interested in protecting the health of the infant, and her concerns will reflect her awareness of its needs (Figure 8-1). The general concerns include the following:

1. Nutritional intake ("Am I gaining too much weight? Too little?")
2. Amount of exercise or travel ("What restrictions are necessary?")
3. Progression of fetal growth ("How big is the baby this month?")
4. Warning signs of problems
5. Changing body image ("How is this reflected in my clothes? Hygiene? Hair? Skin?")
6. Changes in sexual desires ("Are there restrictions? Am I misinformed?")

Signs of Difficulty

Signs of difficulty with second-trimester tasks may include continuing anger and depression because of a lack of acceptance of the pregnancy. A woman who continues to voice physical complaints or who focuses on her own

RESEARCH

PURPOSE OF STUDY

To examine the relationship of daydreaming styles to perception of the maternal parenting role and to maternal-fetal attachment.

LITERATURE REVIEW

Maternal-fetal attachment is thought to begin early in pregnancy and may be initiated by physical changes in body appearance and by psychologic events such as daydreaming. Maternal role attainment is believed to develop in progressive stages that are simultaneous with maternal attachment to the fetus.

METHOD

A sample of 150 women who were experiencing their first full-term pregnancy were used in this study. Participants were asked to complete the Maternal-Fetal Attachment Scale, the Perception of Parental Role Scale, and the Imaginal Processes Inventory.

FINDINGS AND IMPLICATIONS FOR PRACTICE

Individually, the three major styles of daydreaming are not predictive of parenting role and maternal-fetal attachment in first-time expectant women during the third trimester of pregnancy. The use of dream diaries in conjunction with the Imaginal Processes Inventory may provide a greater understanding of the development of themes during pregnancy. Childbirth educators, health professionals, and pregnant women should be aware that daydreaming is especially common during pregnancy and may be used to foster positive parenting and early attachment behaviors.

Kaplan J: *The relationship of daydreaming styles to perception of maternal parenting role and maternal-fetal attachment in first-time expectant women during the third trimester of pregnancy,* Unpublished doctoral dissertation, New York, 1993, New York University.

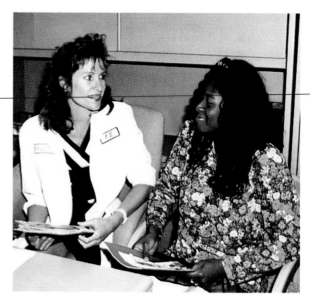

Figure 8-1   Expectant mother and nurse discuss prenatal care concerns. (Courtesy Marjorie Pyle, RNC, *Lifecircle.*)

ences and values. Parents, extended family, and friends who allow the mother to confide in them about the concerns of pregnancy and future mothering demands are helpful resources (Figure 8-2). If signs of depression exist, individual or family counseling should be recommended. See Chapter 26 for a detailed discussion of depression.

Third Trimester

Separation and birth

In the final weeks the mother's task is to prepare for the end of the pregnancy and for the birth itself. As the mother looks forward to the birth, she may again feel considerable ambivalence. She must prepare for *letting go* of the pregnancy and all its warm feelings of fusion and creativity, a process known as *fetal separation.* Conscious or unconscious fears of mutilation, death, or abandonment often surface at this time. Anticipatory anxiety is now considered to be normal and healthy. As the birth nears, the overriding concern is how to cope with the stress of labor and delivery and whether there will be a *safe passage.* While working on understanding what labor and birth will be like, many couples seek out other new parents for advice and questioning and to listen to stories of their birth experiences.

During pregnancy, dependency needs increase, reaching a peak in the third trimester, during labor, and in the early nurturing period after birth. The expectant mother must herself be nurtured so that she can "store up" reserves for the time when she is nurturing the infant. A man also feels a heightened need to have someone dependable to care for him, particularly because the

concerns rather than on thoughts about the fetus may have problems. Clues that a woman may have difficulty parenting are evident when she becomes self-involved or regresses to childish behavior.

The nurse working with the pregnant woman must first assess for any of these signs. A woman who does not follow through with prenatal appointments or who is nutritionally noncompliant (either gaining too little or too much weight) may have problems. Because of the many stressors on the mother, father, and family during this time, the nurse should assess for support needs. Difficulties may be related to the mother's feelings that she is overwhelmed and lacks support or to cultural differ-

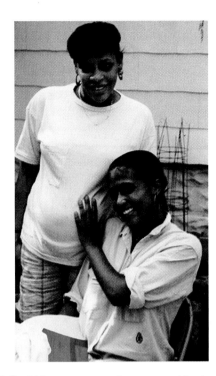

Figure 8-2 When pregnancy is supported in the family, self-esteem grows. (Courtesy Camille Bodden.)

expectant mother becomes more introspective with advancing pregnancy and often withdraws some of the "mothering" attention he usually receives. Family members should be reminded to be especially attentive during these periods.

During the third trimester, a person who is becoming a parent realizes that it is not possible to remain a child in relation to his or her own parents. The new parent will become the provider rather than the recipient of care. In this sense, becoming a parent for the first time means that the new parents can never return to the lack of responsibility experienced in childhood. In addition, it is during the third trimester that the pregnant woman may focus on evaluation and criticism of other parents, including her own mother. According to Rubin (1984) she is *differentiating* herself from others to become the kind of mother she imagines she will be.

Though many couples seek childbirth classes to learn the facts and techniques of childbirth and to receive support (see Chapter 12), most couples still gain information from their friends or families. Those who do not attend classes tend to discuss every aspect with friends, sometimes gaining inaccurate information. The woman is eager to learn any methods to relieve discomforts and to assist her during labor. Information for recovery, self-care, and infant care should be presented in the third trimester because early hospital discharge does not allow adequate time for teaching

Concerns

Almost all expectant mothers express needs in the third trimester in approximately the same ways despite differences in background, educational level, and experience. A woman focuses on the infant, the process of labor, and her own changing physical condition and emotions. Even those with several children have questions about the differences in labor and delivery with each infant, and they may be fearful about the upcoming birth. Concerns expressed in this trimester include the following:

1. The infant's well-being (questions on birth defects, signs of fetal well-being, how birth affects the infant, effects of medication and anesthesia)
2. The costs of having an infant (hospital fees, wages lost during maternity leave, expenses for equipment)
3. The process of labor and delivery (pain, fears, misconceptions, when to go to the hospital)
4. Family (how other children will accept the infant, how to plan for them during hospitalization, how partner will respond to the infant)

During this trimester, the changing contours of the woman's body become more prominent; backaches, leg aches, lower abdominal pressure, ligament pain, fatigue, and extra weight all cause her to be impatient for labor to begin (Table 8-1).

Some women are superstitious about buying anything for the infant before its birth; to do so, they believe, risks death or injury to the child. Acknowledge this belief but be sure to discuss the equipment that the new infant will need, even though purchasing will begin later. Though the father or grandparents may make these purchases during the mother's hospitalization, the mother will want to know how to plan. The important fact to emphasize is that planning should be done before the infant is taken home. Mothers who have limited apartment space or income will usually welcome suggestions on how to economize. Almost all women feel the "nesting" impulse, an urge to prepare for the infant.

Signs of difficulty

Signs of difficulty in the third trimester include the mother's continuing high level of anxiety about herself, labor, or the discomforts of pregnancy. If the woman neglects health practices or cannot prepare for or focus on the needs of the coming infant, she may be indicating that she cannot adjust to what is happening in her body.

Childbirth classes can often be a support for the pregnant woman anxious about the discomforts of pregnancy, labor, and delivery. It is often reassuring to discuss concerns and know that other women are going through the same process. Use of imagery—visualizing a positive outcome—will help prepare the woman for labor and delivery. Progressive relaxation techniques also help reduce anxiety. Both imagery and relaxation techniques enhance the woman's sense of control at a time when she

Table 8-1   **Maternal Tasks, Concerns, and Signs of Difficulties**

Tasks	Concerns	Signs of Difficulties
FIRST TRIMESTER		
To acknowledge pregnancy	Normalcy of symptoms, future changes in lifestyle	Exaggerated discomforts such as nausea, sleeplessness
To begin working through conflicts with own mother	Changes in relationship with partner	Excessive need for reassurance that she is pregnant
To begin developing own mothering role	Cost of care, how to manage	Anger, rejection of idea of pregnancy
To validate and accept pregnancy	Normalcy of ambivalence	Depression, crying, extreme mood swings
		Distance from sexual partner
SECOND TRIMESTER		
To regard fetus as a reality (fetal embodiment)	Nutritional intake	Lack of acceptance of pregnancy
To manage shifts in dependency from the role of daughter to the role of mother	Changing body image	Continuing depression, anger, anxiety
To continue working through conflicts with own parents	Changing lifestyle, sexual needs	Numerous physical complaints, focus on own concerns
To use mimicry, role playing, imagery to help herself to assume the role of mother	Progression of fetal growth	Indications of no family support
	Warning signs of problems	Indication of inability to plan ahead
THIRD TRIMESTER		
To view fetus as a separate individual to be "let go" through birth	Infant's well-being, factors affecting labor and birth	High level of anxiety about self, labor
To accept physical, psychologic changes	Anxiety over possibility of deformed baby	Continued nonacceptance of pregnancy
To prepare for parenting	Expenses	Behavior that neglects health practices
To prepare for labor, birth, and to accept the risk of "safe passage"	Process of labor, delivery	Lack of support from family or spouse
	Acceptance of infant by other children	Lack of preparation for or focus on needs of new infant
	Present discomforts	

may feel very much out of control. If the pregnant woman shows inability to participate in the expected practices to ensure a safe delivery, increased assistance through counseling and home health visits may be warranted.

TEST *Yourself* 8-1 _____

a. Describe three tasks the expectant mother should accomplish during pregnancy.
b. How can imagery help with role attainment? Compare and contrast imagery with visualization.

EXPECTANT FATHER'S TASKS

Although much attention has been focused on the woman, men also undergo parallel experiences. As society changes and more women work outside the home, childrearing and household responsibilities have become more of a partner-

ship. Some men also express a desire to be more involved in fatherhood and to "do things differently from their fathers." Research indicates, however, that men have not been prepared for the ambivalence, anxiety, and increased tension that are common experiences of pregnancy (Donovan, 1995). Men may not be recognized as expectant parents, but instead are thought of more as breadwinners. A man's lack of ease in sharing pregnancy anxieties and concerns may interfere with his validation of the reality of the pregnancy or child (Jordan, 1990).

Like his mate, the expectant father must make the psychologic shift from an idea of himself as a man or boy without children to that of a *man with a child,* a father. The ease with which he is able to make this transition is related to his readiness for the pregnancy and the level of his ambivalence. Antle-May (1982) states that readiness is related to the man's sense of financial security, to stability in the couple relationship, and to his readiness to end the childless state within the couple's relationship. Although his experience lacks the immediacy of the expectant mother's role shift, it follows a similar pattern.

First Trimester

When tests confirm the pregnancy, the couple makes an announcement to family and friends. Jordan (1990) reports that in "laboring for relevance" the first process is *grappling with the reality of the pregnancy and child*. In the first trimester, changes in the mother's behavior and body, such as fatigue or nausea, act as reminders that the pregnancy is real. These changes may cause her to withdraw; the father may feel ignored.

Second Trimester

As the reality of the child becomes more evident by hearing the fetal heartbeat or by visualizing fetal movements on sonography, the father continues to evolve toward his role as parent. The mother plays a critical part in making the father feel as though he has an integral part to play. Jordan (1990) reports that mothers bring their mates into the experience by frequently and openly sharing their physical sensations and emotional responses. Jordan calls this process *struggling for recognition as a parent*. Nurses can be instrumental in this process by including fathers in prenatal visits and by not viewing them simply as maternal supporters.

The expectant father remembers how he was fathered and accepts or rejects that role. Other relationships are examined. He tends to seek friendship with men who have children and to drift away from those who do not.

In terms of the couple's relationship, increased sexual activity is possible as physical discomforts decrease. The couple begins to discuss the degree of involvement that he will have in childbirth and in parenting the child. Though this decision is highly individual, the decision needs to be made by both partners. If a couple's expectations differ, a compromise must be reached before the birth, or unmet expectations may lead to conflict.

Third Trimester

As the third trimester arrives, the expectant father may become more focused on the actual arrival of the baby. Though a father may be reluctant to attend childbirth education classes or to hear repeatedly about plans or ideas about the baby, he may begin to "nest," accumulating equipment and supplies for the baby. The father may be involved in painting the baby's room or rearranging furniture, and this actual "physical doing" may make the father feel for the first time that he is actually a part of the process.

Like the mother, the father may experience heightened anxiety as the birth becomes imminent. He may have fears for his partner's well being and concerns about the health of the baby. He may mourn the loss of his previous role and lifestyle. With the birth of the child, Jordan (1990) reports that fathers slowly develop the role of involved fatherhood. A nurse can assist in this process by supporting and recognizing his struggle for role attainment.

Couvade

The father's adjustment may include a series of health symptoms and complaints termed **couvade**. The term is derived from the French verb *couver,* meaning "to brew, hatch, or sit on eggs." Throughout history and in different cultures, couvade behaviors vary. Expectant fathers may have refrained from eating certain foods or secluded themselves alone or with their partner during pregnancy. Today couvade refers to the male experience of pregnancy. The man's adjustment is seen in the form of behavioral changes that may or may not be socially sanctioned or somatic symptoms for which there is no apparent physiologic cause (Mason, 1995). Symptoms such as intestinal gas pains, nausea, hunger and weight gain, restlessness, sleeping difficulties, and bad dreams may be reported.

It is thought that couvade demonstrates a positive level of identification with the pregnant partner. Longobucco and Preston (1989) found that men who experience symptoms score higher on scales measuring paternal role preparation than men who report no symptoms. Since paternal bonding does begin during the pregnancy, this finding seems logical. One father's experience is recorded below.

One father left the scene of the birth of his first child to cry alone. He shared with me his deep sadness that he could not also bear a child. He has continued to be a very nurturing father.

T E S T *Yourself* 8-2 _____

> a. According to the studies by Antle-May (1982), the expectant father's readiness for pregnancy is related to what factors?
> b. Jordan reports that fathers often "struggle for relevance." How can the mother help her partner with this task?

COPING DURING PREGNANCY

Most women do well with support. Others find pregnancy an additional stress that puts them off balance. With an understanding of the normalcy of body changes, the woman may enjoy her progress. If she is uninformed, she may resent or be fearful of what is happening. If she looks forward to and recognizes the steps of pregnancy, however, she will feel pride and enjoyment. The woman already under stress may feel anger and frustration at her changing body responses. Richardson (1990) identifies four phases of body experience, each related to equilibrium or disequilibrium in body accommodation; these terms refer to the "balance between the demands for self-preservation and the demands for maternal giving to and enduring for the unborn baby."

- From the woman's awareness of pregnancy to her sensing fetal movement (20 weeks), a series of events occurs that causes *disequilibration* in the body. The woman endures these changes (and gives to the fetus) without "knowing" the reality of the fetus who is the cause of the changes. Richardson calls this the *reduction phase.*
- In the brief period between 21 and 26 weeks, all goes well and the sense of fetal movement and real presence provides the first feedback that the woman is nurturing a real person. This *expansion phase* takes place in a state of equilibrium; the woman is "reinforced in her sense of maternal confidence and adequacy."
- The *tension phase* occurs from 27 to 32 weeks. The woman questions her ability to endure "to the end." If complications occur, they often arise in this phase.
- The *stabilization phase* occurs from 33 weeks until birth. Social support is more intense and the woman seeks knowledge about birth and becomes more confident that she can carry through.

Any hindrance in the mother's progress through the developmental tasks and these phases may result in anxiety or conflict that further impedes her ability to form an image of her maternal self. Such impediments can arise from low self-esteem, lack of a maternal role model, or conflicts between the mother-self and career-self roles. When the woman is either quite young or older or when medical or social problems occur, maternal role attainment may be more troublesome.

Nursing Responsibilities

ASSESSMENT

Use the questions in Table 8-2 to elicit information regarding family and individual situations that may precipitate stress during pregnancy. Often when questions focus on what the woman really needs or is concerned about, the presenting need is far from what the nurse assumes it to be. Always *listen* first before giving instructions or advice. See Chapter 27 for a model that has been developed for care of high-risk teenagers and women with psychosocial problems or problems that place mother and infant at risk.

To determine whether the woman has positive role models, ask her with whom she will talk about her pregnancy. Find out if the woman is socially isolated (even within a marriage) by asking her how she spends time with friends or family.

NURSING DIAGNOSES

Whenever a nurse works with expectant parents, the following should be considered for psychologic growth during pregnancy.

- Altered role performance related to adaptations to the pregnancy
- Family coping: potential for growth related to anticipation of parenting
- Individual coping compromised by inadequate family support or disengagement
- Situational low self-esteem related to prior life experiences or level of support during pregnancy

EXPECTED OUTCOMES

Consider these examples of outcomes to patient care.
- Mother seeks assistance from appropriate resources and referrals and works on problem resolution.
- Mother verbalizes changes that are taking place and anticipates the future.
- Mother seeks involvement of the partner in the care process.
- Partner participates in care and preparation for birth.
- Mother appears to be going through developmental tasks smoothly.

NURSING INTERVENTION

The nurse must be perceptive enough to identify some of the subtle indications of problems and must also recognize the importance of psychosocial adaptation in planning care during pregnancy and recovery. The following examples of questions to elicit the woman's perception of her life events are adapted from suggestions by Kleinman and Eisenbergh-Good (1979):
- What do you think caused your problem?
- Why do you think it started when it did?
- What do you think the problem does to you? To your infant?
- How do you think you can resolve this problem?
- Can you express the anxiety that comes from this problem?

The woman often articulates a different emphasis than the health care professional expects. Cultural differences play a significant part in the emphasis placed on the meaning of the problem. If a depressed affect or lack of grooming is evident, the woman should be further evaluated for more severe problems, and appropriate referrals should be made.

Plans to help the mother become more active in her own self-care can be as simple as reinforcing her ability to make appropriate choices. To do this, allow her to make choices about her care and give her the responsibility of carrying them out. Self-care means treating the expectant parents as adults, even when they are adolescents. In addition, refer to

Table 8-2   Initial Questions to Elicit Status Regarding Pregnancy

Questions	Factors Influencing Planning
SUPPORT AVAILABLE	
Length of time living in this location?	An isolated couple will need encouragement to seek support.
Support system in this locality?	Referrals must be considered. Exploration with family about
Who is available to help with siblings or during the early postpartum period?	resources is important.
What emotional supports are available for each partner?	A major component of parenting classes is to foster sharing about these issues.
Financial plans to cover costs of pregnancy?	Location and type of medical service influence available referrals.
What are their needs for assistance?	Working may be beneficial or harmful, depending on risk status.
Are there needs that will keep the woman working throughout pregnancy?	
RESPONSE TO PREGNANCY	
What are the most direct concerns about the idea of being pregnant at this time?	Ambivalence about pregnancy is usual in first months but may be a clue to difficulty if still present toward the end of pregnancy.
What interruptions in life goals?	Partner's responses need to be elicited. His attendance at
What sense of "this is the right time"?	one prenatal visit and at parenting classes is highly recommended.
What are the reactions of other family members to the pregnancy?	Single mothers need extra support, as do those in hostile environments.
Are there strong desires to bear only a son or daughter? Has there been discussion about acceptance of either sex in the infant?	Fixation on sex of infant may hinder bonding after delivery; some opportunity to talk about this aspect is important.
PROCESS	
What information needs do the expectant parents have?	Information giving must be preceded by a determination of what the person already knows.
Fetal growth and development?	
Sexuality during pregnancy?	
Care of woman to promote health?	
Other questions?	
What plans for or fears of delivery are present?	Fears are not easily elicited. Sharing common misconceptions
Which questions need to be asked of physician (anesthesia, type of delivery)?	that other mothers have had may prompt a person to recognize her own fears.
What fears can be identified?	Fearful women need special assisstance and perhaps some
How do they feel information can help?	group discussions before they can openly admit fears.
How much interest in parenting classes is expressed?	Encourage attendance when possible if classes are supportive.
	Provide several options for differing approaches and needs.

REMEMBER: "Parents who are secure, supported, valued, and in control of their lives are more effective parents than those who feel unsure and who are not in control" (Kenniston K, The Carnagie Council on Children: *All our children: the American family under pressure,* New York, 1978, Harcourt Brace Jovanovich.)

social service any woman with stressed life circumstances or economic problems that interfere with adequate nutrition, housing, or future care of the infant and herself.

EVALUATION

Sample questions to evaluate whether the mother has reached outcomes are listed below.
- Did the partners seek to learn about pregnancy and parenting?
- How was her partner to be involved?
- Were clinic appointments kept and outside resources used?

- Did she indicate adequate social support?
- Has she received and followed through on referrals for unresolved problems?

SEXUAL RESPONSES DURING PREGNANCY

Mother's Responses

In the course of prenatal counseling a woman may express anxiety about sexuality during pregnancy and allude to particular problems. Even if she does not, approach the subject in a nonthreatening way, either individually or in prenatal classes. A number of women react positively to their changing body image, feeling less restricted in their sexual expression. Some experience a sense of fulfillment when they are pregnant or feel more attractive than before. For these women, there may be heightened interest in sexual activity. Other women feel less desirable and awkward and express less interest in sexual activity because of discomforts.

Desire. Changes in body image may increase or decrease sexual interest; a woman may be either more tense or more relaxed. If she enjoys her body changes, she will have an increased interest in more frequent intercourse; if the pregnancy brings discomforts, however, sexual desire will be reduced.

Excitement. The phase of physiologic excitement includes vasocongestion of vaginal and labial tissues and clitoral enlargement. Pregnancy increases lubrication and vasocongestion, and excitement may come more quickly. Breasts, too, are already enlarged and may be tender or even sore. Sexual excitement makes nipples erect and may bring discomfort for some; breasts may be a new focus in sex-play because all women have enlargement. In some cases the woman may be increasingly uncomfortable with the enlargement, whereas her partner finds it stimulating.

Plateau and orgasm. The vaginal tract is more engorged and orgasm may be reached more swiftly. There may be several orgasms and some women describe orgasm as "fulminating" during pregnancy (Reamy and White, 1985).

Resolution. The period of decrease in tissue engorgement and relaxation is often changed. Vasocongestion does not diminish quickly. Some women have continuing discomfort and take longer to relax.

Father's Responses

Although many men have no change in sexual desires because of pregnancy, some find the partner's changing body to be newly attractive and feel an increased closeness, intimacy, and eroticism. Other men may find these same changes to be unattractive and less stimulating. Men may express a fear of harming the woman or fetus or have questions about whether intercourse is "right" when the woman is pregnant. A man may have fantasies about the fetus or about being inadequate to satisfy the woman's increased desires. As a result he may withdraw or seek a sexual outlet outside the partnership.

Sexual responses may differ between the woman and her partner (see Chapter 3); she may be more interested, while he may be less. Interest levels also change as the pregnancy progresses. Research studies have shown that each trimester may have a different set of responses. It is important for the couple to communicate their individual sexual needs throughout the pregnancy. In addition to intercourse, sexual needs may be met through kissing, touching, and being held.

Nursing Responsibilities

ASSESSMENT

The nurse working with different ethnic groups should seek information about any cultural sexual taboos during pregnancy and recovery. By seeking this information from each client, the nurse can avoid stereotyping and can plan care that is based on individual needs.

NURSING DIAGNOSES

The few possible diagnoses to use for this concern depend on whether the problems expressed are related to the partner or to the woman or stem from a medical complication during pregnancy.

- Altered sexuality patterns related to differing responses to pregnancy
- Altered individual coping related to symptoms or complications of pregnancy
- At risk for sexually transmitted infection depending on partner's status

EXPECTED OUTCOMES

- Expresses feelings regarding sexual responses during pregnancy
- Incorporates anticipatory guidance
- Protects herself from sexually transmitted diseases (STDs)

NURSING INTERVENTION

The most effective intervention for sexual problems expressed by the client during pregnancy is *anticipatory guidance*. On the basis of current understanding of the physiologic changes of pregnancy, the following may be taught regarding sexual activity during pregnancy (Reamy and White, 1985):

1. There is little potential for injury.
   - The fetus is not injured by normal coitus because it is cushioned by amniotic fluid and protected by the cervix and uterus.
   - In the last few weeks, after the fetal head has descended into the pelvic canal, a woman may find deep thrusting uncomfortable.
2. There is little potential for harm by stimulating uterine contractions.
   - Miscarriage in the first 3 months is rarely caused by coitus. Almost all reasons for spontaneous abortion are intrinsic, related to genetic causes or to poor development of the embryo.
   - If the threat of spontaneous abortion exists, absti-

nence is suggested until it is clear that the pregnancy will continue.

- Prostaglandins in semen may stimulate mild uterine contractions, especially a few days before labor begins. For this reason, women who have a history of preterm labor or premature rupture of the membranes and those who experience strong uterine contractions after orgasm should be advised of the possible risks of coitus after 32 weeks gestation (Kochenour, 1994). Conversely, if the infant is overdue, some encourage the couple to have intercourse in hopes of stimulating labor.

3. STDs and infection have adverse effects on the fetus.
   - STDs should be taken very seriously. Both partners should be treated if an infection is diagnosed (see Chapter 25). Information concerning protection should be provided to the woman and her partner.
   - Women with new partners or multiple partners must insist that partners use a condom for protection. Women whose partners are at risk should always insist on condom use but may not be able to do so (see Chapter 25).

4. Air must never be blown into the vagina during sex-play because there is a rare chance of death due to air embolism (Reamy and White, 1985). Because of the partial dilation of the cervix, air forcibly blown into the vagina may enter the uterus and find a way into maternal circulation through the placenta.

5. Variations in sexual interest are normal and reflect physiologic changes.
   - First trimester: Because of increased blood supply to vaginal tissue and the enlarging uterus, some women have a more total orgasmic response. Nulliparas may have a decreased response, often because of discomforts and fatigue. Multiparas often find it a relief not to need contraception.
   - Second trimester: There is an increase in eroticism and orgasmic response noted by all women. Most women indicate increased interest. The enlarging uterus begins to require changes in position for coitus, including side to side, rear entry, and woman-superior.
   - Third trimester: As the due date approaches, the frequency of intercourse is reduced for most women. Fatigue and discomfort play a part, but women may also be worried about arbitrary instructions by health professionals. Though it is common to hear "6 weeks before and 6 weeks after" as the period of abstinence, such instruction should no longer be provided.

EVALUATION

Evaluation questions that may be asked to determine progress toward the outcomes include the following.

- Did the woman (or couple) ask appropriate questions and indicate understanding of the effects of pregnancy on sexuality?

- Did she state that she used precautions to protect against STDs?
- Did a medical condition during pregnancy cause stress between partners? Were they able to resolve these problems?

INCREASED PSYCHOSOCIAL RISK

When the parent-child relationship is healthy the child learns to socialize with others in the home. He or she becomes an adult who can complete the developmental and pregnancy-related tasks in preparation for becoming a parent and can in turn form bonds to his or her own children. People in today's urban societies often move away from the family of origin, thus extended kinship groups may not exist. The result is that parents often raise children without the support of a group. Without an extended family on which to depend, the parent-child relationship is *absolutely crucial* to the child's psychologic growth. A new mother may have only her own family as a role model or may come from a single-parent family. Choices become limited and the media may have a stronger influence. For these and a number of other reasons, women at either extreme of reproductive age—the older, *mature gravida* and the *adolescent gravida*—are at increased psychosocial risk. These risks vary with and correspond to developmental stages.

Mature Pregnant Women

Many women delay pregnancy until after age 35. The rate of first births to women between the ages of 35 and 39 more than doubled between 1980 and 1992 in the United States. For women between the ages of 40 and 44, the birth rate increased by 40% during the same period (U.S. Bureau of the Census, 1993). An older primigravida may have postponed childbearing until her career was well established or until she felt financially secure. She may have had difficulty finding a suitable partner. Although the child may be wanted and anticipated, she will often have ambivalence and concern about how motherhood will affect her lifestyle and how it will affect her relationship with the father of the baby. If she is newly married pregnancy may cause added stress on the relationship.

The client may be a single woman deciding to have a child on her own, perhaps even by artificial insemination or she may have conceived after treatment for infertility or after in vitro fertilization. She may be having a child later in her childbearing years because of remarriage or by "accident." This child may be much desired or unwelcome. The nurse must ascertain this information because the responses of the woman and her family are closely tied to their feelings. Regardless of the reason for delayed childbearing, a woman over 35 who is expecting her first child is often referred to as elderly primigravida or mature primigravida.

Developmental stage

The woman over 35 may have entered the life stage of *generativity vs stagnation* defined by Erikson (1963) as "primarily the concern in establishing and guiding the next generation." Productivity and creativity are words that embody what is meant by generativity. Though these women seem best prepared psychologically for the demands of pregnancy and parenthood at this stage because their lives are stable, this readiness intensifies their need for nursing care. They are heavily invested in their pregnancies because of the need to have the first, the only, or the last child. They have decided to carry and deliver this pregnancy, perhaps one that is unplanned, because it may be their last chance to have a child. When something goes wrong or threatens to go wrong, the reaction will be intense.

On the other hand, women who have had difficulties moving through previous developmental tasks may find themselves with unfinished psychosexual and psychosocial development; thus they are still in the stage of *intimacy vs isolation*.

Issues particularly important for the woman over 35 are control and past coping behaviors. A woman may have been successful in her career by manipulating situations, but when faced with a situation in which she is not in control and must trust others, severe anxiety may develop. Her past coping behaviors may not be effective, and this will intensify anxiety. She may feel unable to take care of herself and often has little experience in relying on others during times of need. The mature gravida's perceptions of life change, including changes in personal life and in relationships, may correlate with higher stress even 1 year after delivery (Reece, 1993). An important part of *anticipatory guidance* is letting the client know that her old ways of dealing with situations must change during the pregnancy. A newborn will disrupt its parents' lifestyle tremendously, and the client must begin to consider this during pregnancy.

Genetic concerns

Genetic concerns complicate the psychosocial needs of the mature gravida and her family. Genetic counselors can furnish the client with statistics that can put risks into perspective and aid in the decision to either undergo or forego genetic testing (see Chapter 28). The decision to undergo genetic testing is not always easy. Some women are certain that they will abort a genetically defective fetus; others are equally resolute that they will not. These additional concerns are superimposed on normal worries. This phenomenon, called the **tentative pregnancy**, occurs when women are unsure whether they are mothers or "carriers of a defective fetus" (Katz-Rothman, 1986). Many mature gravidas are concerned because there is a higher risk of Down syndrome and other autosomal trisomies when a woman is older.

Medical concerns

Preexisting conditions such as hypertension, obesity, or diabetes may be important factors to consider. Preeclampsia occurs at a higher rate among mature gravidas. Fibroid tumors occur with greater frequency in the mature gravida. Increased estrogen production, particularly in the first trimester, may cause fibroids inside the uterus to increase in size. This may result in premature labor or mechanical difficulties during delivery or it may increase the likelihood of postpartum hemorrhage by preventing the uterus from contracting completely.

Because of these difficulties and the fact that the mature gravida is at higher risk, cesarean birth is chosen more often by obstetricians. This trend of higher cesarean births is an important factor to consider. Reece (1993) reports that the perception of labor and delivery of older primiparas influenced them for as long as 1 year after delivery. Dissatisfaction with the birth experience affected not only her stress level but also the spouse or partner relationship and the mother's satisfaction with her infant and how she accomplished infant care tasks.

Nursing Responsibilities

Assessment of the woman over 35 is similar to the assessment of any pregnant woman, with special attention paid to preexisting physical problems such as diabetes, hypertension, and uterine fibroids. It is important to elicit information regarding family and individual situations that may precipitate stress during pregnancy. The nurse should not assume knowledge but should ask questions to assess understanding of the pregnancy, delivery, and infant care needs. Because of the increased risk of chromosomal abnormalities, the woman will be given information by the physician about available diagnostic tests. Determine the woman's anxiety levels and her understanding of the procedures involved. Marked ambivalence, particularly if career choices in relation to the pregnancy need to be made, should be looked for. Finally, a discussion with the client of how she will cope with the stress of childcare and the demands of work, if and when she returns to the workplace, should be held. Encourage attendance at childbirth classes where the woman and her partner can express any concerns they have about the pregnancy and delivery.

Adolescent Pregnancy

Adolescent pregnancy presents an enormous health and financial burden in society. More than 1 million teenage girls in the United States become pregnant each year, a rate higher than that in most other developed nations. Births to teens aged 10 to 14 have risen, and birth rates for African-American teenagers have been substantially above those for Hispanics or European Americans

(Statistical Bulletin Oct.-Dec. 1994). In addition, nearly one in five teenagers who experiences a premarital pregnancy becomes pregnant again within a year. Within 2 years more than 31% have a repeat pregnancy (Guttmacher Institute, 1991). Of these pregnancies 85% are unplanned; 400,000 choose to have abortions each year. Another 100,000 miscarry, and 500,000 pregnancies are continued to term (Bluestein, 1994). Among adolescents who carry pregnancy to full term, over 90% keep and raise the infant, whereas 10% choose to give the child up for adoption (Steinberg, 1993). The impact of pregnancy and birth often causes the teenager to drop out of school, thus dramatically effecting future employment and income levels. Welfare costs for all families started by teen pregnancies were estimated to be $25 billion, and it is estimated that $10 billion can be saved if those pregnancies are delayed until the mother reaches age 20 (Burnhill, 1994).

The problem of birth control

Sexual activity among adolescents is common, yet many do not use birth control. The most common reasons given are that they (1) do not believe they will get pregnant and (2) did not anticipate having intercourse. On average, teenagers wait almost 1 year to attend a family planning clinic after becoming sexually active. One half of all teenage pregnancies occur in the first 6 months after initiation of intercourse, and 20% occur in the first month alone (Zabin, Kantner, and Zelnick, 1979). If a birth control method was used, it was not the most effective. In one study, oral contraceptives were used by slightly fewer than one half of those surveyed. Condoms were listed as the principal method by 25% of those surveyed (Burnhill, 1994). Girls' first age of intercourse has been another variable studied in adolescent pregnancy. Girls who engaged in intercourse beginning at a younger age increased their likelihood of becoming pregnant (Morgan, Chapar, and Fisher, 1995).

From a psychosocial perspective, some teenagers, either consciously or subconsciously, want to have babies because friends have them, or because they want something they can succeed in doing, something to love, or something to make them feel important or special (Figure 8-3). When adolescents come from intolerable home or living situations, becoming pregnant may be a means of escape. Impoverished teenagers may find the consequences of early childbearing less disturbing than teenagers raised in more fortunate circumstances. For other teenagers, pregnancy may be an important part of the cultural process of becoming an adult (Stevens-Simon, Lowry, 1995; Klerman, 1993). Some teenagers want to keep their boyfriends and fear that refusing sex will drive them away. Some want to gain attention from their parents. These are all adolescent ways of expressing basic needs for belonging, love, and self-esteem.

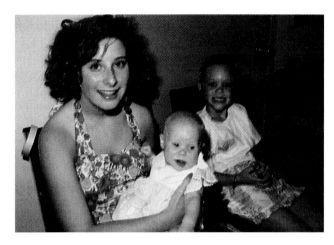

Figure 8-3   The teenage mother may think of her infant as a doll. (Courtesy Marjorie Pyle, RNC, *Lifecircle*.)

♪elf-♩iscovery

Baby-Think-It-Over is a tool that provides a simulation of real infant care demands. The high-tech newborn doll, equipped with a microprocessor, shrieks randomly—day and night—and is quieted only when "fed" or "comforted." To do either, the teenage "parent" who has been assigned 3 full days of care must insert a key into the doll's back and hold it in place for as long as 35 minutes.

Schools are using this doll simulation to help teenagers become motivated to delay pregnancies. Teenagers are reported to come into class exhausted from the demands of the "baby" and to be highly motivated to learn about the requirements of delaying pregnancy with birth control methods. ～

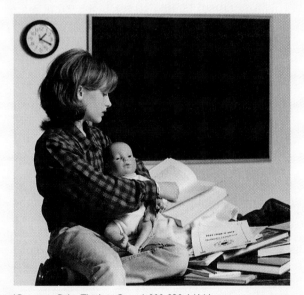

(Courtesy Baby-Think-it-Over, 1-800-830-1416.)

The role of the media may be influential in affecting adolescent sexuality. Television shows, movies, and advertisements often bombard young people with sex and sexual innuendos. Rarely do the media address the issue of responsibility regarding sexual behavior. Although the media have begun to modify their approach to sexuality because of the risk of human immunodeficiency viral (HIV) infection, there is still much to be done. The emphasis must be placed on responsible sexuality, including abstinence and contraception. While the national debate continues about where and by whom sexual education programs should be taught, research is clear: we must begin early and be specific. It is unlikely that the United States will soon develop policies to encourage early sex education programs even though the urgency of the rates of HIV and other STDs and of teenage pregnancy demand it. Experience in other countries where teenage sexual activity is just as prevalent as in the United States shows that the rate of pregnancy can be reduced by making effective contraception readily available. High-quality sex education programs have been found to be useful only if accompanied by provision of supplies (Hatcher et al, 1994).

A nurse's role is twofold: (1) care for adolescent parents and (2) support their parents and teachers in an effort to communicate about responsible sexual behavior before pregnancy occurs and after its termination. Parents and teachers also need education. Fears that talking about sex will encourage earlier sexual activity are unfounded. Adolescents often have distorted ideas about sex and lack knowledge about their bodies and bodily changes. Many parents find it difficult to talk with their children about maturation, sex, birth control, and parenting. Parents may not understand that this information is vital and that it must be given early, *before* the onset of sexual activity. Furstenberg (1980) found that although 59% of mothers frequently talked to their daughters about sex and 92% occasionally talked to their daughters about sex, most of the messages were "Don't get mixed up with boys" or "Don't do anything you will be sorry for later." This is not the information teenagers require. On the other hand, 50% of the young girls whose mothers discussed methods of birth control used contraception at least occasionally.

Developmental tasks

The word "adolescence" comes from the Latin verb *adolescere*, which means "to grow into adulthood." It is a time when one moves from childhood into adulthood. Adolescence is studied in phases: early adolescence refers to the period of time from age 11 through 14; middle adolescence, from age 15 through 18; and late adolescence, from age 18 through 21. During this passage from childhood to adulthood, which is smooth for some and rough for others, many tasks must be accomplished. Biologically, the body undergoes physical changes that are referred to

as puberty. Cognitively, the adolescent begins to develop more sophisticated thinking abilities, and socially he or she is granted more freedom. With each of these changes, the adolescent undergoes profound changes in self-image that have an impact on relationships with peers, family, and society as a whole.

Psychosocial development during adolescence is one of the most important accomplishments of this period. Developing identity, autonomy, and intimacy and expressing sexuality and achievement play an important role (Steinberg, 1993).

Identity. This is the adolescents' quest for who they really are. They begin to experiment with various roles to discover their true self. This experimentation period involves trying on different postures, personalities, and ways of behaving (Steinberg, 1993). This may be a difficult time for parents, who try to adapt to ever-changing moods.

Autonomy. This is the adolescents' struggle to gain independence. During this process they become less emotionally dependent on parents and better able to make independent decisions, and they begin to establish their own set of values and morals (Steinberg, 1993). Thinking becomes more abstract and they begin to understand cause and effect. This is a time to differentiate values, religious beliefs, or political views.

Intimacy. The capacity for intimacy during the adolescent period allows for the formation of trusting and loving relationships. It begins with same sex relationships and progresses to opposite sex relationships during middle adolescence (Steinberg, 1993). These relationships promote growth and support for the many changes occurring at this time. During this period the adolescent also develops a greater capacity to empathize and understand how others are feeling.

Sexuality. This is another psychosocial issue of adolescence since sexual activity usually begins during this period. Sexual development during this period is important because it can change relationships between peers and can have lasting consequences. Sexuality raises many questions and issues of responsibility.

Achievement. Although achievement is a lifelong issue, it is particularly important during adolescence because decisions about school and work are often made during this period. These decisions may have a lasting effect in terms of occupation and socioeconomic status. Feeling good about one's own skills is a key to developing self-esteem.

Since the adolescent has many tasks to accomplish and skills to develop, pregnancy is often a tremendous burden on the adolescent mother. Flanagan et al (1995) report that the young mother's psychosocial and cognitive development is related to her experience of motherhood and the conceptualization of the maternal role. Her phase of adolescence will also have an impact on her needs and abilities. Early adolescents may still be concrete thinkers who have trouble understanding that actions have consequences. In the middle period, adolescents begin to think more abstractly but experiment and struggle with autonomy. This struggle may lead to poor decisions that have undesirable consequences. During later adolescence, young mothers may be more willing to accept adult advice, but discussions must be focused on choices and consequences and on building healthy relationships.

Self-Discovery

Think about when you first learned about sex and birth control. Who gave the information to you? Was the information correct? How did you respond at that time? How would you do it differently for your own child? ∼

Psychosocial concerns

Since adolescence is a key time for growth and development, the challenge of being pregnant is often overwhelming. Many of the developmental tasks cannot be completed as the adolescent struggles to adapt to being pregnant. All aspects of the adolescent's life are changed. Physical changes alter body image. The pregnancy itself effects relationships with friends, boyfriends, and family. Schooling is disrupted. To make sense of all these changes, the adolescent must have a tremendous amount of support.

Adolescents may often deny a pregnancy until the obvious signs can no longer be ignored by family members. It is common for teenagers to diet and wear constricting clothes to hide the pregnancy until it is quite advanced, sometimes even until delivery. The level of denial in some teenagers and their families can be quite high. The nurse must be especially concerned about a teenager who arrives in labor and delivery claiming she did not know that she was pregnant. She may have been brought in by her family, with whom she was living and who also claim they were unaware of the pregnancy. This truly may be denial or a way for her family to hide embarrassment about the pregnancy or the delay in seeking care. The possibility of incest or sexual abuse may exist and must be considered. Nevertheless, the ability of the family to care for the infant in these cases requires the help of an interdisciplinary team.

Many adolescent mothers fail to seek or receive adequate prenatal care. In her study, Lee (1995) reported that those who do seek early care do so because they feel ill, are worried about themselves, want a pregnancy test, or because their mothers insist on prenatal care. Reasons for delayed care include not recognizing pregnancy symptoms, denial of pregnancy, fear of parents' response to the pregnancy, and lack of financial resources.

Because the adolescent mother's needs are many, care for the adolescent must be comprehensive. Programs should include counseling on social services and nutritional issues; education about pregnancy, childrearing, and contraception; reinforcement for staying in or returning to school; and health education on the need to stop smoking, drinking, and using drugs (see Box 8-1). Research shows that programs that provide social and behavioral services and medical care may improve both the health of the mother and the outcome of her pregnancy (Scholl et al, 1994).

▌ *Box* **8-1**   **Content of Classes for Adolescents**

CHANGES IN LIFE OF TEEN WHEN SHE BECOMES PREGNANT
Am I my mother's child or my child's mother?
Will my own parents offer support?
How can I finish school?

CHANGES DURING THE PREGNANCY
What can I do about all these changes?
Is everything I've heard about pregnancy true?
How long does it take to make a baby?
What do I have to eat?

PREPARATION FOR LABOR AND DELIVERY
How does this baby get out?
Who helps me?
Does it hurt too bad?
When will I be thin again?

SEXUALITY AND FAMILY PLANNING
What do I know about sex and menstruation?
How did I learn?
How do birth control things work?
How can I protect myself from HIV? Should we use condoms during pregnancy?
Will anyone want to date me after the baby is born?

INFANT NEEDS AND CARE
How do I care for the baby's physical needs? (bathing, feeding, and dressing the infant, taking its temperature, caring for the cord, creating the proper environment, using equipment properly)
How do I care for the baby's emotional needs? (learning about infant behavior and how to love it)
How does this baby grow? (learning about the infant's feeding needs [breast or bottle] and developmental needs)
Who do I take the baby to see if it is ill?

In the best situation a complete set of classes will be possible.

Data from Roye and Balk, 1996; Scholl, 1994; Fleming, 1993.

Physiologic concerns

Pregnant adolescents may have increased risk for potentially serious medical problems. Because of physical immaturity, inadequate social and economic support, and limited or no prenatal care, a young mother is at a higher risk for problems. Adolescents under age 16 may be at an even higher risk (Scholl et al, 1994). Pregnancy-induced hypertension, which increases the risk of placental abruption, maternal renal failure, and cerebral hemorrhage, is more common in both whites and blacks under the age of 20 years. Although pregnancy-induced hypertension has been studied extensively and the etiology is not yet completely clear, a poor diet with low protein intake may be implicated. Iron-deficiency anemia in teenage mothers, also related to low caloric intake, or a high carbohydrate and low protein diet may increase risks of preterm birth. Because of the immaturity of the maternal pelvis in younger adolescent girls, the disproportion between the fetus and the pelvic size may cause a difficult delivery.

Preterm delivery, which is often associated with the risk of infant low birth weight, is another risk of adolescent pregnancy. It has been associated with inadequate weight gain. Scholl et al (1994) report that preterm delivery risk is diminished in teenagers enrolled in comprehensive care.

Social risk factors

STDs are common in the adolescent mother. Adolescent mothers must be assessed for general vaginal infections, especially herpes, gonorrhea, and chlamydial infections. Information on protecting against STDs is given early in care. Other social factors include whether the adolescent smokes or drinks. Although it is often assumed that teenagers smoke, and consume more alcohol than mature women, this may not necessarily be true of pregnant teenagers. In one study the use of cigarettes, alcohol, and cocaine was all less frequent among pregnant teenagers than among mature women, though the frequency of marijuana use was about the same for both groups (Scholl, 1994).

Adolescent Fathers

Adolescent fathers undergo the same difficulty as their female counterparts. Because of all the changes and responsibilities involved with pregnancy, the young father is often ill equipped to deal with parenting. Even though the developmental tasks of adolescence are unfinished, the young father is expected to make adult decisions. These young men who impregnate adolescent women are more likely than their peers to drop out of school and report feeling anxious and depressed as young adults (Steinberg, 1993). Career choices and earning potential are greatly affected by an incomplete education. Although many factors affect the outcomes of teenage pregnancy, poverty is perhaps the most difficult to overcome.

Because of the spread of AIDS, young people have been encouraged to use condoms. Some school programs have actually made these readily available. Media coverage of paternity issues, particularly those related to the enforcement of child support, have also increased public awareness of unplanned pregnancy. However, the young male adolescent's perception of contraception and paternity may involve other social issues. In a large national study of young men, Marsiglio (1993) found that neighborhood quality, parental education, race or ethnicity, and attitudes about male gender roles affected procreative consciousness and responsibility. Young men living in poor neighborhoods are more likely to be pleased about an unplanned pregnancy than those in better living conditions and are more likely to view impregnating a woman as enhancing masculinity. Young men whose parents have less education and those who hold traditional male gender role attitudes are also more likely than their counterparts to view fatherhood as increasing masculinity (Marsiglio, 1993). The implications of this study show the considerable impact poverty and education have on young men's procreative consciousness and responsibility. Marsiglio also found that sexually active African-American men and Hispanic men are more likely than European American men to have discussed contraception with their last partner, and African-American men are more likely to have used a condom during their most recent intercourse. Young men responsible for a previous pregnancy are less likely than those who reported no pregnancy to have used an effective contraception the last time they had intercourse. This population should be the target for encouragement of future contraceptive responsibility. Programs to boost self-esteem and educate young men regarding gender issues may also be helpful. In general, encouraging openness to talk about sex and contraceptive responsibility is what is most important.

At dinner my 16-year-old daughter related a story of a girl in her class, Nancy, who had announced she was pregnant. My 14-year-old son, Bill, was not interested in this "girl talk." When asked why she wanted a baby, Nancy had given the classic answer: "I wanted a baby so I'll have someone who will always love me." Nancy said she had no intention of marrying her boyfriend. "He didn't even want a baby, so I had told him I was on the pill." After being asked how she was going to support herself and the baby, Nancy responded that she was going to sue her boyfriend for child support. Suddenly Bill was intensely interested and exclaimed, "But she can't do that! She lied!" I assured Bill that Nancy could indeed sue the boyfriend, and the "girl talk" then became a discussion of shared responsibilities, consequences, and maturity.

Concerning fatherhood responsibility, some young men are not involved by their own choice, whereas others may distance themselves because they assume that there is no role to play or that their partner does not need support. They may fear being forced to marry and to provide financial support or being "saddled" with 20 years of child support payments. An adolescent father may be neglected; his family may be angry and ostracize him. In the best situation, both families pool financial, physical, and emotional resources to support the young parents as they care for their infant.

Family support

The family should be involved early, working out detailed arrangements as soon as possible so that the crisis of delivery is less overwhelming. Any nursing interventions or social services should build on and supplement family resources, only substituting for families when it is absolutely necessary.

Families can also be instrumental in providing child care support so the mother can continue her education. Those who returned to school had a lower rate of recurrent early pregnancy (Furstenberg, 1980). Adolescents generally have unrealistic expectations about the abilities and needs of an infant (Figure 8-4). Responsibilities of parenting may be difficult since sacrificing personal pleasure for the needs of another is a developmental growth task not usually completed by this age. With support and guidance, however, teenagers can adapt well. Parenting education classes that focus on increasing the mother's skills and knowledge of child care are necessary.

Studies of interaction between teenage mothers and their infants consistently report that adolescent mothers respond less sensitively to their infants and display less instances of mutual gaze, vocalizations, and touch than do older women. Censullo (1994) reported that coaching adolescents in these interactions increased the level of responsiveness and parental self-esteem.

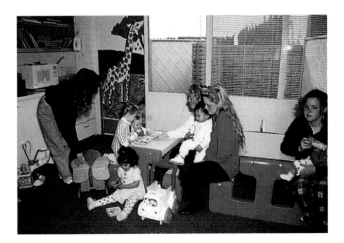

Figure 8-4   Teenage mothers in a day-care facility learn child care. (Courtesy Marjorie Pyle, RNC, *Lifecircle*.)

Box **8-1**

CLINICAL DECISION

Debate whether the following statements should be adhered to:
1. Parents and teachers should be involved in early comprehensive programs about sexuality.
2. Condoms should be provided in a school clinic so that sexually active teenagers can be protected from STDs and pregnancy.
3. Teenagers should be educated about the consequences of early parenting on the success of marriages and careers.

Nursing Responsibilities

NURSING DIAGNOSES

These diagnoses may be included in a complete nursing care plan for the pregnant adolescent or the more mature gravida.
- Individual coping, ineffective related to developmental level or situation in which pregnancy occurs.
- Family coping: potential for growth related to responses to adolescent or mature pregnant woman.
- At risk for sexually transmitted infections related to unprotected intercourse.

EXPECTED OUTCOMES

- Recognizes potential for growth in the situation.
- Chooses to obtain prenatal care and follows through.
- Seeks support for expressed needs and finds family support.
- Recognizes fetal needs for a healthy start and changes lifestyle to provide these needs.

NURSING INTERVENTION

The nurse must gain an understanding of the teenager's situation when she comes in for the first visit. The fact that she has chosen to come in reflects a major decision. She may be afraid to tell her parents and may need assistance, or she may have been brought in by her mother, and the dynamics between them will reveal much about the situation. She and her family may need a variety of assistance programs, such as women infants, and children (WIC) supplemental food programs, public assistance, or general social service. Unless you learn this at the *first encounter,* the young woman may be lost to follow-up. Do not wait for her to volunteer information. It is important to engage her trust, a difficult task because an adolescent may not trust easily and may have difficulty relating to authority figures. The adolescent fears *breach of confidentiality*. A climate of *strict confidentiality* is vital in all nursing situations but is crucial for adolescents. For these reasons, care is best given in a setting that has providers who specialize in adolescent health care.

Respond to the adolescent's *needs* rather than to her behavior. For example, when a teenager is asked how her mother feels about the pregnancy, she may state, "Fine." When probed further, she may get angry and respond, "Why do you care?" Perhaps she is afraid to say that she has not yet told her mother about her pregnancy or that her mother is insisting that she have an abortion. In these situations respond to the need; do not react. For example, say, "Lots of pregnant girls your age have real problems when they tell their parents, and some are even afraid to tell them. Let's talk about that." In this way she is given the opportunity to talk to a provider who shows caring and understanding.

Because the teenager may not want her parents to know where she is going and is concerned that you will call them, she may not give correct information. Also, she will most likely not be able to secure the insurance information on her own. In fact, maternity care for dependents is usually not covered by the family's private insurance plans. Inability to provide insurance information or pay for services should never become a barrier to providing care for adolescents, though social service may have to become involved.

The nurse must identify the girl's readiness to use referrals. Ask her to write down the sequence of what she and the nurse have together planned because later stress may prevent her from remembering what to do. If her family is aware of her condition, follow through with telephone contact when she skips appointments. If she still does not tell them early in the pregnancy, ask her for a way to establish contact. Continue to gently urge full disclosure to the family because her pregnancy will become evident in a very short time. Help her identify other sources of support in her extended family circle.

The key to successful care of the pregnant adolescent is to keep her in the health care system and to keep her in school. Since mothers and infants suffer fewer adverse effects when quality care is provided, such care becomes of prime importance. In the most effective settings, the supportive primary nurse adds the new client to her case load and follows through the pregnancy with her. The impersonal nature of large clinics is counterproductive for the adolescent mother. (See Chapter 27 for a model of care.)

Peer support groups in schools for pregnant adolescents or in clinics are helpful in preparing teenagers to cope with the demands and sacrifices of parenting (Figures 8-5 and 8-6). Educational programs and literature should be geared to teens. Providers must like working with teens and understand their unique problems

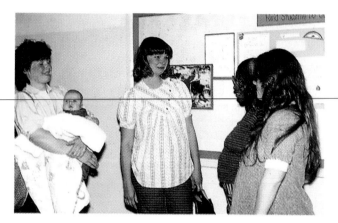

Figure 8-5 Sharing experiences in a prenatal clinic may help ease anxiety for teenage mothers. (Courtesy Marjorie Pyle, RNC, *Lifecircle*.)

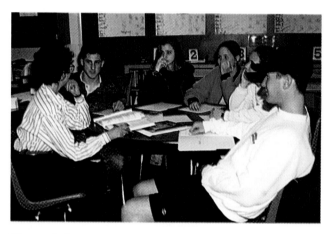

Figure 8-6 Adolescent learning groups where free discussion about parenting may be held. (Courtesy Marjorie Pyle, RNC, *Lifecircle*.)

and responses. The teen father must be involved as much as possible. He should be invited to clinic visits and parenting classes and assisted to see his role in providing physical and emotional support for his partner and his child. The nurse's attitude will influence how well the teen follows through on care (see Nursing Care Plan).

EVALUATION

The results of comprehensive care for a teenage mother would show some of the following:

- Stated she learned a great deal about herself and problem solving.
- Followed through on referrals and obtaining assistance.
- Involved father of child in planning and care of infant.
- Followed guidelines for nutrition and self-care during the pregnancy.
- Attended school and parenting classes.

Nursing Care PLAN | *Adolescent Pregnancy*

CASE:

Sixteen-year-old Cathy was brought to the emergency department by her anxious father. She had vaginal bleeding. On admission, she was found to be in preterm labor. A 32-week-old infant was born in good health. Cathy was upset but more by her parents' angry, blaming response because she had hidden the pregnancy from them. No one could focus on the infant or make plans for her. The infant was to remain in the neonatal intensive care unit (NICU) for 3 to 4 weeks. Cathy would not identify the father of the infant.

Assessment

1. Unprepared for pregnancy, no prior experience or support during pregnancy
2. Evidence of low self-esteem and difficulty with parental communication
3. May be in conflict with mother and father, no siblings
4. Physical condition seems healthy, no signs of high blood pressure, anemia, excessive weight gain
5. Unwilling to identify father of child, potential for relative incest
6. Factors precipitating preterm labor need investigation
7. Infant is preterm, in NICU for 3 to 4 weeks; condition stable

Nursing Diagnosis

1. Role performance, altered, related to keeping secret or lack of affirmation
2. Lowered self-esteem related to teenage pregnancy and potential victimization
3. Parenting, risk for altered, related to prematurity of infant and adolescent, unsupported pregnancy

Expected Outcomes

1. Expresses concerns to health care team member
2. Seeks information about pregnancy and self-care during recovery
3. Shows evidence of self-esteem by following through on recommended self-care activities and referrals
4. Attempts communication with parents
5. Shows evidence of beginning attachment to infant
6. Discusses with NICU nurses potential of infant's future

Nursing Interventions

1. Assign one primary nurse for the whole stay. Assess level of acceptance of infant. Affirm Cathy's need to talk about experience.
2. Assess mood and reactions to birth.
3. Encourage problem solving and provide information about resources.
4. Educate regarding self-care during recovery; include family planning.
5. Involve significant other person if parental anger continues.
6. Collaborate with social service to build a support network involving extended family.
7. Refer to social service counseling because of unwillingness to involve infant's father, financial needs, and outcome for infant.
8. Communicate with NICU personnel regarding infant's status: homegoing, foster care, or adoption.

Evaluation

1. Did Cathy understand and agree to follow through on self-care activities?
2. Did she seek information to prepare herself for the new infant?
3. Has communication with family members improved?
4. Has beginning attachment started?
5. Were resources found in support network or through referrals?

ATTACHMENT AND BONDING

Background of Bonding Theory

As early as 1952, scientists wrote about imprinting behavior in birds and other animals and described a critical period during which attachments between the mother and her young must be formed. Separation during this critical time resulted in rejection of the young. Researchers observed that human mothers who are separated for long periods of time from premature or sick infants often have difficulty in accepting them when the emergency is over; this observation led researchers to wonder whether there was a time for attachment in humans.

Klaus and Kennell (1976) hypothesized that a special period of sensitivity may exist after birth. If this opportunity is missed, the mother-infant pair never bonds. They later revised this statement, though, because attachment is a slow process that occurs over time and short periods of separation do **not** negatively affect attachment behaviors. For example, an infant in the NICU with respiratory problems who has not been initially held by the mother will not be prevented from later attachment behaviors.

Other theorists have hypothesized that maternal-fetal **bonding** begins early in pregnancy and is viewed as a developmental accomplishment (Cranley, 1981; Deutsch, 1945; Gay, 1981; Lo Biondo-Wood, 1985; Rubin, 1977). Knowledge of pregnancy provides the primary stimulus for a connection between the parent and fetus. Increasing fetal movements validate the fetus as a separate entity from the mother and enhance attachment behaviors. There are several attachment scales to use if questions arise (Gay, 1981), and it should be noted that fathers attach to the fetus in a similar way (Figure 8-7).

Changes in maternity care now encourage extended contact between parents and infants. If an infant is high risk or ill and separated from its parents in the ICU, the parents may be anxious about bonding. The nurse can be helpful by assuring them that although the early recovery period is the ideal time for attachment to take place, it is not the only time. The mother who began attachment with visualization early in pregnancy is unlikely to be seriously hindered if initial interaction with her newborn must be deferred. Hormonal stimulation may contribute to the attachment, but social and cultural components play a far more influential role.

Encouraging Attachment during Pregnancy

Around the fourth month of pregnancy the expectant mother becomes increasingly aware of her fetus as a separate individual through movement (see the section on developmental tasks during pregnancy found earlier in this chapter) and begins to develop feelings for it. Before this time, her feelings for it consisted of an abstract notion of what "a baby" is like. From the time of quickening onward, she becomes acquainted with her infant by identifying fetal parts and by noting its response to changes in its environment, such as when she is anxious or taking a warm shower or is listening to loud or soothing music. The more she becomes familiar with her infant's responses to her actions, the more she feels she "knows" the infant before birth. The fact that a mother can form an attachment to her unborn fetus is indicated by her grief if her infant is stillborn.

The nurse can encourage prenatal attachment as she performs her usual care-giving tasks. Ask the woman what she calls her infant; it can be the name that will be put on the birth certificate or an affectionate nickname such as "the lump" or "Thumper." This name helps her to personalize the infant within. Help her to examine behaviors to identify who the infant is "like" in her or her partner's family. When

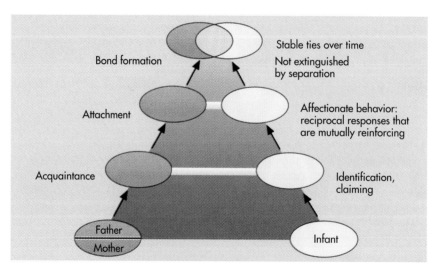

Figure 8-7 Model of the bonding process.

the woman complains that the infant is always moving, ask, "Who in your family is like that?" Encourage her to pay attention to fetal activity and to note what behavior on her part seems to influence the infant to move or kick.

An ability to identify fetal parts can be encouraged by guiding the pregnant mother's hands to identify the hard, round head; the long, curved back; the softness of the rump; the fleeting movements; and a surprisingly large number of prods from heels, toes, knees, shoulders, elbows, and hands. She can be urged to soothe and quiet her infant by massaging, stroking, or rocking.

A Doppler that amplifies fetal heart tones can also be used during prenatal visits to help parents identify the infant's various sounds: the hoofbeat rhythm of the fetal heart tones; the slower, more measured rate of the mother's heartbeat; the swooshing sound as the blood rushes through the umbilical cord; and the gurgling of the mother's intestines. Time spent in this way gives the parents a feeling of increased knowledge and reduced uncertainty.

A sonogram can also be used as an aid for discussion on attachment. Women report that they feel that the infant is real for the first time when they see its features in the sonogram. Encourage parents to request a copy of their infant's "picture." Although women who are concerned for the infant's survival often fear becoming attached to the infant (the tentative pregnancy), those women who have experienced threatened miscarriage or similar problems often express positive feelings for their infants after viewing the sonogram.

By the end of the third trimester a strong attachment should have been formed for the infant (Rubin, 1984). If the mother demonstrates obvious negative behaviors

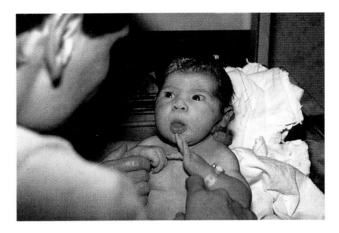

Figure 8-8   Fingertip exploration and eye-to-eye contact are initial responses just after birth. (Courtesy Ross Laboratories, Columbus, Ohio.)

during later pregnancy, closely observe postdelivery interactions. Phases of bonding occur throughout pregnancy and parenting, including the phase of **acquaintance**, with cues of acceptance being exchanged, and the phase of **attachment**, with affection exchanged when parents and the infant are in close contact. Note in Figure 8-8 the eye-to-eye contact and tentative exploration that begin acquaintance. Nursing interventions during prenatal care can be very supportive of the young family. (Strengthening the attachment after the birth of the infant is discussed in Chapter 20.) Keep in mind that bonding will occur in all family-infant groupings, and it is most often a positive, loving relationship that will be able to endure over time and distance.

Key points

- Major developmental tasks of pregnancy follow a step-by-step progression. Any lag will delay the next phase.
- Adjustment to pregnancy proceeds through phases: the mother comes to acceptance of the infant, sees it as separate from herself, and prepares for separation and birth.
- Women seek maternal role models and men seek paternal role models to help them imagine how they will respond as parents. This task is more difficult when there are dysfunctional families or difficult life circumstances.
- Parental adjustments in role responsibility and in self-concept take emotional energy. Expectant parents need support while the psychologic tasks of pregnancy are being achieved. Single mothers may often feel isolated.
- Family networks provide most women with support, but young, single, or older women may need additional support.

- Pregnancy modifies sexual responses. Anticipatory guidance may help the woman to understand and explain these changes to her partner.
- During pregnancy young women and men need to cope with role confusion, with gaining a sense of identity and positive self-esteem, and with understanding what the pregnancy means to them.
- When teaching the sexually active teenager, focus must be placed on the knowledge and use of family planning.
- If the teenage parents are supported and allowed to continue schooling, the outlook for them is positive.
- Bonding occurs throughout pregnancy and parenting. The process goes through phases and is reinforced by nurses who understand the importance of the parent-infant bond.

Study Questions

8-1. Select the terms that apply to the following statements:

  a. The idea that being pregnant becomes part of ones lifestyle and plans is _____.

  b. Thoughts about the "fantasy" child's characteristics and how it will feel to be a parent is _____.

  c. A positive emotional connection that persists over time and distance is _____.

  d. The woman's recognition that the fetus is separate from herself is _____.

  e. The situation in which the father has more physical discomforts during his partner's pregnancy is _____.

  f. The woman's feeling of comfort and competence as a new mother is _____.

8-2. Identify the trimester in which the feelings listed below are most likely to be present.

  a. Decreased sexual desire because of physical discomfort such as nausea and vomiting

  b. Bad dreams about harm to self or fetus

  c. Feelings of inadequacy that she is unable to give enough to the fetus to make it though the pregnancy

  d. Strong need to prepare the "nest" for the new infant

8-3. Anticipatory guidance is usually not effective during pregancy for which of the following events?

  a. Acceptance or incorporation

  b. Giving to and enduring the fetus

  c. Imaging the fetus

  d. Fetal separation or letting go

8-4. Pregnancy in the later reproductive years is becoming more commonplace. The older woman's chances of carrying the pregnancy to term and giving birth to a healthy baby are:

  a. Not the same as younger women because of chronic disease older women carry.

  b. Poorer because the risk of Down syndrome increases to about 1% by the time a woman is 36.

  c. Not significantly different from that of younger women in the same health category.

  d. Better, since older women know how to better care for themselves.

8-5. The best time to teach expectant mothers about parenting is:

  a. During the first trimester because there is enough time to explore all the issues.

  b. During the second trimester because the mother is beginning to realize that the infant is a separate individual.

  c. During the third trimester because the imminent birth gives a feeling of immediacy and a need to get organized.

8-6. The expectant mother's attachment to her infant occurs by:

  a. Visualizing herself as a mother.

  b. Getting to know the infant by identifying its behaviors.

  c. Learning all she can about fetal development.

  d. Trial and error.

Answer Key

8-1: *a*, Acceptance; *b*, visualization; *c*, bonding; *d*, individuation; *e*, couvade; *f*, maternal attainment. 8-2: *a*, First; *b*, second; *c*, second; *d*, third. 8-3: b. 8-4: c. 8-5: c. 8-6: b.

References

*Antle-May K: Three phases of father involvement in pregnancy, *Nurs Res* 31:337, 1982.

Blake R: The pregnancy-related dreams of pregnant women, *J Am Board of Fam Pract* 6:117, 1993.

Bluestein D, Starling ME: Helping pregnant teenagers, *West J Med* 161:140, 1994.

Burk ME et al: Cultural beliefs and health behaviors of pregnant Mexican-American women: implications for primary care, *Adv Nurs Sci* 17:37, 1995.

Burnhill MS: Adolescent pregnancy rates in the US, *Contemp Pediatr* 11:43, 1994.

Calister LC: Cultural meaning of childbirth, *J Obstet Gynecol Neonatal Nurs* 24:327, 1995.

*Classic reference.

Censullo M: Strategy for promoting greater responsiveness in adolescent parent/infant relationships: report of a pilot study, *J Pediatr Nurs* 9:326, 1994.

*Cranley M: Development of a tool for the measurement of maternal attachment during pregnancy, *Nurs Res* 30(5):281, 1981.

Curry M: Validity and reliability testing of the prenatal psychosocial profile, *Res Nurs Health* 17:127, 1994.

*Deutsch H: *Motherhood: psychology of women*, vol 2, New York, 1945, Grune & Stratton.

Donovan J: The process of analysis during a grounded theory study of men during their partners' pregnancies, *J Adv Nurs* 21:708, 1995.

Edge V, Laros RK Jr: Pregnancy outcome in nulliparous woman aged 35 or older, *Am J Obstet Gynecol* 168:2882, l993.

*Erikson E: *Childhood and society*, New York, 1963, W W Norton & Co.

Flanagan P et al: Adolescent development and transition to motherhood, *American Academy of Pediatrics* 6:273, 1995.

Fleming BW et al: Assessing and promoting positive parenting in adolescent mothers, *MCN Am J Matern Child Nurs* 18:32, l993.

*Furstenberg F: The social consequences of teenage parenthood. In *Adolescent pregnancy and childbearing: findings from research,* Pub No 81-2077, Washington, DC, 1980, National Institute of health, Department of Health and Human Services.

*Gay J: A conceptual framework of bonding, *J Obstet Gynecol Neonatal Nurs* 10(6):440, 1981.

Guttmacher Institute: *Facts in brief: teenage sexual and reproductive behavior in the United States,* New York, 1991, Alan Guttmacher Institute.

Hatcher R et al: *Contraceptive technology 1994-1996,* New York, 1994, Irvington.

Hutchinson M.K, Bagi-Azia M: Nursing care of the childbearing muslim family, *J Obstet Gynecol Neonatal* 23:767, 1994.

Imle M: Third trimester concerns of expectant parents in transition to parenthood, *Holistic Nurs Pract* 4(3):25, 1990.

Johnson PA: Teen pregnancy prevention: an afrocentric developmental framework, *Assoc Black Nurs Faculty Journal* 6:11, 1995.

Jordan P: Laboring for relevance: expectant and new fatherhood, *Nurs Res* 39:11, 1990.

*Katz-Rothman B: *The tentative pregnancy,* New York, 1986, Viking Penguin.

*Klaus MH, Kennell JH: *Maternal-infant bonding,* St. Louis, 1976, Mosby.

*Kleinman A, Eisenbergh-Good B: Culture, illness and care: clinical lessons from anthropological and cross-cultural research, *Ann Intern Med* 88:251, 1979.

Klerman LV: Adolescent pregnancy and parenting controversies of the past and lessons for the future, *J Adolesc Health* 14:553, 1993.

Kochenour NK: Normal pregnancy and prenatal care. In *Danforth's obstetrics and gynecology,* ed 7, Philadelphia, 1994, Lippincott.

*Lederman RP: *Psychosocial adaptation in pregnancy,* Englewood Cliffs, NJ, 1984, Prentice Hall.

Lee SH, Grubbs LM: Pregnant teenagers reasons for seeking or delaying prenatal care, *Clin Nurs Res* 4:38, 1995.

*Lo Biondo-Wood G: *The progressions of physical symptoms in pregnancy and the development of maternal-fetal attachment,* unpublished doctoral dissertation, New York, 1985, New York University.

*Longobucco DC, Preston MS: Relation of somatic symptoms to degree of paternal role preparation, *J Obstet Gynecol Neonatal Nurs* 18(6):482, 1989.

Marsiglio W: Adolescent males' orientation toward paternity and contraception, *Fam Plan Perspect* 25:22, 1993.

Mason C: Is there a physiological basis for the couvade and onset of paternal care? *Int J Nurs Stud* 32:137, 1995.

Mattson S: Cultural sensitive perinatal care for Southeast Asians *J Obstet Gynecol Neonatal Nurs* 24:335, 1995.

May J: Fathers: the forgotten parent, *Pediatr Nurs* 22(3):243, 1996.

*Mercer, R: The process of maternal role attainment over the first year, *Nurs Res* 34:198, 1985.

Miller MA: Culture, spirtuality, and women's health, *J Obstet Gynecol Neonatal Nurs* 24:257, 1995.

Morgan C, Chapar GN, Fisher M: Psychosocial variables associated with teenage pregnancy, *Adolescence* 30:277, 1995.

Nichols MR: Paternal perspectives of the childbirth experience, *Matern Child Nurs J* 21(3):99, 1993.

*Reamy KE, White SE: Sexuality in pregnancy and the puerperium: a review, *Obstet Gynecol Surv* 40:1, 1985.

Reece SM: Social support and the early maternal experience of primiparas over 35, *Matern Child Nurs J* 21(3):91, 1993.

Richardson P: Body experience differences in preterm labor, *Matern Child Nurs J* 24(1):5, 1996.

Roye CF, Balk E: Evaluation of an intergenerational program for pregnant and parenting adolescents. *Matern Child Nurs J* 24(1):32, 1996.

*Rubin R: Binding-in in the postpartum period, *Matern Child Nurs J* 6(2):67, 1977.

*Rubin R: *Maternal identity and the maternal experience,* New York, 1984, Springer.

Scholl T et al: Prenatal care and maternal health during adolescent pregnancy: a review and meta-analysis, *J Adolesc Health* 15:444, 1994.

Spector R: *Cultural diversity in health and illness,* Norwalk, Conn, 1996, Appleton & Lange.

Stainton MC, McNeil D, Harvey S: Maternal tasks of uncertain motherhood, *Matern Child Nurs J* 20(3-4):113, 1992.

Starn J, Niederhauser V: An MCN model for nursing diagnosis to focus nursing intervention, *MCN Am J Mat Child Nurs* 15(3):180, 1990.

Statistical Bulletin: Recent trends in teenage childbearing in the United States, Oct-Dec, 1994.

Steinberg L: *Adolescence,* New York, 1993, McGraw-Hill.

Stevens-Simon C, Lowy R: Teenage childbearing: an adaptive strategy for socioeconomically disadvantaged or a strategy for adapting to socioeconomic disadvantage? *Arch Pediatr and Adolesc Med* 149:912, 1995.

*Tanner LM: Developmental tasks of pregnancy. In Bergeson BS, ed: *Current concepts of clinical nursing,* St Louis, 1969, Mosby.

US Bureau of the Census: *Statistical Abstract of the United States 1993,* ed 113, Washington, DC, 1993.

Wayland J, Tate S: Maternal-fetal attachment and perceived relationships with important others in adolescents, *Birth* 20:198, l993.

Zabielski MT: Recognition of maternal identity in preterm and fullterm mothers. *Matern Child Nurs J* 22(1):2, 1994.

*Zabin L, Kantner J, Zelnick M: The risk of adolescent pregnancy in the first months of intercourse, *Fam Plann Perspect* 11:215, 1979.

Zachariah R: Mother-daughter and husband-wife attachment as predictors of psychological well-being during pregnancy, *Clin Nurs Res* 3:371, 1994.

 ## *Student Resource Shelf*

Nance TA: Intercultural communication: finding common ground, *J Obstet Gynecol Neonatal Nurs* 24:249, 1995.
Looks at the relationship of culture to communication.

Leonhardt-Lupa M: *A mother is born,* Westport, Conn, l994, Bergin & Garvey.
A woman's experiences during pregnancy are woven in with information on pregnancy. Focuses in on the woman's inner thoughts and feelings.

O'Brien B et al: Variables related to nausea and vomiting during pregnancy, *Birth* 22:93, 1995.
Looks at relationship of nausea and vomiting to selected variables such as maternal age, occupation, parity, cigarette smoking and infant gender.

Pipher M: *Reviving Ophelia,* New York, Ballantine Books, 1994.
Explores the many aspects of adolescent girls in our society today.

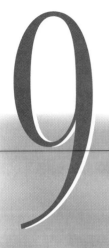

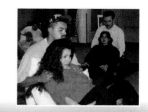

9

The Pregnancy Process & Nursing Care

Learning Objectives

- Explain the relationship of maternal physiologic adaptations to pregnancy and common, minor discomforts of the antepartum.
- Identify significant health history information to be elicited through prenatal interviews, assessments, and screening.
- Correlate appropriate anticipatory guidance by pregnancy trimesters.
- Recognize methods of encouraging self-care for pregnant clients.
- Individualize a nursing care plan for prenatal care, including cultural adaptations.
- Identify referral needs according to a pregnant woman's physical and emotional adjustment.

Key Terms

Anticipatory Guidance
Asymptomatic
  Bacteriuria
Carpal Tunnel
  Syndrome
Changes of
  Accommodation
Colostrum
Coombs' Test
Diabetogenic Response
Due Date (DD)
Erythema
Estimated Date of Birth
  (EDB)
Estimated Date of
  Childbirth (EDC)
Gravidity
Heartburn
Hematocrit
Isoimmunization
Kegel Exercises
Ketosis
Last Menstrual Period
  (LMP)

Leopold's Maneuvers
Leukorrhea
Lightening
Linea Nigra
Lordosis
Mean Arterial Pressure
  (MAP)
Melasma
Mucous Plug
Nägele's Rule
Nocturia
Orthostatic
  Hypotension
Parity
Pruritus
Ptyalism
Relaxin
Striae Gravidarum
Supine Hypotension
  Syndrome (SHS)
Syncope
Vena Caval Syndrome
  (VCS)

$\mathscr{P}$regnancy triggers a complex chain of events. Energy is required to fuel the rapidly dividing fetal cells on their journey of growth and development. At the same time, hormones send messages throughout the body, directing the organ systems in the **changes of accommodation** during pregnancy.

CARDIOVASCULAR SYSTEM

Blood volume expansion is one of the earliest and most basic of changes in pregnancy. An increase of 30% to 50% provides enough blood for circulation to all the developing organs and body parts. To accommodate the expansion, there is vasodilation or relaxation of smooth vascular tissue. This vasodilation is thought to be partly caused by increased amounts of *prostacyclin* (PGI₂), a prostaglandin that is produced in the placental tissue. Soon after conception, the intravascular space expands, allowing greater blood volume. The average increase of 45% may occur as early as 6 weeks after conception (Blackburn and Loper, l992), although it generally rises slowly to reach a peak at 30 to 34 weeks (Table 9-1).

Hematocrit

Most of the increased volume (1200-1600 ml) is plasma, with approximately 250 to 450 ml composed of red blood cells (RBCs). Because of this imbalance the **hematocrit** (ratio of RBCs to plasma) will decrease. This is *hemodilution* of pregnancy and appears to resemble a mild anemia. The ratio decreases from a normal level of 37 to 45 ml in every 100 ml(%) to a ratio of 34% to 42% (Figure 9-1). The RBC count may fall from a prepregnancy count of 4.0 to 5.5 million/mm³ to 3.75 to 4.5 million/mm³ (written on laboratory reports as 3.75⁶, adding six places to the right of the decimal point, which takes its place with a comma—3,750,000). Hemoglobin levels may also drop slightly because of the demand for extra iron. Hemoglobin levels below 10.5 g/dl are considered to indicate true anemia in the second and third trimesters.

Coagulation Factors

The usual equilibrium in the coagulation-fibrinolysis pattern is changed during pregnancy. Plasma fibrinogen increases steadily until the time of birth while activators of plasminogen are reduced (Gilbert and Harmon, 1993).

There is an increase in platelets, fibrin, and other coagulation factors, especially factors VII, VIII, IX, and X, to assist in healing after the birth. However, this hypercoagulability makes the client more susceptible to thrombus development during pregnancy and the *puerperium*, the postbirth period.

White Blood Cells

The normal white blood cell (WBC) count begins to rise during the second month to approximately 10,000 mm³, and by late pregnancy and labor it can reach levels of

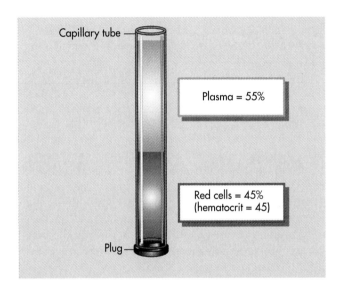

Figure 9-1   After centrifuge, the hematocrit is the volume of red blood cells per 100 ml of whole blood (expressed as a percentage).

Table **9-1**   **Laboratory Values for Cardiovascular System during Pregnancy**

Determination	Value*
Blood volume	+30%-50% (+1500-2000 ml)
Red blood cell (RBC) mass	+30% (250 to 450+), 375⁶ − 4.5⁶/mm³
Hematocrit (Hct)	34%-42% (no less than 32% in second trimester)
Hemoglobin (Hb)	11.0-14 g/dl (no less than 10.5 g in second or third trimester)
White blood cells (WBCs)	5000-16,000/mm³
Heart rate (HR)	+15-20 beats/min
Cardiac output (CO)	+30%-53% (to 6 L/min)
First-stage labor	+60%
Second-stage labor	+80%
Blood pressure (BP): second trimester	90/60-128/79 mm Hg (−5-10 systolic, −10-15 mm Hg diastolic)
Mean arterial pressure (MAP): second trimester	
Adult	<90 mm Hg
Adolescent	<80 mm Hg

*Values will be higher for a multiple pregnancy.

16,000 or more. This count is within normal limits for pregnancy and recovery. An increase in the granulocytes, particularly neutrophils (which are polymorphonuclear [PMN] cells), causes this increase. Neutrophils, which normally constitute more than half of the WBC profile, increase in response to inflammation, pain, anxiety, stress, and labor and delivery. These cells protect against invading organisms, engulfing them through phagocytosis and débride the decidual tissues of dead cells during the healing process.

TEST *Yourself* 9-1

In the prenatal clinic, what additional information should you obtain if a woman's laboratory report at 18 weeks shows the following values: RBC count 3.9⁶/mm³, Hb 11.5 g/dl, and Hct 30%?

Cardiac Output

The heart makes several adaptations to accommodate these changes. Viewed during radiographic examination, the heart is more prominent because of its increased work load; this is temporary cardiac hypertrophy. The *heart rate* (HR) increases by 15 to 20 beats/min (30%); the *cardiac output* (CO), the amount of blood pumped from the heart in 1 minute, increases by 30% to 40% early in the pregnancy, and then slowly increases to 53% more at the time of birth (Sibai and Frangieh, 1995).

CO is determined by multiplying the stroke volume by the HR in 1 minute. The stroke volume, which also slowly increases (+18%), added to the HR changes yields the increased CO. (See Chapter 22 for cardiovascular alterations that result in problems during pregnancy.)

Blood Pressure

In spite of the increase in blood volume and increased intracapillary pressure, *blood pressure* (BP) in the first 24 weeks of pregnancy usually *decreases* 5 to 10 mm Hg systolic and 10 to 15 mm Hg diastolic, producing a widening of the *pulse pressure*. These changes result from (1) relaxation of the vascular smooth muscle layer and (2) formation of new peripheral vascular beds in the breasts, uterus, and placenta. However, by the time labor begins, when influenced by the enlarging uterus and increased venous pressure in the lower extremities, BP levels usually rise to *stabilize at nonpregnancy levels.* Thus when evaluating the significance of the BP, the nurse takes into account the earliest BP reading, which becomes the baseline reading, notes the week of pregnancy, and compares the baseline with the current reading.

Because of vascular changes, during auscultation of the BP, the diastolic sound may be heard as a change in sound and then at a lower reading, the disappearance of sound

may occur at levels as low as 30 or 40 mm Hg or even at 0 mm Hg. *Both* diastolic readings should be recorded (Sabai and Frangieh, 1995).

Mean arterial pressure

To follow the significance of the BP, the **mean arterial pressure** (MAP) is useful. It is computed by the following formula, which uses the systolic (S) and diastolic (D) readings:

$$\text{MAP} = D + \frac{(S-D)}{3} \quad \text{(pulse pressure)}$$

Figure 9-2 shows the Finipres cuff attached to a finger and to the BP monitor with a MAP readout of 103. This is obtained by adding the diastolic, 93, to ⅓ of the difference between the systolic and diastolic numbers, which here is 10, therefore 93 + 10 = 103.

In the second trimester a mean arterial pressure (MAP-2) of more than 90 mm Hg after 24 weeks or a rising MAP of more than 20 points above baseline can be interpreted as a warning of hypertension (Ferris, 1994). A BP elevation of 30 points systolic and 15 points diastolic above prepregnant baseline may also warn of hypertension. These figures are general guidelines; remember that BP readings must be measured against a woman's baseline.

Accuracy of readings can be ensured by consistent measurement on the same arm or finger and, during labor, always *between* contractions. Readings are also influenced by maternal factors such as anxiety, pain, and drug use.

Vena caval compression

The vena cava is less rigid than the aorta, and the enlarging uterus may compress the inferior vena cava, impeding venous return. CO is diminished, the pulse rises, and BP falls. *Vena caval compression* occurs within 30 seconds of a woman lying supine after the fourteenth week of pregnancy (Sabai and Frangieh, 1995). The symptoms are dizziness, light-headedness, nausea, pallor, clamminess of skin, and even **syncope**, or fainting. The **vena caval syndrome** (VCS) or **supine hypotension syndrome** (SHS) occurs more often as the uterus becomes larger and heavier and is aggravated during labor (Figure 9-3). Treatment consists of changing the maternal position from supine to left side-lying or less effectively, placing a wedge under the right hip to maintain a lateral tilt, and explaining to the woman the reason to avoid the supine position.

Femoral venous pressure

An increase in femoral venous pressure is also related to the weight of the uterus. Venous return from the femoral veins is affected by the enlarged uterus and by increased blood volume. Femoral venous pressure rises in the legs from a normal level of below 10 mm Hg to as much as 18 mm Hg. This contributes to a feeling of fullness in the legs

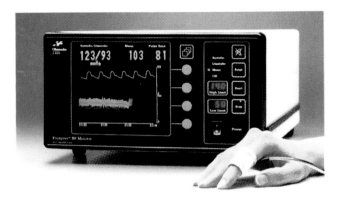

Figure 9-2   New techniques of blood pressure monitoring save time for the nurse. Note that the mean arterial pressure (here, 103) is obtained with each reading on the Finipres cuff. (Courtesy Ohmeda Corp., Englewood, Colo.)

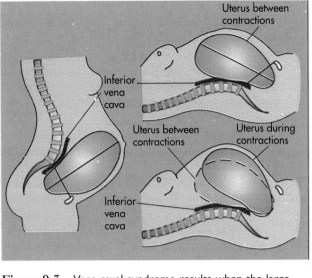

Figure 9-3   Vena caval syndrome results when the large uterus presses on the vena cava as it lies beside the spine. Side-lying position relieves pressure, and blood pressure returns to normal.

and to *dependent edema,* which is more noticeable in the evening or after standing or sitting for a long time.

Positional change to facilitate venous return helps reduce this *gravity-based edema.* The side-lying position during sleep and rest provides maximal kidney blood flow and function. Lower extremity edema that persists is a warning signal that should be reported to the physician.

Varicose veins

Varicose veins may appear early in the second trimester and worsen as pregnancy progresses. Varicose veins of the saphenous system and of the vulva and rectum (hemorrhoids) are affected primarily by the rising venous pressure in the lower extremities. Varicosities are usually more common and pronounced in the multigravida but may occur for the first time in a young primigravida with a family history of varicose veins. In addition to being unsightly, these enlarged superficial veins may be painful and throbbing, especially those in the vulva and rectal-anal area. Walking and positional change to facilitate venous return is helpful. A woman with a tendency toward varicosities should wear support hose during pregnancy to give support and counterpressure to the walls of the distended veins. For other interventions see Chapter 22.

Orthostatic hypotension

A decrease in the CO caused by the interference of venous return can result from the effects of **orthostatic hypotension,** which occurs when a woman moves from a recumbent to a standing position. Normal, uncomplicated pregnancies can usually withstand this stress without harm

to the fetus. However, it might cause problems in pregnancies with borderline placental function. Pregnant women are advised to sit on the side of the bed briefly before rising to their feet.

TEST *Yourself* 9-2

When you teach self-care, how do you explain the physiologic changes underlying the following?
a. Dependent edema
b. Orthostatic hypotension
c. Varicose veins

RESPIRATORY SYSTEM

Changes in the respiratory system result from the increased need for oxygen intake and carbon dioxide (CO_2) discharge. The need for increased oxygen consumption of 20% to 30% during pregnancy results from cardiac work, renal performance, respiratory performance, and breast, uterine, and placental demands.

Progesterone lowers the CO_2 threshold in the respiratory center, increasing sensitivity to CO_2. This hormone also decreases pulmonary resistance, thereby promoting increased alveolar function, allowing the chest wall to expand laterally and the diaphragm to become more mobile. The result is a 30% to 40% increase in tidal volume. Although these events increase the depth of respiration, the rate remains stable, but the lungs have a greater capacity to exchange gases.

Blood Gases

To facilitate CO_2 transfer from the fetus, the pregnant woman is in a state of compensated respiratory alkalosis with a lowered carbon dioxide pressure (PCO_2) and an elevated oxygen pressure (PO_2) (Blackburn and Loper, 1992). Gases are in solution because of their partial pressures. Gas transport and exchange moves from higher to lower concentrations referred to as the *gradient*.

Maternal PO_2 increases to a partial pressure of 100 to 108 mm Hg during pregnancy, from a normal level of 80 to 100 mm Hg. At that level, 100% of maternal hemoglobin is oxygen-saturated, thereby readily allowing maternal RBCs to release oxygen to the fetus. Fetal PO_2 levels are much lower at 25 to 35 mm Hg. Fetal hemoglobin (HbF) has an extremely high affinity for oxygen, and in this way the *maternal-fetal oxygen gradient* promotes fetal uptake.

To promote elimination of fetal waste CO_2, the maternal $PaCO_2$ values decrease from a normal level of 35 to 45 mm Hg to approximately 27 to 32 mm Hg during pregnancy. To maintain a mild alkalosis, the concentrations of sodium bicarbonate ($NaHCO_3$) also become lower in pregnancy, averaging 16 to 20 mEq/L. The maternal pH remains stable at approximately 7.40 to 7.42 because bicarbonate is efficiently eliminated from the kidneys (Table 9-2).

Dyspnea

Approximately 60% to 70% of pregnant women suffer from mild dyspnea, probably related to hyperventilation during pregnancy. The onset is early and becomes more marked as the pregnancy progresses, provoking anxiety. In addition, by the eighth or ninth month, the enlarged uterus crowds the diaphragm sometimes by as much as 4 cm. The discomfort may be temporarily alleviated by a change in position to allow freer excursion of the diaphragm. Some women must sleep in a semi-Fowler's position. Later, discomfort is relieved by **lightening**, or the descent of the presenting part of the fetus as the body prepares for delivery (see Figure 9-10).

Airway hyperemia

Nasopharyngeal congestion occurs as intracapillary pressure rises. Secretions increase, and there is edema, tissue fragility, and sometimes nosebleeds. Because of increased edema in the upper airway, care must be taken to prevent damage or bleeding if any manipulation of the passage is necessary, such as with intubation or suctioning at the time of delivery. A few women complain of chronic nasal stuffiness and may have a hoarse voice. The pitch of the voice may change. These women feel as if they always have a cold. A humidifier may help this discomfort. The symptoms recede without treatment in the postbirth period. Women should be cautioned not to take over-the-counter antihistamines without a recommendation from the physician or midwife.

Table 9-2	Laboratory Values for Respiratory System during Pregnancy

Determination	Value
PaO_2	104-108 mm Hg
$PaCO_2$	27-32 mm Hg
pH	7.40-7.42
Sodium bicarbonate ($NaHCO_3$)	16-20 mEq/L

ENDOCRINE SYSTEM AND METABOLISM

Thyroid Function

In the first trimester the thyroid gland increases in size and is readily palpable. This results in a normal increase in thyroid hormone (triiodothyronine [T_3] and thyroxine [T_4]) synthesis to support gestational growth. In spite of this increase the hypothalamic-pituitary-thyroidal relationship remains stable.

Normal pregnancy mimics a mild *hyperthyroid* state; the basal metabolic rate (BMR), heat intolerance, and emotional lability increase. The BMR increases gradually during pregnancy to 25% above normal. The thyroid hormones function to increase the production of intracellular proteins and energy, which in turn increases the rate of consumption of carbohydrates, fats, and oxygen and results in increased heat production. Because of increased heat production and expanded vascular supply, many women complain of being warm and flushed. This change is normal and subsides after childbirth.

Adrenals

The adrenal glands produce increased amounts of glucocorticoids during pregnancy. Free plasma cortisol levels rise to 2.5 times higher at full term than what they were before pregnancy. Cortisol mobilizes glucose and free fatty acids improving carbohydrate metabolism and influencing insulin production. The adrenals produce increased amounts of renin and angiotensin, which have the effect of counteracting vasodilation. Finally, aldosterone levels are increased to affect sodium reabsorbtion and blood volume (Blackburn and Loper, 1992).

Pancreas

The insulin-producing cells of the pancreas increase in size and number during pregnancy. Because of this an accelerated starvation effect will be produced by maternal fasting. During fasting, the woman's blood glucose levels can drop 15 to 20 mg/dl below nonpregnancy levels because of the steady fetal drain on the maternal supply. The fasting levels of insulin also are lower, resulting in the potential for **ketosis**, the build up of ketones in the body caused by inadequate metabolism of carbohydrates. Ketosis must always be avoided because ketone bodies have been implicated in fetal brain damage.

Alternately, maternal intake of a large meal produces an extreme opposite response. Blood sugar levels rise sharply, as do insulin and triglycerides, and there is decreased tissue sensitivity to the action of insulin. This **diabetogenic response**, or insulin antagonism, is heightened by the action of human placental lactogen (hPL) and, to a lesser extent, is related to the higher levels of estrogen, progesterone, and free cortisols. This is one reason for encouraging six small meals a day in place of three large meals.

Although maternal insulin does not cross the placenta, the fetus relies on facilitated diffusion of maternal glucose for energy needs. If maternal hyperglycemia is present, fetal levels are elevated. (See Chapter 24 for detrimental effects of hyperglycemia on the fetus.)

Parathyroid

Activity of the parathyroid glands decreases gradually during pregnancy. With less parathyroid hormone (PTH) released, the body still is able to absorb more calcium from the gastrointestinal (GI) tract because the placenta produces a similar hormone, *PTH-related peptide* (Sibai and Frangieh, 1995).

Pituitary

Because the menstrual cycle has been interrupted, the anterior pituitary gland ceases its release of follicle-stimulating hormone (FSH) and luteinizing hormone (LH). After birth, prolactin or luteotropic hormone (LTH) will be secreted in response to nipple stimulation and breast-feeding. The posterior pituitary secretes small amounts of *oxytocin* late in pregnancy, which is involved with stimulation of uterine contractions. After delivery, nipple stimulation with breast-feeding triggers release of oxytocin (1) to contract uterine muscles and thus prevent bleeding, (2) to release prolactin, and (3) to contract the ducts, which causes the *let-down reflex* whereby milk is ejected as the infant sucks on the nipple.

Renal

Pregnancy requires a salt-conserving state for the first few months to increase the blood volume (to as much as 8 liters of fluid) (Sibai and Frangieh, 1995). There are increased levels of aldosterone and increased renin activity to counterbalance a tendency to lose sodium. At the same time, the kidneys increase in size and weight to enable greater filtration volume and reabsorption. With these changes, no real increase in volume of output occurs in spite of the 50% increase in flow through the kidneys. The pelves, calyces, and ureters are dilated in response to hormonal stimuli and the physical presence of a more filtered load. In addition, the ureters may loop, which is often more evident on the right side.

Hemodynamic changes

Hemodynamic changes include increases in the *glomerular filtration rate* (GFR), *renal plasma flow* (RPF), excretion of amino acids, and elimination of water-soluble vitamins. Early in pregnancy, glucose and creatinine may be more readily excreted, and there is better reabsorption of sodium, chloride, and water. A trace of *glycosuria* and *proteinuria* may develop; any greater amounts should be investigated because these factors could signal other disorders.

Positional changes affect kidney function. In a similar way to vena caval compression, the uterus presses on renal veins and arteries, reducing effective flow. Best function is produced during rest in a side-lying position (see Figure 24-5).

Frequency of urination

Some common urinary complaints during pregnancy arise from physiologic adaptations. *Urinary frequency* usually occurs in the first and third trimesters. In the first trimester the enlarging uterus presses or impinges on the bladder, stimulating the sensation of needing to void even though the bladder is not full. During the second trimester the uterus rises out of the pelvic cavity and into the abdominal cavity, alleviating pressure on the bladder. Later, during the third trimester when *lightening*, or descent of the presenting part, occurs, the enlarged uterus will again compress the bladder.

Nocturia

The horizontal position for sleep promotes renal flow, with the result that more urine is produced during rest and sleep (**nocturia**). This has a positive benefit in reducing lower extremity edema but may become a problem because of interrupted sleep. The woman can plan to avoid fluid intake after the evening meal to help reduce the number of times she must void during the night.

Urinary tract infections

Although only a small number of women are affected by urinary tract infection with symptoms, many more women may have **asymptomatic bacteriuria**, that is, a count of >100,000 bacteria/mm³ in the urine, without symptoms of an infection. The changes of pregnancy promote growth of bacteria because of obstruction of free flow of urine by the pressure of the uterus on the ureters and decreased muscle tone. The bladder may contain residual urine, and the ureters loop and dilate allowing stasis of urine, and a medium for bacterial growth. (See Chapter 24 for interventions for more severe urinary tract infections.) Nursing interventions include teaching the woman to consume adequate amounts of fluid each day and to report signs and symptoms of urinary tract infections: dysuria, pain, blood in urine, and urgency. Because there may be a strong link with preterm labor, some physicians treat bacteriuria with antibiotics. (See Chapter 21.)

TEST *Yourself* 9-3 _____

Why might any of the following changes in the renal system lead to significant health problems?
a. A dilated and looped right ureter
b. A trace of glucose in the urine
c. Nocturia that leads to voiding twice during the night

GASTROINTESTINAL SYSTEM

Pregnancy causes many changes in the GI system resulting in common discomforts. Hormones of pregnancy affect the whole system, and the growing fetus causes crowding of the surrounding organs. Nursing interventions for GI discomforts are discussed in Chapter 10.

Mouth

Several changes occur in the mouth. The gums become more vascular and are more likely to bleed when the woman brushes her teeth or even eats crunchy foods. Gingivitis has been noted in 55% to 70% of pregnant women. In 2% of pregnant women, *epulis*, or small growths at the juncture of two teeth, may aggravate bleeding from the gums. These recede after birth but may need the attention of a dentist and removal during pregnancy.

General dental care is important, but there is no evidence that dental caries are more common at this time. The production of saliva is unchanged or only slightly more acidic during pregnancy. When nausea occurs, a woman may not swallow saliva as frequently and perceive that there is more. For some women however, **ptyalism**, an increased secretion of saliva, may cause serious discomfort. These women usually experience extreme symptoms of nausea as well (Van Dinter, 1991).

Esophagus and Stomach

The lower esophageal sphincter (LES) has reduced muscle tone that becomes more marked as pregnancy progresses. The enlarging uterus presses upon the stomach, and there may be gastric reflux causing **heartburn**.

Changes within the stomach are the result of smooth muscle relaxation, which decreases motility. Gastric emp-

tying time is slowed. The normal amounts of gastric secretions are somewhat lower in the first and second trimesters but increase dramatically in the third. Throughout gestation, however, mucous production increases, which produces a soothing, protective effect on the gastric lining (Blackburn and Loper, 1992). The mucosa needs this effect because delayed emptying time means that irritating gastric juices remain in the stomach longer. Acid indigestion may include burping and an acidic taste in the mouth.

Nausea and Vomiting

Nausea and vomiting related to early pregnancy affects 50% to 80% of women. The problem begins close to the sixth week of pregnancy and continues until the fourteenth week. The incidence of nausea parallels the curve of human chorionic gonadotropin (hCG) and the increase in steroidal hormones (Figure 9-4). The state of pregnancy increases olfactory acuity, and smells often trigger nausea. Even common odors such as freshly brewed or old coffee, breath and body odors of others, perfumes, room fresheners, cigarettes, soiled diapers, and gasoline fumes may trigger nausea (Erick, 1995).

Approximately two thirds of women with nausea complain only about *morning sickness;* another third have symptoms persisting all day. In some cases, the nausea is severe enough to prevent adequate nutrition and results in weight loss, hypokalemia, and ketosis. A condition of *hyperemesis gravidarum* (HG), or pernicious vomiting of pregnancy, will require hospitalization (see Chapter 10).

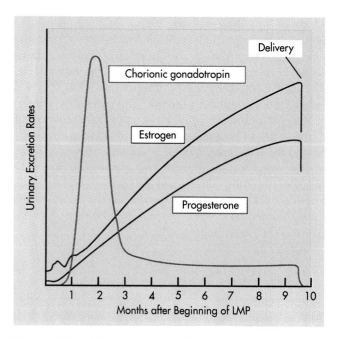

Figure 9-4   Urinary excretion of estrogen, progesterone, and hCG during pregnancy. (From Vander AJ, Sherman JH, Luciano D: *Human physiology,* New York, 1970, McGraw-Hill.)

Intestinal Tract

Motility is reduced in the small bowel. Although absorption of many nutrients is unchanged, the absorption of iron, calcium, glucose, sodium, and certain other substances is increased. Delayed transit in the colon causes increased water absorption and a reduced volume of stool. Flatulence may become a problem and constipation is a common complaint.

Hepatic

The size of the liver and blood flow to it are unchanged during pregnancy. Normal function is altered; serum albumin levels fall gradually. Liver enzymes serum alkaline phosphatase, leukocyte alkaline phosphate, and serum cholesterol levels rise by the end of pregnancy. Serum concentrations of many proteins are also elevated.

Gallbladder

Tone and motility of the gallbladder decrease during pregnancy, leading to various degrees of stasis. The result may be formation of gallstones and a decreased ability to handle cholesterol. If there is a tendency to retain bile salts, itching may be a symptom.

INTEGUMENTARY SYSTEM

Vascular Changes

As a result of higher estrogen levels, there may be superficial vascular changes related to increased blood flow. *Spider angioma,* commonly seen in light-skinned women, consists of tiny vessel networks that appear mainly on the face, chest, and arms. Women may notice **erythema**, or redness of the palms and soles of the feet. In addition, because of increased peripheral circulation, women who may have been intolerant of cold weather are more comfortable. Others feel too warm and flushed.

Striae gravidarum, commonly called stretch marks, appear as pink or purple lines on the breasts, lower abdomen, or thighs. In time, these become brown or silvery but never completely disappear. Striae occur in approximately 90% of white women and less commonly in Asians and blacks. Striae occur in women who are genetically predisposed to these changes, and appearance may be related to increased glucocorticoids, occurring regardless of the amount of weight gained. Recently, topical tretinoin has been reported to be of some aid (Chanco-Turner, 1994).

Pigmentation

The actions of hormones during pregnancy spur increased pigmentation, especially on the nipples and areolae, umbilicus, and genitalia. New scars and pigmented nevi (moles) may darken. On the lower portion of the abdomen, a line between the symphysis pubis and the umbilicus, the *linea alba,* will darken, to become the **linea nigra**. A blotchy, irregular hyperpigmentation of the forehead, cheeks, nose, and upper lip, commonly called the "mask of pregnancy," or **melasma**, occurs more frequently in women with darker complexions (see Figure 22-8). This condition, which formerly was called *chloasma,* fades after delivery, but in some women it never completely disappears.

Glandular Changes

During pregnancy under the influence of estrogen, hair remains in the *anagen,* or growth, phase. After the birth, many of these follicles enter the *telogen,* or resting, phase, and hair is shed in sometimes alarming amounts. Women welcome an explanation and reassurance that most of the shed hair will grow back within a year (Chanco-Turner, 1994).

Sweating and the excretion of sebum increase during pregnancy, requiring more frequent cleansing for comfort. Oily skin and sometimes acne may recur in women with a history of this problem. Other women with normally dry skin appear to have well-lubricated skin during pregnancy. In contrast, some women complain of **pruritus** (itching) relating to dry skin. If it persists, the women should be evaluated for liver function or gallstones.

Itching

Cholestasis of pregnancy results in constant itching, appearing in the third trimester. There may be slight jaundice, and delivery of the infant is the best cure. *Pruritic urticarial papules and plaques of pregnancy* (PUPPP) is another dermatologic condition that may affect a primigravida in her third trimester. The condition is thought to occur in 1 in 200 pregnancies. The rash usually starts as eruptions in the stretch marks (striae) and spreads across the abdomen and buttocks to the arms and legs. The rash resembles poison ivy rash, according to one affected mother. Women affected by this pruritic rash tend to have excessive weight gain. Treatment for both conditions consists of oatmeal baths, topical ointment, and antihistamines, usually diphenhydramine (Benadryl). According to Chanco-Turner (1994), the eruptions usually clear within a few days of delivery. Blackburn and Loper (1992) report spontaneous clearing within 3 weeks after birth.

NEUROMUSCULAR SYSTEM

As pregnancy progresses, the skeleton makes several adjustments to accommodate the growing uterus and to prepare for delivery. To facilitate vaginal delivery, progesterone and the hormone **relaxin** loosen the cartilage and connective tissues all over the body and especially from the symphysis pubis and sacroiliac joints. Such changes can lead to pelvic and back discomfort, particularly in late pregnancy. In addition, there also may be *diastasis* of the rectus abdominis muscle, a central separation of the muscle.

Progressive **lordosis** (abnormal increased degree of forward curvature of the spine) develops to keep the center of gravity over the woman's legs, related to the tilting forward of the pelvis and the heavy weight of the uterus. Although this measure allows her to maintain an upright posture, the abnormal curvature contributes to backache. As a result of these adjustments, the pregnant woman acquires a characteristic carriage and *gait*. Toward the last few weeks she may assume a "waddling" gait.

Leg Cramps and Restless Legs

Muscle cramping is a common complaint for approximately 25% of women. It occurs later in pregnancy and often at night. The gastrocnemius, thigh, and gluteal muscles may be affected. The cause may be related to a change in electrolytes, to an imbalance in calcium and phosphorus, or to uterine pressure on the nerves leading to the legs. Calcium and magnesium levels are checked. Although there is no real evidence that these are effective, women may be treated with calcium lactate or vitamin B complex or are asked to change their milk intake, but no standard intervention exists. Increasing sodium intake has helped some cases (Enkin et al, 1995). For home care, she may stretch the muscle by sitting up and pulling hard on her toes or by standing at the bedside and, with her foot flat, flexing the foot to stretch the calf muscle.

Restless legs may be experienced by approximately 15% of pregnant women. Differing from cramps, the sensation is a creeping, burning ache that develops approximately 20 minutes after lying down. The urge to move the legs back and forth is irresistible (Rosenbaum, Donaldson, 1994). Walking may relieve symptoms, and correcting low folic acid and iron levels has been of some help.

Carpal Tunnel Syndrome

Carpal tunnel syndrome may flare up during pregnancy. The radial side of the hand may be numb or painful. Because of the changes in the neuromuscular system, the median nerve is compressed in the fibrous tunnel through which it passes. Wrist supports are useful, and surgical treatment to moderate the condition is not done until after childbirth because it may disappear spontaneously.

Backache, Neuralgia, and Round Ligament Pain

Strain on weak abdominal muscles and lower back muscles and increased weight of the uterus may cause back-

ache. A few women have a serious problem with backaches or with pain radiating along the nerve to the leg. Sacroiliac joint strain is common, with tenderness over the posterior aspect of the joint (Beischer and MacKay, 1993). Separation of the symphysis pubis is uncommon but distressing. The woman has pain while walking, and the pubic joint is tender. This problem may appear at the time of childbirth, and a client who reports severe pain during ambulation should be examined for symphysis separation. Remember, pain during pregnancy is always a sign of a problem.

Round ligament pain results from tension on the round ligament as it stretches to accommodate the enlarging uterus. Pain is sensed as a grabbing, intense pressure in the groin area. For some women, this pain becomes a major discomfort. Andrews et al (1994) studied the effect of the pelvic (hip) tilt exercise (Figure 9-5), used four times a day and when pain occurred, and found it to be an effective intervention for this particular discomfort.

Exercise to strengthen the lower back and abdominal muscles is basic to improved status. Warmth to the affected area and physical therapy may be advised. Women should be advised to wear low-heel, comfortable shoes, and to strengthen lower back muscles with exercise. Proper body alignment for standing, stooping, and lifting (Figure 9-6) and for walking upstairs (Figure 9-7) is important. Squatting instead of stooping is beneficial; yet women who are unaccustomed to squatting may fall.

To balance and compensate for the weight at the front of the body, the woman moves to the edge of the chair and leans forward until the weight of her body is over the feet.

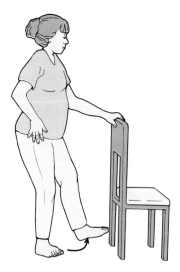

Figure 9-5   Pelvic (hip) tilt exercise. While supporting body with one hand placed on back of chair, lift leg straight only 1.5 to 2 inches off floor, keeping shoulders and bottom of foot parallel to floor. Hold for 6 seconds. Lower leg, and repeat 10 times. Repeat with other leg.

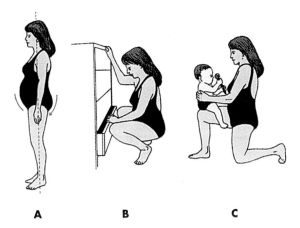

Figure 9-6   Correct posture during pregnancy. **A,** Standing. **B,** Stooping. **C,** Lifting.

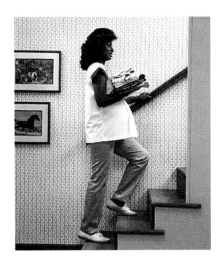

Figure 9-7   Posture while walking upstairs or carrying loads is important to discuss during prenatal teaching. (Courtesy Ross Laboratories, Columbus, Ohio.)

To arise from a bed, she should move to the edge of the bed while lying on her side. She pushes up with her dependent elbow and opposite hand to a sitting position and waits for dizziness to pass before standing upright. (See "Orthostatic Hypotension" discussed earlier.)

Exercise

Wallace (1986) compared exercising women with nonexercising women and found that women who exercised had significantly higher self-esteem and lower ratings for physical discomforts than did the nonexercising group. In most communities, classes are available through fitness centers and childbirth educators. Home videotapes help women who do not attend these sessions. Women who work at jobs away from home or with small children at home feel active but may need to add certain groups of exercises to tone muscles.

Maternal physiologic responses

Exercise physiology is a new field that explores the effects of exercise on pregnancy and the fetus. Current guidelines are based on extensive studies of women who choose to engage in work and fitness programs. The major response is redistribution of blood flow to the skin and muscles by means of vasoconstriction in the vital organs. Because of the increased oxygen consumption and cardiac workload there also is concern about the effects on the fetus of the maternal metabolic demands and the temperature elevation produced during a workout.

Oxygen uptake is increased to meet the demands of the heart and muscles. There is an increase in respiratory rate, metabolic rate, tidal volume, HR, CO, and body temperature. If exercise is prolonged and strenuous, the oxygen supply may be exceeded, leading from an aerobic (with oxygen) to an anaerobic (without oxygen) state. If the latter occurs, metabolic acidosis arises, which may compromise the fetus. Stress also may be placed on joints already loosened by hormonal influence.

Fetal responses to maternal exercise

Fetal responses to maternal exercise can be transitory or long-term. FHR and breathing movements increase with moderate exercise. The fetus is approximately 1° C warmer than the mother and has only a few ways to dissipate heat. Regular strenuous exercise, particularly in the first trimester, could raise the core body temperature sufficiently to manifest the teratogenic effects of heat on the growing embryo. For this reason, moderation is advised (Sternfeld, 1995).

Another concern for the fetus is the adequacy of uteroplacental blood flow. Studies of working mothers and those who have engaged in active fitness programs have shown that birth weights are consistently somewhat lower (Speroff, 1996). Most physicians advise limiting activity for women diagnosed with known uteroplacental deficiency problems such as hypertension or intrauterine growth retardation. In addition, women who engage in strenuous activity should be monitored for signs of compromise before continuing regular exercise throughout the pregnancy (Hatch et al, l993).

Basic exercises

The nurse shares the guidelines of exercise with each client and inquires about her exercise, posture, and fatigue level at each clinic visit. In addition, conditioning exercises for childbirth preparation should be encouraged (see Chapter 12). Basic exercises to strengthen the abdominal muscles and lower back are curl-ups or partial sit-ups and the pelvic tilt. The woman should be taught **Kegel exercises** in preparation for birth and recovery (Pearce, 1994). To perform Kegel exercises, the woman should sit in a

---

Box 9-1   Guidelines for Exercise during Pregnancy

- Maternal HR in general should not exceed 140 beats/min. (Or, pulse greater than 70% of 200 minus the woman's age.) Do not get out of breath while exercising.
- Strenuous activities should not exceed 15 minutes in duration. Always warm up and taper down after exercise.
- No exercise should be performed in the supine position after the fourth month of gestation.
- Exercises that use the Valsalva maneuver (holding breath and pushing) should be avoided.
- Caloric and fluid intake should be adequate to meet not only the extra needs of pregnancy but also of the exercise performed. Avoid hypoglycemia.
- Maternal core temperature should not exceed 38° C (100.4° F). Dissipate heat by light clothing, fluids, environmental controls.

From American College of Obstetricians and Gynecologists: *Exercise during pregnancy and the postnatal period,* 1994, Washington, DC.
Speroff L: Exercise. In Queenan JT, Hobbins JC: *Protocols for high-risk pregnancies,* ed 3, Cambridge, Mass, 1996, Blackwell.

---

chair or lie on her side and alternately tighten and then relax the muscles of the pelvic diaphragm and perineum for 6 seconds at a time.

Guidelines for exercise during pregnancy are listed in Box 9-1. Before a pregnant woman begins a new exercise program or considers a strenuous new activity, risks and benefits must be discussed. For example, the supine position for exercise must be avoided after the fourth month. High-impact aerobics and aggressive contact sports should be questioned. Low-impact aerobics are safer for the pregnant woman and provide equal benefit. Because of use of all the large muscles of the body, swimming is a recommended activity during pregnancy (Figure 9-8). Activities in which atmospheric and oxygen pressure changes occur, such as scuba diving, should be avoided.

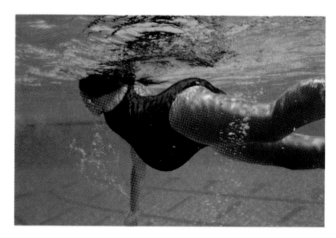

Figure 9-8   Swimming is a recommended exercise during pregnancy. (Courtesy Ross Laboratories, Columbus, Ohio.)

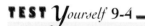

TEST *Yourself* 9-4 —

Jane is accustomed to doing an aerobic workout three times a week. She asks about precautions during the second trimester. What would you tell her? Give rationale.

REPRODUCTIVE SYSTEM

Hormones

Estrogen

Estrogen is secreted by the ovary at the beginning of pregnancy and then by the placental cells. Estrogenic effects on most of the body systems have been discussed in Chapter 3. Acting alone or in conjunction with other hormones, estrogen stimulates the following groups of actions:

- Alters vaginal tissue: more acidic pH and increased glucose levels contribute to increased infections
- Increases uterine size and weight
- Breasts: develops mammary duct in preparation for breastfeeding and changes in nipple consistency and color

- Various skin changes include darker coloration of melana-influenced cells, accelerated hair and nail growth
- Renal system: changes in reabsorbtion-excretion rates
- Increases blood flow to all tissues, stimulated by estrogen

Progesterone

The hormone that maintains the pregnancy is named for its action—progestation. Progesterone inhibits uterine motility increasing potential for implantation and allowing the uterus to contain the fetus. It maintains the decidual lining, relaxes smooth muscle throughout the body, and contributes to vascular changes. The following categories of effects are seen:

- Cardiovascular system: relaxes vessels to allow for blood volume expansion
- Respiratory system: decreases pulmonary resistance
- Renal system: relaxes structures to allow for higher volume

- Liver: decreases levels of serum albumin and increases levels of serum phosphatase and cholesterol
- Pancreas: increases insulin production, which contributes to diabetogenic effects
- GI system: reduces motility

Human chorionic gonadotropin

Human chorionic gonadotropin (hCG) is secreted by the trophoblastic layer of the blastocyst to maintain the corpus luteum until the placental tissue can produce adequate estrogen and progesterone. hCG has been implicated in the cause of morning sickness; nausea of pregnancy closely follows the curve of hCG in the first trimester (see Figure 9-4). hCG levels in urine or serum provide the basis for pregnancy tests. The hormone also may be called *urinary chorionic gonadotropin* (UCG).

Relaxin

Relaxin is secreted during pregnancy, first by the corpus luteum and then by the placenta. It appears to work in conjunction with progesterone, quieting uterine muscle activity and preventing loss of the conceptus. It may contribute to the fatigue and tiredness experienced early in pregnancy. Later in pregnancy it affects the connective tissue, especially in the sacroiliac and symphysis pubis in preparation for labor. Softening of the cervix is also partially attributed to relaxin.

Human placental lactogen

When hPL was first isolated from the placenta, its similarity to both human growth hormone (hGH) and prolactin was noted. Because its effect on the mammary gland is greater than its effect on growth, it is called *hPL*. Later, because it also possesses somatotropic and lactogenic properties, the name *human chorionic somatomammotropin* (hCS) was proposed. Both names are still used.

hPL prepares the body for lactation by stimulating the development of the breast for milk production. Many other possible effects are attributed to this hormone; it may assist hCG in prolonging the life and activity of the corpus luteum. Blackburn and Loper (1992) list other influences of hPL, including enhancement of carbohydrate metabolism, promotion of fat storage, increase of free circulating fatty acids, and stimulation of erythropoiesis (erythrocyte production) and aldosterone secretion.

Prolactin

Prolactin (PRL) is secreted by the chorionic layer of the placenta and the pituitary gland. Its major influence is indicated by its name, pro-lactin (for lactation). The hormone is also known as lactogenic hormone and luteotropic hormone (LTH).

Prolactin affects breast growth, osmoregulation, reproductive activity, integumentary action, synergism with steroids, and lactogenesis. Medications, exercise, and anesthesia can influence its release. Serum levels rise from 30 ng/ml in the first trimester to a high of 200 ng/ml at term. Amniotic fluid contains 5 to 10 times more prolactin than does maternal serum.

Uterus

To accommodate the growing fetus the smooth muscles of the uterus enlarge, stretching to at least eight times their prepregnant size. The once pear-shaped organ enlarges first to a globular shape and then to an ovoid or egg shape weighing more than 1000 g. The total increase in size depends on fetal size, the shape of the placenta, and the volume of amniotic fluid. Most of the increase is in the fundal portion and is due not to an increase in the number of cells but rather to cell size. This hypertrophy contributes to the remarkable changes just after the birth.

Uterine growth follows a pattern, and measurement of the height of the uterine fundus gives clues to deviations that may indicate a problem with pregnancy. By week 12 the uterus is palpable at the symphysis pubis; by weeks 20 to 24 the fundus should reach the umbilicus; by week 36 it should be at the xyphoid process (Figure 9-9). Within 2 weeks of birth, as the fetus settles into position for birth, the uterus shifts position and moves into a more forward angle, relieving pressure on the diaphragm. This final shift in position is known as lightening for the sense of relief that is experienced. Figure 9-10 illustrates the positions of the uterus during pregnancy.

The myometrium is thick and firm and becomes progressively stretched and thinner in the second half of gestation. Toward the end of pregnancy, it is thin enough to allow the fetal head and extremities to be palpated easily.

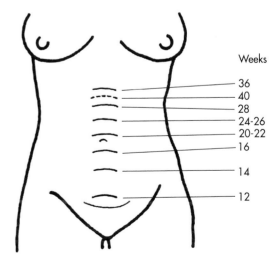

Weeks

- 36
- 40
- 28
- 24-26
- 20-22
- 16
- 14
- 12

Figure 9-9 Expected changes in height of uterine fundus in relation to weeks of gestation.

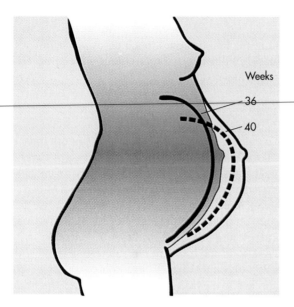

Figure 9-10   Changes in uterine position as lightening occurs. Lordosis may become a discomfort of pregnancy.

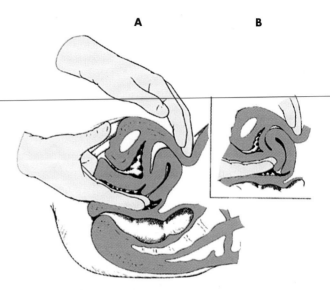

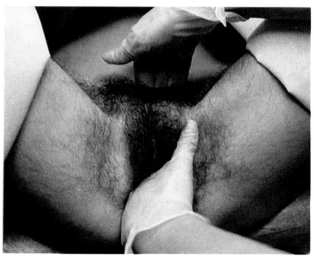

Figure 9-11   Bimanual examination. **A,** Palpation of cervix to determine size, shape, consistency, and its relation to axis of vagina. **B,** Palpation of uterus for size, shape, consistency, mobility, and tenderness; its anterior position is best determined when corpus can be "grasped" between fingers of two hands. **C,** Position of gloved hands for vaginal examination.
(*C,* From Seidel HM et al, eds: *Mosby's guide to physical examination,* ed 3, St Louis, 1995, Mosby.)

The isthmus or juncture between the body of the uterus and the cervix is softened by hormonal influence. By bimanual examination, the isthmus can be compressed to almost paper thinness, a condition called Hegar's sign. Another early sign of pregnancy is *Ladin's sign,* a softening of a spot on the anterior portion just above the uterocervical juncture (Figure 9-11, *B*).

Cervix

The nonpregnant cervix has the firmness and feel of the tip of a nose. Because of expanded blood circulation and hormonal activity, it becomes increasingly soft. The softening is called *Goodell's sign,* one of the early indications of pregnancy. The cervical *os,* or channel into the uterus, is lined with mucous-secreting glands that enlarge to secrete a thick, tenacious mucus that effectively closes the os for the duration of pregnancy. This seal, the **mucous plug,** prevents ascending infection from contaminating the fetus. In the few weeks before birth, the cervix becomes gradually softened, or it ripens. Toward the beginning of labor, it gradually shortens (*effaces*) and begins to open (*dilates*). As the uterus begins the work of labor to open and thin the cervix, the mucous plug (called "show") is expelled from the cervical canal. The show is one of the first indications that effective labor has begun. Because small capillaries in the cervix may be broken, blood mixes with the mucus and hence the term *bloody show.*

Vagina

During pregnancy the vaginal rugae enlarge and become more elastic in preparation for the passage of the fetus and placenta. Because of hormones, especially estrogen, there is increased sloughing of cells from the cervical and vaginal walls, causing increased amounts of vaginal mucus or **leukorrhea.** Leukorrhea may be thin and milky or thick and sticky but should not cause itching or irritation to tissues unless infection, such as *Trichomonas vaginalis* or *Candida albicans,* is present (see Chapter 4). The pH changes from a low of 4 to 5 to a less acidic pH of 5 to 6. This change, with increased glycogen content in cells, may foster growth of organisms in the vagina. Circulation to the vaginal and cervical tissues increases, and the vaginal mucosa and cervix take on a bluish-purple hue; this change is *Chadwick's sign* and can be seen by the eighth week of pregnancy.

Breast

For many women, one of the first signs of pregnancy is a fullness or tingling of the breasts similar to the fullness and tingling experienced during the premenstrual period. During pregnancy, however, the fullness can cause discomfort. Blood vessels in the breast enlarge and become prominent, showing visible, blue, twisting patterns. There is enlargement and mobility of the nipple and darkening and enlargement of the tubercles of Montgomery (see Figure 3-7).

Colostrum, a fluid full of nutrients and antibodies, is secreted in small amounts as early as the second trimester. Most authors do not recommend breast preparation or expression of colostrum during pregnancy. Research studies to assess the value of preparation for breast-feeding have not shown any significant difference through use of Massé cream, massage, or expression of colostrum (Enkin et al, 1995).

Breast stimulation during later pregnancy is not recommended because nipple stimulation triggers the release of oxytocin from the posterior pituitary. Oxytocin is a factor in the initiation of labor.

SIGNS AND SYMPTOMS OF PREGNANCY

Because early symptoms may be confusing, several weeks may pass before a woman suspects she is pregnant. Although fatigue and breast changes often are the earliest symptoms, amenorrhea or a scanty, brief menstrual flow signal to most women a possible pregnancy. Other women report nausea or taste and olfactory changes and frequency as early clues.

Possible Signs and Symptoms

Possible signs are those that indicate a growing embryo but might also occur with another condition. In the past the term *presumptive* referred to signs *most likely* to indicate pregnancy; this distinction no longer is necessary. If pregnancy is suspected, it may be verified by a urine test for the presence of hCG or by ultrasound examination. Table 9-3 summarizes signs and symptoms of pregnancy by trimester.

Subjective signs

Tender breasts. This occurs because of increased blood supply. Many women experience breast tenderness or tingling as one of the first symptoms (Box 9-2). Tender breasts also occur during the menstrual cycle.

Nausea. This is experienced by approximately 50% of pregnant women. It is easy to identify and often occurs on

---

■ *Box* **9-2**   **Signs and Symptoms of Pregnancy**

> **POSSIBLE SIGNS AND SYMPTOMS**
>
> **Subjective Signs**
> Breast tingling
> Nausea
> Frequency of urination
> Fatigue
> Increased abdominal girth
> Quickening
>
> **Objective Signs**
> Breast enlargement
> Amenorrhea
> Changes in uterus and cervix
> Vaginal hyperemia
> Positive pregnancy tests
>
> **Positive signs**
> Ultrasonic visualization of moving embryo or fetus and
>   fetal heart movements
> Auscultation of fetal heartbeat
> Fetal parts or movement palpated by examiner

awakening. With onset at approximately the sixth week, nausea usually lasts until the fourteenth week.

Frequency of urination. This occurs during the first trimester because of compression of the bladder by the enlarging uterus. With no other signs of infection, frequency usually indicates pregnancy.

Abdominal enlargement. This does not become evident until the second trimester. By the sixteenth week a woman will find it difficult to wear her normal waistband size. The rise of the uterus into the abdominal cavity is gradual and reaches the symphysis pubis by the twelfth week. From that time the height of the fundus becomes a guide to the progress of fetal growth. Measurements are changed by obesity, multiple pregnancy, and a smaller or larger than average amount of amniotic fluid.

Quickening. This occurs by the sixteenth to eighteenth week and certainly by the midpoint of pregnancy. A woman will feel the infant move. "Feeling life" is a significant point in pregnancy for many women. Even the woman who is anxiously waiting for the signs may mistake it for flatulence because fetal movement is so slight at the beginning.

Objective signs

Breast enlargement. Enlargement, under the influence of hormones and with increased vascular supply, begins soon after the woman becomes pregnant. By term the breasts may have doubled in size. Superficial veins become more prominent. Nipples and areolae darken and become more prominent. By 14 weeks, colostrum, the precursor of breast milk, is produced.

Table 9-3 **Subjective and Objective Signs during Pregnancy**

Subjective Signs	Objective Signs
FIRST TRIMESTER	
Weeks 1-4	
Fatigue, thought to be due to relaxin	Amenorrhea, but possible spotting at time of
Nausea, peaking 60 to 100 days after conception	expected period
Soreness, tingling of breasts	Elevated hCG levels
	Elevated BBT because of progesterone secretion
Weeks 5-8	
Enlarging uterus causing pressure on bladder and frequency of urination	Breast enlargement, darkening of areolas, enlarged Montgomery's tubercles
Possible decrease in desire for sexual relations	Signs (weeks 5-7):
	Ladin's sign
	Goodell's sign
	Hegar's sign
	Chadwick's sign
	Positive pregnancy test for hCG using isoimmunologic methods
Weeks 9-13	
Nausea subsiding by 13 weeks	Weight gain of 0-3 lb but also possible weight loss
Frequency of urination subsiding by 12 weeks	Fundus at the symphysis pubis, rising approximately 1 cm/wk thereafter
	Detection of fetal pulse by ultrasonic techniques (9-12 weeks)
SECOND TRIMESTER	
Weeks 14-20	
Breast fullness	Colostrum present
Headaches	Mucous plug formation in cervical canal
Light-headedness, postural hypotension begins by 14 weeks	Leukorrhea; report if pruritus or foul order develops: *Candida albicans,* trichomonal infections
	Abdominal appearance of pregnancy
	Height of fundus between symphysis and umbilicus
Weeks 20-24	
Quickening	Fundus at umbilicus (22 weeks)
Often increased sexual desire	Pelvic joints relaxing because of hormone relaxin
	Possible pigment changes in skin: melasma, linea nigra, striae gravidarum
	Increased perspiration, oily secretions
	Dilation of right ureter as a result of pressure from dextrorotated uterus
Weeks 25-28	
Leg cramps may occur	Constipation and hemorrhoids because of slowed peristalsis and pressure of uterus on lower colon and rectum
Fatigue	

BBT, Basal body temperature; *BP,* blood pressure; *hCG,* human chorionic gonadotropin.

Table 9-3	**Subjective and Objective Signs during Pregnancy—cont'd**
Subjective Signs	**Objective Signs**
THIRD TRIMESTER	
Weeks 29-33	
Fatigue Anxiety about future Bad dreams Decrease in sexual desire because of physical discomfort	Heartburn caused by pressure of uterus on stomach, causing mild hiatus hernia and regurgitation of stomach acid into esophagus BP returning to prepregnancy level Braxton Hicks contractions may begin Fundus midway between umbilicus and xiphoid
Weeks 34-38	
Backache, change in gait Impatience for end of pregnancy Mood swings because of ambivalence about future	Increase in shortness of breath and other pressure symptoms (heartburn, feeling of fullness after eating, constipation, varicose veins, dependent edema, hemorrhoids)
Just before labor	
Lightening Aching in lower abdomen	Fundus just below diaphragm until lightening, then appears to tip forward

Amenorrhea. This is a sign that may be caused by other factors such as stress, anemia, illness, and approaching premenopause. Also, some women may not have amenorrhea but have spotting during the early weeks of pregnancy, particularly at the time of implantation or expected menstrual period.

Uterine and cervical changes. These occur as a result of hormonal activity and increased blood supply to these tissues. Hegar's sign, Goodell's sign, and Ladin's sign may be determined. Today, with the use of ultrasound, these tests are used less frequently to assess pregnancy status.

Vaginal hyperemia. This results from increased circulation in the pelvic area that causes the tissues to take on a bluish-purple hue (Chadwick's sign).

Pregnancy tests. Tests based on isoimmunologic reactions are in common use. Because testing kits available over-the-counter (OTC) provide a 85% accuracy rate, these results are listed as "possible." A fresh urine sample is tested together with hCG-coated particles and antiserum. As early as 15 to 20 days after conception, if enough hCG is present in the urine, the particles will not agglutinate. The later the test is performed, the more accurate it will be, with positive results reflecting higher levels of hCG. Monoclonal antibody tests are more accurate but more costly.

Positive signs and symptoms

Visualization. Visualization of the fetus by ultrasonic examination will demonstrate the amniotic sac, fetal parts, and HR movements. It is also used to confirm the expected date of childbirth (see Chapter 11).

Auscultation. Auscultation of a faint fetal heartbeat may be noted at 9 weeks with a Doppler scan (see Figure 11-2). Auscultation with a stethoscope must wait until 18 or 20 weeks.

Palpation of the fetal outline. This is done by the use of **Leopold's maneuvers** (Figure 9-12), which allows the examiner to feel for parts of the fetus, including the head, knees, and back. By week 20 an observer may also see fetal movements by watching the surface of the abdomen when the fetus is active.

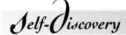

Self-Discovery

Have you been pregnant? Think back to early signs and symptoms or interview a friend about these signs. Which were anxiety producing; which were reassuring? ～

DETERMINING FETAL MATURITY

Classic Definitions of Fetal Maturity

The preterm or premature infant is born after week 20 and before the end of week 37. The term or mature infant has developed for 38 to 41 weeks. The postterm or postmature infant's gestational age is more than 42 weeks. Once the infant is born, physical assessment will be done to confirm the gestational age (see Chapter 18).

The *previable period* extends to week 20; if the pregnancy ends before week 20 the fetal product is termed an abortion, whether termination is by induction or occurs

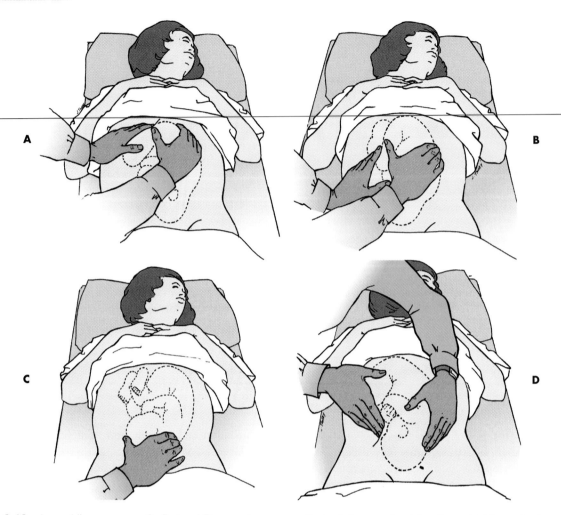

Figure 9-12   Leopold's maneuvers. **A,** *First and,* **B,** *second maneuvers:* Both of the examiner's hands are laid flat and relaxed on the abdomen to assess the contour of the uterus, the lie of the fetus, and the level of the fundus. With the tips of the fingers, the examiner then assesses which part of the fetus occupies the uterine fundus. Then by using the palm, the examiner feels for the back and extremities. **C,** *Third maneuver:* The fetal part above the symphysis pubis is grasped gently but firmly with the thumb and fingers of the right hand. The contour and consistency of the fetal part can then be examined and compared with the opposite part in the fundus. **D,** *Fourth maneuver:* If the presentation is cephalic, the examiner faces the mother's feet and presses with the first three fingers of each hand on the sides of the fetal head, in the direction of the pelvic inlet. (From Lowdermilk DL, Perry SE, Bobak IM: *Maternity and women's health care,* ed 6, St Louis, 1997, Mosby.)

spontaneously (see Chapter 21). To be considered *viable,* or able to live, the fetus must weigh more than 499 g and have a crown-rump (C-R) length of 16 cm or more. Because a fetus older than 20 to 24 weeks is considered potentially viable, any fetus who dies in utero after 20 weeks of gestation must be considered a *stillbirth* to be recorded in the statistics of fetal mortality (Figure 9-13). These facts reinforce the importance of determining the gestational age of the pregnancy.

Estimating Duration of Pregnancy

The duration of pregnancy has been evaluated in a number of large research studies that found with ultrasound dating

that the mean expected time of birth was between 280 to 283 days ±8 days (Mongelli and Opatola, 1995). This more precise estimation is possible by *ultrasound evaluation* of the biparietal diameter of the fetal head and of the length of the femur (see Chapter 11). Early evaluations done between 8 and 13 weeks accurately predict birth time within ±4 days. Later evaluations before 20 weeks predict birth time with a variance of ±10 days (Ott, 1994).

The full-term date of birth is indicated most commonly by the terms **estimated date of childbirth** (EDC), **estimated date of birth** (EDB), or **due date** (DD). It is difficult to be precise about the expected day of birth because (1) the exact day of fertilization rarely is known, and (2) the first half of a woman's menstrual cycle may be longer

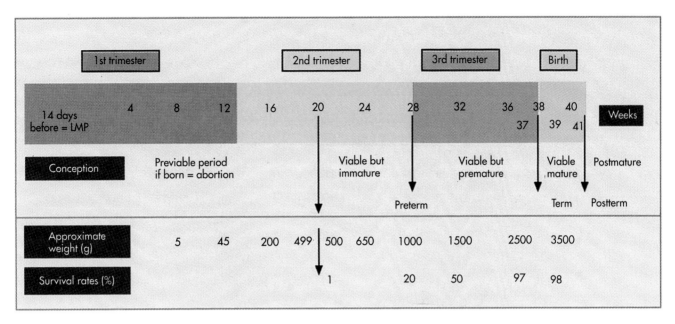

Figure 9-13   Fetal maturity and relative risk.

or shorter than 14 days. Because the **last menstrual period** (LMP) is the most easily remembered marker, calculations are done based on the first day of the LMP although there is a 2 week "error factor." To use the LMP, therefore, approximately 14 extra days must be added to the conception age. All calculations will be based on a 28-day cycle in which ovulation occurs on day 14 ± 2 days after the menstrual period begins. Because 50% of all women have a shorter or longer interval between menses, there will be variation in the actual outcome.

Several methods besides ultrasound are used to calculate the EDC. Using **Nägele's rule** (first formulated in 1812), the EDC is calculated by adding 7 days to the first day of the LMP and then subtracting 3 months from the month of the LMP. Using the LMP date of July 5 the following calculation is made:

	Day	Month (July)
LMP	5	7
	+ 7	−3
	12	4

EDC = April 12

Remember to account for the number of days in a month. For instance if a calculation resulted in the figure July 32, move forward to August 1. A newer method uses + 9 days + 9 months from LMP. This measure is the *method of nines*. Another means to determine EDC is by using the gestational age wheel (Figure 9-14).

A simple guide to the progress of pregnancy is to measure from the symphysis pubis to the top of the fundus (Figure 9-15) and to add 12 weeks to the centimeter reading on the tape. The fundus rises approximately 1 cm a week after the twelfth week. When it reaches the umbilicus, 22 to 24 weeks should have elapsed; when it reaches the xiphoid process, 36 weeks should have elapsed. Fundal height may be altered by the presence of twins, a large fetus, obesity, and the presence of less or more than expected amounts of amniotic fluid.

In any case the woman should know that the EDC by any method is approximate so she will not worry unnecessarily if labor is delayed a few days beyond her estimated date.

TEST *Yourself* 9-5

Using the LMP of May 27, calculate Amy's EDC by Nägele's rule and by the new method of nines. How much variation do you find?

Terminology of Pregnancy

Terms are used in obstetrics to refer to a woman's obstetric history (Box 9-3). **Gravidity** means that a woman has conceived or has been pregnant, regardless of the length of time she is or was pregnant; it refers only to the number of conceptions, not to the number of infants born.

Parity refers to pregnancies carried longer than 20 weeks. Thus if a woman miscarried before week 20 of gestation, it is recorded with her gravidity but not in her parity. Parity does not refer to the number of infants, just the number of times a woman has carried a pregnancy later than 20 weeks. Thus a preterm, full-term, or multiple birth each counts as one parity.

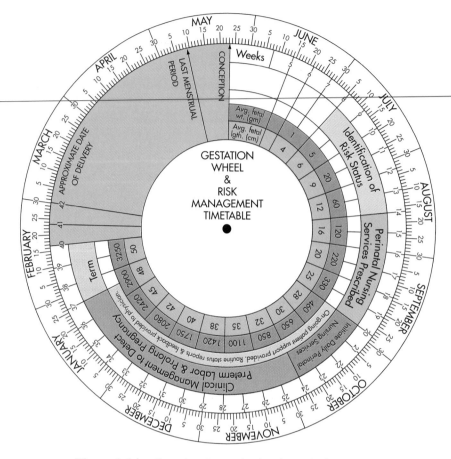

Figure 9-14 Gestational age wheel makes calculation easy.

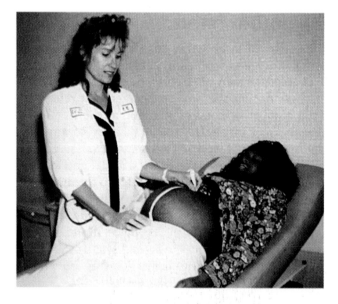

Figure 9-15 Measuring the height of the fundus. A tape measure is used to measure the distance between the symphysis pubis and the level of the uterine fundus. (Courtesy Marjorie Pyle, RNC, *Lifecircle*.)

Box 9-3 Terms Used in Obstetrics

Gravidity: The number of times a woman has been pregnant

Gravida: A pregnant woman

Primigravida: A woman pregnant for the first time (described as gravida 1, para 0)

Multigravida: A woman who has been pregnant more than once

Parity: Number of pregnancies that reached viability and were delivered; infant considered viable (whether alive or stillborn) after 20 weeks gestation

Nullipara: A woman pregnant for the first time but undelivered

Primipara: A woman who has had one delivery of a viable infant

Multipara: A woman who has had two or more deliveries of viable infants

In an effort to clarify and provide more detail in describing obstetric history, a second system was developed. In this system, parity is listed in the following four categories:

- *Full-term* (F/T) birth: 38+ weeks
- *Preterm* (P) birth: 20 to 37 completed weeks
- *Abortion* (A): Loss of pregnancy before viability (spontaneous or elective)
- *Living offspring* (L): Number of children, whether or not living with the family (covers multiple gestations). If a child has subsequently died the notation will seem inaccurate, and additional comments must be made to explain the (L) column. Occasionally a fifth column is added to detail the outcome of multiple pregnancies. Examples of transferring between systems are found in Box 9-4.

𝒩ursing 𝓡esponsibilities

Prenatal Care

The three components of prenatal care have been defined as early and continuing risk assessment, health promotion, and medical and psychosocial interventions with follow up. Thus the goal is health promotion and disease prevention (HPDP).

The concept of prenatal care is being expanded because for many people it is their only adult introduction to health screening. An opportunity to screen and educate women must be expanded to include partners and the family. A *preconception visit* is now considered advisable for counseling about nutrition and environmental hazards and screening for chronic infections or conditions that would have an adverse effect early in the pregnancy. Rubella screening can be done at this time. It also provides an early opportunity to counsel the family on the tasks of preparing for parenting.

Currently less than 80% of pregnant women in the United States obtain early prenatal care, and 6% do not seek care until the third trimester or have no care at all (Groutz and Hagay, 1995). The U.S. Public Health Service's goal for the year 2000 is that at least 90% of women begin care in the first trimester. For this goal to be achieved, there needs to be major changes in the ways women obtain care.

Many women cannot afford the cost of care or live too far from the source of care. Child care is usually not available, and there may be a long wait in the office for a short visit (Maloni et al, 1996).

Psychosocial needs may predominate, but the clinic may address mainly medical issues. Thus low income women, teenagers, immigrants, and socially marginal women may not come to the clinic for care until a problem arises. The advice given may not be useful, may be too "middle class," or may require more money than can be spared.

One of the chief challenges for nurses is to communicate appropriately with each woman who seeks care. Each pregnancy is special for the woman and her partner who bring to the pregnancy their own concepts, feelings,

---

Box **9-4**   **Comparison of Gravidity and Parity**

CASE A:
A woman is pregnant; she has had one delivery at term, and this child is living.

CASE B:
A woman is not pregnant; she has had one delivery at 38 weeks, an abortion (spontaneous), and has one living child.

CASE C:
A woman is pregnant; she has had three deliveries at term, one preterm delivery, and two abortions. She has four living children.

CASE D:
A woman is not pregnant; she has had one preterm delivery (at 33 weeks) and has two living children.

	System I		System 2 (Parity Only)			
Case	Gravidity	Parity	Term	Preterm	Abortion	Living
A	II	I	I	0	0	I
B	II	I	I	0	I	I
C	VII	IV	3	I	2	4
D	I	I	0	I	0	2 (twins)

BRIGHAM AND WOMEN'S HOSPITAL
A Teaching Affiliate of Harvard Medical School
75 Francis Street, Boston, Massachusetts 02115

Ambulatory Services
Monday — Friday 8:00 am to 4:30 pm

Phone: _____

After 4:30 pm and on weekends call
732-5987, ask for

OB _____ on call.

Site: _____   Health Care Provider: _____

LMP: _____   EDC DATES: EDC CORRECTED: _____
EDC U/S:

A

Test	Date	Result	Test	Date	Result	Test	Date	Result
Bld. tpe. & Rh			HCT			3rdΔ HCT		
Anti-bodies			HBsAg					
Serology			Urine C & S					
Rubella			Sickle Prep					
G/C			GLT					
Pap			GTT					
PPD								
AFP								
U/S Dates								
Presen-tation								
Placenta								
Fluid volume								
G.A.								
Wt.								
BPP								
Other								

Figure 9-16   A, The front of the prenatal medical record precis.

Continued.

and, with second or third pregnancies, previous positive or negative experiences. Providing an atmosphere for open communication allows the woman to explore feelings and gain knowledge about self-care and new role demands. Such an increase in knowledge will also benefit her future health care because she will learn the importance of nutrition, exercise, weight gain, and protection from hazards.

The nurse works in partnership to engage the woman in self-monitoring including reporting minor discomforts or warning signals. When women are included in decisions and carry their own medical records with them, the greater sense of control fosters self-confidence and interest in the process of pregnancy (Enkin et al, 1995) (Figure 9-16).

Assessment of cultural differences, whether the woman's practices are neutral, functional, or dysfunctional (see Chapter 2), is especially important. Nurses should also ascertain if the woman would be most comfortable seeing a woman health care practitioner and if the partner wants to participate in childbirth preparation. If the woman can see the same health care professional at each visit, she has the opportunity of developing rapport and may discuss problems, questions, and needs more openly.

The Future

Changes in the delivery of prenatal health care need to incorporate community-based care with satellite clinic

CONTACT THE HOSPITAL AT ONCE IF YOU HAVE__	**PONGASE EN CONTACTO CON EL HOSPITAL SI USED TIENE __**
1. Any vaginal bleeding 2. Persistant severe headaches. 3. Swelling of ankles, legs or face. 4. Nausea or vomiting. 5. When your labor pains come every 10 minutes. 6. If your water breaks even though you are not in labor. 7. If in doubt, phone doctor at hospital.	1. Derrame Vaginal. 2. Dolores de cabeza fuertes. 3. Hinchazon de los tobillos, piernas, o de la cara. 4. Nauseas o Vomito. 5. Cuando le den los dolores de parto cada diez minutos. 6. Si se rompe la bolsa de agua sin tener dolores de parto. 7. Si Tiene Alguna Duda Llame El Medico En El Hospital.

OB HISTORY

# Pregnancies	Illnesses Past Present
OB Problems Past Present	Current Meds Allergies

Other Delivery Needs

☐ MMR Post Partum   ☐ Booked C/S   ☐ Desires VBAC

☐ PPS Signed   ☐ PPS Post Partum   ☐ Rhogam

☐ Social Service _____

B

Figure 9-16—cont'd. B, The back of the prenatal medical record precis. The inside is a duplication of the prenatal flow sheet. (Courtesy Freida B Diamond and Antenatal Diagnostic Center, Brigham and Women's Hospital, Boston, Mass.)

settings and home visits to those who cannot travel long distances. Volunteer women can assist the newly pregnant woman to enter care. All the needed services would be in the same setting, allowing coordination of care and child care to allow the woman freedom to concentrate on instructions. A greater use of nurse-midwives and nurse clinicians would tend to promote holistic care (Enkin et al, 1995). Care after pregnancy should be in the same setting so women are comfortable and look forward to meeting with familiar people. The atmosphere of the care setting that is welcoming, and focused on the needs of the mothers and children will help ensure continuity of care and consistent follow through (Maloni et al, 1996).

ASSESSMENT

Interview

The nurse interviews the client during her first visit to the clinic or office. Because of the wide variation in ethnic groups, the nurse needs to develop considerable knowledge and cultural sensitivity to obtain useful data. If the woman's reading level is adequate, she can respond to a questionnaire to save time. Reluctance to answer some questions will be evident if the woman perceives that the information seems unnecessary to health care. Therefore to gain her cooperation, the nurse can fully explain the purpose and uses of the information.

Data gathered in the interview assist in determining the direction of the client's care. Each woman requires counseling and teaching according to her particular life circumstances without generalizing or making assumptions.

Box 9-1

CLINICAL DECISION

Marie R. comes to the clinic with a friend for her first prenatal visit. She is given a questionnaire to complete but stares at it for a long time without writing. You come back to collect the form and find it empty. What would you do next?

Family history. *Family history* includes ethnic and cultural factors and family problems that may have a genetic or social impact on the woman and her pregnancy. The nurse asks about the current status of the family's health and immunizations, especially if there are children in the home, and whether any family members have chronic illnesses that the woman might develop during her pregnancy, for example, diabetes, hypertension, and certain anemias. In this section of the interview, her birthplace, education, occupation, marital status, and support system are recorded.

Health history. A woman's *health history* includes allergies, medications regularly used, and immunizations and childhood diseases. The physician or midwife will want to know if there has been any injury or surgery in the pelvic or abdominal area. Finally, knowledge of prior health problems in any body system provides aid in screening for current health and well-being.

Reproductive history. The *reproductive history* begins with menstrual history, including onset, duration each month, and interval. If a woman has discomfort with menses or if onset began later than normal, the presence of hormonal imbalances should be considered. The nurse asks about history of prior pregnancies (GP/TPAL), experiences with prior labor and deliveries, and any complications that developed during those pregnancies. The ages and status of any children should be recorded. Her experience with contraception and whether or not this is a planned pregnancy will provide data related to acceptance of the pregnancy. Specific details are important in eliciting history of exposure to STDs.

Current status. A woman's current status includes reasons for seeking care and experience with the present pregnancy. What symptoms does she describe? How does she perceive this pregnancy? What are her expectations of health care?

Social history. Her *social history* includes habits such as customary amount of drinking or smoking and use of drugs. Often this information is asked again at the second visit because the woman may have been tense and unsure about what the interviewer needed to know during the first visit. Information may be elicited about social and family factors that may complicate adjustment during pregnancy.

Physical examination

For many healthy women, this may be the first physical examination as adults. Therefore explanations of each step will ease anxiety. The physical examination is performed by the physician or midwife during the first or second visit. If a confirming pregnancy test is needed, it is performed at the first visit, and the result is made available before the woman leaves.

Overall appearance. During the general examination, the nurse should note the following to get an overview of the whole person:
- Does the woman look happy, sad, or depressed?
- Is she clean or dirty?
- Is she overweight or underweight?
- Is there a sense of alertness or does she seem less alert?
- Does she seem tired, harassed, or upset?

The physical examination begins with the head and proceeds caudally; the pelvic examination is performed last.

Skin and hair. Skin and hair are assessed during the examination. Their condition gives clues to overall health. A skilled examiner can gain a general impression of adequate diet and self-care by observing color, turgor, and condition of the skin and quality of the hair.

Head, ears, eyes, nose, and throat. During a head, ears, eyes, nose, throat (HEENT) examination, funduscopy—examination of the fundus of the eye—may give clues to hypertensive or diabetic changes that may be observed in the blood vessels in the fundus of the eye. Indications of anemia or infection may be seen in mucous membranes of the eyes, nose, and throat. Dental caries or gum problems may be observed while examining the mouth.

Neck and chest. Neck and chest examination yields information about the thyroid gland, lymph nodes of the axillary area, and neck. The breasts are examined for asymmetry, dimpling, and retraction of the nipple or skin surface. With the client supine, the breasts are palpated for masses. Every woman should be taught about breast self-examination (see Chapter 4). If she is first seen later in pregnancy when breasts are enlarged, examination may not be valid, but teaching should take place.

Heart and lungs. The heart and lungs should be auscultated for irregularities in function. These findings and a medical history may permit diagnosis of a borderline cardiac condition.

Extremities. Extremities are examined for varicose veins and edema. Signs of infection or restriction of movement are noted. Pulses and color in the extremities are checked.

Abdomen. Abdominal examination is performed to find any tenderness or masses. The size and shape of the uterus and the fundus are usually measured during each visit to permit recording of the rate of fetal growth (see Figure 9-15). Clients often are tense about abdominal palpation and need help in relaxing.

Pelvic examination. A pelvic examination is performed with the woman placed in the lithotomy position. The external genitalia are examined for lesions, scars, or infection. A vaginal speculum is inserted to provide a clear view of the cervix (see Figure 4-2). The color and condition of cervix and amount of leukorrhea are observed. At this time a Pap smear may be obtained to screen for cervical cancer cells. A specimen of cervical mucus for detection of infections such as gonorrhea is also taken. The speculum is removed, and a bimanual examination is performed to determine pelvic and uterine size.

TEST *Yourself* **9-6**

During the physical examination at 14 weeks, the midwife determines that the uterine fundus is 2 cm above the symphysis pubis. Which other physical findings should accompany a normal pregnancy at this stage?

Pelvic measurements. Pelvic measurements are obtained, including the *biischial diameter*, the distance between the ischial tuberosities (normally 8 cm or more), and the *diagonal conjugate*, the distance between the lower margin of the pubic bone to the promontory of the sacrum (normally 11.5 cm or more). (Measurements of the birth canal are discussed in detail in Chapter 13.)

There is controversy about the frequency of cervical examinations during pregnancy. Routine cervical examinations at later visits had been used to determine the risk of premature labor, however, recent studies show no difference in preterm births between those with more or less frequent examinations. Currently, a pelvic examination is done on the first visit and then not until the last

month of pregnancy, unless factors indicate a need to evaluate leukorrhea or cervical condition.

After completion of the physical examination, the health care provider will discuss the findings with the woman and make recommendations for self-care. Screening tests will be arranged and referrals made for anticipatory instruction, nutritional care, or social service involvement. It is important to encourage the woman to voice her concerns.

Vital signs

The nurse records vital signs during every visit. BP is the most important indication of a potential problem. An early baseline reading is essential for comparison with later changes. A drop in pressure is expected in the first half of pregnancy, with a return to normal or slightly above baseline in the last trimester. An elevation above a baseline of 30 points systolic and 15 points diastolic or an elevated MAP reading may indicate hypertension or preeclampsia. If BP is elevated, the nurse checks for signs of headache, dizziness, epistaxis, and increased edema in the extremities (see Chapter 22).

Screening tests

Problems will be detected by screening tests performed during prenatal visits. Table 9-4 lists the most frequently performed tests.

Blood tests. Blood tests include a complete blood count. Hematocrit is repeated in the last trimester and as indicated. If the reading is 32% or less, a work-up is performed for anemia and intestinal ova and parasites. Folic acid and ferrous gluconate may be prescribed (see Chapter 10).

Blood factor incompatibility. Blood is tested for A, B, or O categories and the Rh factor. The partner's type should be ascertained if possible because of the potential for incompatibility of type between mother and fetus.

Maternal-fetal blood incompatibility occurs when there is an antigen-antibody reaction to the mixing of minute amounts of fetal blood into the maternal circulation, an event that occurs at times during pregnancy. The mechanism of becoming sensitized or forming antibodies against antigens from the same species is **isoimmunization.** These antibodies may cross the placenta to attack fetal erythrocytes. The mechanism of Rh incompatibility is discussed in detail in Chapter 23. The **Coombs' test** is used to determine the level of reaction and will be ordered on the first visit and again several times during the pregnancy for Rh-negative women with an Rh-positive partner. If antibody titer is negative, RhD immune globulin is given and will be repeated at 28 or 34 weeks (Box 23-1).

Genetic screening. Screening for genetically carried diseases is performed routinely for sickle cell trait and for

Table 9-4   **Screening Tests during Pregnancy**

Test	Results and Comments
COMPLETE BLOOD CELL COUNT	
Hemoglobin	Measured as g/dl. May drop to 11.5 g/dl later in pregnancy because of increase of plasma in ratio to red blood cells (RBCs).
Hematocrit	Volume of RBCs in 100 ml blood, measured in a percentage; 33% is lowest acceptable level.
Mean corpuscular volume	Average volume of individual RBC; below average indicates some types of anemia.
RBC count	Number of RBCs in each microliter of blood. In pregnancy, hemodilution level may drop to 3.75 million/mm^3.
WBC count	Neutrophils (50%), lymphocytes (21%-35%), monocytes (4%), basophils (0.3%), eosinophils (2.7%). Total count is 7000-10,000/mm^3. Rises to 16,000 by late pregnancy.
Platelets	>150,000/mm^3
Hemoglobin electrophoresis	Determines sickle cell trait.
MATERNAL SERUM ALPHA-FETO PROTEIN (MSAFP)	Elevated levels or low levels cause concern. Done between 15-20 weeks.
GLUCOSE	
Hemoglobin A$_{1c}$	Less than 3.5% is normal; if above, indicates hyperglycemia within the last 6 weeks.
1-hr 50-g glucose load test	Load at 28 weeks; if 1-hr level less than 140, is normal. If above, then glucose tolerance testing is done.
BLOOD TYPE (ABO)	
Rh factor	Check partner's blood type and potential for incompatibility.
Coombs' test	Indirect Coombs' test should remain negative. Retested at 28 weeks in Rh-negative woman.
INFECTION*	
Rubella titer	If less than 1:8, immunize after birth. If titer more than 1:128 in early pregnancy, repeat test.
Syphilis	Venereal Disease Research Laboratory (VDRL) or fluorescent treponemal antibody absorption (FTA-ABS) test; repeat at 32 weeks for high risk.
Vaginal and cervical smear Gonorrhea	Gram stain or enzyme-linked immunosorbent assay (ELISA) test; repeat at 28 weeks.
Chlamydia	Direct examination of smear on slide.
Gram-positive *Streptococcus*	Direct slide examination.
Hepatitis B surface antigen	Vaccination advised.
Tuberculosis	Screen for tuberculosis. Skin tests: tine, Mantoux. Radiographic examination after positive finding.
URINE	
Glucose, ketones, albumin	Dip-stick test each visit.
Cells: leukocyte, RBCs, bacteria casts	Urinalysis performed first visit and as necessary. Catch clean, midstream specimen for culture if cells present.
Specific gravity	

*Some physicians also check all women for toxoplasmosis. See Chapter 25 for a complete discussion of infection.

other problems such as *thalassemia* and *glucose-6-phosphate dehydrogenase* (G-6-PD) *deficiency* (see Chapter 23).

Glucose. In spite of the fact that no benefit has yet been established for glucose screening during pregnancy (Enkin et al, 1995), all women continue to be tested in the clinic at 28 weeks with a 1-hour *glucose load test* to determine if gestational diabetes is developing (see Figure 24-3 and Chapter 24 for complete discussion). If glucose levels are more than 140 mg/dl on this test, the woman is required to have a 3-hour *glucose tolerance test.*

If there is a history of diabetes or if any risk factors are present, the woman may also be tested for elevated *hemoglobin A$_{1C}$* levels, which would indicate a history of hyperglycemia within the past 6 weeks. If the test result is positive, the woman will be referred for a work-up for diabetes.

Urine tests. During each visit, a fresh urine specimen is obtained for evaluation by a dip-stick (which may be performed by the woman herself as part of her participation in care). Dip-stick screening for glucose and protein provides approximate results (25% inaccuracy for trace protein) but indicates if further testing is required. This simple test, repeated at every prenatal visit, is a source of essential information in screening for glucose intolerance or hypertension.

For routine urinalysis in pregnancy, a clean midstream specimen is always desirable because of the presence of leukorrhea. Urinalysis determines cells, casts, and specific gravity. If there are any signs of infection, a careful midstream, clean-catch voided specimen for testing is preferable to a catheterized specimen.

Infection screening. There are various screens for infections (see Chapter 25). A rubella titer below 1:10 indicates that the woman is susceptible to rubella. She must be immunized after the pregnancy is over and avoid exposure to children with German measles. Recently the number of tuberculosis cases has risen. It is especially important that women in susceptible populations be screened by skin test, with a chest radiograph obtained if the test result is positive. Finally, the presence of any STD must be discovered. Syphilis, gonorrhea, and chlamydia tests are done routinely. Human immunodeficiency virus (HIV) tests are recommended, with consent, especially for high-risk persons. Routine toxoplasmosis screening during pregnancy is not currently recommended unless definite exposure has occurred (see Chapter 25 for complete discussion of infections affecting pregnancy).

NURSING DIAGNOSES

Nursing diagnoses relating to the pregnancy process include the following:

- Health-seeking behaviors related to self-care during pregnancy and for fetal health
- Sleep-pattern disturbance related to discomforts of pregnancy
- Altered pattern of urinary elimination
- Risk for activity intolerance related to fatigue, musculoskeletal adaptations, work requirements
- Risk for injury related to environmental toxins, drug use, accidents, or pregnancy complications

EXPECTED OUTCOMES

The following examples of expected outcomes of prenatal care are discussed in this chapter:

- Participates in prenatal care and follows through on referrals
- Incorporates health practices that demonstrate new knowledge
- Manages variations in sleep patterns, elimination, and activity
- Recognizes and reports occurrence of warning signs
- Describes ways of avoiding potential hazards during pregnancy; reports the faithful use of seat belts
- Evidences preparation for birth and infant care; involves partner

NURSING INTERVENTION

To perform self-care, the client must know what is important for health. A woman in her first pregnancy is usually unaware of health maintenance unless she has read literature or is a member of an extended family and has observed other pregnant women. She needs **anticipatory guidance** about the events of each trimester and the growth patterns of the baby. People learn in different ways, and learning may be inhibited for a number of reasons. The skill to work with women of various backgrounds or with those who speak English as a second language is a requirement for a nurse.

Women are asked to monitor themselves, and the nurse emphasizes these self-monitoring activities, including regularly weighing themselves and noting and reporting any difficulties. They are taught requirements for food and fluid intake and encouraged to report difficulties (see Chapter 10). Questions about labor onset or fetal condition are addressed in the last trimester, and the woman is taught to self-monitor contractions and fetal movements (Box 9-5). Women do best in self-care activities when they are asked to take responsibility. Effective compliance with clinic visits has been demonstrated by women who were given copies of their medical screening records (Diamond, 1990). The results of each visit's activities (e.g., vital signs, urine tests, weight changes, fetal assessment) are recorded. The woman receives the record at the first visit, and it is

Box 9-5

TEACHING PLAN *for* HOME CARE

Prenatal Care

FIRST TRIMESTER

Describe Pregnancy Changes and Minor Discomforts
• Nausea, vomiting, ptyalism
• Breast tenderness and care
• Fatigue, rest and activity, frequency

Explain Safety Concerns
• Hazards in home and workplace, seat belts
• Smoking, drugs, and alcohol cessation
• Over-the-counter (OTC) drugs and vitamin precautions
• Hot tubs and dangers of hyperthermia

Discuss Schedule of Clinic Visits and Clinic Resources
• Calculate expected date of childbirth (EDC); discuss weight, nutrition
• Screening tests: tuberculosis, blood, urine

Interpret Psychosocial Adjustment and Concerns
Identify Warning Signs
• Spotting, bleeding, cramping, pain
• Infection signs and symptoms

SECOND TRIMESTER

Describe Pregnancy Changes and Minor Discomforts
• Backache, constipation, hemorrhoids, varicose veins
• Hygiene, leukorrhea
• Breast changes and care

Discuss Fetal Growth and Development
Discuss Nutrition and Weight Management
Explain Safety Concerns
• Seat belts and travel
• Employment
• Exercise and activity

Identify Reasons for Screening Tests
• MSAFP, ultrasound, glucose load test

Interpret psychosocial concerns
• Sexuality and partner's concerns

Identify Warning Signals
• Bleeding, pain, leaking membranes
• Preterm labor signs and symptoms
• Hypertension
• Pain

THIRD TRIMESTER

Describe Pregnancy Changes and Minor Discomforts
• Pressure symptoms; dependent edema, leg aches, leg cramps, round ligament pain
• Dyspnea, frequency, pyrosis

Identify Screening Tests
• Nonstress test (NST), biophysical profile

Discuss Preparation for Childbirth
• Planning for siblings, classes for siblings
• Exercises, breathing, relaxation
• Birth plans
• Emergency arrangements for transport, child care

Explain Safety Concerns
• Signs of preterm labor, true labor
• Balance, rest, activity, travel, seat belts
• Body mechanics/posture/positions in bed

Interpret Psychosocial Concerns
• Sexuality and partner's concerns
• Support system for homecoming and care

---

used at each visit, including any emergency visits (see Figure 9-16).

Warning signs

An important part of helping the woman to self-monitor progress is to provide a clear description of the warning signals of potential complications (Box 9-6). Warning signals of problems other than normal minor discomforts should be taught early. If the warning signs are not taught, a

woman may not report a pathologic change in her condition under the assumption that it is supposed to happen (see Box 9-5).

1. **Bleeding.** Bleeding during pregnancy is abnormal. In the first trimester, it may warn of impending abortion or a poorly implanted placenta. Later it may signal placenta previa, a sudden separation of the placenta, or preterm labor. A few women have vaginal bleeding from cervical erosion caused by chronic infection (see Chapter 21).

Box **9-6**

WARNING SIGNS

Pregnancy

Vaginal bleeding: From spotting to frank hemorrhage
Infection: Fever, chills, dysuria, burning on urination, frequency
  Cough with chest pain
  Localized infection, or warm, swollen extremity
Pain: Can be present anywhere
Preeclampsia: Persistent headache, generalized edema, dark scanty urine, visual disturbances, epigastric pain
Preterm labor: Increased vaginal discharge, menstrual-like or rhythmic cramping or backache, heavy feeling in pelvis
Severe vomiting: Continues after 3-4 months, weight loss

2. **Infection.** Signs of infection in any part of the body are warning signals, but during pregnancy, conditions that might affect fetal condition are especially serious. Fever, chills, may be accompanied flank pain, which are signs of kidney infection. Bladder infection may show dysuria, burning on urination, frequency, and cloudy urine (see Chapter 24). Vaginal infection should be reported for interventions (see Chapters 4 and 26). Signs of upper respiratory infections and influenza should be reported.

3. **Pain.** Pain is usually abnormal. Exceptions are the abdominal aching and perineal pressure of prelabor or a brief pain in the side caused by a pulling sensation of the round ligament. Occasionally, pain radiates through the groin or down the line of the sciatic nerve as a result of pressure on the nerves in the pelvic region.

4. **Preeclampsia.** Signs and symptoms related to developing preeclampsia are severe continuous headache; edema in the face, hands, or legs on arising in the morning; scanty, concentrated urine; visual disturbances; and epigastric pain. Any of these symptoms must be reported at once because severe hypertension may develop rapidly (see Chapter 22).

5. **Premature labor.** This may be signaled anytime in the last trimester by menstrual-like aching or thigh cramps, rhythmic backache, pelvic ache or uterine contractions, and increased vaginal discharge of mucus or watery, blood-tinged fluid. Interventions may delay labor if the woman is seen promptly for contraction monitoring and diagnosis (see Chapter 21).

6. **Severe nausea and vomiting.** This may escalate. Treatment for *hyperemesis* is important to prevent ketosis, dehydration, and fetal deprivation of nutrients (see Chapter 24).

Sleep patterns

Causes of sleep disturbance vary according to the trimester. Early in pregnancy, fatigue related to relaxin and other hormonal effects may lead the woman to take naps and then to be wakeful at night. Later, discomforts of pregnancy interrupt rest. Nasal congestion is a major problem for some because of increased peripheral circulation to nasal tissues. Excessive use of antihistamines is not advised. Humidified air may relieve breathing. When positional dyspnea occurs, the woman may use the semi-Fowler's position for sleep. Use of extra pillows helps her to maintain a side-lying position. During later pregnancy the supine position must be avoided to prevent SHS (see Figure 9-3).

If fatigue is related to anemia, the cause should be corrected, if possible. If fatigue is related to night wakefulness, the woman should be asked about feelings of anxiety, dreams, environmental noise, overfatigue during the day, muscle cramping, and nocturia.

A woman may have a life situation, such as work or several small children, that prevents a rest period during the day. She should be encouraged to analyze her situation to determine how to obtain additional rest. In this way she learns coping skills and may be able to solve the problem. Unfortunately, social support does not include mother's helpers for fatigued pregnant women.

Hygiene

Hygiene during pregnancy may be a problem for some women because of increased oil and perspiration, and for some, because of inadequate bathroom facilities. Safety during bathing should be emphasized. The most important point to discuss is maintaining balance. Tub and shower baths may be taken up to the time of birth, but a woman may find it awkward to move in and out of a tub because of the altered center of gravity.

Reinforcing good dental hygiene is important. Dental plaque should be removed by flossing at least once a day and teeth brushed with a soft toothbrush to prevent injury to tender or bleeding gums.

Preventing hazards

Every pregnant woman should be informed regarding the dangers of self-medication (see Chapter 16) and cautioned that home remedies may contain substances that can affect the infant. She should be asked to list any over-the-counter and prescription medications she takes.

Over-the-counter drugs. Drugs for pain relief are available OTC. *Acetaminophen* is the analgesic medication recommended during pregnancy and lactation. It works as an antiprostaglandin but has less antiinflammatory effect than aspirin or ibuprofen. It is also an antipyretic, producing peripheral vasodilation through action on the heat-regulating center. Listed in risk category B (see Table 16-1), the drug should not be taken in high doses because it is metabolized in the liver, crosses the placenta, and is then metabolized by the fetal liver as well. Drug interactions must be observed. With caffeine combinations, central nervous system stimulation is increased. Laboratory test readings for glucose may be reduced, and prothrombin time and bilirubin concentrations may be increased.

Acetylsalicylic acid (ASA) may be found in many OTC combinations (more than 400). This drug is not recommended in adult doses during pregnancy and is classified as risk category C (see Table 16-1) because of potential harm to the developing fetus. When the drug crosses the placenta, its anticoagulant action may result in a reduction in clotting time and in fetal bleeding. The antiprostaglandin action may promote closure of the ductus arteriosus before birth and may prolong gestation and labor. In addition, the mother may have an anticoagulation effect and extra bleeding after delivery. However, in low doses (60 to 80 mg) ASA is proving useful in certain women with preeclampsia (see Chapter 22).

Nonsteroidal prostaglandin inhibitors (*ibuprofen*) inhibit prostaglandin synthesis and decrease inflammation by inhibiting local inflammatory responses. Women have discovered the effectiveness of these drugs for menstrual cramping and may be inclined to continue to use them during pregnancy. These drugs are not recommended because they prolong gestation and labor and may prematurely close the fetal ductus arteriosus, acting somewhat like ASA.

Women should be encouraged to read the labels on all drugs and taught self-care and avoidance of drug-related hazards. OTC medications should be cleared with the physician before use. A woman will be more sensitive to drug effects because of pregnancy changes, therefore she should check dosages with the physician.

Women may have read about teratogenic substances and may ask about drug safety. In addition, substances and chemicals in the work and home environment are a source of concern. (See Chapter 10 for discussion of cigarettes, alcohol, and coffee and Chapter 27 for hazards of drug abuse and teratogens.)

Work precautions. Despite the fact that 60% to 65% of women between the ages of 18 and 64 have jobs, there is still no uniform policy on pregnancy and recovery leave in the United States. Therefore work during pregnancy is a major issue. Working conditions for women vary throughout the country, and each job causes potential difficulties. Women who work on assembly lines and farms, for example, may have to perform heavy lifting and may also be exposed to chemical and environmental hazards. Saleswomen, teachers, nurses, and other health-related workers spend most of their day standing. Even a "safe" position as a secretary or an office worker may cause problems because of long periods of sitting and standing or working at computer terminals. Neck, back, and eye strain are major complaints, and there is growing concern about possible effects on the fetus of low-level magnetic field emissions emanating from elements that coat video display terminals (Blackwell and Chang, 1988). See Chapter 28 for reproductive hazards in the workplace.

It is now acceptable for a woman to continue work while pregnant. This may be a satisfying or an exhausting experience for the woman, depending on physical fitness, discomforts, and stress of the job. Many women worry about endangering or even losing their positions when they need to take extra time off for complications or even normal maternity leave. Often it is only when this extra time is needed that the woman finds that her job does not provide enough sick leave. This may be especially true for women with prior health problems or low-income work situations that traditionally offer few or no health care benefits. For the woman whose financial situation demands work, stress and fear of losing her job may prevent compliance with prescribed regimens of rest and treatment (Figure 9-17).

The woman should be asked about her job, including its responsibilities, environment, and sick and maternity leave policies. She should be encouraged to plan realistically to maintain her financial security while caring for herself and her child. If there is or may be a serious problem, referral to social services for assistance and guidance is appropriate.

Rest periods with the legs elevated whenever possible should be encouraged, and support hose should be worn when the woman must stand for long periods. If she sits for most of the day, she should change position frequently, walk, or elevate her legs on a stool.

Box 9-2
CLINICAL DECISION

During the prenatal visit at 24 weeks, Hannah asks whether she should continue working as a secretary. Give the rationale for and debate the pros and cons of the following statements:

a. Sitting without moving or walking at intervals adversely affects venous circulation in the lower extremities.

b. If a woman is able, she needs time at home to adapt to the developmental tasks of pregnancy.

c. Women today are in better condition than ever, and working is not a health hazard as long as the woman gets enough rest.

d. Pregnant women are self-involved in the last part of pregnancy and do not concentrate well for long periods.

Hyperthermia. Heat may be a hazard to the developing embryo in the first trimester because it cannot be dissipated if the mother has hyperthermia. The fetus already is 0.5° to 1° F warmer than the mother; thus a fever could cause adverse fetal effects. Offspring of laboratory test animals that had suffered hyperthermia developed smaller brains and learning dysfunction (Smith, Edwards, and Upfold,

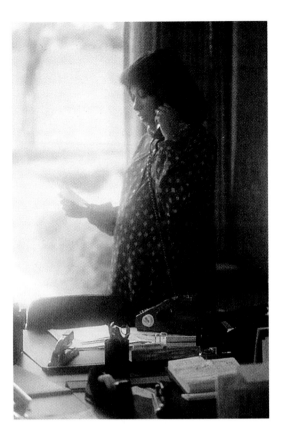

Figure 9-17   Many women work throughout the entire pregnancy. Rest periods are important and provide a chance to elevate the legs several times during the day. (Courtesy Ross Laboratories, Columbus, Ohio.)

1986). Thus a woman should not allow a temperature elevation above 103° F (38.9° C) especially during the critical time of organogenesis, the first 12 weeks of pregnancy (Smith, Edwards, and Upfold, 1986).

Hyperthermia may result from excessive aerobic exercise, extended use of a sauna or hot tub, and fever. Speroff (1996) recommends no more than 10 minutes in a sauna or hot tub with a temperature set at less than 102° F. Normally, as a result of vasodilation, pregnant women report that they feel warmer and usually do not choose to voluntarily become warmer. In climates that are humid and warm, however, special efforts should be taken to maintain a lower temperature. Antipyretics such as acetaminophen and cooling sponge baths are used to reduce body temperature during illness.

Infection. Women must understand that infection may adversely affect the fetus. Information should be provided from the beginning regarding STDs, other vaginal infections, and urinary infections. Primary prevention avoids exposure to infectious diseases (see Chapter 25).

Immunizations should be checked. If a woman is unprotected against rubella, she should be scheduled for inoculation after childbirth and should avoid exposure during pregnancy, particularly in the first trimester. Exposure is more common than would be expected because so many children are not immunized adequately. She will not be immunized during pregnancy with vaccinations that contain live attenuated preparations. (See Appendix 3 B.)

Because of vaginal changes during pregnancy, the presence of *Lactobacillus* species increases and anaerobic bacteria decrease. Increased vaginal secretions may become a problem. The woman may have to wear a pant liner because of leukorrhea. If leukorrhea is odorous, discolored, or causes itching or pain, the physician should be notified and treatment prescribed. Douching should not be done without the physician's recommendation, and tampons, feminine deodorants, and suppositories are prohibited. Perineal care should relieve any discomfort.

During each visit the woman should be queried about the status of vaginal or urinary infections because recurrence is common. The common vaginal infections, *Trichomonas* and *Candida,* are most troublesome during pregnancy (see Chapter 4). Friederick and Phillips (1988) reported that monilial spores are not destroyed by normal laundry temperatures and thus may remain on underwear to reinfect the woman. These findings lead to recommendations for microwaving wet cotton underwear (for 5 minutes on a high setting) or using a hot iron before wear when a monilial infection is being treated.

Travel and accidents

After midpregnancy, trips of more than 2 to 3 hours by car, train, or plane are unwise because of prolonged sitting. If a trip must be made, the woman should change positions frequently and, when possible, walk to promote circulation. Prolonged sitting or standing is related to a marked increase in sodium retention, a change initiated by the postural effect on renal blood flow. Sodium retention leads to water retention and edema. Compression of the veins leading from the legs also occurs, with elevated femoral venous pressure and edema.

Automobile accidents are the leading reason for maternal mortality unrelated to pregnancy. The woman restrained by a seat belt comes to a stop with the car, rather than leaving the seat and flying through the windshield or door. This force is dissipated more evenly when a seat belt is used correctly (see the discussion on trauma, Chapter 23).

Seat belts. It is possible to sustain injury in an accident from the improper use of seat belts. Lap belts or shoulder belts should not be used alone. Lap belts used alone or not fastened below the abdominal bulge may cause injury from the pressure of the buckle; sudden flexion may cause injury to the intestines, spleen, kidneys, pancreas, stomach, bladder, and uterus. Shoulder belts used alone may injure the ribs, spine, neck, or sternum.

In contrast, injuries tend to be minor with the three-point belt. These injuries include lacerations on the shoulder area, thighs, or chest. The three-point belt is by far the safest restraint system. In addition to use of this belt, the headrest should be adjusted correctly to avoid whiplash (American College of Obstetricians and Gynecologists, 1991).

Every pregnant woman should be told about the correct method of applying a seat belt. The restraint should be a lap belt worn as low as possible over the pelvic bones and below the abdominal bulge. The strap across the shoulder, chest, and upper abdomen should be firm but comfortable. A pad may be attached to the shoulder strap if the belt touches the side of her neck (Figure 9-18). The woman should be questioned about consistent seat belt use and introduced to guidelines for infant car seats (see Chapter 20).

Referrals

Before the end of the first or second visit, women receive referrals to the dentist to provide dental screening for those whose teeth may be neglected, to prevent decay if sufficient calcium is not ingested and to obtain an assessment of dental health from the beginning of pregnancy. Dental health contributes toward her total health status.

In clinic care, referrals are made to the social worker for assistance with family or economic concerns. The nutritionist also is available for women who are overweight or underweight and for those with chronic diabetes, hypotension, hypertension, or anemia (see Chapter 10).

Revisits

The interval for subsequent visits may vary. The American College of Obstetricians and Gynecologists (ACOG) guidelines for prenatal care include a visit as early as possible in pregnancy and intervals of 4 weeks until week 28, after which visits are scheduled according to the woman's progress. Most physicians schedule weekly visits during the last few weeks. (For psychosocial care see Chapter 8, and for nutritional care see Chapter 10.) One preconceptual visit is now being recommended to every couple anticipating pregnancy within a year.

Summary of nursing interventions during prenatal care

- Introduce yourself to the client and partner, and welcome them to the beginning of prenatal care. Help them feel that care will be individualized.
- During the interview, listen to the woman's responses to identify unspoken concerns. Foster communication between staff members and couple.
- Ask personal and potentially awkward questions (about family matters, use of adverse substances) in a nonthreatening, nonjudgmental manner.
- Explain sequences of the visit and all procedures. Begin care plan.
- Stay with the woman during the vaginal examination if the physician is a man. Find a female caregiver if the woman indicates that care by a man is unacceptable.

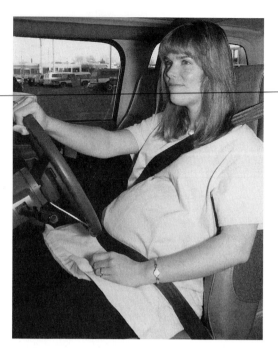

Figure 9-18 Proper use of seat belt and headrest.
(Courtesy Michael S Clement, MD, Mesa, Ariz.)

Protect her privacy, and identify cultural roots of any problems she expresses concerning the examinations.

- Be aware of cultural differences that may affect care in pregnancy and labor. Discuss these with the client, making sure she understands instructions that do not counteract her cultural patterns. If practices conflict with her customs or practices, work with her to find neutral practices to substitute for routine instructions on nutrition, activities, and hygiene.
- Describe self-care activities such as urine testing and weighing. Include rationale for monitoring during pregnancy. Begin prenatal record for client to keep.
- Explain warning signals. Provide the client with the clinic telephone number and 24-hour telephone number.
- Discuss minor changes of accommodation and discomforts. Discuss nonpharmacologic interventions she may use.
- See partners together some time during each visit to answer questions and observe responses. Elicit from partner his feelings about participation in labor and birth support.
- Make referrals to other health professionals, dentists, nutritionists, and social workers. Set up appointments while the client is in clinic.
- Refer the client and partner to childbirth education classes or provide them in your setting. Give literature in client's own language.
- Discuss labor plans with couple. Determine if making a birth plan is important to them.

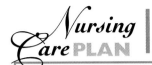

Early Prenatal Care

CASE

Mary, 18, and Leonard, 20; first pregnancy. LMP September 1; vital signs: temperature, pulse, respiration: 98.8/80/24; BP 106/74; ht. 5 ft 6 in, wt. 106 lb; complains she is nauseated for a few weeks; wants to sleep all the time; takes naps after work, and finds it hard to sleep at night between running to the bathroom and restlessness. Works at local fertilizer plant. Eats out often at fast food restaurants (mainly french fries and hamburgers). Has lost 2 lb in the last month. Smokes one pack/day. Drinks beer with coworkers after work.

Assessment

1. History
   Patient's age, parity
   Knowledge of pregnancy
      Signs and symptoms of pregnancy
      Determine EDB
   Role expectations
   Support systems and family history

2. Knowledge of self-care for minor discomforts in pregnancy
3. Knowledge of nutrition, diet habits
4. Knowledge of safety habits
   Employment setting
   Smoking
   Alcohol

Nursing Diagnoses

1. Health seeking behaviors regarding self-care related to first pregnancy
2. Sleep-pattern disturbance related to daytime nap and nocturia
3. Altered nutrition: less than body requirements related to inadequate food intake as a result of nausea and poor eating habits
4. Injury, risk for, related to nicotine, alcohol, and possible chemical toxicity in workplace

Expected Outcomes

1. Actively participates in pregnancy-related care; monitors progress, and reports warning signs promptly
2. Adjusts activities of daily living (ADL) to gain sufficient rest and sleep
3. Reports intake of adequate nutrients for sufficient weight gain
4. Reports reduction or cessation of smoking and drinking; negotiates work responsibilities and schedule to minimize hazards

Nursing Interventions

1. Prenatal education
   - Discuss signs and symptoms of pregnancy and changes during pregnancy that precipitate minor discomforts.
   - Discuss nonpharmacologic remedies during pregnancy.
   - Discuss warning signals of pregnancy. Encourage prompt reporting.
   - Discuss available support systems.
   - Make referrals to appropriate departments.
2. Assist client to modify ADL, including nap times, limiting fluid intake in the evening, and work schedule.
3. Nutrition
   - Obtain complete nutritional and diet history.
   - Discuss nutritional requirements of pregnancy.
   - Collaborate to develop a diet plan that will encourage adequate intake.
   - Refer to nutritionist and WIC food program if necessary.
4. Education to prevent injury
   - Explain dangers of smoking and alcohol and possible workplace hazards to self and fetus.
   - Encourage reduction or elimination of hazards, use of seat belts.
   - Encourage client to seek assistance as needed for these problems (such as Alcoholics Anonymous [AA]), and make referrals to appropriate agencies as needed.

Evaluation

1. Did she monitor self-care and report problems promptly?
2. Does she report that she got adequate rest?
3. Does dietary diary indicate a nutritionally adequate diet as evidenced by appropriate weight gain, hemoglobin, and hematocrit?
4. Does she report reduction in or elimination of her smoking and drinking behaviors?
5. Does she report employer cooperation regarding work environment and schedule?

- Introduce the need to make decisions about breast-feeding and infant circumcision. Provide literature.
- Keep the client informed of progress and results of testing.

- Were guidelines for health maintenance followed?
- Were deviations from normal promptly reported?
- Did dietary intake and exercise result in adequate weight gain and nutritional status and soft stools?
- Did the client state that hazards were avoided and seat belts used at all times?
- Were plans discussed for labor and birth and recovery support?

EVALUATION

These questions can be asked to evaluate the outcomes of the course of prenatal care:

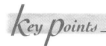

Key points

- Changes in pregnancy are accomplished by the delicate balancing of bodily functions, that is, the changes of accommodation.
- Every body system is affected by the pregnancy and is under the influence of hormones of pregnancy.
- Minor discomforts occur as a result of the changes of accommodation, and women benefit from instruction that teaches them how their bodies work.
- Each woman should be taught self-monitoring techniques and given information that includes warning signs and record keeping.

- Increasing women's participation in self-care increases compliance with health maintenance behaviors and prenatal clinic visits.
- Safety from hazards related to employment, travel, home environment, and drug use is an important part of prenatal teaching.
- Warning regarding self-medication with OTC drugs should be given early in pregnancy.
- Individual instruction on activity and exercise is an important part of prenatal care.

Study Questions

9-1.   Select the terms that apply to the following statements:
   a. Darkened streaks on the abdomen or breasts
   b. Low bacterial levels present in urine, without discomfort
   c. Change in posture to keep balance during late pregnancy
   d. Change in BP that causes light-headedness when getting up
   e. Patchy, darkened pigmentation on the face during late pregnancy
   f. Exercise to strengthen the perineal floor
   g. Number of times a woman ever has been pregnant
   h. Need to void more than once during the night

9-2.   Hemodilution of pregnancy leads to the following signs in the woman:
   a. Slight elevation of BP   c. Supine hypotension in later pregnancy
   b. Decrease in Hct levels by the second trimester   d. Reduction in pulse rate and CO

9-3.   If at 34 weeks the client complains of flushed face, reddened palms, and nasal congestion, your counsel depends on knowledge of the following:
   a. These signs indicate increasing hypertension.
   b. All women do not get melasma, which will recede postpartum.
   c. This is an unusual complaint during pregnancy and needs follow-up.
   d. Symptoms result from increased peripheral circulation.

9-4.   Your anticipatory guidance during the first trimester will be based on the understanding that:
   a. Pregnant women are eager to learn about growth and development.
   b. Nutritional balance is difficult to achieve during pregnancy.
   c. Pregnant women generally are anxious to follow health guidelines.
   d. Women often resent detailed questioning about their family situations and future plans.

9-5.   Maria shows that she has understood your guidance about her skin changes when she states:
   a.   "This lotion is really working on those ugly stretch marks."
   b.   "I'm glad feeling so hot and sweaty will go away when the baby comes."
   c.   "I don't have to use sun screen when I'm pregnant."
   d.   "Everyone comments on how good I look. I'm glad it lasts after the baby is born."

9-6.   You would note problems in vital signs in the first trimester if one of the following was present:
   a. BP: 10/5 mm Hg below baseline   c. MAP: 105 mm Hg
   b. Pulse: 20 beats/min above baseline

9-7.   Jane would be demonstrating automobile safety if at 28 weeks she told you that she always followed this pattern in the car:
   a.   Sat in rear seat and elevated her legs frequently
   b.   Fastened the lap belt below the bulge of the uterus
   c.   Adapted the shoulder belt so it did not touch the uterus
   d.   Used shoulder and lap belt during every ride

9-8.   In the last trimester a pregnant woman should not wait for her regular appointment a week later to report one of the following:
   a.   Shortness of breath while climbing stairs with a load of laundry
   b.   Increased whitish vaginal mucus that required use of a vaginal pad
   c.   Bloated feeling and blurring of vision
   d.   Constipation with new hemorrhoids

9-9.   During the last trimester, it is most important to teach self-monitoring of which of the following?
   a.   Fatigue levels and interrupted sleep patterns   c.   Heartburn and inability to take large meals
   b.   Patterns of edema in lower extremities   d.   Changes in mild contraction frequency

Answer Key

9-1. *a,* Striae; *b,* asymptomatic bacteriuria; *c,* lordosis; *d,* postural hypotension; *e,* melasma; *f,* Kegel exercise; *g,* gravidity; *h,* nocturia.
9-2: b. 9-3: d. 9-4: c. 9-5: b. 9-6: b. 9-7: d. 9-8: c. 9-9: d.

References

American Academy of Pediatrics, American College of Obstetricians and Gynecologists: *Guidelines for prenatal care,* Washington, DC, 1992.

American College of Obstetricians and Gynecologists: *Automobile passenger restraints for children and pregnant women,* Technical bulletin 151, Washington, DC, January 1991.

American College of Obstetricians and Gynecologists: *Exercise during pregnancy and postpartum period,* Technical bulletin 189, Washington, DC, February 1994.

American College of Obstetricians and Gynecologists: *Preconceptional care,* Technical bulletin 205, Washington, DC, May 1995.

Andrews CM et al: Use of pelvic tilt exercise for ligament pain relief, *J Nurse Midwifery* 39(6):370, 1994.

*Barry M, Bia F: Pregnancy and travel, *JAMA* 261:728, 1989.

Beischer NA, MacKay EU: *Obstetrics and the newborn,* ed 3, Philadelphia, 1993, Harcourt, Brace, Jovanovich.

Bernhardt JH: Potential workplace hazards to reproductive health, *J Obstet Gynecol Neonatal Nurs* 19:53, 1990.

Blackburn ST, Loper DL: *Maternal, fetal, and neonatal physiology,* Philadelphia, 1992, WB Saunders.

*Blackwell R, Chang A: Video display terminals and pregnancy, *Br J Obstet Gynaecol* 95:466, l988.

Breart G: Antenatal care, *Curr Opinion Obstet Gynecol* 7:417, l995.

*Brucker MC: Management of common minor discomforts in pregnancy: part II, managing minor pain, *J Nurse Midwifery* 33:25, 1988.

*Brucker MC: Managing gastrointestinal problems in pregnancy, *J Nurse Midwifery* 33:67, 1988.

Chanco-Turner ML: The skin in pregnancy. In Burrow A, Ferris TF, eds: *Medical complications during pregnancy,* ed 4, Philadelphia, 1995, WB Saunders.

Delaney J: Participation in sports and exercise during pregnancy, *Int J Childbirth Educ* 10(3):721, 1993.

Diamond FB: Patients' prenatal medical record precis, *J Obstet Gynecol Neonatal Nurs* 19:491, 1990.

Dilorio C et al: Recommendations by clinicians for nausea and vomiting of pregnancy, *Clin Nurse Res* 3(3):209, 1994.

*Doshi ML: Accuracy of consumer performed in-home tests for early pregnancy detection, *Am J Public Health* 76:512, 1986.

*Dougherty MC et al: The effect of exercise on the circumvaginal muscles in postpartum women, *J Nurse Midwifery* 34:8, 1989.

Enkin M et al: *A guide to effective care in pregnancy and childbirth,* Oxford, 1995, Oxford University Press.

Erick M: Hyperolefaction and hyperemesis gravidarum: what is the relationship? *Nutr Rev* 53(10):289, 1995.

Ferris TF: Hypertension and preeclampsia. In Burrow A, Ferris TF, eds: *Medical complications during pregnancy,* ed 4, Philadelphia, 1995, WB Saunders.

Fiscella K: Does prenatal care improve birth outcomes? A critical review, *Obstet Gynecol* 85(3):468, 1995.

*Friederick EG, Phillips LE: Microwave sterilization of Candida on underwear, *J Reprod Med* 33:1, 1988.

Gilbert ES, Harmon JS: *Manual of high risk pregnancy and delivery,* St Louis, 1993, Mosby.

Gobe LI: Pregnancy and movement disorders, *Neurol Clin* 12(3):479, 1994.

Groutz A, Hagay ZJ. Prenatal care: an update and future trends, *Curr Opinion Obstet Gynecol* 7:452, l995.

Hatch MC et al: Maternal exercise during pregnancy, physical fitness and fetal growth, *Am J Epidemiol* 137(10):1105, 1993.

Mongelli M, Opatola B: Duration and variability of normal pregnancy, *J Reprod Med* 40(9):645, 1995.

*Classic reference.

National Institutes of Health: *An evaluation and assessment of the state of the science. Pregnancy, birth and the infant,* Washington, DC, 1992, National Institutes of Health.

*Nesler CL et al: Effects of supine exercise on fetal heart rate in the second and third trimesters, *Am J Perinatol* 5:159, 1988.

Ott, WJ: Accurate gestational dating: revisited, *Am J Perinatol* 11:404, 1994.

Parsons C: Back care in pregnancy, *Mod Midwife* 4(10):16, 1994.

Pearce KL: Kegel exercises: levels I and II, *Nurse Pract Forum* 5(3):146, 1994.

Rosenbaum RB, Donaldson JO: Peripheral nerve and muscular disorders, *Neuro Clin* 12(3):461, 1994.

Sampselle CM: Changes in pelvic muscle strength and stress urinary incontinence associated with childbirth, *J Obstet Gynecol Neonatal Nurs* 19:371, 1990.

Schick-Boschetto B, Rose NC: Exercise in pregnancy, *Obstet Gynecol Surv* 47:10, 1991.

Schiene LA et al. Urinary tract infection during pregnancy: its association with maternal morbidity and perinatal outcome, *Am J Public Health* 84(3):405, 1994.

Sibai BM, Frangieh A: Maternal adaptation to pregnancy, *Curr Opinion Obstet Gynecol* 7:420, 1995.

*Smith MSR, Edwards MJ, Upfold JB: The effects of hyperthermia on the fetus, *Devel Med Child Neurol* 28:203, 1986.

Speroff L. Exercise. In Queenan JT, Hobbins JC: *Protocols for high-risk pregnancies,* ed 3, Cambridge, Mass, 1996, Blackwell.

*Classic reference.

Sternfeld B et al: Exercise during pregnancy and pregnancy outcomes: sports and exercise, *Med Science* 27(5):634, 1995.

Van Dinter MC: Ptyalism in pregnant women, *J Obstet Gynecol Neonatal Nurs* 20(3):206, 1991.

Van Lier D et al. Nausea and fatigue in early pregnancy, *Birth* 20(4):193, 1993.

*Wallace AM: Aerobic exercise, maternal self-esteem and physical discomforts of pregnancy, *J Nurse Midwifery* 31:255, 1986.

Zellis S Et al: When the pregnant woman experiences itching, *Dermatol Nurs* 5(5):380, 1993.

Student Resource Shelf

Davis DC: The discomforts of pregnancy, *J Obstet Gynecol Neonatal Nurs* 25(1):73, 1996.
Discussion of selected discomforts of pregnancy with interventions.

Maloni JA et al: Transforming prenatal care: reflections on the past and present with implications for the future, *J Obstet Gynecol Neonatal Nurs* 25(1):17, 1996.
Historical overview of prenatal care that is focused on preventing preeclampsia, with recommendations for changes that more readily will accomplish the goals of the year 2000.

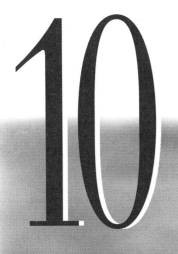

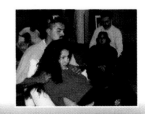

10

Nutritional Guidelines *during* Pregnancy, Lactation, *&* Recovery

Learning Objectives

- Describe the caloric and nutritional requirements for pregnancy.
- Determine nutritional additions on the basis of a woman's weight gain pattern and dietary assessment.
- Identify the point at which cultural differences in diet become dysfunctional.
- Describe possible signs of pica, bulimia, and anorexia.
- Describe the harmful effects of smoking, caffeine, and alcohol on the client's nutritional health.
- Identify nutritional needs for the recovery period postbirth and during lactation.

Key Terms

Anorexia Nervosa
Body Mass Index (BMI)
Bulimia
Fetal Alcohol Effect (FAE)
Fetal Alcohol Syndrome (FAS)
Fetal Tobacco Syndrome
Gingivitis
Hyperemesis gravidarum
Hyperolefaction
Hyponatremia
Ketoacidosis
Lactose Intolerance
Pica
Ptyalism
Pyrosis
Recommended Dietary Allowances (RDAs)

Good nutrition before and during pregnancy builds a healthy fetus and protects the woman's own nutritional health. From conception the fetus relies on nutrients in correct amounts for its development. Studies are currently being done to determine if the origin of certain diseases in the adult, such as cardiovascular disease, hypertension, or chronic lung disease, stem from inadequate fetal growth (Goldberg and Prentice, 1994). In a society where food is abundant, many women do not take in a minimum of the **recommended dietary allowances** (RDAs) or follow dietary guidelines. The desire to be underweight, to eat fast food, or skip meals is common, especially among adolescents.

Because the first prenatal clinic visit usually occurs late in the fetal development timetable (at more than 8 weeks), women need to prepare for conception. Women must be informed that the use of alcohol, drugs, or cigarettes during pregnancy will reduce the weight gain of the fetus unless such activities stop or diminish and their nutritional intake improves. Other potential damage from these substances is discussed in Chapter 28.

The objective of dietary management is to equalize caloric intake with caloric expenditure, thus preventing use of maternal fat stores. When maternal stores are mobilized, a state of **ketoacidosis** is produced. Studies have shown a high association of ketoacidosis with low birth

219

weight (LBW) and mental retardation (Catalano and Hollenbeck, 1992).

Pregnancy is the best time to offer nutritional guidance. In many busy settings, unfortunately, the woman is simply handed a pamphlet on food guidelines. Instead, time should be taken to assess the woman's diet and the current weight and to provide dietary instruction for optimal weight gain and fetal growth.

A great deal of attention has been placed on the correct weight gain during pregnancy. Women often have misconceptions about how much weight is appropriate. When patterns do not match the "average," anxiety levels can rise. Therefore weight gain patterns should be understood before a discussion of nutrients can be meaningful.

WEIGHT GAIN

Recommendations about weight gain in pregnancy have undergone significant changes in the past few decades. It is now recognized that inadequate weight gain poses a higher risk to the pregnant woman (premature labor, anemia, infection) and to her fetus (LBW, small-for-gestational age infants) than excessive weight gain.

The components of the weight gained during pregnancy are listed in Table 10-1 and shown in Figure 10-1. The nurse can explain that in the first half of pregnancy while the fetus is still small, most of the weight is gained in body fat and circulating fluids. Weight gain in the second half of pregnancy goes primarily toward growth of the fetus, uterus, and placenta (Blackburn and Loper, 1992).

The rate of gain should not be linear; the average gain should start gradually in the first trimester while the embryo is small, about 0.8 lb/wk, then rise to about 1.0 lb (0.4 kg)/wk in the second and third trimesters. Other factors also determine the amount of weight a woman should gain. Women carrying more than one fetus should be encouraged to gain liberally, at least 35 to 45 lb. Teenagers within 2 years of menarche are advised to gain about 5 lb more than mature women.

Determining Baselines

The amount of weight to be gained is based on the assessed nutritional status and **body mass index** (BMI). See Figure 10-2 for method of determining the BMI using prepregnant weight. A sample showing the percent over and under weight for the medium frame appears in Table 10-2. Frame type can be determined by using Table 10-3.

Low weight: Less than 90% of the ideal standard weight for height or a BMI of less than 19.8. Recommended weight gain: 28 to 40 lb, with at least 0.5 kg/wk during the first two trimesters.

Table **10-1**	**Distribution of Weight Gained during Pregnancy**
Body Part	**Weight (lb)**
Breasts	1.0-1.5
Blood	3.0-4.5
Extra water	4.0-6.0
Stores of fat	4.0-6.5
Uterus	2.5-3.0
Placenta	1.5-2.0
Amniotic fluid	2.0-3.5
Infant	7.0-8.0
Total	25-35 lb

Modified from Dimperio D: *Prenatal nutrition: clinical guidelines for nurses,* White Plains, NY, 1988, March of Dimes Birth Defects Foundation, p 21.

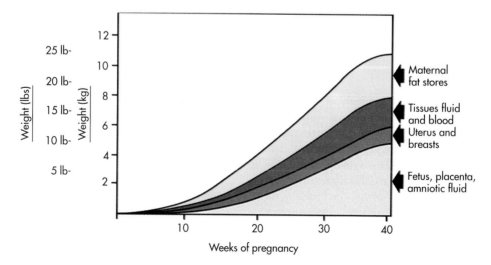

Figure 10-1   The components of weight gain in pregnancy. A weight gain of 25 to 35 lb is recommended. Note the various components total about 25 lb. (From Wardlaw GM, Insel PM: *Perspectives in nutrition,* ed 2, St Louis, 1993, Mosby.)

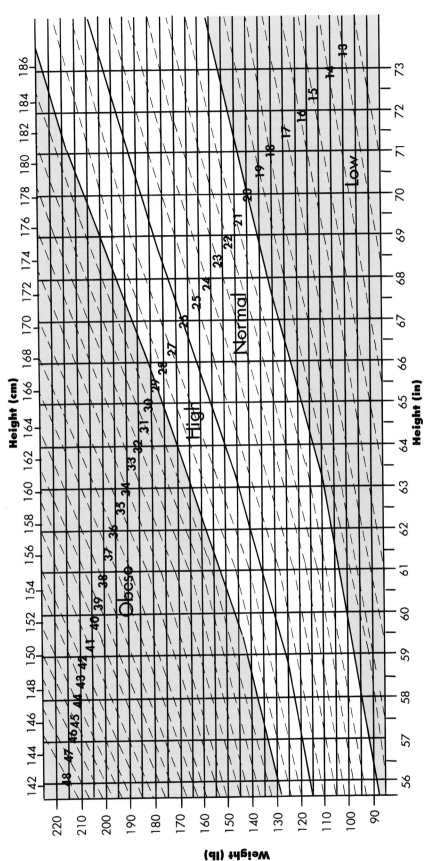

Figure 10-2   Chart for estimating body mass index (BMI). Find the point where height and weight intersect. Read the bold number on the dashed line closest to this intersection. (From National Academy of Sciences: *Nutrition during pregnancy and lactation; an implementation guide*, Washington, DC, 1992, National Academy Press.)

| Table 10-2 | **Height and Weight for Women (Medium Frame)*** | | |

Weight in Pounds
(indoor clothing, no shoes)

Height	A (90%-100%)	B (101%-119%)	C (120%-139%)
4'10"	103	103-123	124-143
4'11"	106	106-126	127-147
5'0"	109	109-130	131-152
5'1"	112	112-132	133-156
5'2"	116	116-137	138-161
5'3"	120	120-142	143-167
5'4"	124	124-147	148-173
5'5"	128	128-152	153-178
5'6"	132	132-156	157-184
5'7"	136	136-161	162-189
5'8"	140	140-166	167-195
5'9"	144	144-171	172-201
5'10"	148	148-176	177-206

Modified from Metropolitan Life Insurance Co.
*Weight in column A is at or below the ideal. Weight in column B is considered 1% to 19% over the ideal. Weight in column C is 20% to 39% over the ideal.

Self-Discovery

Find both your frame type and actual weight for height. What is your BMI? ~

Weight Variations

Rapid fluctuations in the weight-gain pattern indicate that the client needs careful reassessment. Although there is cause for concern, this signal does not mean that the client is in danger, only that her status may have changed.

| Table 10-3 | **Determination of Body Frame by Height and Wrist Circumference for Women (Medium Frame)** | | |

Height (in) (without shoes)	Wrist Circumference (in)	(cm)
<63	5-6	14.3-15.8
63-65	5-6	14.8-16.3
66-67	6	15.3-16.8
68-69	6	15.8-17.3
70-71	6-7	16.3-17.8
>71	6-7	16.8-18.3

From Alton I, Caldwell M, eds: Health and Human Services: *Guidelines for nutritional care during pregnancy*, Chicago, 1990, U.S. Public Health Service Region V.
Lower measurement = small frame. Higher measurement = large frame. With palm facing up, measure right wrist with insertion tape or nonflexible measuring tape distal to styloid process (toward fingers from wrist bone).

Weight loss

During early pregnancy many women experience weight loss from vomiting. Because the weight loss is partially the result of dehydration, the nurse can quickly address the problem by stressing increased fluid intake. A moderate weight increase followed by a weight loss can result from diuresis after water retention. Weight loss related to other factors must be determined by close questioning, laboratory tests, and physical examination.

Inadequate weight gain

Inadequate weight gain is a gain of 2.2 lb (1.0 kg) or less *per month* in the second or third trimester. A client may have an ideal weight for height at the onset of pregnancy but then demonstrate insufficient weight gain during pregnancy.

Many women are driven by a fear of "becoming fat" and thus do not eat properly. Others are undernourished for a variety of reasons, including economic circumstances or lifestyle behaviors. Smoking has a detrimental effect on weight gain; other substances that influence weight gain are caffeine, alcohol, and drugs of abuse. Stressors of living also prevent adequate gain, including increased family tension, high levels of activity, or even exposure to the cold. In all instances of inadequate gain, contributing reasons must be determined. Appropriate referrals should be made for counseling to modify detrimental lifestyle behaviors. If economic problems exist, women should be referred to available food subsidy programs and other social services.

Inadequate food intake does not provide essential nutrients for mother and fetus. If sufficient calories are not provided for maternal and fetal growth, the woman's

Normal weight: At or near ideal weight for height or a BMI of 19.8 to 26.0. Recommended weight gain: 25 to 35 lb.
High weight: More than 120% of the standard weight for height or a BMI of more than 26.0 to 29.0. Recommended weight gain: 15 to 25 lb with 0.3 kg/wk during the last two trimesters.
Obese: More than 135% of the standard weight for height or a BMI over 29.0. Recommended weight gain: at least 15 lb, with 0.3 kg/wk during the last two trimesters.

The preceding numbers are recommendations, not absolute cut-off figures. Each woman should try to gain *at least the lower* of the figures in the range of weight for her baseline.

own body proteins will be mobilized for calories. Dieting and fasting during pregnancy will lead to more rapid development of ketoacidosis and hypoglycemia than in nonpregnant women. Ketoacidosis is poorly tolerated by the fetus and can lead to neurologic impairment.

If a woman with inadequate weight gain appears for prenatal care only near the end of her pregnancy, it is unrealistic to expect her to gain enough weight to catch up with total desired weight. The goal for weight gain from the point of entry into care should be *double the weight gain* recommended for the particular gestational age (i.e., 2 lb instead of 1 lb/wk) (ACOG, 1993).

Sudden increase in weight

The most common weight concern during pregnancy is a sudden weight increase. After establishing the accuracy of the weight, determine whether the increase is the result of prior counseling to increase caloric intake, stop smoking, or drink more liquids. A physical assessment to rule out twins or an excess of amniotic fluid may also be needed. Blood pressure measurement, edema assessment, and urine test strip analysis for proteinuria would indicate whether the woman is developing pregnancy-induced hypertension (PIH). One of the warning signs of this condition is fluid retention and thus weight gain beyond the normal rate. Edema may also be caused by insufficient protein and caloric intake or by unrecognized cardiac disease.

High weight gain pattern

Although some women are within the normal weight range during the first trimester they gain weight rapidly during pregnancy. A gain of *more than 2 lb/wk* in the second and third trimesters is considered excessive weight gain. A careful evaluation must be made of each client (Box 10-1). It is important to be sensitive to the client's perception of the weight gain. Some clients will fast, use diuretics or laxatives, or even avoid prenatal visits if they are worried about gaining too much weight. Encouragement to avoid these practices and a supportive exploration of the cause of the gain can be helpful. The client may then be able to plan her own interventions. Most importantly the client should not be made to feel guilty about the subject of her weight.

If a client appears for prenatal care having already gained excessive weight for gestational age, it is unwise to limit her intake. Going hungry only results in nutritional deficiencies for mother and fetus. Instead, analyze the types of food in her diet; a diet history will provide insight into the problem. Goals for the remaining weight gain should be set according to the phase of pregnancy (i.e., gain approximately 1 lb/wk in second and third trimesters).

Many normal pregnancies have been marked by gains of 50 to 60 lb; in these instances some of the weight is attributed to a greater increase in the plasma volume, which results in hematocrit and hemoglobin levels in the

Box 10-1	**Possible Causes of High Weight Gain Pattern**

Excess calories
High fat or sugar intake
Infrequent, large meals
Low activity level
Emotional eating
Weight gain after loss in early pregnancy
Smoking cessation
Pica (e.g., laundry starch, cornstarch, ice)
Undetected multiple birth
Fluid retention

low normal range and accompanying edema of the feet and ankles. Because the excess gain is due to fluid retention, these women need support and comfort measures rather than further limitation of calories.

DIETARY GUIDELINES

The Dietary Guidelines are issued every 5 years, and the 1995 version is the basis for the Food Guide Pyramid, which illustrates the balance between foods (Figure 10-3). When teaching dietary balances, place emphasis on variety, moderation, and ratios between foods (Achterberg et al, 1994).

Variety means eating a wide selection of food within a group and preferring no single group over another.

Moderation means eating reduced amounts of fats, oils, and sugars and eating food in recommended serving sizes (which are smaller than most clients imagine).

Ratios or *proportionality* means choosing more foods from the larger groups and less from the smaller groups.

Note that fruits and vegetables are now in separate categories, for the purpose of adding more complex carbohydrates and fiber to the normal diet.

Three other guidelines are provided in addition to those from the Food Guide Pyramid.

1. Use salt and sodium in moderation,
2. If alcohol is consumed, do so in moderation,
3. Maintain a healthy weight.

During pregnancy the guidelines change to discourage alcohol intake (see discussion in this chapter), but salt and sodium intake are not restricted. Changes in food intake are minor and are listed in Box 10-2.

NUTRITIONAL REQUIREMENTS

Calories

It has been estimated that 60,000 to 80,000 calories are required to complete the pregnancy or approximately 300 cal/day beyond the normal intake. The sedentary pregnant woman expends less energy than the active woman.

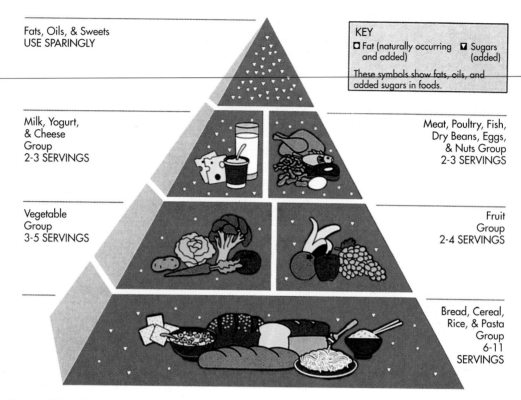

Figure 10-3   The Food Guide Pyramid includes guidelines for healthy nonpregnant people. Pregnant women should base diet modifications upon this food guide.

| *Box* **10-2**   **Minimum Daily Food Intake during Pregnancy** |

DAIRY PRODUCTS

4 servings (5 for adolescents)

Provides calcium, vitamin D, riboflavin, vitamin A, and protein

Serving size: 8 oz milk, I cup cottage cheese or ice cream, or I½ oz cheese

PROTEIN FOODS

3 servings (3-4 for adolescents)

Provides protein, vitamin B, and minerals

I serving from animal source: 2-3 oz meat, fish, or poultry (I egg = I oz lean meat)

I serving from vegetable source: ½ cup cooked beans or ½ cup nuts or 2 Tbsp peanut butter

FRUITS

2 servings

I serving from vitamin C source

I serving = I cup berries, I orange or apple, 6 oz juice

VEGETABLES

3 servings

Provides folic acid and vitamin A

I serving: Leafy dark-green or deep-yellow vegetables: Asparagus, broccoli, brussels sprouts, cabbage, dark leafy greens, carrots, squash, yams

Provides vitamins A, B, and C and fiber

2 servings: Other vegetables:

Serving size: ¾ cup raw or ½ cup cooked (cooking destroys folic acid)

BREAD, CEREAL, RICE, PASTA

6 servings

Provides vitamin B and iron (whole grains provide more vitamin B, additional minerals, and fiber)

Serving size: ½ - ¾ cup or I slice of bread

From Worthington-Roberts and Williams, 1993.

Table 10-4	**Functions and Sources of Major Nutrients**

Functions	Sources	Functions	Sources
PROTEIN		**NIACIN**	
Builds and repairs all tissues	Meat, poultry, fish	Aids in fat synthesis, tissue respiration, and use of carbohydrate	Peanuts, peanut butter
Helps build blood, enzymes, hormones, and antibodies	Eggs Milk, cheese		Meat (especially liver) Milk
Supplies energy: 4 cal/g	Dried beans, peas Nuts Breads, cereals	Promotes healthy nervous system	Enriched or whole-grain breads and cereals
		Promotes healthy skin, mouth, and tongue	Beans, peas
CARBOHYDRATE		Aids digestion and fosters normal appetite	
Supplies energy: 4 cal/g	Breads, cereals		
Unrefined products supply fiber for regular elimination	Potatoes Corn Dried fruits (smaller amount in fresh fruit)	**PYRIDOXINE (VITAMIN B$_6$)**	
		Aids in metabolism of protein	Meat, poultry, fish Whole-grain products
	Sugar, syrup, jelly, honey	Assists absorption of protein across intestinal wall	Legumes Potatoes, sweet potatoes Bananas
FAT			
Supplies energy: 9 cal/g	Shortening, oil	**VITAMIN B$_{12}$**	
Supplies essential fatty acids	Butter, margarine, cream	Assists in protein metab-	Meat, poultry, fish
Provides and carries fat sol-uble vitamins A, D, E, and K	Salad dressing Sausage, bacon Fat in meat	olism, including DNA synthesis and red blood cell formation	Small amounts in dairy products and eggs (supple-ments are required for vegans)
VITAMIN A		Functions in metabolism of fatty acids	
Assists formation and maintenance of skin and mucous membranes, thus increasing resistance to infection	Liver Dark-green and deep-yellow (orange) vegetables Deep-yellow (orange) fruits (e.g., peaches, cantaloupe)	**PANTOTHENIC ACID**	
		Aids in transmission of nerve impulses	Meat Milk, cheese, eggs
		Functions in production of energy	Whole-grain products Legumes
Functions in visual processes; promotes healthy eye tissue and eye adaptation in dim light	Butter, whole milk, cream Cheddar cheese Ice cream	Aids in synthesis of fatty acids and cholesterol	Peanuts Broccoli
		Functions in the formation of hemoglobin	Mushrooms Corn Sweet potatoes
Helps control bone growth			
THIAMINE (VITAMIN B$_1$)		**BIOTIN**	
Promotes use of carbo-hydrate	Pork, other meats Eggs	Assists in protein and carbohydrate metabolism	Organ meat Egg yolk
Contributes to normal functioning of nervous system	Enriched or whole-grain breads and cereals Dried beans, peas	Aids in synthesis of fatty acids	Legumes Peanuts Mushrooms
Promotes normal appetite and digestion	Nuts Potatoes, broccoli, collard greens	**FOLACIN (FOLIC ACID)**	
		Assists in DNA synthesis	Dark-green, leafy vegetables
RIBOFLAVIN (VITAMIN B$_2$)		Aids transmission of nerve impulses	Meat (especially organ meat) Nuts
Aids in use of oxygen and production of energy within body cells	Milk, cheese, ice cream Enriched or whole-grain breads and cereals	Assists in maturation of red blood cells	Legumes Whole-grain products
Promotes healthy skin, eyes, tongue, and lips	Meat (especially liver) Eggs	Plays role in prevention of neural tube defects (NTDs)	Yeast Asparagus
Helps prevent scaly, greasy skin around mouth and nose	Green, leafy vegetables		

From Buckley K, Kulb N: *Handbook of maternal-newborn nursing,* New York, 1983, John Wiley; modified from Gazella JG: *Nutrition for the childbearing years,* Wayzata, Minn, 1979, Woodland; Green ML, Green JH: *Nutrition in contemporary nursing practice,* New York, 1981, Wiley; National Dairy Council: *Nutrition source book,* Chicago, 1970, The Council.

Continued.

Table 10-4   **Functions and Sources of Major Nutrients—cont'd**

Functions	Sources	Functions	Sources
VITAMIN C (ASCORBIC ACID)		**PHOSPHORUS**	
Aids in production of cementing materials that hold cells together, thus strengthening blood vessel walls, hastening healing of wounds and broken bones, and increasing resistance to infection	Citrus fruits Strawberries Cantaloupe Tomatoes Broccoli, green peppers Mango, papaya Raw or lightly cooked greens and cabbage	Is a constituent of all body cells Regulates transport of chemicals into and out of cells; participates in energy production Participates in regulation of acid-base balance Aids in use of B vitamins	Milk products Meat, poultry, fish Nuts Whole-grain products Legumes
Aids in use of iron Helps regulate cholesterol level of blood			
VITAMIN D		**IRON**	
Aids in absorption and use of calcium and phosphorus, both of which are required for normal bone mineralization, muscle contraction, and conduction of nerve impulses	Fish liver oil Milk fortified with vitamin D Sunshine on skin (nondietary)	Combines with protein to form hemoglobin Functions as part of enzymes involved in tissue respiration Increases resistance to infection	Liver, other red meat Eggs Dried beans, peas Enriched or whole-grain breads and cereals Green, leafy vegetables
VITAMIN E		**SODIUM**	
Helps maintain integrity of cell membrane "Spares" vitamins A and C	Vegetable oils: corn, soybean, safflower, cottonseed	Participates in regulation of water balance Aids transportation of nutrients across cell membranes Aids maintenance of acid-base balance Participates in transmission of nerve impulses Participates in muscle contraction	Table salt Milk Meat, poultry, fish Eggs Green, leafy vegetables Swiss chard Celery Watermelon
VITAMIN K			
Is a factor in blood coagulation	Green, leafy vegetables Pork liver Eggs Vegetable oils		
CALCIUM		**POTASSIUM**	
Helps build bones and teeth Assists in blood coagulation Functions in normal muscle contraction and relaxation Functions in normal nerve transmission Helps regulate the use of other minerals in the body	Milk Yogurt Cheese Sardines and salmon with bones Turnip, mustard, and collard greens Kale Broccoli	Participates in regulation of water balance Required for protein formation Aids in converting glucose to glycogen Aids in transmission of nerve impulses Aids in muscle contraction	Meat, poultry, fish Whole-grain products Legumes Prunes Leafy vegetables Bananas Oranges, grapefruits Tomatoes Potatoes

Eating primarily *nutrient-dense* foods can make a dramatic difference in nutrition. Recommendations for nonpregnant women (shown in Figure 10-3) should be compared with the increases recommended for adult and adolescent pregnant women (see Box 10-2). Table 10-4 lists the functions and major sources of nutrients needed during pregnancy.

Protein

Protein is needed for building and repairing all maternal and fetal tissue and for the increase in blood volume and products, the growth of the placenta and fetus, and the formation of amniotic fluid. More than 20 different amino acids combine in different ways to form proteins. Eight *essential amino acids* are not synthesized by the body and must be supplied by diet. If a dietary protein contains all eight of the essential amino acids, it is a *complete protein*. Most complete proteins come from animal sources such as meat, eggs, or milk. Most vegetable sources of protein are *incomplete* and require combination with another source that will supply the missing essential amino acids (see Table 10-6).

During pregnancy the American Dietetic Association (ADA) recommends that adult women have at least four servings of milk or foods made from milk and three servings of meat or other protein foods each day. Adolescents, who have higher protein requirements because their bodies are still growing, may have the least protein in their diets. The ADA recommends five servings of milk foods and three or four servings of protein foods every day for the pregnant adolescent.

Carbohydrate

Carbohydrates are the main sources of energy in the diet. Most carbohydrates should come from *complex carbohydrates* such as whole grain breads, cereals, and vegetables. These foods have the benefit of containing other nutrients, as well as fiber. Fiber intake helps combat constipation, a frequent complaint in pregnancy. *Simple carbohydrates* should come from naturally occurring sources such as fruit and fruit juices rather than from sweets. Getting high-quality carbohydrates into the adolescent's diet may be a challenge. A discussion of better choices in fast foods may be more helpful than expecting a teenager to adhere to an ideal diet.

Fat

Fat has more than twice the calories by weight as carbohydrates. In addition to supplying energy, fat provides the essential fatty acids for myelinization of nerves and for membrane synthesis. Fat also supplies and carries the fat-soluble vitamins A, D, E, and K. Fat-deficient diets are rare in the United States; the common problem is a high intake of fat at the expense of other nutrients. If a pattern of high weight gain seems to be linked with caloric intake, a diet history often reveals high fat choices.

Vitamins

Vitamins help regulate the metabolism of carbohydrate, fat, and protein. Since most vitamins are not manufactured by the body, dietary sources are important. A balanced diet will supply most of the necessary vitamins and minerals, with the possible exception of iron and folic acid. As a precaution against deficiencies, vitamin and mineral supplements sometimes are prescribed. It is important that the pregnant woman take only supplements that are designed for use during pregnancy and are appropriate to her nutritional needs because an overdose can be as harmful as a deficiency. See the recommended changes in dietary allowances during pregnancy in Figure 10-4.

Fat-soluble vitamins

Vitamins A, D, E, and K are stored in the body, and thus large doses can be harmful. Megadoses of vitamins A and D have been shown to cause teratogenic effects. Excesses of

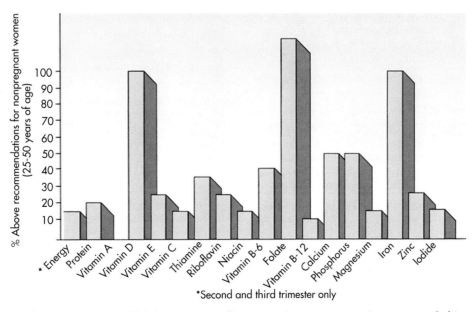

Figure 10-4   Changes in the RDA for pregnancy. During pregnancy, many nutrients are needed in greater amounts than at other times; these include vitamin D, folate, and iron. (From Wardlaw GM, Insel PM: *Perspectives in nutrition*, ed 2, St Louis, 1993, Mosby.)

these vitamins usually come from supplements rather than from diet. *Vitamin A,* which helps form and maintain skin and membrane tissues, is important in the mineralization of the fetal skeleton and in tooth bud formation. Too much vitamin A (more than 10,000 IU) can cause spontaneous abortion and fetal malformations. *Vitamin D* can be produced by the body when skin is exposed to sunlight, but it is also readily available in fortified foods such as milk. Certain Asian women and those living in the northern zones may be vitamin D deficient. They may need to take additional vitamin D because of a lack of sunlight and dietary patterns of low intake of milk products (Enkin et al, 1995). *Vitamin E* helps maintain the structure of cell membranes and increases absorption of vitamin A. *Vitamin K* is necessary to form prothrombin for normal blood clotting. Deficiencies of A, E, and K vitamins are seldom seen.

Water-soluble vitamins

Vitamin C and the *B-complex vitamins*—thiamine (B_1), riboflavin (B_2), niacin (B_6), folacin (folic acid), and B_{12}—are not stored in the body, and thus deficiencies are more common with these vitamins. *Vitamin C* is necessary for collagen formation, for tissue growth, and to increase iron absorption. Stress or infections increase the requirement for vitamin C, but megadoses are not advisable during pregnancy because cases of *rebound scurvy* can occur in the neonate when it is cut off at birth from high levels of vitamin C in the mother's blood.

The *B-complex vitamins* function mainly as coenzymes, working with other enzymes in metabolic reactions in the body. *Thiamine* helps in carbohydrate metabolism; *riboflavin* and *niacin* aid in the metabolism of fat, carbohydrate, and protein; *folic acid* assists in DNA and RNA synthesis; B_{12} helps in protein metabolism.

Folic Acid. The MRC Vitamin Study Research Group (1991) has proved that folic acid deficiency can result in defects in the development of the neural tube of the fetus (anencephaly or spina bifida). All women capable of childbearing or planning it are now encouraged to take 0.4 to 0.8 mg folic acid daily. If this is not done daily, a minimum folic acid intake of 0.8 mg with multivitamins, should begin 1 month before conception and continue until 3 months after conception. This precaution reduces the risk of a neural tube defect by two thirds and significantly reduces all congenital malformations (Enkin et al, 1995). To ensure that folic acid is taken by pregnant women, the U.S. Public Health Service is currently planning to require the addition of folic acid to flour (MMWR, 1995).

A woman who has previously had a child with neural tube defects is at higher risk for having another baby with the same problem. She is advised to continue to take 4.0 mg folic acid daily (which is 10 times the normal dose) if she intends to have another pregnancy. Exceptions are women taking the anticonvulsant valproic acid or women with vitamin B_{12} deficiency (Enkin et al, 1995).

Minerals

Iron

Iron is necessary for the formation of hemoglobin. A total intake of about 1000 mg is needed during pregnancy because of the increase in maternal blood cell volume, the formation of fetal blood, the creation of fetal iron stores for early infancy, and the loss of blood during delivery. The fetus needs about 350 mg of iron and is born at term with 75 mg/kg of iron stores (Institute of Medicine, 1990). Iron deficiency anemia is widespread internationally, but it is not common in a woman with a balanced diet. Because anemia increases the chances of LBW and perinatal mortality, women are screened for a hematocrit lower than 31% to 33% or a hemoglobin less than 10.5 to 11 g/dl, depending on the trimester (see Table 9-1). Chapter 23 discusses in detail the more severe anemias that may have an impact on pregnancy.

Iron absorption from the diet increases from the usual 10% to 20% to as high as 50% during later pregnancy, and some iron is conserved in the first trimester because there is no menstruation. Even so, it may be difficult to meet the later requirement for iron (5 to 6 mg/day). The National Research Council (1989) recommends an oral iron supplement of 30 mg/day in the second and third trimesters. Truly anemic women may be prescribed up to 60 mg/day. Other authorities do not recommend *routine* iron supplementation unless the blood studies show a clear indication of deficiency; in fact heavy iron intake and a high hematocrit have been associated with an increase in preterm birth and LBW (Enkin et al, 1995).

Recent studies that find weekly doses of oral iron are as effective as daily doses may change the methods of administration, decreasing side effects and increasing compliance. Box 10-3 lists teaching points to enhance iron intake during pregnancy.

Box 10-3	**Ways to Enhance Iron Intake**

Iron is absorbed best when taken between meals or at bedtime.

Absorption is decreased by 40%-50% if it is taken with meals.

Iron should be taken with fluids other than coffee, tea, or milk. Calcium binds iron.

Vitamin C sources enhance iron absorption, but it is not necessary to take iron with a citrus juice.

An iron skillet should be used to stir fry or simmer foods.

Iron is best absorbed when it is not enteric coated.

Childproof bottles should be used, since iron poisoning is the most common cause of pediatric poisoning.

Side effects of nausea, heartburn, bloating, and constipation are managed by reducing the iron dose or taking it at bedtime.

Modified from Engstrom JL, Sittler CP: Management of iron deficiency during pregnancy, *J Nurse Midwifery* 39(2):205, 1994.

Calcium and phosphorus

Calcium plays a major role in regulating nerve excitability, muscle contraction, and blood coagulation. Calcium and phosphorus facilitate mineralization of the fetal skeleton and deciduous teeth. The fetus acquires most of these minerals in the last month of pregnancy. If the woman is to have sufficient stores to meet the demand, she must increase her intake during the entire pregnancy. If the mother's stores are inadequate, the fetus is supplied but *demineralization* of her own bones may occur. Demineralization, particularly with frequent pregnancies, can contribute to osteoporosis later in life. Recent studies also indicate that calcium supplements may lower blood pressure and have a value in preventing or modifying gestational hypertension (Levenson and Bockman, 1994).

Calcium affects absorption of iron, and calcium absorption is itself blocked by aluminum-containing antacids. Anticonvulsant medications and corticosteroids that affect vitamin D metabolism will reduce calcium availability (Levenson and Bockman, 1994). Women who are not exposed to sunlight or who live in the far north must be assessed for calcium and vitamin D needs. The RDA for calcium during pregnancy is 1200 mg/day, an amount easily obtained by drinking a quart of milk each day.

Iodine

Iodine is a necessary component for the thyroid to regulate growth, metabolism, and reproduction. Iodine deficiency can cause retarded mental and physical development in the fetus. In areas where the iodine content in the water is low, use of iodized salt provides adequate intake.

Zinc

Zinc is a component of insulin, helps maintain the acid-base balance in tissues, and is important in RNA and DNA synthesis. Meats and other protein foods have a fairly high zinc content; thus a diet with adequate protein intake should have adequate zinc. Because the safe upper limit of zinc supplementation has not been established, use of zinc supplements is not advisable.

Sodium

Because fluid retention increases in a normal pregnancy, a *slightly larger* amount of *sodium* is needed to maintain an adequate blood volume. Therefore severe restriction of sodium is detrimental as it may cause neonatal **hyponatremia** (low blood sodium), as well as problems for the mother. Moderate intake of salt-seasoned and sodium-rich foods is appropriate during pregnancy. Sodium intake should be *2 to 3 g/day*, a goal easily reached in most American diets (Worthington-Roberts and Williams, 1993).

Supplements

A woman may think she is "ensuring" adequate nutrition by taking extra supplements. It is important for her to know that self-medicating with megadoses of vitamins or minerals may harm the fetus or herself. Multivitamin dosage regimens should be specifically designed for prenatal use and discussed with the client's health care provider. The best source of vitamins, minerals, and other nutrients is a varied, well-chosen diet.

High protein supplements are not recommended during pregnancy because there is no evidence of a benefit to the fetus, and in some cases there has been a higher incidence of small-for-gestational age infants (Enkin et al, 1995).

Fluids

Water is a vital component of a nutritious diet, aiding in digestion, absorption of nutrients, excretion of wastes, and maintenance of blood volume. Water also helps maintain body temperature. The pregnant woman should drink at least 6 to 8 servings (8 oz each) of fluid a day. The best choices are water, milk, and juices rather than soft drinks or caffeine-containing drinks. A compromise may be reached when habits are ingrained. A woman may agree to use juice in sparkling water rather than soda, cut down on her caffeine intake, or drink milkshakes made with milk, ice, and fruit if plain milk does not appeal.

Some women may perceive herbal teas and remedies as "healthy" or at least harmless. However, some can induce labor, harm the fetus, or act as a diuretic or emetic. The effect of many herbal preparations is simply unknown. A moderate amount of mint or rose hip tea is probably safe, but more exotic preparations should be avoided.

CULTURAL FOOD VARIATIONS

Culture has an impact not only on what we eat but also on how we think about food. Pregnancy is a time when many cultures advocate avoiding or including special foods. Some of these practices may be helpful, such as eating the traditional Chinese fish soup that is high in calcium made for pregnant women. Others may be problematic or *dysfunctional*, such as the belief of some Mexican-American women that animal-protein foods should be avoided during pregnancy. Other food preferences are *neutral*, meaning their use does not change nutritional balance (see Chapter 2 for cultural variations).

Examples of dietary considerations are seen in the Hispanic culture, in which certain foods are classified as hot or cold. It is believed that a balance between these two types of food is important. This can be a neutral food practice because there are many types of food in both groups. However, some Hispanic women avoid certain protein foods for fear of "marking" the baby. Alternative protein sources must be found. Milk consumption is often low, with soda, fruit drinks, and coffee being preferred. Calcium intake can be enhanced by increasing cheese intake or using nonfat dried milk in preparing homemade tortillas. See Figure 10-5 showing where hard-to-place Mexican-American foods fit into the Food Guide Pyramid.

The Chinese diet during pregnancy may vary widely depending on the region of the diet's origin. One common *dysfunctional* practice is washing enriched rice before cooking, which causes the loss of nutrients. Scanty milk intake can also be a problem, but soybean curd can be used in many ways and is a good source of calcium and protein. Vegetables are commonly stir fried, which is an *efficacious* practice minimizing nutrient loss (Kaufman-Kurzrock, 1989).

Table 10-5 summarizes some of the food preferences of various ethnic groups; these generalizations vary according to the woman's regional background and the degree to which she has adopted a generic "American" diet. In assessing the diet of an ethnic group it is important to find out which foods from each food group are acceptable to the woman and which beliefs influence her choices.

TEST *Yourself* 10-1

a. Contrast the methods of cooking vegetables in Table 10-5. Why is boiling vegetables for a long time a *dysfunctional* practice?
b. What might be the result of excessive sodium intake during pregnancy?

Vegetarians

Women who are vegetarians may need special help obtaining a balanced protein intake. Tables 10-6 and 10-7 indicate the modifications for vegetarians who add milk and eggs to the diet or use only milk products. If only meat is excluded, complete protein can be obtained by combinations of foods plus dairy products and eggs. If eggs or milk are excluded, more careful planning will be needed to obtain complementary protein from plant sources (see Table 10-6).

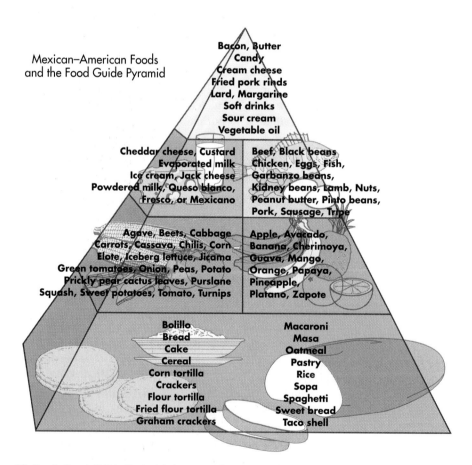

Figure 10-5   A Food Guide Pyramid showing where some hard-to-place Mexican-American foods fit.
(From Pyramid Packet, Penn State Nutrition Center, 417 East Calder Way, University Park, Pa. 16801.)

Table 10-5   **Cultural Food Patterns**

Milk	Meat	Fruits and Vegetables	Breads and Cereals	Possible Dietary Problems
NATIVE AMERICAN (MANY TRIBAL VARIATIONS; MANY "AMERICANIZED")				
Fresh milk	Pork, beef, lamb,	Green peas, beans	Refined bread	Obesity, diabetes, alcoholism,
Evaporated milk for	rabbit	Beets, turnips	Whole wheat	nutritional deficiencies
cooking	Fowl, fish, eggs	Leafy greens and other	Cornmeal	expressed in dental
Ice cream	Legumes	vegetables	Rice	problems and iron-
Cream pie	Sunflower seeds	Grapes, bananas, peaches,	Dry cereals	deficiency anemia
	Nuts: walnut, acorn,	other fresh fruits	"Fry" bread	Inadequate amounts of all
	pine, peanut butter	Root vegetables	Tortillas	nutrients
	Game meat			Excessive use of sugar
AFRICAN-AMERICAN				
Milk	Pork: all cuts (plus	Leafy vegetables	Cornmeal and hominy	Extensive use of frying
Ice cream	organs, chitterlings)	Green and yellow	grits	or simmering
Cheese: longhorn,	Beef, lamb	vegetables	Rice	Fats: salt pork, bacon
American	Chicken, giblets	Potato: white, sweet	Biscuits, pancakes,	drippings, lard, and gravies
	Eggs	Stewed fruit	white breads	High consumption of sweets
	Nuts	Bananas and other	Puddings: bread, rice	Insufficient citrus
	Legumes	fresh fruit		
	Fish, game	Vegetables often boiled		
		with pork fat, salt		
CHINESE (CANTONESE MOST PREVALENT)				
Milk in small	Pork sausage	Many fresh vegetables	Rice, rice flour	Tendency of some immigrants
amounts	Eggs and pigeon eggs	Radish leaves	products	to use large amounts of
	Fish	Bean, bamboo sprouts	Cereals, noodles	grease in cooking
	Lamb, beef, goat		Wheat, corn, millet	Limited use of milk
	Fowl: chicken, duck		seed	and milk products
	Nuts			Often low in protein, calories,
	Legumes			or both
	Soybean curd (tofu)			Soy sauce (high sodium)
SOUTHEAST ASIAN (VIETNAMESE, CAMBODIAN)				
Milk is generally	Fish (daily): fresh,	Seasonal variety:	Rice: grains, flour,	Poultry and eggs may be
not taken	dried, salted	fresh or preserved	noodles	limited
Coffee with con-	Poultry and eggs: duck	fruits and vegetables	French bread	Meat considered "unclean"
densed cow's milk	chicken	Green, leafy vegetables	"Cellophane" (bean	is avoided
Plain yogurt	Pork	Yams	starch) noodles	Preference for a diet high in
Ice cream (rare)	Beef (seldom)	Corn		salt and pepper, as well as
Soybean milk	Dry beans			rice and pork
	Tofu			High intake of monosodium
				glutamate (MSG) and soy
				sauce
FILIPINO (SPANISH-CHINESE INFLUENCE)				
Flavored milk	Pork, beef, goat,	Many vegetables and	Rice, cooked cereals	Tendency to prewash rice
Milk in coffee	rabbit	fruits	Noodles: rice, wheat	Tendency to have only small
(limited otherwise)	Chicken	Salads		portion of protein foods
Cheese: gouda,	Fish			
cheddar	Eggs, nuts, legumes			

From Lowdermilk DL et al: *Maternity and women's health care,* ed 5, St Louis, 1996, Mosby.

Continued.

Table 10-5　Cultural Food Patterns—cont'd

Milk	Meat	Fruits and Vegetables	Breads and Cereals	Possible Dietary Problems
JAPANESE (ISEI, MORE JAPANESE INFLUENCE; NISEI, MORE WESTERNIZED)				
Not common, increasing amounts being used by younger generations	Pork, beef, chicken Fish Eggs Legumes: soya, red, lima beans Tofu Nuts	Many vegetables and fruits Seaweed, rich in minerals Salad	Rice, rice cakes Wheat noodles Refined bread, noodles	Excessive sodium: pickles, salty crisp seaweed, MSG, and soy sauce May use prewashed rice
HISPANIC, MEXICAN-AMERICAN				
Milk Cheese Flan, ice cream	Beef, pork, lamb, chicken, tripe, hot sausage, beef intestines Fish Eggs Nuts Dry beans: pinto, chickpeas (often eaten more than once daily)	Spinach, wild greens, tomatoes, chilies, corn, cabbage, avocado, potatoes Pumpkin, zapote, peaches, guava papaya, citrus	Rice, cornmeal Sweet bread, pastries Tortilla: corn, flour Vermicelli *(fideo)*	Limited meats primarily because of cost Limited use of milk and milk products Large amounts of lard Abundant use of sugar Tendency to boil vegetables for long periods
PUERTO RICAN				
Limited use of milk products Coffee with milk *(café con leche)*	Pork Poultry Eggs (Fridays) Dried codfish Beans *(habichuelas)*	Avocado, okra Eggplant Sweet yams Starchy vegetables and fruits *(viandas)*	Rice Cornmeal	Small amounts of pork and poultry Excessive use of fat, lard, salt pork, and olive oil

Table 10-6　**Vegetarian Food Guide: Complementary Plant Protein Combinations**

Amino Acids Deficient	Samples of Complementary Protein Foods	Amino Acids Deficient	Samples of Complementary Protein Foods
IN GRAINS		**IN NUTS AND SEEDS**	
Isoleucine Lysine	Rice + legumes Corn + legumes Wheat + legumes, peanuts, or milk	Isoleucine Lysine	Peanuts + sesame + soybeans Sesame + beans or wheat Peanuts + sunflower seeds
IN LEGUMES		**IN VEGETABLES**	
Tryptophan Methionine	Legumes + rice Beans + wheat or corn Soybeans + rice + wheat Soybeans + peanuts + wheat + rice	Isoleucine Methionine	Lima beans Green beans Brussels sprouts Cauliflower Broccoli } + Sesame seeds, Brazil nuts, or mushrooms Greens + millet or rice

Modified from Lappe FM: *Diet for a small planet,* New York, 1971, Friends of the Earth/Ballantine.

Table 10-7   Modified Food Guide for Vegetarian Diets during Pregnancy

	Recommended Servings Per Day	
Food Group	Lactovegetarian*	Lacto-ovovegetarian†
Milk, yogurt, cheese	5	5
Protein		
Eggs (1 = 1 serving)	0	1
Legumes	3	3
Nuts	1	1
Fruits and vegetables (total)	9	8
Vitamin C	3	3
Vitamin A	2	2
Breads, rice, grain products	8	7

From Bobak IM, Jensen MD, Zalar MK: *Maternity and gynecologic care: the nurse and the family,* ed 4, St Louis, 1993, Mosby.
*Lactovegetarian: uses milk products but not eggs.
†Lactoovovegetarian: adds eggs to above diet.

The woman should use calcium supplements and vitamin D, which should be in prescribed doses. Protein and iron come from legumes, seeds and nuts, and dark-green, leafy vegetables. Whole-grain breads and cereals also supply vitamin B₆, iron, and protein. Fruits and vegetables supply vitamins A and C and minerals. The woman must adhere to the amounts recommended in Table 10-7. Vegetarians are motivated to achieve a healthy diet and may already have numerous resources. Low pregnancy weight and low weight gains can be problems in this group; thus high-energy foods can be recommended to help weight gain and to spare protein. Anemia may also be a problem for some vegetarian women.

TEST *Yourself* 10-2 _____

Mrs. Sharma is a vegetarian who does not eat eggs. What combination of foods should she eat to get enough complete protein in her diet if her main staple is rice?

Lactose Intolerance

Many people have difficulty digesting *lactose* (milk sugar) because they lack a sufficient amount of the enzyme *lactase* in the small intestine. This condition is known as **lactose intolerance.** When milk or milk products are ingested, gas forms in the large intestine and causes abdominal cramping, diarrhea, bloating, and flatulence. Lactose intolerance is more common in Hispanic, African-American, Asian, Arabic, and native American populations (see Chapter 28).

If a person merely dislikes the taste of milk, it can be incorporated into the diet in many ways, such as the addition of powdered milk to casseroles or liquid milk to soups, custards, and other foods. Because of slowed intestinal motility during pregnancy, the lactose-intolerant woman may find that she is more able to tolerate milk and some cheeses that are lower in lactose. Alternative sources of calcium can be supplied by legumes, nuts, dried fruits, and dark-green, leafy vegetables such as kale, cabbage, and turnip greens.

The lactase-deficient woman should consume as many dairy products as she can tolerate, taking Lactaid or similar enzyme preparations, but she should consume no more than 500 mg of these preparations at a time with meals. Calcium balance may need observation (Levenson and Bockman, 1994).

Fast Food

Fast food is available in almost every community in the United States, and many families visit fast food restaurants regularly. This habit is likely to continue throughout a woman's pregnancy, and especially in the case of adolescent pregnancy. It is unrealistic to expect women to totally avoid fast foods; it may be more helpful to educate them about more nutritious fast food choices. For instance, having a roast beef sandwich or plain hamburger rather than a superburger loaded with special sauce can mean 200 fewer calories and 5 teaspoons less fat. Choices that increase nutritional value include selecting baked potatoes rather than french fries, fruit juice or milk instead of soft drinks, frozen yogurt rather than cookies or pies, pizza rather than fried chicken, grilled items instead of those that are fried, milk products rather than sweets, and ketchup and mustard instead of sauces. Because fast food consumption often has a strong social function for the adolescent, it is important that she feel comfortable making healthy choices and that she receive support and praise for doing so. She is preparing to make nutritional choices for her child as well; thus supportive education can extend beyond the pregnancy.

NUTRITIONAL RISK FACTORS

A number of women are at nutritional risk because of lifestyle choices, poverty, adolescence, or eating disorders (Box 10-4). Severely underweight or obese women need evaluation for underlying medical problems (see Chapter 24). Certain elements are known to affect fetal health or growth, and clients, often partially informed, have many questions. Smoking, alcohol use, and drug abuse clearly affect maternal nutrition and fetal health. Pregnancy may motivate the woman to seek help in

Box 10-4   Significant Nutritional Risk Factors

ADOLESCENT
Increased nutritional needs, possible poor food habits
Frequent pregnancies or breast-feeding in past year
Depleted nutrient stores, especially iron and calcium

OVERWEIGHT
Increased incidence of pregnancy complications, possible poor food habits

UNDERWEIGHT OR POOR WEIGHT GAIN
Increased incidence of pregnancy and neonatal complications
Increased number of low birth weight (LBW) infants

CHRONIC MEDICAL CONDITIONS
(diabetes, phenylketonuria [PKU])
Need specially tailored diets to meet nutritional requirements and decrease complications

COMPLICATIONS OF CURRENT PREGNANCY
(anemia, hyperemesis gravidarum, preeclampsia, gestational diabetes)
Additional nutritional intervention needed for adequate nutrition

DYSFUNCTIONAL DIETARY PATTERNS
(pica, abuse of alcohol, use of drugs or tobacco)
May interfere with appetite, may displace nutrients

SOCIOECONOMIC FACTORS
(poverty, ethnic and language differences)
May interfere with ability to obtain nutritious food and with accessibility to nutritious resources

PSYCHOLOGIC FACTORS
(bulimia, anorexia, depression)
May have severe impact on food intake or absorption

withdrawal or tempering intake. Chapter 27 discusses in greater detail the woman with increased-risk social practices, and Chapter 28 discusses the potential for birth defects from these substances.

Caffeine

Heavy caffeine use appears to affect fetal weight on a dose-response scale; the more caffeine, the smaller the fetus. In one large study heavy users of caffeinated drinks had four times the risk of intrauterine growth-retarded infants (Fenster et al, 1991). Caffeine is found in coffee, tea, and cocoa. Tea also contains theophylline and cocoa contains theobromine. All three chemicals—caffeine, theophylline, and theobromine—have similar behavioral and physio-

logic effects (McKim, 1991). Many people do not realize that there are many other foods and drinks with caffeine-like substances. Most colas, including some clear-looking fluids like Mountain Dew, contain caffeine.

Warnings about teratogenic effects are based on studies of laboratory rats in which the equivalent of 80 cups of coffee were fed to pregnant rats. It may be reasonable to conclude that the usual adult intake of caffeine cannot cause structural birth defects. The important points are that caffeine *half-life* (the time when approximately half of the active drug is metabolized to be excreted) varies, and it has the longest duration in the last two trimesters (13 to 18 hours). Thus a pregnant woman who continues her prepregnancy caffeine intake schedule may receive a cumulative dose because caffeine is being excreted so slowly. The half-life in the newborn is even longer, about 4 days. Thus asking about caffeine consumption is important for the admission interview at labor time. Some fetal heart arrhythmias have been attributed to maternal coffee intake just before labor. The newborn may also experience withdrawal from caffeine in the initial recovery days.

London (1988) has shown that daily maternal intake of the caffeine equivalent of three cups of coffee, cola, tea, or cocoa poses no risk. This information should be used to counsel the pregnant woman who may have no desire for coffee but who may be controlling her weight by drinking numerous diet colas.

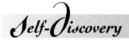

Self-Discovery

Analyze your daily intake of caffeine. Which foods containing caffeine do you take and in what amounts? ～

Smoking

There is much written about the adverse effects of smoking on the human body. Chronic stress is placed on the fetus, probably from hypoxemia; evidence is seen in its higher-than-normal hemoglobin level at birth. There is sound evidence that smoking causes biochemical toxicity. Nicotine, carbon monoxide, and hydrogen cyanide cross the placenta and enter the fetal blood, limiting oxygen access (Ventura et al, 1995). Severe vascular changes occur in cells of the inner wall of placental capillaries and major arteries, changes that may account for placental insufficiency and a reduction in the exchange of nutrients, oxygen, and carbon dioxide.

The rate of smoking during pregnancy for white women is currently 17% and is 13% for African-American women. Women without a high school diploma are more likely to smoke than women who complete high school (Ventura et al, 1995). Infants of smokers have twice the risk of LBW (<2500 gm). Reduced birth weight may be related to smoking's potential to decrease maternal nutrition (smoking affects the mother's appetite) or to the vascular changes in the placental tissue. If the mother stops smoking *before the third trimester,* the birth weight may assume the normal curve; other changes may not be improved (CDC, 1994).

The **fetal tobacco syndrome** includes weight reduction of 150 g to 300 g and premature birth. Lowered mental scores may result. Women who smoke are more likely to use caffeine and alcohol (Bottoms, 1996), and though the combination may obscure the signs of each, it may increase the risk for poor fetal and newborn health. Finally, passive smoking affects the infant. There is increased risk for sudden infant death syndrome, asthma, respiratory infection, and attention deficit disorder (Bottoms, 1996).

Prevention

Early in the pregnancy the woman should be taught the risks of smoking and should be encouraged to stop. If she cannot do so, she should cut back to no more than four cigarettes a day. If the woman increases her nutritional intake but does not reduce cigarette number, the fetal effects persist. If she stops or reduces the number and eats well, the fetus will gain more weight than expected. Therefore smoking cessation groups are an important part of prenatal care.

Alcohol

Confusion about alcohol in pregnancy occurs because studies indicate different results. It is clear that heavy alcohol use (six or more drinks a day or a single binge in the first trimester) results in the **fetal alcohol syndrome** (FAS), including overt signs of intellectual impairment with IQ as low as 40, neuromuscular disability, lag in growth, developmental delays, and facial characteristics recognizable at birth. These problems result from poor nutrition and the additive effects of caffeine and nicotine, since most heavy alcohol users also smoke and drink coffee (Aaronson and Macnee, 1989). Ethanol primarily disrupts neural development, affecting migration of neural and nonneural brain cells (there may be large holes in the brain tissue). Alcohol also affects brain cell size, resulting in a smaller mass of tissue. Finally, it changes acid-base balance and metabolism (Barbour, 1990). (Effects of alcohol on and care for the newborn are discussed in Chapter 27.)

Since 1981 the U.S. Surgeon General has advocated alcohol abstinence during pregnancy, and signs are posted where alcoholic beverages are sold. This action has raised the public awareness, which is critical to correcting the problem. In the early 1980s the FAS rate in the United States was 1:800 among users of alcohol. In France and Sweden it was 1:300. As has been done in the United States, both France and Sweden launched intensive drives to educate women about pregnancy and alcohol use.

Fetal alcohol effect

Moderate use of alcohol has been connected with a variety of learning deficits, and the widespread alcohol use in the United States may have contributed to the increased number of learning disabilities seen during the school years. The group of neurologic factors that contribute to learning deficits from alcohol are labeled the **fetal alcohol effect** (FAE).

Prevention

Prevention education must begin before pregnancy; it is in the early weeks of development that the most severe damage occurs. Questions about use must be asked of every pregnant woman early in prenatal care. Box 10-5 shows the measurement of alcoholic drinks and Box 10-6 presents nonthreatening questions with which to begin such conversations. It is important for the pregnant woman to know that structural defects that occur during the period of organogenesis cannot be reversed, but abstinence or a reduction in alcohol intake can bring a significant improvement in the size of the fetal brain cells. With improved nutrition, decreasing cigarette use, and abstinence from alcohol, the fetal brain has a better chance to grow. (See Chapter 27 for discussion of care of the increased-risk alcohol user during pregnancy.)

Pregnant Adolescents

Many adolescents enter pregnancy underweight or with diets deficient in iron, calcium protein, vitamins A, D, B_6, and folic acid. Factors that influence the adolescent diet

---

> *Box* **10-5**   **Alcohol Measurement**
>
> Single drink = 15 ml (¹/₂ oz) ethanol
> Approximate amount of alcohol the nonpregnant body can metabolize in 60 minutes:
>   12 oz beer
>   4 oz wine
>   1.2 oz 80-proof liquor

> *Box* **10-6**   **Introductory Questions to Ask About Alcohol Use**
>
> How do you use alcohol?
> Are you used to having some alcohol every day?
> Has your pattern of use changed over this year?
> Has your pattern changed since you have known about the pregnancy?
> Are you aware of the reasons alcohol is restricted when you are pregnant?

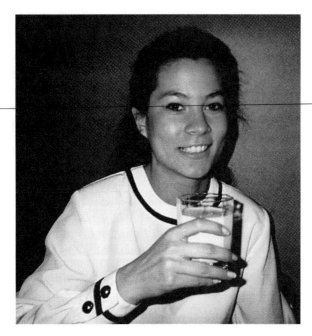

Figure 10-6   Five servings of milk products per day are recommended for pregnant adolescents.

often include the desire to be slim, peer group food practices, and irregular eating habits; more than 60% skip breakfast or eat poor breakfasts. Fast foods and nonnutritious snacks may be mainstays of their diet. The teenager may not have total control of her diet if someone else does the cooking and shopping in her household. Substance abuse and bulimia are more common in adolescents and may be hidden factors that influence diet. Because adolescent pregnancy is more common in low-income groups, economic problems may limit food choices.

When counseling a pregnant adolescent, the nurse must remember that the adolescent is likely to be under a greater amount of stress than an older woman. She may not have the support of her family, the father of the baby, or her peer group. Discovering what foods she typically eats and likes, identifying any food groups lacking in her diet, and negotiating with her about adding needed nutrients are good starting points (Figure 10-6). Options for supplying breakfast may have to be "creative," such as a piece of pizza or a bowl of frozen yogurt. If a supportive relationship can be established, the teenager is more likely to ask questions or admit problems such as substance abuse or bulimia. Because it is unlikely that a nurse will routinely have time to spend with the pregnant adolescent, the teenager needs support groups in her community that may be able to meet more of her informational and emotional needs. A referral to WIC (the special supplemental food program for women, infants, and children) should be initiated for all pregnant adolescents whose income limits their ability to buy nourishing food.

Eating Disorders

Bulimia

Bulimia is a food binge followed by self-induced vomiting, taking laxatives or diuretics, or compulsive exercise. The behavior is seen especially among adolescents, although the rate has been estimated to be 4% in all women (Muscarini, 1996). Current research is focused on the role of the biochemical imbalance of serotonin and other factors connected to feeding and hunger.

The problem may not be evident because bulimic women tend to be secretive about their behavior and feel intensely guilty about it. Binge eating and vomiting creates for the fetus a detrimental biochemical environment characterized by unbalanced nutrition. In addition, bulimic women often abuse laxatives, which can cause malabsorption of nutrients.

Because bulimic women tend to be near normal weight, they are more likely to be fertile than anorexic women. Their weight gain in pregnancy may cause panic, thus increasing episodes of vomiting. Some will be able to stop vomiting and purging but will continue to binge, gaining large amounts of weight.

Because bulimia is a complex and resistant problem, the nurse's primary intervention is to participate in detecting the problem and making appropriate referrals. Appealing to the bulimic woman to take care of herself will not be effective because she is already struggling with that issue. Education about the nutritional needs of the fetus and feedback on the infant's growth (as indicated by fundal height measurements) may help reinforce the need to provide the fetus with nutritional support.

Undiscovered bulimia can be confused with hyperemesis gravidarum, but the distinction usually can be made during hospital management of a vomiting crisis. The person who truly wants to eat and gain weight will respond to physical interventions, whereas the woman with bulimia requires antidepressants and psychologic interventions.

Anorexia nervosa

Anorexia nervosa is characterized by rejection of food, extreme weight loss, and low metabolic rate. Because of the severe impact of anorexia on the body, fertility is reduced greatly. Women with anorexia are rarely able to conceive or carry a pregnancy. If a pregnant woman has had a borderline case of anorexia or a history of it, she could have special needs because of being underweight and having depleted stores of vital nutrients. She may also need psychologic support to eat appropriately, since her perception of her body's growth may be exaggerated.

Pica and cravings during pregnancy

Pica is a persistent compulsion to ingest nonfood substances that have little or no nutritional value. Although reported more commonly in pregnant women who are African-American, live in rural areas, and have a family history of pica, the practice of pica is found in all regions, races, and economic groups (Cooksey, 1995). Women who have pica report craving ice, freezer frost, clay, flour, dirt, or laundry starch. Other substances include burnt matches, charcoal, cigarette ashes, mothballs, antacid tablets, baking soda and powder, coffee grounds, and plaster. Sometimes substances are only held in the mouth or sucked, such as pieces of the inner tubes of tires or gravel, whereas at other times large quantities of substances may be ingested. In addition to displacing needed nutrients, some pica substances may contain toxic compounds, such as lead in wall plaster. Other complications have been fecal impaction after clay ingestion, parasitic infection from contaminated soil, and small bowel obstruction from excessive ingestion of laundry starch. In rare cases pica has been associated with LBW and maternal and fetal death.

All pregnant women should be screened for pica on initial assessment. Iron deficiency and poor nutrition and weight gain may be seen in women who practice pica. Pregnant women who are anemic should be questioned about pica in case it was missed initially. The woman who practices pica will need education and counseling about the effects of her habit, but it may first be helpful to determine her reasons for the practice. Many have attributed their behavior to reasons based on superstition or custom that has been passed from mother to daughter (Cooksey, 1995). Women may be secretive and reluctant to "confess" their cravings. A matter-of-fact discussion may help women talk about their cravings.

Olfactory cravings, sometimes occurring alone or in combination with pica, can be harmful or neutral practices. **Hyperolefaction,** or a heightened sense of smell, is demonstrated in women who crave certain odors during pregnancy. Cooksey (1995) found a large sample of women who described cravings for odors from gasoline, bleach, ammonia, aerosol air freshener, pine oil cleaner, body powder, nail polish remover, and many other substances. Women may feel embarrassed by these desires, yet may find an irresistible need to indulge. The nurse must be a listener, realizing that these cravings will continue. The goal is to educate and assess nutritional intake. As Cooksey states, "Caregivers have an opportunity and responsibility to relieve women of their burdens of secrecy, shame, and guilt surrounding pica and craving for certain odors" (1995).

Nursing Responsibilities

ASSESSMENT

When the nurse assesses nutritional status, the measurement of height and weight and the determination of *body* *frame* size provide a baseline for evaluating weight gain throughout the pregnancy. A woman may find it helpful to plot her weight gain on a grid as long as she is aware that real gains will rarely fall exactly on the recommended line every time (Figure 10-7). It is important not to *scold* the woman but to *encourage* her by teaching and noting her progress.

Questions about food intake and culture should be asked; food preferences, nondietary intake (pica), and special eating habits or routines are all important. The home situation should be explored. Is there enough money to buy food? Are there adequate food preparation facilities? Does she have control over food selection?

The woman should be questioned about her intake of caffeine, alcohol, over-the-counter (OTC) medications, recreational drugs, and cigarettes. Her usual daily routine and activity level are important in planning to meet energy requirements for optimal weight gain.

A woman's physical appearance also provides clues about nutritional deficiencies; for instance, pallor, pale conjunctiva, and spoon-shaped, ridged nails may indicate iron deficiency. Many other signs of nutritional deficiencies are often nonspecific. Thus they are not reliable indicators by themselves and must be confirmed with laboratory tests and diet history.

Box 10-1
CLINICAL DECISION

A woman is 7 months pregnant and has gained only 10 lb over her prepregnant normal baseline.
a. What gain would you recommend for the remaining period of pregnancy and what are some strategies to achieve that goal?
b. List questions you might ask to elicit why weight gain has been so low.

Screening tests

Routine laboratory testing of hemoglobin and hematocrit levels is used to evaluate the woman's iron status. Hemoglobin, hematocrit, and serum ferritin measure iron deficiency. Urinary glucose and ketones screen for diabetes or insufficient intake. Folacin, albumin, total serum protein, and vitamin B_{12} levels may also be measured as nutritional indicators.

NURSING DIAGNOSES

Suggested nursing diagnoses include the following:
• Knowledge deficit regarding pregnancy-related nutritional needs
• Altered nutrition: at risk for more or less than body requires

Prepregnancy BMI <19.8(   ), Prepregnancy BMI 19.8–26.0 (Normal Body Weight) (   ), Prepregnancy BMI >26.0 (   )

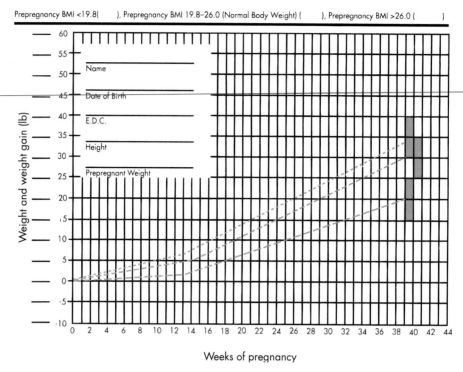

Figure 10-7   Prenatal weight gain chart. (From National Academy of Sciences: *Nutrition during pregnancy and lactation: an implementation guide,* Washington, DC, 1992, National Academy Press.)

- Altered health maintenance related to lifestyle, socio-economic status, age-related factors, or gastrointestinal (GI) discomforts

EXPECTED OUTCOMES

The following list provides samples of expected outcomes:
- Exhibits weight gain pattern consistent with expected parameters
- Identifies foods from each of the food groups in her diet and states plans for adding missing nutrients
- Hemoglobin and hematocrit levels remain within normal range
- States which nonpharmacologic interventions she will use for GI discomforts of pregnancy
- Seeks assistance from her health care provider if non-pharmacologic interventions fail to provide adequate relief

NURSING INTERVENTION

In the middle of the second month of gestation, the woman begins to notice taste and olfactory alterations. Her preferences for salty, sweet, and sour foods change. Often she will not be able to tolerate coffee or heavy desserts, and she may become nauseated. Some women state that these changed preferences were the first indication of pregnancy.

Interventions for nausea and vomiting

Although nausea and vomiting of pregnancy (NVP) is commonly called "morning sickness," the episodes can occur throughout the day. Nausea may be linked to patterns of activity, such as work routines. In most instances the problem is not serious enough to compromise nutritional status, though the duration of the episodes seems endless to the woman. The usual time of remission is by the end of the fourth month.

NVP is on a continuum with **hyperemesis gravidarum** (HG), the more extreme form that continues after 16 weeks and includes metabolic disturbance, carbohydrate depletion, dehydration, and electrolyte imbalances.

Ambivalent maternal feelings about the pregnancy is a psychologic component that may play a considerable role in HG. Interventions should be early, and women should know when to notify the caregiver about this more serious form of NVP. Fortunately, HG occurs in only 0.3% to 1.0% of pregnancies. Hospitalization is required for rehydration and medication and for the gradual reintroduction of foods into the diet. Parenteral nutrition may be required for a period of time.

Erick (1995) postulates that hyperolefaction contributes to NVP and HG. The nurse can inquire about which smells seem to trigger nausea and can encourage the woman to avoid these odors if possible. Among many other odors, cigarettes and ash, soiled diapers, and gasoline fumes can trigger nausea.

Supportive treatment is usually sufficient for NVP. Nonpharmacologic interventions are preferable and these include taking dry carbohydrates in the morning before arising, such as crackers, potato chips, toast, or pretzels; reducing fats, spices, and sweets in the diet; spacing food intake throughout the day in small, frequent meals to avoid having the stomach completely empty; drinking liquids between meals; and eating a high-protein snack before sleep. In addition, ginger ale, fruit juices, milk, and sour substances such as lemonade and pickles appear to reduce nausea. Cold foods seem to be tolerated better than lukewarm foods. The woman should choose what works.

Diet should be low in fat and should include proteins and carbohydrates that can be easily digested. Eating every 2 to 3 hours maintains blood glucose levels and prevents gastric distention. Supplemental iron should not be given until NVP has subsided (Davis, 1996). Because prenatal vitamins with folic acid are important, the woman should speak with the caregiver if she is having difficulty taking the daily doses.

Acupressure for nausea

Acupressure is effective for treating nausea. Using the first two fingers, pressure can be applied to the P-6 point on the wrist for 10 minutes 4 times a day and during episodes of nausea (Belluomini, 1994). The point is located 2 inches proximal to the wrist crease and between the tendons. The woman can also use Sea-Bands, elasticized wrist bands with a button that is placed over the point (Figure 10-8). One band is worn on each wrist (Beal, 1992). Women may complain, however, that the bands are uncomfortable and often slip.

Antiemetics

The standard antiemetic, Bendectin, was very effective and was taken by millions of women worldwide. Even though the danger of using it was never proved, it was removed from the market because of litigation. Sahakian et al (1991) showed that oral doses of vitamin B_6 (pyridoxine), significantly improved the condition of those with severe nausea and reduced vomiting in all the subjects.

For severe nausea, one of the antiemetics in the Drug Guide in Box 10-7 may be prescribed, but information on side effects and the benefit-to-risk ratio for potential effects on the fetus should be offered, and informed consent should be obtained.

Interventions for ptyalism

The woman with **ptyalism** experiences excessive saliva and typically has a dry, swollen tongue with swollen salivary glands, irritated perioral skin, and speech difficulties. Ptyalism affects the woman's normal eating patterns because of increased nausea associated with swallowing saliva. Interventions include having small frequent meals, chewing gum, and using oral lozenges or hard candy. The woman should use mouthwash frequently and wipe her mouth with nonirritating tissue. She should also be questioned about pica (Horner, Lackey, Kolasa, 1991; Van Dinter, 1991).

Interventions for gingivitis

Gingivitis, bleeding and tender gums, is related to increased peripheral circulation and will last throughout the pregnancy. Self-care includes increasing vitamin C intake through fruits and vegetables and avoiding trauma to gums. Careful brushing and flossing are important. A visit to the dentist may reassure the woman.

Interventions for heartburn and acid indigestion

The enlarged uterus may displace the stomach upward in the later part of pregnancy, causing a slight hiatal hernia (affecting 5% of women) that results in increased discomfort after meals. Heartburn, or reflux esophagitis, results from regurgitation of stomach contents into the esophagus, where gastric acids "burn" the lining. Heartburn is

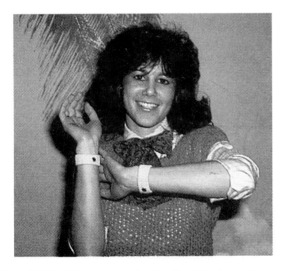

Figure 10-8   Woman wearing Sea-Band that exerts pressure on the P-6 point. (Courtesy Sea-Bands of Solon, Ohio.)

▌ *Box* **10-7**   Drug Guide for Antiemetics*

Vitamin B_6 (Pyridoxine) 25 mg PO QD
Promethazine (Phenergan) 12.5-25.0 mg Q6 hr PO or
    rectally
Hydroxyzine (Vistaril) 25-50 mg Q6 hr PO or rectally
Trimethobenzamide (Tigan) 200 mg Q6 hr PO
Perchlorperazine (Compazine) 5-10 mg Q6 hr or 10 mg
    IM Q4 hr, or 25 mg suppository Q12 hr rectally

From Scially AR: Nausea and vomiting. In Queenan JT, Hobbins JC, eds: *Protocols for high-risk pregnancies,* Cambridge, Mass, 1996, Blackwell Science.

*In *rare* cases there have been minor fetal defects after high doses of these drugs. Informed consent is advised.

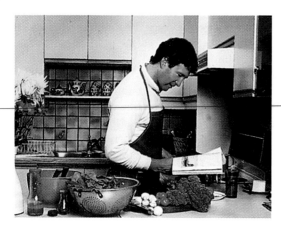

Figure 10-9 Nutrition is a family affair. (Courtesy Ross Laboratories, Columbus, Ohio.)

related to the relaxation of the lower esophageal sphincter (LES) and may increase in the last trimester. It is aggravated by large meals, spicy foods high in fat, citrus juices, and alcohol, and certain body positions (stooping or lying recumbent), heavy lifting, or straining at stool.

Acid indigestion is **pyrosis** and may include burping and an acidic taste in the mouth. A number of nonpharmacologic remedies are available for these two problems. In addition to the interventions for nausea, the woman should separate solid foods from liquids; avoid overfilling the stomach, rapid swallowing of cold liquids, ingesting gastric irritants (coffee, alcohol, tobacco), chocolate, and acidic juices; and recognize and limit gas-producing foods.

In addition, sitting up for an hour after meals, eating supper at least 3 hours before bedtime, and sleeping with a wedge under the mattress help prevent reflux into the esophagus. If these interventions do not seem to work, medication should be prescribed. Prescribed antacids contain combinations of magnesium and aluminum and/or simethicone (antiflatulant), since magnesium by itself causes diarrhea and aluminum compounds cause constipation and interfere with iron absorption. Histamine$_2$-blockers, cimetidine and ranitidine, have been used. Questions about the safety of the fetus exist when cimetidine is used, since it has an antiandrogenic effect on experimental animals. Ranitidine 150 mg in the evening is sometimes prescribed.

Interventions for constipation and hemorrhoids

Pregnancy is an appropriate time to teach health maintenance related to the intestinal tract. For instance, a high-fiber diet is known to be part of prevention of later colon cancer. The use of habit-forming OTC laxatives must be discouraged. Instead, the use of nonpharmaceutic interventions such as increasing daily fluid intake to at least eight glasses, adding prune or apple juice to the diet, increasing fiber and complex carbohydrates in the diet,

increasing regular exercise (especially walking), drinking warm fluids in the morning, and establishing a regular stooling time should be encouraged. If the medication is needed, the prescribed laxatives may be bulk-forming agents or emollients. Stimulants or lubricants such as mineral oil should be avoided. Suppositories to lubricate and soothe the anal area may be used if hemorrhoids are painful. Sitz baths or a tub bath in 6 inches of very warm water is also soothing.

When the pregnant woman's energy is reduced because of GI discomforts, the father may help with meal preparation (Figure 10-9).

Each woman should work out additions to her diet for healthy weight gain. Figure 10-10 is a sample dietary assessment form she can use to analyze her diet. She should keep a record of intake for a minimum of 3 days and check off what is missing from the four food groups. Although she may bring this record to the next prenatal visit, she can begin at once to add the missing ingredients. The nurse and client together should review the diet analysis at the visit and then continue to check diet progress during each subsequent visit (Figure 10-11). A registered dietitian (RD) is available for referral in some settings. The RD should receive referrals for all difficult situations that require more extensive counseling.

Women with socioeconomic problems may have a deficient diet because of the lack of education or money. For this reason, the women, infants, and children (WIC) federal supplemental nutritional program was established. The nurse should ensure that these women are enrolled during their first visit by initiating a WIC referral (Dobson, 1994).

Self-Discovery

Use the nutrition assessment form in Figure 10-10 to analyze your diet this week. Are there elements missing? How much fluid do you regularly drink each day? ~

Refer to Box 10-8 for a teaching plan for nutrition and GI discomforts. A nurse or dietitian conducts a class and distributes literature. The nurse in prenatal care should ensure that each woman receives information and should then assess the woman's understanding of how to achieve a balanced diet. An informed client can cooperate and gain self-confidence in her own choices.

EVALUATION

Evaluation of appropriate dietary intake takes place at each prenatal visit. The following questions may be asked in the process of evaluation:

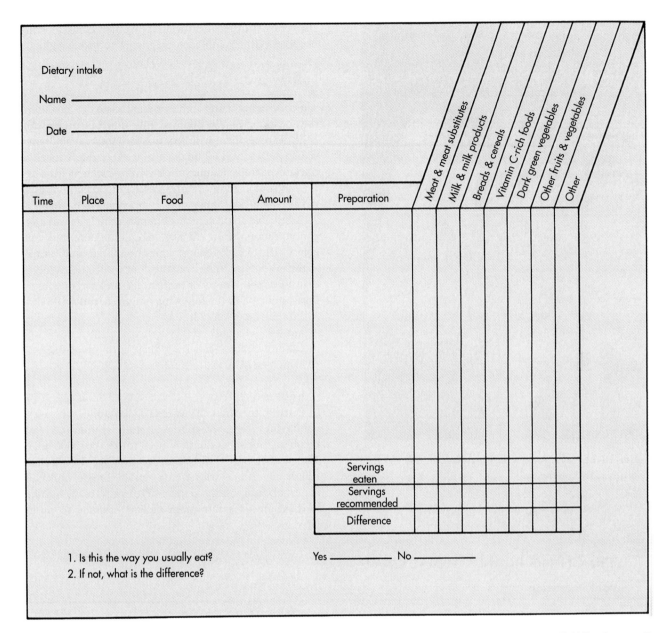

Figure 10-10 Dietary assessment form. (From Buckley K, Kulb N: *Handbook of maternal-newborn nursing,* New York, 1983, Wiley; Dimperio D: *Prenatal nutrition: clinical guidelines for nurses,* White Plains, NY, 1988, March of Dimes Birth Defects Foundation.)

- Was weight gained in a pattern appropriate to woman's status?
- Were woman's nutritional requirements met by adaptations in diet?
- Are there signs of anemia during pregnancy?
- Were gastrointestinal discomforts relieved without the use of OTC medications?
- Were referrals made for specialized nutritional requirements?
  The postnatal evaluation focuses on the newborn:
- Was the infant of normal weight and development?

MATERNAL NUTRITION DURING RECOVERY AND LACTATION

The postbirth period is a time for a woman to regain her prepregnant ideal weight. Nutritional requirements are generally the same as in the nonpregnant state, depending on body weight, height, and frame size. Since fat was stored for the lactation period, weight loss may be more difficult when a woman is not lactating. The amount of exercise a woman gets, the physical demands of child care, and her home situation will influence the rate at which

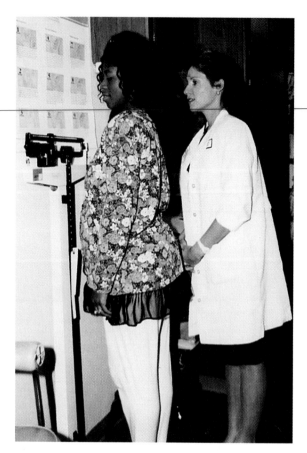

Figure 10-11   Weighing in during a clinic visit. (Courtesy Marjorie Pyle, RNC, *Lifecircle*.)

she returns to her ideal weight. Women complain that it becomes harder with each pregnancy to lose weight.

Lactation

The nutritional status of the mother has no direct relation to the nutritional *quality* of breast milk; if her nutritional intake is inadequate, there will be *less milk* but its quality remains stable. A lack of fluid intake also leads to the reduced production of milk. Human milk is very different from cow's milk in composition; all formulas are modified to be as similar as possible to human milk components (see Table 17-5). A remarkable characteristic of human milk is its variation in concentration during the day. In addition, fore milk (available at the start of feeding) varies from hind milk (available at the end). Hind milk contains four to five times more fat than fore milk. Levels of protein, fat, and carbohydrates in breast milk are in the following ranges (Bertino, 1981):

Protein—0.6-1.5 g/dl
Fat—2.1-3.3 g/dl
Carbohydrates—6.9-7.2 g/dl (in form of lactose)
Water—87%-95%

Calories

During the first 2 weeks of lactation, an average volume of 600 to 650 ml/day of milk is produced. As the infant matures, production rises to 950 to 1000 ml/day. The mother needs 30 calories to produce 30 ml of milk (there are 20 calories in 30 ml of breast milk). The maternal basal metabolic rate increases by 60%, and therefore she needs a minimum of 750 kcal/day to produce

 Box **10-8**

TEACHING PLAN *for* HOME CARE

Prenatal Nutrition

GOAL FOR WOMEN	INTERVENTIONS
Achieve desired weight gain for height each trimester. Track weight gain and graph weekly weight.	Record weight on chart and discuss rate of weight gain. Assess progress and nutrition plan during each visit. Explain causes of delayed or accelerated weight gain.
Use self-care steps to prevent or minimize each discomfort affecting nutritional state. Report discomforts as needed. Follow directions for interventions. Use over-the-counter remedies only if prescribed. State food groups and prepare a diet history to analyze her own diet.	Provide anticipatory guidance on self-care to minimize each discomfort affecting nutritional state. Emphasize avoidance of self-medication. Provide reason for increase in specific food groups and nutrients. Assist in diet analysis: teach substitutions for limited budget; refer for nutrition counseling or supplement food program when appropriate.
Recognize danger to fetus as a result of poor nutrition, smoking, and alcohol.	Explain risk of low birth weight and prematurity. Refer to smoking cessation group, if available; make other referrals. Clarify need to gain extra weight if unable to stop smoking.

enough milk for the infant (Blackburn and Loper, 1992). During the first 3 months of lactation, 200 to 300 kcal are provided from fat stores, allowing the woman to experience gradual weight loss without the need to take extra nutrients. After the desired weight is lost, the woman must add those 300 cal/day to her diet if breast-feeding. Even more is needed if she is breast-feeding twins or if she is underweight.

Protein

Lactation requires an increase in protein to 65 g/day, an amount obtained by the extra milk intake recommended during lactation. The daily milk requirement is 4 cups, which will provide all the extra calories, protein, and calcium required for lactation. If the woman does not like milk or is sensitive to it, other sources of protein and calcium can be used, and she should drink an equal amount of fluid. The nurse should encourage her to include a variety of alternative sources of protein in her diet.

A thin or malnourished woman may use extra milk to increase her protein and calcium intake. Since protein needs may pose a problem for vegetarians, many vegetarians allow protein increases when they understand the importance of the increase (see Table 10-7).

Other nutrients

Consumption of citrus fruits, vegetable oils, and dark-green, leafy vegetables satisfies the increased need for ascorbic acid, iron, vitamin E, and folic acid. Dark-green and yellow vegetables provide vitamin A. The breast-feeding mother may continue to take prenatal vitamins.

Fluid intake

Because the lactating woman produces 900 ml or more of milk per day, she should receive at least that amount of extra fluid through her normal intake. The importance of fluids to a new mother should be stressed. See Table 10-7 for fluid and nutritional recommendations.

Precautions

A mother often asks whether she should omit any foods during lactation. There is no physiologic basis for avoiding certain foods, such as curry, garlic, or small amounts of chocolate. Foods tolerated by the mother are generally tolerated by the infant. If there is a question about a food, the health care provider may advise omitting it on a trial basis (see Research Box).

Alcohol is also secreted in milk. Empiric data indicate that a small glass of wine or a light beer is unlikely to affect the nursing infant, and in a tired mother, it may assist the let-down reflex by increasing relaxation. Excessive amounts of alcohol, however, may inhibit milk ejection, and in alcohol abusers, inadequate nutrition will inhibit milk production and deplete the mother. Larger quantities of alcohol have a dose-response effect on the infant.

RESEARCH

PURPOSE OF STUDY

To assess the relationship among components of maternal diets and the presence of colic symptoms in exclusively breast-fed infants aged less than 4 months.

LITERATURE REVIEW

Approximately 10% to 40% of infants in the United States are diagnosed with colic. Colic is recurrent spasms of abdominal pain that begin 2 to 3 weeks after birth and usually abates after 4 months.

METHOD

Members of La Leche League were mailed questionnaires inquiring about the presence of colic symptoms in infants and the maternal intake of 15 foods, including cabbage, brussels sprouts, broccoli, and cauliflower. Women were also asked if they avoided certain foods because they thought the foods caused discomfort in their infant.

RESULTS AND IMPLICATIONS FOR PRACTICE

A positive relationship was identified between colic symptoms and cruciferous vegetables, cow's milk, onions, and chocolate. It was recommended that a trial elimination of cruciferous vegetables, onions, cow's milk, and chocolate be implemented for mothers whose infants experienced colic symptoms. A diet journal should be maintained to identify other foods that may also contribute to colic symptoms.

Lust K, Brown J, Thomas W: Maternal intake of cruciferous vegetables and other foods and colic symptoms in exclusively breast-fed infants, *J Am Diet Assoc* 96(1):46, 1996.

Smoking should be curtailed or eliminated during lactation. Passive smoking has been recognized as a major health problem, especially for young infants, because of the rapid absorption of smoke through the infant's lungs. Smoking also reduces the volume of milk produced by affecting the release of prolactin and oxytocin.

Caffeine in large quantities can cause the mother and infant to be jittery, wakeful, and irritable. Caffeinated beverages (coffee, tea, soda) should be limited to two servings a day. (See Chapter 16 for a complete discussion of drugs and lactation.)

TEST *Yourself* **10-3**

a. What factors inhibit adequate lactation?
b. How much fluid over baseline does a lactating woman need and why?
c. What are the dietary recommendations for lactating adolescents?

Key Points

- Adequate weight gain lessens the woman's chance of having an LBW infant who is at greater risk of morbidity and mortality than an infant of normal weight.
- Prepregnancy weight and height influence the amount of weight a woman should gain during pregnancy.
- Excessive weight gain in pregnancy is not always caused by excessive eating but may reflect increased body water.
- Megadoses of vitamins and minerals are harmful to the fetus and should never be taken during pregnancy.
- Moderation and variety are key principles in achieving a healthy diet. Frequent small meals are preferable.
- A woman's diet may or may not follow the common practices of her ethnic group; she can learn to assess her own dietary needs.
- Pregnant adolescents typically are at higher nutritional risk because of poor food habits and emotional and environmental factors.

- Eating disorders increase the risk of poor pregnancy outcomes, and interventions must be specific and consistent.
- A woman may overcome the adverse effects of smoking and alcohol abuse by discontinuing their use and increasing balanced nutrition.
- Morning sickness usually subsides by week 14 to 16; until then acupressure and vitamin B_{12} may be helpful. Antihistamines are prescribed as needed.
- GI discomforts require intervention to allow adequate nutritional intake during pregnancy.
- An informed client will be able to meet her self-care needs and gain self-confidence during pregnancy.

Study Questions

10-1. Select the terms that apply to the following statements:
   a. Inability to digest milk is caused by an inadequate amount of _____ in the small intestine.
   b. To have a balanced diet, _____ amino acids must be ingested.
   c. A common problem for a vegetarian is getting enough _____ and _____ in her diet.
   d. A compulsion to ingest unsuitable substances during pregnancy is _____.
   e. The fixed desire to remain thin by not eating is _____.
   f. Vomiting after eating large amounts is called _____ behavior.

10-2. Which factors increase iron absorption?
   a. Taking enteric-coated capsules
   b. Using milk and calcium supplements
   c. Taking iron supplements with citrus at bedtime
   d. Taking iron supplements with meals

10-3. Decide whether the following statements are *true* or *false*.
   a. Self-medication with therapeutic vitamins and minerals is permissible in some situations.
   b. Salt on foods and prepared foods with extra salt should be completely avoided during pregnancy.
   c. If a woman gains the amount of weight appropriate for the week of pregnancy, it is safe to assume her nutrition is adequate.
   d. Pregnant women should drink at least six glasses of fluid per day.

10-4. If a woman experiences heartburn, she should do the following:
   a. Lie on her left side after eating.
   b. Take a mild antacid in between meals.
   c. Assume a high Fowler's position when resting.
   d. Eat 6 to 8 small meals instead of a few large ones.

Answer Key

10-1: *a*, Lactase; *b*, essential; *c*, protein, iron; *d*, pica; *e*, anorexia nervosa; *f*, bulimic. 10-2: *c*. 10-3: *a*, False; *b*, False; *c*, false; *d*, true. 10-4: *d*.

References

*Aaronson LS, Macnee CL: Tobacco, alcohol, and caffeine use during pregnancy, *J Obstet Gynecol Neonatal Nurs* 194:279, 1989.

Abrams BF et al: Nutrition during pregnancy and lactation, *Prim Care* 20(3):585, 1993.

American College of Obstetricians and Gynecologists (ACOG): *Nutrition during pregnancy*, Technical Bulletin 179, Washington, DC, 1993.

American Dietetic Association (ADA): Position on nutrition care for pregnant adolescents, *J Am Diet Assoc*, 94(4):449, 1994.

Barbour BG: Alcohol and pregnancy, *J Nurse Midwifery* 35(2):78, 1990.

Beal MW: Acupressure and related modalities. II: application to antepartal and intrapartal care, *J Nurse Midwifery* 37(4):260, 1992.

Belluomini J et al: Acupressure for nausea and vomiting of pregnancy: a randomized blinded study, *Obstet Gynecol* 84(7):245, 1994.

*Bertino JS: The pharmacology of human milk, *Birth* 8(4):19, 1981.

Blackburn ST, Loper DL: *Maternal, fetal, and neonatal physiology*, Philadelphia, 1992, WB Saunders.

Bottoms SF: Smoking. In Queenan JT, Hobbins JC, eds: *Protocols for high-risk pregnancies*, ed 3, Cambridge, Mass, 1996, Blackwell.

Carruth BR, Skinner D: Practitioners beware: regional differences in beliefs about nutrition during pregnancy, *J Am Diet Assoc* 91:435, 1991.

Catalano M, Hollenbeck T: Energy requirements in pregnancy: a review, *Obstet Gynecol Surv* 47:368, 1992.

Centers for Disease Control and Prevention (CDC): Cigarette smoking among women of reproductive age—United States: 1987-1992, *MMWR* 43(43):789, 1994.

Cooksey N: Pica and olfactory craving of pregnancy: how deep are the secrets? *Birth* 22(3):129, 1995.

Davis DC: The discomforts of pregnancy, *J Obstet Gynecol Neonatal Nurs* 25(1):73, 1996.

Dawes MG, Grudzinskas JG: Repeated measurement of maternal weight during pregnancy: is this a useful practice? *Br J Obstet Gynaecol* 98:189, 1991.

Dobson B: A WIC primer, *J Human Lact* 10(3):199, 1994.

Editorial, Calcium supplementation prevents hypertensive disorders of pregnancy, *Nutr Rev* 50:233, 1990.

Engstrom JL, Sittler CP: Nurse-midwifery management of iron-deficiency anemia during pregnancy, *J Nurse Midwifery* 39(2):20(S), 1994.

Enkin M et al: *A guide to effective care in pregnancy and childbirth*, Oxford, 1995, Oxford University Press.

Erick M: Hyperolfaction and hyperemesis gravidarum: what is the relationship? *Nutr Rev* 53(10):259, 1995.

Fenster et al: Caffeine consumption during pregnancy and fetal growth, *Am J Public Health* 81:458, 1991.

Goldberg GR, Prentice AM: Maternal and fetal determinants of adult diseases. *Nutr Rev* 52(6):191, 1994.

Horner RD, Lackey CJ, Kolasa K: Pica practices of pregnant women, *J Am Diet Assoc* 91(1):34, 1991.

Institute of Medicine (IOM): *Nutrition in pregnancy*, Washington DC, 1990, National Academic Press.

*Classic reference.

Jackson R et al: Alcohol consumption guidelines: relative safety vs absolute risks and benefits, *Lancet* 346(8977):716, 1995.

*Kaufman-Kurzrock DL: Cultural aspects of nutrition, *Top Clin Nutr* 4(2):1, 1989.

Knowledge and use of folic acid by women of childbearing age—United States, 1995, *MMWR*, September 29, 1995.

Levenson DI, Bockman RS: A review of calcium preparations, *Nutr Rev* 52(7):221, 1994.

McKim EM: Caffeine and its effects on pregnancy and the neonate, *J Nurse Midwifery* 36(4):226, 1991.

Merlin R: Understanding bulimia and its implications in pregnancy, *J Obstet Gynecol Neonatal Nurs* 21(3):199, 1992.

MRC Vitamin Study Research Group: Prevention of neural tube defects: results of the Medical Research Council vitamin study, *Lancet* 338:131, 1991.

Muscarini ME: Primary care of adolescents with bulimia nervosa, *J Pediatr Health Care* 10(11):17, 1996.

*National Research Council, Food and Nutrition Board: *Recommended dietary allowances*, Washington, DC, 1989, National Academy of Sciences.

Newman V, Fullerton JT: Role of nutrition in the prevention of preeclampsia: review of the literature, *J Nurse Midwifery* 35:282, 1990.

Newman V, Fullerton JT, Anderson PO: Clinical advances in the management of severe nausea and vomiting during pregnancy, *J Obstet Gynecol Neonatal Nurs* 22(6):483, 1993.

Report of the Dietary Guidelines Advisory Committee: Dietary guidelines for Americans: 1995, *Nutr Rev* 53(12):376, 1995.

Sahakian et al: Vitamin B_6 is effective therapy for nausea and vomiting of pregnancy: a randomized, double-blind placebo-controlled study, *Obstet Gynecol* 78:33, 1991.

Ventura SJ et: Advance report of final natality statistics 1993, *Monthly Vital Statistics Report* 44(3S):2, 1995.

Worthington-Roberts B, Williams SR: *Nutrition in pregnancy and lactation*, ed 5, St Louis, 1993, Mosby.

Student Resource Shelf

Achterberg C, McDonnell E, Bagby R: How to put the food guide pyramid into practice, *J Am Diet Assoc* 94(9):1030, 1994.
Clearly presents methods of making the Food Guide Pyramid understandable to the lay person. Describes why the change was made from the Basic Four Food Groups to the Food Guide Pyramid.

Horner RD, Lackey CJ, Kolasa K: Pica practices of pregnant women, *J Am Diet Assoc* 91(1):34, 1991.
A summary of current knowledge about pica practices during pregnancy that concludes that pica is more prevalent than commonly believed.

Van Dinter MC: Ptyalism in pregnant women, *J Obstet Gynecol Neonatal Nurs* 20:206, 1991.
Discussion of ptyalism in pregnant women, including case studies and comfort measures.

11

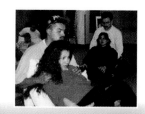

Assessment *of* Fetal Health

The recent advances in fetal assessment and testing are both comforting and disturbing. Although these methods of assessment can help couples increase their chances of having a healthy infant, the options provided lead to difficult choices.

Highly technical methods of assessment can distance nurses from clients. The nurse can lessen that distance by remembering that a thorough assessment begins with hands-on clinical skills such as listening and touching. The ability to blend "high-touch" with "high-tech" will con-

tribute to the client's comfort and well-being. Nursing care includes thorough preparation and support of parents during this time. Therefore the nurse must be familiar with all methods of fetal assessment.

Basic assessment begins with assessment of maternal health and family history (see Chapter 9). Many clients receive some type of antepartum testing. In fact, use of antepartum monitoring and ultrasonography has become a standard of care in most areas of the United States.

FETAL WELL-BEING AND MATURITY

Fetal health can be determined by fetal well-being and fetal maturity. **Fetal well-being** describes the fetus whose growth is appropriate for length of gestation and who has normal form and structure (morphology), metabolic functions, and adequate oxygenation and perfusion. **Fetal maturity** usually refers to pulmonary maturity, but neurologic, gastrointestinal, and metabolic maturity are also vital to survival after birth. Although prenatal care focuses on the prevention of prematurity, postmaturity also poses a threat to fetal and neonatal well-being.

Assessment of fetal maturity, or dating of the pregnancy, provides initial necessary information. Baselines for future evaluation of fetal growth and development are established by several clinical methods.

Fetal Movements

Historically, fetal movements have provided reassurance of fetal well-being to the pregnant woman and her health care practitioner. Movements provide the first subjective confirmation of pregnancy and are still used in the clinical estimation of gestational age. Fetal movement is discernible by ultrasound as early as 7 to 8 weeks of gestation, but fetal movements are not perceived as quickening (felt by the mother) until weeks 16 through 22.

Fetal movements may be an early alarm system in the last few months of pregnancy. These movements will decrease or disappear when the fetus is compromised. No standard exists because of the wide range of normal movements. Each woman needs to sense her own fetus's pattern and evaluate movements against that pattern. Daily fetal movement counts are now being used worldwide because no cost is involved. However, results are difficult to interpret and may lead a woman to come in for unnecessary testing (Enkin et al, 1995).

There are several patterns used to count fetal movements. The woman is taught one pattern suitable to her lifestyle that she uses at a convenient time of day. The Sadovsky method requires counting for 60 minutes three times a day. The Cardiff method requires a woman to begin at the same time every day and count 10 movements before she stops. The start and stop times are recorded. The following changes should be reported for follow-up evaluation:

1. Less than 10 movements in 12 hours
2. Lack of movement for 8 hours
3. Sudden increase in violent movements, especially if followed by reduced movement

During the ultrasound examination, increased movements may be seen. Objective assessment of fetal movements is included in the **Biophysical Profile Score** (BPS).

BIOCHEMICAL ASSESSMENT

Triple analyte screening is used to identify certain birth defects and chromosomal anomalies during the antepartum period. Triple analyte screening includes three tests: (1) levels of *unconjugated estriol* (uE3) and (2) levels of human chorionic gonadotropin (hCG) are compared with normal standards and low or high levels related to various problems, and with levels of (3) **alpha-fetoprotein** (AFP), which is produced by the fetal yolk sac and liver. As the liver matures, the levels of AFP fall. AFP enters the amniotic fluid through fetal urine and enters the maternal circulation as amniotic fluid is recycled. Normally AFP is detectable in maternal serum at approximately 7 weeks of gestation and rises steadily to its peak level at 30 weeks. Normal ranges exist for each week of pregnancy, therefore correct dating of pregnancy is vital to interpret the significance of levels (ACOG, 1994) (Figure 11-1). Maternal serum alpha-fetoprotein (MSAFP) screening is now being offered to all pregnant women between 16 and 21 weeks gestation. Any woman at risk will be offered further testing.

Neural Tube Defects

MSAFP levels obtained at 16 to 18 weeks gestation are used to screen for neural tube defects. When MSAFP

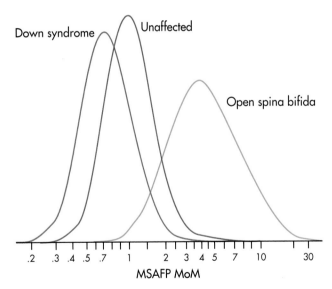

Figure 11-1 Maternal serum alpha-fetoprotein (MSAFP) curve. Distribution of MSAFP values expressed as multiples of median (MoM) for fetal Down syndrome (*blue line*) and unaffected pregnancies (*red line*), generated using data from Cuckle et al (1984). The distribution of MSAFP values for open spina bifida (*green line*) was generated using data from the United Kingdom Collaborative Study presented for comparison (1990). (From Knight GJ et al: Use of maternal serum alpha-fetoprotein measurements to screen for Down syndrome, *Clin Obstet Gynecol* 31(2):307, 1988.)

levels are high, further investigation for neural tube defects may be done with ultrasound examination and analysis of amniotic fluid for acetylcholinesterase, an enzyme found in fetal spinal fluid. Approximately 90% of anencephalic fetuses and 50% of those with open defects of the spine are identified by maternal screening followed by amniotic fluid analysis (Box 11-1).

Down Syndrome

A low level for MSAFP has been shown to be associated with Down syndrome. However, the relatively low sensitivity of this test as a screening test for Down syndrome (trisomy 21) has resulted in the addition of two other biochemical markers highly associated with trisomy 21. Low levels of unconjugated estriol (uE3) and elevated levels of hCG are also associated with Down syndrome. An algorithm (comparative table of values) based on age, race, and analyte values for these three tests has been used to calculate a client specific risk for trisomy 21 (Simpson and Sherman, 1994; Reece et al, 1992).

TEST *Yourself* 11-1 _____

a. Distinguish between fetal well-being and fetal maturity.
b. Before AFP results are evaluated, it is important to consider which factors?

BIOPHYSICAL ASSESSMENT

Ultrasonography

Ultrasound waves are intermittent sound waves at a frequency beyond the highest range of audible sound. These waves are emitted by a transducer placed on the maternal abdomen. A clear gel is placed on the transducer before it is used to facilitate the transmission of these waves.

Types

Several kinds of ultrasound are used in obstetric **ultrasonography**; each produces a different type of image and therefore has different clinical applications.

A-mode ultrasonography. *A-mode ultrasonography* uses pulse-echo information to move the tracing made on the oscilloscope upward in an amount proportional to the intensity of the echo. Thus A-mode images will look like peaks and valleys from a baseline.

B-mode ultrasonography. With *B-mode ultrasonography* or brightness mode, the strength of the echo determines the brightness of the dots displayed on the screen, resulting in a two-dimensional image. Although the presence or absence of structures can usually be determined by B-mode ultrasonography, it is difficult to detect fine differences between them.

■	*Box* 11-1	**Conditions Related to Abnormal Levels of Alpha-Fetoprotein**

ELEVATED MATERNAL SERUM ALPHA-FETOPROTEIN (MSAFP)
Open neural tube defects
Fetal distress and death
Multiple gestation
Maternal diabetes mellitus
Rh isoimmunization

LOW MSAFP, LOW ESTRIOL, AND ELEVATED HUMAN CHORIONIC GONADOTROPIN (hCG)
Down syndrome
Maternal hypertensive

DECREASED MSAFP
Maternal hypertensive states

Gray-scale imaging. *Gray-scale imaging* relates echo amplitudes to varying intensities of gray, somewhat like a black-and-white television. Strong echoes are brighter, whereas less intense ones are a softer gray. Details of many placental and fetal characteristics become visible when this method is used (Figure 11-2).

If many serial gray-scale images are taken, these images will run together in real time and show movement (much like how the motion picture is a series of still photographs). Therefore the function of structures (such as fetal breathing movements and cardiac motion) can also be evaluated by *real time imaging*.

Risks versus benefits

Ultrasonic examination appears to present little risk of injury to the mother or fetus. There is little client discomfort. Results can be seen immediately and further studies, interventions, or reassurance offered promptly.

Uses in the first trimester

The early diagnosis of pregnancy by ultrasonic examination aids in the determination of the estimated due date (EDD) (Box 11-2). Ultrasonography is also used to determine the presence of an intrauterine contraceptive device (IUD). For the client who has signs of an ectopic pregnancy, ultrasonography offers confirmation for quick diagnosis and treatment. Clients who have had a previous pregnancy loss as a result of an ectopic implantation may be reassured by an early ultrasonic examination.

Diagnosis of multiple gestation is advisable because changes in the antepartum and intrapartum care of women with multiple fetuses can improve outcome. It is important to also know fetal size.

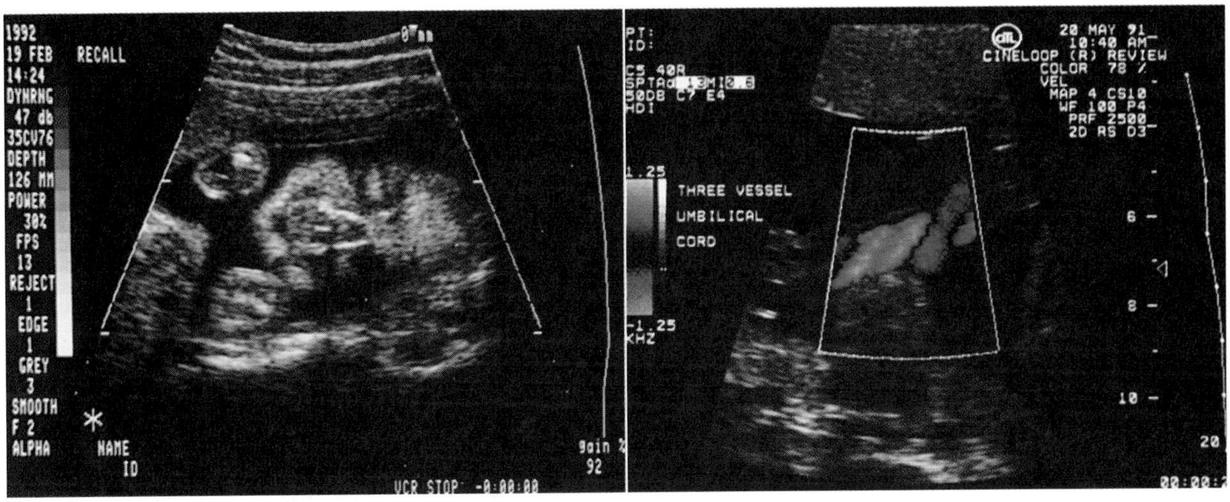

Figure 11-2 Two views of the fetus using ultrasonography. **A,** Fetal face (20 weeks). **B,** Umbilical cord (26 weeks). (Courtesy Advanced Technology Laboratories, Bothell, Wash.)

Box 11-2	Ultrasonography Uses in the First, Second, and Third Trimesters

FIRST TRIMESTER

Early dating and confirmation of pregnancy
Detection of an intrauterine contraceptive device (IUD)
Diagnosis of ectopic pregnancy
Diagnosis of multiple gestation
Assessment of placental location

SECOND AND THIRD TRIMESTERS

Assessment of placenta
Assessment of fetal body structure
Assessment of fetal growth
Visualization of fetus, placenta, and amniotic cavity during amniocentesis
Assessment of fetal position and presentation
Diagnosis of fetal viability
Biophysical Profile Score

Assessment of placental location is vital if the client experiences vaginal bleeding. Location of a low-lying placenta may be made through ultrasonic examination. The client is monitored closely during pregnancy because the placenta may "move up" the uterine wall as the uterus grows or may remain in the lower segment, possibly requiring cesarean delivery (see Chapter 21).

Uses in the second and third trimesters

During the second trimester, assessment of the placenta is done for clients who experience vaginal bleeding (see Box 11-2). Because ultrasonography detects soft tissue

location (in contrast to radiographic studies), placental condition may be assessed (Figure 11-3). The placenta may also be examined for grading, which is the detection of maturational changes caused by increasing calcification (Enkin et al, 1995). Changes in the appearance of the placenta are noted in the following areas: the chorionic plate, placental substance, and basal layer. Grading is used by some in the BPS.

Assessment of fetal defects by ultrasound allows identification of congenital problems and thus helps the family make a decision about the management of the pregnancy. In addition, advances in neonatal intensive care have given many infants with congenital anomalies a chance for survival. Interventions that begin before birth can maximize these chances. Ethical, religious, and legal issues influence the family's decision to continue or terminate the pregnancy (see Chapter 30).

Assessment of fetal growth is important because many maternal and fetal conditions can cause alterations. Because these conditions affect fetal well-being, oxygenation, and growth, their detection before fetal compromise is essential. If a fetus shows signs of growth retardation, further testing is done to assess its well-being. Serial ultrasonic examinations of fetal growth are more accurate than a single measurement. Several parameters of fetal physical growth should be examined and a **growth profile** determined. This consists of measurements of head and trunk size, soft tissue mass, length, weight, and proportions of body parts to one another.

Diagnosis of fetal viability is important for the woman who reports decreased or absent fetal movements. She will need confirmation of fetal viability or death as soon as possible. Real-time ultrasonic examination of the fetal heart will immediately reveal the presence or absence of cardiac activity.

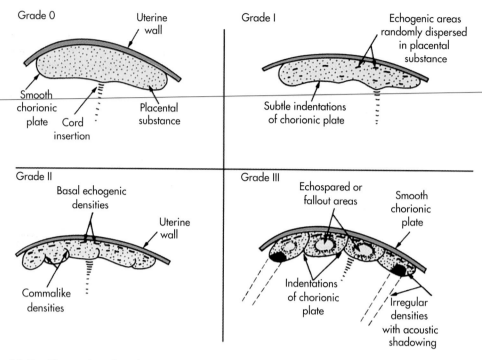

Figure 11-3 Placental grading demonstrates how the placenta ages. It can be used to assist in evaluating readiness or need for delivery. (From Grannum PA, Berkowitz RL, Hobbins JC: The ultrasonic changes in the maturing placenta and their relation to fetal maturity, *Am J Obstet Gynecol* 133:916, 1979.)

Doppler Velocimetry

Doppler ultrasonography, the basis of external fetal monitoring, has been applied to detecting the speed of blood flow through the umbilical vein and arteries. In *Doppler velocimetry* the systolic (S) rate of flow is compared with the diastolic (D) rate. The normal S/D ratio should be at least 3:1 after 30 weeks of gestation (Gregor, Paine, and Johnson, 1991). The time averaged mean velocity (V) is used to calculate the volume of blood flow (Q), or the cardiac output (CO). Abnormal CO may be seen in a fetus with a cardiac defect. Abnormal flow through umbilical vessels, and either vein or arteries can be seen when the fetus is affected by intrauterine growth retardation (IUGR) or placental abnormalities such as those found in severe hypertension (Reed, 1996).

If there is no diastolic end flow, impaired uteroplacental or umbilical circulation exists, and the fetus is in jeopardy. A high S/D ratio indicates preeclamptic changes in the placental vascular pressure (see Chapter 22). Doppler velocimetry is not performed routinely, but it is useful in conjunction with the BPS if complications are suspected.

Transvaginal Sonography

The technologic basis of **transvaginal sonography** is ultrasound, but the route is through the vagina with a probe that contains the sound wave source (Figure 11-4). It is

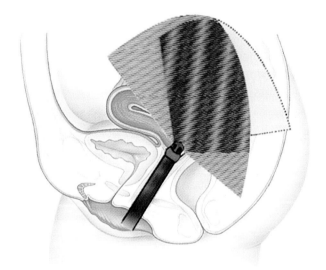

Figure 11-4 The major scanning planes of the transducer. Horizontal and vertical. (Redrawn from Modica MM, Timor-Tritsch: Transvaginal sonography, *J Obstet Gynecol Neonatal Nurs* 17(2):89, 1988.)

aimed at the deep pelvic tissues and is especially useful early in pregnancy; detection of the amniotic sac is possible by 4 weeks and 3 days (Timor-Tritsch et al, 1996). The transvaginal route allows the detection of ectopic pregnancy and is easier for the woman undergoing removal of ova for fertilization. Transvaginal ultrasonography can be used in cases of possible preterm labor, to detect if the cervix has changed shape and consistency (see Chapter 21).

Amniocentesis

Amniocentesis is the collection of amniotic fluid and its cellular components for antepartum identification of birth defects, genetic diseases, and fetal pulmonary maturity; evaluation of progress in pregnancies with isoimmunization; and treatment of polyhydramnios. When amniocentesis was initially performed in the 1930s, it was used to manage the fetus with Rh isoimmunization. Prenatal determination of fetal sex became possible in the 1950s by examination of cells found in amniotic fluid. In 1966 the technique for culturing amniotic fluid cells was perfected and yielded enough cells for analysis of chromosomes and biochemical study.

Uses

Amniocentesis can be used for genetic studies. It is offered to families at risk for specific genetic disorders and birth defects (see Chapter 27). For this purpose, it is performed from 15 to 18 weeks for genetic testing. The specimen contains sloughed fetal cells from the skin, bladder, and amnion, which are placed in a culture medium to grow. The culture takes 2 to 3 weeks, which creates the uncomfortable "tentative period" for the parents. Parent-infant attachment, which begins prenatally, is disrupted for the family who spends much time speculating about the test results and their choices; they must decide to continue or end the pregnancy if the results are abnormal (see Chapter 21).

Later, in the third trimester, amniocentesis may be performed to assess fetal status. Fetal pulmonary maturity indicates a rate of **surfactant** production adequate for pulmonary function. This state is usually achieved by week 35 of gestation, but the timing is variable.

Ultrasound is a valuable adjunct to amniocentesis. Before ultrasound, amniocentesis was performed without direct visualization of the fetus, placenta, and amniotic cavity. Accidental trauma to the fetus, placenta, or umbilical cord was common. The addition of real-time ultrasound during amniocentesis has made it safer to aspirate amniotic fluid.

Lung profile. Analysis of the lung profile is based on the lecithin/sphingomyelin ratio (L/S), phosphatidyl glycerol (PG) levels, and desaturated phosphatidylcholine (DPC) levels.

Lecithin and *sphingomyelin* are phospholipids produced by the type II alveolar cells. The L/S ratio increases with gestation (Figure 11-5), and a ratio of 2:1 indicates lung maturity. There are several potential problems with this ratio; thus other parameters must also be measured. Meconium or blood in amniotic fluid alters the ratio.

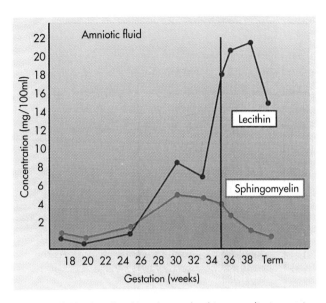

Figure 11-5   Levels of lecithin and sphingomyelin in amniotic fluid at increasing gestational ages. Note sharp rise in lecithin production at 35 weeks. (From Gluck L et al: Diagnosis of the respiratory distress syndrome by amniocentesis, *Am J Obstet Gynecol* 109:441, 1971.)

Biologic maturation of surfactant production can be assumed when PG, also a pulmonary phospholipid, appears in amniotic fluid after week 35. Maternal diabetes or contamination of the amniotic fluid with blood or meconium does not influence the reliability of PG as a predictor of fetal lung maturity.

Evaluation of fetal maturity can also be determined by amniotic fluid creatinine levels. *Creatinine* is excreted by the fetal kidneys when growth occurs. Creatinine amniotic fluid levels of more than 2 mg/dl reflect more mature renal function and muscle growth.

Amniocentesis can be used to evaluate pregnancies complicated by isoimmunization (see Chapter 23). As the excess unconjugated bilirubin produced by the affected fetus is only partially metabolized by the mother, much of it seeps into amniotic fluid, which is analyzed to determine the degree of fetal involvement.

This method can also be used to treat effects of *polyhydramnios*. Polyhydramnios complicates pregnancy when excess amniotic fluid causes uterine overdistention with increased pressure on surrounding organs. Unusual amounts of amniotic fluid are associated with specific fetal malformations. Amniocentesis may be performed several times during pregnancy to drain excess fluid and thereby relieve pressure.

Method

To undergo amniocentesis the client is instructed to wear comfortable pants and a blouse; the pants will be only partially removed during the procedure. Written consent is obtained. The woman is asked to empty her

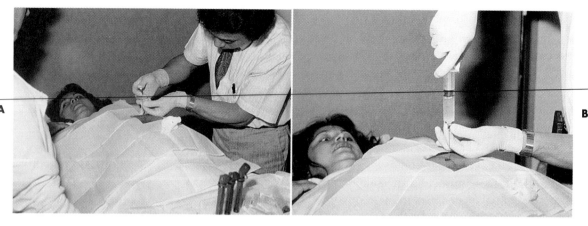

Figure 11-6   A, Under sterile conditions, a 10-cm, 20-gauge spinal needle is introduced through the abdominal wall into the amniotic cavity. **B,** As the needle stylet is removed, clear amniotic fluid slowly wells out and can be aspirated by a syringe. (Courtesy Marjorie Pyle, RNC, *Lifecircle*.)

bladder. She is positioned in the supine position; a rolled towel is placed for slight lateral tilt to prevent supine hypotension. As required by policy, maternal and fetal vital signs are monitored. A prepackaged sterile tray contains necessary equipment.

An initial ultrasound scan is performed to confirm fetal viability and gestational age, to identify gross structural anomalies, and to locate the placenta or pockets of amniotic fluid in relation to the fetus.

The following steps are performed to obtain amniotic fluid (Figure 11-6):

1. A site for needle insertion is chosen to avoid the placenta and fetus and yield an adequate amount of amniotic fluid.
2. The maternal abdomen is prepared with the antiseptic, and the sterile drape is placed.
3. Local anesthesia is optional. A 3-inch, 20-gauge spinal needle, attached to a 20-ml syringe, is inserted; when fluid begins to flow, the syringe is changed to avoid contaminating the fetal specimen with maternal cells.
4. Approximately 20 ml of amniotic fluid is collected for analysis.
5. The client is informed that she will feel pressure as this is done.
6. The needle is withdrawn. Monitoring of maternal and fetal vital signs continues for approximately one-half hour.
7. The Rh immunoglobulin (RhoGAM) is given to any mother who is Rh negative and not sensitized.

Risks

The client should know that she may experience cramping or local soreness. However, she should notify her physician or midwife if any of the following signs appear:

- Leakage of amniotic fluid at the site or in the vagina
- Localized or generalized signs of infection
- Decreased or increased fetal movement (when amniocentesis is performed after 20 weeks)
- Bleeding
- Persistent uterine contractions

Spontaneous abortion is a complication of amniocentesis in 0.25% to 0.5% (1/400 to 1/200) of women who undergo the procedure (MMWR, 1995). This rate is adjusted for the normal rate of spontaneous abortion during these weeks.

Chorionic Villus Sampling

Chorionic villus sampling (CVS) is performed early (10 to 12 weeks) for identification of genetic disease. Because it is possible to analyze the cells more rapidly, this procedure greatly reduces the waiting time. Results are available in 1 to 2 weeks.

Method

By means of ultrasound a transcervical catheter is introduced, and 15 to 30 mg of chorionic villi are aspirated from several sites into a 20-ml syringe. Alternately, a spinal needle may be used to aspirate placental tissue, via the amniocentesis approach (Figure 11-7). When the procedure is completed, the Rh-negative client is given Rh immunoglobulin prophylactically.

Risks

Complications of CVS are similar to those of amniocentesis and include amniotic fluid leakage, infections, bleeding, fetal death, and Rh isoimmunization. After adjustment for the normal rate of spontaneous abortion in the first trimester, the risk of abortion after CVS is re-

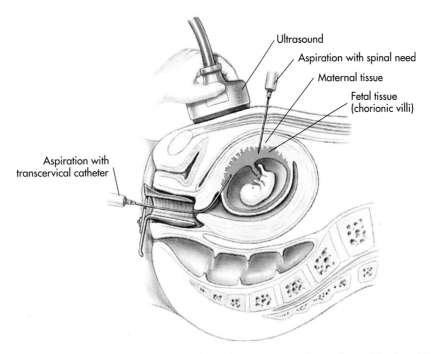

Figure 11-7   Chorionic villus sampling involves taking chorionic tissue for analysis of fetal problems. (Courtesy Medical and Scientific Illustration, Crozet, Va.)

ported to vary from 0.5% to 1.0% (1/200 to 1/100) (MMWR, 1995). Because the catheter must be passed transvaginally, the risk of infection seems to increase with the number of catheter passages needed to obtain the sample, leading some centers to limit this number to no more than three.

The infection rate with either amniocentesis or CVS is approximately <0.1% (MMWR, 1995). A higher rate of failure and infection is seen in primigravidas because of more resistance to passage of the catheter. There is also the potential for diagnostic error during CVS, especially if maternal tissue is analyzed by error or if a multiple gestation is unnoticed.

Limb defects caused by chorionic villus sampling. There have been reports of groups of infants born with transverse defects of entire limbs (in contrast to absence of parts of the fingers or toes) after CVS early in gestation. Some of these infants also have anomalies of the lower jaw, tongue, or both. The severity of the defect is directly related to the timing of the sampling, with risk for major limb defects being highest for infants who have undergone sampling before the ninth week of gestation (MMWR, 1995). The biologic mechanism for these defects is disruption of critical vascular supply to developing limb and jaw structures. Delaying CVS until the eleventh week of gestation appears to decrease the risk for these major defects, but the risk for defects of the digits (which are still developing) remains. Clients need to be aware of the benefits and risks of both CVS, which allows for earlier and safer termination of pregnancy, and amniocentesis.

Fetoscopy

Fetoscopy is a high-risk procedure for the visualization of the fetus. It has been replaced largely by ultrasound. Because of advances in technology, the use of ultrasound has made fetoscopy safer when it must be used for fetal blood and tissue sampling (Figure 11-8, *A*).

Fetoscopy is used to diagnose problems and treat the fetus in utero. Diagnosis may be obtained by direct visualization of fetal structures or analysis of samples of fetal tissue or blood.

Cordocentesis

Percutaneous umbilical blood sampling (PUBS) is a puncture of the umbilical cord (a cordocentesis) to obtain a blood sample while using ultrasound (Figure 11-8, *B*). It may be used to evaluate fetal blood components for diagnosis of anemias, blood incompatibility, and genetic problems. Also, a transfusion to the fetus is delivered through this route rather than into the peritoneal space.

Method

The cordocentesis begins with sonographic examination to locate the placenta and umbilical cord and to assess fetal growth and development. A flexible, small-bore "needlescope" (endoscope and needle) is passed through the maternal abdomen into the uterus and to the fetus or umbilical cord under ultrasonic guidance. Samples of fetal skin or blood are obtained for diagnosis of fetal genetic disorders. Intrauterine blood transfusion may be performed if

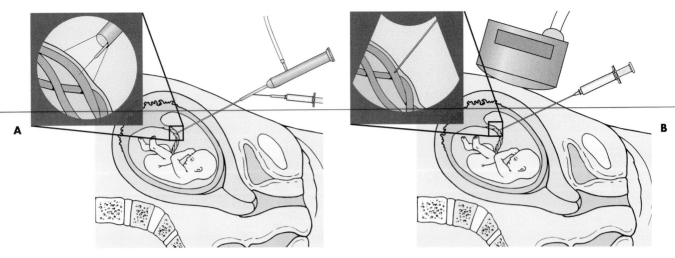

Figure 11-8   A, Fetoscopy has been used in the diagnosis of small fetal malformations (such as facial cleft or digital defects in families at risk for specific genetic syndromes), and for the visual guidance for fetal blood sampling, skin, and liver biopsy. **B,** Cordocentesis has now superseded fetoscopy for fetal blood sampling and fetal blood transfusions.

the fetus is severely anemic as a result of blood incompatability. After the procedure is completed, the **fetal heart rate** (FHR) is monitored to detect a nonreassuring FHR.

Risks

Infections, bleeding, and preterm labor occur in less than 1% of women who undergo cordocentesis.

TEST *Yourself* 11-2 _____

> a. How would you explain the use of ultrasound to a client with first-trimester vaginal bleeding?
> b. What is meant by the "tentative period" of pregnancy?
> c. Name three complications common to amniocentesis and CVS.

ELECTRONIC FETAL MONITORING

The introduction of **electronic fetal monitoring** (EFM) provided the opportunity to monitor continuous fetal response. Before its development, FHR monitoring was limited to sporadic auscultation, usually 30 seconds after the end of a contraction. Auscultation, however, cannot demonstrate periodic changes in heart rate patterns, baseline variability, objective assessment of uterine activity, and other parameters. Many devices have been used as fetoscopes, including hollow, wooden, cone-shaped devices and regular and specialized stethoscopes.

Antepartum Monitoring

Antepartum FHR monitoring is now more commonly used to establish fetal well-being. In general, testing is not begun until after approximately 25 weeks of gestation because FHR accelerations only become apparent by 25

weeks. However, earlier gestations of less than 30 weeks demonstrate more nonreactive testing because of immaturity of the fetal central nervous system, not because the infant is compromised. For this reason, FHR monitoring is not routinely done in most centers before 30 to 33 weeks.

Nonstress test

The **nonstress test** (NST) is used to identify the compromised fetus. During the NST the FHR is monitored for **accelerations** in relation to fetal movements. These accelerations are a sign of an intact and well-oxygenated central and autonomic nervous system. Most tertiary centers perform an NST as part of the BPS. Situations for which monitoring is recommended are found in Box 11-3.

Repeated monitoring by the same nurse or nurses in the NST unit allows the woman to establish a much-needed supportive relationship (Procedure 11-1). In addition, staff members familiar with subtleties of each individual's monitor strip will be better able to identify significant changes. A support person (family member or friend) may be present. Every effort is made to explain the procedure and its significance. In some centers, written consent is obtained.

Reactive nonstress test. A baseline FHR tracing is analyzed for baseline rate, changes, and variability in relation to fetal activity. The test is considered **reactive** if, during a 10- to 20-minute period, there are two FHR accelerations, each of at least 15 beats above baseline, lasting at least 15 seconds, and occurring simultaneously with fetal movements. A reactive NST (Figure 11-9, *A*) is considered a good predictor of fetal well-being for 1 week, although in some centers women with multiple risk factors may be tested two or three times a week. In some instances daily testing is indicated.

Nonreactive nonstress test. Lack of fetal movement during the test may indicate fetal sleep. The nurse should

| **Box 11-3** | **Indications for Antepartum Monitoring** |

MATERNAL INDICATIONS
Maternal diabetes
Maternal hypertension, essential or pregnancy induced
Maternal collagen or vascular disease
Drug use (therapeutic, tobacco, alcohol, or recreational)
Poor uterine or placental growth
Rh isoimmunization
Maternal heart or renal disease
Previous stillbirth
Vaginal bleeding in second and third trimesters
Premature rupture of membranes
Postterm pregnancy
Maternal age more than 35 years

FETAL INDICATIONS
Intrauterine growth retardation
Multiple gestation
Oligohydramnios or polyhydramnios
Assessment of fetus after amniocentesis
Decreased fetal movement
Selected fetal anomalies

---

attempt to rouse the fetus by gently manipulating the maternal abdomen (Figure 11-9, *B*). Fetal movements may also begin after maternal ingestion of fruit juice. The test period may be extended for an additional 20 minutes, or acoustic stimulation may be added. The healthy fetus who is not compromised by uteroplacental insufficiency will usually respond to these measures. Failure to elicit any FHR accelerations during the test may result from maternal drug use or fetal age of less than 32 weeks (this fetus may fail to exhibit accelerations because of immaturity of the central nervous system). Other factors affecting a false positive rate are aortocaval compression, lowered uterine blood flow, and recent maternal smoking (Goodman, Visser, and Dawes, 1984).

If the fetus fails to fulfill the criteria for a reactive test, uteroplacental reserve must be further evaluated. Figure 11-9, *B*, illustrates a **nonreactive** NST.

Acoustic stimulation test

Vibroacoustic stimulation, or the **acoustic stimulation test** (AST), by means of an artificial larynx sound has been used to stimulate the fetus who appears to be sleeping when the NST is performed. The sound is transmitted through the maternal abdomen and "wakes up" the fetus. According to the monitor record, within 5 minutes after the stimulus the fetus with a well-oxygenated central nervous system will show reactivity for a 10-minute period of two fetal heart accelerations of at least 15 beats above baseline lasting 15 or more seconds. Some infants are startled into a long period of active movement with a long period of accelerated

FHR. Because there is an increase in baseline rate and in tachycardia in infants younger than 36 weeks, vibroacoustic stimulation is used less often in the early third trimester.

In many units the AST has largely replaced the longer NST. The test may take only 10 minutes, whereas the NST may take 30 to 60 minutes. Thus the AST may be more efficient in the physician's office or the antepartal testing area (Miller-Slade et al, 1991). The AST may also be used during labor to check fetal responses when abnormal tracings appear. Research is still in progress, however, to confirm that the current levels of abrupt sound will not cause hearing loss in the fetus.

Contraction stress test

When a nonreactive NST is recorded, a few centers still may elect to do a **contraction stress test** (CST). An intravenous (IV) line is inserted, and increasing amounts of dilute oxytocin are infused for long enough to cause three contractions within 10 minutes. This may take 1 to 2 hours. A positive CST reaction means that significant FHR changes, such as late decelerations or bradycardia, result from poorer circulation to the placenta when the contractions occur. If the fetus cannot tolerate these mild contractions, intense labor may cause fetal distress, and a cesarean delivery may be considered. The value of CST is not considered worth the risk to the mother or fetus, and its use is being discontinued and replaced by the AST.

Mammary stimulation test

The basis of the **mammary stimulation test** (MST) is that nipple stimulus results in a release of oxytocin from the posterior pituitary. Because oxytocin receptors in the uterus increase just before labor, this test is more valid later in the third trimester. If oxytocin receptors have not developed in the uterus, the uterus will not respond in either case. The MST was developed on the basis of these factors, primarily to avoid IV oxytocin.

The test takes at least 20 minutes and requires no medication. The fetal monitor and tocotransducer are positioned, and a baseline strip is observed for 10 minutes. If uterine activity is present, it is evaluated for premature labor characteristics and the MST is *not done*. If uterine activity is *not present*, the woman lightly stimulates one nipple though her clothing for 2 minutes. She then rests for 2 minutes. The stimulation may be repeated once if there is no contraction response.

A major reason not to use this test is that if contractions become strong, endogenous oxytocin may not "switch off" as quickly as can be done with an IV flow. Contraindications to the use of CST and MST include premature rupture of membranes and threatened premature labor, third trimester bleeding, multiple gestation, and any complication in which fetal perfusion may be threatened. For these reasons the CST and MST are done much less often than formerly.

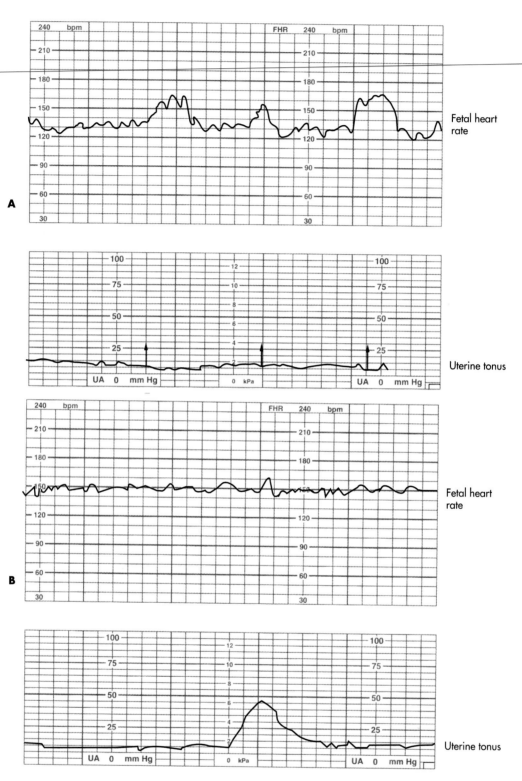

Figure 11-9   A, Reactive nonstress test (NST) (FM). Arrows indicate fetal movement with acceleration. **B,** Nonreactive NST. No fetal movements or accelerations are seen. (From Fields LM, Haire MF, Troiano NH: *Current concepts in fetal monitoring,* Pleasantville, NY, 1987, PPG Biomedical Systems, Inc.)

PROCEDURE 11-1

Nonstress Testing

Nonstress testing (NST) consists of the following steps:

1. The woman is asked to empty her bladder because confinement to bed or chair for at least 1 hour is probable. Fasting is not necessary; in fact, maternal hypoglycemia may adversely influence fetal activity.
2. She may choose the semi-Fowler's position with a lateral tilt or left lateral position; either will ensure adequate uterine blood flow.
3. Baseline maternal vital signs are obtained and reassessed regularly.
4. The tocodynamometer is placed over the fundus of the uterus. The ultrasound transducer is positioned over the point of maximal impulse (PMI), which is determined by finding the shoulder of the fetus by Leopold's maneuvers (Figure 11-10, A). (See Figure 14-2 for points on the abdomen to obtain the FHR.)
5. The woman is asked to record fetal movements by pushing a button on a cable (similar to a call bell) that signals the monitor pen to mark the tracing. (See placement of tocotransducer and ultrasonic transducer in Figure 11-10, B and C.)

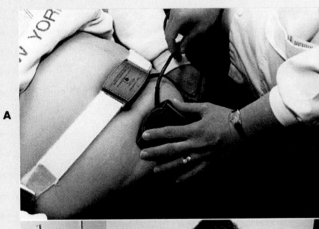

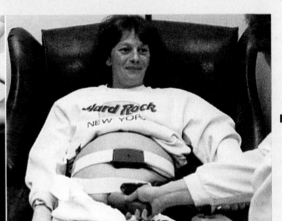

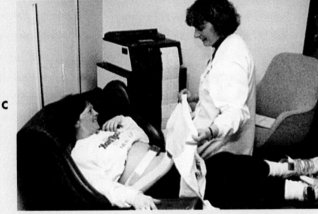

Figure 11-10   A, Beginning the nonstress test (NST) by locating the best fetal heart sound. **B,** Applying acoustic stimulation to measure reactivity. **C,** Comfortable position for NST. (Courtesy St John's Mercy Medical Center, St Louis, Mo.)

BIOPHYSICAL PROFILE SCORE

The BPS was developed by Manning and Platt in 1980 in an effort to better identify the compromised fetus. The BPS consists of five items: four observations made during ultrasonic examination—fetal muscle tone, movements, breathing movements, and amniotic fluid volume—plus the results of the NST. Some medical centers add placental grading to the five original parameters in the BPS so that a perfect score is 12. Table 11-1 illustrates this scoring of the BPS.

Scores of 8 or more are considered *reassuring,* and repeat testing is indicated within the week. Scores of 7 and under are *equivocal* and require retesting within 24 hours. Scores of 4 or less are considered *abnormal and worrisome* and indicate the need to consider delivery, especially because a score in the lower range rarely increases when the fetus is retested. The BPS is an accurate predictor of a

Table 11-1 **Biophysical Profile Scoring**

Criteria	Score		
	2	1	0
Fetal muscle tone (FT)	One episode of flexion/extension of fetal spine, limbs, or hand in 30 min	One episode of extension with return to flexion of extremities or spine	Extremities/spine in extension or slow return after slow extension
Fetal movements (FM)	Three or more episodes of fetal movements/rolling in 30 min	Two or less gross movements with 30-min observation	Absence of fetal movements within 30-min observation
Fetal breathing (FBM)	60 sec of continuous breathing within 30 min	One episode of FBM lasting from 30-60 sec during 30 min of observation	Absent respiratory effort or no episodes of >30 sec within 30 min of observation
Nonstress test (NST)	Two accelerations of 15 beats above baseline ×15 sec within 10 min of testing	One fetal heart rate (FHR) acceleration during 40 min of testing	No FHR acceleration during 40 min of testing
Amniotic fluid volume (AFV)	One or more pockets of fluid >2 cm in vertical diameter	Pocket less than 2 cm but larger than 1 cm in vertical diameter	Fluid pockets < 1 cm or absent, or polyhydramnios
Placental grading	Grade 0, I, or II	Placenta posterior and difficult to evaluate	Grade III

Data from Manning FA et al (1993) and Vintzileos et al (1983).

compromised fetus (Platt and Walla, 1996). It can detect the development of intrauterine infection and is performed to track onset of infection if preterm rupture of membranes occurs. Note that NST results are considered in relation to other parts of the BPS, and the decision to deliver the fetus with abnormal responses will be based on the entire BPS.

TEST *Yourself* 11-3 _____

a. Compare reactive versus nonreactive NST. What parameters would lead you to conclude that an NST was reactive or nonreactive?
b. Name and describe the areas assessed in the BPS.

Nursing Responsibilities

ASSESSMENT

Nurses manage NST and CST preparation and testing and may assist the physician with several other tests. In some settings, ultrasonography and BPS may be managed by nurses. The nurse must recognize reassuring, borderline,

and nonreassuring results and report these accurately to the physician. Legal problems can arise if the test is read incorrectly (see Chapter 14).

NURSING DIAGNOSES

A nurse involved with antepartum testing should consider the following nursing diagnoses:

- Risk for ineffective coping related to adverse findings
- Fear related to fetal health or illness
- Anxiety related to fear of the unknown and possible discomfort as a result of the procedure
- Risk for fetal injury related to hypoxia or specific invasive procedure

EXPECTED OUTCOMES

Because normal results of all fetal testing parameters do not always occur, families need to find healthy ways of coping with negative results and the decisions they must make based on those results. The following outcomes demonstrate the fulfillment of these needs.

- Family members will support each other during this experience.
- Client will demonstrate understanding of purpose and procedure of relevant assessment techniques.

Box 11-4   Antepartum Electronic Fetal Monitoring

NURSING PRACTICE COMPETENCIES

The nurse who will have responsibility for performing antepartum testing should demonstrate competency in intrapartum fetal heart rate (FHR) monitoring and subsequently complete an educational program to develop competency in antepartum electronic fetal monitoring (EFM). Before assuming responsibility for antepartum monitoring, the nurse should be able to do the following:

1. Describe antepartum testing criteria and indications for testing
2. Provide client education regarding the procedure and its purpose
3. Prepare the client by performing complete assessment using Leopold's maneuvers, palpating the fundus, and applying external EFM
4. Recognize contraindications to the use of oxytocin and nipple stimulation
5. Conduct the prescribed antepartum test
6. Communicate the content of EFM data for final interpretation in accordance with institutional policy
7. Document appropriate entries in the written or computerized client record and the EFM tracing or storage disk
8. Discontinue EFM according to institutional policy, procedure, or protocol
9. Communicate appropriate follow-up information to the client

From *Nursing practice competencies and educational guidelines: antepartum fetal surveillance,* Washington, DC, 1991, Nurses Association of the American College of Obstetricians and Gynecologists.

- Family members will express feelings about testing procedures, results, and their effects on the progress of the pregnancy.
- Threats to fetal well-being will be recognized and their effects minimized.

NURSING INTERVENTION

Antepartum fetal monitoring requires that the nurse understand the physiology regulating fetal heart responses. The nurse will need to seek additional education to develop the competencies listed in Box 11-4. The American College of Obstetricians and Gynecologists (ACOG) and the Nurses Association of the American College of Obstetricians and Gynecologists (NAACOG) (now AWHONN) published a joint statement that describes practice competencies for nurses involved in antepartum EFM (Box 11-4).

Support for the woman undergoing testing is a major nursing intervention. Without exception, women will be anxious about the results of the test and will need to discuss their concerns. Although the physician is responsible for obtaining the consent for any invasive procedure, the nurse will ensure that consent is informed and that the woman's questions are answered. The nurse monitors vital signs before and after such procedures.

EVALUATION

The opportunity to evaluate supportive nursing interventions varies with the work setting. When a woman has repeated testing, a more thorough evaluation may be done.

- Are reactions of family members appropriate to the situation and accepted by other members?
- Does the client verbalize concerns and ask questions?
- Were the fetal response and condition identified and potential injury minimized?

Key Points

- Rapid growth has occurred in the technology of fetal assessment. Techniques valued today may later be abandoned for safer and more accurate tests.
- Effective fetal therapy is already being used in some centers.
- All women are offered the option of testing for triple analyte screening in mid-second trimester, with follow-up triple analyte testing and amniocentesis if values are abnormal.
- Use of technologic advances may distance the woman from health care workers; therefore it is important to provide thoughtful interaction and explanations.
- Ultrasonography is a valuable tool to assess fetal well-being, growth, congenital anomalies, and general condition.
- The NST is performed for every woman with any risk factor. It may be repeated as often as three times a week in high-risk situations.
- NST is part of the BPS and can indicate when the fetus is compromised.
- Nursing interventions can smooth the path for women who must have testing because the fetus is at risk.

Study Questions

11-1. Select the terms that apply to the following statements:
   a. Protein produced by the fetal yolk sac and liver that enters the maternal circulation through the placenta and the amniotic fluid through fetal urine
   b. Intermittent sound waves produced at a high frequency
   c. Collection of amniotic fluid and its cellular components by needle tap
   d. Fetal heart accelerations occurring with fetal movements during a measured period of monitoring
   e. Aspiration of cells from the placenta for examination
   f. Startling the fetus into a response by means of sound pulse

11-2. At 36 weeks' gestation, Jane is instructed to count fetal movements. Using the Cardiff method, she should count the first 10 fetal movements beginning at the same time each day and note which of the following:
   a. Where the infant is kicking her
   b. If position change makes a difference
   c. A change in strength and frequency of movements
   d. Fetal sleep periods

11-3. Mary's MSAFP was unusually elevated at 17 weeks. To what conditions might this be attributed?
   a. Fetal hypoxia
   b. Open defects of the spine
   c. Down syndrome
   d. Maternal hypertension

11-4. Choose whether the following are true or false statements.
   a. A compromised fetus is one whose well-being is threatened by intrauterine environmental factors.
   b. Only fetal cells may be cultured from CVS.
   c. The tentative period after amniocentesis includes the time spent discussing alternatives to the final diagnosis.
   d. CVS carries half the risk of amniocentesis as far as causing abortion.

Answer Key

11-1: *a,* AFP; *b,* ultrasound; *c,* amniocentesis; *d,* NST; *e,* CVS; *f,* AST. 11-2: *c.* 11-3: *b.* 11-4: *a,* True; *b,* true; *c,* false; *d,* false.

References

Afriat CI et al: Electronic fetal monitoring competency—to validate or not: the opinions of experts, *J Perinatal Neonatal Nurs* 8(3):1, 1994.

American College of Obstetricians and Gynecologists: *Antepartum fetal surveillance,* Technical bulletin No. 188, Washington, DC, 1994.

American College of Obstetricians and Gynecologists: *Fetal heart rate patterns: monitoring, interpretation and management,* Technical bulletin No. 207, Washington, DC, 1995.

American College of Obstetricians and Gynecologists: *Assessment of fetal lung maturity,* Technical bulletin No. 230, Washington, DC, 1996.

Devoe LD: Automated methods of fetal assessment, *Clin Perinatol* 21(4):823, 1994.

Eden RD, Sokol RJ: Predicting prematurity: the mammary stimulation test, *Clin Perinatol* 19(2):291, 1992.

Enkin M et al: *A guide to effective care in pregnancy and childbirth,* Oxford, 1995, Oxford Univ Press.

Ferguson JE et al: Transcervical chorionic villus sampling and amniocentesis—a comparison of reliability, culture findings, and fetal outcome, *Am J Obstet Gynecol* 163(3):926, 1990.

*Goodman JDS, Visser FGA, Dawes GS: Effects of cigarette smoking on fetal trunk movement, fetal breathing movements and the fetal heart rate, *Br J Obstet Gynaecol* 91:657, 1984.

Goodwin L: Home fetal assessment, *J Perinatal Neonatal Nurs* 5(4):33, 1992.

Gregor CL, Paine LL, Johnson TRB: Antepartal fetal assessment, *J Nurse Midwifery* 36(3):153, 1991.

Gregor CL, Paine LL: Antepartum fetal assessment techniques, *J Perinat Neonat Nurs* 5(4):1, 1992.

Haddow J, Palomaki G: Maternal protein enzyme analyses. In Reece EA et al: *Medicine of the fetus and the mother,* Philadelphia, 1992, Lippincott.

Johnson TRB: Maternal perception and Doppler detection of fetal movement, *Clin Perinatol* 21(4):765, 1994.

Leerentveld RA et al: Accuracy and safety of transvaginal sonographic placental localization, *Obstet Gynecol* 76(5):759, 1990.

Lin CC, Verp M, Sabbagha R: *The high-risk fetus: pathophysiology, diag-nosis and management,* New York, 1993, Springer-Verlag.

Manning FA et al: Fetal biophysical profile score, VI: correlation with antepartum venous fetal pH, *Am J Obstet Gynecol* 169:755, 1993.

Miller-Slade D et al: Acoustic stimulation-induced fetal response compared to traditional nonstress testing, *J Obstet Gynecol Neonatal Nurs* 20(2):160, 1991.

Morbidity and Mortality Weekly Report: Use of CVS and amniocentesis, 44(RR-9):2, July 21, 1995.

Phelan JP: Labor admission test, *Clin Perinatol* 21(4):879, 1994.

Platt LD, Walla CA: Fetal biophysical profile. In Queenan JT, Hobbins JC, eds: *Protocols for high-risk pregnancies,* Cambridge, 1996, Blackwell Scientific.

Policy statement: Maternal serum alpha-fetoprotein screening, *Am J Public Health* 81(2):241, 1991.

Reece EA et al: *Medicine of the fetus and the mother,* Philadelphia, 1992, Lippincott.

Reed K: Clinical use of Doppler. In Queenan JT, Hobbins JC, eds: *Protocols for high-risk pregnancies,* Cambridge, 1996, Blackwell Scientific.

Simpson J, Sherman E: Prenatal diagnosis of genetic disorders, *Maternal-fetal medicine: principles and practice,* ed 3, Philadelphia, 1994, WB Saunders.

Smith CV: Vibroacoustic stimulation for risk assessment, *Clin Perinatol* 21(4): 797, 1994.

Timor-Tritsch IE et al: Can a "snapshot" view of the cervix by transvaginal ultrasonography predict active preterm labor? *Am J Obstet Gynecol* 174:990, 1996.

*Vintzileos AM et al: The fetal biophysical profile and its predictive value, *Obstet Gynecol* 62:217, 1983.

 ## *Student Resource Shelf*

Antenatal Fetal Assessment, *Clin Perinatol* 21(4), 1994.
   The entire issue addresses current status of antenatal fetal assessment.
Tucker SM: *Fetal assessment and monitoring,* ed 3, St Louis, 1996, Mosby.
   A handbook describing each of the methods of assessment.

*Classic reference.

12 Childbirth Preparation

Learning Objectives

- Describe basic philosophy and concepts of preparation for childbirth.
- Compare expectations of the woman in labor and her coach in selected methods of childbirth preparation.
- Explain the rationale for neuromuscular conditioning for labor.
- Demonstrate recommended exercises, relaxation techniques, and breathing patterns for labor.
- Relate the value of childbirth education to a couple's sense of control as they approach birth.
- Summarize the role of the nurse as health teacher in preparation for birth.

Key Terms

Birth Plans
Cues
Effleurage
Fear-Tension-Pain Cycle
Focal Point
Hydrotherapy
Hypnosis
Locus of Control
Nonpharmacologic Analgesia
Open-Glottis Pushing
Valsalva's Maneuver

*P*reparation for the birth of an infant takes several forms. Because couples may not have a supportive extended family from which to learn, childbirth education assumes increased importance. Nursing interventions can change perceptions of the childbirth experience, even for an unprepared couple. Therefore it is important that the nurse understand the support and teaching roles in childbirth education.

The availability of formal programs of prenatal education is a modern phenomenon. Girls and boys have always been educated informally for their roles as parents, and depending on culture and family setting, this education varies in its positive and negative qualities. Because of the changes in family structure, the nuclear family does not have the support system of the extended family that includes mother and father, cousins, aunts, and uncles. Pregnant couples that approach parenting without a clear notion of what it entails often seek preparation for childbirth.

METHODS OF PREPARATION

The two major approaches to preparing for childbirth in the United States are the *psychophysical method* and the *psychoprophylactic method*. The psychophysical method evolved from the natural childbirth movement in the 1940s and was founded on the writings and work of Dick-Read (Great Britain) and Thomas and Goodrich (United States). This program of education and exercise is directed toward breaking the **fear-tension-pain cycle** in which fear is replaced by knowledge, tension is replaced by relaxation, and pain is reduced by decreasing the perception of pain.

Gate-Control Theory of Pain

According to the gate-control theory of pain, pain is the result of interactions among three specialized neural systems. Melzack and Wall (1965) proposed that a mechanism in the dorsal horn of the spinal column functions as a gate that increases or decreases the flow of nerve impulses through the spinal cord to the brain. The gate can be closed, thus interrupting the flow of pain impulses by substituting other impulses such as tactile stimulation. Childbirth education must teach the couple techniques such as backrubs, effleurage, and sacral pressure, plus conditioning and other distraction methods, which are believed to interfere with pain impulses and thus modify pain sensations.

Because past experiences, attitudes, and emotions may also influence pain perception, discussing and sharing anxieties in the classes often relieve some of these concerns. Most courses now incorporate prenatal education with specific techniques that interfere with pain and thus provide some comfort during labor. Many courses also add a postpartum class, as requested by parents uncertain of their infant-care skills.

Each method of preparation for childbirth provides the couple with the means to cope effectively with the stress

Table 12-1   Comparison of Methods of Childbirth Preparation

	Psychophysical Methods		Psychoprophylactic Methods (Lamaze)	
Dick-Read	**Bradley**	**Kitzinger**	**Adapted**	**Classic**
RATIONALE				
Designed for women negatively influenced by cultural conditioning with the need to break fear-tension-pain cycle	Attempts to imitate other mammals' instinctive conduct in labor through intelligent reasoning	Mental and physical harmony produce a creative childbirth experience	Behavioral conditioning of mother produces reliable, constructive responses to demands of labor	Pavlovian conditioning raises threshold of pain by creating a zone of inhibition in cortex
PROVISION OF SUPPORT FOR MOTHER				
Medical labor attendants	Husband, physician	Husband or significant other	Husband or significant other Medical labor attendant	Medical labor attendants, including a "monitrice" or specialized labor attendant
PRENATAL PHYSICAL EXERCISE				
Strenuous physical exercise inherent to preparing the body for labor	Rigorous exercise based on rationale of athletic qualities of labor	None specifically prescribed	Nonstrenuous program of physical fitness to increase comfort in pregnancy	"Body-building" exercise to prepare for "athletic event" of labor
LABOR TECHNIQUES				
Creation of positive mental attitude Use of abdominal breathing for most of labor Use of panting	Imitation of sleep through position and use of abdominal breathing	Rhythmic breathing: slow to shallow as labor progresses	Rhythmic breathing: slow to shallow but not panting or rapid	Diaphragmatic breathing: slow and rapid; use of panting and vigorous blowing
Passive relaxation exercise	Deep mental relaxation	Refined relaxation technique	Refined active relaxation and body awareness	Neuromuscular disassociation exercises
Pushing technique	Pushing technique	Detailed pushing technique and exercise stressed	Detailed pushing technique	Pushing technique
COMMENTS				
Mystical overtones Diluted in practice by others from Read's original premise	Absolutes in methodology Domineering role of husband Role of techniques secondary	Adaptive approach to teach women to approach labor with confidence	Flexible but structured to integrate physical, emotional, and mental responses during labor	Often practical with rigid and dogmatic qualities

brought about by the last weeks of pregnancy, the birth of the infant, and the early postpartum period. The psychophysical and psychoprophylactic methods (Table 12-1) are based on the following three important areas:

1. Presence of accurate information to reduce anxieties and fears that accentuate pain
2. Acquisition of specific techniques of relaxation, muscular control, and respiration to reduce pain
3. Creation and maintenance of a calm and supportive environment so the woman believes she can "go with" the process, using her learned techniques

Maternity Center Association Concept

The psychophysical family-centered approach of preparation for birth was pioneered in New York by the Maternity Center Association. The Maternity Center encourages physical and mental preparation for birth, emphasizing the inclusion of the expectant father, the creation of a warm, supportive environment during labor, and the use of specific activities such as abdominal and chest breathing for the management of labor. Focus is placed on the alternative settings for birth in the Maternity Center's nurse-midwife–directed birthing center. Women attend prenatal care sessions with a midwife in the birthing center, and preparation classes are held there for the couple. Families are welcome to attend the birth, and the woman is prepared to go home within 6 to 12 hours after birth. Freestanding birth centers across the country follow a similar pattern as the one established by the Maternity Center Association, including backup obstetric support for complications that may develop.

Bradley method

Bradley (1974) based his method on observations of animal behavior during birth. Most of the techniques for labor are derived from this "imitation of nature." Bradley asserts that these techniques meet the woman in labor's need for the following:

1. Darkness and solitude
2. Quiet
3. Physical comfort and relaxation
4. Controlled breathing
5. Closed eyes and the appearance of sleep

Bradley pioneered the rejection of the typically passive role of the expectant father. Instead, the expectant father acts as one who directs the woman's labor preparation and conduct. This emphasis on the partner, however, may be interpreted by contemporary women as paternalistic and overbearing. Often the class may seem "rule-bound" to women. Furthermore, pregnant women without traditional marital partners feel excluded. The transference of the dominant male authority figure from physician to partner may neglect in part the woman's need to take responsibility for her own behavior.

Kitzinger method

The writings of the British childbirth educator Sheila Kitzinger (1980) blur the distinction between psychophysical and psychoprophylactic methods. Her program is structured to achieve a rhythmic coordination and harmony of the body during labor.

Kitzinger's approach advocates an elaborate system for relaxation that includes the father as a helper. The system was developed from the "method school" of acting and includes training in active relaxation. Although it does not claim to be part of an active conditioning process, Kitzinger's approach creates a new type of adaptive behavior for the mother. She uses breathing techniques, starting with slow breathing and progressing to shallow, rapid breathing, during the final phase of labor.

Psychoprophylaxis: Lamaze Method

Through the efforts of Marjorie Karmel and her book, *Thank you, Dr. Lamaze* (1959), the Lamaze method became popular in the 1960s. Lamaze, working in Paris, applied Pavlov's classic conditioning techniques to the process of birth. Known as the Lamaze method, psychoprophylaxis was originally a rigid and dogmatic approach to childbirth. Today it is used less rigidly throughout the world, though it is still *highly structured* and based on *conditioning, discipline,* and *concentration.* It is believed that the woman must undergo a period of disciplined training to substitute new responses to the stimulus of labor contractions. The support of a knowledgeable coach is recognized, and sound prenatal education is aimed at reducing psychic tension.

Although all these methods incorporate what is referred to as **nonpharmacologic analgesia,** various types of anesthetics can be used as circumstances indicate. Criticism of these methods centers on the "structured, goal-oriented attitude that encourages couples to go into labor as into combat" (Noble, 1981).

Hypnosis

Hypnosis is an effective approach to reduce the discomfort of labor, but it is not practical in hospital settings because it requires trained physicians or hypnotherapists to be available during the irregular schedule of childbirth. Hypnotherapy is more often used in a home birth setting along with complementary modalities of pain control such as aromatherapy. With training in hypnosis, the woman learns to enter a trancelike state, focusing on the therapist or on a prearranged self-hypnotic suggestion. It is possible to go through labor and birth, even by cesarean delivery, and remain completely comfortable because this trance significantly reduces attention to outside stimuli.

Leboyer Method

During the 1970s, attention was given to Leboyer's method. Leboyer (1975) wanted to create a more satisfying birth experience through environmental changes. Although he did not advocate a new method of childbirth, he recommended the creation of a warm, human, and gentle environment for birth. The Leboyer method, unlike other methods, is not a form of childbirth education but rather a method of delivery.

Leboyer sought to minimize what he considered to be the trauma of birth, and he appealed to the physician to take responsibility for reducing this trauma by eliminating unnecessary stimuli and by encouraging the maternal-infant bond. The Leboyer philosophy includes patience, emotional support, good communication, and education as integral parts of obstetric management. Leboyer emphasizes a gentle, controlled delivery, one which specifically avoids placing stress on the infant's craniosacral axis. He suggests that such stress interferes with the baby's well-being, particularly with the initiation of breathing, and may cause irritability and other central nervous system (CNS) problems. He advocated a gentle, warm water bath at birth to restore lost body heat, relax the infant physically, and thus place the newborn in harmony with its environment. One problem with the Leboyer method is neonatal delayed breathing caused by reduced stimulation after birth.

Elements of Leboyer's approach have been integrated into many current popular methods of preparation. The emphasis, however, is on the physiologic and emotional needs of the mother and child at the birth rather than on prenatal preparation.

General Education

A few physicians teach childbirth classes as part of prenatal care. Most physicians who take the time to provide education for their clients find that there is a reduction in the number of questions and a heightened sense of cooperation on the part of the couple. In fact, most prenatal classes are taught by nurses who are either part of a hospital-based program or are childbirth educators in private practice. General education uses most of the basic knowledge of the psychophysical method, but it may be much less structured.

EXPANDING SCOPE OF CHILDBIRTH PREPARATION

A considerable number of pregnant adolescents need prenatal and childbirth education. Their needs are based on their unique developmental requirements and other issues, such as their ability to continue their education, receive economic support, and learn parenting skills. The traditional 6-week course for childbirth education is not adequate for these mothers. A number of research reports show that more extensive preparation is effective in reducing the fear-tension-pain cycle in adolescents (Hetherington, 1990; Slager-Ernest, Hoffman, and Beckmann, 1987).

For women delaying childbirth until their careers are established, childbirth preparation creates another kind of challenge. These women bring expectations that may or may not be realistic. They are accustomed to controlling and directing the details of their lives. Some are eager for the changes that parenting will bring; others are unrealistic about the demands of childbirth and parenting. Childbirth preparation classes afford a format in which these issues may be explored. An alternative to weekly classes for busy career couples has been a 1-day seminar or a weekend series (see the Research Box below).

RESEARCH

PURPOSE OF STUDY

To determine whether there is a difference in the amount of knowledge retained following three different class formats.

LITERATURE REVIEW

Many studies related to childbirth education have been conducted. Findings from these studies indicate that women who attend childbirth education classes use fewer medications, are more self-confident and self-controlled during their labor and delivery experience, and demonstrate an overall increase in their knowledge base.

METHOD

A sample of 61 mothers and 45 partners attended childbirth education classes over periods of 2 weekends, 4 weeks, or 5 weeks. Content of the class and total amount of time in class were the same for all formats. Each participant completed a demographic data tool that asked age, education, number of children, and reasons for attending the classes. A knowledge tool was administered to participants a total of three times.

FINDINGS AND IMPLICATIONS FOR PRACTICE

Learning occurred in all three formats, although more learning did occur in the 4- and 5-week formats than in the weekend classes. No significant differences were found between the 4- and 5-week series. Traditional classes are often structured to meet the needs of the educator. Because class participants are diverse in terms of age, learning ability, and time availability for class attendance, it becomes more important for educators to meet the needs of the learners.

Bradley D, Shira M: A comparison of three childbirth education class formats, *J Perinat Educ* 4 (3):29, 1995.

Preconceptional and First Trimester Classes

These classes may include couples in early pregnancy and those planning for pregnancy. Participants learn about nutrition, the need for adequate rest and exercise, fetal development, maternal gestational changes, self-care, and sexuality. Discussions of types of health care providers and birth plans are also included. When both parents acquire knowledge related to common discomforts of pregnancy and their relief measures, as well as the psychologic changes that occur in pregnancy, a positive start to the pregnancy is likely for both. Preconceptional classes and visits to health care providers are now highly recommended (ACOG, 1995).

Sibling Classes

Classes to prepare a sibling for the birth of an infant have a positive effect on both the child and the family (Figure 12-1). The whole family attends, but the focus is on the child. It has been demonstrated that the use of a combination of techniques, such as charts and the child's own drawings, dolls, and group activities, will keep interest. Films and stories may be used to enhance enjoyment and learning. Snacks are served. The brother or sister can ask questions and learn to anticipate the new "rival" with less apprehension (Spadt, Martin, and Thomas, 1990). Involvement of the grandparents makes the event special, and visits to the nursery add excitement (Figure 12-2).

Breast-feeding Preparation

Women may elect to attend an extra class for breast-feeding preparation. Reading about breast-feeding and planning for it appear to promote successful lactation. Women learn the benefits of early and frequent feedings and can insist on early access to the infant if they will not be in a labor-delivery-recovery (LDR) setting.

TEST *Yourself* **12-1**

Select three examples of social changes that have affected the scope of childbirth education.

EVALUATION OF CHILDBIRTH EDUCATION

Benefits of Preparation for Childbirth

The prepared woman knows how to concentrate during labor. This response is in contrast with that of the unprepared woman who remains out of focus, finds the physical responses to labor overwhelming, and becomes incapable of rational thought (Figure 12-3). The training principles for learning either basic athletic skills or a new subject apply to childbirth. In addition, practice in relaxation and concentration has been shown to be beneficial in other

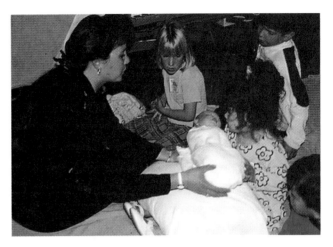

Figure 12-1 Siblings learn about infant care. (Courtesy Marjorie Pyle, RNC, *Lifecircle*.)

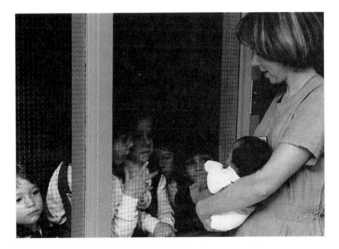

Figure 12-2 Siblings get a chance to visit the newborn nursery. (Courtesy St John's Mercy Medical Center, St Louis, Mo.)

medical areas (Mast et al, 1987). Through disciplined learning and applied techniques, the prepared woman recognizes her responses and resists the inclination to panic; she works *with* the process of labor. She learns to minimize fatigue by reducing tension, fearful anticipation, and heightened perception of pain. Thus the need for analgesics, anesthetics, and obstetric interventions may be reduced. During birth the prepared woman works more efficiently than the unprepared woman and is able to cooperate with the powerful forces of the second stage.

It is important to remember that the childbirth educator is not usually present when the couple comes to the labor area. Therefore the couple must know basic questions to ask and how to state their desires for support and analgesics. Shearer (1990) states that despite prenatal classes, it is the staff members who help or hinder the childbirth process: "Bedside practices can make prenatal education appear to be effective, or to have made no difference,

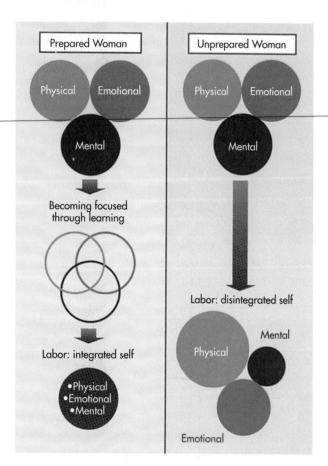

Figure 12-3 Results of childbirth education. Woman learns to integrate physical, emotional, and mental activity to remain focused and in control during labor. In the conditioning process, she substitutes learned responses to stimuli (contractions) for tension responses.

or to have actually caused harm to the patients." It is difficult to evaluate the effectiveness of childbirth classes because of this random factor that is not acknowledged by most researchers. Two studies, for example, report different results: the physicians' study found no extra benefit (Sturrock and Johnson, 1990); the nurse's study found significant benefit (Hetherington, 1990).

Barriers to Childbirth Education

Barriers against preparing for childbirth do exist; consequently, the woman's culture, education, attitude, family, and economic status must be considered. In certain cultural groups, the *lack of interest* by the woman's husband or family or their overt opposition to her interest in childbirth preparation is a strong enough factor to deter her from considering of childbirth preparation programs, unless such preparation is an integral part of her prenatal care.

Other *cultural, social, temperamental,* or *maturational factors* influence the woman's involvement. Preparation for childbirth may violate sexual taboos, cultural expectations, or family structure. If the woman has unresolved conflicts

about her sexuality, pregnancy, or motherhood, she usually will not participate. A woman may be unaware of the availability of classes in her community, and lacking strong motivation, she may fail to seek such information. A single woman may hesitate to join a class because of her anticipation of criticism by others.

The woman may be *uninformed* about the basic concepts of childbirth preparation, especially if she is a member of a lower socioeconomic group.

Fatigue and other physical factors may seriously affect the woman's ability and motivation to seek out and attend classes. If a woman's anxiety level is extremely high, she may avoid the counseling and education that would help her cope. When possible these particular deterrents must be significantly modified by the accurate presentation of the purpose and availability of classes to the whole community.

Other factors are influential; classes must be made available at convenient times and locations for the couple, and the cost must be reasonable for all socioeconomic groups. Childbirth educators in private or group practice must make known their willingness to accept reduced fees if low-cost programs are not otherwise available. Costs range from free for clinic classes to more than $100 for six lessons by a private educator.

Selection of the Health Care Provider

Expectant parents may select their physician, midwife, clinic, and hospital on the basis of the cooperation of the health care providers in childbirth preparation. Most women desire the atmosphere of a family-centered maternity care unit as a continuation of their prenatal and labor education. Many women today are choosing home birth or a freestanding birth center with nurse-midwives. Each option should be presented by the childbirth educator.

The nurse engaged in private or group practice as a childbirth educator is one of the most important sources for classes. Parents usually find an educator through referral by a friend, nurse, midwife, or physician. Clinic care through public hospitals and health maintenance organizations (HMOs) now includes childbirth classes. Unfortunately, classes may be large, with videotapes or films substituting for more personal interaction with the childbirth educator.

Goals of Childbirth Education

The central goal of parent education is the *reduction of anxiety and fear* through dissemination of accurate information (Box 12-1). When presenting factual information, the educator directs the discussion to the level of the group. The direction and depth of information required may be assessed by a brief period of asking couples to share prior experiences or by having the parents write a list of questions and concerns.

The content must be relevant and easily understood, with enough detail to give the couple an accurate and realistic picture of labor. Effective learning will take place if self-esteem is enhanced and anxiety is lessened by a positive approach.

Another goal of the educator is to *create informed and assertive consumers.* Too often the couple is passive in the childbirth experience, allowing health care providers to do almost anything without questioning them. There are still many degrees of acceptance by those in the medical profession of the couple's involvement in the childbirth process; not all physicians welcome it. A couple should be encouraged to consult their chosen physician or nurse-midwife about possible childbirth methods and together make a tentative *birth plan* for labor, including potential use of analgesics or anesthetics.

Birth plans

Helping couples create meaningful **birth plans** means offering a careful and reasoned exploration of traditional and nontraditional approaches to birth. The nurse must not place unreasonable expectations on the couple and must know the likelihood of newer methods being used in a particular community. Birth plans help the couple form a realistic view of the approaching events and can provide continuity in care when several health care persons are involved (Kitzinger, 1992).

Self-Discovery

Create a birth plan for yourself. ～

Birth partners

Practitioners of prepared childbirth have always advocated the active participation of the father as a labor support person. In situations in which the father is unavailable, a substitute is sought. The woman in labor desperately wants to help herself (which facilitates preparation), but she also needs a caring person with her. The presence of a caring person knowledgeable about what

should be done for support and control has a discernibly calming effect during this time of stress and challenge. The term labor "coach" has been used, but because of its sports overtones, it is being replaced by "support person" or "partner."

In studies of birth in which the father is an active participant, the couple's relationship as partners and as parents is found to be enhanced. Each speaks of the other in new appreciation; the bond seems to be strengthened, and couples gain new perspectives on their marital and parenting roles. Objective, controlled studies demonstrate the validity of these observations (Westrich et al, 1991).

The anxieties of pregnancy are not limited to the pregnant woman but extend to the father as well, thus creating a *pregnant couple.* Parent education in preparation for childbirth must deal with these anxieties. Such preparation seeks not only to present the father with the same factual information as the woman but also to give him a sense of importance and relevance during the birth. He gains an appreciation of the physical effort of birth and the assurance that he, too, will be prepared to function in specific and definite ways as part of the team.

My boyfriend isn't sure if he wants to be with me when I have the baby. My sister said she would be my coach. When we went to birthing classes, I was afraid that I'd have to choose between them. But the teacher welcomed them both. She made my boyfriend feel so much better, he's even saying he might come in the labor room with me.

Childbirth educators provide opportunities for the exploration of feelings, thus involving partners in nonthreatening ways. From the very first session, the partner is introduced as the chief support person, and as the class progresses, his or her importance in the process is emphasized. The educator should be sure to indicate that the birth partner can be any "significant other" and women without male partners are encouraged to choose a close friend or relative to be their support person.

Childbirth educators encourage mutual respect for the roles of father and mother during the childbirth experience and foster the concept of birth as a family experience (Figure 12-4). Through this learning experience, the partners feel more independent and develop increased self-confidence. **Locus of control** is enhanced as they learn to manage a stressful situation. The result of childbirth preparation extends beyond the specific techniques used during labor; the family can be strengthened with an emotional readiness for parenthood.

CONTENT OF CLASSES

Introductory Class

During the first class (Box 12-2), group interaction is facilitated by making introductions, which should be limited to simple information such as name, parity, due date, community, and choice of site for birth.

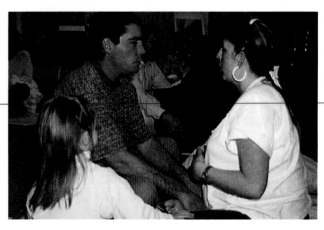

Figure 12-4　Learning relaxation exercises with the whole family. (Courtesy Marjorie Pyle, RNC, *Lifecircle.*)

TEST *Yourself* 12-2

How can a childbirth educator assist couples in the following?
a. Coping with the physical challenges of labor and thereby of maintaining control
b. Changing the perception of pain
c. Fostering self-esteem by a sense of being able to participate in childbirth and to manage self during labor

The educator makes general comments about the purpose of the course, presents realistic goals, and introduces basic concepts. Parents must understand that they can establish their own goals as the class evolves.

Because the class is still a collection of persons and not yet a group, couples respond more readily to concrete and factual details. Pertinent information about conception and the trimesters of pregnancy is enhanced by the use of visual aids. Discussion of fetal development and maternal changes reinforces the reality of the infant. The use of words such as "Now your baby's heart can be heard" helps the couple identify their baby, particularly if it is their first. Comments such as "Many women feel very tired at this point" or "You may feel the need to talk over each detail" enhance maternal self-awareness.

Exercises

Introducing physical conditioning exercises is appropriate to this first class, since couples are eager to do something. These prenatal body conditioning exercises increase the woman's sense of well-being and her physical comfort during pregnancy. They are directed not toward developing muscular strength but toward improving circulation, ventilation, body awareness, and posture. Strengthened muscle tone prepares the body for birth and enhances restoration of muscle tone after birth. Exercise videotapes and pregnancy conditioning classes in exercise

clubs are available. (See Chapter 9 for restrictions on exercise.) The following are commonly taught body conditioning exercises.

Tailor press. Instruct the pregnant woman to sit on the floor, placing the soles of her feet together. With the palms of her hands on her knees, she is instructed to exert slight downward pressure, then release. She should feel the muscles pull on the insides of her thighs. Repeating this exercise in groups of ten will stretch the muscles of the inner thighs. This exercise should be performed daily. The tailor position is a useful one during labor.

Pelvic tilt. Pelvic tilt or pelvic rocking improves abdominal muscle tone and helps prevent or decrease back strain. The pelvic tilt exercise can be performed in a chair, on the floor, on hands and knees, or while standing with the back against the wall.

Lying supine on the floor with her knees slightly bent, the woman presses her spine against the floor, flattening the curvature in her back, and then relaxes. Buttocks and abdominal muscles should be tightened at the same time. This exercise can be repeated in groups of ten repetitions.

Kegel exercise. This perineal muscle-tightening exercise strengthens the pubococcygeus muscle and increases its elasticity. The woman can identify the correct muscle group to be exercised by stopping the flow of urine midstream. Instruct her to squeeze her vagina and then rectum, as if she were preventing a bowel movement. The exercise is most effective when the muscle is contracted, held for a count of six, and released. Upon release, it is important to relax the entire body. This exercise should not be done routinely while voiding because it may result in urinary stasis and infection. This exercise can be done while sitting in the car, standing in lines, watching television, or at any other time. Kegel exercises should be repeated at least 20 to 30 times a day.

Practicing good posture

Good posture is important because it decreases strain on abdominal and back muscles. It will also decrease fatigue. It is also important to instruct the pregnant woman to rise from a lying position by keeping her legs parallel and rolling to one side. She can then use her hands to support herself and then push herself into a sitting position.

Conditioning Techniques

Progressive relaxation is the foundation on which all other techniques are applied. As the woman begins to develop awareness of bodily changes, she learns how to be comfortable, to detect tension in her body, and to facilitate relaxation. Her partner begins to learn to detect tension in her by touch and observation. Together they concentrate on achieving the active (versus passive) relaxation necessary for control during labor. The partner is encouraged to touch and stroke her in ways to enhance relaxation and rest. Stroking always accompanies the verbal cue "relax" so that stroking itself soon becomes a signal for relaxation.

To begin progressive relaxation exercises, the woman should lie on her back on the floor, with a pillow under her head and another pillow under her knees. Each exercise should begin and end with a "cleansing breath." The cleansing breath is achieved by taking a deep breath, then exhaling and relaxing the entire body. The birth partner should assess the arms and legs for relaxation. The birth partner continues with the exercise by giving the command to contract the right arm. The partner should assess for contraction of the right arm and relaxation of the remainder of the body. The next command is to release the right arm. These exercises progress through a series of commands: right arm, release; left arm, release; right leg, release; left leg, release; right arm and leg, release; left arm and leg,

release. These exercises should be practiced at least once a day. Relaxation exercises enable the woman to become aware of her body, prepare her for labor, and establish a pattern of teamwork between the woman and her partner.

Managing Pain

Childbirth education encourages alternatives to pharmacologic means to lessen pain. Pain is modified or inhibited when the person is able to have a specific focus of attention; when anxiety, fatigue, and muscle tension are reduced; and when there is an increase of controlled sensory input (see section on pain in Chapter 16).

In an effort to relieve local irritability through the creation of organized controlled sensory input, **effleurage** (light stroking) may be administered by the woman

---

▌ *Box* **12-2**   **Sample Class Outline***

INTRODUCTORY CLASS
Introduce self and class participants.
Discuss basic purpose and goals of the course.
Present common terms.
Discuss highlights of conception, fetal development, maternal reactions, and physical changes.
Teach physical conditioning exercises and rationale:
  Tailor press
  Tailor stretch
  Tailor reach
  Pelvic tilt
  Bent-leg lift
  Perineal control (Kegel exercise)
Teach basics of controlled relaxation:
  Achieving comfort
  Facilitating relaxation
  Detecting tension and relaxation in self
  Detecting tension and relaxation by support person
  Using touching and stroking methods to enhance relaxation
  Using precise verbal cues

INTERMEDIATE CLASSES
Practice relaxation techniques.
Introduce and develop the mechanism of labor.
Discuss related maternal reactions and emotional responses to the mechanism of labor.
Teach various labor techniques in which the couple must become proficient:
  Integration of controlled relaxation
  Rationale for respiratory techniques
  Rhythmic chest breathing: slow and modified rates
  Shallow breathing: combined with rhythmic chest breathing (modified rate) and rhythmic pattern of shallow breathing and short puff-blows
  Managing back labor

Discuss ways to recognize, prevent, and deal with hyperventilation.
Teach expulsion techniques, such as overcoming fear of pushing, integrating controlled relaxation (especially perineal), using abdominal muscles effectively in directing pushing effort, and correcting position to enhance the effort.
Teach open-glottis pushing.
Introduce couple to community resources, such as baby care classes, visiting nurse services, and family planning services.
Acquaint couples with local hospital facilities and policies of birthing centers.

CONCLUDING CLASS
Complete review of mechanism of labor, maternal reactions, labor techniques, and partner's role.
Discuss immediate postpartum period:
  Physical recuperation
  Emotional responses
  Emotional needs
Present hospital facilities, such as labor-delivery-recovery (LDR) area, postpartum unit, and nursery.
Discuss newborn's appearance at birth.
Teach care of infant in delivery room.
Point out characteristics of newborn during first few days.
Discuss the infant's need for mother's physical contact.
Teach infant feeding if pertinent to class needs.
Discuss postpartum period at home:
  Physical changes, nutrition, fluids, constipation
  Emotional needs and responses
  Simple exercises to improve muscle tone and sense of well-being
Discuss partner's needs and role.

*The instructor uses visual aids, demonstration, questions and discussion, group participation, role playing, and tours in the class.

herself or by the support person. While concentrating on the sensation at the skin level, she may be able to disregard the more diffuse sensation from the pain fibers of the uterus or cervix. When the woman performs alternate activities such as breathing in specific patterns or relaxing in learned ways, she may further modify pain transmission. Mental rehearsal and imagery activate concentration and improve performance.

Hydrotherapy (water therapy)

Immersion in water may be used during labor and birth or only during specific times of labor. **Hydrotherapy** includes the use of baths, whirlpools, and specially designed birth pools. It is thought that the relaxing effects of water may accelerate labor, decrease blood pressure, decrease perineal trauma, increase the mother's control over the birth environment, and reduce the use of pharmacologic methods of pain relief (Aderhold and Perry, 1991).

Critics of hydrotherapy suggest that there may be an increased risk of infection for both mother and infant, increased risk of trauma to the infant, and a greater incidence of postpartum hemorrhage. Limited criteria have been devised to guide hydrotherapy practice (see the Research Box at right).

Imagery

Imagery, or visualization, is often used in conjunction with relaxation and breathing exercises. During labor the woman visualizes the birth in a positive manner. For example, she may think of her cervix opening like a flower bud to allow for easy passage of the fetus. She may bring a picture to provide a focal point.

Aromatherapy

Aromatherapy refers to the use of essential oils such as lavender, rose, chamomile, and sage. Oils can be massaged into the skin, dropped onto the skin, applied with a hot face cloth, or placed on a ceramic ring around a heat source such as a candle or a lamp. Some oil aromas are thought to be calming, whereas others are believed to strengthen contractions by relieving stress and tension.

Music and audioanalgesia

Music can be used to create a peaceful and relaxed atmosphere during labor and delivery. Music can also block out distracting or unpleasant sounds. Music may enhance rhythmic breathing patterns and massages, and may facilitate visualization and hypnosis, thus reducing pain in some women (Figure 12-5).

The woman is encouraged to respond to labor in a variety of ways. She may assume several positions, breathe in any comfortable way, employ methods of nonpharmacologic analgesia, and ask for assistance (see Figures 12-6 and 13-16).

RESEARCH

PURPOSE OF STUDY
To determine if hydrotherapy decreases labor pain.

LITERATURE REVIEW
Research on the effects of hydrotherapy in labor is extremely limited. It is thought that the hydrothermic effect is caused by the water's ability to conduct heat, which results in dilation of peripheral vessels and improves venous return. The additional hydrokinetic effect produces weightlessness and relaxation.

FINDINGS AND IMPLICATIONS FOR PRACTICE
Women laboring in a bath are more relaxed, have less pain, use less pain medication, and have shorter labors. The rate of infection does not increase even when membranes are ruptured. A few cases of infant drownings were reported in other studies, as were increased perineal lacerations.

WATERBIRTH PROTOCOL
- Gestational age more than 37 weeks, cephalic presentation, and no fetal distress
- No maternal intrapartal complications
- Spontaneous onset of labor
- Single gestation
- No known active genital herpes or active AIDS
- No history of drug or alcohol use
- Adequate prenatal care
- Water temperature between 90° F and 101° F
- Infants not underwater for more than 20 seconds after delivery

Nichols F: The effects of hydrotherapy during labor, *J Perinat Educ* 5(1):41, 1996.

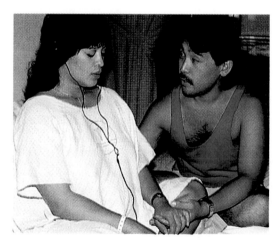

Figure 12-5 Music provides an alternate stimulation during labor and any comfortable position may be assumed. (Courtesy Marjorie Pyle, RNC, *Lifecircle*.)

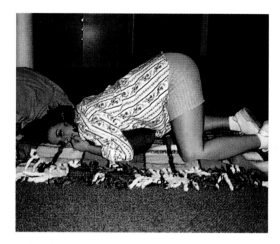

Figure 12-6   Knee-chest position is taught for changing infant position if necessary or if cord problems occur. (Courtesy Marjorie Pyle, RNC, *Lifecircle*.)

TEST *Yourself* 12-3 _____

Listed are three factors that help diminish pain perception. An example is provided for each. List other actions that would help a woman reduce pain sensations.
* *Focused attention:* Example—provide education that teaches mother to tune in to her body rather than yield to panic.
* *Reduction of anxiety, fatigue, muscle tension:* Example—provide consistent reassurance.
* *Increased controlled sensory input:* Example—woman or partner strokes abdomen.

Intermediate Classes

Building on the information and rapport of the introductory class, subsequent classes are expanded in a logical progression. In teaching the second stage, for instance, the instructor must be alert to the couple's anxiety about and fear of giving birth. Attitudes toward sexuality, fears about safety, misconceptions about labor, and inaccurate information contribute to these fears of pain and injury held by both the woman and her partner. The couple must gain an accurate and positive understanding of the mechanism of birth and a realistic expectation about their ability to work with the birth process.

Breathing techniques

To enhance relaxation and remove the focus from the contraction, breathing rhythms can be altered. Breathing normally is automatic; humans do not think about breaths at all. Learning new techniques takes practice and an interest in self-help. Childbirth education teaches various breathing patterns for use during labor stages. These tech-

niques may be practiced in front of a mirror or with the partner timing the "practice" contraction. At the onset of labor, the couple should tell the nurse which sequences of breathing they have been practicing. Classic Lamaze technique has been modified by most teachers and includes the following basic aspects.

1. Chest breathing is believed to diminish diaphragmatic interference on the uterine fundus and is used throughout the birth process. The woman feels as though she is breathing higher and higher in the chest as she progresses with the techniques.
2. A deep breath initiates and concludes each contraction. Also, the deep breath clears carbon dioxide and increases oxygen levels. This is an important signal for the woman and her partner. She has learned to relax consciously as she exhales this breath. These beginning and ending breaths make each contraction a single entity, as opposed to a series of endless contractions.
3. A **focal point** increases the woman's concentration and diminishes distraction. It serves to direct her attention to dealing with the contraction constructively. The point of focus may change from time to time.
4. Verbal and nonverbal **cues** are used to indicate when the woman should use a particular breathing technique (e.g., "contraction begins . . . contraction ends"). At times these cues may be used by the partner during labor if the woman has become drowsy, tired, or uncertain about the actual onset of each contraction.
5. A comfortable position is important for effective relaxation and efficient respiration. The supine position will interfere with the progress of labor and cause undesirable intraabdominal pressure on the large blood vessels. The woman is encouraged to use a tailor-sitting, side-lying, or a more upright position in the bed or chair (Liu, 1989).

Early phase. The first respiratory pattern is *rhythmic chest breathing* at the slow rate of about eight breaths per minute (bpm). The woman inhales through the nose and exhales through the mouth; exhalation is stressed and slightly prolonged. In rhythm with the breathing, she can apply a circular stroke over the abdominal area, using her fingertips. Stroking may be done with one or both hands or by her partner. This type of breathing is continued as long as it is effective.

As the phase progresses and dilation advances, the woman may also need to progress in breathing activity. She modifies the rhythmic chest breathing by increasing the rate to 16 or 20 bpm, continuing rhythmic stroking (Figure 12-7, *A*).

Active phase. To deal with the intensity of labor, the woman progresses to a combined pattern of modified rhythmic chest breathing and *shallow chest breathing*. She matches the increment and decrement of the labor contraction with the rhythmic chest breathing pattern; she uses the lighter, faster, shallow breathing for the acme and

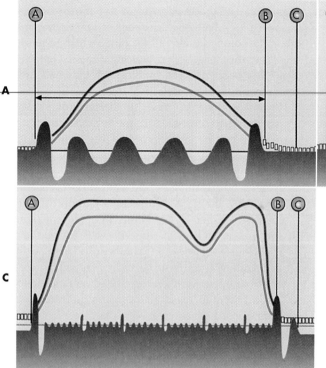

Figure 12-7 **A,** Latent phase contractions contrasted with rhythmic chest breathing. Duration (*A to B*) is 30 to 45 seconds; interval (*A to C*) is 10 to 5 minutes, and intensity is mild to moderate. Rhythmic chest breathing is at a rate of eight breaths per minute. Deep breath begins and ends each contraction. **B,** Active phase contraction contrasted with shallow chest breathing. Duration (*A to B*) is 50 to 60 seconds; interval (*A to C*) is 5 to 3 minutes, and intensity is moderate to strong with well-defined peaks. Shallow chest accelerated-decelerated breathing is matched to contraction intensity. **C,** Transition phase contraction. Duration (*A to B*) is 60 to 90 seconds; interval (*A to C*) is 2 to 3 minutes and intensity is strong with several peaks and rising tonus; shallow chest breathing is encouraged, alternating with blow (puff) breaths.

the deeper cleansing breathing to begin and end each contraction. Rhythmic stroking is continued if she finds it soothing. As contractions demand, she may use shallow breathing for the entire contraction, permitting greater flexibility in rate and depth. When using this technique, she breathes lightly and evenly, inhaling and exhaling through her slightly opened mouth. The rate is just fast enough to ensure respiratory exchange (as opposed to simply moving tidal air) with minimal effort and depth of respirations (Figure 12-7, *B*).

Transition phase. To handle this difficult period, a woman must use specific strategies. She uses a rhythmic pattern of shallow chest breathing with short puffs, which requires concentration and promotes a sense of control. The sequence is usually two or three breaths, alternating with a puff. These patterns are altered in response to the intensity of each contraction. Speeding up the pattern to one shallow breath and one puff is particularly useful in controlling intense peaks, sensations of pressure, or the urge to push (Figure 12-7, *C*).

Expulsion phase. Technique at this phase focuses on controlled relaxation and voluntary bearing down. Recent research studies have made it clear that expulsion techniques should avoid sustained breath holding. The woman learns to use her oblique abdominal muscles and

a fixed diaphragm to bear down. By pushing as though she is going to quickly empty her bladder, she will direct her efforts through the vagina and not the rectum. Conscious release of the perineum reduces resistance to the head. Positioning herself into a C shape, whether semisitting or upright, will allow the woman to favorably influence the axis of the birth canal. The position of her body and legs influences the relaxation of the perineum, further reducing resistance to the baby's head as it emerges (Figure 12-8).

The woman learns to push during the peak of each contraction, permitting the contraction to build by taking two deep breaths. Then she is encouraged to bear down repeatedly, tuning in to her body.

To sustain the work, to increase the efficiency of that effort and the efficiency of her ventilation, and to avoid **Valsalva's maneuver** (a forcible exhalation effort against a closed glottis), the woman learns to use a series of breaths, holding for a moment to start the push and then bearing down vigorously as she exhales slowly; this is **open-glottis pushing.** She can say a word such as "push" or "out" or grunt to control the release of air as she maintains her pushing efforts. She may alternately hold her breath and bear down without the controlled exhalation as long as she avoids sustained breath holding.

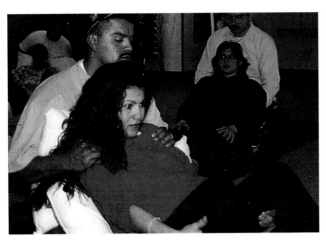

Figure 12-8   Practice with the pushing position during class. (Courtesy Marjorie Pyle, RNC, *Lifecircle*.)

Valsalva's maneuver. Holding breath and bearing down for more than 5 or 6 seconds is associated with a lowering in maternal blood pressure and a decrease in placental circulation. Like a domino effect, fetal pH and oxygen pressure (PO_2) decrease and carbon dioxide pressure (PCO_2) and fetal heart rate (FHR) increase. Thus bearing down should be brief, accompanied by open-glottis pushing with air release (Roberts et al, 1987). Although this technique has been known since 1980, many labor and birth units continue to insist that the woman do forceful sustained pushing during the second stage of labor. *Here is an area for nurse advocacy for the health of the woman in labor.*

Concluding Class

The couple's proficiency in labor technique and knowledge must be reviewed and evaluated in the concluding class. The instructor can introduce material pertinent to the postpartum period. Couples need a basic awareness of the physical changes and emotional and social adjustments of the recovery period. They also must be prepared for the "unfinished" qualities of the newborn, as well as the infants' demands and needs. First-time parents must to be aware that they will not suddenly be transformed into the romanticized image of a parent but will grow into their new role.

Many primigravidas are unprepared for various aspects of physical recovery. A brief discussion of what to expect aids understanding of the physiology of the recovery period and provides a few practical suggestions for dealing with this recuperative period. Because couples share in each others' excitement and learning, new friendships may start. The childbirth educator often offers to hold a "reunion" at a reasonable time in the future.

Cesarean Birth Preparation

When cesarean birth is expected, couples may attend classes that omit the emphasis on self-help during labor. Although preparation details may differ, basics remain the same. Box 12-3 lists topics that are helpful to the couple. Not all women take advantage of such classes, and the nurse will care for women who are unprepared for cesarean birth or did not expect a cesarean birth. In these cases the list in Box 12-3 will be useful for teaching the woman about cesarean birth upon her admission to the birthing area.

 Box 12-3

TEACHING PLAN *for* HOME CARE

Cesarean Birth

Reasons for cesarean birth and safety and risks of the procedure
Couple's prior experiences with cesarean birth
Potential for vaginal birth in the future after cesarean delivery
Policies regarding cesarean birth in various facilities
Costs of the procedure
Preparation before and procedures on admission
Anesthetic choices and recovery process
Couple's understanding of their choices
Relaxation responses that help calm anxiety—breathing, imagery
Role of physician, anesthesiologist, nurse
Signs of labor onset and what to do if early labor ensues

Actual cesarean procedure (films)
Role of support partner before and after birth
Parent-infant contact opportunities
Neonatal care in delivery area, pattern of care in hospital
Recovery process, intravenous lines, catheters, pain management, fluids, food
Involution patterns and recovery expectations
Discharge timing and choices
Home care opportunities
Managing at home
Infant feeding choices, lactation support
Expected emotional response, integration of experience
Possibilities of a cesarean support group

Key Points

■ Information and support reduce the fear-tension-pain cycle of labor. Birth partners enhance the feeling of security and support for the woman in labor.

■ Pain may be reduced through use of alternative methods of stimulation that incorporate the gate-control theory of pain.

■ The couple in labor functions best when they have discussed the birth plan with health care providers and feel a sense of trust in them.

■ Effects of childbirth education may be diminished by unsupportive hospital personnel.

■ Barriers to childbirth preparation should be recognized, and arrangements should be made to facilitate classes for all women.

■ Exercises and breathing practice develop a sense of self-care and foster self-esteem.

■ Valsalva's maneuver can occur with incorrect bearing down; mother and fetus need protection by informed nurses.

■ Those who plan a cesarean birth have as much or more need for childbirth preparation.

Study Questions

12-1. Select the terms that apply to the following statements:
  a. A perineal exercise that strengthens perineal muscles is _____.
  b. Control commands given to mother before a contraction are _____.
  c. A breathing technique to enhance relaxation is _____.
  d. A light stroking of woman's skin as a counterstimulus is _____.

12-2. Which observation of the couple helps you make an assessment of potential coping skills?
  a. Expressions of anxiety
  b. The manner in which the couple interacts
  c. The skill demonstrated in performing learned techniques
  d. Comments about prior experiences

12-3. Select one important value of having a birth partner.
  a. The partner feels needed in the birth experience.
  b. Labor is usually shorter when the partner is present.
  c. The expectant mother retains a better sense of control.
  d. Less nursing attention is needed during labor.

12-4. Choose true or false for the following statements:
  a. Tactile stimulation such as backrubs, pressure on sacrum, and effleurage may interrupt pain impulses through neural gates.
  b. A cleansing breath should only be used at the end of a contraction.
  c. Open-glottis pushing is key for the expulsion phase.

12-5. Valsalva's maneuver will result in:
  a. Maternal dizziness.
  b. Change in fetal acid-base balance.
  c. Increased placental blood flow.
  d. An extended second stage of labor.

Answer Key

12-1: *a*, Kegel; *b*, cues; *c*, slow chest; *d*, effleurage. 12-2: *b*. 12-3: *c*. 12-4: *a*, true; *b*, false; *c*, true. 12-5: *b*.

References

Aderhold K J, Perry L: Jet hydrotherapy for labor and postpartum pain relief, *MCN Am J Matern Child Nurs* 16(2):97, 1991.

American College of Obstetricians and Gynecologists: *Exercise during pregnancy and the postpartum period,* ACOG Technical Bulletin 189, Washington, DC, 1994.

American College of Obstetricians and Gynecologists: *Preconceptional Care,* ACOG Technical Bulletin 205, Washington, DC, May 1995.

*Bing, E: *Six practical lessons for an easier childbirth,* New York, 1967, Bantam Books.

Bradley D, Shira M: A comparison of three childbirth education class formats, *J Perinatal Educ* 4(3):29, 1995.

*Bradley R: *Husband coached childbirth,* New York, 1974, Harper & Row.

*Carty EM, Tier DT: Birth planning: a reality-based script for building confidence, *J Nurse Midwifery* 34(3):111, 1989.

Chapman L: Expectant father's roles during labor and birth, *J Obstet Gynecol Neonatal Nurs* 21:114, l992.

Enkin M, Keirse M, Renfrew M: *A guide to effective care in pregnancy and childbirth,* Oxford, 1995, Oxford University Press.

Hetherington SE: A controlled study of the effect of prepared childbirth classes on obstetric outcomes, *Birth* 17(2):86, 1990.

Hodnett E: Nursing support of the laboring woman, *J Obstet Gynecol Neonatal Nurs* 25(3):257, 1996.

Jimenez SL: Para dar la luz: reaching Hispanic women, *Childbirth Instructor* 2(2):42, 1992.

*Johnsen NM, Gaspad ME: Theoretical foundations for a prepared sibling class, *J Obstet Gynecol Neonatal Nurs* 14(3):237, 1985.

*Karmel M: *Thank you, Dr. Lamaze,* New York, 1959, Dolphin Books.

Kennel J et al: Continuous emotional support in a U.S. hospital: a randomized controlled trial, *JAMA* 265:2197, 1991.

Kitzinger S: Birth plans, *Birth* 19(1):36, 1992.

Koehn M: Effectiveness of prepared childbirth and childbirth satisfaction, *J Perinatal Educ* 1(2):35, l992.

*Lamaze F: *Painless childbirth,* New York, 1972, Simon & Schuster.

*Leboyer F: *Birth without violence,* New York, 1975, Alfred A. Knopf.

*Liu YC: The effects of the upright position during childbirth, *Image J Nurs Sch* 21(Spring):14, 1989.

Mattson S, Smith S, eds: *Core curriculum for maternal-newborn nursing,* Philadelphia, 1993, Saunders.

*Melzack R et al: Severity of labor pain: influence of physical as well as psychologic variables, *Can Med Assoc J* 30(3):580, l984.

Nichols R: The effects of hydrotherapy during labor, *J Perinatal Educ* 5(1):41, 1996.

*Noble E: Controversies in maternal effort during labor and delivery, *J Nurse Midwifery* 26(2):13, 1981.

Ottani P: When parents ask: what about waterbirth? *J Perinatal Educ* 4(3):1, 1995.

*Roberts JA et al: Effects of maternal position on uterine contractibility and efficiency, *Birth* 10:243, 1983.

*Roberts JA et al: The effects of a lateral recumbency and pitting on the first stage of labor, *J Reproductive Med* 7:477, 1984.

*Roberts JA et al: A descriptive analysis of involuntary bearing-down efforts, *J Obstet Gynecol Neonatal Nurs* 16(1):48, 1987.

Schuler W: Home birth, freestanding birthing center, or hospital birth—is there another option? *J Perinatal Educ.* 1(1):11, l992.

*Classic reference.

Shearer MH: Effects of prenatal education depend on the attitudes and practices of obstetric caregivers, *Birth* 17(2):73, 1990.

*Slager-Ernest SE, Hoffman SJ, Beckmann CJA: Effects of specialized prenatal adolescent programs on maternal and fetal outcomes, *J Obstet Gynecol Neonatal Nurs* 16(6):422, 1987.

Sturrock WA, Johnson JA: The relationship between childbirth education classes and obstetric outcome, *Birth* 17(2):82, 1990.

Westrich R et al: The influence of birth setting on the father's behavior toward his partner and infant, *Birth* 18(4):198, 1991.

*Yeates DA, Roberts JE: A comparison of two bearing down techniques during the second stage of labor, *J Nurse Midwifery* 29(1):3, 1984.

Student Resource Shelf

Carrington B et al: Modifying a childbirth education curriculum for two specific populations: inner-city adolescents and substance-using women, *J Nurse Midwifery* 39(5):312, 1994.
> *Research study that discusses the need to individualize childbirth education for different populations.*

*Mast D et al: Relaxation techniques: a self-learning module for nurses, *Cancer Nurs* 10(3):26, 1987.
> *A student can learn these techniques used for cancer patients to better support the woman in labor.*

Spadt SK, Martin KR, Thomas AM: Experiential classes for siblings-to-be, *MCN Am J Matern Child Nurs* 15(3):184, 1990.
> *Outlines an innovative approach for sibling preparation classes.*

Resources

Teacher Preparation Courses

Psychoprophylaxis
Council of Childbirth Education Specialists
8 Sylvan Glen
East Lyme, CT 06333

Psychophysical
Maternity Center Association
48 East 92 Street
New York, NY 10028

Parent-Teacher Groups

American Society for Psychoprophylaxis in Obstetrics (ASPO)
1523 L Street NW
Washington, DC 20005

International Childbirth Education Association (ICEA)
P.O. Box 5852
Milwaukee, WI 53220

National Association of Parents and Professionals for Safe Alternatives in Childbirth (NAPSAC)
P.O. Box 1307
Chapel Hill, NC 27514

Three

Labor, Birth, & Recovery

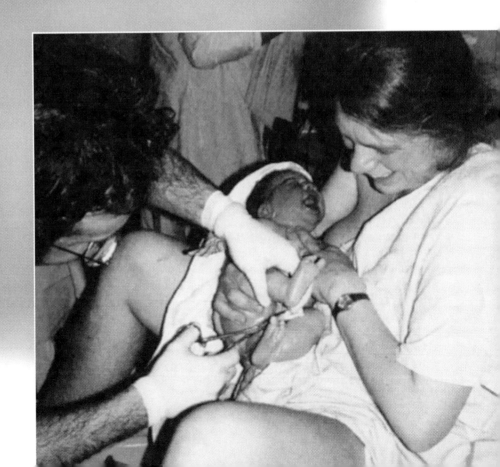

13

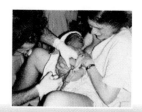

The Labor Process
& Nursing Care

This chapter reviews the activities that occur during the labor process. Normal labor requires that the *powers* be sufficient to expel the fetus, the *passage* be of adequate size to allow descent and expulsion of the fetus, and the *passengers* be of average size. The *psyche* also plays an intricate part during labor.

Labor is the process that allows the fetus to be born. It is accomplished by rhythmic contractions of the uterus that cause the cervix to open wide enough to allow passage of the infant's body, the placenta, and the membranes through

the vagina. The beginning of forceful labor is on a continuum from ineffective, widely spaced uterine contractions (Braxton Hicks contractions) to increasingly forceful contractions. Coordinated contractions of sufficient pressure usually begin after 35 to 38 weeks of gestation.

THE PSYCHE

Today women seek positive birth experiences that are physically safe and emotionally gratifying. Women who are not prepared in childbirth techniques may be assisted by nurses and may find control during labor more difficult to achieve. Today's focus of care must (1) be centered on a model that includes the client and her family, (2) be based on ethnic and cultural values and lifestyle and psychosocial assessment (Kowalski, 1996), and (3) emphasize the positive experience of childbirth.

Levine (1973) describes four basic principles of nursing management that apply to supporting the birth experience: conservation of (1) energy, (2) personal integrity, (3) social integrity, and (4) structural integrity, which includes safety during birth. These principles serve as a framework for determining appropriate nursing care during all stages of labor and facilitate nursing assessment, analysis, planning, implementation, and evaluation.

Conservation of Energy

During the inevitable stress of labor the woman may seem to regress to a more dependent state. She will be sensitive to indifferent or negative interpersonal exchange. Often she may not talk about this experience until the infant is born. Nurses can set a positive tone for the labor experience simply by introducing themselves, asking the client the name she prefers to use, and orienting her carefully to the space she will occupy. Establishing interpersonal trust is important because the woman is vulnerable in an entirely new way during the hours of labor and birth.

Hospital protocols may be ineffective, routine, or even harmful and can diminish a woman's sense of self-control during labor. Three such examples include routine frequent vaginal examinations, routine intravenous (IV) fluids, and requiring bedrest during labor. Research studies are being implemented to change these outdated protocols (Enkin et al, 1995). Providing the woman with information and interpreting labor data and treatments help her conserve energy. Words of encouragement, affirmation, and validation diminish fatigue.

The father or birth partner plays a significant role in the labor and birth process. Whether or not the partner is trained as a coach in a prepared childbirth class, studies show that labor is completed with greater self-fulfillment when a partner is present. The birth partner contributes significantly to whether the woman experiences achievement and self-control or has a sense of loss of control, anxiety, fear, and fatigue (Chapman, 1991).

The nurse remains alert to expressions of concern and anxiety by the woman through verbal and nonverbal behavior. Remember that routine nursing care is unique to both the laboring woman and her partner. The woman needs reinforcement to use learned adaptive responses to labor. She is now experiencing the "real thing," and application of techniques may need validation. The partner requires accurate information, clarification, and guidance.

Conservation of Personal and Social Integrity

Instead of directing the woman while controlling all aspects of management and the environment, the nurse and physician should balance care and interventions with participation by the expectant mother and her partner. The couple should be appropriately involved in decision making. Changes in the attitude toward parental decision making are shown by the extent to which expectant parents have become involved in formulating birth plans, discussing types of birth, following indications for surgical interventions, following procedures, and involving the partner.

Interpersonal skills that support the couple are important. Respectfully praising their involvement, preserving human dignity in care, and demonstrating regard for the individual are as important as technical skills. Nursing interventions such as comfort measures and clear explanations of procedures, combined with a friendly demeanor, will convey a sense of well-being and security to the client.

Support and comfort

The goal of labor support is to help the woman achieve her self-imagined outcomes during this life-changing event. Several factors must be carefully considered because the laboring woman will remember her childbirth experience for the rest of her life (Hodnett, 1996). Regardless of the type of labor (long, short; normal, complicated) the type of support can make the difference in whether she recalls her experience as *disembodied* (just another faceless labor client) or as one that increases her feeling of self-worth. The professional supportive behavior of caregivers can provide encouragement and has measurable benefits on the outcomes of labor and birth (Hodnett, 1996). The use of eye contact, chosen name, and spoken communication that transmits a message of shared responsibility must be incorporated into care. Clear communication about procedures benefits the woman's sense of control if she is asked to respond by verbal consent before being touched (Bergstrom et al, 1992).

Studies indicate that there are various levels of need for support during labor (Kowalski, 1996; Thornton, 1994). In one study, women with prepared labor partners required and expected minimal nursing involvement (Mackey and Locke, 1988). These women saw the nursing role as competence in technical tasks, monitoring, and evaluating labor progress. The nurse was viewed as a source of information and someone who would provide support as follows:

- Respect their wishes
- Let them do what they wanted
- Leave them alone with their partner
- Not interrupt during a contraction

In contrast, Bond (1996) found that pregnant women who were unable to have family or significant others present expected the nurse to be a constant companion.

These women reported a range of emotions—from nervousness to dread to fear. They considered the labor experience to be lonely and noted that receiving detailed information related to the labor processes and procedures was helpful. The nurse's presence was experienced as a continuous source of comfort and reassurance.

Another study found that nurses spent only 9.9% of the shift providing supportive care (McNiven et al, 1992). Supportive care included physical care, emotional support, instruction, information, and advocacy. All other direct and indirect care activities took 81.4% of the caregiver's time. These activities included performing physical assessments, assisting with techniques, documenting care, and participating in other activities occurring in the unit.

Support by touch. Support by touch has been extensively studied (Kowalski, 1996; Kintz, 1987). Weaver (1990) defined touch as "physical contact, usually made with the hands, in a transactional activity within a nurse-patient relationship." Bond supports this definition and includes touch as having value as a sign of a "compassionate human presence."

How do you assess which woman will need extensive support? Direct discussion of the woman's need for assistance is the best way to discover her need for support. Birth plans may give some indication of anxiety or preparedness. Needs change as labor progresses, and questions such as, "Are there ways I could be of more assistance?" or reflective statements such as, "You must be feeling that this part of labor is overwhelming," may open up further discovery of needs for support.

In a busy labor unit it is easy to view labor as mechanistic. Obstetric technology may seem to result in an engineering approach that views the client as a complex machine. Nurses must recognize the need for "high touch" in maternal infant nursing, integrating advanced technology with "hands-on" care for the benefit of the mother, the partner, and the newborn.

THE POWERS FOR LABOR

Uterine Contractions

Uterine contractions provide the *primary* (involuntary) *powers* to dilate the cervix. During the second stage, the woman adds *secondary* (voluntary) *powers* by using bearing-down pushing efforts for the last few inches of fetal descent.

Uterine contractions originate in the fundus, the active segment where the greatest concentration of muscle cells is located. The contraction spreads into the lower portion, or passive segment (Figure 13-1). (See Chapter 3 for structure of the muscle layers.) This lower portion of the uterus is stretched by the pressure of the fetus and amniotic sac and does not rhythmically contract in the same way. The smooth muscle myometrium has two qualities:

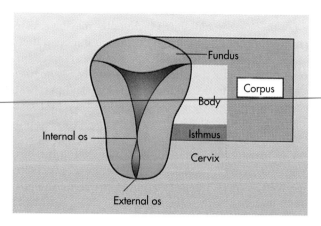

Figure 13-1   Anatomic landmarks of uterus that are important during labor.

(1) elasticity, which allows it to stretch, maintain tone, and shrink after birth, and (2) contractility, which allows it to shorten and lengthen in a synchronized pattern.

Each contraction has three parts: an *increment* (increasing intensity), an *acme* (peak intensity), and a *decrement* (decreasing intensity). Note in Figure 13-2 that the increment is steep and rapid whereas the decrement is more prolonged and gradual. The contraction follows a bell-shaped curve.

The degree of relaxation between contractions is important because this period allows the fetus and the uterine muscles to recover from the stress of the contraction. **Resting tone** is the lowest intraamniotic pressure between contractions. This tonus is 10 to 15 mm Hg and rises in late labor. Because the intense contractions have completely stopped circulation to the placenta for the length of the contraction, if the tonus rises too high, refilling (perfusion) will be inadequate, and the fetus will begin to suffer from lack of oxygen. Hypertonic contractions exist when there is uncoordinated uterine activity without a normal resting phase. On the other hand, the uterus that cannot contract effectively has *hypotonic* contractions.

An abnormally slow or nonprogressive labor pattern is called **dystocia**. If the uterus is incapable of the necessary powers to allow progress of labor, the result is a prolonged labor phase caused by uterine dysfunction.

Monitoring contractions

Assessing intensity may be done by palpation of the fundus, external contraction monitoring, or internal pressure monitoring (see Chapter 14). Contractions must be assessed for **frequency, intensity,** and **duration** (see Figure 13-2).

- *Frequency* is the time from the beginning of one contraction to the beginning of the next (usually recorded in minutes).
- *Intensity* is the force of the contraction (the strength) and is recorded as mild, moderate, or strong.

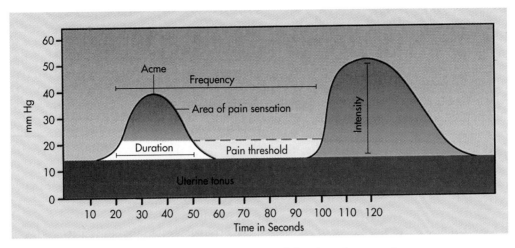

Figure 13-2   Measurement of frequency, intensity, and duration of contractions.

- *Duration* is the time from the beginning to the end of each contraction (usually recorded in seconds).

The nurse notes this information after palpating several contractions or observing the strip paper of the external or internal monitor record. Although recognizing that the external tocodynamometer gives only an approximation, contractions may be recorded as mild, moderate, or strong by palpation:

Palpation	Internal Monitor
Mild	Below 40 mm Hg
Moderate	40-70 mm Hg
Strong	Above 70 mm Hg

Why do contractions change during labor?

During pregnancy, contractions are mild, irregular, and nonsynchronized. To be coordinated (synchronized), **gap junctions**, or cell-to-cell communication points, must develop between smooth muscle cells. This process suddenly boosts the energy in the muscle cells. Communication is almost instant. As pacemakers signal a contraction, a wave of tightening, beginning at the top, is experienced throughout the uterus.

These gap junctions gradually increase in size and number during the last weeks of pregnancy and then develop rapidly *during labor*. The length of latent labor varies from woman to woman and is believed to be the time needed for gap junction formulation, oxytocin receptor enhancement, and collagen changes (Steinman, 1991). Once the process has begun, it is difficult to stop. For instance, it is almost impossible to stop preterm labor once the cervix reaches 3 to 4 cm dilation or the woman reaches the end of the latent period of labor (see the discussion on preterm labor in Chapter 21).

Theories. Labor onset is thought to be a complex combination of factors working together. The following descriptions are based on reports by Blackburn and Loper (1992), Steinman (1991), and Huzar and Naftolin (1984).

1. Genetic factors have a role perhaps in influencing hormonal levels and patterns of labor.
2. An increase in availability of estrogen and a decrease in progesterone occurs in the myometrium. (Progesterone suppresses uterine contractions.) Estrogen fosters gap junctions, increases oxytocin receptors, and stimulates prostaglandin production. Some estrogen originates in the fetal adrenal glands so that fetal hormonal activity helps to trigger labor onset.
3. Prostaglandin PGE_2 contributes to cervical changes and prostaglandin PGF_2 contributes to contractions and formation of gap junctions. These prostaglandins increase calcium ion flow in the cells, which strengthens contractions. The effects of prostaglandins are seen indirectly in that antiprostaglandin agents such as aspirin and indomethacin will delay labor onset.
4. Oxytocin receptors increase 100 to 200 times by term. Thus oxytocin will effectively stimulate labor in full-term pregnancies but has less effect earlier.
5. Relaxin is present throughout pregnancy and probably works with progesterone to block uterine contractions. Its role during labor is unclear, but it may be involved with connective tissue changes.
6. Overstretching of the uterine wall related to multiple pregnancy or polyhydramnios often ends with preterm labor.

Cervix during Labor

Normally the cervix is firm, resembling the consistency of the tip of one's nose. For labor to be effective, the cervix must become soft or "ripe," be tipped forward in the vagina, and be partially effaced. These changes often occur within the few weeks before labor onset.

Effective contractions lead to further changes in the cervix. With each contraction, the cervix is drawn slowly up into the lower uterine segment. This shortening and thinning of the cervix is called **effacement**. The force of the contractions with the pressure of the fetus causes cervical **dilation** (opening). The first time this process takes place requires the most time. A primigravida may begin to efface several days before dilation begins; a multigravida may have effacement and dilation occuring together and may not have completed effacement before dilation is completed (Figure 13-3). The progress of effacement and dilation is determined by internal vaginal examination (see Procedure 13-1).

THE PASSENGERS

The passengers are the fetus, the placenta, the umbilical cord, and the amniotic fluid and membranes.

The Fetus

The size of the head of the fetus affects the progress of labor. Because the bones of the head are separated by membranous interspaces (the sutures [Figure 13-4]), the bones are slightly moveable and assume a more elongated shape to fit through the tight passage. This **molding** is seen in Figure 18-18. The anterior and posterior fontanelles will be palpable landmarks, depending on the position of the head. The landmarks of the fetal head are as follows:

- **Occiput:** area of head containing occipital bone, below posterior fontanelle
- **Mentum:** fetal chin
- **Bregma:** area around the anterior fontanelle
- **Sinciput:** anterior area (the brow)

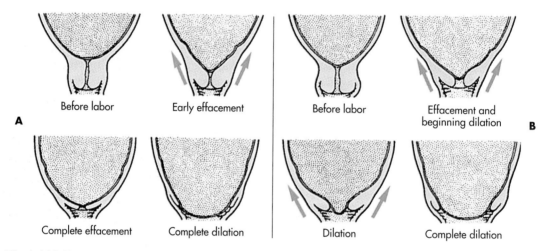

Figure 13-3 Degrees of effacement and dilation. **A,** Primigravida. **B,** Multigravida. (From Clinical Education Aid: *The phenomena of normal labor*, Ross Laboratories. Courtesy Ross Laboratories, Columbus, Ohio.)

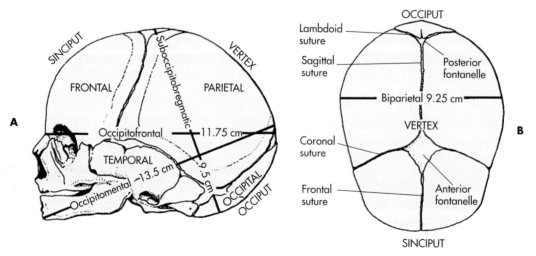

Figure 13-4 Fetal skull. **A,** Side view. **B,** Vertex view. (From Clinical Education Aid: *The phenomena of normal labor*, Ross Laboratories. Courtesy Ross Laboratories, Columbus, Ohio.)

- **Vertex:** lies in front of the posterior fontanelle
- **Anterior fontanelle:** where anterior cranial sutures intersect
- **Posterior fontanelle:** where posterior cranial sutures intersect

The diameters of the fetal head are illustrated in Figure 13-4.

Fetal lie

Lie is the relationship of the long axis of the fetus to the long axis of the mother. The lie is either longitudinal or transverse (sideways). The fetus in Figure 13-5 is in a longitudinal lie. The final presentation is assumed in late pregnancy; until the ninth month, the fetus will have changed lie many times. The fetal **attitude** is the pose assumed within the uterus, usually the *fetal position* with the arms and legs flexed on the abdomen and the head flexed with the chin almost touching the chest.

Fetal presentation

Lie and presentation are similar. **Presentation** identifies the portion of the fetus coming first to the cervix. There are three major presentations: vertex or cephalic (head first [95%]), breech (buttocks first [3.5%]), and shoulder (actual shoulder or arm first [0.5%]). Presentations other than vertex can result in a longer labor or more difficult delivery (see the discussion on dysfunctional labor in Chapter 15).

Vertex or cephalic presentation. The head is sharply flexed, and the posterior fontanelle is the presenting part in a **vertex presentation** (the cephalic or vertex area lies just in front of the posterior fontanelle). Rarely, a face presentation is seen (see Figure 15-9), or a brow presentation may occur.

Breech presentation. Classification of **breech** is made according to the position of the thighs and legs (see Figure 15-11). There may be an attempt made to change breech presentations to vertex to facilitate vaginal delivery (see Chapter 15).

Shoulder presentation. All transverse presentations are called shoulder presentations, but the arm or abdomen may be presenting into the birth canal. Of course, it is not possible to deliver the fetus this way, therefore either the fetus must be turned or a cesarean delivery is done.

Fetal position

Position refers to the relation of the fetal presenting part to the four quadrants of the maternal pelvis. With each presentation there may be a variety of positions—right, left or transverse, and anterior or posterior (Table 13-1). Note that when the term "transverse" is used with fetal positions, it refers to the part presenting to the maternal birth canal, not the fetal lie.

The fetus is commonly in the left occiput transverse (LOT) position at engagement and rotates to left occiput anterior (LOA) position as it descends through the pelvis. With the fetus in LOA position, the suture lines that should be palpated are shown in Figure 13-6. The six possible occiput (vertex) positions are illustrated in Figure 13-7. Fetal position and presentation can be assessed by Leopold's maneuvers (see Figure 9-12), by vaginal examination during labor, and with ultrasonography. Any variation in position, lie, or presentation may adversely affect the progress of labor. Attempts to change the fetal position by changing

Table **13-1**	**Possible Variations in Position**	
Presenting Part	**Fetal Point of Reference**	**Maternal Relationship**
Vertex	Occiput (O)	Anterior or posterior (A or P)
Face	Mentum (M)	
Brow	Brow (B)	Right or left side (R or L)
Buttocks (breech)	Sacrum (S)	
Feet	Sacrum (S)	Transverse (T)
Shoulder	Scapula (Sc)	

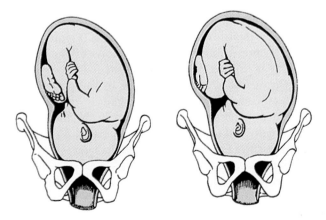

Figure 13-5 Longitudinal lie with fetus in left occiput transverse (LOT) and left occiput anterior (LOA) positions. (From *Clinical Education Aid* No. 18, Ross Laboratories. Courtesy Ross Laboratories, Columbus, Ohio.)

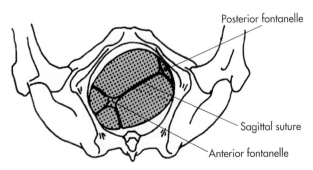

Figure 13-6 Position of suture lines and fontanelles in left occiput anterior (LOA) position.

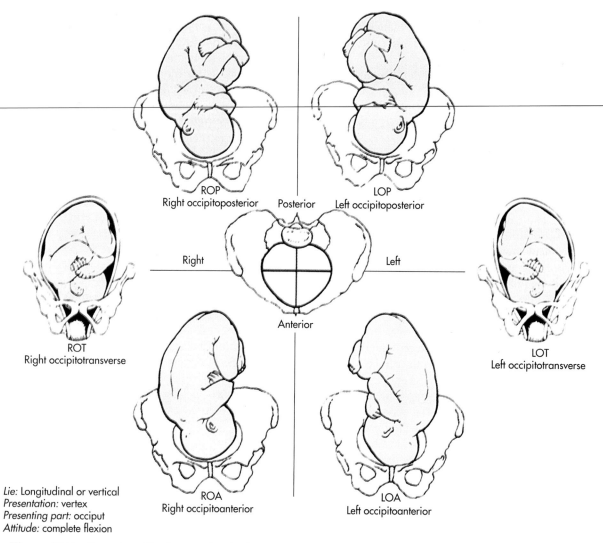

Figure 13-7   Examples of fetal vertex (occiput) presentations in relation to front, back, or side of maternal pelvis. (Modified from Iorio J: *Childbirth: family-centered nursing*, ed 3, St Louis, 1973, Mosby.)

maternal positions and ambulation are made before or during early labor. An occiput transverse (OT) or occiput posterior (OP) position may be influenced by standing, kneeling, leaning on the hands and knees, or using the lateral Sims position (Roberts et al, 1983). There is a trend toward using external version (turning) to change the breech to vertex and thus facilitate vaginal delivery (see the discussion on dysfunctional labor in Chapter 15).

TEST *Yourself* 13-1 ⎯⎯⎯⎯⎯⎯

a. Using Leopold's maneuvers, if you palpate a soft, irregular mass in the fundus and firm irregularities on the right lower anterior side of the abdomen, what would be the position of the fetus?
b. Where could you best hear the fetal heart for this position?

Station

Station refers to the relationship of the presenting part to the ischial spines of the pelvic midplane (Figure 13-8). When the presenting part is at the level of the ischial spines, it is said to be at zero (0) station or engaged. Engagement indicates that the ring of the pelvic inlet encircles the head, and the head is relatively *fixed* into the pelvic canal. The stations above and below the ischial spines are divided into fifths of approximately 1 cm each. As the presenting part descends from the inlet toward the spines, the stations would be -5, -4, -3, -2, -1, and 0 station. Below the spines, the fetal presenting part descends through $+1$, $+2$, $+3$, $+4$, and $+5$, which is the pelvic outlet. If the presenting part has not descended and is freely moveable in the inlet, it is *floating*. If during labor the presenting part cannot make the descent through all stations, it is "arrested," and a cesarean birth may be indicated. (See the discussion on dysfunctional

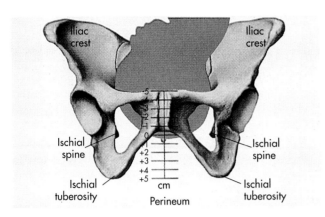

Figure 13-8   Station in relation to descent of fetal head. (From Clinical Education Aid: *The phenomena of normal labor,* Ross Laboratories. Courtesy Ross Laboratories, Columbus, Ohio.)

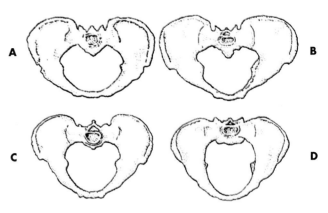

Figure 13-9   Types of pelves. **A,** Platypelloid. **B,** Android. **C,** Gynecoid. **D,** Anthropoid. (Redrawn from Ullery JC, Castallo M: *Obstetric mechanisms and their management,* Philadelphia, 1957, FA Davis Co.)

labor in Chapter 15.) Station is determined by means of a vaginal examination.

Amniotic Sac and Fluid

The **membranes** of the amniotic sac normally remain intact until the middle or late stages of labor. Amniotic fluid provides space for symmetric fetal growth, maintains a constant temperature, and protects and cushions the fetus while allowing free movement. A pocket of fluid, the forewaters, cushions the presenting part and is considered to protect the head from the pressures exerted by the cervix and uterine muscle.

In some cases, the amniotic sac or bag of waters (BOW) may rupture spontaneously before or during labor. If the site of the spontaneous rupture of membranes (SROM) is high, there may only be a trickle of fluid during a contraction. If there is any question about rupture, nitrazine paper is used. The test paper turns dark blue in the presence of alkaline amniotic fluid. Fluid may also be placed on a glass slide to dry; a fernlike crystallization of sodium chloride will appear (see Figure 6-2).

During labor, artificial rupture of membranes (AROM) may be done by the midwife or physician. The presenting part must be well engaged and active labor well established. If rupture is accompanied by a gush of fluid and the head is not engaged, the umbilical cord may be washed downward and compressed between the presenting part and the cervix (see the prolapsed cord in Figure 14-9).

The fetal heart rate must be checked after membrane rupture, and fluid should be observed for color, odor, and amount. These observations should be charted. Normally the fluid is a clear, straw color with flecks of *vernix caseosa* (cheesy coating of fetal skin). If it is brownish green, it contains *meconium,* fetal stool. Note the color and consistency of fluid that contains meconium to determine whether it is thick or thin, dark or light green. Meconium at the vaginal entrance (introitus) is considered normal in

a breech presentation because pressure on the infant's abdomen causes stooling. If the fluid is yellow, it indicates the presence of bilirubin. Any blood would indicate fetal hemorrhage, but this is rare. Amniotic fluid has a characteristic odor. A foul-smelling odor indicates an infectious process, **chorioamnionitis.**

Umbilical Cord

Normally the umbilical cord floats in the amniotic fluid that surrounds the fetus. It may become entangled or compressed against the fetal body during contractions, resulting in fetal hypoxia. If the fetal monitor is in place, compression appears as variable decelerations in the heart rate pattern. A change in maternal position may relocate the cord and alleviate cord compression.

The Placenta

The placenta is essential to fetal well-being during labor. Because placental perfusion and oxygenation are always reduced during contractions, careful observations are made of fetal responses to contractions. Transient fetal hypoxia is normally overcome when the healthy placenta refills after a contraction. Placental problems are discussed with fetal distress in Chapter 14. The placenta separates within minutes of the birth of the infant and is delivered through the birth canal during the third stage of labor (see Chapter 15).

THE PASSAGE

Labor depends on the accommodation of the fetus moving through the passage. The pelvis plays an important part in the process. It differs in size and shape in women and men. Each pelvis is classified according to the shape of the inlet (Figure 13-9). The *gynecoid* pelvis is ideal for birth because its shape allows the presenting part to enter more easily. The *platypelloid* shape allows the fetus to enter only in an

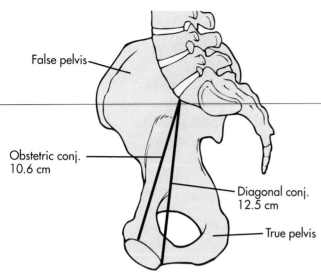

False pelvis

Obstetric conj.
10.6 cm

Diagonal conj.
12.5 cm

True pelvis

Figure 13-10   Diameters of pelvic planes.

OT position because the anteroposterior diameter is too narrow. The *android* pelvis, a usual male pelvic shape, forces the fetal head to engage in an OP position, as does the *anthropoid* shape. These three pelvic shapes result in a long labor and may require an instrumental or cesarean delivery.

Diameters of the Pelvis

The pelvic diameters are assessed by the midwife or physician in early physical examinations. The importance of these measurements is to indicate the type of pelvis shape and whether there is adequate room for descent of the presenting part.

Figure 13-10 illustrates two of the following obstetrically important measurements.

- **Obstetric conjugate:** the shortest distance between the promontory of the sacrum and internal top edge of the symphysis pubis (10 cm or more)
- **True (vera) conjugate:** measures the inlet from the promontory of the sacrum to the internal center of the symphysis pubis
- **Diagonal conjugate:** measures the distance from the promontory of the sacrum to the lower margin of the symphysis. If greater than 11.5 cm, vaginal delivery is usually possible if fetal size is average.
- **Interspinous diameter:** 10 cm or more
- **Plane of the outlet:** distance between the ischial tuberosities (8 cm or more)
- **Angle of the pubic arch:** at least 90°

The midplane can only be assessed by radiographic examination. The diagonal conjugate, the sacrum, and the coccyx and ischial spines can be palpated with the examiner's fingers. The coccyx should be slightly movable. Problems may be suspected if ischial spines are too prominent, if pelvic side walls are narrow, or if the curve of the sacrum is shallow.

THE MECHANISMS OF LABOR AND BIRTH

To negotiate the bony pelvis, the fetus must go through the mechanisms of labor, the *cardinal movements*. The mechanisms of labor for the LOA position are illustrated in Figure 13-11.

1. **Descent** continues throughout the process. If descent does not take place, none of the other mechanisms can occur. Descent is measured in stations above or below the ischial spines.
2. **Engagement** indicates that the presenting part has reached the level of the ischial spines and is encircled by the bony pelvic inlet. The part descends in a transverse position so that the largest diameter of the pelvis will accept the largest diameter of the head.
3. **Flexion** must occur now for the other mechanisms to follow. The head and neck flex as a result of the resistance met in the passage. This allows the smallest diameter of the head to come first. Flexion is maintained until the last step, when the head extends as the neck unflexes.
4. **Internal rotation** is the crucial next step and may be prolonged. From the transverse position the head may rotate to the anterior or posterior position; the direction is based on the structure of the pelvic canal and cannot be certain until rotation is in progress. Then to pass the ischial spines, the head must rotate 45 degrees to the right or left position. After more descent, as the fetus becomes ready for the last phase, the head again rotates to bring the occiput in alignment with the anterior or posterior center point of the pelvic outlet.
5. **Extension** allows the head to pass under the pelvic arch. It is at this point that the infant's scalp is seen at the vaginal opening. The head then moves through the vaginal opening.
6. **External rotation** involves two movements. After the head is delivered, it turns to realign with the shoulders, which are still in a transverse position in the vagina. Then the shoulders rotate to the anteroposterior position to permit the body to emerge through the vaginal opening. During this time the head appears to "untwist."
7. **Expulsion** of the rest of the body follows as the anterior shoulder moves under the symphysis pubis. The posterior shoulder is carefully delivered first to prevent perineal tearing.

To accomplish these maneuvers, proper coordination of the passengers, passage, and powers must exist. If the presenting part is too large or the lie is transverse, engagement cannot occur. If the position is OP, the head does not apply equal pressure on the cervix, and labor is slowed. If contractions are too weak or irregular, the force does not propel the fetus through the pelvic canal. If the measurements of the pelvis are too small, the fetus cannot pass through the canal.

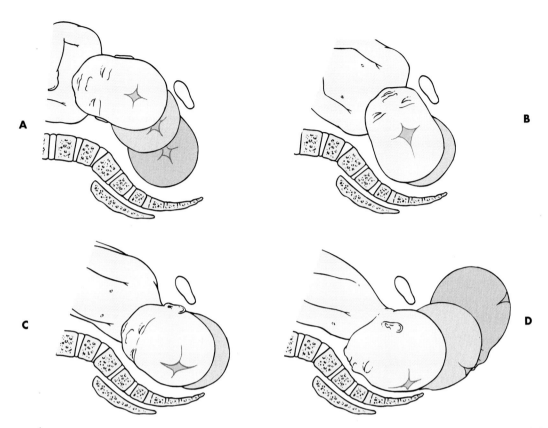

Figure 13-11   Mechanism of labor for a vertex presentation in the left occipitotransverse position. **A,** Flexion and descent. **B** and **C,** Continued descent and commencement of internal rotation. **D,** Completion of internal rotation to the occipitoanterior position, followed by delivery of the head by extension. (Modified from Hacker MH, Moore JG, and Meyer J: *Essentials of obstetrics,* Philadelphia, 1992, WB Saunders.)

INITIATION OF EFFECTIVE LABOR

Labor is equated with the onset of regular contractions and cervical effacement and dilation. Evaluations show that some effacement and dilation usually take place in the last weeks of pregnancy. Because this period is an integral part of the process, it is no longer called "false labor" but rather *prelabor.* Few women enter true labor without some dilation. Those who have not achieved adequate dilation usually have a potential labor problem or have come in for assessment too early. On the other hand, a client unaware of contractions may report for a routine appointment and be found to have a cervix almost fully effaced and partially dilated.

Readiness for labor is the key factor in how long the body will take to accomplish the work of the first stage of labor. Some of the preparatory work has characteristic early signs.

Signs of Early Labor

During the last weeks before labor, contractions will be felt as a painless tightening. These contractions rarely exceed 20 mm Hg or last longer than 60 to 80 seconds. All women should have been instructed on the signs of premature labor (see Box 21-1). They should be instructed when to come in for evaluation of true term labor. Differentiating signs are as follows:

Prelabor	Effective (true) Labor
Uterine contractions:	
Irregular, less than 4 in 20 min	Irregular progressing to regular, > 8/hr
Disappear on ambulation	Intensify with ambulation
Do not increase in duration, frequency, or intensity	Increasing in duration, frequency, or intensity
Cervix:	
No significant dilation/effacement	Increasing dilation/ effacement
	Increased blood-tinged vaginal mucus
Other:	
Discomfort in lower pelvis	Discomfort in lower back, around to abdomen, may feel heavy pressure in groin
	May have diarrhea, ruptured membranes

Lightening

The settling of the fetus into the pelvic cavity is characterized by relief of pressure on the diaphragm and stomach and increased pressure on the bladder. The woman usually experiences the ability to inhale more deeply, with more ease in breathing. Now there is an increase in urinary frequency. This is called **lightening**, which usually occurs 10 to 14 days before labor for primigravidas and at the time of labor for multigravidas. The fundus moves downward and shifts forward. The decrease in fundal height may be noticeable, causing some to say, "it looks as if your baby has dropped."

Bloody show

Changes that occur in the cervix during pregnancy result in increased vascularity. At or near the onset of labor, the mucous plug that has obstructed the cervical canal is expelled because of cervical dilation. The mixture of mucus and a small amount of capillary blood is called the *bloody show.*

Other signs

During the week before labor, a woman may experience increasing pressure sensations throughout the pelvic area. Multiparas particularly complain of perineal or groin pressure. A characteristic "pregnancy waddle" can be observed as the woman walks.

One or two days before onset of labor there may be a weight loss of 1 to 3 pounds. There will be varying energy levels experienced by the pregnant woman, although at the same time, there is a flurry of trying to finish the preparations for the infant.

FIRST STAGE OF LABOR

The first stage of labor traditionally is divided into the latent, active, and advanced active (transition) phases.

Latent (Early) Phase

The **latent phase** extends from the beginning of effective labor (progressive effacement and dilation) until 3-cm dilation has been achieved. Often the start of latent labor is not known. Membranes are usually intact. However, if the woman's membranes rupture spontaneously before regular contractions are established, this is usually considered the beginning of the latent phase. Contractions become increasingly intense, more regular, and more frequent, starting approximately 15 to 20 minutes apart and progressing to 4 to 5 minutes apart. This sequence, when counted, is approximately four contractions an hour and increases to 10 to 12 contractions an hour. Duration of each contraction is 30 to 60 seconds, and intensity is described as mild to moderate.

Active Phase

The **active phase** of labor is the period in which the cervix completes most effacement and dilates to 8 cm. Contractions are more regular, more intense, and more frequent. Although labor patterns show some variation, active labor contractions are 3 to 5 minutes in frequency, last 50 to 75 seconds in duration, and are moderate to strong in intensity. During this phase, cervical dilation should occur rapidly or be *accelerated*.

Advanced Active (Transition) Phase

The **advanced active (transition) phase** is the most difficult period. The cervix opens the final 2 cm, dilating from 8 to 10 cm. Painful, intense, erratic contractions occur every 2 to 3 minutes in frequency with an intensity that is moderate to severe. The woman finds this phase particularly difficult. The **tonus** rises, and there is little time to recover from the painful contractions. Intense contractions persist for 75 to 90 seconds. As the cervix is stretched the last few centimeters, small capillaries may break, and vaginal fluids may be bright red. However, active bleeding or blood containing clots should not occur. As the phase ends, the dilation rate *decelerates* or slows down.

Friedman's phases

Friedman (1985), describes dilation in two phases: latent and active (Figure 13-12). Friedman suggests that the latent phase extends from the onset of labor to the beginning of active dilation. The active phase of labor is divided into three parts: an acceleration phase, a phase of maximum slope, and a deceleration phase. Table 13-2 compares the classic phases of labor with those of Friedman.

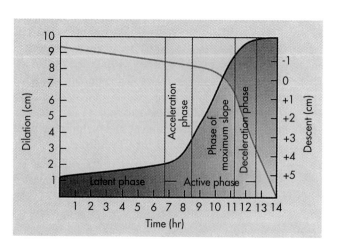

Figure 13-12 Friedman's labor curve and divisions of labor. (From Friedman E, Greenhill JP: *Biological principles and modern practice of obstetrics,* Philadelphia, 1975, WB Saunders.)

Table 13-2	Comparison of Classic Labor and Friedman's Phases of Labor

Classic Description	Friedman's Phases
FIRST STAGE	
Latent (0-3 cm)	Latent (0-2 cm)
Active (3-8 cm)	Active (3-10 cm)
Transition (8-10 cm)	Acceleration (3-4 cm)
	Maximum slope (5-8 cm)
	Deceleration (9-10 cm)

Friedman's study indicates the time for the latent phase for the nullipara to be from 8 to 10 hours but not more than 20 hours. The time for the multipara should be 3 to 5 hours but not more than 14 hours. In assessing the progress of dilation, Friedman used centimeters per hour (cm/hr) rather than total number of hours, making it possible to recognize any problems in a timely fashion. During active dilation, the nullipara averages 3 cm/hr and not less than 1.2 cm/hr, whereas the multipara averages 5.7 cm/hr, and not less than 1.5 cm/hr. A graph of a client's labor (Figure 13-13) provides a much clearer picture of labor progress than do separate recordings. Note that the normal pattern is an **S**-shaped curve. Also note the normal curve of descent. A significant variation in the shape of the patterns reflects difficulty that requires further assessment.

Each woman has a different pattern, and Friedman's graph is only an average. In some cases the graph has been used too literally, and a small delay was used as an indication of operative delivery. Many practitioners do not use the labor curve rigidly, and as long as progress is made and the infant and mother are responding well, labor is continued.

 Box **13-1**

CLINICAL DECISION

Mary, a 26-year-old primipara, was admitted with her husband at 10 PM. Her status on evaluation was as follows: membranes ruptured at 6 PM; contractions every 5 minutes, 40 seconds of mild-to-moderate intensity; cervix 4 cm, 100% effaced, bloody mucus observed; vertex presentation, at −1 station.

At 2 AM Mary's contractions are strong, occurring every 3 minutes and lasting 60 seconds. Vaginal examination shows dilation of 5 cm, but the vertex is still at −1 station. Use the accompanying graph to chart her progress.

At 4 AM Mary is comfortable after regional anesthesia. Her station is 0, and dilation is at 5 cm. What might be reasons for her slow progress? What interventions might be helpful?

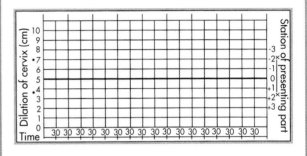

SECOND STAGE OF LABOR

The major function of the second stage is the descent and expulsion of the fetus. Today there are second-stage guidelines that limit the amount of time the woman in labor should remain in this period (for the nullipara, 2 hours and not more than 3; for the multiparas, 1 hour and not more than 2). (With epidural analgesia the time is

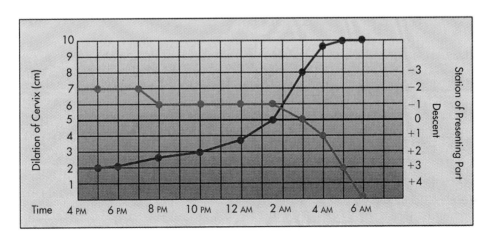

Figure 13-13   Graphic labor record.

increased by 1 hour for both nulliparas and multiparas.) Friedman defined the normal time limits of descent to enable recognition of early problems and to serve as a guide for normal presentations uncomplicated by malposition or other problems. For the nullipara whose birth canal has not been previously distended, the fetus can be expected to descend at least 1.5 cm/hr but in most cases at 3 cm/hr. In the multipara the fetus usually progresses faster than 2.1 cm/hr and most often at approximately 5 cm/hr. The average duration of second stage labor for the multipara is 20 minutes compared with 50 minutes for nulliparas (Cunningham et al, 1993).

For the infant to be born, the resistance of the vaginal canal must be overcome. The pelvic floor, composed chiefly of the levator ani muscles and fasciae, must be displaced downward and outward by the fetal head. The resistance is variable and can be evaluated during vaginal examination. The folds (rugae) of the vagina form a lining membrane. The fascial layers are thinned as they stretch, making vaginal tissue susceptible to tears. The client must add her voluntary expulsive efforts during contractions to achieve the pressure needed for this process. See Chapter 12 for the techniques of open glottis pushing with abdominal muscles.

THIRD STAGE OF LABOR

After the birth of the infant, the height of the uterine fundus and its consistency are assessed. It should remain firm with no unusual bleeding. Watchful waiting is done until the placenta is separated, which usually occurs approximately 5 to 20 minutes after delivery. No massage is performed; the hand is simply rested on the fundus to make certain that the uterus does not become atonic and filled with blood behind a separated placenta (Cunningham et al, 1993).

As the uterus contracts down, the placental site becomes smaller causing separation. The woman must then bear down to move the placenta into the vaginal canal and expel it. Indications that the placenta has separated include the following:

- Uterus becomes smaller and spherical
- Blood gushes from the vagina
- Umbilical cord lengthens by several inches
- Uterus may be displaced upward in the abdomen

The placenta is examined for fragments, and then the fundus is gently massaged to promote contraction and hemostasis.

Nursing Responsibilities

Chapter 14 discusses fetal assessment during labor. Chapter 15 includes nursing care during the second, third, and fourth stages of labor and birth and complications of the labor and birth process.

During labor nursing care changes from hour to hour, and the nurse must respond appropriately to these maternal and fetal changes. Nursing responsibilities are summarized at the end of each phase in the next section of the chapter.

As the nurse plans and provides care, the plan's effectiveness is measured against the degree to which goals are accomplished. Box 13-1 lists nursing diagnoses to consider for low-risk labor clients.

Universal precautions

Nurses attending women and their infants during labor, delivery, and immediately after the birth are frequently exposed to blood and body fluids. Nurses should also be aware of the fact that mandatory human immunodeficiency virus (HIV) testing is virtually unenforceable. This testing probably would drive away from the health care system individuals who are most in need of prenatal assessment (Zuspan et al, 1994). It should also be known that the HIV epidemic has now increased to the point that HIV infection in pregnancy has a prevalence in the low-risk population of 1 in 1000. In high-risk populations, the prevalence may approach 1% to 2%, and in no geographic locale is the client population immune (Zuspan et al, 1994). Three mechanisms for transmission of HIV to health care professionals are parenteral inoculation of blood by needle stick or puncture wound, blood contamination of nonintact skin, and splash exposures to mucous membranes.

Because blood and body fluids are known to be reservoirs for hepatitis and HIV, exposure is a special hazard for health care personnel (see Chapter 25 for a complete discussion). During labor, it is nursing's responsibility to see that universal precautions are observed consistently. Strategies for prevention of blood-borne infection include barrier protec-

---

Box **13-1**	**Nursing Diagnoses to Consider during Labor**

- Fear or anxiety related to lack of knowledge or prior negative experiences
- Ineffective individual or family coping related to couple's age, prior negative experiences, or problems during labor
- Ineffective breathing pattern related to difficulty with labor breathing techniques or no prenatal classes
- Pain related to status of mechanisms of labor and size of fetus
- Caregiver role strain in companion, related to long or difficult labor
- Sleep-pattern disturbance related to long latent period or long labor
- Altered nutrition related to limited oral intake during labor
- Potential for reduced fetal perfusion and distress related to type of labor contractions
- Potential for infection related to duration of rupture of membranes

tion, good infection control technique, and common sense (ACOG, 1997). Gloves must be used for any contact with body fluids, and double gloving is recommended for nurses who scrub for cesarean section or perform vaginal examinations. Waterproof gowns, masks, caps, and eye shields are used for splash exposure and should be worn during procedures such as AROM, vaginal delivery, cesarean section, or other procedures that may cause droplets of blood or amniotic fluid to splash (Zuspan et al, 1994; Acosta et al, 1992). Finally, mechanical suctioning devices should be used to remove secretions and meconium from the neonate's airway (Zuspan et al, 1994). The best line of defense against transmission of disease is good hand-washing technique.

Violations of universal precautions are approximately 48% in the labor areas (Ginsberg, 1990), even though these universal precautions are reviewed on a regular basis for all staff members. Perinatal nurses must be vigilant in their care. They should use the Centers for Disease Control (CDC) guidelines in the care of all clients. Studies have shown that most HIV-infected women are unaware of their HIV status. (Acosta, 1992). The current rate of an HIV-negative status becoming a positive status after a needle stick or cut is 1 in 200 (0.5%). For hepatitis B virus (HBV), it is 30% to 70% (Ginsberg, 1990). Fortunately, vaccination is now available for HBV, and every person who works in the maternity area should be immunized (Box 13-2).

> *Box* 13-2   **Universal Precautions to Reduce Risk of HIV, HBV, and Other Blood Pathogens Transmitted in Obstetric Care**

BODY FLUIDS

Body Fluids to which Universal Precautions Apply

- Fluids known to transmit HIV or HBV infection
  Blood, semen, vaginal secretions
  Other visibly bloody secretions
  Amniotic fluid
- Fluids with unknown risk of transmission for HIV or HBV infection
  Cerebrospinal, synovial, pleural, peritoneal, or pericardial fluids
  Saliva

Body Fluids to which Universal Precautions do not Apply

- Risk of transmission of HIV or HBV infection is extremely low or nonexistent in these fluids:
  Feces, nasal secretions, sputum, sweat, tears, urine, vomitus (Some of these secretions represent potential sources for other pathogens; recommendations for prevention of transmission are available)
  Breast milk is a rare source of perinatal transmission but is not implicated in transmission to health care workers. Health care workers may wish to wear gloves if they have frequent exposure to breast milk.

PRECAUTIONS

- Use appropriate barrier precautions to prevent skin and mucous membrane exposure when contact with blood or body fluid from any client is anticipated.
  When caring for all clients, gloves should be worn for the following:
  - Contact with blood (venipuncture, finger stick, intravenous insertion; changing perineal pads, chux, linen)
  - Contact with body fluids (changing saturated pads, chux, linen, or clothing after rupture of membranes)
  - Contact with mucous membranes (vaginal examination)

Contact with nonintact skin
Handling items soiled with blood or body fluids (soiled pads, chux, bedding, clothing)
- Gloves should be changed after contact with each client and between client contacts.
- Medical gloves (vinyl or latex sterile surgical or nonsterile examination gloves) should not be washed and reused. Washing with surfactants may enhance penetration of liquids through undetected holes in gloves.
- Masks, protective eyewear, face shields, and fluid-resistant gowns should be worn during procedures that commonly cause splashes of blood or body fluids onto mucous membranes of mouth, nose, or eyes.
  Vaginal or cesarean birth
  Cutting umbilical cord between infant and placenta
  Possible AROM under pressure
- Gowns and gloves should be worn by health care workers handling placenta or the infant until blood and amniotic fluid have been removed from the infant's skin by bathing. Gloves should be worn for care of umbilical cord after delivery.
- Removal of infant nasopharyngeal secretion at delivery should use mechanical suction (not with De Lee suction apparatus).
  Resuscitation should use resuscitation bags or other ventilation equipment.
- Gloves torn or punctured by needle stick or other injury should be removed and replaced as promptly as possible.
- Precautions should be taken to prevent injury from needles and surgical instruments.
  Needles should not be recapped, bent, broken, or removed from disposable syringes.
  After use, needles, scalpel blades, and other sharp items should be placed in puncture-resistant containers for disposal. Surgical instruments should be carefully cleaned to avoid injury.

Occupational Safety and Health Administration (OSHA): Blood-borne pathogens, the final standard, *Federal Register* 56(64):175, 1991.
Centers for Disease Control: Update: universal precautions for prevention of transmission of human immunodeficiency virus, hepatitis B virus and other blood-borne pathogens in health care settings, *MMWR* 37(24):377, 1988.

ADMISSION TO LABOR

When a client comes to the labor area, the initial assessment taken by the nurse should be a quick overview. The essential points will reveal any urgent problems. This is a form of **triage** that determines priorities in care (Angelini et al, 1990). To prioritize care, the following information is needed:

1. When labor started
2. What is the current contraction pattern
3. When, or if, membranes ruptured
4. Baseline vital signs and fetal heart rate (FHR)
5. Woman's parity and type of prenatal care
6. Birth plan, which must include any problems affecting progress in labor

Usually the external fetal heart monitor is attached to obtain a short tracing as a baseline reading. Findings are documented on the admission form.

Labor care begins with the client's admission into the triage area. The orientation through this triage area follows an ordered sequence as the nurse performs the following procedures:

1. Introduces herself or himself to the client, using the woman's preferred name at all times, avoiding the use of terms such as "Mommy" or "Dearie"
2. Communicates effectively, making sure to include the client and her significant other
3. Explains the sequence of the admission procedures and gives supportive instructions if the woman needs to wait for admission
4. Obtains a complete admission history and nursing systems assessment, including vaginal examination, which is compared with the baseline history from the physician's chart
5. Applies the external fetal monitor to assess the FHR and the tocodynamometer to assess the woman's contraction patterns; makes a careful assessment of the fetal monitor strip to determine the status of the fetus. Makes a note of any signs of abnormalities; determines the frequency and duration of contractions
6. Detects any high-risk conditions requiring immediate medical attention and notifies the physician or midwife. The response time of the medical staff must be documented.

7. Reviews the prenatal chart data and includes pertinent points in the admission notes
8. Initiates an individualized nursing care plan and documents all care and treatments on the client's chart
9. Uses universal precautions in all care

After the initial assessment, the nurse notifies the physician of the woman's arrival and whether there is need for additional prenatal information. After the nurse assesses whether the woman has experienced the rupture of her membranes (ROM), specific priorities are established depending on these initial findings.

Vaginal Examination

The nurse converses with the woman, instructing her in breathing and relaxation techniques as she performs or assists with the obstetric examination (Procedure 13-1) (see Chapter 4). Her gentle manner and careful explanations of findings are important.

The vaginal examination is an important procedure to assess progress of cervical dilation, pelvic adequacy, and fetal descent. Unfortunately, it also may provide access for ascending infection. Even with aseptic technique, vaginal bacteria will be tracked up into the cervical canal. Therefore examinations must be kept to a minimum and performed quickly. After AROM or SROM, vaginal examinations should be minimized and each examination documented. (If a later infection of the endometrium develops, quality assurance and the infection control team may track the relationship of the number of examinations. This will be compared with onset and severity of maternal or newborn infections [see Chapter 25].)

Vaginal examinations are *never* done when there is frank vaginal bleeding, known low placental location, or early ROM. A sterile speculum examination may be performed in these cases to visualize the vagina and cervix and to verify rupture of the membranes. (Follow the steps for preparation as discussed in Chapter 4.)

Once the sterile, lubricated, gloved hand is inserted in the vaginal canal, it should not be removed until the assessment is completed. Because findings during a contraction may be compared with findings during the resting phase, the duration of the vaginal examination may seem long to the woman.

The *Bishop score* may be used to determine readiness for labor. After the vaginal examination a score of 0, 1, 2, or 3 is given for each of the following:

- Consistency of the cervix (firm to soft)
- Position of the cervix (posterior to anterior)
- Effacement of cervix (up to 80% effaced)
- Dilation of cervix (up to 5 cm)
- Station of presenting part (from floating down to +2)

A total score of less than 5 to 7 indicates that the cervix is not completely ready for labor.

PROCEDURE 13-1
Vaginal Examination during Labor

1. Examine the perineal area.
2. Look for signs of health, intact skin, and proportions.
3. Look for signs of inflammation or infection on perineum.
4. Note any fluid leaking or bloody show. If a nitrazine test is indicated, it should be done before sterile vaginal examination (SVE) because lubricant can affect nitrazine.
5. Note any strong odor to fluids and their color and consistency.
6. Note any scars indicating episiotomy or prior perineal surgery.
7. Apply sterile lubricating jelly to a sterile latex glove.
8. Part the labia to slip the first two fingers into the vagina.
9. Direct fingers to the back of the vagina.
10. Move fingers up to contact the cervix.
11. Place the opposite hand over the abdomen.
12. Palpate during a contraction, pushing down slightly in the direction of the perineum (Figure 13-14).

Assess the cervix for the following criteria:

Position: Is the cervix directed toward posterior, midposition, or anterior?

Consistency: Is the cervix firm, medium, or soft?

Effacement: Recorded as a percentage as follows:

%	Result
Not begun	2-cm long and thick
25	1.5-cm long and softened
50	1-cm long and very soft
75	0.5-cm long
100	Feels very thin; ready to be pulled up into the lower uterine segment

Dilation: Recorded as a range up to 10 cm (fully dilated); measurement is approximate and depends on the examiner's finger size.

Closed or fingertip	Cannot insert fingertip into canal
2	1 fingerwidth can be inserted into canal
3-4	2 fingerwidths can be inserted into canal
4-5	3 fingerwidths can be inserted into canal
5-6	Finger moves easily from side to side of fetal presenting part before touching cervix
7-8	Cervix is felt like a low, smooth ridge surrounding the curve of the presenting part
8-9	Ridge of encircling cervix is stretched taut, with more vaginal bleeding as capillaries are broken in the cervix
9-10	Cervix flat, almost pulled up around presenting part; may still be felt as an anterior or posterior rim or lip
Complete	Cervix cannot be felt as fetal part slips through, enters the vagina, descends through the stations

Station: Assess the level of descent of the presenting part by locating the ischial spines on either side of the canal and assessing the relative location of the fetal part to these spines (see Figure 13-11).

Explain findings to woman, and make her comfortable after examination procedure is concluded.

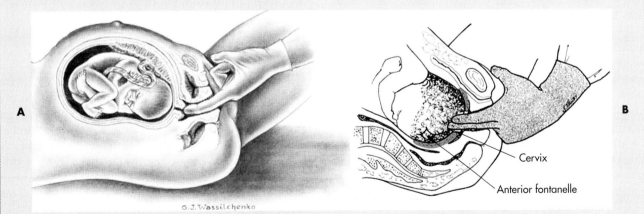

Figure 13-14   Vaginal examination. **A,** Undilated, uneffaced cervix; membranes intact. **B,** Palpation of sagittal suture line. Cervix effaced and partially dilated. (From Lowdermilk DL, Perry SE, Bobak IM: *Maternity and women's health care,* ed 6, St Louis, 1997, Mosby.)

OPTIONAL ACTIVITY

Write a sample nursing note correctly documenting the performance of this procedure.

Protocols for "Walk-In" Clients

Women who have not received prenatal care may arrive at the labor area. Often they are women with varying degrees of psychosocial and personal struggles. To single out one group of individuals would be difficult. Women who lack fluency in English may find it difficult to enter the obstetric unit. An interpreter may be needed, a role that the partner may be able to fill. Other reasons why women do not receive prenatal care include lack of access to care, lack of financial resources or transportation, or abuse of drugs.

Nursing responsibilities

Every attempt must be made to decrease the woman's fear. This client may be in advanced labor on admission. The nurse must assess quickly to determine priorities and potential complications, a form of **triage**. Each assessment step must be documented. Assessment and support are especially critical because of time constraints and need for information.

In addition to the usual admission steps, if a woman in labor has not received prenatal care, the physician performs a physical examination to determine the presence of any impending obstetric or medical complications. Blood is sent to the laboratory for screening for sexually transmitted infections, HBV, anemia (hemoglobin and hematocrit values), Rh antibodies, rubella antibodies, and white blood cell and platelet counts. Urine for glucose and albumin is obtained.

CARE DURING LATENT LABOR PHASE

The latent phase extends from the beginning of effective dilation to 3-cm dilation. Contractions begin to be effective with progress in frequency from approximately 3 to 4/hr to 10 to 12/hr (20 minutes apart progressing to 4 to 5 minutes apart). Contractions are mild at first with an acme below 35 mm Hg, increasing to moderate, or an acme between 50 and 60 mm Hg (Figure 13-15). The contractions may not be sensed as painful, but as the phase progresses, the woman begins the pattern of slow chest breathing. Cervical changes become evident during this period because contractions will almost complete effacement and bring dilation to 3 cm. Usually the presenting part gradually moves deeper into the pelvis. The ROM does not profoundly influence labor during this early phase.

Mood

During the latent phase the woman's reactions vary. She is comfortable, but she also may be excited, ambivalent, or anxious. Her mood parallels the ambivalence of the first trimester. Her confidence in herself and her coach is reinforced as she appropriately applies the techniques she has learned.

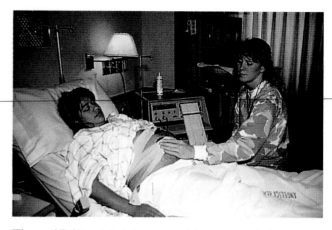

Figure 13-15   Admission to the labor area includes orientation and a period of time for contraction and fetal heart monitoring. (Courtesy Marjorie Pyle, RNC, *Lifecircle*.)

Coach/Partner

The woman needs the support of the partner during the latent phase to indicate caring and concern. The partner supports and encourages the woman by assisting, reinforcing, directing, and clarifying the techniques and supportive strategies she has learned. The childbirth preparation assists in increasing her self-esteem and personal strength (Lowe, 1996).

The unprepared woman's perceptions may be drastically altered by anxiety. Relaxation and self-directed activities may be difficult because concern for her own and her infant's well-being increases as her anxiety heightens. As a result, perception of contractions may be felt as more acute pain (Hodnett, 1996). The nurse should provide praise and encouragement with contractions, stay with the laboring mother as much as possible, and provide a calm, quiet environment.

Comfort Measures

The prepared couple should be encouraged to view the woman's work during labor as a close parallel to that of a long-distance runner or swimmer. After the warm-up, the race begins. Runners pace themselves with controlled effort, coordinated muscular effort, and rhythmic breathing patterns.

At the beginning of the early phase, the woman usually is at home and may continue diversional activities, interspersed with rest periods. She should urinate often to prevent bladder distention. Her diet usually is restricted to liquids that will sustain her for labor. If she awakens with mild contractions, she should be encouraged to get up, take a warm shower, drink a cup of tea, and then try to sleep. If she is unduly apprehensive, she can use *controlled relaxation:* She takes a deep breath as the contraction begins, relaxes her body completely as she exhales, concentrating on the contraction. She may breathe normally as she permits the contraction to work. If needed, she can begin controlled breathing activities.

Nursing Approach

The nurse who is available for consultation during the earlier phases of labor can offer suggestions about techniques and will boost the couple's self-confidence. She can also validate their appraisal of labor and interpret instructions from the physician in a positive and supportive manner.

As long as membranes remain intact, the well-informed couple should stay at home during the latent phase of labor. With the approval of the physician or nurse midwife, the nurse should encourage activity during this phase. If the woman does come in and the active phase has not yet begun, she may be encouraged to walk in hospital corridors or her room and should not be put to bed in a recumbent position. For example, one birthing center sends the woman in this phase out for a light meal at a local restaurant. On the other hand, many hospitals and physicians discourage their clients from eating full meals in early labor.

If they have come to the hospital too early, the couple should not be sent home with an abrupt dismissal. The nurse can underscore the need for rest and the maintenance of fluid balance and energy reserves and remind them of the nature of the labor process. The couple at this point may see themselves as amateurs and appreciate specific directions relevant to their needs.

Box 13-2

CLINICAL DECISION

Mary and Jim arrive in the labor unit at 4 AM for their first birth. She has had mild labor for 6 hours. They had two classes but did not find time to practice consistently. Mary is anxious; Jim looks "blank" and wants to be with Mary but looks as if he does not know what to do. How would you work to smooth the transition into their being a "laboring couple"?

Vital signs during labor

The nurse should always be aware of baseline readings obtained from the last prenatal visit. The labor admission chart may reveal a false reading because the woman may be excited on admission. The pulse rate should be considered in terms of excitement, impending fever (pulse rises first), or alteration in cardiac output related to blood volume or drugs. Maternal tachycardia also may influence the FHR (see the discussion on intrapartal fetal assessment in Chapter 14). The external monitor is applied, and FHR characteristics are observed (see Figure 13-15).

The blood pressure is perhaps the most significant indicator of maternal cardiovascular status (see Chapter 9). It is abnormal for any young woman to have a diastolic pressure above 80 mm Hg. Therefore if a comparison of pressures with the baseline readings for the last trimester reveals an elevation—even if not above 80 mm Hg—further assessment includes checking the urine for albumin. Blood pressure during labor is taken only with the woman in a lateral position, sitting, or with a wedge tilt to the side to avoid supine hypotension. The same arm should be used for each reading. Each unit has a protocol for timing of vital signs. Usually temperature, pulse, and respiration are obtained every 4 hours unless there is an elevation of temperature or membranes are ruptured. Blood pressure is taken every 4 hours in early labor, every hour when active labor begins, and every 30 minutes in second-stage labor.

Temperature can begin to rise for several reasons during labor. First, the woman may have not received adequate fluids and may be dehydrated. A check of urine concentration will determine if this condition exists. If membranes have ruptured more than 8 to 12 hours before the onset of labor, it is possible to have ascending infection, with inflammation of the chorion and the uterine endometrium (see Chapter 25). The temperature will rise slowly. Any temperature above 99° F should be checked more frequently (Table 13-3). Finally, if epidural anesthesia is used, there may be an elevated temperature (see Chapter 16).

Summary of Nursing Responsibilities

The client and her partner should be greeted courteously when they come to the labor unit. The nurse performs the initial evaluation, and in some settings the physical examination is done by the nurse midwife or physician. After evaluation, it may be determined that they have come too

Table 13-3   **Vital Signs during Low-Risk Labor and Birth**

Sign	Cervical Progress		
	Latent	Active	Second Stage
Blood pressure	q4h	q1-2h	q30-10min
Fetal heart rate	q1h	q30min	q15min
Temperature	q4h	q4h	q4h
After ROM	-	q2h	q2h
If elevated	q1h	q1h	q1h
Pulse	q4h	q2-4h	q2-4h
Respirations	q4h	q4h	Not done— pushing

Follow unit protocol. Record signs on flow sheet and, if fetal monitoring in place, on strip chart.

early and would be more comfortable at home until labor is more well established.

Labor and delivery place several stressors on the maternal-fetal system, which may increase the risk of unforeseen complications. Alterations in the physiologic and psychologic processes can have a significant impact on the well-being of both, therefore a complete assessment and evaluation must be carried out to lessen the chance of problems that can be avoided.

The following steps must be completed once the woman is admitted into the labor suite:

1. Obtain prenatal history; ask about immediate events such as onset of labor, status of membranes, and bloody show.
2. Assess phase of labor and condition of woman; obtain vital signs, and perform physical assessment, including Leopold's maneuvers.
3. With external fetal tocodynamometer and ultrasound transducer, run a monitor strip for 20 minutes. This enables assessment of contraction strength and frequency, and fetal heart responses to contractions.
4. By means of vaginal examination, assess station, cervical status, and condition of external perineal tissues.

In some settings, the nurse decides if the woman is.in active labor or if there are reasons for her to be admitted. In other settings, she is initially examined by the physician. If she is to go home temporarily, she should be given careful instructions about activities during the next few hours and when to return. Once the decision is made about admission, the following further steps are taken.

1. Continue with admission activities after determination of status. Establish the presence of any risk factors. Complete the nursing history, and attach the mother's identification band.
2. As ordered, ensure that blood is drawn for admission tests, usually complete blood cell count, type, and crossmatch (kept for use by blood bank if needed), plus any other specimens. Some units use a heparin or saline lock for drawing blood and administering needed IV fluids.
3. Note where woman's belongings are placed.
4. Assist couple to settle into the labor room. Establish a relaxed atmosphere. Explain equipment, and orient them to routines of checking vital signs and monitors and physician's visits.
5. Determine couple's birth plan, type of childbirth preparation, and expectations for nurse involvement in support. Assure them that you will be flexible in your interventions for support.
6. Promote comfort by showing them positions to assume during labor, where to obtain ice chips, and how to use comfort equipment.
7. Evaluate couple's response to this phase of labor. Document all findings.

CARE DURING ACTIVE LABOR PHASE

The active phase includes a period of accelerated, progressive dilation with well-defined contractions at frequent intervals and a **transition phase** immediately before complete dilation.

At the midpoint of this phase, contractions become strong and more consistent in interval and duration, with shorter rest intervals. This phase demands the total concentration of the laboring woman and the encouragement of those attending her if she is to remain confident.

The cervix is effaced further while rapid dilation to 8 cm occurs. The dilation may plateau or seem to stop at 5 cm, but this phase is short. The increase in bloody show may begin. The woman becomes increasingly uncomfortable and fatigued.

CULTURAL AWARENESS

HISPANIC MOTHER

In my family, when you hurt, you make noise. Every time I moaned or cried out in labor, the nurse offered me pain medication. When I refused, she'd tell me to use the breathing I'd learned in class to help me stay in control. Making noise *was* my way of staying in control. She also kept asking my mother and sisters to leave the room. She didn't understand that this birth wasn't just happening to me, it was happening to my whole family. I needed them with me.

Mood

The woman's confident, talkative mood during the latent phase is quickly replaced by an intense, total absorption in labor. As this phase continues and fatigue increases, the woman's confidence may begin to waver; if so, she always requires active supportive measures.

The unprepared woman may exhibit a disorganized pattern of behavior. Apprehension increases, and sentences become fragmented. She may become irritable, unable to cope if left alone, and beg to be put to sleep.

Coach/Partner

The need for coaching increases with the active phase. As contractions heighten and occur more frequently, the woman's perspective becomes distorted. She needs to be reminded to take one contraction at a time. Her coach may help her to focus by counting each 15-second interval with the contraction. Other women are irritated by these reminders.

Comfort Measures

The woman must now direct her conscious efforts to controlled relaxation. She becomes aware of the importance of concentration as she deals with contractions. It is during this phase that analgesics may be needed. (See Chapter 16 for types of drugs and routes of administration.)

The woman should be encouraged to be ambulatory when possible (see Box 13-3). The use of comfort devices such as rocking chairs, birthing beds, and hydrotherapy conserves energy.

Hydrotherapy, either in a bathtub or shower may facilitate labor, either through relaxation or position changes (see Chapter 12). The woman's position in the bathtub may be leaning on the hands and knees, resting in a side-lying position, or floating with the abdomen down

CULTURAL AWARENESS

The transcultural committee at our hospital learned that 84 Kurdish refugees from northern Iraq would be settling in the area. Members educated themselves about Kurdish cultures and the Muslim faith and held workshops for the staff to prepare them should the Kurds need hospital services. Consequently, when a Kurdish mother arrived with her own midwife for her first hospital experience and her ninth birth, personnel made every effort to accommodate her customs. There were only female attendants, including a female translator, and the mother chose to deliver the infant in the hands-and-knees position to which she was accustomed. She also kept her head and the infant's head covered at all times.

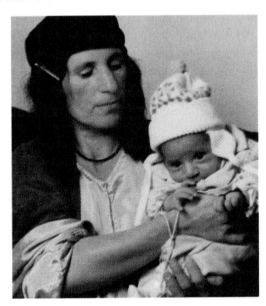

Muslims in the United States are estimated to be 2 to 3 million in population. Islamic laws governing modesty *(hijaab)* and diet *(halal)* are important to Muslim women. Nurses must also be aware that Muslim women are not to be alone in the presence of a man other than her husband or a male relative *(mahram)*.

(Aderhold and Perry, 1991). Because "failure to progress" in labor is a leading reason for cesarean births, nursing measures that conserve energy, prevent fatigue, encourage the efficiency of the process, and encourage the woman's stamina are important.

Positions for labor

The woman's position during labor can affect the physical comfort and the physiologic processes of birth. Traditionally, each culture has promoted a position for labor and birth (see Cultural Awareness box). In this country until the last few years the labor position has been recumbent: supine with slightly elevated head and shoulders. Table 13-4 compares the advantages and disadvantages of selected positions for labor and delivery. Position during labor is influenced by cultural factors, obstetric practices, place of delivery, technology, and health care practices, according to Blackburn and Loper (1992). Although recumbent (flat) position during the labor process offers advantages for the caregiver, when supine, the woman may experience a decrease in the strength of uterine contractions and will develop vena caval compression, late decelerations, and a decrease in the newborn's Apgar scores (Andrews, 1990).

Research has shown that the upright position—high Fowler's, sitting in chair, or ambulating during active labor—shortened the phase of maximum slope (4 to 8 cm) by an average of 90 minutes (Roberts et al, 1983). More recent findings state that the upright (standing, sitting, squatting, kneeling) positions (versus supine) were associated with more regular and intense contractions and shorter duration of first and second stages and total labor (Blackburn and Loper, 1992). Although changes in pain perception or fetal outcome did not occur, contractions were more efficient, intense, and frequent. In addition, dilation possibly was increased because of the effects of gravity. Maternal mobility and choice of position during labor have been found to be beneficial forms of care with clear evidence from controlled trials (Enkin et al, 1995). Such a finding should be implemented into standard labor nursing practice (Figure 13-16). The woman may prefer sitting or walking during early labor but later may choose the semi-recumbent or side-lying positions with pillow support as labor progresses. Women may choose to change positions many times during labor (Box 13-3).

Fluids during labor

Routine withholding of food and drink during labor has been a controversial issue, with individuals opposed to food and fluids arguing that, although rare, aspiration has devastating consequences and can still occur. Those advocating ignoring current restrictions have noted that general anesthesia has been replaced by regional anesthesia, and the incidence of maternal aspiration in normal labor is rare (Blackburn and Loper, 1992). Research studies have found that both psychologic and physiologic problems can arise

Table 13-4   Positions for Labor

Advantages	Disadvantages
RECUMBENT	
Supine	
Convenient for fetal monitoring, vaginal examination, treatments, and palpating contractions; familiar resting position	Decreases strength of contractions. Increases risk of supine hypotension; increases length of labor (Liu, 1989)
Lithotomy	
Facilitates a standing or sitting position for physician; exposes perineum widely for vaginal examination; used for fetal monitoring; helpful in hemorrhage, emergency	Increases venous return and central blood volume when legs higher than heart. Adverse effects: tachycardia, increased blood pressure
Left Lateral	
Comfortable for woman; more intense, less frequent contractions (Roberts et al, 1983). Prevents vena caval compression. Allows birth in relaxed position for woman; reduces potential for perineal lacerations	More difficult to obtain consistent fetal heart rate; longer labor than upright position (Roberts et al, 1983)
UPRIGHT	
High Fowler's, In Chair, Ambulating	
Facilitates efficient and more intense contractions; cervical dilation assisted by gravity effect	May need position change as woman gets fatigued; fetal monitor tracing more difficult to obtain

Box 13-3   Appropriate Activity during Labor for Low-Risk Mothers

- Early labor: ambulating, upright
- Active labor: ambulating, if desired; if in bed, upright, lateral; sitting
- Bed rest after ROM unless fetal head is well engaged and danger of cord prolapse is negligible
- Second stage: sitting, semi-sitting, squatting, left lateral

from fasting during labor. Potential physiologic effects of fasting include increased ketones and fatty acids with decreased alanine, glucose, and insulin. Psychologic effects include increased anxiety and stress.

In the earliest periods of labor, women are instructed to drink clear liquids frequently and to eat simple foods such as tea, gelatin, frozen sicles, and toast and jelly. After labor is well established, liquids may be continued. Fluids by mouth, especially fruit juices, help the woman to maintain appropriate colloid osmotic pressure. In general, infants have fewer problems with hypoglycemia, jaundice, and weight loss when the mother had adequate liquids during labor (Ludka and Roberts, 1993).

Although in some settings nothing by mouth during labor is still the fixed rule, more physicians and most midwives in hospitals do not follow this practice. Some have advocated for a relaxation of these current restrictions because: (1) aspiration of stomach contents in normal labor is rare; (2) gastric emptying is not significantly altered in normal women who have not received narcotics; (3) the use of intravenous (IV) fluid administration is increased; and (4) prolonged fasting during labor has adverse effects. (See Chapter 16 for reasons why fluid use during labor remains controversial.) When IV fluids are given, physiologic fluids without glucose are used. Care must be taken with the flow rate because too rapid of an infusion may result in circulatory overload. The normal rate of flow is 125 ml/hr. The exception is the increased IV rate used before a regional anesthetic when the rate is changed and monitored by the anesthesiologist. Some labor units use only a heparin or saline lock for IV access, which is used as a precaution if there is hemorrhage.

Monitoring intake and output. It is important to understand why intake and output recording are necessary during labor. First, activities of labor lead to dehydration, which is revealed by dry mucous membranes, slight elevation of temperature, and dark concentrated urine. Second, fluid restrictions in some units or liberal oral fluids in others will change the normal voiding patterns. (IV fluid overload is a key iatrogenic [treatment-caused] problem in labor, especially if epidural anesthetics are used). Third, a full bladder hinders descent of the fetus, and fetal pressure may injure the stretched urethra and bladder tissues. All of

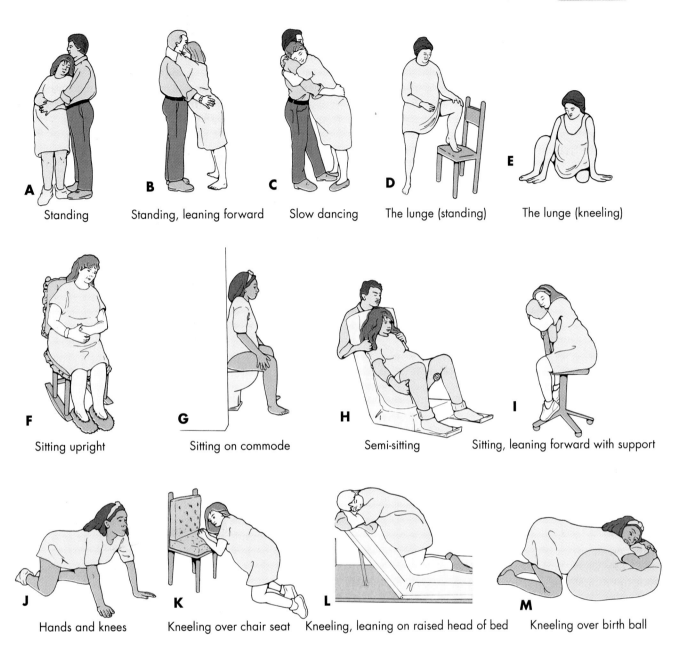

Figure 13-16 Positions helpful during labor. *Top row,* upright positions; *Second row,* sitting positions; *Third row,* kneeling positions. (Redrawn from Ancheta R, Simkin P: *Labor progress handbook: early interventions for the prevention and treatment of dysfunctional labor,* 1994.)

A Standing

B Standing, leaning forward

C Slow dancing

D The lunge (standing)

E The lunge (kneeling)

F Sitting upright

G Sitting on commode

H Semi-sitting

I Sitting, leaning forward with support

J Hands and knees

K Kneeling over chair seat

L Kneeling, leaning on raised head of bed

M Kneeling over birth ball

these problems are avoided by careful monitoring and appropriate interventions by the nurse.

Bladder care during labor

The bladder is checked for fullness every 2 hours, and the woman is encouraged to void. Concentrated urine indicates dehydration. On occasion, with the use of an epidural anesthetic, the woman may not be able to void; therefore a Foley catheter is placed. This catheter should be removed before the pushing phase of labor because the inflated balloon may traumatize

bladder tissue. It also causes discomfort and inhibits pushing efforts. The bladder should be emptied by straight catheterization just before application of forceps or vacuum extractor or if the fetal head is having difficulty descending.

Before a cesarean section, a Foley catheter is placed to empty the bladder and minimize risk of surgical trauma. The lower uterine segment is attached to the bladder by fascia; it must be dissected away before the incision into the uterus is made. If the bladder is not empty, there is danger of cutting into it during surgery.

Checking urine during labor. Upon admission, each woman may be requested to void so that urine may be checked for albumin, ketones, glucose, and leukocytes. Because of the vaginal fluids, the initial specimen must be a midstream, clean-voided specimen. The presence of urinary albumin levels above +1 may indicate pregnancy-induced hypertension. If the leukocyte count is high, a straight catheterization may be ordered to obtain a specimen for culture and sensitivity. Counts greater than 100,000 colonies/mL indicate bacteriuria. Unless blood in the urine is marked, its presence usually is believed to result from red blood cells in the bloody show. Ketones and glucose are checked on admission, and later, if the woman has diabetes, capillary glucose will be used to follow her blood glucose levels. Ketones are checked on each voiding for a diabetic client because ketones may be present in spite of a normal serum glucose (see Chapter 24).

Box 13-3

CLINICAL DECISION

Sara is in the accelerated period of the active phase. She was admitted at 4 cm of dilation and is now at 6 cm. This is her first pregnancy, and dilation is progressing at a rate of approximately 1 cm/hr. She and her husband, Rick, have participated in childbirth preparation classes. They have begun to call for you frequently. Describe four appropriate interventions.

Back labor

A woman may experience "back labor" because of a posterior position of the fetus or a focus of tension. While using appropriate breathing techniques, she should direct her concentration on releasing tension, specifically in the sacrum, perineum, buttocks, and thighs. She avoids lying on her back; instead, her coach can apply firm *counterpressure* to the sacral area. The partner should not rub the skin because over the hours of labor the skin will become irritated by friction. Some women find relief from having cold or warm compresses or lotion applied to the sacrum. The *pelvic rock exercise,* in which the woman rounds the back and tilts the pelvis forward, may also provide some relief for back labor.

Hyperventilation

If a woman begins to **hyperventilate,** a respiratory imbalance of decreased carbon dioxide (CO_2) levels will develop. She may rebreathe exhaled air from her cupped hands, or O_2 can be administered to corect symptoms of **hyperventilation,** including dizziness, light-headedness, and tingling. Nursing interventions can prevent hyperventilation by encouraging slow breathing and tension reduction.

Nursing Approach

Although the couple has learned various skills, discomfort still occurs. Ensure that the couple understands medication, anesthetics, and other obstetric techniques that may be indicated for the birth. If they have not attended childbirth classes, explanations are important so the partners may discuss options.

In observing labor and reactions, the nurse must rely on the woman's judgment of her comfort. She may appear to be in distress when she is concentrating and working hard. Note that cultural variations may significantly change labor responses. Comments such as, "You're working very hard," "Having a baby is hard work. You're doing a good job," or "That contraction was not easy, but you managed it" underscore appreciation of the work of labor and the effectiveness of her efforts.

The unprepared woman with no partner needs special encouragement. Ideally, provision should be made for a nurse to remain with her on a one-to-one basis. This is not often possible because of staffing limitations. The woman needs to be informed of her progress and the infant's condition in terms she can understand. The nurse's direct and positive manner and use of simple terms can help the woman with relaxation and breathing techniques.

Summary of Nursing Responsibilities

The active phase of labor requires the nurse to be increasingly involved. As the phase progresses, fetal responses may change, and the woman's coping abilities are tested. Besides continuing the supportive care of the first phase, the nurse performs the following functions:

1. Monitors woman's responses by checking vital signs, assessing contractions by palpation or internal pressure catheter
2. Monitors progress of cervical dilation and fetal descent, remembering to avoid frequent vaginal examinations after membranes rupture
3. Assesses fetal responses to phase of labor, checks heart tones in relation to contractions, and documents per protocol
4. Maintains woman's hygiene for comfort; observes vaginal fluids for any changes in show or rupture of membranes during this phase
5. Promotes positions of comfort, supports coach in using comfort measures, and notes mood changes and coping abilities
6. Interprets labor progress to couple and affirms their coping abilities
7. Assists with analgesic or regional anesthetic administration if needed
8. Monitors intake and output
9. Evaluates nursing interventions and makes necessary modifications

10. Documents all findings, and informs midwife or physician of labor progress.

CARE DURING THE ADVANCED ACTIVE (TRANSITION) PHASE

As cervical dilation nears completion, the woman enters the most intensive and demanding part of the first stage. Fatigue, the inconsistency and discomfort of contractions, and the intensities of labor make self-control difficult. Most of this period is in the *pelvic phase* as the fetus finishes its descent through the pelvis in preparation for entry into the vaginal canal. Internal rotation occurs.

Contractions

Contraction intervals shorten from 3 to 2 minutes. There is little rest, and tonus may rise. Contractions build rapidly into strong peaks that last approximately two thirds of each contraction. Contractions may show multiple peaks. The contraction also subsides quickly, but the woman often feels as though these never completely disappear. Her body is being bombarded with stimuli, and she is highly sensitized.

With contractions, the cervix now dilates fully, from approximately 8 to 10 cm. This may produce a heavy show because more cervical capillaries rupture. The presenting part may cause strong sensations of pressure in the rectum, back, groin, or perineum. A woman may feel as though she is going to have a bowel movement and may call for a bedpan. In the multipara, dilation may progress dramatically from 8 to 10 cm in a few minutes.

Mood and Physical Reactions

The woman may become agitated and intense during this period. The physiologic changes of labor and fatigue make her irritable, discouraged, panicked, and restless. Her reactions are like those of a marathon runner "hitting the wall" at the 20-mile mark. She finds it difficult to cope with contractions. Relaxation during the brief rest intervals is almost impossible without special strategies. She may sweat profusely, become chilled, or alternate between these reactions. She may be nauseated and briefly vomit. Her legs may tremble and cramp. She may feel overwhelmed and discouraged; she may want to give up. Her perspective may be severely distorted.

Coach/Partner

Coaching must be specific and direct. The woman's reactions frequently require active and continual direction. The partner may have to touch the abdominal area lightly to help her discern the absence of a contraction. Verbal and nonverbal communication is important to her ability to remain in control (Figure 13-17).

Comfort Measures

To assist efforts to relax between contractions, restore respiratory balance, and foster a sense of well-being, the woman uses the rhythmic chest breathing. She should be instructed to perform the slowest rate, 8 breaths/min, during the brief intervals and puff-blows in rhythms of 4-1, 3-1, 2-1, and 1-1 during the contractions (see Chapter 12).

Effleurage is irritating and distracting during the advanced phase, but the woman may find relief in supporting the lower abdominal area with her hands. The coach may hold her hand, embrace her, or give counterpressure to the lower back (Figure 13-18). (See Chapter 16 for other comfort techniques.) Position changes may be helpful.

Nursing Approach

The woman's need for reassurance intensifies. The nurse continues to interpret progress of labor through

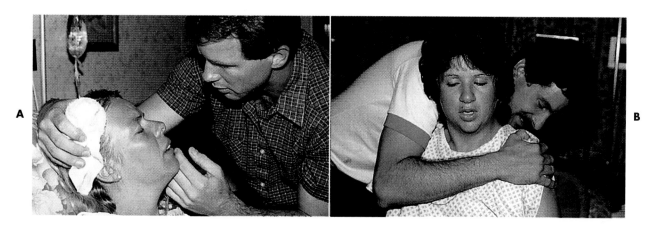

Figure 13-17   Transition is the most difficult phase. **A,** A cold washcloth helps. **B,** The coach offers support. (Courtesy Marjorie Pyle, RNC, *Lifecircle.*)

vaginal examinations, monitoring readings, palpation, and observation. The woman must not be left alone at this phase. At the same time, preparations for the birth phase need to be organized. The couple needs to know when and if the woman will be moved to another room for the birth. In a labor-delivery-recovery room (LDR), the nurse will already have checked supplies and equipment so there will be no interruption of nursing support. The fetal condition will be checked every 30 minutes as a minimum standard of care for low-risk labor. The nurse remains alert to sudden changes in the position and station of the presenting part, particularly with multipara.

Summary of Nursing Responsibilities

1. Assess the woman's condition and the progress of the phase of labor.
2. Assess fetal response to accelerated labor every 30 minutes.
3. Monitor intake and output.
4. Maintain perineal hygiene and a dry underpad.
5. Take appropriate action in assisting physician or midwife.
6. Prepare the birthing room.
7. Evaluate woman's responses to interventions.
8. Support partner as he or she helps with breathing and coping activities and using various comfort measures.
9. Document all observations.

Table 13-5 summarizes all the phases of labor. A sample care path for vaginal birth follows.

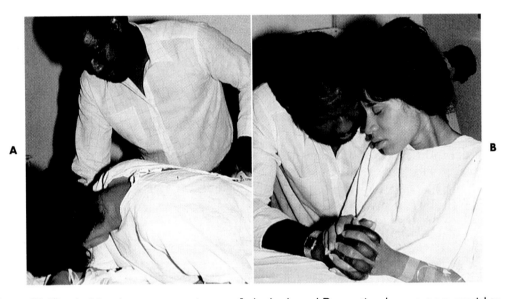

Figure 13-18   As labor becomes more intense, **A,** backrubs and **B,** emotional support are crucial to coping. (Courtesy Marjorie Pyle, RNC, *Lifecircle*.)

Table **13-5   Labor Summary***

Phase	Recommended Coping Techniques	Partner Activities
LATENT: EARLY		
Duration: Nullipara, 8.6-20 hr*; multipara, 5.6-14 hr*	Conserve energy. Call physician; emphasize degree of comfort.	Time contractions; note progress every hour. Support her efforts.
Contractions: Mild to moderate, 30-45 sec long, 20-10 min, then 10-5 min apart, more regular	Take clear fluids as permitted. As necessary: use controlled relaxation.	Help with relaxation. Monitor her breathing techniques.
Work: Effacement and dilation to 3 cm	For control, use rhythmic chest breathing: slow rate at 8 breaths/min	If at home, help with organizing household; assist general relaxation.
Mood: Talkative, comfortable, excited, ambivalent	and modified rate at 16-20 breaths/min.	Notify obstetrician/midwife.

*This pattern reflects an average labor for a first birth. Duration of contractions is determined here *by palpation;* the maternal tocotransducer may indicate a longer duration.

TENS, Transcutaneous electrical nerve stimulation.

Table 13-5   Labor Summary*—cont'd

Phase	Recommended Coping Techniques	Partner Activities
ACTIVE: ACCELERATED *Duration:* Average 2-3.5 hr *Contractions:* Strong, 50-60 sec, 5-3 min apart *Work:* Dilate from 3 to 8 cm *Mood:* Very intense, concentrated; if membranes break, contractions increase in strength	Conserve energy. For control, use controlled relaxation, combined breathing pattern (rhythmic chest or shallow). If necessary, use shallow, accelerated-decelerated with contraction. Usually go to hospital. Take sips of clear liquid, if allowed.	"Count down" contractions. Use mouth rinses, cool cloth to woman's hands and face. Touch and stoke her arms and legs. Talk to her; encourage her efforts. Remind her that contractions are intermittent. Monitor her breathing.
ACTIVE: TRANSITION *Duration:* 20-60 min but not more than 2 hr for primipara *Contactions:* Erratic, intense, 60-90 sec, 3-2 min apart *Work:* Dilate 8-10 cm *Mood:* Irritable, discouraged, overwhelmed *Physical sensations:* Nausea, vomiting, chills, trembling, profuse sweating, pressure sensations, difficulty in relaxing ***Special considerations*** *Hyperventilation:* Tingling, dizzy, light-headedness, apprehension, out of rhythm *Back labor:* Strong discomfort in small of back; difficulty in relaxing; contractions erratic; increase in tension	Use controlled relaxation. Use shallow breathing: pant-blow 3/1, 2/1, 1/1 as contraction demands. Use for rectal pressure: 1/1 pant-blow rhythm. Use for urge to push: repeated blows. Use rhythmic chest breathing between contractions. Rebreathe exhaled air between contractions; slow rate of breathing. Prevention: keep breathing lightly and rhythmically. Lie on side. Focus on progressive relaxation throughout each contraction. Warm or cold compresses; TENS. Constant pressure to small of back.	Give specific directions. Insist that she take one contraction at a time. Remind her that infant is almost here. Encourage her. Monitor her breathing. If she uses repeated "blowing" or has the urge to push, summon nurse. Monitor her breathing. Correct technique—mark cadence, breathe with her. Talk through contractions. Apply counterpressure. Encourage her.
SECOND STAGE *Duration:* Multipara 20-60 min; nullipara, primipara up to 120 min *Contractions:* Rhythmic, strong, 90 sec, 2-4 min apart *Work:* Descent and birth of baby *Mood:* Refreshed, sense of work, cooperative *Physical sensations:* Vaginal fullness, pressure in rectum; burning, stretching *Episiotomy:* Painless, "unzipped"	Avoid Valsalva's maneuver. Use correct open-glottis pushing. If instructed to stop pushing at birth of head, use pant-blow.	Coach efforts: in, out/in, out/in, hold, relax key areas, push (count slowly to 10), push while releasing air (repeat); several deep breaths at end of each effort. Change positions as she desires.
THIRD STAGE *Delivery of placenta:* 5-20 min *Contractions:* Moderately strong *Mood:* Thinking of infant *Work:* Placenta expelled	Push as directed. Enjoy infant.	Enjoy infant together. Praise her efforts.

Care PATH | *First Stage of Labor*

Category	Parameters	Interventions
PHYSICAL ASSESSMENT		
1. The woman will maintain normal progress through stages/phases of labor. • Vital Signs	• Vital signs q1h Temperature q4h unless ruptured membranes Admitting BP_____ TPR_____	• TPR in early labor q4h After membrane rupture, q2h, or if rising temperature, q1h BP q1h and q15-30 min elevation.
• Status of membranes	• Presence of mucous plug/bloody show. Fluid is clear without meconium, blood, or foul odor. Volume is adequate by ultrasound Time of membrane rupture_____ FHR_____	• Assess status of membranes. Use nitrazine paper, ferning if question of rupture. If AROM, estimate volume lost, quality of fluid, plus FHR before/after. • Attach contraction and fetal heart monitor for 10-20 min on admission, and intermittently or as ordered.
• Contractions • Cervical dilation/effacement	• Latent phase: Active phase: Advanced/transition phase: • Progressive dilation to fully dilated and effaced at end of transition phase	• Evaluate/document contractions and uterine tonus q30-60 min during first stage. Detect hypotonic/hypertonic labor. • Initial vaginal examination if membranes intact. Limit examinations thereafter.
• Descent of presenting part/station • Laboratory reports WNL	• Engagement progresses to internal rotation and ++ station by end of stage one • Admission status: Hemoglobin_____ Hematocrit_____ WBC_____ ABO_____ Rh_____ STD: pos_____ neg_____ Proteinuria_____ Any other signs?_____ PIH?_____ Recent drug abuse?_____	• Encourage descent by positioning, walking, sitting, high Fowler's position. • Relate laboratory findings to care. Follow up with repeat measurements as required.
PSYCHOSOCIAL ADJUSTMENT		
2. The process of labor and birth will be experienced as a positive experience by woman and her partner. • Obtain history	• Demographic data, prenatal course, previous obstetric history, and attendance at childbirth classes. Gestational age, any psychosocial factors affecting the labor experience.	• Explain, interpret each step in labor and procedures. Explain caregiving activities. Anticipate questions.
• Support client and partner	• Psychosocial adjustment to pregnancy. Cultural beliefs related to birth. Language/education level. Is there a birth plan? Relationship with support person.	• Involve support person in care. Assess receptivity to instruction. Find interpreter as needed.
FACILITATION OF LABOR		
3. Client and partner demonstrate ability to cope with discomforts and tension of labor. • Emotional status and coping ability	• Anxiety and fear cause tension and delay progress. Encourage verbalization. Support coping methods, keep partner informed.	• Apply comfort measures. Evaluate causes of excessive anxiety. • Maintain empty bladder. • Assist with breathing/relaxation/visualization
• Pain and fatigue	• Excessive pain results in fatigue, panic, and poor coping	Teach partner techniques for promoting relaxation:

Care PATH | *First Stage of Labor — cont'd*

Category	Parameters	Interventions
FACILITATION OF LABOR—cont'd • Pain and fatigue—cont'd	Identify nonpharmacologic methods with client. Epidural analgesia_____ IV analgesia_____ PO Stadol_____ PO and IV fluids per order	effleurage_____, application of heat or cold_____, massage, counterpressure_____ Other_____ Administer analgesia. Monitor effects.

FETAL STATUS DURING LABOR
4. The fetal well-being is maintained throughout labor.
• Reassuring rate and patterns
	• Assess for reassuring FHR patterns
	Intermittent auscultation/fetal monitor:
	  Consistent baseline 110-160 bpm
	  Transient acceleration or deceleration
	  Good variability
	And after the following:
	  Rupture membranes, SROM or AROM
	  Change in contraction patterns
	  Regional analgesia/anesthesia
	  Vaginal examination/OB procedure
	  Medication
		• Evaluate and document normal rates:
		  Early labor q60 min
		  Active labor q15-30 min
		  Second Stage q10-15 min or after contraction

• Early detection of and interventions for nonreassuring rates and patterns	*Continuous fetal monitoring:*
	  Baseline >160 bpm or tachycardia
	  Average variability
	  Nonreassuring patterns
		• Report indications of nonreassuring patterns
		Intervene by position change, D/C oxytocin, O_2 by mask
		Monitor progressive descent of presenting part.

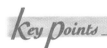

Key points

- Parturition is the process of giving birth, and coordination of the psychologic and physiologic components must interact in a dynamic whole.
- Support for the woman in labor takes several forms depending on the birth plan and process of labor and must involve both the woman and her partner.
- Women are sensitive to indifferent or negative interpersonal exchanges. Studies have shown beneficial results from a woman-centered individually focused and family-centered plan of care.
- Alterations in the psyche, the powers, an inadequate passage, or too large of a passenger may change the processes of normal labor.
- An intact amniotic sac will cushion the fetal head and prevent ascending infections; prolonged ROM may lead to infection.
- There are several theories of how labor begins. Causes of labor, however, are largely unknown.

- Women should be taught signs of effective term labor and when to seek evaluation of symptoms of early labor.
- The phases of the first stage of labor have distinct characteristics. Timing, however, may vary widely.
- Universal precautions are mandatory when handling blood and body fluids.
- Nursing management of labor includes conservation principles that reflect the today's paradigm shift toward "high touch" and "high tech" nursing care.
- Position in labor facilitates or hinders the labor process. The nurse must assess the variables related to comfortable positioning for the woman in labor.
- Fluids usually are permitted in labor unless a complication is present. Epidural anesthesia is more commonly used than general anesthesia, lessening the chance for aspiration during labor and birth.
- Competence and confidence in labor nursing care is mandatory. Serious legal implications accompany lack of knowledge in this area.

Study Questions

13-1. Select the terms that apply to the following statements:
   a. Changes in the infant's head shape as a result of birth pressure _____
   b. Relationship of a fixed point on the fetus to the right or left side of the maternal abdomen _____
   c. Cervical changes that allow dilation to progress _____
   d. Opening up of the cervix _____
   e. Rate of descent measured as _____
   f. Imbalance of oxygen and carbon dioxide because of rapid breathing _____
   g. Muscle tension of the uterus when there are no contractions _____

13-2. For a primigravida with adequate pelvic measurements, match the description of labor progress with the appropriate phase of labor in which the signs occur.

Signs of progress	Phase of labor
a. Mild contractions occurring approximately 10 minutes apart, lasting 40 seconds, cervix 2-cm dilated, partial effacement	1. Latent phase
b. Contractions building into intense peaks every 2 to 3 minutes, cervix 8-cm dilated and effaced	2. Active, accelerated phase
c. Strong contractions occurring 4 to 5 minutes apart, lasting 60 seconds, cervix 6-cm dilated	3. Active, transition phase

13-3. To determine the duration of contractions, you should measure the time interval between:
   a. The beginning of one contraction to the acme of that contraction.
   b. The acme of one contraction to the end of the same contraction.
   c. The beginning of one contraction to the end of the same contraction.
   d. The beginning of one contraction to the beginning of the next contraction.

13-4. At the end of the first stage of labor, an increase in the bloody show primarily results from:
   a. Placental bleeding.
   b. Small tears in the vaginal mucous membranes.
   c. Capillary bleeding from the final stretching of the cervix.
   d. Onset of minor clotting deficiency as labor ends.

13-5. Contractions were noted at 3- to 4-minute intervals and at 50 mm Hg pressure on the monitor strip. This describes contraction:
   a. Intensity and duration.
   b. Frequency and interval.
   c. Duration and frequency.
   d. Frequency and intensity.

13-6. Effacement is the process by which the cervix is:
   a. Opened to its widest diameter
   b. Pulled up into the lower uterine segment
   c. Freed of the mucous plug
   d. Forced to move into the upper vagina

13-7. The rationale for waiting until the head is well engaged to rupture membranes includes which two reasons?
   a. To ensure that a small amount of amniotic fluid is left in the uterus to lubricate the birth canal
   b. To speed the labor process after being sure the fetus is flexed
   c. To prevent prolapse of the cord with a gush of fluid
   d. To cushion the fetal head as long as possible

13-8. Ann and Joe have not attended classes to prepare for the birth of their second child. As transition progresses, Ann becomes very anxious, hyperventilates, and cries out that this labor is much worse than her first delivery. Joe is upset and turns to you for help. Your first response should be:
   a. "Tell me what happened in your first labor."
   b. "Calm yourself, Ann; your rapid breathing may make the baby distressed."
   c. "Ann, I can see that you are really making progress. I'll stay to help Joe help you."
   d. "Do you want pain medication at this point?"

13-9. The first stage of labor is considered to have ended when:
   a. Regular 3-minute contractions have been established.
   b. The membranes have been ruptured.
   c. The cervix is completely effaced and dilated.
   d. Pushing is an overwhelming need.

Answer Key

13-1: *a*, Molding; *b*, position; *c*, effacement; *d*, dilation; *e*, station; *f*, hyperventilation; *g*, resting tone. 13-2: *a*, 1; *b*, 3; *c*, 2. 13-3: *c*. 13-4: *c*. 13-5: *d*. 13-6: *b*. 13-7: *c* and d. 13-8: *c*. 13-9: *c*.

References

Acosta Y et al: HIV disease and pregnancy, part 2: antepartum and intrapartum care, *J Obstet Gynecol Neonatal Nurs* 21(2):97, 1992.

Aderhold KJ, Perry L: Jet hydrotherapy for labor and postpartum pain relief, *MCN Am J Matern Child Nurs* 16(2):97, 1991.

American College of Obstetricians and Gynecologists: *Human immunodeficiency virus infections in pregnancy,* Technical bulletin #232, 1997, The College.

Andrews CM, Chrzanowski M: Maternal position, labor and comfort, *App Nurs Res* 3(1):7, 1990.

Angelini DJ et al: Toward a concept of triage for labor and delivery: staff perceptions and role utilization, *J Perinat Neonatal Nurs* 4(3):1, 1990.

Bergstrom L et al: "You'll feel me touching you, sweetie:" vaginal examinations during the second stage of labor, *Birth* 19(1):10, 1992.

Blackburn ST, Loper DL: *Maternal, fetal, and neonatal physiology,* Philadelphia, 1992, WB Saunders.

Bond, ML: The ideal nurse for the relinquishing mother: lesson from the labor room, *MCN Am J Matern Child Nurs* 20(3):156, 1996.

*Caldeyro-Barcia R: Influence of maternal position on the time of spontaneous rupture of the membranes, progress of labor, and fetal head compression, *Birth Family J* 6(1):7, 1979.

Chapman L: Searching: expectant fathers' experiences during labor and birth, *J Perinatal Neonatal Nurs,* 4(4):21, 1991.

Chez R: Cervical ripening and labor induction after previous cesarean delivery, *Clin Obstet Gynecol,* 38(2):287, 1995.

Cunningham FG et al: *Williams obstetrics,* ed 19, Norwalk, Conn, 1993, Appleton & Lange.

Elkington KW: At the water's edge: where obstetrics and anesthesia meet, *Obstet Gynecol* 77:304, 1991.

Enkin M et al: *A guide to effective care in pregnancy and childbirth,* ed 2, Oxford, 1995, Oxford Univ Press.

*Friedman E: Failure to progress in labor. In Queenan J ed: *Management of high-risk pregnancy,* Oradell, NJ, 1985, Medical Economics Books.

Ginsberg R: Occupational exposure to bloodborne pathogens: the new OSHA regulations, *Pediatr AIDS & HIV infect: fetus to adolescent* 2(1):37, 1990.

Hill WC et al: Let's get rid of the term Braxton Hicks contractions, *Obstet Gynecol* 75(4):709, 1990.

Hodnett E: Nursing support of the laboring woman, *J Obstet Gynecol Neonatal Nurs* 25(3):257, 1996.

*Hodnett E, Osborn R: Effects of continuous intrapartum professional support on childbirth outcomes, *Res Nurs Health* 12:289, 1989.

Hopko-Sharts NC: Birth in the Japanese context, *J Obstet Gynecol Neonatal Nurs* 24(4):343, 1995.

Hutchinson MK: Nursing care of the childbearing Muslim family, *J Obstet Gynecol Neonatal Nurs* 23(9):767, 1994.

*Huzar G, Naftolin F: The myometrium and uterine cervix in normal and preterm labor, *N Engl J Med* 311:571, 1984.

Johnson N, Johnson VA, Gupta JK: Maternal positions during labor, *Obstet Gynecol Surv* 46(7):428, 1991.

Jordan PL: Laboring for relevance: expectant new fatherhood, *Nurs Res* 39(1):11, 1990.

Kennel J et al: Continuous emotional support in a US hospital: a randomized controlled trial, *JAMA* 265:2197, 1991.

*Kintz D: Nursing support during labor, *J Obstet Gynecol Neonatal Nurs* 16(6):126, 1987.

Kowalski K et al: The high-touch paradigm: a 21st century model for maternal-child nursing, *MCN Am J Matern Child Nurs* 21(1):43, 1996.

*Levine M: *Introduction to clinical nursing,* Philadelphia, 1973, FA Davis.

*Liu Y: The effects of the upright position during childbirth, *Image J Nurs Sch* 21(1):14, 1989.

Lowe NK: The pain and discomfort of labor and birth, *J Obstet Gynecol Neonatal Nurs* 25(1):82, 1996.

Ludka LM, Roberts CC: Eating and drinking in labor, *J Nurse Midwifery* 38(4):199, 1993.

Lydon-Rochelle MT et al: Perineal outcomes and nurse-midwifery management, *J Nurse Midwifery* 40(1):13, 1995.

*Mackey MC, Locke SE: Women's expectations of the labor and delivery nurse, *J Obstet Gynecol Neonatal Nurs* 17(6):505, 1988.

Mattson S: Culturally sensitive perinatal care for Southeast Asians, *J Obstet Gynecol Neonatal Nurs* 24(4):335, 1995.

McNiven P et al: Support of women in labor: a work sampling study of the activities of labor and delivery nurses, *Birth* 19(1):3, 1992.

*Classic reference.

Menticoglou FM et al: Perinatal outcome in relation to second-stage duration, *Am J Obstet Gynecol* 173(3):906, 1995.

Metzger BL, Therrien B: Effect of position on cardiovascular response during the Valsalva maneuver, *Nurs Res* 39(4):200, 1990.

Newell ML et al: Risk factors for mother-to-child transmission of HIV-1, *Lancet,* 339(4):1007, 1992.

Nichols DH: *Clinical problems, injuries and complications of gynecologic and obstetric surgery,* ed 3, Baltimore, 1995, Williams & Wilkens.

Nichols F: The effects of hydrotherapy during labor, *J Perinat Educ* 5(1):41, 1996.

*Nurses Association of the American College of Obstetrics and Gynecology (NAACOG): *Standards for obstetric, gynecologic, and neonatal nursing,* Washington, DC, 1986, The Association.

Oakley A: The best research is that which breeds more, in supporting women in labor, *Birth* 19(3):8, 1992.

Oxhorn H: *Human labor and birth,* ed 6, New York, 1997, Appleton-Century-Crofts.

Prendiville W et al: The third stage of labour. In Enkin M et al, eds: *Effective care in pregnancy and childbirth,* Oxford, 1993, Oxford Univ Press.

Reece E et al: *Handbook of medicine of the fetus and mother,* Philadelphia, 1995, JB Lippincott.

*Roberts JA et al: Effects of maternal position on uterine contractibility and efficiency, *Birth* 10:243, 1983.

*Roberts JA et al: A descriptive analysis of involuntary bearing-down efforts, *J Obstet Gynecol Neonatal Nurs* 16(1):48, 1987.

Sleep J et al: Monitoring progress of labour. In Enkin M et al, eds: *Effective care in pregnancy and childbirth,* Oxford, 1993, Oxford Univ Press.

Steinman G: Forces affecting the dynamics of labor, *J Reprod Med* 36(12):868, 1991.

Thornton, JG: Active management of labour: current knowledge and research issues, *Br Med J* 309(6951):366, 1994.

Weaver DF: Nurses' views on the meaning of touch in obstetrical nursing practice, *J Obstet Gynecol Neonatal Nurs* 19(2):157, 1990.

Weber SE: Cultural aspects of pain in the childbearing woman, *J Obstet Gynecol Neonatal Nurs* 25(1):67, 1996.

Zuspan FP et al: *Current therapy in obstetrics and gynecology,* ed 4, Philadelphia, 1994, WB Saunders Co.

Student Resource Shelf

Albers LL et al: Birth settings for low-risk pregnancies—an analysis of the literature, *J Nurse Midwifery* 36(4):215, 1991.
Helpful analysis of the many settings for birth.

Arrabal P: Is manual palpation of uterine contractions accurate?, *Am J Obstet Gynecol* 174(1):217 1996.
This study assesses the accuracy of uterine contraction palpation, determines whether the accuracy of palpation improves with experience, and records whether mild, moderate, or strong compares with the documented recorded findings.

Callister LC: Cultural meanings of childbirth, *J Obstet Gynecol Neonatal Nurs* 24(4):328, 1995.
Nursing practice is benefiting from the efforts made to move the care of the childbearing unit from the perspective of one-dimensional streamline care to the aspect of cultural differences and sensitivity to each individual family. Gaining an understanding of the cultural meanings of childbirth enhances the role of the nurse.

Kennel J et al: Continuous emotional support in a US hospital: a randomized controlled trial, *JAMA* 265:2197, 1991.
The United States is the only country that has until recently kept women from having support ad lib during labor. Now the physician team that studied bonding goes a step further to find the benefits of support so that the mother has emotional energy to bond with her infant.

Kowalski K et al: The high-touch paradigm: a 21st century model for maternal-child nursing, *MCN Am J Matern Child Nurs* 21(1):43, 1996.
As a result of high technology, clients were isolated, families alienated, and the "high-tech–low touch" paradigm was characterized by minimal human support and caring relationships. The shift is beginning, and future maternal-child nursing will be affected by this change in the focus of care.

Ramer L: Culturally sensitive caregiving and childbearing families: nursing issues for the 21st century, *March of Dimes Module 1,* p 35, 1992.
To keep a balance or harmony in life, nursing care must reflect a basic understanding of culture-specific caregiving. Issues outlined in this module include samples of general cultural information, clinical applications for assessing ethnicity in the childbearing family, a self-assessment, and activities for group discussion.

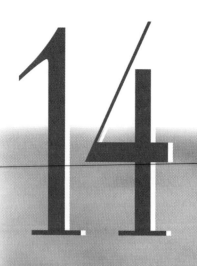

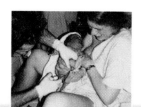

14

Fetal Assessment *during the* Intrapartum Period

Learning Objectives

- Recognize when electronic fetal monitoring can be useful.
- Describe fetal physiologic responses to labor.
- Differentiate between reassuring and nonreassuring fetal heart rate patterns.
- Recognize normal and abnormal patterns of uterine activity.
- Relate nursing interventions to physiologic factors underlying selected patterns.
- Describe methods of documentation of fetal assessments.
- Explain uses of monitoring and fetal assessment tests to the laboring woman and her support partner.

Key Terms

Accelerations
Amnioinfusion
Asphyxia
Baseline Fetal Heart Rate
Baseline Variability
Beat-to-Beat Variability
Bradycardia
Cord Compression
Early Decelerations
Electronic Fetal Heart Rate Monitoring
Fetal Compromise
Increased Baseline Variability
Intraamniotic Pressure
Intrauterine Resuscitation
Late Decelerations

Long-term Variability
Meconium Aspiration Syndrome (MAS)
Nonreassuring Fetal Heart Rate Pattern
Nuchal Cord
Prolapse of Umbilical Cord
Reassuring Fetal Heart Rate Pattern
Short-term Variability
Sinusoidal Pattern
Tachycardia
Umbilical Cord Compression
Uteroplacental Insufficiency
Variable Decelerations

*L*abor and birth are periods of physiologic stress for the fetus. **Electronic fetal heart rate (FHR) monitoring** and uterine activity monitoring are methods to assess the fetal response to the labor and birth processes. Electronic FHR monitoring is commonly used during active labor in most labor and birth units. Some institutions require that a woman be monitored continuously from the time of admission until birth, whereas other institutions routinely use intermittent monitoring during labor. Many research studies have compared electronic FHR monitoring with intermittent auscultation with a stethoscope. Although there is contro-versy as to whether continuous electronic fetal monitoring (EFM) is the best method of fetal assessment, approximately 98% of women in the United States will be monitored via EFM for at least some time during labor and birth. Much of the controversy is related to the expectations for neonatal outcomes when EFM is used continuously during labor.

When EFM was first introduced in the late 1960s, there was hope that the incidence of cerebral palsy would be dramatically reduced with the use of this technology. This initial expectation has not been realized, primarily because it is now known that events that cause cerebral palsy usually occur in the prenatal period, well before labor and birth (Nelson et al, 1996). When EFM is used to predict a healthy fetus and thus a good neonatal outcome, the data are sound. The positive predictive value of EFM—the likelihood that a reassuring FHR tracing means the fetus is healthy and tolerating labor well—is high. The issue is what to do when the FHR pattern is nonreassuring. In general, a nonreassuring fetal heart rate pattern is the basis for interventions and in some cases, an operative birth. Regardless of one's professional opinion or choice in method of fetal assessment during labor and birth, EFM has improved fetal outcomes simply by increasing the attention of perinatal healthcare providers and researchers to FHR as an indicator of fetal status (Menihan, 1996).

EFM is used continuously or intermittently during labor. It is important to involve the woman in labor and her support person as decision makers in the plan of care. As with any nursing intervention, the nurse should clearly explain how the monitor works and the rationale for its use before initiation. If the woman in labor does not wish to be confined to bed and there is evidence of fetal well-being via a reassuring FHR tracing, EFM can be used periodically during labor. A woman can be encouraged to walk around the room or in the hall and try different positions during labor. Newer EFM units have the ability to monitor FHR and uterine activity via telemetry.

Therefore the monitor can be used while a woman is walking or taking a shower. Because the physiologic benefits of an upright position and ambulation are important to enhance a successful birth outcome, the monitor can be reapplied periodically or the nurse can listen to the FHR at selected intervals. A woman-centered policy for fetal assessment during labor may influence whether the woman perceives fetal monitoring as a positive part of the childbirth process. One of the factors that can contribute to a positive childbirth experience is that hearing and seeing the FHR as it is displayed on the monitor may provide reassurance of fetal well-being for the woman and her support person.

The frequency for assessing the FHR is determined by the stage of labor and the presence of risk factors. In the absence of maternal-fetal risk factors, the FHR is assessed at least every 60 minutes during the latent phase, increasing to every 30 minutes as the active phase of labor progresses, and then every 15 minutes during the second stage of labor. However, when risk factors have been identified, the FHR is assessed every 15 minutes during the active phase of the first stage of labor and every 5 minutes during the second stage (American College of Obstetricians and Gynecologists, 1995).

Box 14-1 summarizes the potential benefits and risks of intrapartum monitoring, including the consideration that its use may tend to dehumanize the birth experience.

| *Box* 14-1   **Risks and Benefits of Intrapartum Fetal Heart Rate Monitoring**

RISKS

Increased Cesarean Birth Rate

Increase is caused by easier identification of compromised fetus plus lack of physician experience in discriminating between fetal compromise and normal variations.

Increased Maternal Infection

Increased rate of artificial rupture of membranes to facilitate internal monitoring increases the potential for infection.

Uterine Perforation

The intrauterine pressure catheter may rarely perforate the uterus.

Fetal Scalp Infection

Scalp infection is a possible but rare complication of an internal fetal scalp electrode.

Dehumanization of Birth

A woman in labor may perceive that the machine receives more attention than she does unless the nurse takes steps to ensure that this does not happen.

BENEFITS

Decreased Intrapartum Stillbirths

Careful monitoring will reduce the incidence of stillbirth, especially for women in high-risk groups.

Decreased Neonatal Mortality and Morbidity

Monitoring can identify the compromised fetus before profound asphyxia occurs.

Assistance in Labor Management

Staff can more easily recognize hypertonic or ineffective labor patterns.

Influence on Malpractice

Reassuring FHR tracing during labor can serve as evidence of fetal well-being.
Monitoring provides continuous readout with a permanent record.

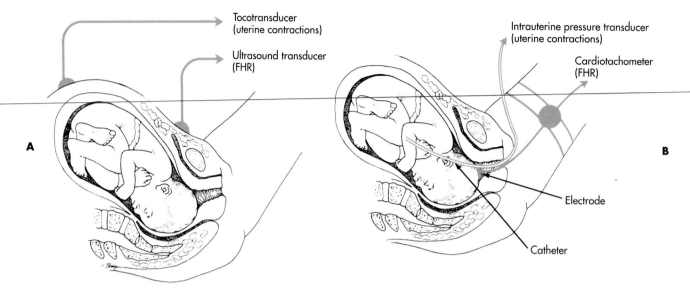

Figure 14-1   Intrauterine pressure monitors. **A,** External noninvasive fetal monitoring with tocotransducer and ultrasound transducer, with ultrasound transducer placed below umbilicus and tocotransducer placed on uterine fundus. **B,** Internal fetal monitoring with intrauterine catheter and spiral electrode in place (membranes ruptured and cervix dilated). (From Lowdermilk DL, Perry SE, Bobak IM: *Maternity and women's health care,* ed 6, St Louis, 1997, Mosby.)

ASSESSMENT OF UTERINE ACTIVITY

Electronic assessment of uterine activity can be performed by two methods: externally, by placing a tocodynamometer on the maternal abdomen, and internally, by inserting an intrauterine pressure catheter (IUPC) that directly measures intraamniotic pressure into the uterine cavity. Manual assessment of uterine activity is determined by palpation. Frequency of contractions is recorded in minutes. Duration of contractions is recorded in seconds. When contraction intensity or strength is measured by palpation, it is usually recorded as mild, moderate, or strong. When assessing contraction intensity via an IUPC, **intraamniotic pressure** is measured in millimeters of mercury (mm Hg).

Methods

Tocodynamometer

The tocodynamometer is an external monitoring device that is applied over the uterine fundus and secured with an elastic belt around the woman's abdomen. As a contraction builds, increasing pressure is transmitted from the uterus through the maternal abdominal wall to the pressure-sensitive device. The "toco" sends the signal to the recorder, which provides a continuous record of contractions (Figure 14-1, *A*).

Intrauterine pressure catheter

An IUPC may be inserted when there are clinical indications for more accurate assessment of intraamniotic pressure. Use of an IUPC is invasive to the woman in labor, so this method is not used routinely. The cervix must be dilated at least 2 to 3 cm and membranes ruptured before internal monitoring is possible. The catheter is passed through the cervix and along the presenting part into the uterine cavity (Figure 14-1, *B*). The increasing intraamniotic pressure that occurs during a contraction is transmitted through the catheter to the recorder, which provides a continuous record of contractions.

Interpreting Uterine Activity Patterns

Uterine activity is assessed externally or internally. The monitor records uterine contractions on the lower segment of the graph paper. The intrauterine baseline pressure, or *resting tone,* is assessed between contractions. Normal resting tone varies with the stage of labor; however, it does not usually exceed 15 to 20 mm Hg. Frequency, duration, and intensity are assessed according to unit protocol and then recorded (Figure 14-2). These assessments may be performed by direct palpation. The nurse places her hand over the fundus and palpates uterine activity. The frequency of contractions (time from the beginning of one until the beginning of the next) and the duration of each (time from the beginning to the end of one contraction) can be assessed through external electronic monitoring. The intensity, or strength, of contractions, however, *cannot be accurately assessed* by the tocodynamometer because it only detects abdominal wall changes. Abdominal wall changes may occur for reasons other than uterine contractions (including maternal muscle tension during movement such as vomiting or coughing or during fetal movement). It may be difficult to adequately monitor uterine

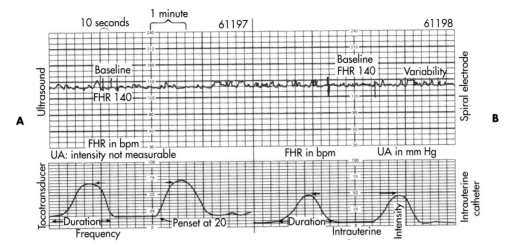

Figure 14-2   Display of fetal heart rate (FHR) and uterine activity (UA) on monitor strip. **A,** External mode: ultrasound and tocotransducer are the signal sources. **B,** Internal mode: spiral electrode and intrauterine catheter are the signal sources. Other significant information is supplied. (From Tucker SM: *Fetal monitoring and assessment,* ed 3, St Louis, 1996, Mosby.)

activity in women in labor who are obese because of the amount of adipose tissue between the fundus and the abdominal wall. Women who are in preterm labor also present a challenge because many of the monitors presently in use are not equipped with tocodynamometers that are sensitive enough to detect preterm labor contractions. Therefore the method of monitoring uterine activity is based on each clinical situation. If accurate assessment of intraamniotic pressure is necessary and there are no contraindications to amniotomy, the best method is the IUPC. However, most women in labor will do well with external electronic monitoring palpation of uterine activity.

It is important to remember that the tocodynamometer cannot replace hands-on nursing assessment. Palpation of uterine contractions should be done frequently to compare and validate the data provided by the external tocodynamometer. Often a laboring woman states that her contractions are stronger than those seen on the monitor. Although her perceptions may sometimes be inaccurate, they require evaluation. Contractions that seem stronger than what the recording shows should always be palpated, as should those accompanying a labor pattern that does not seem to correlate well with the tracing. Readjusting the tocodynamometer may enhance electronic tracing accuracy.

PHYSIOLOGIC BASIS FOR FETAL HEART RATE MONITORING

FHR monitoring during labor is based on the premise that the FHR reflects fetal oxygen status. Many factors can influence fetal oxygen status, including maternal medical and obstetric complications, maternal position, cardiac output, and the oxygen-carrying capacity of the blood. Any factor that influences maternal blood flow to the pla-

centa will potentially have an impact on fetal oxygenation. Complications of pregnancy that adversely affect maternal vascular status, such as diabetes, hypertension, systemic lupus erythematosus (SLE), or cardiac disease, can result in chronic decreased blood flow to the placenta. Conditions that lead to vascular changes in the placenta cause a decreased blood flow through the placenta and subsequent decreased maternal-fetal oxygen exchange. Respiratory conditions such as asthma or pulmonary edema that may affect maternal oxygen status can influence fetal oxygen status. Acute maternal events also have the potential to influence maternal-fetal exchange. Decreased maternal cardiac output resulting from maternal hemorrhage, hypovolemia, and hypotension will in turn lead to decreased placental perfusion. Supine maternal position can cause compression of the aorta, superior and inferior vena cava, internal iliac arteries, and the uterus. A lateral maternal position during labor enhances maternal-fetal blood flow and oxygen exchange. Previously it was thought that the left lateral position was best for maternal-fetal exchange, but now it is known that both the right and left lateral positions work equally well; the key is to avoid the supine position.

In addition to maternal status, there are a number of fetal factors that influence regulatory control of the FHR. These factors and their location, action, and effect on the FHR are summarized in Table 14-1.

Methods of Assessing the Fetal Heart Rate

Intrapartum monitoring may be performed externally (indirectly) or internally (directly). Both methods provide the nurse with valuable information about the fetal response to labor.

Table 14-1   Factors Regulating Fetal Heart Rate

Factors Regulating Fetal Heart Rate	Location	Action	Effect
Parasympathetic division of autonomic nervous system	Vagus nerve fibers supply sinoatrial (SA) and atrioventricular (AV) node	Stimulation causes release of acetylcholine at myoneural synapse	Decreases FHR Maintains beat-to-beat variability
Sympathetic division of autonomic nervous system	Nerves widely distributed in myocardium	Stimulation causes release of norepinephrine at synapse	Increases FHR Increases strength of myocardial contraction Increases cardiac output
Baroreceptors	Stretch receptors in aortic arch and carotid sinus at the junction of the internal and external carotid arteries	Responds to increase in blood pressure by stimulating stretch receptors to send impulses via vagus or glosso-pharyngeal nerve to midbrain, producing vagal response and slowing heart activity	Decreases FHR Decreases blood pressure Decreases cardiac output
Chemoreceptors	Peripheral—in carotid and aortic bodies	Responds to marked peripheral decrease in O_2 and increase in CO_2	Produces bradycardia, sometimes with increased variability
	Central—in medulla oblongata	Central chemoreceptors respond to decreases in O_2 tension and increases in CO_2 tension in blood and/or cerebrospinal fluid	Produces tachycardia and increase in blood pressure with decrease in variability
Central nervous system	Cerebral cortex	Responds to fetal movement Responds to fetal sleep	Increases reactivity and variability Decreases reactivity and variability
	Hypothalamus	Regulates and coordinates autonomic activities (sympathetic and parasympathetic)	
	Medulla oblongata	Mediates cardiac and vasomotor reflex center by controlling heart action and blood vessel diameter	Maintains balance between cardioacceleration and cardiodeceleration
Hormonal regulation	Adrenal medulla	Releases epinephrine and norepinephrine with severe fetal hypoxia producing sympathetic response	Increases FHR Increases strength of myocardial contraction and blood pressure Increases cardiac output
	Adrenal cortex	Low fetal blood pressure stimulates release of aldosterone, decreases sodium output, increases water retention, which increases circulating blood volume	Maintains homeostasis of blood volume
	Vasopressin (plasma catecholamine)	Produces vasoconstriction of non-vital vascular beds in the asphyxiated fetus	Distributes blood flow to maintain FHR and variability
Blood volume/capillary fluid shift	Fluid shift between capillaries and interstitial spaces	Responds to elevated blood pressure by causing fluid to move out of capillaries and into interstitial spaces	Decreases blood volume and blood pressure
		Responds to low blood pressure by causing fluid to move out of interstitial space into capillaries	Increases blood volume and blood pressure

From Tucker SM: *Fetal monitoring and assessment*, ed 3, St Louis, 1996, Mosby.

Table 14-1	Factors Regulating Fetal Heart Rate—cont'd		
Factors Regulating Fetal Heart Rate	Location	Action	Effect
Intraplacental pressures	Intervillous space	Fluid shift between fetal and maternal blood is based on osmotic and blood pressure gradients; maternal blood pressure is about 100 mm Hg and fetal blood pressure about 55 mm Hg; therefore balance is probably maintained by some compensatory factor	Regulates blood volume and blood pressure
Frank-Starling mechanism	Based on stretching of myocardium by increased increased inflow of venous blood into right atrium	In the adult the myocardium is stretched by an increased inflow of blood, causing the heart to contract with greater force than before and pump out more blood; the adult then is able to increase cardiac output by increasing heart rate and stroke volume; this mechanism is not well developed in the fetus	Cardiac output is dependent on heart rate in the fetus: ↓ FHR = ↓ cardiac output ↑ FHR = ↑ cardiac output

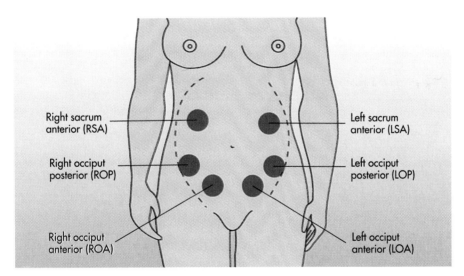

Figure 14-3 Position at which the fetal heart rate is best heard varies with fetal position. The nurse should try to listen over the fetus' back. (From Hamilton PM: *Basic maternity nursing*, ed 6, St Louis, 1989, Mosby.)

External monitoring

Doppler ultrasound (external) monitoring requires the use of an ultrasonic transducer applied to the maternal abdomen and held in place with an elastic belt or tape. The transducer is placed over the area yielding the most consistent and continuous FHR. Figure 14-3 illustrates the various points at which to auscultate the FHR. These areas vary with fetal position. Because the thin layer of air between the transducer and the maternal abdomen hinders the transmission of sound waves, ultrasound gel is placed on the transducer before it is positioned. The transducer emits high-frequency sound waves, which are directed toward the fetal cardiac valves and are then bounced back to the transducer at frequencies that reflect the FHR. During labor, the fetus may change positions, thus requiring readjustment of the external monitor to get the best signal.

Internal monitoring

Internal monitoring is invasive to the laboring woman and fetus; however, in certain clinical situations it is necessary to obtain a more accurate assessment of fetal status. The cervix must be dilated at least 2 to 3 cm, and membranes must be ruptured. An internal fetal electrode is a thin, spiral needle that will be attached in the subcutaneous tissue of the presenting part, usually the fetal scalp (Figure 14-4). A grounding circuit is attached to a small, metal leg plate to which electrocardiographic gel is applied, then the plate is placed on the mother's thigh. In this way a direct tracing of the FHR may be obtained without interference from maternal or fetal movement. An internal fetal monitor is useful for direct assessment of the FHR when the external ultrasound transducer is unable to provide a continuous tracing or when the FHR pattern tracing is uninterpretable or nonreassuring.

Interpreting Fetal Heart Rate Patterns

The nurse should develop a systematic method of interpretation that includes assessment of the FHR baseline rate, variability, periodic patterns, and uterine activity. The FHR is recorded on the upper tracing of the graph paper. Note the markings on the tracing paper in Figure 14-2.

Baseline rate

To determine the **baseline fetal heart rate**, the nurse observes a tracing during 10 minutes of monitoring (Figure 14-5). The baseline rate is assessed *between* any contractions or accelerations or decelerations. The average FHR ranges from 110 to 160 beats per minute (bpm), although each fetus is an individual and thus has its own baseline rate. This average rate *decreases* with increasing gestational age because of maturation of the parasympathetic nervous system. Therefore there is sometimes a slightly higher baseline rate for a preterm fetus than for a full-term fetus, although in most cases the healthy fetus does not have a rate above 160 bpm. The normal rate may change during labor in response to physiologic stress or maternal drug administration. Figure 14-6 illustrates fetal **tachycardia** and **bradycardia**. Table 14-2 lists reasons for baseline rate changes.

Bradycardia

FHR bradycardia is a condition in which the FHR baseline is below 110 bpm for 10 minutes or more or is

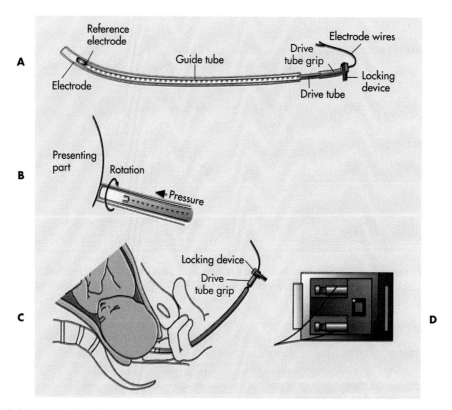

Figure 14-4　Internal fetal heart rate (FHR) monitor. **A** to **C,** Spiral electrode used for internal (FHR) monitoring. **D,** Attached to leg plate. (Courtesy Corometrics Medical Systems, Inc.)

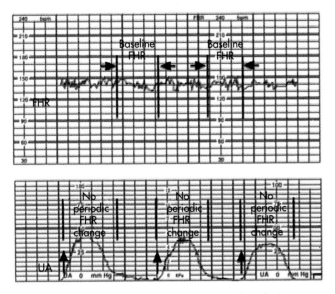

Figure 14-5 Baseline fetal heart rate is identified between uterine contractions. (From Tucker SM: *Fetal monitoring and assessment,* ed 3, St Louis, 1996, Mosby.)

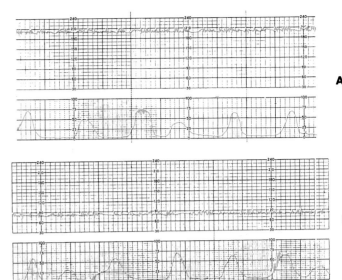

Figure 14-6 **A,** Fetal tachycardia. **B,** Fetal bradycardia.
(From Tucker SM: *Fetal monitoring and assessment,* ed 3, St Louis, 1996, Mosby.)

Table 14-2   **Causes of Fetal Tachycardia and Bradycardia**

Causes of Fetal Tachycardia		Causes of Fetal Bradycardia	
Fetal hypoxia	Fetus attempts to compensate for reduced blood flow by increase of sympathetic stimulation or release of epinephrine from adrenal medulla, or both.	Late (profound) fetal hypoxia	Myocardial activity becomes depressed and lowers heart rate.
Maternal fever	Fever accelerates metabolism of fetal myocardium; increases sympathetic cardioacceleration activity up to 2 hours before the mother is febrile.	Beta-adrenergic blocking drugs (e.g., propranolol)	Epinephrine receptor sites in the myocardium are blocked by these drugs, permitting unopposed vagal tone and a decreased heart rate.
Parasympatholytic drugs (e.g., atropine, scopolamine, hydroxyzine [Vistaril, Atarax], phenothiazines)	Drugs block the parasympathetic division of the autonomic nervous system.	Anesthetics (epidural, spinal, and pudendal)	Bradycardia may develop indirectly because of a reflex mechanism or because of maternal hypotension produced by maternal supine position, insufficient preanesthesia hydration, or the response to the anesthetic agent.
Betasympathomimetic drugs (e.g., terbutaline and ritodrine)	These tocolytic drugs, given to control labor, have a cardiac stimulant effect similar to that of epinephrine.	Maternal hypotension	Maternal supine position causes uterine compression of the vena cava, which results in hypotension syndrome (a decrease in cardiac output and blood pressure with a subsequent decrease in FHR).
Ilicit drugs (e.g., cocaine and methamphetamines)	Epinephrine/norepinephrine response that causes increased maternal and fetal heart rates (FHR)	Prolonged umbilical cord compression	Cord compression triggers sensitization of fetal baroreceptors, resulting in vagal stimulation and decreased heart rate.
		Fetal cardiac dysrhythmias	FHR can be low (70 to 90 bpm) with bradyarrhythmias (complete heart block).

From Tucker SM: *Fetal monitoring and assessment,* ed 3, St Louis, 1996, Mosby.

Continued.

Table 14-2	**Causes of Fetal Tachycardia and Bradycardia—cont'd**

Causes of Fetal Tachycardia		Causes of Fetal Bradycardia	
Amnionitis	Increased heart rate can be the first sign of developing intrauterine infection (as with prolonged rupture of membranes).	Hypothermia	Maternal (and therefore fetal) hypothermia reduces myocardial metabolism, decreases oxygen requirements, and decreases heart rate.
Maternal hyperthyroidism	Long-acting thyroid-stimulating hormones (LATS) probably cross the placenta and increase the FHR, if maternal hyperthyroidism is controlled.	Maternal systemic lupus erythematosus	Complete atrioventricular dissociation associated with connective tissue disease produces persistent bradycardia.
Fetal anemia	FHR increases in an effort to increase cardiac output and tissue perfusion.	Cytomegalovirus (CMV)	Structural cardiac defects may occur with CMV infection, resulting in congenital heart block expressed as fetal bradycardia.
Fetal heart failure	The fetal heart attempts to compensate for failure by concurrently increasing rate and cardiac output; can occur as a result of tachyarrhythmia.	Prolonged maternal hypoglycemia	Maternal and subsequently fetal hypoglycemia can potentiate hypoxemia with a depression of myocardial activity and decreased heart rate.
Variations in Variability Appearance and Cause	**Clinical Significance/Intervention**	Congenital heart block	Congenital heart block of first, second, or third degree can result in bradycardia. First degree block does not require treatment in the fetus and has not yet been reported in the literature. In second-degree block not all the impulses from the sinoatrial node in the atria are conducted to the ventricles. Mobitz type I block is evidenced by a progressive lengthening of the PR interval and is rarely of any significance. Mobitz type II block occurs infrequently but is more serious and often a percursor to third-degree heart block.
Fetal cardiac dysrhythmias	Tachyarrhythmias and variations of normal sinus rhythm may occur (e.g., paroxysmal atrial tachycardia [PAT], atrial flutter, and premature ventricular contractions [PVCs]); congenital cardiac anomaly may be present; FHR in excess of 240 bpm cannot be followed by monitor because this exceeds FHR range parameters.		

decreased from the previous baseline rate by 20 bpm for 10 minutes or longer (AWHONN, 1993). There are many possible chronic and acute causes for bradycardia. Chronic fetal conditions that lead to hypoxemia or acidemia can result in bradycardia. Acute events that are associated with stimulation of the vagal nerve or parasympathetic system or prolonged compression of the umbilical cord will also cause a decrease in the FHR.

Prolonged bradycardia is associated with acidemia, which may decrease responsiveness to resuscitative measures. Newborns depressed from analgesic or anesthetic medications that have crossed the placental barrier tend to respond more slowly or need resuscitation. The choice of medications and the timing and dosage are therefore extremely important (see Chapter 16).

Tachycardia

FHR tachycardia is a condition in which the FHR baseline rate is above 160 bpm for 10 minutes or more or is increased from the previous baseline rate by 20 bpm for 10 minutes or longer (AWHONN, 1993). The cause of tachycardia may be sympathetic stimulation, early fetal hypoxemia, maternal drug use or administration, intraamniotic infection, maternal temperature elevations, or fetal vibroacoustic stimulation (see Figure 14-6). A rising baseline during labor requires careful assessment because an elevation of the baseline rate by more than 20 bpm indicates *beginning tachycardia*, even though the actual number may be within the normal range. For example, a rising FHR baseline sometimes precedes an elevated maternal temperature in the presence of intraamniotic infection.

Variability of the Fetal Heart Rate

The interaction between the sympathetic and parasympathetic divisions of the autonomic nervous system results in variability of the FHR. The sympathetic system stimulates the fetal heart to increase rate, and the parasympathetic system stimulates the fetal heart to decrease rate. This continual interaction is thought to be reflective of an intact, well-oxygenated fetal central nervous system (CNS). The changes in the FHR occur from one beat to the next, resulting in **beat-to-beat variability**, or short-term FHR variability. FHR variability is usually evidence of fetal well-being. The **baseline variability** is the irregularity of the FHR tracing as assessed in between uterine activity over a 10-minute time period.

Baseline variability

The baseline variability may be short or long term; however, the changes are interdependent and therefore should be considered together. **Short-term variability** is seen as the monitor records the intervals between one heartbeat and the next, which usually vary from 2 to 3 bpm to 10 bpm. **Long-term variability** is seen as the monitor records wavelike fluctuations in FHR. These rhythmic changes do not occur from one beat to the next but instead occur from two to six times per minute.

Short-term variability and long-term variability tend to increase and decrease simultaneously; therefore these are usually described together. It is important to note that there is no nationally agreed upon terminology to describe FHR patterns, including variability and periodic pattern changes. The nurse must therefore be aware of the terminology used at each institution so all members of the team are using the same descriptive terminology. Some institutions use a beat-per-minute range to describe variability, whereas others use descriptive terms such as "absent" or "present." One way to describe variability is presented here.

Range in bpm	Assessment of variability
0-2	None
3-5	Minimal
6-10	Average
11-25	Moderate
>25	Marked

A comparison of FHR variabilities is shown in Figure 14-7. It is sometimes difficult to assess variability during external monitoring because of *artifact*, interference with transmission or reception of the signal. Most of the newer monitors, however, have improved technology allowing

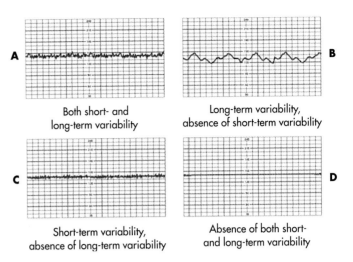

Both short- and long-term variability

Long-term variability, absence of short-term variability

Short-term variability, absence of long-term variability

Absence of both short- and long-term variability

Figure 14-7   A-D, Variations in short- and long-term variability. (Modified from Tucker SM: *Fetal monitoring and assessment,* ed 3, St Louis, 1996, Mosby.)

detection of FHR changes, which closely approximate the FHR variability that would be recorded if an internal electrode was in place. The inability to detect FHR variability during external tracing may be an indication that more accurate assessment via internal monitoring is necessary.

Sinusoidal patterns

Sinusoidal patterns have a wavelike appearance, with alternating small accelerations and decelerations centering around the baseline. There may be little or no fetal movement, and short-term variability is decreased. This is a rare pattern, but it may be seen in the severely anemic fetus. The fetus with a sinusoidal heart rate pattern needs immediate attention, so the primary health care provider must be notified at once.

Fetal Heart Rate Changes

Next, *periodic heart rate* changes in the fetus are examined. These are short-term changes, lasting from a few seconds up to 1 to 2 minutes, occurring *with* uterine contractions. The FHR provides data to assess fetal status during and after contractions and will show either a **reassuring fetal heart rate pattern** or a **nonreassuring fetal heart rate pattern**.

Accelerations

FHR **accelerations** are usually associated with fetal movement. These are transient elevations that may rise 5 to 15 bpm from the baseline, stay elevated for several seconds to minutes, and then return to the baseline rate. Accelerations indicate that the cardiac control center in the medulla is functional; the rise in heart rate seen with fetal movement is similar to a rise after physical activity. Accelerations with fetal activity may be less marked in a premature fetus. The presence of accelerations with fetal movement is a *reassuring* sign and the basis of the nonstress test (NST) (see Figure 11-12, *A*).

Decelerations

FHR **decelerations** may indicate fetal compromise or may not be clinically significant. Decelerations are classified as early, late, and variable. The differences in the three are related to their *shape* and *timing* in relation to uterine contractions (Figure 14-8).

Early decelerations. **Early decelerations** result from a *vagal response to head compression.* They have a smooth, U-shaped form and *begin and end when the contraction begins*

and ends. The lowest point of the deceleration occurs at the highest point of intensity of the contraction. For this reason, they are said to "mirror" contraction shape (Figure 14-8, *A*). During early decelerations, the FHR is almost always within the normal range of 110 to 160 bpm. These decelerations do not indicate fetal compromise; in fact, the fetus is showing healthy response to head compression. Nursing interventions for early decelerations are not required because early decelerations are a benign pattern.

Late decelerations. When the fetus is experiencing hypoxia the fetal heart may demonstrate **late decelerations** in relation to the contraction. This pattern is thought to be the result of decreased uteroplacental perfusion, which is sometimes referred to as **uteroplacental insufficiency** (Figure 14-8, *B*). The decrease in uteroplacental blood flow may be chronic as occurs with maternal conditions that cause placental deterioration (diabetes, hypertension, SLE), or it can be the result of an acute event such as maternal hypotension, hypovolemia, or excessive uterine activity. As

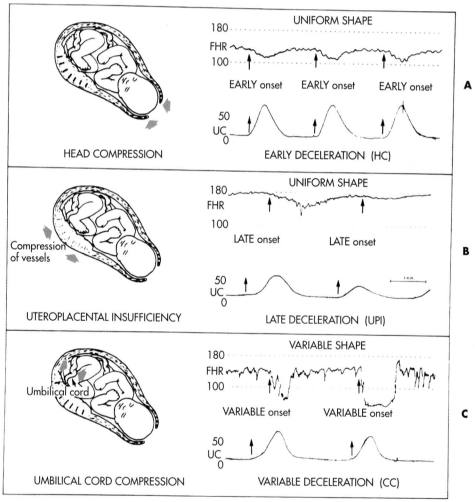

Figure 14-8 Mechanisms of fetal heart rate patterns. **A,** Head compression (HC), usually observed only during transition and second stage. **B,** Uteroplacental insufficiency (UPI), present when blood flow to fetus is compromised. **C,** Umbilical cord compression (CC), returning to normal heart rate only when pressure is relieved. (From Hon EP: *An introduction to fetal heart monitoring,* Hartford, 1968, Harty Press.)

with early decelerations, late decelerations usually remain within the normal FHR baseline range. Some late decelerations can be deceptively subtle. They may appear similar to early decelerations; being smooth and U-shaped, but there is an important difference in the timing of the deceleration. A late deceleration starts when the contraction is at its peak, reaches its low point when the contraction is almost over, and does not return to baseline until well after the contraction has ended. It starts *late* and resolves *late*. Late decelerations caused by uteroplacental insufficiency (see Figure 14-8, *B*) may occur in the following instances:

1. Pregnancies in which placental abnormalities such as infarctions or calcifications are present, which have a negative impact on maternal-fetal exchange
2. Labor patterns with intense contractions occurring at intervals less than 2 minutes apart for a prolonged period of time (a type of pattern that may be an iatrogenic effect of oxytocin administration)
3. Maternal hypotension from hypovolemia
4. Epidural or general anesthesia that decreases blood pressure and uteroplacental perfusion

It is common to see late decelerations, a rising baseline rate, and decreased baseline variability together because hypoxemia depresses the cardiac control center in the medulla. The presence of late decelerations is always *nonreassuring* and necessitates immediate investigation into the cause, as well as appropriate interventions to enhance fetal oxygenation. Late decelerations also require notification of the primary health care provider. Late decelerations that are the result of acute conditions are more likely to respond to nursing interventions such as maternal position changes, medications to reverse hypotension, and intravenous (IV) hydration to treat hypovolemia.

Nursing interventions for late decelerations

Nursing interventions for late decelerations are based on the entire clinical picture. For example, it is important to consider whether the decelerations are repetitive and if they are associated with loss of FHR variability. Generally the approach is to alleviate the physiologic stress on the fetus that has caused the late deceleration pattern. Nursing interventions for late decelerations include encouraging the woman to move to a lateral position, giving oxygen by face mask at 8 to 12 liters per minute, increasing IV fluids, discontinuing oxytocin if infusing, and notifying the primary health care provider. These interventions are collectively referred to as **intrauterine resuscitation.**

When signs of fetal compromise related to uteroplacental insufficiency appear, assessment may reveal the possible causes. Because blood supply may be affected on the maternal or fetal side, it is important to look first for the most common causes:

- Maternal hypotension, with or without low blood volume, may be caused by

—Vena caval compression.
—Dilation of lower extremity vessels after epidural or spinal anesthesia.
—Bleeding (hidden or overt) that depletes blood volume.

- Hypertonic uterine contractions may be caused by excessive response to oxytocin or the result of naturally hypertonic contractions, later in labor.
- Poor placental perfusion as a result of changes caused by preeclampsia, hypertension, diabetes, premature separation of placenta, or inadequate placental size may cause intrauterine growth restriction (IUGR).

Based on the assessment data, interventions are directed to correct the most likely causes of late decelerations, beginning with the least complicated interventions and observing the fetal response.

1. Change maternal position, since vena caval compression by the heavy uterus can occur in a lithotomy, in supine or semi-Fowler's position, or in a slight right or left lateral tilt. Turn the woman completely to the left or right side.
2. Increase mainline IV solution if the problem could be related to low cardiac output because of hypotension related to anesthesia or bleeding. Note exactly when and how much fluid is given during this period.
3. At the same time, observe the character of the contractions. Are they hypertonic for the stage of labor?
4. Is oxytocin infusing in a secondary line? If oxytocin is infusing, the IV pump should be turned off to stop the flow.
5. Begin administration of oxygen by face mask at 8 to 10 L/min.
6. Check maternal blood pressure and pulse to see whether they are affected by recent activities such as regional anesthesia and examinations.
7. Notify the physician or midwife of the FHR pattern and the results of intrauterine resuscitation interventions. Document time of notification and response on the medical record. If late decelerations do not resolve after interventions, the physician or midwife will make plans for an operative birth.

TEST *Yourself* 14-3

If working alone, list the logical sequence of actions you will choose in response to a nonreassuring FHR pattern.

Variable decelerations. Variable decelerations are caused by **umbilical cord compression,** which inhibits blood flow to and from the fetus (see Figure 14-8, *C*). These decelerations are variable in shape and timing with respect to contractions. Variable decelerations appear different from early and late decelerations and often appear different from each other. The FHR decreases sharply, stays down for a

Box 14-1

CLINICAL DECISION

Karen T has been in labor for 4 hours. The cervical dilation is now 6 cm and the following is seen on the fetal monitoring strip.
What would you do next?

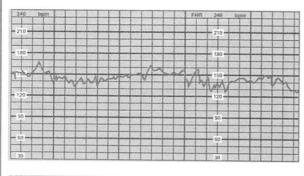

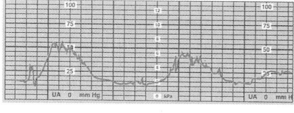

variable number of seconds, and then usually returns to the baseline rate as sharply as it descended (Figure 14-8, *C*).

It has been hypothesized that occlusion of the umbilical cord first causes compression of the umbilical vein, interrupting blood flow from the placenta to the fetus. In response, the FHR increases. As the occlusion progresses, it interrupts blood flow through the umbilical arteries, causing an increase in peripheral resistance. Stimulation of fetal carotid sinus and aortic arch baroreceptors follows; parasympathetic fibers then cause the fetal blood pressure and FHR to decrease. As the pressure is released and blood flow in the umbilical cord is restored, the FHR increases. Some fetuses overcompensate, however, and sometimes there may be an acceleration of the FHR over the baseline rate before the FHR returns to the previous baseline rate.

Nursing interventions for variable decelerations

Because variable decelerations are related to cord compression, they usually respond to changes in maternal position, which alleviate compression of the umbilical cord. Though some experts advocate oxygen administration to the woman during variable decelerations, the problem is not due to oxygen-deficient blood; rather it is the result of a mechanical compression of the umbilical cord, which causes a temporary decrease in blood flow. Although occasional periods of variable decelerations are

benign, repetitive decelerations require notification of the primary health care provider. Repetitive variable decelerations that do not respond to maternal position changes can result in fetal hypoxemia and acidemia. One indication of fetal compromise is loss of baseline variability as the variable decelerations continue. Variable decelerations are often seen toward the end of labor after rupture of membranes, when cord compression accompanies fetal descent and expulsion.

Many labor patterns show variable decelerations in the second stage. These can lead to fetal compromise if they occur during every maternal effort to push. If the FHR returns promptly to the baseline and variability is maintained, this is an indication that the fetus has time to recover. It is important to note the fetal response to pushing and adjust the timing of expulsive efforts, based on how the fetus is tolerating the second stage of labor. Some of the possible reasons for variable decelerations are listed:

1. Cord is caught between fetus and uterine wall.
2. Cord is being pulled tightly around fetal neck, a **nuchal cord,** or around an arm, shoulder, or other part as fetus descends through the birth canal.
3. There is a true knot in the cord that tightens during labor.
4. Occult (hidden) or frank (obvious) **prolapse** of the **umbilical cord** occurs through the cervix.
5. There is pressure on the cord because of insufficient amniotic fluid (oligohydramnios).
6. *Long or short cord* exists. Knots or loops in the cord occur if the cord is excessively long (>100 cm). These knots may be pulled tighter during labor; when the cord is looped around the neck (*nuchal cord*), it may become stretched and narrowed as the fetus descends the birth canal. A *short cord* (<32 cm) is also likely to show signs of traction, with narrowed umbilical vessels during descent.

Cord Prolapse

When the cord lies beside the presenting part or below it, the pressure of the head or buttocks will occlude circulation (Figure 14-9, *A*). *Cord prolapse* will result in varying degrees of cord compression and variable decelerations or in complete loss of heart beat. Complete cord compression occurs most frequently with premature rupture of membranes when the fetal presenting part is not engaged or when there is a footling or complete breech presentation. If cord prolapse cases occur at home with ruptured membranes, there is an increased risk of fetal death. A vaginal inspection might show the bluish shiny cord protruding through the cervix.

Interventions for prolapsed cord

Prevention of prolapsed cord is important. When artificial rupture of membranes (AROM) occurs, the fluid

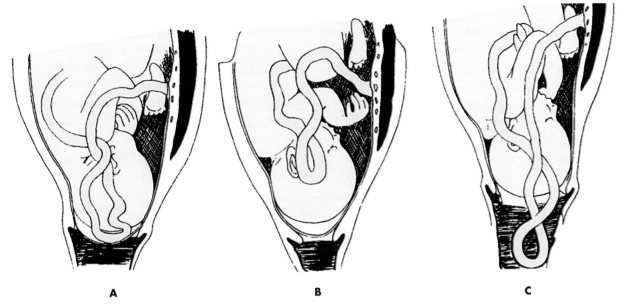

Figure 14-9   Prolapse of cord. **A,** Partial (trapped beside presenting part). **B,** Hidden. **C,** Complete (demonstrating cord visible in vagina).

should be released very slowly and the vaginal area inspected immediately. Monitoring or auscultation should continue before and after the procedure. If variable decelerations are noted, a change in maternal position should be tried first to relieve pressure.

1. Use the lateral Sims' position first. Rotate to the other side if no effect is achieved. If the cord is not through the vagina, it may be between the internal os and the head.
2. Discontinue oxytocin if infusing.
3. A knee-chest position may then help move the fetus off the cervix.
4. If the cord is prolapsed and visible in the vagina, the only recourse is to put on a sterile glove and manually push the presenting part off the cord so that circulation can continue while preparations are made for emergency cesarean birth.
5. Call for help and make sure the health care provider is notified and the appropriate team is assembled for a cesarean birth, including those with skill in newborn resuscitation.
6. Continue EFM.

FETAL COMPROMISE

A reassuring FHR is a rate between 110 and 160 bpm with average short- and long-term variability. Accelerations with fetal movement are additional reassuring signs. During labor it is important to assess the fetal response to uterine activity. The FHR pattern provides data about how well the fetus is tolerating contractions.

A nonreassuring FHR pattern may be a sign of increasingly poor tolerance to the physiologic stress of labor. This stress is imposed by uterine contractions, during which the blood flow to the placenta is greatly decreased. If the fetus is otherwise well-oxygenated, the 60- to 90-second contraction period without free flow of uteroplacental circulation is not harmful. Most fetuses tolerate contractions lasting 60 to 90 seconds every 2 to 3 minutes, as long as there is a period of rest and uterine relaxation between contractions (Figure 14-10).

When patterns indicate **fetal compromise**, the FHR may change in the following ways: changes in FHR baseline, such as tachycardia or bradycardia; late decelerations of the FHR or repetitive persistent variable decelerations of the FHR; and loss of short- and long-term FHR variability. Fetal compromise may be *chronic*, occurring during the course of pregnancy, or become *acute*, usually occurring during labor if the woman is hypotensive or hypovolemic.

Without interventions for these nonreassuring patterns such as intrauterine resuscitation or expeditious birth, the compromised fetus that is not tolerating the physiologic stress of labor may become increasingly hypoxemic and acidemic and may be slow to recover at birth. After prolonged fetal compromise, the fetus may suffer permanent injury and is at increased risk for neonatal death. Figure 14-11 illustrates a decision tree when nonreassuring fetal responses are evident.

Meconium Fluid

In utero, meconium passage is generally seen only after 34 weeks of gestation and therefore is considered a maturational sign. Although it is sometimes associated with

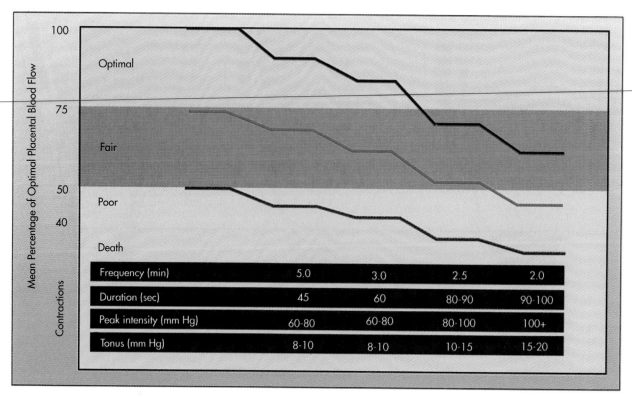

Figure 14-10   Effect of myometrial contractions on mean placental blood flow (PBF). As the duration and frequency of contractions increase, PBF progressively decreases. Even mild contractions may cause fetal distress or death when PBF is poor. (Modified from Spencer JAO, ed: *Fetal monitoring,* Philadelphia, 1989, FA Davis.)

Box 14-2

CLINICAL DECISION

Asha A is a 32-year-old primigravida in early labor. Your admission assessment reveals that her membranes have been ruptured for 17 hours, her cervix is 2 cm dilated and 70% effaced, and contractions are irregular. She has chronic hypertension; blood pressure upon admission is 170/90. Describe the risk factors for fetal compromise and how they may manifest in the FHR tracing.

fetal compromise, many full-term infants may pass meconium as a normal physiologic event. A fetus in breech position usually passes meconium during the descent phase. About 11% to 22% of all infants have meconium in the amniotic fluid at birth (Weitzner et al, 1990). Most of these infants will not be depressed at birth. Meconium is feces that is usually dark green to black and is full of bilirubin, which has a strong yellow-green color when diluted (see Figure 19-14). The concentration of meconium is directly related to the volume of amniotic fluid. Assessment of the characteristics of meconium-stained fluid is critical because thick meconium is more likely to

cause respiratory problems in the newborn. If a compromised fetus, stimulated by hypoxemia, takes deep gasping breaths before birth, the meconium-stained fluid can be aspirated into the lower portion of the lung and can partly obstruct airways if it is thick. **Meconium aspiration syndrome** (MAS) may lead to further cardiorespiratory problems (see Chapter 29).

Asphyxia

Asphyxia is the metabolic state of hypoxia and acidosis. It is important to distinguish the difference between hypoxemia and hypoxia and between acidemia and acidosis. *Hypoxemia* is a deficiency of oxygen in the blood, whereas *hypoxia* is a deficiency of oxygen in the tissues. *Acidemia* is the accumulation of excess acid in the blood, whereas *acidosis* is the accumulation of excess acid in the tissues. Objective data to evaluate fetal status are limited for the most part to assessment of the blood, such as by capillary scalp blood sampling or umbilical cord blood sampling. The cycle of events leading to fetal asphyxia begins with the lack of oxygen (O_2) and excess buildup of carbon dioxide (CO_2). These events may occur because the balance of production and elimination of CO_2 is upset. CO_2 must be released across the

Decision TREE | Nonreassuring Fetal Heart Rate Pattern

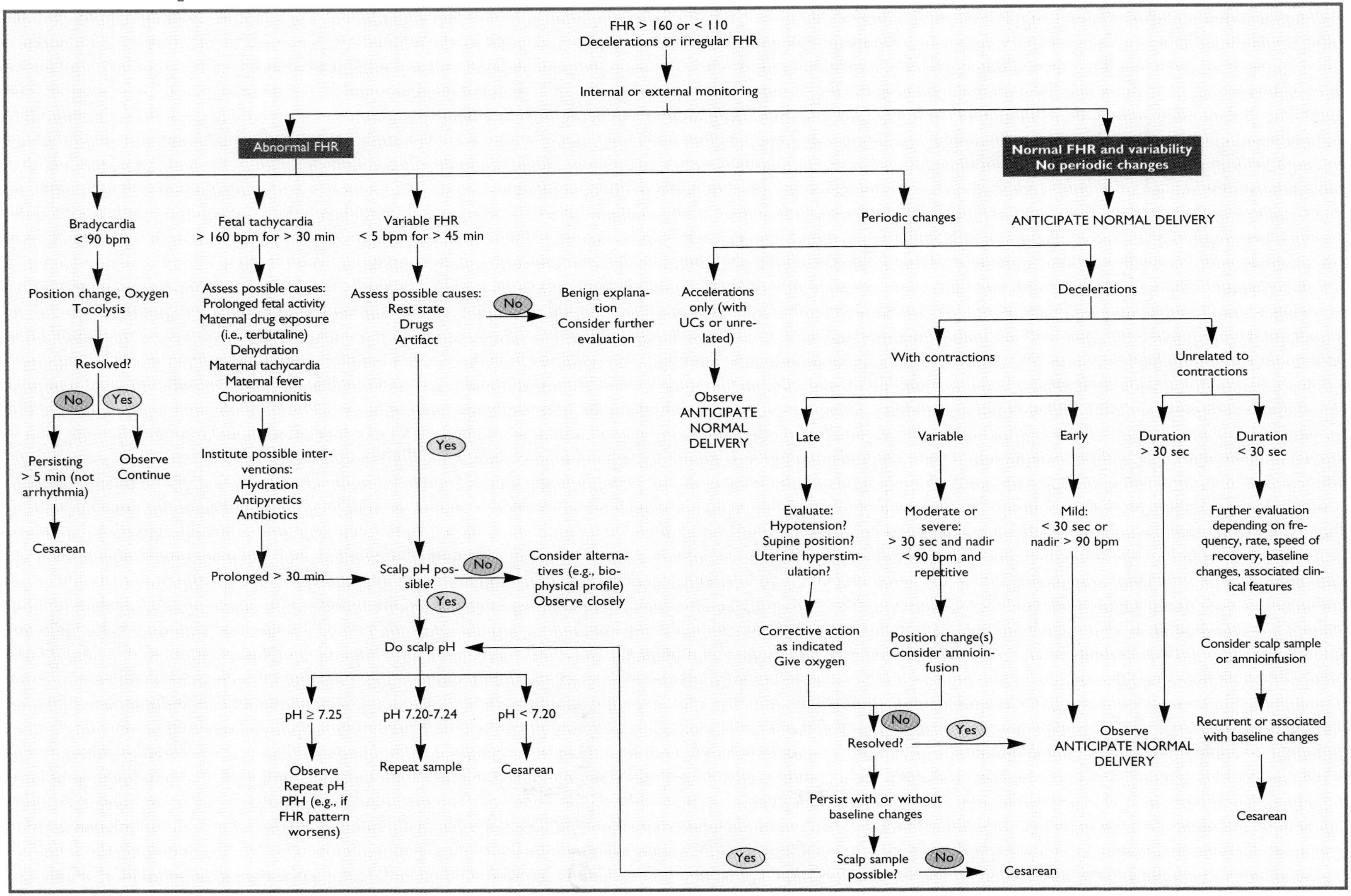

Figure 14-11 Decision tree for nonreassuring fetal heart rate (FHR) pattern. (Modified from Simpson KR, Creehan PA: *AWHONN: perinatal nursing*, Philadelphia, 1996, Lippincott.)

placenta to the mother, and oxygen must be taken up; the O_2 and CO_2 *gradient* between mother and fetus greatly affects placental perfusion and exchange across the placenta.

Respiratory acidosis begins first as CO_2 increases. As O_2 levels fall, further energy production converts from aerobic to anaerobic paths, causing lactic acid to accumulate. The result is a mixed respiratory and metabolic acidosis. (Figure 14-12 shows how lactic acid begins rising rapidly at a certain point in the sequence, with pH dropping quickly. See Chapter 29 for resuscitation of the asphyxiated infant. Normal and low fetal pH levels are listed in Box 14-2.) Further management of labor varies with the progress of labor and other fetal or maternal conditions. Operative delivery will be arranged quickly to prevent further damage in an asphyxiated infant. If there is continued evidence of fetal compromise, birth by the quickest method possible is necessary.

Umbilical cord blood samples are sometimes obtained to evaluate acid base status when there has been evidence of fetal compromise via a nonreassuring FHR pattern.

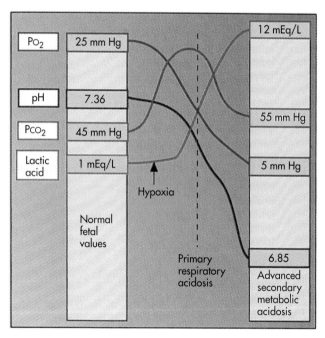

Figure 14-12 A sample pattern of fetal blood gases, pH, and lactic acid with fetal compromise caused by hypoxemia. (Modified from Spencer JAO, ed: *Fetal monitoring,* Philadelphia, 1989, FA Davis.)

▌ *Box* 14-2   **pH Range of Fetal Scalp Samples**

Normal: more than 7.25 (mild hypoxemia normally accompanies labor)
Borderline: 7.20-7.25
Worsening acidemia: 7.19 and below
Severe acidemia: 6.90 and below

These values provide objective data related to fetal status. The arterial pH from a cord artery is 0.05 to 0.07 below that of the umbilical vein pH.

Testing fetal oxygenation

In some institutions, additional data about fetal status may be obtained via fetal scalp blood sampling. In this procedure a small amount of fetal scalp capillary blood is obtained and evaluated for acid-base status. If the results indicate that the fetus is not acidemic, labor can continue. The disadvantages of this technique are that it is invasive to the mother and fetus, is subject to error related to sampling, and reflects fetal assessment at only one point in time. Fetal scalp blood sampling reached peak popularity during the late 1980s as an adjunct method of fetal assessment in the case of nonreassuring FHR patterns. However, this procedure is no longer used in most institutions. Currently under investigation in the United States is a new method for fetal status assessment that can be used when the FHR is nonreassuring. This method is fetal oxygen saturation monitoring, a technologic advance based on the oxygen saturation monitoring known as pulse oximetry. Fetal oxygen saturation monitoring via pulse oximetry has been successfully used in European research studies, but it is not widely available for clinical use in the United States. This method involves inserting a small device through the cervix until it is next to the fetal cheek or forehead. It is held in place by pressure of the uterine wall against the fetal part. Membranes must be ruptured and the cervix dilated at least 2 to 3 cm. One advantage to this method of fetal assessment is that it provides real time data about fetal status as it relates to oxygenation. Like EFM, the data are continual. Fetal oxygen saturation monitoring during labor will be useful in clinical situations where more accurate assessment of fetal oxygen status is required.

Amnioinfusion

When there is less amniotic fluid than normal, the cord may be compressed (see Chapter 7 for normal volumes). If variable decelerations are not improved by other interventions, **amnioinfusion**—instilling a normal saline or lactated Ringer's solution into the uterine cavity by catheter—can have a beneficial effect. Amnioinfusion may sometimes be used to flush out thick meconium fluid to decrease the risk of MAS. When this procedure was first introduced, it was thought that the fluid had to be prewarmed and that it was best to use an IV infusion pump. Over the last decade, amnioinfusion has been studied by multiple researchers.

TEST *Yourself* 14-4 _____

a. What is the lower limit for normal fetal blood pH?
b. Describe how poor placental perfusion can cause fetal acidosis.

PROCEDURE 14-1

Amnioinfusion

1. Encourage the woman to assume a lateral position.
2. Hang I L of normal saline or lactated Ringer's solution and attach IV tubing to IUPC catheter tubing and flush tubing with solution.
3. Insert an intrauterine pressure catheter (IUPC), if one is not already in place.
4. Infuse the solution at approximately 15-20 ml/min until the variable decelerations have resolved.
5. Carefully assess amount of fluid returned. If there is little return of fluid after infusing 600 ccs, discontinue the infusion until the fluid has returned.
6. Monitor uterine resting tone via palpation or IUPC (see figure at right). (A double-lumen IUPC can be used simultaneously to administer the amnioinfusion and to monitor intraamniotic pressure.) Ultrasound may be used to evaluate fluid volume before and after procedure, but this is usually not necessary.
7. Support the woman during the tense time, when many tubes and wires are inserted into her vagina; she will be concerned for fetal well-being.

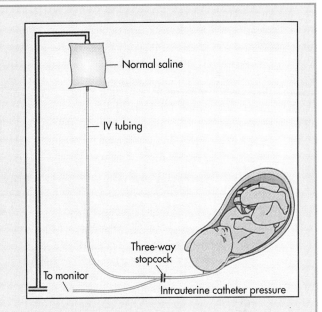

OPTIONAL ACTIVITY

Write a sample nursing note that correctly documents the performance of this procedure.

Most practitioners do not prewarm the solution or use IV infusion pumps. The infusion can be administered at room temperature using a gravity flow device (Glantz and Letteney, 1996).

SUMMARY OF FETAL HEART RATE PATTERNS

Reassuring patterns provide information that suggests the fetus is well-oxygenated and thus placental perfusion is adequate. The average baseline rate is between 110 and 160 bpm. Baseline variability is most accurately assessed during internal monitoring; an average of 6 to 10 bpm is reassuring. Normal periodic changes include accelerations with fetal movements and early decelerations during the later phases of labor. The nurse's intervention for reassuring patterns is continued observation.

Other FHR patterns suggest possible alterations in fetal oxygenation or placental perfusion. The baseline rate may be near the upper or lower limits of normal. Mild bradycardia (100 to 120 bpm) may be normal if no other problems are present and the baseline heart rate has not changed significantly. Mild tachycardia may be related to prematurity, intraamniotic infection, chronic or early fetal hypoxia, maternal or fetal anemia, maternal fever, anxiety or hyperthyroidism, or administration of beta-sympathomimetic or parasympatholytic drugs. **Increased baseline variability** (over 25 bpm) is associated with fetal

movement but may be an early sign of fetal hypoxemia. Finally, variable deceleration patterns with an FHR decrease no lower than 80 bpm for less than 30 seconds, with average variability, and that respond to maternal position changes may be related to transient umbilical cord compression.

Nonreassuring patterns indicate significant alterations in fetal oxygenation or perfusion; bradycardia is especially concerning when associated with late decelerations, variable decelerations, or loss of variability. Decreased baseline variability (less than 3 to 5 bpm) may be related to maternal drug administration (meperidine and other analgesics, magnesium sulfate), fetal sleep, prematurity, anomalies of the central nervous system, or fetal tachycardia or hypoxemia. Decreased variability is nonreassuring if fetal stimulation does not elicit an acceleration or increase in variability.

TEST *Yourself* 14-5 _____

Describe three nonreassuring FHR patterns on the EFM strip.

Nursing Responsibilities

In 1986 the American College of Obstetricians and Gynecologists (ACOG) and the Association of Women's Health, Obstetric and Neonatal Nurses (AWHONN) (known at that time as the Nurses' Association of the American College of Obstetricians and Gynecologists [NAACOG]) published a joint statement describing practice competencies for care providers involved in intrapartum EFM. Since then, both the ACOG and AWHONN have published other guidelines and standards on this topic. A recent ACOG publication is the technical bulletin "Fetal Heart Rate Patterns: Monitoring, Interpretation, and Management" (1995). A recent AWHONN publication is "Didactic Content and Clinical Skills Verification for Professional Nurse Providers of Basic, High Risk, and Critical Care Intrapartum Nursing"

(1993). Box 14-3 lists intrapartum FHR monitoring competencies as revised in 1991 by AWHONN.

The perinatal nurse plays an important role in assessing the fetal response to labor and birth. Skill in EFM pattern interpretation and knowledge of EFM equipment are expected perinatal nursing competencies. The institution is responsible for ensuring that nurses who use EFM are competent. Competency validation involves both clinical skills verification and knowledge base evaluation. Nurses must also take the initiative and seek out continuing education in this area. Although intrapartum fetal monitoring

---

Box 14-3   Intrapartum Fetal Heart Monitoring

NURSING PRACTICE COMPETENCIES

To function competently in the use of intrapartum fetal heart monitoring, the nurse should demonstrate competency in the application and use of auscultatory and electronic fetal monitoring equipment and interpretation of data. The intrapartum nurse should therefore be able to:

A. Implement the appropriate fetal heart monitoring method based on patient status, hospital policy, and current standards of practice recommended by professional organizations.

B. Explain the principles of the chosen method of fetal heart monitoring to the patient and her support person(s).

C. Identify the limitations of information produced by each method of monitoring.

D. Demonstrate competency in fetal heart monitoring by auscultation.
1. Perform complete assessment including Leopold's maneuvers to determine fetal position, and palpate the fundus to determine appropriate site for auscultation.
2. Apply fetoscope or Doppler device to the appropriate site.
3. Palpate uterine contractions for frequency, duration, and intensity; confirm uterine rest between contractions; determine if abnormal findings are present.
4. Identify and determine the baseline fetal heart rate and rhythm.
5. Identify the presence of fetal heart rate changes with or between uterine contractions.
6. Determine if findings are reassuring or nonreassuring and implement appropriate nursing interventions, including additional fetal monitoring methods.
7. Identify the clinical situations, based on fetal heart monitoring findings, in which immediate notification of the primary health care provider is appropriate.
8. Communicate the findings from auscultation, interpretation of findings, and resulting nursing intervention(s) in written and verbal form in an appropriate and timely manner.
9. Document appropriate entries on the written or computerized patient record.

10. Demonstrate appropriate maintenance of auscultation equipment.

E. Demonstrate use of electronic fetal monitor.
1. Perform complete assessment including Leopold's maneuvers, palpate the fundus, and auscultate the fetal heart rate prior to application of the transducers.
2. Apply external transducers and adjust the electronic fetal monitor accordingly.
3. Prepare the patient, set up equipment, and complete connections for fetal electrode with and without intrauterine pressure catheter.
4. Calibrate the monitor for the use of the intrauterine pressure catheter.
5. Identify technically inadequate tracings and take appropriate corrective action.
6. Obtain and maintain an adequate tracing of the fetal heart and uterine contractions.
7. Interpret uterine contraction frequency, duration, intensity, and baseline resting tone as appropriate based on monitoring method, and determine if abnormal findings are present.
8. Identify baseline fetal heart rate and rhythm, variability, and the presence of periodic and nonperiodic changes.
9. Determine if findings are reassuring or nonreassuring and implement appropriate nursing interventions.
10. Identify the clinical situations, based on fetal heart monitoring findings, in which immediate notification of the primary health care provider is appropriate.
11. Communicate the content of electronic fetal monitoring data, interpretations of data, and resulting nursing intervention(s) in written and verbal form, in an appropriate and timely manner.
12. Document appropriate entries in the written or computerized patient record and on the electronic fetal monitoring tracing or storage disk.
13. Demonstrate appropriate maintenance of electronic fetal monitoring equipment.
14. Demonstrate appropriate storage and retrieval of fetal heart monitoring data.

Association Women's Health, Obstetric and Neonatal Nurses (AWHONN): *Nursing practice competencies; intrapartum fetal heart monitoring,* Washington, DC, 1991.

is associated with more litigation than other aspects of nursing care, this issue should not be the primary reason for maintaining EFM competency. The perinatal nurse has an ethical and moral obligation to the mother and fetus to provide the best possible care based on the current knowledge that is available (see Chapter 30).

Documentation to Avoid Liability

Many of the recent malpractice claims in the United States involve the use or misuse of EFM. Cases include failure to monitor the fetus during labor and just before birth, failure to accurately interpret the FHR pattern, or failure to respond appropriately to the FHR pattern tracing, especially a failure to initiate a cesarean birth in a timely manner in response to fetal compromise (Simpson and Chez, 1996). The health care provider may have monitored the fetus carefully and responded correctly, but there may be little documentation in the medical record to support these interventions. It should be kept in mind that in most cases, *"If it is not written, it is considered not to have been done."* The importance of documentation is heightened because in most states, cases may be filed up to 21 years after the birth; most nurses cannot remember details for so long. Thus nurses must take special care to document observations, interventions, and notification of the primary health care provider. It is especially critical to document events when the primary health care provider does not respond in an appropriate or timely manner. If the chain of command is initiated, careful and complete documentation of who was called and when the call was made is essential.

A flow sheet should be kept at the bedside for noting the important assessments, such as vital signs, contraction characteristics, amniotic fluid status, vaginal examinations, cervical status and station, and FHR and FHR reactivity. Medications, procedures, and anesthetics are also noted on the flow sheet. It may not be necessary to document events and critical assessments in more than one place; in fact, duplicate documentation can lead to error. Therefore if the interventions are documented with the correct times on the labor flow record, it is not necessary (unless required by the unit's protocol) to repeat documentation directly on the EFM tracing. The EFM tracing is an important part of the medical record. Unit policy should be followed in providing information on the tracing so it can be identified readily. Generally, at least the date and the woman's name and medical record number should be noted on the strip. Some institutions no longer save EFM tracings in paper form because they can be stored on computer disks and retrieved if needed at a later date.

Each unit has a protocol for FHR monitoring management. It is important to be aware of your unit protocol and follow it as much as possible. If *artifact* causes a poor FHR signal, it should also be noted. Sometimes it is difficult to obtain an adequate external FHR reading for an obese patient. Contraction characteristics, as well as variability and periodic changes, that appear on the strip must be noted on the flow sheet. In the current legal climate, documentation is essential to the practice of "defensive nursing." It is also important to list the times of physician or nurse-midwife notification and response. Avoid vague phrases such as, "Physician (or nurse-midwife) called." Years later, who called whom may be unclear. Instead, if the nurse initiates a call to the primary health care provider, it is best to note which physician (or nurse-midwife) was notified. When the primary health care provider does not respond promptly or appropriately, nursing actions should be taken. The nurse who notes inadequate physician or midwife response or intervention is legally required to initiate the *chain of command* to obtain satisfactory follow-up. Therefore it is important to be aware of the chain of command policy for the unit. The staff nurse will usually notify the charge nurse who should notify the next appropriate person until the issue is resolved. There are nursing, medical, and administrative chains of command. Nurses have been involved in lawsuits because they did not follow through in advocating for the mother or fetus in the case of a nonreassuring FHR pattern, even though they knew there was evidence of fetal compromise.

ASSESSMENT

The nurse gathers information from the prenatal history and physical assessment that accompanies the family, and determines the following:
- Whether the woman has had prior experience with antepartum or intrapartum fetal monitoring
- The woman's parity and previous fetal losses and whether they were close to term or during labor
- Whether the couple or woman has attended childbirth preparation classes
- Whether there are factors that place this pregnancy at risk (prematurity or postmaturity, intrauterine growth restriction, hypertension, diabetes mellitus, or other chronic conditions) and how they might affect the fetus' ability to withstand the stressors of labor
- Whether the maternal vital signs are within normal limits
- Whether the baseline FHR and variability are within normal range
- The significance of any periodic changes in FHR, including decelerations or accelerations and whether they are associated with maternal medications, fetal movement, or changes in maternal position

NURSING DIAGNOSES

Examples of nursing diagnoses include the following:
- Maternal anxiety related to fetal health or prior experience

- Impaired gas exchange related to decreased placental perfusion

EXPECTED OUTCOMES

- Couple will be kept informed and will participate in decision making.
- Fetal injury will be avoided or minimized by prompt interventions.

NURSING INTERVENTION

- The nurse maintains a birthing setting that is as natural as possible during intrapartal monitoring. The woman should be encouraged to ask questions and to remain mobile as long as possible. The nurse keeps the family informed of all changes and proposed interventions in a timely manner and encourages their input when possible.
- The mother should not be separated from her support person, even when problems arise, and childbirth techniques should be reinforced.
- Nursing interventions should always minimize the potential for fetal hypoxemia while maintaining the woman's comfort and sense of control. Simple measures such as avoiding the supine position can prevent fetal compromise.
- The nurse observes the monitor tracing every 15 to 30 minutes and records findings on the bedside labor flow chart. When a nonreassuring FHR pattern is noted, the nurse tries various interventions and notes response. If differences in opinion about the significance of findings occur among personnel, consultation should be sought. Maternal-fetal status may change quickly, and all staff members must be ready to intervene as needed. When a depressed fetus is about to be born, persons who are skilled in newborn resuscitation must be present (see Chapter 29).

EVALUATION

To evaluate outcomes during fetal monitoring, the nurse asks questions such as the following.
- Did the couple participate in decision making? Was anxiety kept to a minimum by information and support?
- Was fetal oxygenation maintained as evidenced by FHR and Apgar scores?
- Was communication with the physician appropriate and timely?

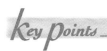
Key Points

- Monitoring contractions and fetal status during labor is a standard of care.
- If EFM is not used, auscultation must be performed on the same schedule.
- In most settings, nurses have the management responsibility for application of the monitor, interpreting and reporting patterns, and documenting findings.
- Adequate placental perfusion and fetal oxygenation are the basis for a reassuring FHR tracing. The nurse looks for causes of interrupted blood flow, which results in uteroplacental insufficiency.
- Intrauterine resuscitation includes all the corrective steps to reverse fetal compromise.
- Cord compression is a mechanical problem, and many times it can be resolved by maternal position changes or, in some cases, by amnioinfusion. Otherwise, the fetus with severe cord compression must be delivered as quickly as possible.
- Fetal acid-base status indicates whether there is fetal compromise. Direct assessment of fetal acid-base status may be performed by the physician or midwife by means of scalp sampling or pulse oximetry.
- If a nonreassuring pattern cannot be resolved, the caregiver's responsibility is to always initiate interventions to prevent asphyxia or to rescue the fetus.
- Maintain communication that supports the couple because interventions may be abrupt and anxiety-producing.

Study Questions

14-1. Select the terms that apply to the following statements:
   a. A result of cord compression during labor is _____.
   b. Variable decelerations can be caused by a tight cord around the neck or a _____.
   c. The average rate during 10 minutes of FHR monitoring is _____.
   d. FHR of less than 110 bpm for 10 minutes is _____.
   e. FHR of more than 160 bpm for 10 minutes is _____.
   f. Pattern caused by fetal head compression and stimulation of the vagal nerve is _____.
   g. Pattern caused by uteroplacental insufficiency is _____.

14-2. Ms. P has been admitted to the labor and delivery unit. External monitoring is initiated. Choose four parameters assessed when you interpret the tracing of uterine activity.

    a. Interval of contractions   d. Intensity of contractions

    b. Frequency of fetal movements   e. Duration of contractions

    c. Resting tonus   f. Reaction of fetus to labor

14-3. Choose four parameters assessed when you interpret the FHR pattern tracing.

    a. Baseline rate   d. Periodic changes

    b. Response to fetal movements   e. Baseline variability

    c. Intensity of uterine contractions

14-4. In the second stage of labor, if variable FHR decelerations occur with each contraction, the nursing intervention should be to do which of the following?

    a. Change pushing position to a side-lying position and observe response.

    b. Notify the primary health care provider.

    c. Call the anesthesiologist.

    d. Coach for more effective pushing.

14-5. Which procedure may be used to correct variable decelerations caused by cord compression as a result of oligohydramnios?

    a. Amnioinfusion   c. Maternal oxygen administration

    b. Cesarean birth   d. Stimulation of labor

Answer Key

14-1: *a*, Variable deceleration; *b*, nuchal cord; *c*, baseline heart rate; *d*, bradycardia; *e*, tachycardia; *f*, early decelerations; *g*, late decelerations. 14-2: a, c, e, f. 14-3: a, b, d, e. 14-4: a. 14-5: a.

References

Afriat CI et al: Electronic fetal monitoring competency—to validate or not: the opinions of experts, *J Perinat Neonat Nurs* 8(3):1, 1994.

American College of Obstetricians and Gynecologists: *Fetal heart rate patterns: monitoring, interpretation, and management,* ACOG Technical Bulletin 207, Washington, DC, 1995.

American College of Obstetricians and Gynecologists: *Umbilical artery blood acid-base analysis,* ACOG Technical Bulletin 216, Washington, DC, 1995.

Association of Women's Health, Obstetric, and Neonatal Nurses: *Didactic content and clinical skills verification for professional providers of basic, high risk, and critical care intrapartum nursing,* Washington, DC, 1993.

Beischer NA, MacKay EV, eds: *Obstetrics and the newborn,* ed 3, Philadelphia, 1993, WB Saunders.

Blackburn ST, Loper DL: *Maternal, fetal, and neonatal physiology,* Philadelphia, 1992, WB Saunders.

Cibils LA: On intrapartum fetal monitoring, *Am J Obstet Gynecol* 174:1382, 1996.

Cusick W, Smulian JC, Vintzileos AM: Intrapartum use of fetal heart rate monitoring, contraction monitoring, and amnioinfusion, *Clin Perinatol* 22(4):875, 1995.

Glantz JC, Letteney DL: Pumps and warmers during amnioinfusion: are they necessary? *Obstet Gynecol* 87:150, 1996.

*Hon E, Quilligan EJ: The classification of fetal heart rate: II, a revised working classification, *Conn Med* 31:779, 1967.

*Classic reference.

Lameier LY, Katz VL: Amnioinfusion: a review, *Obstet Gynecol Surv,* 48: 829, 1993.

McNamara HM: The effect of uterine contractions on fetal oxygen saturation, *Br J Obstet Gynaecol* 102:644, 1995.

Menihan CA: Intrapartum fetal monitoring. In Simpson KR, Creehan PA eds: *AWHONN's perinatal nursing,* Philadelphia, 1996, Lippincott.

Naeye RL, Localio AR: Determining the time before birth when ischemia and hypoxemia initiated cerebral palsy, *Obstet Gynecol,* 86:713, 1995.

Nelson KB et al: Uncertain value of electronic fetal monitoring in predicting cerebral palsy, *N Engl J Med,* 334:613, 1996.

Simpson KR, Chez BF: Professional and legal issues. In Simpson KR, Creehan PA eds: *AWHONN's perinatal nursing,* Philadelphia, 1996, Lippincott.

*Spencer JAO, ed: *Fetal monitoring,* Philadelphia, 1989, FA Davis.

Tucker SM: *Fetal assessment and monitoring,* ed 3, St Louis, 1996, Mosby.

Weitzner JS et al: Objective assessment of meconium content of amniotic fluid, *Obstet Gynecol* 76(6):1143, 1990.

Student Resource Shelf

Tucker SM: *Pocket guide to fetal monitoring and assessment,* ed 3, St Louis, 1996, Mosby.

The most useful pocket handbook on the subject of antepartum and intrapartum fetal assessment.

15

The Birth Process & Nursing Care

Learning Objectives

- Compare management of normal birth in the hospital setting with management of normal birth in an unexpected location.
- Relate principles of conservation of energy and integrity to the second stage of labor.
- Explain the rationale for choosing different positions for labor and birth.
- Explain the rationale for using specific breathing methods for labor and birth.
- Identify essential safety measures necessary when labor is induced.
- Anticipate the need for operative interventions during birth
- Discuss the protocols for episiotomy use and nursing care.
- Discuss feelings of guilt and failure experienced by some women after surgical birth
- Recognize that there are a variety of culturally diverse responses to the pain of labor and to the stress of childbirth.

Key Terms

Bearing-Down Efforts (BDEs)
Breech Presentation
Caput Succedaneum
Cephalhematoma
Cesarean Birth
Crowning
Dystocia
Episiotomy
Forceps
Hypertonic Contraction
Induction
Laceration
Open-Glottis Pushing
Reorganization
Vacuum Extraction
Vaginal Birth After Cesarean (VBAC)
Valsalva's Maneuver
Ventouse

Several interrelated factors are necessary for a successful outcome of the labor and birthing process. In keeping with the advances in family-centered nursing care, the expectant couple must be encouraged as "co-laborers" in the work of second-stage labor and birth. During this time a number of activities will be happening simultaneously.

THE PROCESS OF THE SECOND STAGE

The structure component of the second stage centers on the rapid physiologic changes and is called the *pelvic phase* of labor. The cervix is now fully stretched to provide adequate dimension for the head of the fetus to slip through. When the cervix is fully dilated, the forces of labor shift to effect descent of the fetus through the vaginal canal. As the fetus passes through the obliterated, or "taken up," cervix and maneuvers through the pelvic outlet, it will then distend the vaginal orifice, pass through the perineal muscles and labia, and emerge.

Once the presenting part is through the cervix, the uterine contractions are insufficient to effect descent; the woman's controlled bearing down efforts must complete the process. **Bearing down efforts** (BDEs) add a force of 120 mm Hg in a lateral position and 150 mm Hg in a sitting position (Roberts et al, 1987).

The erratic quality of contractions in the transition phase now changes to a more rhythmic pattern. The pattern will show strong, intense contractions lasting at least 90 seconds. Rest intervals, depending on parity, may have an interval of 2 to 4 minutes. Some women may briefly fall asleep between contractions, whereas others remain alert and concentrate intently on the process.

Aderhold and Roberts (1991) have published numerous articles from *Phases of the Second Stage of Labor,* a study that indicates ways of working with women during the second stage. The second stage of labor has been divided into three phases that reflect the three phases of the first stage of labor. Recognition of these subdivisions of the second stage will facilitate a change in traditional care. The Aderhold and Roberts study also identifies the nursing care that accompanies each phase (Box 15-1). Since three phases are accepted in the first stage, it should not be difficult for caregivers to recognize these three second-stage phases, although they are perhaps less clearly defined and happen more rapidly. These phases need different and individualized interventions and sensitive guidance from a caring, knowledgeable support person.

Phase One: Early or Latent Phase

The latent phase occurs after full dilation of the cervix. There can be a dramatic shift from the agitation of transition to a calm, or a lull, when the woman may briefly drop off to sleep. Contractions occur less frequently and are not as strong or painful. This first phase may be thought of as a period of **reorganization** as the body prepares for expulsion. The woman may be anxious and may also complain of back and leg aches. During the 10- to 30-minute period of reorganization that follows complete dilation, she should be encouraged to relax and to rest her legs and body. The caregivers should not force the woman to push as soon as full dilatation is reached, although this is the current practice in many settings. Nurses, nurse midwives, and childbirth educators must allow the body's normal mechanisms of labor to take place spontaneously.

Phase Two: Descent or Active Phase

Phase two has often been understood as the *start* of the second stage, and it is described as the active phase of descent of the presenting part through the vagina. During this phase the mother will cooperate as she senses progress. The Ferguson reflex (the urge to push), brought on by the release of stretch receptors in the pelvic floor, has been researched. The urge to push is more influenced by the fetal station than by cervical dilation, and it can occur before or after full dilation (Cosner and deJong,

---

| *Box* **15-1**   **Second-Stage Phase Boundaries**

PHASE 1 LATENT—RESTING

Duration of Phase
From complete dilation until the urge to bear down becomes frequent and rhythmic

Maternal Responses
Eager to follow simple directions from one labor support person

PHASE 2 ACTIVE—DESCENT

Duration of Phase
Nulliparas—50 minutes
Multiparas—20 minutes
From onset of rhythmic bearing down efforts (BDEs) until crowning; presenting part becomes visible

Duration of Contractions
Uterine contractions and the accompanying expulsive forces may last 1½ minutes and recur at times after a myometrial resting phase of no more than 1 minute

Maternal Responses
Highly variable; depend on parity, pelvic accommodations. Sedation will lengthen the second stage

PHASE 3 TRANSITION—PERINEAL

Duration of Phase
Highly variable; a short phase lasting five to seven contractions or 8 to 12 minutes; from crowning until the birth of the infant

Maternal Responses
Silent pauses in conversation; prepares for and is excited about birth; small particles of feces expelled; area cleaned with soapy sponge, downward strokes away from the vagina; variable maternal position

Modified from Aderhold KJ, Roberts JE: Phases of the second stage of labor, *J Nurse Midwifery* 36(5):267, 1991.

1993). Studies show that the mother needs to learn how to recognize when to begin BDEs and how to push during this second phase (Evans, 1995).

Pushing or BDEs must follow the dictates of the woman's own urges. Unless she has been given an epidural anesthetic, the woman has an urge to push rhythmically with each contraction. She enters fully into BDEs and may make grunting noises. These noises should be encouraged because a noise with BDEs indicates that the **open-glottis pushing** technique is being used. See Chapter 12 for ways to avoid the adverse effects of **Valsalva's maneuver** (breath

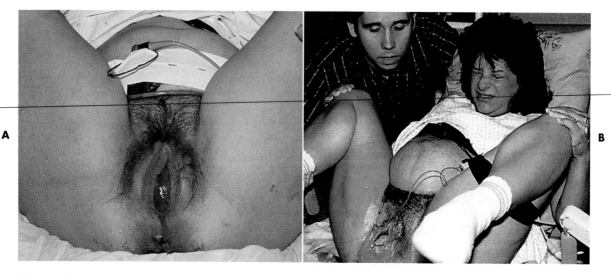

Figure 15-1   A, Crowning. **B,** Bulging of the perineum just before birth. (**A,** From Lowdermilk DL, Perry SE, Bobak IM: *Maternity and women's health care,* ed 6, St Louis, 1997, Mosby. **B,** Courtesy Marjorie Pyle, RNC, *Lifecircle.*)

holding while bearing down, resulting in changes in the mother's blood pressure and acid-base balance).

Approximately midway through the descent phase, the presenting part may be seen at the vaginal opening (introitus). The labia gradually separate until the fetal scalp is seen (Figure 15-1). Between contractions, the fetal head is forced back by the elasticity of the muscles of the pelvic floor. After a few contractions, the labia flatten with distention, and the head maintains the perineal opening during the relaxation phase; this is **crowning.** Crowning means that the presenting part stays visible when the contraction is over and the largest diameter of this part is encircled by the vaginal opening.

Phase Three: Perineal Phase

Phase three is short, lasting approximately 5 to 12 minutes. The perineum begins to bulge, the anal area dilates, and the stool may be expelled. Contractions are frequent and intense. A woman often worries about "ripping open" but should be encouraged to use positive affirmations, such as, "My body knows how to deliver my baby" or "I am opening up like a flower."

Birth

The skin over the perineum glistens as it is stretched to its limit. If there are adequate tissue elasticity and outlet dimensions, the occiput progresses with the head in flexion, until the largest area is encircled. The occiput emerges and then, by extension of the head, the face and chin slip out over the perineum (Figure 15-2).

Delivery of the head should not be hurried. If progress seems too fast to adequately stretch the perineum, the mother can be coached to pant rather than push during contractions. The physician or midwife may then ask her to exert some pressure between contractions to ease the head out under better control. Forcible pressure must never be put on the head to restrain its progress. Although this maneuver is simpler than the one originally described by Ritgen (1855), it is designated the Ritgen maneuver, or the modified Ritgen maneuver (see Figure 15-28). It allows the physician or midwife to control the delivery of the head.

When the head emerges, the nose and mouth are cleared of mucus and amniotic fluid to prevent aspiration when the infant first breathes. The physician or nurse midwife feels for the cord. If it is wrapped around the neck, an attempt is made to slip it over the head. If this cannot be done, it is clamped and cut. Occasionally, when immediate delivery may be advisable, the sides of the head are held with two hands and a *gentle* downward traction is applied until the anterior shoulder appears under the pubic arch. Then, by an upward movement, the posterior shoulder is delivered (Figure 15-3). The physician or nurse midwife delivers the posterior shoulder while carefully watching the perineum and applying steady traction to the presenting part of the infant, then the rest of the body slips out.

There are differences of opinion regarding whether the cord should be cut before or after draining the residual blood contained in its vessels. The prevailing opinion is that this extra blood increases the likelihood of hyperbilirubinemia in the neonatal period (see Chapter 29). Therefore the infant is held at the level of the perineum until cord pulsation has ceased or the cord is clamped. If an infant is held too high above the perineum, blood may be drained through the cord back into the placenta, and

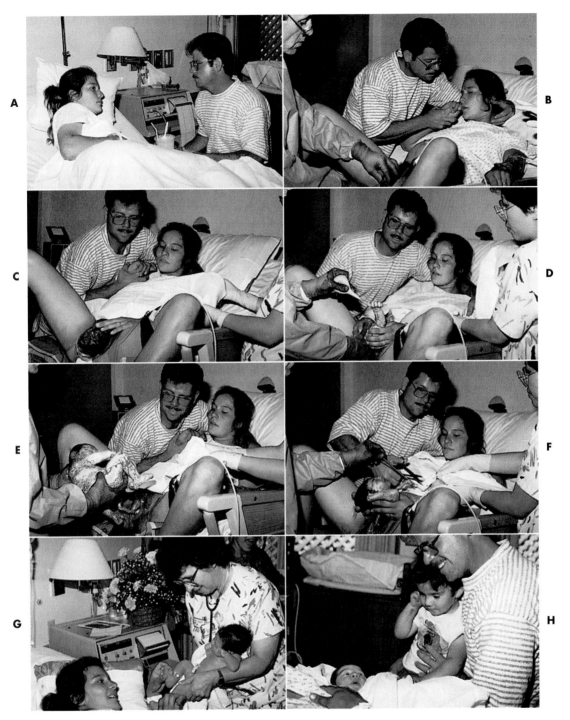

Figure 15-2 **A,** Woman chooses side-lying position between contractions; coach facilitates relaxation. Note monitor. **B,** Second stage of labor; vertex presentation. **C,** Delivery of head. **D,** Mother supports infant while physician clears nose of mucus with bulb syringe. **E,** Infant fully delivered. **F,** Nurse and physician assist as father cuts clamped cord, with infant supported on mother's abdomen. **G,** Cleansed and with identification bands in place, newborn is returned to mother. **H,** Sibling is encouraged to become acquainted with new family member. (Courtesy Marjorie Pyle, RNC, *Lifecircle.*)

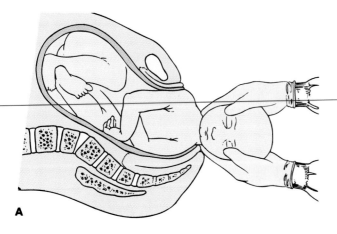

A

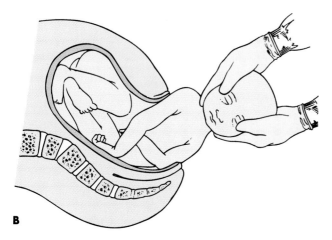

B

Figure 15-3   Delivery of the shoulders. (From Hacker N, Moore JG: *Essentials of obstetrics*, Philadelphia, 1992, WB Saunders.)

the infant may be anemic because of a low blood volume during the recovery period.

Mood

The irritability, discouragement, and agitation that mark the final hour of the first stage of labor disappear at full dilation. The woman's mood during phase one is similar to her mood during latent labor. The woman's cooperative efforts begin as she prepares for the sensations that accompany expulsion. These changes include distention of the vaginal tissue (increasing pressure on the perineum), rectal pressure, and absence of the perception of the contraction itself with the pushing effort. As the woman frequently asks about her progress, the support person can help calm her fears and build her self-confidence with positive statements (Cosner and deJong, 1993). During this phase, a nurse can make a difference in the fear-tension-pain triangle by reducing the tension throughout the woman's body, and by offering support for the father. Preparations for the birth are carried out and

will progress according to the needs of the mother. For a multipara, this phase may involve only one or two contractions, so the nurse should move quickly.

In phase two, emotional intensity parallels the transitional phase of the first stage. Encouraging the woman to sustain her immense pushing effort is very important. Although she becomes oblivious to peripheral activity, she is susceptible to confusion if conflicting directions are given or if there are several people attempting to direct her. Moreover, the unprepared woman may completely lose control, and she may utter loud screams at the peak of the contraction. She is often unable to follow directions unless given in simple commands that are repeated; otherwise she cannot process the messages being sent.

Coach/partner

The father's presence at the birth can be a profound experience for the new parents and can make them aware of parenthood as a shared effort. As the partner, the father is encouraged to remain at the woman's side, speaking directly into her ear if needed (see Figure 13-18). A partner will be of great help during these few minutes. Women can get "out of control," crying out and feeling panicked. Thus they need direct statements of encouragement, instructions on how to use the pant-blow breathing techniques, and assurances of support. If the labor partner has learned the correct pushing technique, he or she can encourage the woman's efforts. During practice and during the delivery of the infant, cue words should be used, such as *breathe—in, out; in, out; hold* (your breath); *relax* (key areas, such as jaw, mouth, and perineum); *push out* (use the abdominal muscles; push out through the vagina, while releasing air and grunting). The coach should include open-glottis pushing instructions, which allows grunting sounds with the mouth open. Remind the labor partner that open-glottis pushing is not associated with changes in maternal blood pressure, probably because of less sustained intrathoracic pressure elevations.

Labor support persons should repeat the sequence of these instructions several times for each contraction and should count slowly to help the woman sustain each push for up to 6 to 8 seconds at a time, repeating until the contraction subsides. Between contractions, the woman should be encouraged to relax and should be spoken to in soothing tones, stroked, or given a cool washcloth. The woman will appreciate anything that increases her comfort, such as wiping her face, giving her ice chips, or adjusting the birthing bed to a higher position (see Figure 15-4). During the second phase, the coach may also assist in placing a warm, wet towel over the perineum to relax the tissues, or an ice compress may be placed over the clitoris during crowning to reduce the pain.

TEST *Yourself* 15-1 _____

> a. What comfort measures would Joe use for Ann as her coach during the second stage?
> b. What are two measures the nurse as a caregiver can implement, as contrasted with two measures used by a labor support person?

Nursing approach

By recognizing the mother's progress through the phases of the second stage and changing interventions as needed, the nurse serves as a back up to the father or labor partner. Studies have shown that the nurse provides one of the most important intrapartum roles, with measurable effects on the outcomes of labor and birth (Hodnett, 1996, Stover, 1994).

Nursing care does not replace the labor support person or coach. Support from the nurse enhances the care given and is different from the support a woman receives from her partner. Nursing support supplies supervision during BDEs, encouragement to the woman while she rests between contractions, and knowledgeable directions to the partner. This nursing support helps keep the woman and her partner relaxed. It is important to control the number of people giving directions because too many voices will confuse her. Only one person should take the lead, with turns taken by another. The woman should not be left alone to push. If the second phase lasts more than an hour, the coach will be fatigued and needs comfort, too, and explanations.

Birth positions. The woman's *positioning* during birth is extremely important. One cannot push in the supine position. Squatting or holding on to a bar (if the setting includes such equipment) has been used by some women. Squatting is the usual birthing position for women in many developing countries; it opens the passage as widely as possible. Squatting in the second stage of labor enlarges

CULTURAL AWARENESS

Women who have migrated from parts of Africa north of the equator or from parts of the Arab world may have been ritually circumcised to sexually desensitize them (Lightfoot-Klein et al, 1991). This involves removal of the clitoris and/or infibulation (removal of the inner layer of labia majora), with a flap of skin pulled down over the urethra, resulting in a median scar. Health care personnel working with these women must understand the requirements for cutting the skin flap—where to incise if an episiotomy is necessary and how to resuture. Catheterization, if necessary, is difficult but possible; it is done by gently raising the flap with one finger. Lightfoot-Klein's article is mandatory reading for personnel in contact with ritually circumcised women.

pelvic dimensions, a fact supported by direct radiologic measurement of the interspinous distance (Johnson and Johnson, 1991). In Europe many births are in the side-lying position. Pushing can be done effectively in this position; the upper knee may be held by the coach. The side-lying position may slow descent but appears to relax the perineum, thereby reducing the need for an episiotomy (Gardosi et al, 1990). Other positions for second stage are illustrated in Figure 15-4.

Positioning for the third phase had routinely been in the lithotomy position, with the legs higher than the trunk and head. However, this has been researched and found to be uncomfortable and unsafe (Hodnett, 1996; Blackburn and Loper, 1992; Johnson and Johnson, 1991). When the legs are put high into the leg holders, approximately 2000 ml of blood are autotransfused into the central system, increasing cardiac workload (Odent, 1990). Since BDEs

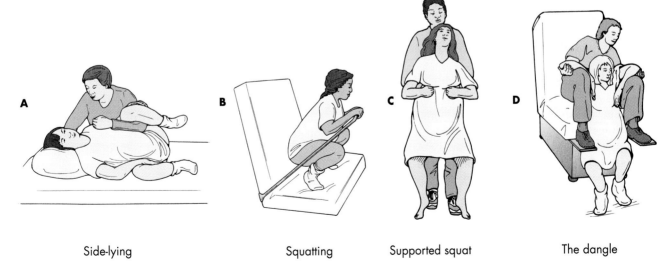

| Side-lying | Squatting | Supported squat | The dangle |

Figure 15-4   Positions for second stage of labor. (Copyright Ruth Ancheta as printed in *Birth* 22:3, 1995.)

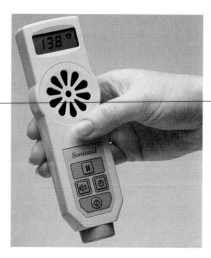

Figure 15-5   Portable doptone. (Courtesy Oxford Instruments, Oxon, England.)

also affect cardiac function, a woman with hypertension or cardiac problems will be compromised by such a position (Odent, 1990). Hodnett (1996) notes that if progress is slow, the woman should be helped into a different position, one that makes maximum use of gravity (squatting) or maximizes the width of the pelvis. A birthing bed allows a moderate semi-Fowler's position, with the knees and legs lower than the heart. With a birthing bed, it is possible to adjust the woman's legs.

Monitoring. Throughout the second stage, the low-risk fetus is monitored with observation every 15 minutes as a standard of care. The high-risk fetus must be monitored with observation made every 5 minutes. Auscultation or electronic fetal monitoring (EFM) is used and must be continued until birth (see Chapter 14). In units where the woman is moved to a delivery room, a portable Doptone may be used to obtain the fetal heart rate (FHR) (Figure 15-5). Findings must then be carefully documented, since nonreassuring FHR may occur under the stress of second-stage labor.

Summary of nursing responsibilities

1. Assess the phases of the second stage, changing comfort measures as indicated.
2. Position the woman according to her preference whenever possible, and encourage and assist her with her BDEs.
3. Support the coach and remind him or her of verbal instructions regarding when the woman is to push and when she is to rest.
4. Observe fetal responses every 15 minutes for low-risk fetuses, and notify physician or midwife of any observable signs of non-reassuring FHRs.
5. Be alert to the woman's verbal cues, vital signs, comfort level, and any early signs of impending problems that may occur suddenly. Document findings.
6. Assess contractions for frequency, intensity, duration, and resting tone. Document findings carefully.
7. Maintain a safe environment.
8. Use universal precautions against body fluids to protect self and staff.
9. Maintain hygiene, offer fluids, and encourage voiding. Catheterize if bladder is full and the mother is unable to void.
10. Prepare birth equipment.
11. Explain each step of the activities—position, monitoring, and preparations for the birth.
12. Evaluate the woman's response to interventions.
13. Assist physician or midwife during the birth.
14. Fill in all records of the birth and condition of the baby. (See Chapter 19 for immediate care of the infant after birth.)

TEST *Yourself* 15-2 _____

a. List the signs of each phase of the second stage of labor.
b. Correlate these signs with fetal station and position.

THIRD STAGE OF LABOR

The placenta, after completing its intricate life-sustaining function, separates from the wall of the uterus after it contracts. Signs of separation include the following:

- Lengthening of the cord as it protrudes out of the vaginal opening
- Change in position of uterus; rises up in a globular shape
- Gush of blood from the vagina

The placenta is expelled as the mother pushes for the last time. The physician may ask her to bear down to deliver the placenta. If she is anesthetized, mild fundal pressure may be exerted. Controlled cord traction may be used to facilitate delivery after separation has occurred. Cord traction and fundal pressure must be performed with great care to avoid inversion of the uterus and avulsion of the placenta. Inversion of the uterus (turning inside out) is one of the grave complications associated with delivery (Cunningham et al, 1993). As the placenta delivers, it presents the shiny fetal side (Schultze mechanism) or the rough maternal side (Duncan mechanism). The Schultze mechanism is more common. The only significance of this fact is that the Duncan mechanism may be associated with complications such as retained fragments of the membrane (Figure 15-6).

After the placenta is delivered, it must be inspected to be certain that no segments or membranes have been left in the uterus. Medications such as oxytocin 10-20 U in an IV solution may be routinely given intravenously after the delivery of the placenta to aid uterine contraction and

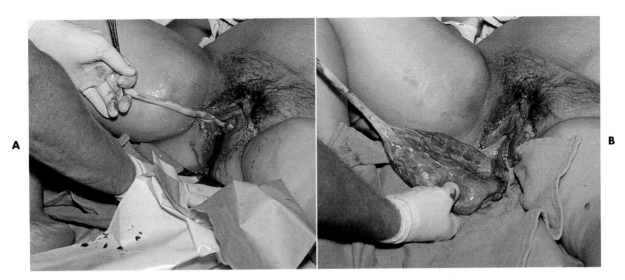

Figure 15-6   Placental delivery with slight controlled traction. **A,** The woman pushes the placenta out of the uterus into the vagina by controlled bearing down. **B,** Here, the Schultze mechanism is seen. (Courtesy Michael S Clement, MD, Mesa, Ariz.)

decrease the risk of hemorrhage. However, putting the infant to the mother's breast may provide the necessary stimulation for uterine contraction in most cases because stimulation of the nipple releases oxytocin from the posterior pituitary (see Figure 17-12).

Complications of the third stage include hemorrhage and retention of the placenta or placental fragments. Risk factors associated with these complications are listed in Box 15-2. In cases in which separation is delayed or does not occur, there may be considerable bleeding. If there is a delay in separation of the entire placenta or if the placenta is incompletely expelled, the placenta or fragments must be manually separated and removed carefully with meticulous asepsis. The woman must be anesthetized while the placenta or the fragments are removed because the procedure is very painful; a light, general, or regional anesthetic must be available. After the procedure, the cervix and vagina must be carefully inspected for lacerations so that these can be repaired to prevent further blood loss.

A placenta does not have to be removed immediately if there is no danger to the mother. In a setting where there is no anesthetic or intravenous fluids, manual removal is dangerous. The fundus should not be massaged but instead observed at intervals for the characteristic changes of separation. Up to 1 hour may elapse before the placenta is considered to be *retained*.

Mood

After the birth of the infant, the mother may be exhilarated and talkative, despite the length or intensity of the labor and delivery process. She may feel very close to the father; she may reach out physically and emotionally for her infant. Her prevailing reaction may be elation, tempered by the new responsibility of parenthood. Other

---

Box 15-2	**Risk Factors Associated with Complications of the Third Stage**

Dysfunctional uterine activity during labor (hypotonic contractions)
Extended oxytocin induction
Overdistention of the uterus
Dehydration
Exhaustion
Full bladder

---

mothers may be exhausted and not have the energy to reach out. This may be a temporary effect or may be a sign of future difficulty with attachment, especially if the parents react negatively to the sex of the infant (Figure 15-7).

If the woman is not given the opportunity to hold her infant, she may experience a sense of deprivation and loss. Most progressive hospitals make certain this opportunity is provided, even for cesarean births, to diminish her sense of loss and increase her feeling of well-being.

More women are asking to breast-feed immediately after delivery. The infant's sucking reflex is very strong at this point, although the infant may just lick the nipple. Breast-feeding creates a strong maternal bond with the infant, and helps the new mother feel a sense of accomplishment and connectedness with the infant (Figure 15-8).

Summary of nursing responsibilities

1. Assign an Apgar score at 1 and 5 minutes. Adjustment of the infant and immediate adaptation are discussed in Chapters 18 and 19.

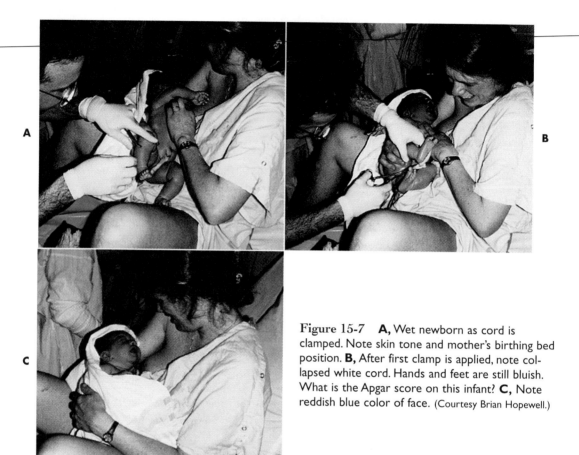

Figure 15-7　**A,** Wet newborn as cord is clamped. Note skin tone and mother's birthing bed position. **B,** After first clamp is applied, note collapsed white cord. Hands and feet are still bluish. What is the Apgar score on this infant? **C,** Note reddish blue color of face. (Courtesy Brian Hopewell.)

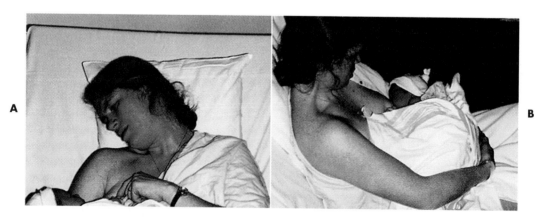

Figure 15-8　**A,** First breast-feeding. Note "en face" position. **B,** Note head covering and extra blankets to keep the infant warm. (Courtesy Brian Hopewell.)

2. With the infant under a warmer or on the mother's abdomen, clear nasal and oral passages with small suction bulb (for alternate suctioning, see Chapter 19).

3. Dry the infant and wrap in a warmed blanket.

4. Assess the mother's immediate condition. If she is stable, spend the first few minutes preparing the infant for an extended visit with his or her parents.

5. Apply a plastic clamp to the cord and cut off the excess using the sterile aseptic technique.

6. Identify the infant with the mother according to protocol.

7. Encourage both parents to hold and become acquainted with the infant.

8. Wait for placental separation. Administer ordered medication.

9. Check maternal vital signs, fundus, and amount of vaginal bleeding.

10. Document events while physician or midwife is completing sutures of episiotomy, if performed.

11. After all procedures are completed, make the woman comfortable with dry clothing, perineal pad, and linens. Adjust body or bed position. Provide nourishment. Some units monitor recovery for an hour before offering fluids.

12. If the infant's condition is stable, encourage family interaction and acquaintance by providing privacy. The mother may place the infant on her breast soon after birth to start breast-feeding techniques (see Figure 15-8).

FOURTH STAGE OF LABOR

The first hour after delivery is a critical period for the mother. The blood vessels and myometrium are intertwined in such a way that natural ligatures are created when the uterus contracts. Assessments every 15 minutes must be made—assess lochia, visually observe the perineum, check blood pressure, and see that firm contraction of the fundus is maintained to prevent hemorrhage. The uterus is palpated to assess the degree of contraction. The fundus should be firm, at the level of the umbilicus or below and in the midline. The perineal pad and bed pads are observed for lochia, color, clots, and amount. Normally the lochia is bright red and may contain small clots. The amount of lochia should not saturate more than one pad per hour. The perineum and, if present, the **episiotomy** (enlargement of the vaginal opening), should be inspected for hematomas and swelling. An ice pack should be routinely applied to the perineum to decrease swelling, alleviate discomfort, and promote healing. Ice may be placed in a glove that is banded and wrapped in a paper or cloth covering. Many units use a prepared chemically-activated cold pack.

Potential for Hemorrhage

The major complication of the fourth stage is hemorrhage. Hemorrhage from the placental site is controlled by contraction of the uterus. Anything interfering with the normal contraction of the uterus, including a full bladder, may result in hemorrhage (see Chapter 21 and Figure 17-4).

Displacement of the uterus upward or laterally indicates a full bladder. The woman should be encouraged to void, and if unable to do so, she may require catheterization. If the fundus is not firmly contracted (boggy), it should be gently massaged until it becomes firm. Despite the presence of a well-contracted uterus, if there are large clots or excessive bleeding, there may be soft-tissue lacerations caused by the trauma of delivery or retained placental fragments. In either case, the woman may need to be reexamined by the physician for detection and repair of lacerations. If retained placental fragments or membranes are suspected, these must be manually removed by the physician.

Box 15-1

CLINICAL DECISION

Examine this picture. Which nursing interventions could improve the parent-infant acquaintance just after birth?

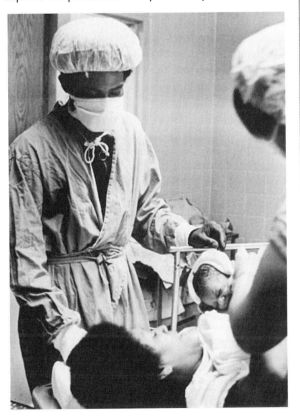

ASSISTANCE WITH LABOR

Although the majority of women in the United States experience normal labor, 60% to 75% receive some type of medical or surgical intervention to assist labor and birth. These rates have been identified in studies related to the duration of the second stage of labor and to routine episiotomies, respectively (Menticoglou, 1995; Thorp and Bowes, 1989). Women must be aware of the possibility that an episiotomy may be needed, but efforts must be made to decrease the number of these operative interventions in the second stage of labor. Studies have shown that operative interventions are not always warranted merely because some particular number of hours has elapsed (Menticoglou, 1995).

To gain cooperation from the woman in labor, full explanations related to specific procedures should be part of the informed consent. Too often, problems and treatments are simply announced or performed without helping the woman take in the information and ask questions. The woman's natural alarm is engendered but then quickly silenced by guilt-producing statements such as, "Don't you want to help your baby?" or "If we don't do this, you and your baby will be in trouble." Labor nurses must protect the parents against such insensitive and negative statements. There is no single technique that helps all women or even the same woman throughout the entire labor process. Assistance during labor will produce positive results if the nurse support person seeks feedback from the woman in labor about what she is experiencing, provides positive encouragement, and makes a real effort to individualize her care. This type of nursing support will improve labor and birth outcomes, reduce risks, and help the woman in labor during one of life's most challenging and memorable experiences (Hodnett, 1996).

Stimulation of Contractions

Stimulation of uterine contractions requires careful control and monitoring. Under ordinary circumstances, the blocks to uterine contractility in pregnancy are very effective. Progesterone blocks the effect of oxytocin; therefore it may be difficult to start labor "from scratch." Nonpharmacologic methods, including exercise, enemas, and castor oil, have always been tried. Walking stimulates labor after it has begun; an enema in early labor clears the lower intestinal tract and may occasionally stimulate contractions. More recently, amniotomy or artificial rupture of the membranes (AROM) was tried, but rupturing the membranes early placed the mother at risk for ascending infection.

Induction is the initiation of labor by artificial means (see Chapter 16 for full discussion).

The processes of prelabor—movement of the head into the pelvic inlet to engagement, stretching of the lower uterine segment and upper vaginal wall, and softening (ripening) of the cervix—are effectively accomplished in a few hours with induction. The woman goes through the same work of labor, often over a shorter period of time.

Labor may need to be *stimulated* when there is ineffective progress through the phases of labor. The method for stimulation uses oxytocin in a method similar to that used for induction.

Importance of monitoring

Whenever oxytocic stimulation or induction of labor is used, there is increased need for careful monitoring of labor. Oxytocin sensitivity varies from person to person, and the dose must be titrated with the woman's individual response. The chief negative response is **hypertonic contractions**, too long and too intense for the phase of labor. The result is extra discomfort for the woman and reduced placental blood flow and thus poor oxygenation for the fetus. FHR monitoring is mandatory, therefore, throughout the period that oxytocin is used. See Chapter 16 for procedure and protocols.

Dysfunctional Labor

Several factors may contribute to dysfunctional labor. The quality of contractions and the fetal position and size in relation to the pelvic canal may be the major causes of difficulty in the birth process.

Uterine dystocia occurs when labor contractions are ineffectual, erratic, or unable to dilate the cervix or cause fetal descent. Dysfunctional labor patterns are described as follows:

1. A *prolonged latent phase* lasts for more than 20 hours in a nullipara or more than 14 hours in a multipara. If the latent phase is truly prolonged (the mother was not admitted during the prodromal phase), reasons underlying the delay may be an unready cervix or ineffective power in the hypotonic contractions.

2. *Prolonged active labor*, slower rates of cervical dilation, or fetal descent may result from malpositions, ineffectual contractions, or cephalopelvic disproportion (CPD). If second-stage descent problems are present, position changes may improve progress. For instance, the supine position forces the fetal head to move against gravity, up and over the pelvic outlet. Consequently, birthing chairs and beds and a high-Fowler's position or semisitting position may facilitate descent.

3. *Hypertonic contractions* may occur in labor. If hypertonic contractions occur (contractions stronger and longer than expected for the phase of labor), labor may progress rapidly to a precipitate birth or labor may be prolonged. In either case, the uterine muscle will be exhausted, and postbirth bleeding is possible. The oxygen supply to the infant may be diminished during labor, causing potential fetal perfusion problems (hypoxia).

4. *Arrest of the head* may occur during late active transition just as the deceleration phase (second stage) should begin. In this case the head is too large to rotate through the ischial spines and appears to be "stuck on the spines" in the occiput transverse (OT) position. The cervix may be fully dilated, but the station remains at −1, 0, or +1.

5. *Arrest of the shoulders* may occur with a large baby during the second stage. As dilation is completed, the fetal head rotates and enters the vagina. The mother may push effectively, but the head does not move farther down the canal. A prolonged second stage (protracted descent) lasts more than 3 hours for a nullipara and more than 1 hour for a multipara. It is extremely important to ascertain whether fetopelvic disproportion is the problem. The head has descended, but the shoulders are unable to follow. Sometimes the mother becomes exhausted from pushing and simply cannot push a large infant the last few inches. Then even forceps or operative delivery is difficult.

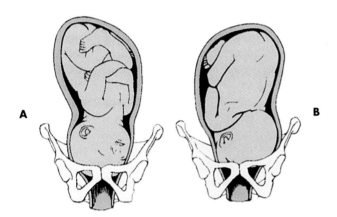

Figure 15-9   A, Brow presentation. **B,** Face presentation. (Courtesy Ross Laboratories, Columbus, Ohio.)

For operative delivery to occur when the head is firmly lodged, the head must be pushed back up the birth canal to be extracted from the lower uterine incision. To do this, one physician inserts a sterile gloved hand into the vagina and firmly pushes while another physician pulls the infant's shoulders and body from the uterus via a cesarean incision, a potentially stressful delivery for both mother and infant.

6. *Dystocia* may occur with malposition of the head. When flexion has not occurred as expected, a persistent *brow or face presentation* may result (Figure 15-9, *A*). The infant cannot be delivered with a brow presentation because the largest diameter of the head will be coming through the birth canal. When hyperextension rather than flexion has occurred at engagement, the face is the presenting part (Figure 15-9, *B*). Because the face presents a smaller diameter than the brow, the infant could be delivered, but trauma to facial tissues and the extreme backward molding of the occiput are potentially injurious to the infant. Face presentation is initially difficult to diagnose because the face becomes edematous and may be confused with the buttocks of a breech presentation. These infants are almost always delivered by cesarean birth (Figure 15-10).

Occiput posterior position

When the vertex presentation changes to a posterior position during internal rotation, second stage may be prolonged (see Figure 13-7). A larger arc of 180 degrees must be crossed over the sacral curve, rather than simpler extension under the symphysis. The woman experiences considerable back pain and may feel that her coccyx is being "sprained." Some women will experience difficulty coping with this fetal position without analgesia or transcutaneous electrical nerve stimulation (TENS) and a great deal of emotional support (see Chapter 16).

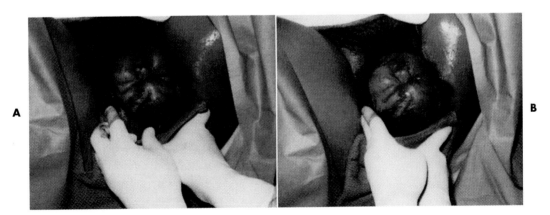

Figure 15-10   A and **B,** Unusual vaginal birth of a face presentation. Note how edematous the face is. Several days will elapse before edema and bruising will resolve. (Courtesy Marjorie Pyle, RNC, *Lifecircle*.)

TEST *Yourself* 15-3 _____

> a. A multipara in the second stage has been pushing for 1 hour. The infant is in occiput posterior position and is still at +1 station. What do the findings indicate?
> b. Which maternal position changes might facilitate this birth?

Breech presentation

When engagement of the buttocks takes place, it may occur in one of three ways (Figure 15-11):

1. Frank breech, in which the thighs are flexed and knees are extended so the feet are beside the head (Figure 15-11, *A*)
2. Complete breech, in which the infant appears to be sitting cross-legged (Figure 15-11, *B*)
3. Incomplete or footling breech, in which one leg is extended so the foot is the leading part. (Figure 15-11, *C*)

Breech presentations can be delivered vaginally, but these carry a higher risk. A preterm infant or the second or third infant of a multiple pregnancy will often present in this way. Small infants are not as difficult to deliver as larger infants (greater than 8 lb). The larger infant may have shoulder or head dystocia, and the body may protrude before full dilation of the cervix. The head then becomes trapped by the tight cervical rim. In addition, there is a higher rate of cord prolapse, premature rupture of membranes (PROM), trauma to the infant, and fetal distress.

Risk. Before cesarean sections were performed as frequently for breech deliveries, an infant mortality rate of 10% to 20% was related to breech presentation. Now the mortality rate is much lower. The overall incidence of breech presentation is about 3% to 4%. Because breech presentation is more common in a premature birth and can be associated with congenital anomalies, risks are multiple in these cases.

Clinical management. More than 75% of breech presentations are delivered by cesarean methods. Presentation is usually settled in the last few weeks before birth. A number of birthing centers are reporting success with maternal positions that facilitate fetal turning. The knee-chest position or having the woman on her hands and knees with her abdomen hanging loosely has been shown to reduce pressure on the fetus and allow turning, even when amniotic fluid is somewhat diminished (Dierker, 1994).

External cephalic version. External cephalic version (ECV) may be attempted at 37 to 38 weeks in the fetal evaluation unit. A *nonstress test (NST)* is first performed to determine the fetus' ability to withstand the procedure. The woman may receive a tocolytic (*terbutaline hydrochloride*), to relax the uterine muscle. She is placed in Trendelenburg position, and by gentle pressure, the vertex (head) is pushed toward the pelvis while the breech (buttocks) is pushed toward the fundus. Powder is used on the woman's skin to smooth the movement of the examiner's hands. After the procedure, an NST is performed and the fetus is observed for responses. In approximately half of such cases, the fetus will remain in the vertex position, whereas the others move back to a breech position or lodge in a transverse presentation, requiring a cesarean delivery (Beischer and MacKay, 1993).

Vaginal birth. When vaginal delivery is chosen for a breech, the procedure follows a careful pattern (see Figure 15-11). Since the body is smaller in diameter than the head, it may be easily born. However, the head must come down through the cervix and vaginal canal with chin flexed on the chest. To facilitate these move-

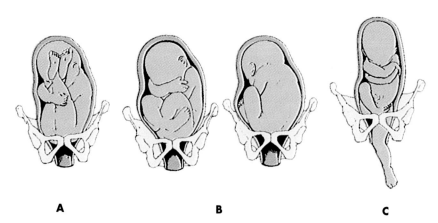

A   **B**   **C**

Figure 15-11   Breech presentation. **A,** Frank breech. **B,** Complete breech. **C,** Incomplete breech or footling. (Courtesy Ross Laboratories, Columbus, Ohio.)

ments, piper forceps may be applied for the "after coming head". An assistant supports the body during this maneuver, taking care not to unduly flex the spine. Meconium passage is normal with the breech birth because of pressure on the abdomen. (Figures 15-12 and 15-13.)

ASSISTANCE WITH BIRTH

Episiotomy

An episiotomy is a surgical incision made into the perineal area to enlarge the introitus for the birth of the infant. This incision, which is made between the vagina and rectum to

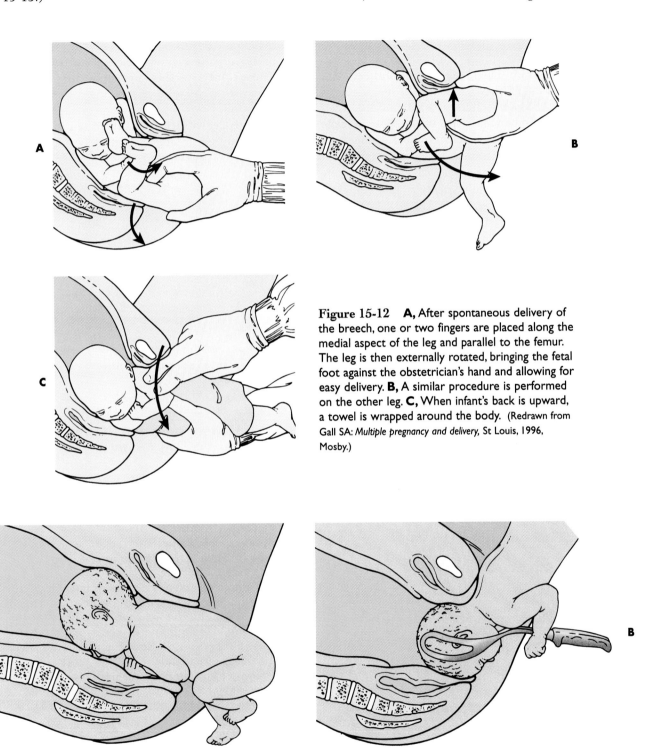

Figure 15-12   **A,** After spontaneous delivery of the breech, one or two fingers are placed along the medial aspect of the leg and parallel to the femur. The leg is then externally rotated, bringing the fetal foot against the obstetrician's hand and allowing for easy delivery. **B,** A similar procedure is performed on the other leg. **C,** When infant's back is upward, a towel is wrapped around the body. (Redrawn from Gall SA: *Multiple pregnancy and delivery,* St Louis, 1996, Mosby.)

Figure 15-13   **A,** The infant's back must be upward all the time. **B,** Piper's forceps may be applied to the after-coming head and used to initially pull downward, then slowly and gently upward until the head is born.

widen the birth area, has been performed in the United States on 90% of first time mothers and 62% of all vaginal deliveries (Thorpe, 1995). This practice is now the focus of debate because these incisions have been associated with tears (**lacerations**) to or through the rectum and with urinary and fecal incontinence (Klein-Kaye, 1994). The most frequently used incision is made midline between the vaginal introitus and anus (Figure 15-14, *B*). The rationale for a midline episiotomy is that because less tissue is incised, there should subsequently be less discomfort, and recovery is more rapid. A mediolateral incision (Figure 15-14, *A*) may be indicated when a forceps delivery is required or when there is a posterior fetal position, a breech birth, or a very large infant. More tissue is cut, but potential extension into the anal sphincter is

avoided. A new modification has been suggested to avoid the anal area (Figure 15-15, *C*).

Only since the 1920s has routine use of an episiotomy been practiced. Today, such routines must be questioned because many studies have shown that supposed benefits are cancelled by adverse effects on the woman's future perineal integrity (Box 15-3). It has been suggested that overstretching of perineal muscles could later lead to pelvic relaxation and the development of a prolapse of the bladder or rectum (cystocele or rectocele) (Menticoglou, 1995).

There is little evidence to support the routine use of episiotomy to prevent this perineal trauma; in fact, recent studies demonstrate that the incidence of third- and fourth-degree lacerations increased in women who had midline episiotomies (Klein-Kaye, 1994; Thorpe,

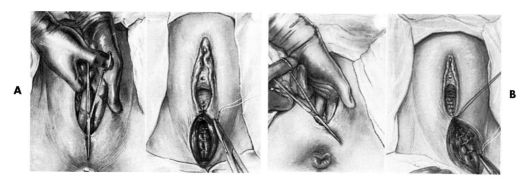

Figure 15-14 **A,** Anatomic location of midline episiotomy. **B,** Anatomic location of mediolateral episiotomy. (From Willson JR et al, eds: *Obstetrics and gynecology*, ed 8, St Louis, 1987, Mosby.)

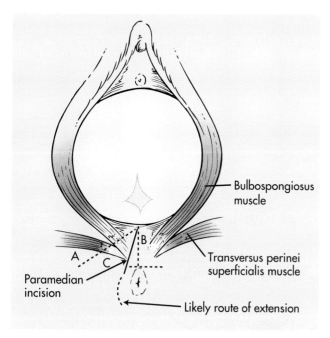

Figure 15-15 Shown are **(A)** mediolateral, **(B)** median, and **(C)** modified median episiotomies. (From Delfs ER, *Contemporary OB Gyn* 40:11, Nov 1995.)

| Box 15-3 | **Risks and Benefits of Episiotomy** |

RISKS

Blood loss up to 300 ml
Potential for hematoma
Infection
Potential for poor repair
Sexual dyspareunia (60%) lasting up to 6 months
Temporary loss of libido
Healing accompanied by moderate to severe pain
Higher risk of third- or fourth-degree laceration if midline

BENEFITS

If done before tissue overstretched, possible benefit of expediting second stage
Reduces pressure on fetal head in last phase
Useful with forceps or malpositions of fetus
Easier to repair; more regular scar than a jagged laceration of same degree

1995). Without an episiotomy, these lacerations may be first- and second-degree lacerations. However, with better birth positions, more women will be able to deliver over an intact perineum.

Delivery position influences whether an episiotomy is performed; the incidence of episiotomy is higher in the lithotomy position and lower in Sims' position. Episiotomies have been routinely performed more often by physicians than midwives. The use of anesthesia, either epidural or pudendal, also raises the incidence of episiotomy, perhaps reflecting the difficulty of delivery. Thorpe (1995) suggests that informed consent be obtained specifically for this surgical procedure because the result of poorly performed or poorly timed episiotomies can be lifelong perineal dysfunction. The woman's autonomy is protected if she understands the risks and benefits of episiotomy and signs an informed consent to indicate her willingness to have the procedure performed. Protocols routinely practiced, such as episiotomies, that are risky and often unsatisfactory must be questioned and require a rapid shift to more physiologic practices (Evans, 1995; Sheil, 1995).

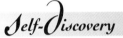

Self-Discovery

What are some of the changes you foresee in delivery of labor care during the next 10 years? Review some recent articles that challenge obstetric routines. ∼

Lacerations

Lacerations of the perineum and vagina may occur with or without an episiotomy. These lacerations are classified as first, second, third, and fourth degree. Box 15-4 describes the types and locations of lacerations that may occur. Lacerations may result in excessive bleeding and the development of a hematoma (see Chapter 21). Episiotomies and lacerations are repaired with chromic sutures, which dissolve several weeks after delivery.

Avoiding lacerations

An episiotomy may be thought of as a second-degree laceration. Even a carefully conducted, slow birth with full maternal cooperation may result in first- or second-degree lacerations around the vaginal opening or near the urethra (periurethral) or in the upper vagina (sulcus tear). Position has been found to be important; those positions with relaxed perineum have the lowest incidence of lacerations. In addition, women who had practiced Kegel exercises and perineal massage in preparation for birth were able to better relax the perineal muscle group and had more positive outcomes (Dougherty, 1989). During the last phases of the second stage, the physician or nurse midwife can gently massage the lower perineal tissue to stretch the opening. Finally, a slow, controlled exit of the fetus allows for a delivery that maintains an intact perineum in many cases. A woman without an episiotomy is capable of getting up and walking to the bathroom or chair without pain or discomfort. This type of recovery may be contrasted with one that involves extensive suturing, swelling, and pain in the perineal area. In the latter, a woman may not be comfortable for several days and may have dysuria and painful bowel movements.

Nursing responsibilities

1. During labor, reinforce how the woman may cooperate with the process of labor and how to use BDEs (Evans, 1995).

▌ *Box* 15-4   **Types of Lacerations**

PERINEAL LACERATIONS	SULCUS TEAR
First-Degree Skin, mucous membrane of posterior fourchette, and proximal vagina	Folds of the vagina torn, often over the ischial spines **PERIURETHRAL TEAR** Tissues around the urethra torn, sometimes the urethra itself
Second-Degree Same as first-degree laceration plus muscles and fascia up to anal sphincter	**CERVICAL TEAR** Any degree, from small, shallow tears to deep lacerations through entire cervix into the lower uterine segment
Third-Degree Same as second-degree laceration, continuing through anal sphincter	**UTERINE TEAR** Usually in lower uterine segment, which is thinner during later pregnancy; especially possible if multifetal gestation, site of placenta previa, or precipitate labor
Fourth-Degree Same as third-degree laceration plus torn anterior rectal wall	

2. Position the woman for best perineal outcome and monitor BDEs to coordinate with her own involuntary urge to push (Roberts and Wooley, 1996.)
3. Offer warm compresses to the perineum during BDEs and an ice pack to clitoris during crowning.
4. Encourage side-lying position or semi-Fowler's position with legs positioned so tension on the perineum is avoided. Change positions as the woman desires.
5. For actual birth, legs should be lower than the heart. (For care after birth, see Chapter 17.)

Forceps Delivery

Forceps may be used to shorten the second stage of labor. If there are complications such as ineffective BDEs caused by the anesthetic or fatigue, if there are malpositions, or if the infant is large, forceps can be an effective way to assist the birth. If there is fetal distress, the last phases of labor may be shortened by the use of forceps.

Forceps are curved metal blades shaped to grasp the head of an infant in a way that allows the physician to apply controlled traction (Figure 15-16). Forceps deliveries are classified as low forceps or midforceps. A *low forceps* delivery is performed when the head is on the perineum. A *midforceps* delivery is done to rotate the head from a left occiput anterior (LOA) or right occiput anterior (ROA) to an occiput anterior (OA) position. The head is at the level of the ischial spines and may have an arrest of internal rotation. This delivery is difficult and can be traumatic to the mother and infant. The mother *must be anesthetized* to tolerate a midforceps delivery because the pressure created is intense. If the head is unengaged, a high forceps delivery is no longer performed; a cesarean birth is the method of choice. Box 15-5 lists indications for the use of forceps.

Before forceps can be applied, several requirements must be met. The cervix must be fully dilated, the head must be engaged, the position of the head must be known, the pelvis must be adequate to allow passage of the infant, and the membranes must be ruptured. After the forceps are applied to the head, pressure is applied in a downward direction to bring the head under the symphysis pubis. As the head rotates around the pubic bone and then crowns, the forceps are gently removed and the rest of the birth is accomplished (Figures 15-17 and 15-18).

Risk

Complications of forceps deliveries may include injury to the cervix, vagina, rectum, and bladder. There may be additional severe pain for the woman if anesthesia is partial. Soft-tissue injury for the fetus is not uncommon. Forceps marks may leave bruised areas over cheekbones that heal quickly. More serious damage to the facial nerve, with resulting facial palsy, may occur from pressure on the facial nerve. The skull may sustain a fracture in very rare cases of midforceps trauma.

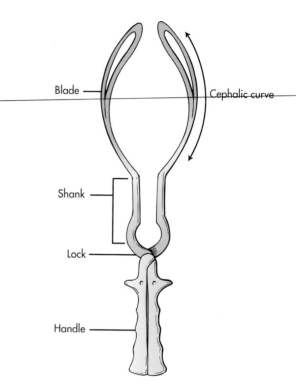

Figure 15-16   Parts of the obstetric forceps (Neville-Barnes).

| Box 15-5 | **Indications for Use of Forceps** |

FETAL PROBLEMS
- Arrested descent
- Arrested rotation
- Abnormal presentation
- Face or brow
- Breech (forceps for head)
- Fetal distress in late second stage
- Preterm infant (to protect fragile head)

MATERNAL PROBLEMS
- Uterine inertia in late second stage
- Inability to push effectively resulting from exhaustion, regional or general anesthesia, mild cephalopelvic disproportion, or poor position for pushing
- Chronic disease requiring the least possible stress during delivery (e.g., cardiac or chest disease, hypertension)

Vacuum Extraction/Ventouse

A safer alternative to forceps birth is delivery with a soft cup made of pliable plastic (Silastic, Mityvac), a procedure referred to in the United States as a **vacuum extraction** (VE). In Europe it is referred to as a **ventouse** (from

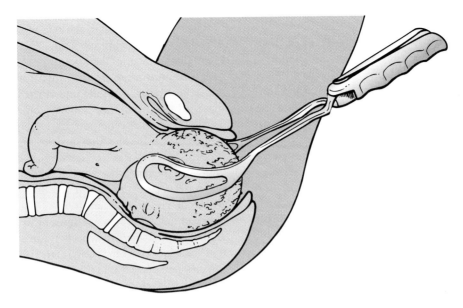

Figure 15-17   Forceps-assisted extraction of the head. Note relation of curve of pelvis to curve of forceps.

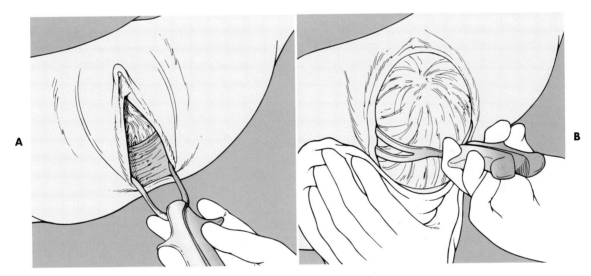

Figure 15-18   A, The mother is encouraged to bear down with the onset of the next uterine contraction, and simultaneous traction is applied on the fetal head. **B,** During delivery of the head, the perineum is supported with a gauze pad, holding the perineum back and preventing further distention; at the same time, traction is directed upward away from the perineum.

French, literally meaning "soft cup") (Cunningham et al, 1993). The vacuum from a suction pump is used after the cup has been placed on the presenting part (vertex). Usually the infant is delivered with three to four pulls. Sometimes during pulling, the cup detaches and must be reapplied again. If undue suction is used, the cup falls off the fetal scalp (Figure 15-19). The procedure is indicated in failure of the fetus to rotate, arrest or delay in the second stage, fetal distress, borderline CPD, and maternal indications for a shortened second stage (cardiac disease, respiratory disease, and severe hypertension). The prerequisites for its use are a vertex presentation, ruptured membranes, no presence of CPD, and completely dilated cervix. The national rate in 1994 for VE use was 5.7% of vaginal births (MMWR, 1996) and is now used more often than forceps (3.8%).

Risk

Vacuum extraction allows for safe rotation of the fetal head. Less force is applied to the head because traction is applied only with the contraction (Williams, 1995). Neonatal findings with VE show **caput succedaneum,** scalp edema and bruising in a circular area (called the chignon) under the cup. This raised edematous area usually resolves within 24 to 48 hours, but bluish or reddened areas may darken and take several days to resolve (Figure 15-19, *B*). **Cephalhematomas,** bleeding between periosteum and bone that does not spread across the bony plate, may develop in the first few hours after birth and are more common with a VE than with a forceps birth (see Chapter 18).

Cesarean Birth

In 1994, nearly one quarter of all births in the United States were by the **cesarean birth** route, a major surgery that requires a longer hospital stay and longer healing time than a vaginal birth. Studies show the incidence of cesarean dilivery is stabilizing in recent years, the result of increased effects by health providers and physicians to lower this rate (Chez, 1995).

Although cesarean birth accounts for approximately one fourth of births in the United States today, one third of these births are by women who have had a prior cesarean delivery. In some high-risk tertiary centers, the rate is even higher because of more complicated pregnancies and labor outcomes.

The overall increase in the rate of cesarean birth, from 4.5% in 1965 to approximately 21.2% in 1994, is the result of a number of factors (MMWR, 1996). First, pregnancy problems can be identified earlier by ultrasound and fetal testing. Second, rates increase with advancing maternal age, and more older women are being seen. Third, Friedman's computerized labor pattern has led physicians to declare that a delay in labor ("failure to progress") can be a reason for surgical birth. The care with which the average labor pattern is followed affects the rate of cesarean births in a particular delivery suite. However, the labor grid is only an *average,* not a rigid pattern. A cesarean delivery can sometimes be avoided by providing a labor support person who is trained to provide consistent bedside coaching (Hodnett, 1996; Stover, 1994). Practitioners have found that not using a predictive curve, coupled with close observation of the FHR to make certain it remains in a good range, can result in a normal vaginal birth (Cosner and deJong, 1993). Continuous electronic monitoring, although not risky in itself, is estimated to double the chances of a woman having a cesarean delivery, with no improvement in the birth outcome (see Chapter 14).

A concern about malpractice suits has led obstetricians and gynecologists to be more cautious about refraining from operative intervention. Herbst (1989) states that 70% of obstetricians and gynecologists have had at least one malpractice suit, often with no fault in their performance. This experience is a painful one for the physician and fosters cautious responses. (Issues related to litigation

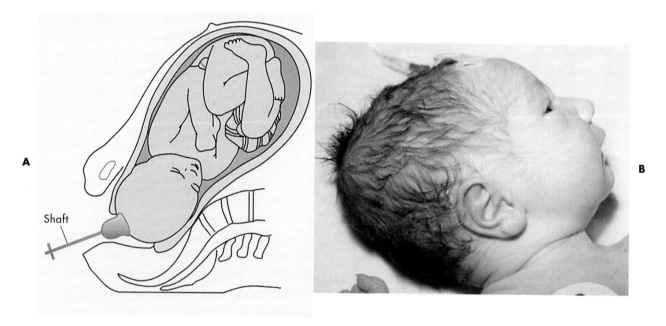

A Shaft **B**

Figure 15-19 Vacuum extraction. **A,** Position. **B,** The chignon is seen in profile; it usually disappears within 24 to 48 hours. (**B,** From Zitelli BJ, Davis HW: *Atlas of pediatric physical diagnosis,* ed 3, 1997, Mosby-Wolfe.)

are discussed further in Chapter 30.) Herbst states that major factors in litigation include a breakdown in communication and respect between the patient and the physician (angry people sue) and a client's unreasonable expectations for a healthy infant even when she has been told the truth about the infant's condition. For these and other reasons, the client must be fully informed about the benefits and risks of an operative delivery and must sign the consent only after indicating an understanding of the reasons for the surgery (Lescale et al, 1996).

Risk

The goal for operative birth is the same as that for vaginal birth—the safe delivery of a healthy infant. However, surgical procedures and anesthesia always entail risk; a large survey concluded the risk was four times that of a vaginal birth (Chez, 1995, Dierker, 1994). Both casarean and vaginal births have very low mortality rates, but the morbidity rate of 5% to 10% in operative delivery is higher than it should be. Wounds and urinary and uterine infections continue to be problematic. Hemorrhage is at a higher rate than with vaginal birth (see Chapter 21), and trauma to bladder and bowel with some later-developing adhesions must be avoided by good surgical technique. Finally, pulmonary emboli and vascular emboli and clotting defects such as disseminated intravascular coagulation (though rare) can occur (see Chapter 22).

Neonatal outcomes with elective (scheduled) surgery depend on two circumstances: preterm birth, if estimate of gestational age was inaccurate and the infant is delivered too early and problems sustained by a term infant delivered without labor. Normal labor supplies the necessary forces the infant needs for an adequate initial respiratory effort. The forces of labor and birth actually compress the chest, a factor not present during a cesarean birth. Thus more infants have respiratory difficulty after a cesarean delivery than after a vaginal delivery. In emergency situations, there are also maternal and fetal stressors present that result in conditions that may cause the infant to be compromised.

Clinical management

The surgery may be planned as an elective procedure or done as an emergency just before or during labor when it is evident that the infant will not tolerate vaginal birth. The abdominal route is chosen when additional hypoxic stress must be prevented, when pelvic dimensions are inadequate, or when some pathologic condition is causing excessive maternal or fetal distress. Box 15-6 lists indications for cesarean birth. Emergency cesarean sections are performed for complications such as placenta previa, premature separation of the placenta, severe infection of the uterus or pelvis, inadequate labor, and fetal distress that occurs during labor. Surgery is *planned* when the following occur:

- Prenatal testing indicates there is disproportion between the fetal size and the pelvic canal
- Prenatal testing reveals a preexisting sexually transmitted disease in the woman, such as herpes simplex, that may be transmitted to the infant during passage through the vagina.
- There are malpresentations such as a breech or transverse lie.
- Multiple fetuses are in poor position.
- Ultrasound reveals that the placenta is located in a low lying position (placenta previa).
- Severe hypertension or diabetes exists.
- Fetal jeopardy is shown by prenatal assessment.
- A preterm infant is very early, requiring rapid birth.

Finally, in about one third of cases, women who have had previous cesarean deliveries are likely to have a repeat procedure. However, when the pelvic measurements are adequate, vaginal delivery may prove successful, and the rate of **vaginal births after cesarean**

Box 15-6   Indications for Cesarean Birth

DELAY IN LABOR
In preparatory period: no response to oxytocin, postmaturity
In active phase: arrest of dilation, prolonged active phase, uterine inertia
In descent phase: cephalopelvic disproportion (CPD), cervical dystocia, uterine inertia

ABNORMAL PRESENTATIONS
Brow, mentum, poor flexion of head, occiput posterior position in a primipara
Transverse position
Breech position, especially in primigravida

FETAL DISTRESS
Chronic: poor environment demonstrated by at-risk pregnancy
Acute: during labor, severe changes of uteroplacental insufficiency (UPI), cord compression (CC), loss of fetal heart tone or falling pH level

MATERNAL ILLNESS
Placental dysfunction, placenta previa, abruptio placentae, herpes progenitalis (active)
Diabetes, if uncontrolled
Chronic hypertension, severe preeclampsia
Cancer of cervix or uterine fibroids

OTHER
Repeated stillbirths with no known cause
Elderly primigravida with other problems
Previous cesarean delivery unless VBAC is possible

SKIN INCISION   UTERINE INCISION

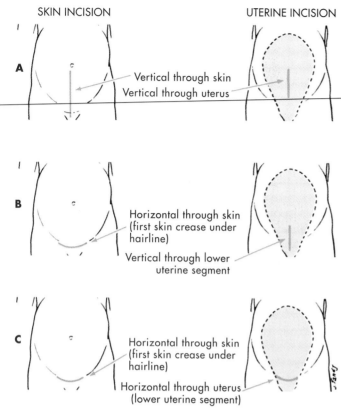

A, Vertical through skin
Vertical through uterus

B, Horizontal through skin
(first skin crease under hairline)
Vertical through lower uterine segment

C, Horizontal through skin
(first skin crease under hairline)
Horizontal through uterus
(lower uterine segment)

Figure 15-20   Cesarean delivery: skin and uterine incisions. **A,** Classic vertical incisions. **B,** Low cervical incision. **C,** Low cervical incision of skin and uterus. (From Lowdermilk DL, Perry SE, Bobak IM: *Maternity and women's health care,* ed 6, St Louis, 1997, Mosby.)

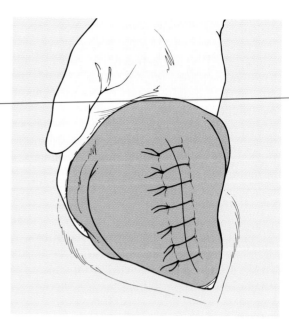

Figure 15-21   Suture on vertical uterine incision.

(VBAC) has increased in the United States. (See section on VBAC found later in this chapter.)

Types of incisions. The type of uterine incision is determined by the fetal presentation or fetal distress and by the condition of the woman before surgery. It is important to realize that the type of abdominal incision *does not indicate* the type of uterine incision. The woman should be informed about her incisions and possible outcomes. One of the first questions asked by the woman having to undergo an unexpected cesarean is, "Do I always have to have surgery for other children?" Only by checking various factors, one of which is the type of uterine incision that has been made, can a correct response be offered.

An abdominal approach to the uterus may be a *vertical* one with a subumbilical or midline incision, or a *transverse* incision made through skin, muscle, and fascia, usually at the crease just above the mons pubis (Figure 15-20). A uterine incision can be *classic,* in which the upper segment is incised, a common approach in an emergency. The incision can be a *lower*

uterine incision through the less muscular, more inactive portion of the uterus. This lower uterine incision may be transverse or vertical and has the advantages of resulting in less bleeding and less tissue repair. However, to reach the lower uterine segment, the bladder must be dissected away because it is attached by fascia to the site. Later it must be resutured. (This illustrates why a Foley catheter is used to deflate the bladder and how it is possible to nick the bladder during surgery.) Figure 15-21 shows sutures on a vertical incision of the uterus.

Initially, an incision is made on the outer skin. Once the skin is incised, the first blade is discarded and a second sterile scalpel is used to proceed through the next layers. Once the incision is made through the uterus, the physician then inserts a hand to grasp the presenting part (Figure 15-22) and pulls the infant only partially up and out of the uterine opening. Suction must be available to clear the infant's oropharyngeal airway. (Figure 15-23 shows the prepared setup for cesarean delivery.) The infant is then carefully and gently lifted out of the uterus. With sterile Kelly clamps, the cord is clamped in two places and then cut using sterile scissors, and the infant is immediately placed in the waiting hands of the pediatrician or the circulating nurse (Figure 15-24 and Chapter 19).

The placenta is then extracted manually and checked to ensure that all pieces are intact. If the uterus has been lifted out of the abdomen, it is carefully replaced inside the abdomen and sutured (from the inner to outer layers) with absorbable sutures. A final instrument and sponge

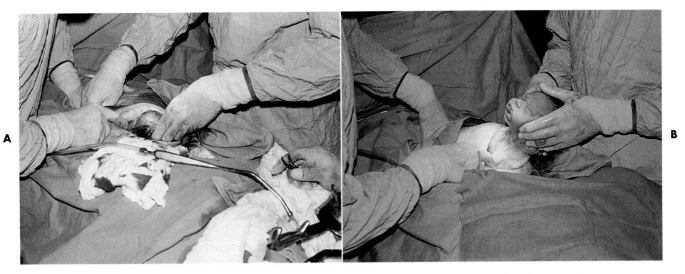

Figure 15-22 Cesarean section delivery. **A,** The surgeon's hand is inserted under the infant head, which is levered out through the uterine wound. The infant's nostrils and mouth are cleared by suction as soon as the head is delivered. **B,** The rest of the infant is delivered by the application of traction on the infant's head. The cord is clamped and cut between two artery forceps, and the infant is passed to the attending pediatrician. (Courtesy Marjorie Pyle, RNC, *Lifecircle.*)

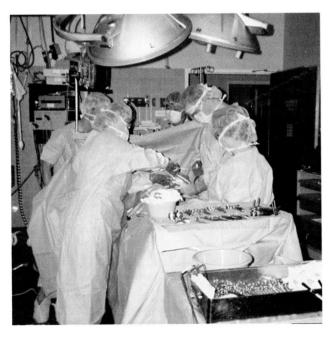

Figure 15-23 Operative setup for cesarean birth. (Courtesy R. Trapp.)

count is performed to prevent accidentally leaving a foreign item inside the woman's abdominal cavity, and then fascia, muscle, and skin layers are closed.

A few women have cesarean hysterectomies. The reason may be related to excessive hemorrhage (thus it is a lifesaving action), or the woman may have known that

> *Box 15-7* **Examples of Criteria for Trial of Labor for Vaginal Birth after Cesarean**
>
> Previous cesarean with low transverse uterine incision
> No cephalopelvic disproportion (CPD) or fetal complications
> Fetal size under 4000 g
> Physician or midwife in constant attendance
> Continuous fetal monitoring during active labor
> Uterine pressure gauge for monitoring contractions, if oxytocin used

this final step would be taken because she has multiple myomas (fibroids) or carcinoma and this will be the last planned birth.

Vaginal Birth after Cesarean

A VBAC may be considered in every case, but especially if the previous cesarean section was the result of unforeseen causes such as prolapse of the cord or fetal distress, or in instances in which there is an adequate pelvic dimension but the previous infant was very large. If the woman has no pathologic problems or constricted pelvic bony structure, she should have a trial of labor (Box 15-7). The major concern is that the scar tissue on the uterus will not be flexible enough to withstand contractions and thus may possibly separate from the muscle. Scar separation, if it occurs, may be insidious, or in rare cases, it may be rapid. For this reason, VBAC is contraindicated for women who have had vertical incisions into the body of the uterus with a classical scar. Since the majority of incisions today are lower uterine, VBAC has become much more common (Chez, 1995, Lie-Nielsen, 1994).

ACOG (1991) has produced guidelines concerning VBAC and with the National Institutes of Health has encouraged physicians and midwives to allow a trial of labor in every possible previous cesarean case. Each hospital unit formulates a protocol to be followed. These procedures include presence of a physician or midwife during labor, fetal and uterine monitoring, and extremely careful use of oxytocin or Prostin gel. Oxytocin may be used for labor stimulation but protocols must be carefully followed.

There has been a varied response when physicians are committed to VBAC. *MMWR* reported rates for VBAC were 26.3% of all women with previous cesarean births (1996).

Risk of uterine rupture

The chief complication of VBAC is uterine rupture along the line of the scar. Uterine rupture can be differentiated from uterine scar *dehiscence* (separation of the suture line). The latter is an asymptomatic event that is discovered on direct visualization of the uterus at laparotomy or found on digital exploration of the uterus after vaginal delivery. It is not associated with either fetal or maternal death or morbidity. Dehiscence occurs in approximately 1% of women who have had previous cesarean delivery at full term with or without labor (Braun, 1996). In contrast, uterine rupture is a tear in the integrity of the uterine wall associated with maternal and fetal morbidity and/or mortality. It occurs in 0.7% of trial of labor (TOL) clients and may occur unexpectedly in early or late labor (Chez, 1995) (see Chapter 21).

Signs of uterine scar separation are an irregular change in contractions or uterine outline, increased vaginal bleeding, and poor labor progress (see Chapter 21). The most common initial sign is escalating fetal distress.

Preparation for Operative Birth

Parents must be aware of the possibilities of planned or emergency cesarean delivery during labor. The childbirth education class will review indications and choices. For planned surgery, preparation includes a conference with the anesthesiologist and a tour of the surgical and recovery areas (see Chapter 12 for a prenatal teaching plan). The woman must know the types of treatments that will be used and the recovery care (Box

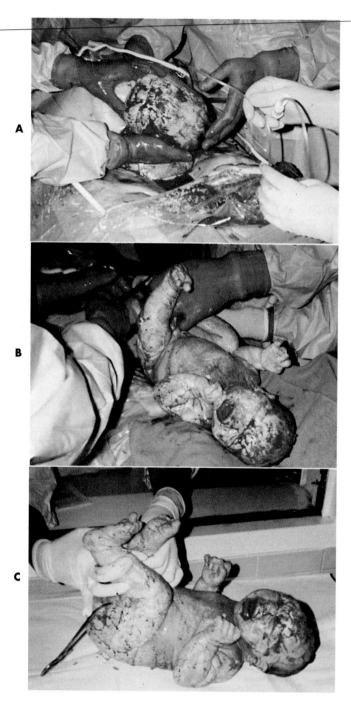

Figure 15-24 Sequence of birth after abdominal incision. (Courtesy R. Trapp.)

15-8). The birth partner may wish to be present during the entire delivery, at least until the time of surgery and directly after to experience the excitement of the birth (Figure 15-25).

Regional anesthesia is used for planned cesarean deliveries almost universally. The woman is usually awake with epidural or spinal anesthesia and her partner sits at the head of the bed; thus both see the infant at birth.

When a woman is to have a cesarean delivery after labor has been in progress, the nurse must recognize that the woman and her partner will experience some or all of the following (Donovan and Allen, 1977):

1. Relief, if the labor was long, difficult, and painful
2. Anxiety and fear that something will happen unexpectedly to the woman or infant as a result of surgery
3. Guilt related to the woman's behavior during labor or any activity in the weeks before
4. Anger directed, in general, at the childbirth educator for not giving a more complete understanding of the possibility of a cesarean delivery; at the physician for a perceived lack of communication; or sometimes at the infant for being too small or too big or for causing her such trouble
5. Feelings of bewilderment, sadness, or loneliness or feelings of failure, frustration, and regret because of a lost normal experience
6. Feelings of helplessness and dependence that rob parents of their sense of control

These feelings may continue well into the first year. See Chapter 17 for further discussion.

Anxiety may inhibit the couple's ability to understand information. They should not go into the recovery period without a clear explanation of the reasons for the decision for the operative birth. This anxiety may be accentuated if they were expecting an unmedicated vaginal birth. See Chapter 17 for Care Path on cesarean birth. The results of these feelings may be loss of self-esteem and emotional distress, which are discussed in depth in Chapters 17 and 26. Explanations and support may reduce the intensity of the sense of loss. Emphasize positive care of the infant. Encourage and make provisions for positive acquaintance with the infant as soon as possible after birth. The father may be involved in the cesarean delivery to the same degree that he would have been for a vaginal birth; he stays by the mother and may assist with infant care, as seen in Figure 15-26. When the mother returns to the LDR room, siblings may visit promptly (Figure 15-27).

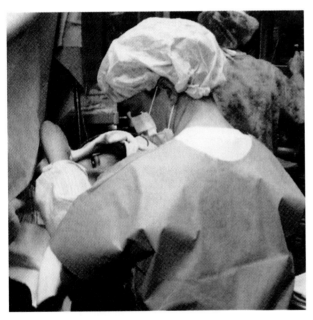

Figure 15-25 Parents' first look at the new infant during the cesarean. (Courtesy St John's Mercy Medical Center, St Louis, Mo.)

Box **15-8**

TEACHING PLAN *for* HOME CARE

Preparation for Cesarean Birth

PROCESS OF PREPARATION AND PROCEDURES	POSTOPERATIVE SELF-CARE: DEMONSTRATE TECHNIQUES
Blood work	Cough and deep breathing methods
Skin preparation	Splinting and supporting incision
Bladder care	Positioning for sleep, breast-feeding infant
Use of intravenous line	Becoming ambulatory
Anesthesia choice discussed with anesthesiologist	Isometrics
Presence of partner and when both will see infant after birth	Pain and other medications
	Process of involution and self-care in home recovery

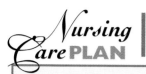

Nursing Care PLAN | Unexpected Cesarean Birth

CASE

Angela M, Para 1001, and her partner, Bruce, entered the LDR room at midnight, 1 hour after Angela's membranes ruptured. Their birth plan indicated no analgesia and an early discharge. Contractions slowed overnight, and at 8 AM oxytocin drip was started to stimulate labor. At 10 AM, when her cervix was 6 cm and station +1, an epidural was started. Five hours later, station was still +1 and dilation was 8 cm. However, nonreassuring fetal heart patterns appeared and worsened despite interventions. Because fetal pH showed falling readings and there was a maternal temperature of 100° F, a cesarean delivery was indicated.

Assessment

1. Childbirth education classes taught possibility of cesarean. Parents are anxious about fetal status. Support by partner is positive.
2. Position and station indicate delayed descent and signs of distress. Factors leading to infection are possible.
3. Epidural is in place, and analgesia is effective. Oxygen is by mask. Hydration is adequate as shown by output. Oxytocin is stopped because of variables. Woman positioned on left side.
4. Antibiotics administered by intermittent infusion.

Nursing Diagnoses

1. Knowledge deficit, regarding anesthesia and postoperative care.
2. Risk for reduced fetal and maternal perfusion, related to anesthesia and evidence of maternal complications.
3. Infection, risk for, related to extended labor and ruptured membranes.
4. Anxiety and fear for self and infant, related to surgical procedure.
5. Altered self-esteem, related to not following birth plan.

Expected Outcomes

1. Fetal and maternal perfusion is maintained; newborn Apgar score is above 7.
2. Infection is prevented or controlled by interventions.
3. Effective coping skills are used to reduce anxiety and fear for self.
4. Adjustment after birth to fact of surgical birth progresses normally.

Nursing Interventions

1. Maintain side-lying position and oxygen by mask. Monitor vital signs every 30 minutes. Record maternal fluid intake and response to regional anesthesia. Insert Foley catheter before surgery. Monitor FHR every 5 minutes.
2. During preparations for cesarean delivery, maintain continuous monitoring of heart rate and contractions. Assist with fetal blood sampling. Monitor IV fluids as indicated.
3. Determine whether couple understands the reasons for surgical intervention. (Is consent informed?) Encourage verbalization of feelings. Use positive reinforcement of coping strategies. Ensure that support person remains with woman during preparation and in delivery room.
4. Use positive reinforcement of cesarean as an alternative birthing method. Focus on infant's need for a safe birth. Diffuse any anger by answering all implied or frank questions.

Evaluation

1. Was maternal and fetal perfusion maintained adequately?
2. Did the mother tolerate surgery without complications?
3. Was infant healthy? Were Apgar scores above 7?
4. Was a positive self-image maintained despite change in birth plan? Does Angela understand that there may be lingering mixed feelings during the first year?

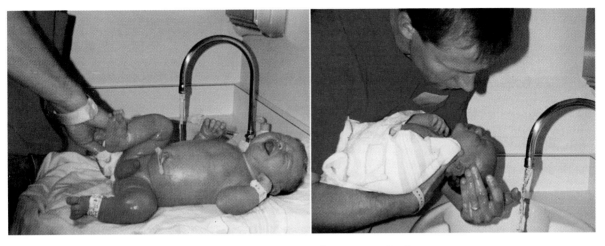

Figure 15-26   Father participates in immediate infant care after cesarean birth. (Courtesy R. Trapp.)

UNEXPECTED BIRTH

Any birth occurring outside a planned, prepared environment is considered unexpected. Before the rise in the emphasis on home births, an emergency delivery was considered any delivery outside the delivery room of a hospital. Today many births take place in alternative settings, with preparation, supervision, and backup provisions if complications occur.

Unexpected birth occurs when labor progresses rapidly, usually in less than 4 hours; often this birth is referred to as a *precipitous* delivery. Women who deliver this way generally fall into a number of groups: those with unusually rapid preterm labor, those with rapid progressions through stages of term labor and with a high threshold for pain, those who are grand multiparas, and those who are uninformed or do not understand ways to seek help (for example, a woman with a language barrier, a terrified teenager, a woman who is mentally retarded or disabled, a substance abuser, or a migrant farm worker). Unexpected birth may occur at home, in a clinic, in the hospital, during transport, or in a public place. Birth en route to the hospital may be caused by external events, such as a traffic jam or car breakdown. Health personnel must be informed about steps of support and care during emergency delivery. If a rescue unit is available, a resource packet will include plans and strategies, information on cultural differences, and the forms necessary for appropriate documentation of details of the unexpected birth.

Birth in a Disaster Setting

Birth during an emergency or disaster may result when the pregnant woman is sequestered in a shelter or

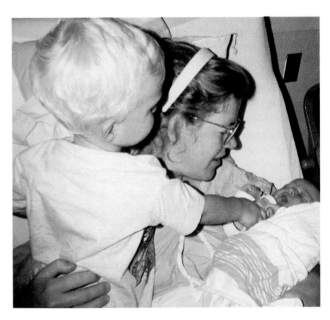

Figure 15-27   Earliest sibling visit to the LDR room (Courtesy R. Trapp.)

marooned in an isolated place. If birth is in a disaster setting, everyone usually protects the woman and infant. Follow the basic guidelines, remembering that the recovery care must include fluids for mother and infant, maintenance of a clear airway for the newborn, and aseptic technique. If there is no way to sterilize a knife, select the cleanest material to tie off the cord. Do *not* cut the cord with a dirty tool; neonatal tetanus may result. Monitor mother and newborn for thermoregulation, fluid balance, and nutrition. See Box 15-9 for information to record after the birth.

Box 15-9	Information to Record for Unexpected Birth

Fetal position and presentation
Color and any unusual odor of the amniotic fluid
Whether the cord was around the neck
Number of loops in the cord
Time of delivery of entire body
Estimate of Apgar score
Resuscitation efforts
Condition of infant
Sex of infant
Time of placental birth and appearance, with amount of
bleeding noted
Woman's condition, including interventions to control
bleeding, condition of perineum

Birth in a Public Place

The environmental setting dictates what is available to aid in a delivery. For example, in a public place, water may be available as a fluid to use for rinsing hands and the perineum and newspaper may be placed under the woman's back. The following interventions apply to birth in a public place and may be modified for other settings:

1. Labor *always* progresses through a step-by-step pattern to delivery. In many emergency cases, labor progress is merely more rapid through phases than it is in a controlled environment (hospital, birthing center, home birth). Therefore the phase of labor must quickly be assessed:

   How frequent are contractions?
   How long and strong are they?
   Does the woman have an urge to push?

2. The most knowledgeable person should take charge. Send volunteers for equipment and help. Maintain a calm atmosphere. Get the woman to focus on her present condition, and encourage proper breathing techniques. Help her into as comfortable a position as possible.

3. Cooperate with the natural forces of labor. Do not do vaginal assessments of dilation; external signs are clearly recognizable.

4. Position the woman to facilitate delivery: a semisitting or squatting position to push and a Sims' position or semisitting for delivery. Position the woman to allow space at the perineum to manipulate the infant's shoulders during the final moments of birth.

5. The infant must be protected against respiratory dysfunction and cold stress; anticipate and provide for the fluid and nutritional needs of the mother and infant.

6. Put the infant to the nipple to stimulate oxytocin release. Skin-to-skin contact, with the infant covered by the woman's clothing, helps prevent chilling.

Nursing Responsibilities

NURSING DIAGNOSES

Although nursing diagnoses are not written in this emergency, consider which of these would apply.

- Fear related to setting, lack of preparation, loss of control, unfamiliar environment
- Increased risk for altered maternal-fetal perfusion related to rapid birth
- Increased risk for altered tissue integrity, bleeding, or infection related to trauma of birth and lack of asepsis
- Ineffective thermoregulation related to environmental temperature

EXPECTED OUTCOMES

- Woman is cooperative and responsive to nursing assistance.
- Maternal-fetal perfusion is maintained as evidenced by a high Apgar score.
- Trauma is minimized, and postbirth bleeding is within normal parameters.
- Infant exhibits consistent body temperature between 97° F and 98° F.

NURSING INTERVENTION

In making a decision about the timing of birth, determine the available options. Evaluate the location. Enlist someone to get help, someone to control a potential crowd, and someone to get equipment. Suggested types of equipment are listed below.

For cleansing the mother: Use water with dishwashing liquid or wipe her down with her underclothes.

For padding or protection during delivery: In a public space, use newspapers (unused), or at home, use large plastic bags, old sheets, towels, or a shower curtain.

To clear infant's airway: Use an ear bulb syringe or meat basting syringe, and manually milk nose and throat.

For the cord: Use strong yarn, a new razor blade, or scissors or knife (flame sterilized), only if no help is available. *Do not* cut the cord if the woman will be transported.

To warm the infant: Use mother's clothes, skin-to-skin contact, blanket, towel, sheet, clean newspapers, and/or a padded box.

To feed the infant (if no help is available): Use milk powder, bottled water, bottle, and nipple. Encourage breastfeeding.

Fluids for the mother: Use any available fluids.

As much as possible in the setting, use precaution with blood and body fluids. When the birth occurs in a health care facility or an ambulance, a birthing pack is available for a precipitous birth. When birth is outside a facility, use what is available.

For the delivery process, follow the mechanisms of labor. It is extremely important to provide a controlled birth. Have the woman pant so she does not push until directed to do so. To avoid a laceration, massage the perineum if sterile gloves are available, with first finger inside the vagina, helping to stretch out the labia. When the head crowns, support the perineum with gentle back pressure to prevent lacerations. If the head has difficulty emerging, use the modified Ritgen maneuver. Follow Figure 15-28 to note the hand positions for the delivery of the head and shoulders.

When the head emerges, the amniotic sac will usually rupture if it has not already. If it does not, puncture it and remove membranes (the caul) from the infant's face so breathing may start. Check for loops of the umbilical cord around the neck. Slip the loop over the head and pull the slack to slip it over the shoulder. If the cord is tight and needs to be clamped while in place, use the two clamps provided in the delivery kit and cut between those clamps. *If there is no equipment,* gently stretch the cord to slide the loop over the head.

Wipe any blood and mucus off the face using towels or the woman's clothing. Clear the mouth of mucus with a cloth over fingers or a suction bulb if available. "Milk" the nose and throat by applying moderate stroking pressure on the throat in the direction of mouth if no suction equipment is available. In the same way, gently squeeze and expel mucus from the nose.

Delivery of the shoulders proceeds by first pulling the anterior shoulder under the symphysis pubis and then carefully easing the posterior shoulder out by gently pulling the head upward (see Figure 15-28). An assistant may apply gentle but steady pressure above the symphysis if the shoulders seem difficult to deliver. The slippery body will quickly follow. Grasp the body securely, supporting the head and trunk with one arm. The infant must be immediately dried off and should be placed on the woman's abdomen with the head in a slightly dependent position to drain mucus. Protect the infant from cold by drying and covering him or her with the woman's clothing, and have the woman hold the infant (skin-to-skin) close to her body. Observe the infant's respirations, color, and activity. Estimate an Apgar score for later documentation (see Box 15-9).

Do not rush to tie and cut the cord. The infant's first breath will close fetal circulation; therefore the cord *does not* have to be tied and cut if no sterile equipment is available. Only if no help will be forthcoming should the cord

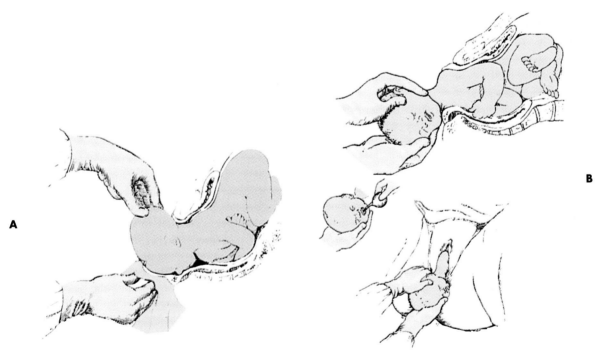

Figure 15-28   A, Assistance may be needed if head does not extend smoothly (Ritgen's maneuver). Exert hand pressure downward on occiput with forward pressure applied to obstetric perineum, just between vaginal and anal openings. Feel for chin, and exert forward pressure on it through perineal tissue. For emergency delivery, use article of mother's clothing (cleanest material available) because skin will be slippery. **B,** Infant's head is gently directed downward to help in partial delivery of anterior (upper) shoulder to "park" it under the symphysis pubis. Then proceed with delivery of lower shoulder by pulling up on the head. (From Willson JR: *Atlas of obstetric technic,* ed 2, St Louis, 1969, Mosby.)

be cut, after it has been tied. Use clean technique whenever possible and be sure the knife or razor blade has been sterilized. Neonatal tetanus may occur if unclean instruments are used to cut the cord.

The placenta will usually be ready for birth a few minutes after birth of the infant. A gush of blood will precede lengthening of the cord at the vagina. It is appropriate to wait up to an hour for separation of the placenta, but separation most often occurs within 30 minutes. The infant should be put to the breast to lick or suck the nipple while waiting for separation. When the uterus rises up into a globular shape and the cord lengthens at the vagina, ask the woman to push down to expel the placenta.

Have a newspaper ready to catch the placenta; wrap it after briefly examining it for missing pieces. Then ask the woman to rub her fundus. Keep the infant at the mother's breast to stimulate oxytocin release. Save the placenta for complete examination if the woman is to be transferred to a health care facility.

Assess the state of the perineum. If lacerations have occurred, obtain ice if possible; wrap it in plastic and then in a paper towel or a piece of clean sheeting, and apply pressure at the perineum to assist with hemostasis. Watch the uterus for atony, and assess the amount of bleeding. Obtain assistance as necessary to move the woman for observation and follow-up care.

An unexpected birth can be a pleasant, successful experience or a frightening one for the woman. The person in charge makes the difference. Remember the predictability and naturalness of the event while remaining alert for evidence of problems.

EVALUATION

Ask the following questions to evaluate care:
- Did any injury occur to mother or infant? Was there a normal Apgar score?
- Was the woman supported during the process?
- Was bleeding controlled?
- Did recovery of mother and infant proceed normally?

Key points

- The nurse maintains attentiveness to the woman by remaining at her bedside, supporting her coach, and assessing her coping ability.
- Carefully monitor the mother's BDEs and her progression through the step-by-step process of labor and birth, and keep her well informed.
- Women who have an attentive nurse have less tendency to lose control and are able to cooperate during the second stage of labor.
- Recognizing how cultural factors affect the outcome of labor for the woman is essential for helping her maintain her composure, reduce her anxiety, and prepare her for the naturalness of labor and birth.
- The Friedman graph describes the "average" labor; some women progress faster, whereas many progress in a normal slower pattern.
- BDEs do not need to begin as soon as the cervix is fully dilated. Instead, allow the reorganization of the first phase to occur, and follow the woman's own involuntary BDEs. Remember to prevent Valsalva's maneuver and the adverse effects of extended breath-holding.

- The woman's position in labor and for birth is a crucial nursing responsibility and promotes an intact perineum.
- Discuss caput, cephalhematoma, head molding, or scratches on the head with the new parents when ventouse or forceps are used or if a scalp pH is done to allay fears of deformity or injury.
- Women who are prepared for a cesarean birth recover faster than unprepared women, with less guilt and sadness. Those who have emergency intervention may grieve over the loss of a "normal" birth and wonder what they did wrong in the process.
- VBAC is now considered for all women who have had a cesarean delivery, unless there are accompanying complications, CPD, or a vertical uterine incision.
- When birth takes place in public places or during a disaster, the mother and infant must be protected from injury, infection, cold, stress, and hemorrhage. The most knowledgeable person should take charge.

Study Questions

15-1. Select the terms that apply to the following statements:
   a. The condition in which the fetal head remains encircled by the vaginal opening between contractions is
   _____.
   b. A delayed descent that requires assistance with birth is _____.
   c. A tear resulting from the extreme stretching of the perineum is a _____.
   d. The maneuver that causes blood pressure to fall and affects fetal perfusion is _____.
   e. A pushing technique that fosters good oxygenation of the fetus is _____.

15-2. Ann needs instruction on the breathing pattern for second-stage pushing. Which of the following is an example of correct breathing during a contraction?
   a. Hold breath and push toward vagina, release air at 30 seconds, and repeat until contraction is over.
   b. Push down at the diaphragm and hold breath for as long as possible during contraction.
   c. Inhale and push down while very slowly releasing air and repeat this every 15 seconds for duration of contraction.
   d. Push down ad lib, as if to defecate, when the involuntary urge to push is felt.

15-3. A woman, para 0020, is bearing down with contractions. The nurse notes caput at the introitus. After calling for assistance, the next most appropriate action would be to:
   a. Ask the woman to pant with the next contraction and prepare her for transfer to delivery room.
   b. Tell her to stop pushing while preparing her for the birth.
   c. Turn her on her left side.
   d. Stay with her and provide reassurance.

15-4. Descent, flexion, internal rotation, and extension allow normal birth. These movements:
   a. Shorten the second stage of labor.
   b. Ease the passage of infant through the birth canal.
   c. Allow the smallest presenting diameter to pass through first.
   d. Allow the infant to be born in an occiput position.

15-5. Match the phase of second-stage labor with the signs listed below.
   a. Contractions change character and become regular (3 to 5 minutes apart).
   b. Anus bulges and perineum distends.
   c. Fetal part may be seen at introitus, even between contractions.

   1. Phase one
   2. Phase two
   3. Phase three

Answer Key

15-1: *a,* Crowning; *b,* dystocia; *c,* laceration; *d,* Valsalva's maneuver; *e,* open glottis. 15-2: *c,* d. 15-3: *d.* 15-4: *c.* 15-5: *a,* Phase one; *b,* phase three; *c,* phase two.

References

Aderhold KJ, Roberts JE: Phases of the second stage of labor, *J Nurse Midwifery* 36:267, 1991.

Alison M et al: Pregnancy, abortion and birth rates among U. S. adolescents—1980, 1985, and 1990, *JAMA* 275(13):989, 1996.

American College of Obstetricians and Gynecologists: *Operative vaginal delivery,* Technical Bulletin No 196, Washington, DC, 1994.

American College of Obstetricians and Gynecologists: *Dystocia and the augmentation of labor,* Technical Bulletin No 218, Washington, DC, 1995.

Arrabal P: Is manual palpation of uterine contractions accurate? *Am J Obstet Gynecol* 174(1): 217, 1996.

*Classic reference.

Beischer NA, MacKay LV: *Obstetrics and the newborn,* ed 2, Sydney, 1993, Harcourt, Brace, Jovanovich Group.

Bergstrom L et al: "You'll feel me touching you, sweetie": vaginal examinations during the second stage of labor, *Birth* 19(1):10, 1992.

Blackburn ST, Loper DL: *Maternal, fetal, and neonatal physiology,* Philadelphia, 1992, WB Saunders.

Braun TE: Wound dehiscence. In Queenan JT, Hobbins JC, eds: *Protocols for high-risk pregnancies,* Cambridge, 1996, Blackwell Science.

*Caldero-Barcia R: Influence of maternal position on time of spontaneous rupture of membranes, progress of labor and fetal head progression, *Birth Family J* 6:7, 1979.

Callister L: Cultural meanings of childbirth, *J Obstet Gynecol Neonatal Nurs* 24(4):327, 1995.

Chez R: Cervical ripening and labor induction after previous cesarean delivery, *Clin Obstet Gynecol* 38(2):287, 1995.

Combs CA et al: Prolonged third stage of labor—morbidity and risk factors, *Obstet Gynecol* 78:893, 1991.

Cosner RK, deJong E: Physiologic second-stage labor, *MCN Am J Matern Child Nurs*, 18(1):38, 1993.

Cunningham F et al: *Williams Obstetrics,* ed. 19, Norwalk Town, Conn, 1993, Appleton & Lange.

Dierker LJ: Breech delivery. In Zuspan F, Quilligan E, eds: *Current therapy in obstetrics and gynecology,* ed 4, Philadelphia, 1994, WB Saunders.

*Donovan B, Allen RM: The cesarean birth method, *J Obstet Gynecol Neonatal Nurs* 6:37, 1977.

*Dougherty MC et al: The effect of exercise on circumvaginal muscles in postpartum women, *J Nurse Midwifery* 34:8, 1989.

Evans S: Maternal learning needs during labor and delivery, *J Obstet Gynecol Neonatal Nurs* 24(3):235, 1995.

Flamm BL et al: Vaginal birth after cesarean delivery—results of a five-year multicenter collaborative study, *Obstet Gynecol* 76:750, 1990.

Floyd-Davis E: Ritual in the hospital: giving birth the American way, *Special Delivery* 18(2): 2, 1995.

Freda C: Arrest, trial, and failure, *J Obstet Gynecol Neonatal Nurs* 24(5): 393, 1995.

Gardosi J et al: Alternative positions in the second stage of labour, randomized controlled trial, *Br J Obstet Gynaecol* 96:1290, 1990.

*Green JR et al: Factors associated with rectal injury in spontaneous deliveries, *Obstet Gynecol* Part 1, 73:732, 1989.

*Herbst AL: Medical professional liability and obstetric care: the Institute of Medicine report and recommendations, *Obstet Gynecol* 75:705, 1989.

Hodnett E: Nursing support of the laboring woman, *J Obstet Gynecol Neonatal Nurs* 25(3): 257, 1996.

Johnson N, Johnson VA et al: Maternal positions during labor, *Obstet Gynecol Surv* 46(7):428, 1991.

Klein-Kaye V et al: The use of fundal pressure during the second stage of labor, *J Obstet Gynecol Neonatal Nurs* 19:511, 1990.

Kowalski K, MacMullen N et al: The high-touch paradigm: a 21st century model for maternal-child nursing, *MCN Am J Matern Child Nurs* 21(1): 43, 1996.

Lambert M: Migrant and seasonal farm worker, *J Obstet Gynecol Neonatal Nurs* 24(3):265, 1995.

Lancashire J: National Center for Health Statistics data line, *Public Health Rep* 110(1):105, 1995.

*Laufer A et al: Vaginal birth after cesarean section: nurse-midwifery management, *J Nurse Midwifery* 32:41, 1987.

Lescale KB et al: Conflicts between physicians and patients in nonelective cesarean delivery: incidence and adequacy of informed consent, *Am J Perinatol* 13(2):171, 1996.

Lie-Nielsen C: Something's wrong here: increasing acceptance of cesarean section as childbirth method, *Special Delivery* 18(1):12, 1994.

Lightfoot-Klein H et al: Special needs of ritually circumcised women patients, *J Obstet Gynecol Neonatal Nurs* 20:102, 1991.

Lowe NK: The pain and discomfort of labor and birth, *J Obstet Gynecol Neonatal Nurs*: 25(1): 82, 1996.

Lyndon-Rochelle MT et al: Perineal outcomes and nurse-midwifery management, *J Nurse Midwifery* 40(1):13, 1995.

*Classic reference.

Mahomed K et al: External cephalic version at term—a randomized controlled trial using tocolysis, *Br J Obstet Gynaecol* 98:8, 1991.

Mattson S: Culturally sensitive perinatal care for southeast Asians. *J Obstet Gynecol Neonatal Nurs* 24(4):335, 1995.

Menticoglou S: Perinatal outcome in relation to second-stage duration. *Am J Obstet Gynecol* 173(3): 906, 1995.

Morbidity and Mortality Weekly Report *(MMWR),* 44(11S):1, 1996.

*Nodine PM, Roberts JE: Factors associated with perineal outcome during childbirth, *J Nurs Midwifery* 32:123, 1989.

Odent MR: Position in delivery, *Lancet* 335:1166, 1990.

O'Mara P: A medley of birth positions (adapted from the Homebirth Australia Newsletter, no 36) *Mothering* 73: 28, 1994.

Paine LL, Tinker DD: The effect of maternal bearing-down efforts on arterial umbilical cord pH and length of the second stage of labor, *J Nurse Midwifery* 37(1):61, 1992.

Prendiville W et al: The third stage of labour. In Enkin M et al, eds: *Effective care in pregnancy and childbirth,* Oxford, 1993, Oxford University Press.

*Roberts J et al: A descriptive analysis of involuntary bearing-down efforts, *J Obstet Gynecol Neonatal Nurs* 16:48, 1987.

Robertson PA: Head entrapment and neonatal outcome by mode of delivery in breech deliveries from twenty-four to twenty-seven weeks of gestation, *Am J Obstet Gynecol* 173(4):1171, 1995.

Rosen MG et al: Vaginal birth after cesarean—a meta-analysis of morbidity and mortality, *Obstet Gynecol* 77:465, 1991.

Sheil E: Concerns of childbearing women: maternal concerns questionnaire as an assessment tool, *J Obstet Gynecol Neonatal Nurs* 24(2):149, 1995.

Stover J: Professional labor support: use of childbirth educators, *Special Delivery* 18(1):16, 1994.

*Thorpe JM, Bowes WA: Episiotomy: can its routine use be defended? *Am J Obstet Gynecol* Part 1, 160:1027, 1989.

Thorpe JM: Patient autonomy, informed consent and routine episiotomy, *Contemp OB Gyn* 40(9):92, 1995.

Thronton J G: Active management of labour: current knowledge and research issues, *Br Med J* 309(6951):366, 1994.

Williams MC: Vacuum-assisted delivery, *Clin Perinatol* 22(4):953, 1995.

Zuspan FP, Quilligan E: *Current therapy in obstetrics and gynecology,* ed 4, Philadelphia, 1994 WB Saunders.

 Student Resource Shelf

Hopko-Sharts NC: Birth in the Japanese context, *J Obstet Gynecol Neonatal Nurs* 24(4):343, 1995.
This article offers a qualitative study of the experiences of 20 American women who gave birth in Japan. Childbearing in the cross-cultural context is stressful, and nurses must understand the impact of these experiences as seen through newcomer's eyes.

J Nurse Midwifery 40(6):1995. (Entire issue)
Considerations when couples are prepared for home birth and then certified nurse midwife (CNM) guidelines for birth and newborn health.

Roberts J, Woolley D: A second look at the second stage of labor, *J Obstet Gynecol Neonatal Nurs* 25(5):415, 1996.
Review of the descent and birth phases by authors involved in the primary research of second stage labor.

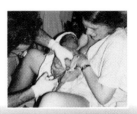

16

Perinatal Guidelines
for Drugs *&* Anesthesia

Learning Objectives

- Identify drug risks and precautions in relation to the phases of pregnancy, labor and birth, and lactation.
- Correlate physiologic changes of pregnancy with drug absorption, metabolism, and excretion.
- Identify the significant membrane barriers regulating drug passage to the fetus and newborn.
- State the rationale for and precautions of oxytocic use during labor.
- Relate the precautions of drug and anesthesia use during the transitional period of labor.
- Explore complementary therapies to enhance comfort during labor and birth.
- Describe nursing interventions when analgesics and anesthetics are used because of altered comfort.

Key Terms

Analgesia
Anesthesia
Benefit-to-Risk Ratio
Cricoid Pressure
Effect
Endorphin
Enterohepatic Recycling
Epidural
Equigesic Doses
Equilibrium
Gradient
Half-Life ($t_{1/2}$)
Ionization
Loading Dose
Membrane Barriers

Minimum Effective
  Concentration (MEC)
Nociception
Nociceptors
Patient-Controlled
  Epidural Analgesia
  (PCEA)
Somatic Pain
Teratogens
Time-Dose Interval
Transcutaneous Electric
  Nerve Stimulation
  (TENS)
Visceral Pain

DRUGS AND PREGNANCY

Nurses administer medication and provide counseling for women regarding drug effects. Women should be counseled regarding the anticipated use of any drug during pregnancy with a health professional. The word "drug" is used to mean prescription or nonprescription medications, chemical and food additives, and environmental agents. The desired effects and possible side effects of these substances on the woman, the pregnancy, and the fetus require careful consideration before initiating use. Knowledge of basic pharmacokinetics and the therapeutic and potential adverse effects of drugs during each phase of pregnancy will enable the nurse to provide safe care and

client teaching. Nurses should review medication basics and apply this knowledge to the welfare of the woman and the fetus.

The 9 months of pregnancy should be viewed as a constantly changing, complex interaction between the woman and fetus. Regardless of the route of administration, most drugs taken by the mother cross the placenta and achieve **equilibrium** (a state of balance) in both the fetus and the woman. In some cases there may be an even higher concentration in fetal circulation than in maternal circulation.

Today many women avoid medications during pregnancy. However, many uninformed women still self-medicate (Fitzgerald, 1993). The most commonly used drugs are analgesics, antacids, antibiotics, antiemetics,

361

antihistamines, diuretics, iron and vitamin supplements, sedatives, alcohol, and cigarettes (Briggs, Freeman, Yaffee, 1994). Over-the-counter (OTC) drugs are a special concern because of the variable doses women may take; too often the OTC drug has been on the home medicine shelf past its expiration date, or OTC drugs may contain substances that have adverse effects on the fetus if taken in unregulated doses. Examples include aspirin taken in adult doses that interfere with prostaglandin synthesis or heavy use of antacids (see Chapter 10). Common household remedies for heartburn include sodium-containing antacids such as baking soda and sodium citrate, which may increase the risk of electrolyte imbalance.

Inadvertent exposure to environmental chemicals may affect both the woman and the fetus. Household insecticides, cleaning products, and pollutants in the environment are examples discussed in Chapter 28. These substances may be **teratogens**, substances that adversely affect fetal growth, development, or health.

Current interest in self-medication with herbal remedies and minerals require education to avoid substances that may be harmful. Most health food stores carry lists of herbal remedies to avoid. Lists are available on the Internet as well. Women should be advised to check intake carefully.

Benefit-to-Risk Ratio

The **benefit-to-risk ratio** estimates if the benefit of the medication to the fetus is greater than the known or unknown risk of side effects of the drug on the mother and fetus. The benefit-to-risk ratio takes into account a worsening maternal condition or fetal compromise without the drug and must be considered because of the side effects of some drugs. Table 16-1 lists the Food and Drug Administration (FDA) categories for drug labeling to indicate risk during pregnancy. A drug with some risk still may be prescribed with the woman's informed consent.

Informed consent

A woman who needs to receive a prescribed drug during pregnancy should give her informed consent. She should understand the benefit-to-risk ratio and agree to be medicated. It is a violation of the woman's rights to withhold this information from her or not to ensure that she understands the language in which the information is given. Although the physician or midwife is legally responsible to obtain informed consent, nurses are legally required to evaluate the client's knowledge and confirm if the client exhibits a clear understanding of any proposed therapeutic action. See Chapter 30 for a full discussion of informed consent.

PHARMACOKINETICS

Drugs are used (1) to replace a missing or deficient substance (vitamins), (2) to counteract physiologic imbalance (antacids), (3) to cause a physicochemical alteration (anesthetics), and (4) to alter body function by combining with receptors in the body to enhance body function, inhibit function, or mimic function (mimetics). The majority of drugs fall into this last major category of altering body function.

Table 16-1	Food and Drug Administration Categories for Labeling Prescription Drugs to Indicate the Risks of their Use in Pregnancy

Category	Risks
A	Controlled studies in women fail to demonstrate a risk to the fetus in the first trimester, and the possibility of fetal harm appears to be remote.
B	Animal studies do not indicate a risk to the fetus and there are no controlled studies in humans, or animal studies show adverse effects on the fetus, but controlled studies in humans have not shown a risk to the fetus.
C	Animal studies have shown the drug to be embryocidal or teratogenic, but there are no controlled studies in humans, or no studies are available in animals or humans.
D	Definitive evidence of risk to the human fetus exists, but the benefit in certain situations (e.g., life-threatening situations in which safer drugs are unavailable or ineffective) may justify the use of the drug despite the risks.
X	Studies in animals or humans have demonstrated fetal abnormalities, or there is evidence of fetal risk based on human experience, or both, and the risk clearly outweighs the possible benefits.

Data from Pregnancy labeling, *FDA Drug Bull* 9:23, 1979.

These biologic responses to drugs are a result of an alteration of normal physiologic processes and are related to the form and concentration of the drug in the specific tissue. There are variables that control the speed and extent to which an active drug causes effects. These variables include (1) rate of transfer across body membranes, (2) pH and ionization of the drug and the body fluids in each compartment, (3) the degree to which the drug is bound to protein or other body tissue, and (4) the rate of metabolism and excretion. Figure 16-1 shows in a schematic way how drugs move across membrane barriers.

Effects of Pregnancy of Pharmacokinetics

The physiologic changes of pregnancy affect a woman's response to drugs. Normal alterations in hormonal levels, body water, fatty tissue, plus the increased blood volume and reduced albumin levels influence drug absorption, distribution, metabolism, and excretion. Specific alterations are discussed with each of these topics. Maternal nutrition and chronic or acute diseases also may influence the effect of drugs on the woman and the fetus. The gestational age of the fetus is important in calculating maternal drug effects, especially during labor.

Mechanisms that regulate placental drug transfer across body membranes and, after delivery, movement of agents across the membranes separating maternal blood and breast milk are particularly relevant to the pregnant woman and later to her infant.

Crossing Body Membranes

One of the transfer mechanisms—facilitated diffusion, active transport, filtration, or phagocytosis and pinocytosis—is needed to allow a drug or albumin molecule to be moved across body membranes; the mechanisms are similar in the nonpregnant state.

Body membranes are made of lipid (fat) and protein molecules and contain small pores through which water and some water-soluble substances can move. Active transport allows a solute to cross in spite of a difference in concentration on the other side of the membrane. Facilitated diffusion is similar to active transport without the chemical or electrical differences on either side. Large molecules or proteins move by *pinocytosis* (transferring droplets of extracellular fluid) or *phagocytosis* (transferring particles of solid material). It is by these two mechanisms that substances such as maternal antibodies or bacteria cross body membranes.

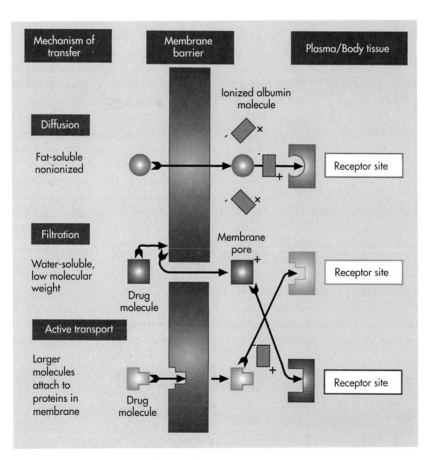

Figure 16-1   How medications cross body membranes. (Modified from Dickason EJ, Schult MO, Morris EM: *Maternal and infant drugs*, New York, 1978, McGraw-Hill.)

The degree of **ionization** of a drug (i.e., having an electrical charge) influences its ability to be absorbed and excreted. *Fat-soluble drugs* tend to be nonionized and are absorbed more easily. *Water-soluble drugs* tend to be ionized and absorbed less easily. Drugs can be altered to become more or less ionized in different pH environments. Acid drugs become more ionized in an alkaline pH, such as that found in the small intestine. Alkaline drugs become more ionized in an acidic environment, such as in the stomach or duodenum. Breast milk also is slightly more acidic than maternal plasma allowing alkaline drugs to move slowly into breast milk. In Figure 16-1, note the different "shapes" indicating different bonding into different tissues; note also the electrical (ion) charges.

Membrane barriers of importance during pregnancy are the placental barrier, the blood-brain barrier, and, during lactation, the blood-milk barrier.

Placental barrier

The so-called placental barrier is not a solid barrier; rather it is like a sieve made up of the chorionic cells that line the villi in the placenta. Usually, within minutes of maternal intake of a drug, the free, unbound portion of the drug crosses over to the fetus. This permeability allows the drug to move from the maternal bloodstream into fetal circulation. If the **gradient** (the difference in concentration of the drug in the mother's serum compared with that in the fetus) is higher in the maternal serum, movement will be in the direction of the lower concentration. Because drugs tend to reach equilibrium, the movement will be in the direction of lower concentration (i.e., "downhill") until the concentration on both sides of the barrier is similar. (Technical measurements of maternal-fetal ratios are given with the number one as the maternal measurement. A ratio of 1:0.8 indicates that the fetal concentration is 80% of that of the drug in the mother's serum.)

All drugs of molecular weight between 100 to 500 daltons (Da) will cross the placental barrier readily. Lipid-soluble drugs are transferred especially rapidly and reach 50 to 100% of the maternal level within minutes of maternal intake. Substances with weights between 600 to 1000 Da cross more slowly, and those drugs with molecular weights >1000 Da usually cannot cross the placenta (e.g., heparin and insulin) (Ward and Mirkin, 1994). The thickness of the barrier diminishes from 25 to 2 mµ during pregnancy, meaning that permeability increases as the fetus approaches birth.

Blood-brain barrier

The blood-brain barrier is made up of several membranes; the lipoid (fatty) sheath of myelin around the capillaries and glial cells that separate brain tissue from extracellular fluid (ECF). After penetrating this barrier into the ECF, the drug must cross the neuronal cell membrane to enter nervous tissue (Blackburn and Loper, 1992). These membranes have no pores. Because capillaries are covered with a tight lipoid sheath, drugs that are lipid-soluble and nonionized will more rapidly cross the blood-brain barrier. Anoxia and trauma will increase the permeability of the blood-brain barrier, a point important to remember for high-risk infants.

During fetal life a higher proportion of blood flow is distributed to the fetal brain. The results can be seen in the effects of opioids and barbiturates, which concentrate in higher amounts in the fetal brain than in the maternal brain. This is one of the reasons for depressed newborn responses if birth is too close to the time of maternal sedative intake.

Because the myelin sheath develops gradually, the degree of permeability is related to gestational age; that is, the younger the fetus, the more easily drugs may enter the fetal brain. Because of this increased permeability, a preterm infant is more affected by maternal sedation than a full-term infant. You will observe that when there is a preterm labor, the mother may not be given normal doses of analgesics for this reason.

Blood-milk barrier

The blood-milk barrier is similar to the blood-brain barrier in that it is difficult to cross by active transport and diffusion. It is made up of the linings of the alveoli and capillaries. Increased circulation to the breast and the variation in milk production make it hard to predict the amount of a drug that will cross the blood-milk barrier. Fat-soluble, nonionized drugs enter breast milk easily. Water-soluble drugs of low molecular weight enter milk by filtration through spaces between alveolar epithelial cells.

The pH of milk ranges between 6.9 and 7.0, which is slightly more acidic than plasma; therefore basic drugs pass more easily than acidic ones (Anderson, 1993). In addition, some drugs are metabolized in the alveolar cells themselves, and some are bound to milk proteins and, although taken in by the infant, are not absorbed or are destroyed in the gastrointestinal tract (Figure 16-2). Additional factors make it difficult to determine how much of the medication is ingested by the infant. The low volume of milk taken by the neonate in the first week reduces potential drug intake during the first week after birth (Rivera-Calimlim, 1987).

Only free drug molecules, unbound in maternal plasma, are able to enter the milk. In general, only 1 to 2% of the maternal dose reaches the milk. This percentage is only a fraction (less than 0.5%) of the standard doses of the same drugs prescribed for infants in the high-risk nursery or pediatric units (Rivera-Calimlim, 1987). For the status of specific drugs see Appendix 3A, and see Chapter 17 for time-dose intervals and safety principles for drug intake while breast-feeding.

Absorption through the Gastrointestinal Tract

The rate of absorption of a medication taken orally is affected by the dose and form (e.g., liquid, tablet, span-

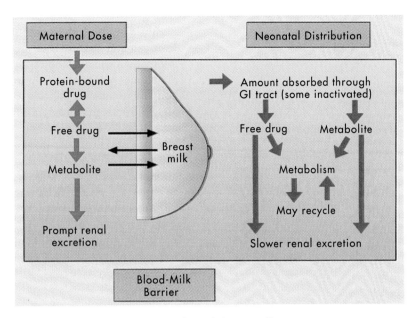

Figure 16-2   Drug distribution through breast milk.

sule, enteric coating), gastrointestinal motility, presence and type of food in stomach, and the pH of the stomach, duodenum, and intestine. Medication taken together with certain foods may enhance or inhibit absorption; for instance, iron compounds are inhibited by milk and enhanced by citrus juice. For rapid absorption, certain drugs must be taken with a glass of water to dissolve the dose and wash it into the intestine.

During pregnancy the digestive tract changes in many ways. Reduced formation of hydrochloric acid leads to slower absorption when a drug needs an acidic environment. In addition, slower gastric emptying delays movement and, if absorption is only in the duodenum or intestine, delays onset of effect.

Parenteral Absorption

During pregnancy, circulation time is faster, blood volume and cardiac output are increased, and renal clearance is faster. If medications are injected intravenously, they always must be diluted and injected slowly. A *bolus* is required for only a few drugs. All intermittent infusions should follow the time schedule and be diluted with at least the minimum amount indicated by the manufacturer. Drugs that are continuously infused maintain an almost equal serum level on both sides of the placental barrier. Therefore when a medication is continuously infused, the level in the fetus may be higher than when drugs are given orally or by intermittent infusion.

Dermatomucosal Absorption

During pregnancy, all mucous membranes and skin have enhanced blood supply therefore drugs are absorbed more

quickly than in the nonpregnant state. Mucous membranes of the respiratory tract have a rapid rate of absorption because of the rich blood supply. Because of augmented circulation to the lung tissue and some hyperventilation during pregnancy, use of general anesthetic gases will result in more rapid induction of anesthesia. In the same way, absorbtion through skin is enhanced by the increased circulation to the skin (Ward and Mirkin, 1994).

BIOAVAILABILITY: DISTRIBUTION AND METABOLISM

After drug absorption, bioavailability is the sum of the speed and the amount of the drug that reaches the circulation free (e.g., unbound) and able to act at the receptor site. Drugs produce their effects by combining with enzymes or cell components. The initial result of the interaction is the *action,* and the result of that action is the **effect.** The action precedes and produces the effects. Indeed, the effects might be far from the site of action.

Many factors influence how long the drug may affect the fetus before being returned to the maternal circulation to be metabolized and excreted by the mother. These factors are tissue and protein binding, the state of ionization of the drug, the pH of the fluids and acidity of the drug, the half-life of the drug, and whether the drug is excreted into the amniotic fluid.

Protein Binding

Only a *free drug molecule* (i.e., unbound) will be able to move to the receptor site. Binding is a reversible process in which a drug is stored temporarily in a body tissue or

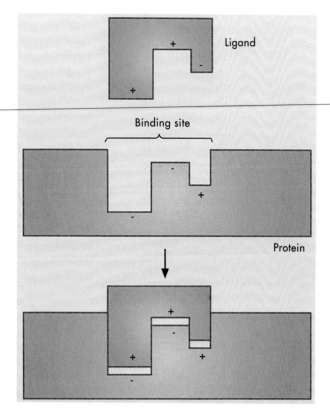

Figure 16-3   Complementary shapes of ligand and protein binding site determine the chemical specificity of binding.

linked to proteins. When drug molecules (the ligand) are linked to albumin molecules or to other proteins, such as nucleoproteins, blood erythrocytes, globulins, or lipoproteins, little may be available. Most bound drugs are linked to an albumin molecule by ionic bonds (Figure 16-3), which may easily be reversed. Binding of a drug molecule is limited by the available number of albumin molecules and by the specific binding sites available for that certain drug.

Unbound drug + Albumin = Drug-albumin complex

When all binding sites are filled up with the drug, the rest of the free molecules seek the receptor sites and cause the effects. There is constant binding and unbinding and movement to and from the receptor site and to the liver for metabolism before excretion by the kidney. Only 5 to 20% of many drugs will be left unbound at one time. In these cases higher doses may be needed to obtain initial action. This higher initial **loading dose** may be ordered to obtain enough free drug to be active, and then the subsequent doses are lower.

Two drugs may compete for the same binding site; one may displace the other, allowing the other to circulate in the free form in greater amounts.

During pregnancy there is increased competition for protein-binding sites because of the following:

- Plasma albumin is decreased.
- Estrogen and progesterone are strongly protein bound, taking up available binding sites.
- Metabolic sources of energy are altered to conserve carbohydrates and fatty tissue.
- Metabolism is increased, resulting in a rise in free fatty acids, triglycerides, cholesterol, and phospholipids, all of which are carried in the plasma attached to proteins.

Without readily available binding sites a larger percentage of the drug will be free to move to receptor sites or to cross the placental barrier. Thus normal doses of some protein-bound drugs will be *more effective* during pregnancy because more of the drug is free to go to the receptor site (Simone, Derewlany, Koren, 1994).

Tissue Binding

Drugs may have an affinity for other body tissues such as bones, hair, nails, and fatty tissue. Tissue binding may lead to storage of large amounts of the drug, and *saturation* in that tissue must be reached before there is free drug to attach to receptor sites. When a tissue-bound drug is no longer given, tissue deposits release shares slowly, causing a persistence of drug effect (e.g., sedatives, hypnotics, and general anesthetics that leave a "hangover" because of slow release). Pregnancy, because of increased fatty tissue, may cause a persistent effect of tissue-bound drugs that are deposited in fatty tissue.

TEST *Yourself* 16-1 _____

a. When a drug is 80% protein bound, how does its journey differ in a pregnant woman?
b. Absorption of drugs through mucous membranes will change in which ways during pregnancy?

Half-Life (t₁/₂)

Half-life ($t_{1/2}$) is the time in which half the absorbed dose is metabolized or made inactive. In each $t_{1/2}$ the blood concentration is reduced again by half (Ward and Mirkin, 1994). Protein or tissue binding determines the $t_{1/2}$. If a drug is tightly bound and only slowly released as free drug molecules, the $t_{1/2}$ will be prolonged. If it is not bound the $t_{1/2}$ may be as short as several minutes. For example, a drug such as oxytocin requires continuous intravenous infusion to be effective because of a $t_{1/2}$ of 3 to 6 minutes. Knowledge of the drug's $t_{1/2}$ especially affects the timing of doses during transition labor and the newborn period. The $t_{1/2}$ may be in minutes or in hours, and it directly influences the minimum effective concentration in the circulation.

Minimum effective concentration

One way to measure medication absorption, distribution, and metabolic breakdown rate is by determining the

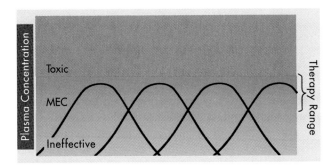

Figure 16-4 Minimum effective concentration (MEC) is achieved by giving a drug at specific intervals determined by its rate of metabolism.

level of **minimum effective concentration** (MEC) in the blood. Doses should be given at intervals close enough to maintain the correct MEC but not close enough to allow the concentration to enter the toxic range. In addition, the dosage should not be too low or too infrequent, which would result in an ineffective blood level. Rapidly metabolized medications, with a short $t_{1/2}$, must be given at closer intervals. Other drugs, such as magnesium sulfate, have a narrow therapeutic range and without careful monitoring may easily reach too high a serum concentration and thus rise to toxic levels.

Medications that are highly tissue or protein bound take longer to reach the MEC and may need to be given only once or twice a day. Such drugs may need a loading dose to bring the blood level up into the MEC more quickly (Figure 16-4).

BIOTRANSFORMATION

Drug action usually is terminated by metabolism and excretion or by leaving the receptor and moving to other tissues. Some medications are inactivated on the first pass through the liver; others are metabolized much more slowly because of protein and tissue binding.

The metabolic process continues until the drug is completely altered into an active metabolite or into an inactive product. The process works toward making the drug molecule more water soluble *(hydrophilic)* with weaker ionization and thus less able to bind to protein, to cross membranes, or to be reabsorbed by the kidney.

The microsomal portion of the liver produces many of the enzymes active in drug metabolism. These enzymes may be induced or stimulated, resulting in faster metabolism or may be inhibited, thus slowing metabolism. Certain functions of the microsomal portion of the liver are further slowed during pregnancy, which delays metabolism of some medications. In addition, the gallbladder becomes hypotonic in response to the effect of estrogen. This effect may delay excretion of certain drugs that pass through the bile.

Drugs not completely metabolized may be excreted through bile into the intestine and then reabsorbed into

the circulation to pass a second time through the liver. This **enterohepatic recycling** is responsible for the delay in excretion of many drugs in the newborn infant, as well (Ohning, 1995b).

Metabolism in the Placenta

The placenta has a role in metabolism, especially of endogenous hormones (e.g., androgen to estrogen, maternal cholesterol to pregnenolone and then to progesterone). In a few cases drugs that compete for metabolic activity in the placenta may alter steroid production enough to interrupt the function of important hormones that control fetal development (Ward and Mirkin, 1994).

EXCRETION

In addition to feces, a major route of excretion is via the kidneys into the urine. Drugs also are excreted through saliva, respired air, and perspiration, but these are relatively minor pathways. An increase of 50% in renal circulation occurs by the second trimester. The rate is altered by body position (the supine position reduces blood flow to the renal arteries). In addition, the glomerular filtration rate is increased even more during pregnancy, a factor that allows increased excretion of waste products without changing the urine volume. Because of increased circulation to the kidney, drugs that are normally excreted in an unaltered state may be lost from the body more quickly during pregnancy.

It is interesting that a drug may be excreted by the fetus into amniotic fluid. From there it may slowly diffuse back across the amnion or may accumulate in amniotic fluid. The drug in the amniotic fluid may also be swallowed by the fetus and reabsorbed into fetal circulation, then passed across the placenta to finally be metabolized and excreted by the mother. For example, penicillins and meperidine have been found in higher amounts in amniotic fluid than in maternal or fetal blood (Simone, Derewlany, Koren, 1994).

TEST *Yourself* 16-2 _____

a. Which types of drugs move most easily across membrane barriers?
b. What are the implications of drug equilibrium on both sides of the placenta, especially during the late labor phase?

TRANSITION PRECAUTIONS FOR THE NEWBORN

All during pregnancy, the woman's body completely handles drug metabolism and excretion for the fetus. If labor begins when a woman has an active, free drug in her system, depending on the serum concentration and the time of birth in relation to her last dose, the infant may be born with nearly the maternal serum level. Newborn pharmacokinetics are different from the adult. Drugs may undergo enterohepatic recycling and in the infant usually take many hours longer to be metabolized and excreted. Thus a maternal dose is always many times too great a dose for the newborn system to handle alone (Ohning, 1995b). Therefore, in the transition period of labor and birth, doses must be spaced in relation to expected time of birth. The $t_{1/2}$ is compared with the expected time of birth to determine when the medication (usually analgesia) should be given. This is an example of the **time-dose interval.**

It is important to remember that if the woman receives medications by continuous intravenous infusion, levels at birth will be almost equal in mother and infant. Fortunately, because of fetal circulation patterns, the fetal brain is somewhat protected. However, delayed infant responses to drugs during recovery will be assessed by Apgar scores, acid-base values, and later by neurobehavioral testing (Datta, 1995).

Negative Effects of Certain Drugs on the Fetus

Drug effects during labor may be detected by changes in fetal heart rates and rhythms. After birth, reflex responses and muscle tone are inhibited by sedatives, analgesics, and magnesium sulfate. Infants may have normal respiratory responses at birth and then in the nursery may become depressed in tone and vital signs. The infant must metabolize the maternal dose on its own and may take up to a week or more to do so.

Anesthetics

Depending on the time-dose interval, most anesthetics cross the placenta and exert a sedative effect. The time-dose interval is critical with general anesthetics. Subtle newborn neurobehavioral changes have been extensively documented for anesthetics and for narcotic analgesics.

Anticoagulants

Warfarin and coumarin are not used during pregnancy. Heparin does not cross the placental barrier so it is considered safe. Doses should end shortly before birth to protect the mother. Aspirin in large doses may precipitate fetal bleeding or delay labor.

Antidiabetic agents

Insulin does not cross the placenta, but fetal hyperglycemia with fetal production of insulin will precipitate *hypoglycemia* in the first few hours after birth.

Antithyroid agents

The fetal thyroid gland may be sensitive to maternal medications (iodides, propylthiouracil) that may cause thyroid imbalance in the fetus. All newborns are tested for thyroid levels because mental retardation may result from low levels.

Psychotropic agents

No psychotropic drug has been proven entirely safe for use during pregnancy. Because the blood flow to the fetal brain is higher and the lipoid sheath is less restrictive, fetal exposure to these drugs may be rapid and complete. The neonate may have tachycardia, tachypnea, urinary retention, irritability, tremors, and even convulsions. *Lithium* may lead to hypotonia and cyanosis in the newborn. The dose should be reduced as labor begins and serum levels monitored closely in the mother and newborn.

Diazepam and *chlordiazepoxide* may depress the neonate and lead to hypotonia, poor suck and listlessness. Diazepam doses above 30 mg lead to hypothermia. *Phenothiazines* are used during labor as adjuncts to narcotic analgesia. In low doses there probably is no adverse effect on the infant.

Drugs of abuse

Alcohol, heroin, cocaine, crack, or methadone if present in high levels during the transition period will lead to withdrawal signs in the newborn. See Chapter 27 for details on the care of the infant exposed to these drugs during the prenatal period.

USE OF OXYTOCICS DURING LABOR

Oxytocin

Oxytocin is a normal body hormone synthesized in the hypothalamus and secreted from the posterior pituitary. Its effect is blocked by progesterone so that as the end of pregnancy nears, a gradual reduction in this block is noted. Contractions are slowly strengthened in proportion to the decrease in progesterone from the "aging" placenta. Oxytocin is inactivated by *oxytocinase,* making its $t_{1/2}$ 10 to 12 minutes in early pregnancy and 1 to 6 minutes in late pregnancy (Shyken and Petrie, 1996).

Oxytocin receptors are found in the myometrium and mammary epithelium. These receptors increase progressively and rapidly to a peak during the second stage of labor. Naturally occurring amounts are present during labor (2 to 3 mU/min), and the fetus contributes oxytocin as well. Based on this physiology, external synthetic oxytocin must be administered in very dilute concentrations when used during labor. Oxytocin receptors become saturated within approximately 40 minutes of the start of the infusion (Brodsky and Pelzar, 1991). With excessive doses, uterine muscle fibrillation and uterine hyperstimulation will reduce oxygen to the fetus, and fetal distress will occur. Oxytocin also has a relaxing effect on vascular smooth muscle. Therefore bolus administration or rapid, high doses may initiate hypotension and tachycardia in the woman in labor (see Drug Profile 16-1).

Induction

Labor is started (induction) or, when inadequate contractions are present, labor is intensified (stimulated) by oxytocin. For induction, the processes of prelabor, which normally take several weeks, occur over several hours and up to a few days. The cervix must efface and begin dilation. With induction, the total pressure needed to dilate the cervix completely is the same as for spontaneous labor. But the contractions may be more intense, more frequent, and longer in duration.

There should be medical reasons for induction. Induction for convenience—"babies by appointment"—is not good practice. Medical induction done for fetal or maternal reasons may rescue a fetus from a poor uterine environment. The most usual indications are fetoplacental insufficiency caused by preeclampsia, hypertension, diabetic or renal disease, prolonged pregnancy of more than 42 weeks, mild antepartal hemorrhage, intrauterine growth retardation or death, and Rh sensitization.

Labor may be stimulated when uterine contractions are inefficient after labor has begun. The method for labor stimulation is similar to that for induction (Procedure 16-1). There is a great deal of controversy about the "active management" of labor. This approach uses early artificial rupture of membranes and frequent, higher incremental doses of oxytocin in an attempt to speed fetal descent. Uterine hyperstimulation occurs significantly more often in the high-dose group and cesarean delivery is required more often for fetal distress (Shyken and Petrie, 1996). Currently, the low-dose method appears to be physiologic and follows the natural pattern of oxytocin release during labor.

When using oxytocin induction the nurse needs to consider the following points:

- Because of increased discomfort, few clients can tolerate oxytocin-augmented contractions and remain in control. Therefore some type of analgesia may be needed.
- Oxytocin sensitivity depends on the number of receptors and varies markedly from person to person and from phase to phase of labor.
- Labor may be substantially shortened and may move toward delivery more rapidly than expected. Therefore close observation and use of the contraction monitor is mandatory.
- There will be more pressure on the presenting part, less recovery time between contractions, and a greater possibility of fetal distress. Close observation of the fetal monitor strip is important.

Prostaglandin Preparation of the Cervix

The starting dose of oxytocin may be low because prostaglandin E_2 (PGE_2) is used to prepare the cervix. Instillation of low-dose PGE_2 gel at the cervix will ripen it (thin and soften) in preparation for induction. Prostaglandin F_2 (PGF_2) and PGE_2 are normal body hormones active in

Box 16-1

DRUG PROFILE

Oxytocin (Pitocin, Syntocinon)

ACTION

Naturally occurring hormone from posterior pituitary, blocked by progesterone until approaching labor. Acts on oxytocin receptor sites in myofibrils of uterus. Receptor sites rapidly proliferate as labor approaches and during labor. Acts on myoepithelial cells during breastfeeding to trigger let-down reflex. Inactivated by oxytocinase with short $t^1/_2$.

DOSAGE AND ROUTE

Stimulation and Induction during Labor

Diluted: 10 U (1 mL) in 500-1000 mL normal saline or Ringer's lactate solution. By secondary line and controlled by IV pump. Initial rate of 0.5 to 1.0 mU/min. Doubled dose rate q40-60min until reach 8 mU/min. Never more than 20 mU/min. Must be titrated with client response.

Prevention Postbirth Hemorrhage

10 to 20 U in 1000 mL IV solution at no more than 250 ml/hr, or IM, *but not both.*

SIDE EFFECTS AND ADVERSE EFFECTS

During Induction

Hypertonic contractions cause reduced placental perfusion, fetal distress, and maternal pain. May require emergency cesarean delivery. If fetal distress: d/c Pitocin at once, position woman on side, give O_2 by mask, notify physician.

Postbirth

With too rapid infusion, tachycardia and hypotension or hypertension may occur. Antidiuretic effect of oxytocin may cause oliguria and fluid overload or arrhythmias, water intoxication, poor output, n/v headache. Follow I & O carefully, vital signs.

d/c, Discontinue; *IM,* intramuscular; *I & O,* intake and output; *IV,* intravenous; *n/v,* nausea and vomiting.

initiating and sustaining labor. The $t^1/_2$ of prostaglandins is short, but initially when higher oral doses were used for induction, adverse effects of uterine hypertonic contractions occurred. Therefore high doses of PGF_2 are limited to late abortion or cases of intrauterine fetal death (see Chapter 21 and Drug Profile 16-2). Nevertheless, to avoid the potential of uterine hyperstimulation even with the current low-dose preparatory period, the start of oxytocin-infusion should not begin until after 4 hours of the last PGE_2 gel application (Shyken and Petrie, 1996).

PROCEDURE 16-1

Induction

1. Prepare solution of either 500 or 1000 mL Ringer's lactate or normal saline solution by adding 10 U (1 mL) oxytocin (depending on unit protocol).

2. Flush secondary line tubing and thread through IV pump chamber. Label bag with dose, date, and time.

3. Calculate flow rate, remembering there are 1000 milliunits (mU) in 1 unit of oxytocin. Use the following formula for a 10 U in 1000 mL solution with a 0.5 mU/min starting rate.

$$\frac{0.5\ mU}{1\ min} \times \frac{1\ U}{1000\ mU} \times \frac{1000\ mL}{10\ U} = 0.05\ mL/min$$

4. Be sure induction permit is signed and order is written. (Many units require the certified nurse midwife [CNM] or attending physician to initiate dose and increments and to be on call in the maternity unit in case of adverse effects.)

5. Initiate the secondary oxytocin flow after evaluating contractions and fetal heart rate and the initial procedures in the protocol are completed.
   - Medical reasons are determined and documented by the physician or CNM.
   - A baseline monitor strip is obtained, evaluated, and documented.

6. Evaluate at 15 and 30 min after initial dose and then as unit protocol requires.

7. Each increase by physician, CNM, or nurse must follow step-by-step increments. Never skip a step.

8. Check bedside monitor for at least 20 min to evaluate contraction response. When effective labor rate reached, stop increments. Never more than 20 mU/min.

9. Reduce increments or stop Pitocin flow at any sign of late decelerations, variable decelerations, or reduced variability in FHR.

10. Documentation on monitor strip includes time of start, each increase, and stop. Observations q15min initially, then q30min during active labor.

11. Documentation on bedside notes include: maternal vital signs, examinations and results, procedures, position changes, and maternal activity interfering with tracing. Note time physician or CNM notified of changes and time of response. Check maternal BP every hour or with each dose increase.

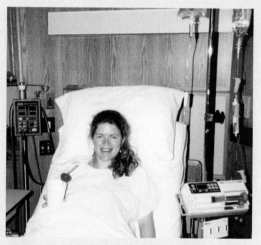

Woman in labor receiving stimulation with oxytocin. Note oral fluid intake and set up of piggyback oxytocin infusion and pump.

OPTIONAL ACTIVITY

Write a sample nursing note correctly documenting performance of this procedure.

Beginning with a solution of 10 U of oxytocin in 1000 mL of lactated Ringer's solution, via volumetric pump, the piggyback tubing is connected to the most proximal port on the mainline IV. (This precaution allows immediate cessation of the flow by turning off the pump if adverse reactions occur). The rate of flow begins at 0.5 milliunits per minute (mU/min). At intervals of 40 to 60 minutes, the rate is doubled until 8 mU/min rate is reached. Then, at the same intervals, increments of 2 to 4 mU/min are set by the physician or nurse midwife. The peak dose will rarely be >20 mU/min. The oxytocin dose is titrated during induction (adjusted in relation to the client's response). The desired contraction rate is the following:

- Frequency 2 to 3 minutes
- Intensity between 40 and 90 mm Hg
- Duration between 40 and 90 seconds
- Resting tone < 15 to 20 mm Hg

When labor is stimulated later in the first stage or early second stage, the same guidelines apply. Each labor unit has a protocol that must be followed to avoid adverse effects. More *is not* better in oxytocin usage. In fact, many patients can have oxytocin infusion decreased or discontinued after active labor is well established (Box 16-1).

If an adverse effect occurs, discontinue the piggyback flow by turning off the pump (remember the short $t_{1/2}$).

Box 16-2

DRUG PROFILE

Prostaglandin E₂ (Prostin E₂ Gel, Dinoprostone)

ACTION

Mediates cervical effacement through connective tissue changes. Prepares cervix for induction. Used when Bishop score < 4.

DOSAGE AND ROUTE

For Cervix Prelabor Preparation

Prostin E₂ gel 0.5 mg placed into cervix by syringe with flexible catheter or into posterior fornix of vagina. Physician or CNM reapplies q8h for a total of three doses as needed. Client must remain recumbent for 30-60 min after application and FHR must be monitored.

To Induce Labor in Case of Second Trimester Abortion or IUFD

Vaginal suppository dinoprostone 20 mg placed into posterior fornix q3h until labor established.

SIDE EFFECTS AND ADVERSE EFFECTS

Rare: hypertonic contractions within 1 hr after application. To treat: swab vagina with gauze sponge. May need tocolysis with terbutaline 0.25 mg SC/IV plus oxygen and position change to support fetal oxygenation. Nausea and diarrhea may be treated with prochlorperazine or kaolin.

IUFD, Intrauterine fetal death.

Intervene as described in Chapter 14 with position changes, oxygen by mask, and an increase in mainline IV fluids. Observe results of interventions. Notify the obstetrician or midwife of these actions and the client's responses. Terbutaline as a *tocolytic* may be used if excessive uterine contraction frequency or intensity *(hypertonus)* persists (see Chapter 21).

TEST *Yourself* 16-3

There is a concentration of 20 U oxytocin in 500 mL of IV fluid. The order reads: Increase infusion rate to 3 mU/mL. For the client to receive this amount, set the pump rate for the secondary line to give ___ mL/min or ___ mL/hr.

PAIN DURING LABOR

Each woman's pain perception is unique, and women's responses vary widely. There always have been nonpharmacologic "complementary therapies" for labor pain. Only in the last 100 years has the idea of a pain-free labor begun to be a reality.

Box 16-1

WARNING SIGNS

Adverse Effects of Oxytocin

Warning signs of adverse effects in the first stage of labor include the following:
- Contractions more frequent than every 2 minutes
- Intensity >90 mm Hg
- Duration >90 seconds
- Rising resting tone >20 mm Hg
- Fetal tachycardia, bradycardia, or altered beat-to-beat variability

Responses to Labor Pain

Pain studies have shown changes in pain intensity and location during labor; these changes vary from hour to hour. In addition, Melzack et al (1984) found the following:

1. A correlation exists between history of severe menstrual pain and more pain in the first and subsequent labors.
2. Childbirth preparation tends to allow a woman to cope, to remain in control, and thus to be able to describe her pain as more manageable, even though it may be as intense as that experienced by an unprepared woman.
3. Usually primiparas complain of more painful labors than do multiparas. If, however, a woman weighs more than usual and has a larger baby than expected, pain levels may be increased.
4. Finally, there is no correlation of pain levels with duration of labor unless fatigue occurs.

Pain threshold

A high pain threshold may be explained somewhat by the opiate peptides, beta-endorphins, and enkephalins (Blackburn and Loper, 1992). These substances are natural analgesics. Cahill (1989) suggests that beta-endorphins do not eliminate but blunt the perception of pain. Just before labor, endogenous **endorphin** levels normally rise. A woman who enters labor at term, is knowledgeable about the procedures and process, and is accompanied by a support person often can tolerate labor discomfort well.

Cultural expectations seem to affect pain behaviors and a person's perception of the intensity of pain (Lowe, 1996). Cultural responses may override "normal" pain responses; some women are taught to be stoic while others are taught to cry out. Nurses must not impose their own cultural assumptions on their clients and should not be misled by client responses about the phase of labor and the pain intensity (Weber, 1996). Cultural comfort with the caregiver is enhanced if the nurse acknowledges cultural variations and is culturally competent for the different populations encountered in the care setting. This competence includes learning body language, spoken language, and preferences for labor support.

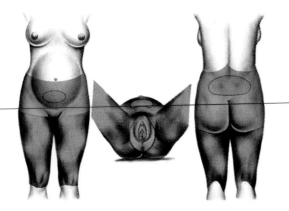

Figure 16-5   There are changing areas and intensities of pain sensations during labor. Transition phase is the most difficult. (From Lowdermilk DL, Perry SE, Bobak IM: *Maternity and women's health care,* ed 6, St Louis, 1997, Mosby.)

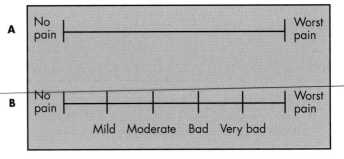

Figure 16-6   Visual analog scale (VAS) **(A)** and a combined verbal and visual analog scale **(B).** Usually 10 cm, this scale is smaller here. (Redrawn from Jorgenson Dick MJ: Assessment and measurement of acute pain, *J Obstet Gynecol Neonatal Nurs* 24(6):843, 1995.)

It is difficult to assess the level of pain from observation because people respond differently to altered comfort. Using a visual analog scale (VAS) (see Figure 16-6) allows the woman to compare and describe her degree of pain (Jorgenson Dick, 1995). According to Moore (1983), responses to labor-related pain may be influenced by the following factors:

- Usual level of anxiety and responses to stress
- Feelings of self-worth and femininity
- Significance of pregnancy (welcomed or not)
- Feelings passed on to the woman by her mother
- Experience with a previous childbirth
- Anxiety about risk factors or illness
- Level of education and preparation for childbirth
- Actual progress through labor phases
- Presence of a support person
- Perceived support of health care personnel

Sleep loss and exhaustion influence pain perception. The young adolescent may have less pain tolerance because of these factors and especially high anxiety, feelings of low self-worth, lack of maturity and knowledge, and fear for self. Finally, researchers have recognized that a history of sexual abuse influences a woman's responses to labor and birth (see Chapter 27).

Model of pain

Loeser's model of pain (1982) may help the nurse support a woman in labor. Loeser uses four parameters for pain analysis: nociception, pain, suffering, and pain behavior. **Nociceptors** are free nerve endings that generate pain impulses. Therefore the term **nociception** indicates the causative factors for pain impulses. Use of this model requires consideration of the following factors during pain assessment:

Nociception: What are the physiologic causes that initiate pain signals? Assess the phase of labor and any abnormality in progress or position. Is the pain visceral or somatic?

Pain: What is the client's description of what she feels?
    Subjective: Have her describe location and intensity.
    Objective: Check changes in vital signs, intensity of contractions, and restlessness.

Suffering: What are her responses to pain, and what significance is attached to it? Is she angry, upset, guilty, stoic, or crying? What is her emotional response to the pain?

Pain behaviors: How does she act? How does she express tension? What brings her relief?

The nurse might provide an outline of the body similar to those in Figure 16-5 and ask the woman to point to where it hurts and describe the pain. The nurse can also use the visual analog scale (VAS) (Figure 16-6). Then comfort measures can be made specific.

Physiologic Factors

Stress produces a rise in cortisol and catecholamine levels. All nurses have observed anxious women who are tense, restless, and frightened. Hypertension, hyperventilation, and increased oxygen use may occur during severe stress and will increase sympathetic activity and norepinephrine release (Blackburn and Loper, 1992). Thus stress leads to a lowering of the pain threshold. Labor always exerts stress on the woman. For these reasons the nurse uses supportive measures that calm the woman.

Two different kinds of pain occur during labor. **Visceral pain** generally is experienced during active dilation and is related to cervical stretching and uterine contraction intensity. **Somatic pain** is related to pressure on and stretching of the birth canal as descent occurs. There is an overlapping of sensations, but observation of a woman in labor reveals changes in her perception of pain.

Visceral pain

Visceral pain may be transmitted slowly (through unmyelinated fibers) and felt as dull, diffuse, persistent, or

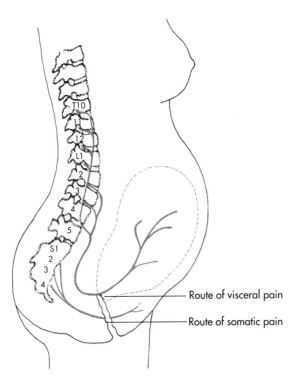

Figure 16-7   Pathways of pain during labor. (Courtesy Abbott Laboratories.)

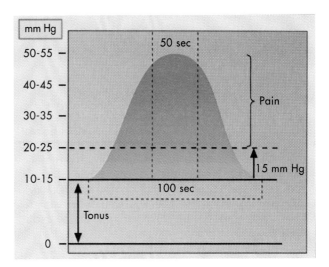

Figure 16-8   Pain is felt when the contraction pressure rises above 15 mm Hg resting tone.

aching sensations. Pain sensations conveyed through myelinated fibers travel more rapidly and are perceived as sharp, localized sensations. During the first stage of labor the nerve impulses enter the sympathetic chain at L1 to L5 and then travel to the posterior roots of the tenth, eleventh, and twelfth thoracic nerves and up the spinal cord to the thalamus (Figure 16-7).

There also may be *referred pain* through the dermatomes of the same nerves. Pain is felt in the skin, thighs, lower back, hips, and "hot" spots of generalized aching. Part of this pain is pressure induced; some may be related to fatigue and hypoxia of the uterine muscle. During labor, these areas of referred pain change location. If labor is prolonged, uterine fatigue factors will increase pain sensations.

Pain caused by contractions is felt when the contraction intensity rises 15 to 20 mm Hg above the resting tonus (Figure 16-8). Therefore one looks for pain at intensities above 25 mm Hg pressure on the monitor strip. (External contraction monitoring does not give an accurate picture of the actual intensity of the contraction. Sometimes the mother appears not to be in effective labor and yet is having painful contractions.) There should be less discomfort during rest periods. If there is continuing acute discomfort, the problem should be investigated.

Somatic pain

Somatic pain usually begins during the transition phase because descent increases the pressure of the fetus on the cervical, vaginal, and perineal tissues. First felt by the woman as a need to bear down, this sensation may become overpowering. These pain sensations travel primarily via pudendal nerves through the dorsal roots of the second, third, and fourth sacral nerves.

Application of the gate control theory of pain. The gate control theory states that a neural mechanism in the dorsal horn of the spinal cord can control the flow of neural impulses to the brain. The degree with which stimuli through the larger nerves override more diffuse stimuli from smaller nerves will allow the "gate" to inhibit the transmission of pain sensations. Sensations from massage, effleurage, pressure, heat, and cold can be used to inhibit transmission of pain sensations. However, the large nerve fibers become "habituated," and techniques need to be *rotated* or changed as labor progresses (Blackburn and Loper, 1992).

 Box **16-1**

CLINICAL DECISION

Jenny is in labor and experiencing a considerable amount of discomfort. Choose the word from the Loeser model of pain to describe each of the following:
a. Jenny is restless, moaning, and turning from side to side.
b. She has been recently examined and is 7-cm dilated; contractions occur every 3 minutes and last 70 seconds. Station is +1.
c. She cries out and says, "My tail bone is breaking!"
d. She clings to her partner's hand saying, "Don't leave me!"

CULTURAL AWARENESS

CRYING DURING LABOR

Some Indian women cry throughout labor. In India, men were nearby but never in the room during childbirth. Here the partner may be at the bedside, perhaps against his real inclination and cultural values. (The nurse should remember that he needs support and explanations of the labor process.) The opposite extreme is found in some Asian women who control crying or any sound, although their pain may be intense. The Asian father may refuse to be at the bedside, because birth is thought to be exclusively women's territory.

Complementary Therapies to Enhance Comfort

Transcutaneous electric nerve stimulation

Transcutaneous electric nerve stimulation (TENS) during labor has been used in some settings and is commonly used in Canada and Europe. The emphasis on continuous fetal monitoring may have limited its adoption for labor in this country. TENS does not interfere with monitoring unless used at a high intensity (Benden, 1993). TENS is effective with chronic pain by stimulating release of beta-endorphins. It allows the client to control the level of stimulation, which helps her to cope. Clients oriented before labor are more comfortable with its use (Figure 16-9).

One pair of electrodes is applied to either side of the spine at T10 to T11 for uterine pain in the first part of labor. For later labor and transition, the electrodes may be moved to S2 to S4. For the second stage, the electrodes may be kept at the sacral level and another pair applied suprapubically. During a contraction the woman or her partner control the intensity of the stimulus until a tingling occurs. TENS is said to have the analgesic effect of 75 to 100 mg of meperidine. It is more effective in active labor than in transition, according to one study (Grim and Morey, 1985). Because it is especially effective for back pain, it may be the choice for labor when the fetus is in a posterior position.

Pressure and touch

The use of touch in a purposeful way to bring reassurance or reduce pain sensation has been used in varying childbirth methods. *Effleurage,* light stroking of the skin, is an accepted method of alternative sensation (see Chapter 12). Touch as a means of reassurance has been used by placing a hand on the fundus of the uterus while questioning the woman about her feelings and sensations (Simkin, 1995). Comfort of touch by the birth partner is reassuring (see Chapter 13).

Acupressure has been effective during labor. There are three points: first, as seen in Figure 16-10, between the first and second metacarpal bones on the dorsum of the

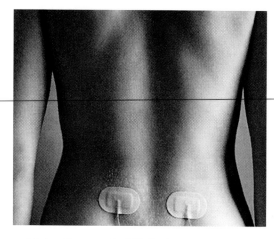

Figure 16-9 One site for TENS electrode placement during labor. (Courtesy 3M HealthCare, Minneapolis, Minn.)

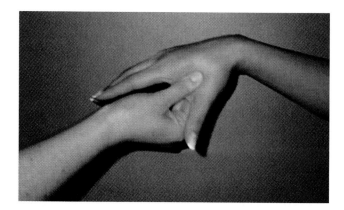

Figure 16-10 Site of one acupressure point for labor pain.

hand; second, behind the tibia; and third, below the tibial tuberosity (Belluomini, 1994).

Counterpressure to the sacrum can be applied by means of the heel of the hand, a clenched fist, or a tennis ball. Firm pressure or deep massage can be applied to the sacrum, the symphysis pubis, or over the borders of the ilium when the pain has shifted downward in late labor.

Acupuncture is a branch of Asian medicine not in common use for labor in this country. However, acupuncture has been used to augment or lessen labor contractions and provide analgesia. In China, cesarean delivery has been conducted under acupuncture anesthesia.

Other therapies

Heat and cold. Hot or cold compresses are useful during labor. Heat may be applied on the abdomen, groin, or perineum. Icepacks may be applied to the area over the bladder to stimulate voiding, or to the area over the clitoris, anus, or entire perineum to reduce the sensations during final pushing. Currently, the use of *hydrotherapy,* a warm bath or shower during parts of the labor process, is popular (see Chapter 12).

Imagery, visualization, and meditation. The use of meditation to enhance focus during labor has been helpful to many women. Those women from cultures familiar with meditative techniques should be encouraged to prepare themselves to use this method for pain relief. A woman can bring a visual focal point with her to the labor area or imagine a scene in which pain does not exist. Nursing intervention may be to suggest imagery. These techniques need to be practiced, as does biofeedback, before the time of birth (Geden et al, 1989; Duchene, 1989).

Distraction. Essentially, the breathing techniques and relaxation responses learned during childbirth education are a basic form of distraction or *alternate attention*. The nurse needs to support the specific learned methods and not try to correct the woman's technique. Audioanalgesia, which uses earphones and favorite music, acts as a distractor (Geden et al, 1989).

Finally, basic comfort measures aid in increasing tolerance for labor discomfort. Cleanliness, a dry bed, frequent changes of position including ambulation (see Figure 13-16), encouragement to void frequently, adjustment of lights, and reduction in noise will all aid the laboring woman. Biofeedback has been explored to reduce tension during labor (Bernat et al, 1992; Duchene, 1989).

PHARMACOLOGIC METHODS OF ANALGESIA

The term **analgesia** indicates a reduction of pain without loss of consciousness. Until recently, analgesia during labor had resulted in many side effects for the mother and infant because significantly high doses were given IM or IV. The effect of large doses may cause reduced fetal movements and poor beat-to-beat variability as seen on the fetal monitor. These drugs pass easily to the fetus and more readily pass the blood-brain barrier. The younger the fetus, the more it will be depressed. Now, with the advent of newer drugs such as fentanyl and bupivacaine, effective doses are smaller and side effects much less evident.

Drugs are chosen for labor analgesia on the basis of the duration of action so that the time-dose interval may be better controlled before delivery. The timing of analgesics in labor is important. The drug should be timed to allow metabolism and excretion before delivery. When this has not happened, a narcotic antagonist may need to be given to the infant to reverse respiratory depression.

Opioid Analgesics

All opioids cause approximately the same analgesic effect in **equigesic doses**. Opiates vary widely in dosage but may cause nausea and vomiting, itching, hypotension, and respiratory depression.

Morphine is the analgesic whose effectiveness in alleviating pain is the standard against which synthetic narcotics are measured. This classic drug is effective as a central nervous system depressant. It may trigger the vomiting center. Morphine may be administered through the epidural catheter for labor analgesia or via the intrathecal route for postoperative analgesia in small doses, but it is not given IM or IV during labor because effective doses depress the infant's respiratory center.

Morphine is used most often as a postepidural "morphine wash." A small dose (0.1-0.3 mg) is inserted into the epidural catheter before it is removed. Analgesia is provided for 12 to 18 hours after a cesarean birth. Follow the precautions listed with epidural analgesia, later in this chapter.

Meperidine (Pethidine, Demerol) acts in many ways like morphine, although it is less effective in relieving severe pain (see Drug Profile 16-3). It has equally depressant effects on respirations at equal analgesic doses. It depresses fetal activity and slightly increases the fre-

Box 16-3
DRUG PROFILE

Meperidine (Pethidine, Demerol)

ACTION

Depresses pain impulse transmission at the spinal cord via opioid receptors. Works best with visceral pain. Slight relaxant effect on intestinal and vascular smooth muscle. $t_{1/2}$ is 1-2 hrs depending on route. Time-dose interval is important when used in labor. Almost always is given with antianxiety agent to potentiate small dose and counteract nausea when given IM or IV.

DOSAGE AND ROUTE

Labor: 25 to 50 mg IM with promethazine 12.5 to 25 mg. If given IV, dilute same dose in 5 mL saline, and give slow IV push over 4 to 5 min.
Postoperatively: cesarean, give 75 to 100 mg q2-3hr IM. Smaller doses via epidural or PCEA.

SIDE EFFECTS AND ADVERSE EFFECTS

Labor dose: hypotension, dizziness, confusion, headache, euphoria; nausea and vomiting, blurred vision; rash, diaphoresis, flushing. Delays stomach emptying. Equilibrium with fetus within 6 min IV dose. Respiratory depression may occur in neonate but rarely in woman. Naloxone is the antidote.

PRECAUTIONS

Additive with other narcotic agents, recreational drugs, alcohol, sedatives, and general anesthesia. Check monitor carefully for signs of contractions or fetal distress because changes may occur. Bedrest for an hour after IM or IV single-dose use. Maintain side rails if there is no attendant.

PCEA, Patient-controlled epidural analgesia; $t_{1/2}$, half-life.

quency and duration of contractions (Zimmer, Divon, and Vadasz, 1988).

Meperidine works best on visceral pain and has a slight relaxant effect on intestinal and vascular smooth muscle. Hypotension and nausea tend to occur, especially when it is given IV. Postural hypotension and tachycardia also may occur, and voiding may be inhibited.

Meperidine has been studied extensively. Its IV onset is within 5 minutes with its peak at 1 to 1½ hours after administration. Only low doses are used during labor (25-50 mg), often combined with an antianxiety agent because high doses of meperidine depress newborn respirations. The highest amount of the drug is found in the fetus 2 to 3 hours later, and *normeperidine,* a metabolite with depressive effects, is at the highest level at 4 hours after larger maternal doses (Kuhnert et al, 1979).

If the dose is timed correctly to enable the drug to be almost completely metabolized and excreted by the mother before birth, meperidine may be useful during labor. Some women do not react well; if the woman gets more restless and does not obtain adequate relief, further doses of the drug are not given, and an alternate analgesic is used. Meperidine also is currently used in epidural and intrathecal analgesia in combination with a local anesthetic.

Fentanyl (Sublimaze) is a narcotic analgesic 100 times more potent than meperidine: 1 mg is equivalent to 10 mg morphine or 100 mg meperidine. Onset is rapid and duration of action is 1 to 2 hours. It may be used IM or IV but is most commonly used now as part of the epidural analgesic or anesthetic dose. If respiratory depression occurs, Naloxone is the antagonist.

Sufentanil (Sufenta) is 10 times as potent as fentanyl and is used only in epidural and intrathecal doses. It acts rapidly and has a short duration. See Drug Profile 16-4.

Butorphanol tartrate (Stadol) is used commonly in this country. This mixed agonist-antagonist analgesic with a duration of effect of 1 to 3 hours crosses the placental barrier but does not cause excessive residuals in the infant because metabolites are inactive (see Drug Profile 16-5). Some centers do not use butorphanol because there may be transient sinusoidal fetal heart rhythms (Datta, 1995). Observe for respiratory depression. Naloxone is the antidote.

Nalbuphine (Nubain) has been used in a similar way as butorphanol and belongs in the same agonist-antagonist class of drug. In a single 10-mg dose IV, or in increments of 3 mg via patient-controlled analgesia (PCA), nalbuphine in the first stage of labor gives better maternal analgesia than butorphanol (Datta, 1995). Observe for respiratory depression. Naloxone is the antidote.

Antianxiety Agents

Antianxiety agents may be used during labor to calm the client and to potentiate (increase the strength of) analgesic effects. When combined, the analgesic dose may be reduced at least by half. Several of these medications have

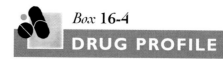

Box 16-4

DRUG PROFILE

Fentanyl (Sublimaze) and Sufentanil (Sufenta)

ACTION

Fentanyl (Sublimaze) is 100 times more potent than morphine or meperidine. Rapid-acting, short duration, up to 2 hr IM or 1 hr IV. Drug of choice for epidural analgesia with bupivacaine. Minimal motor blockade.

DOSAGE AND ROUTE

IM: 50 to 100 μg, IV 25 to 50 μg. Epidural route: 1 to 2 μg with bupivacaine 0.125% at rate of 8-10 mL/hr. May also be used for intrathecal analgesia by anesthetist.

SIDE EFFECTS AND ADVERSE EFFECTS

Dizziness, drowsiness, allergic reactions, rash, respiratory depression. Naloxone is antidote. Few side effects with epidural anesthesia.

ACTION

Sufentanil (Sufenta) is 10 times more potent than fentanyl and in the same class of action and effects. Has rapid onset and short duration.

DOSAGE AND ROUTE

Only as adjunct to anesthesia and used in epidural and intrathecal analgesia. 1 μg sufentanil combined with bupivacaine 0.125% at 10 mL/hr for epidural infusion during labor.

an antiemetic effect, as well. If given too close to the time of birth, the infant may have reduced muscle tone and a slightly lower temperature and respiratory rate. In small doses, however, no lasting effect has been recognized in the newborn infant (see Drug Profile 16-6).

Diazepam (Valium) is only used during the actual birth because of its effects on the fetus.

Opiate Antagonists

Naloxone (Narcan) is the current drug of choice of an antagonist to the depressing effects of narcotic analgesics (see Drug Profile 16-7). It lacks the morphinelike qualities that other antagonists have shown. Currently, it is used in a woman who has recently given birth to combat adverse effects of intrathecal or epidural analgesics. It acts to combat central nervous system and respiratory depression and reduces pruritis related to the narcotic dose.

The depressed newborn may be given 0.1 mg/kg ET or IV through the umbilical vein. The dose may be repeated while resuscitation is performed. The neonate should be observed carefully for a return of depression for as long as 6 to 8 hours later because naloxone metabolism is more rapid than that of the analgesics. Narcotic antagonists

Box 16-5

DRUG PROFILE

Butorphanol Tartrate (Stadol) and Nalbuphine (Nubaine)

BUTORPHANOL TARTRATE (STADOL)

Action

Depresses pain impulses by interacting with spinal cord opioid receptors. A mixed agonist-antagonist analgesic. Widely used for labor pain because metabolites are inactive in fetus. Peak at $^1/_2$ hr, duration: IM 3-4 hr, IV 2-3 hr. Crosses placenta and milk barriers. Time-dose interval is important. Naloxone is antidote.

Dosage and Route

IM 1-2 mg (deep injection) q3-4h or IV 0.5-1 mg q3-4h. Dilute IV dose with NS and give slow push as contraction subsides. IM onset 10-30 min. IV onset 1 min, duration 2-4 hr.

Side Effects and Adverse Effects

Nausea and vomiting, clamminess. Rarely headache, dizziness, tinnitus, lethargy, palpitation, slow pulse, and rash. Diminished urine output. Respiratory depression. Transient sinusoidal-like FHR rhythms.

Precautions

Increases effects of other narcotics, sedatives, skeletal muscle relaxants, and alcohol. Check I&O, vital signs, and fetal responses. Use side rails.

NALBUPHINE (NUBAIN)

Dosage and Route

10 mg IV, or in 3-mg increments via PCEA gives good analgesia during labor.

Side Effects and Adverse Effects

Similar to butorphanal tartrate, except does not have the side effect of sinusoidal FHR.

FHR, Fetal heart rate; *I&O,* intake and output; *NS,* normal saline; *PCEA,* patient-controlled epidural analgesia.

Box 16-6

DRUG PROFILE

Tranquilizers as Adjuncts to Analgesics

PROMETHAZINE (PHENERGAN)

Dosage

25-50 mg IM, onset 15-20 min, duration 3-4 hr
25 mg IV, onset 3-5 min, duration 2-3 hr

Maternal Effects

Antihistamine action adds extra sedation with narcotic; potentiates narcotic, allowing lower doses; stimulates respiration; decreases nausea and vomiting; some disorientation and hypotension; possible tachycardia; no effect on labor progress.

Fetal Effects

Central nervous system depression: equilibrates with maternal level within 15 min of IV solution; transitional effects depend on dosage.

DIAZEPAM (VALIUM)

Dosage

5-10 mg IM, onset 10-15 min, duration 5-7 hr
5-10 mg IV diluted in 5 ml NS injected slowly for 5 min, onset 2-3 min, duration 5-6 hr
Might be used by anesthetist if a difficult assisted vaginal birth or during cesarean.

Maternal Effects

Not used during labor, but may be given IV during delivery only. Potentiates any analgesic. Not recommended if mother is breast-feeding in early recovery period.

Fetal Effects

Will concentrate in fetus. Higher doses (>30 mg) affect thermoregulation in newborn for as long as 1 week. Observe vital signs during recovery.

NS, Normal saline.

---

reverse signs of drug use such as heroin or cocaine for a short time. Therefore it is important to observe early onset of severe withdrawal signs (see Chapters 19 and 27).

For the woman, *naltrexone,* 6 mg po, and *nalmefene,* 0.4 mg/70 kg IV, have been used with success to counteract side effects of epidural or intrathecal opiates.

ANESTHESIA

Anesthesia is a condition of lack of pain with or without loss of consciousness. Anesthetics may provide local or regional numbness, with loss of sensation to pain, or the result may be general muscle relaxation and loss of sensation and consciousness because of varying degrees of central nervous system depression.

Because the maternity client has special considerations for anesthesia, a prepared anesthesiologist should be on staff in birth centers. There is a variation in practice depending on the size of the hospital, the economic class of the client (Datta, 1992), and the availability of complete anesthesia coverage. Because births are unscheduled, it is not always possible to have an obstetric anesthesiologist present.

A woman entering the birth area may have heard of problems with anesthesia. Her concerns should not be dis-

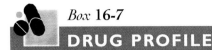

Box 16-7

DRUG PROFILE

Opiate Antagonists

NALOXONE (Narcan)

Action

Combats opiate central nervous system and respiratory depression by competing for receptor sites. Short acting, $t^1/_2$ I hr, therefore depression may reoccur. Useful combating respiratory depression associated with epidural narcotics intrapartum and postpartum and for neonatal respiratory depression.

Dosage and Route

Maternal

IV/SC/IM 0.4-2 mg, repeat q2-3min x 2, or 0.5 mg/hr in infusion.

Neonate

If asphyxiated at birth, 0.1 mg/kg into umbilical vein or endotracheal route; may repeat dose x 3 q2-3min. May also give IM or SC.

Side Effects and Adverse Effects

Maternal hypertension, tachycardia with high dose. Pulmonary edema if preexisting CV problems or other CV drugs are in use. Nausea and vomiting. Delay lactation until narcotics and naloxone out of system.

Precautions

Be sure client is not using other drugs of abuse. Reversal may be abrupt with tremulousness, sweating, nausea and vomiting, tachycardia, and hypertension.

NALTREXONE (Trexan) AND NALMEFENE (Cervene, revex)

Action

Used to counteract effects of epidural or intrathecal morphine. More commonly used to treat opiate addiction and overdose.

Dosage and Route

Naltrexone, 6 mg po. Rapid onset, $t^1/_2$ 4 hr. Excreted in breast milk.
Nalmefene 0.4 mg/70 kg IV.

CV, Cardiovascular; *PO,* by mouth; *SC,* subcutaneously; $t^1/_2$, half-life.

---

missed; rather, every effort should be made to be sure that she understands what medications she will be receiving.

The nurse who works in the birthing area needs to be particularly aware of types of anesthesia; expected and adverse reactions; and the roles of anesthesiologist, nurse anesthetist, obstetrician, and midwife. In addition, it is vital to understand the nurse's role and responsibilities in preparation for and care of the mother during and after anesthesia.

Local Anesthetics

Chemicals used as local anesthetics have the suffix *-caine* in the names. Preparations such as lidocaine, mepivacaine, dibucaine, and bupivacaine are *amides,* which are metabolized slowly and are protein bound and yet may slowly cross the placental barrier. Esters—procaine, chloroprocaine, tetracaine, and cocaine—are metabolized swiftly and are not commonly used in obstetrics. Local anesthetics are used in lower concentrations and in smaller doses for birth than in other operative situations because the fetus may be affected, depending on the rate of transfer across the placenta. Adverse effects in the infant are inhibited muscle tone and responsiveness, with metabolites continuing in the infant's system for long periods (Datta, 1995).

Infiltration

Local infiltration provides a pain-free area for episiotomy or repair of lacerations. A few minutes for absorption must be allowed before the procedure begins. The woman will sense the tugging and pulling of surrounding tissue and will expect to feel pain. A simple explanation may help her to relax during suturing.

Adverse Maternal Reactions

Local anesthetics cause varying degrees of vasodilation. Depending on the location and concentration of the medication, hypotension may occur. Mild reactions include dizziness, palpitations, and headache. In rare instances, if the solution enters the circulation in significant amounts, excitement, apprehension, tachycardia, disorientation, tremors, and, rarely, convulsions may occur. The fetus may show bradycardia. Some persons have hypersensitivity ranging from allergic dermatitis to bronchospasm to anaphylactic reaction. Because of these possibilities, a *test dose* is always given before administration of the full dose, and the smallest effective amount is chosen. The client always should be asked about prior experiences with local anesthetics in her dental visits.

REGIONAL ANESTHESIA

Local anesthetics may be injected to block a group of nerves leading to a region of the body. Medication is injected into or around a nerve pathway or at the plexus of the nerve.

Pudendal Block

The pudendal block provides effective regional anesthesia for the second stage of labor and for delivery. The pudendal nerve plexus lies just above and behind the

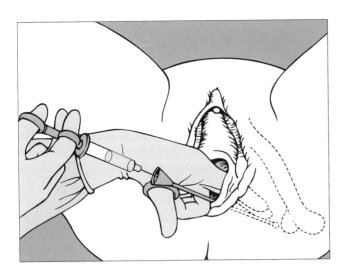

Figure 16-11   Pudendal block. (From Lowdermilk DL, Perry SE, Bobak IM: *Maternity and women's health care,* ed 6, St Louis, 1997, Mosby.)

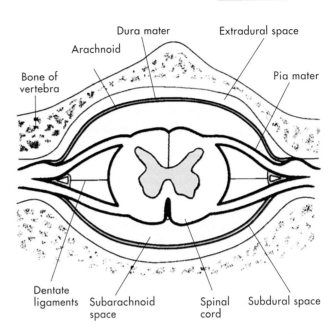

Figure 16-12   Cross-section through spinal cord and its membranes. (From Luciano D, Vander AJ, Sherman JH: *Human anatomy and physiology,* New York, 1983, McGraw-Hill.)

ischial spines, and the nerve itself supplies sensation to the whole perineal area. A block eliminates most of the *somatic pain* of tissue pressure and stretching, but the woman will still feel the *visceral pain* of contractions and is still able to bear down. The block must be done 5 to 10 minutes before delivery to gain the full effect. If time is not sufficient, the delivery may be painful, but later suturing will be painless. Pudendal block usually is sufficient for low forceps delivery but not for more extensive manipulation. A pudendal block may be administered by the midwife or obstetrician (Figure 16-11).

Because the area is vascular, anesthetic absorption may slightly affect vital signs. There is no limitation on movement after delivery. The anesthetic should wear off in less than an hour. Observe for bladder distention because some lingering anesthetic effect may inhibit voiding during the immediate recovery period.

Epidural Anesthesia

The term **epidural** is applied to either a lumbar or caudal insertion site. The epidural (extradural) space runs the length of the spine and is located between the dura mater and the periosteal layer (Figure 16-12). There are blood vessels in the space, and during pregnancy the veins running through this space are slightly dilated from increased blood volume. As a result, less medication must be used, and there is a slightly greater risk of injecting one of these vessels.

The anesthetic fluid should encircle the dura mater, affecting the nerves that exit to the lower body. Just after the fluid is inserted, positioning is critical to promote its movement in the correct directions. If there are malformations in this area, a client may get a one-sided or partial effect. There may be an inadequate block, a unilateral

block, or just one area left unanesthetized. The woman will be informed of these possibilities. In addition, if manipulation is required to extract the infant at the time of birth, the mother may feel pressure sensations and equate it with pain. This sensation can be compared with a tooth being pulled while under local anesthesia.

Depending on the dosage, epidural administration may be used for analgesia during labor or for anesthesia for vaginal or cesarean birth. If a cesarean delivery is needed, the anesthetic must circulate high enough to affect the thoracic nerves at T6 and T7, and a larger dose will be administered than is usual for labor analgesia (Figure 16-13).

Approach

The lateral or sitting position may be used for an epidural block. The neck and knees are slightly flexed. The lumbar area remains fairly flat, not rounded as in a spinal tap. The client must be able to breathe freely and stay absolutely still during the puncture. The sitting position is used when the anesthesiologist prefers it. In this position, the woman supports her feet on a chair. The hands should be resting on the thighs or on an over-bed table, a position that is difficult to hold when in labor.

The lumbar epidural is approached at the L4 and L5 interspace between the spinous processes. The technique is more difficult than a spinal tap; avoiding puncturing the dura mater takes special skill. Because a short but wider gauge needle is used, if the dura mater is punctured, there is more loss of spinal fluid than with a subarachnoid block technique. For a *continuous epidural* the needle is withdrawn after the thin flexible catheter inserted through the

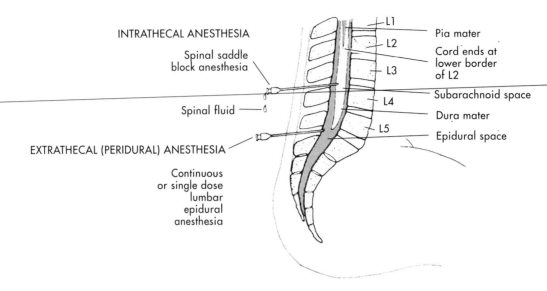

Figure 16-13 Sites of intrathecal and extrathecal anesthesia and analgesia. (Modified from Bobak IM, Lowdermilk DL, Jensen MD: *Maternity nursing,* ed 4, 1995, Mosby.)

needle is located properly. Then the catheter is taped in place with a strip of tape up the back and over the shoulder. Additional doses are given through an entry port at the end of the catheter.

Nursing responsibilities

Epidural anesthesia is effective for labor and vaginal and operative birth. The woman with epidural anesthesia is comfortable, unstressed by pain, awake and aware at birth, able to see and hold her infant, and able to initiate breast-feeding. However, to gain this effect, some motor blockade results. Blockade increases through time and interferes with bladder function and sensations underlying the urge to push during the second stage. Motor blockade also does not permit ambulation, therefore the client receiving epidural anesthesia for labor cannot assume an upright position. As a result, there is a slightly higher risk of birth by cesarean because of motor inhibition causing a prolonged second stage (Arkoosh, 1995).

Major complications are uncommon, yet the nurse should be prepared to assist when problems arise and to participate in monitoring and assessment after administration. Because of vasodilation at first, *hypotension* is always expected because of blood "pooling" in the legs. With hypotension, perfusion to the fetus is reduced, therefore the following preventive measures always precede epidural administration:

1. A loading dose of IV fluid, (usually Ringer's lactate solution) to support blood volume (500 to 1000 ml within 30 minutes) is regulated by the anesthesiologist.
2. Turn off any oxytocin infusion during administration.
3. Prevent vena caval compression by correct positioning. Then follow directions of anesthesiologist regarding

position change after the first test dose and then as the therapeutic dose and further doses are given.

4. Monitor blood pressure (BP) after test dose every minute and then until the woman is stable (usually within 30 minutes) monitor BP every 5 minutes. If stable, then assess routinely every 15 minutes throughout the rest of the labor and delivery (Datta, 1995). Automatic BP measurements are useful, but results must be read at these intervals.
5. Continuously monitor the FHR to note fetal response. Contractions may be inhibited for a short period after insertion of the therapeutic dose.
6. Document on monitor strip and nursing chart the time of start and finish of the procedure and the doses administered, including client and fetal heart responses to doses and increments.
7. If the woman complains of ringing, circumoral numbness, a metallic taste, dizziness, high sensory anesthesia, or excessive motor blockade, notify the anesthesiologist. The epidural catheter may have been displaced from the desired location.

Depending on the dose during labor, the mother may not sense bladder distention and may be unable to void. Monitor the bladder status and encourage voiding. If usual methods to promote voiding are ineffective, a straight catheterization should be performed. The bladder should be emptied before delivery, especially if forceps or ventouse will be used. If a Foley catheter is in place, it must be removed before bearing-down efforts become strong because the balloon may traumatize the bladder.

Depending on the dose, the bearing-down reflex may be numbed, and the mother may not push effectively during the second stage. Therefore epidural doses usually are timed so that some feeling is present during this stage. Coaching will be required (see Chapter 15), and the second stage may be somewhat prolonged.

Epidural administration calls for frequent assessment of vital signs, FHR, bladder distention, and assistance and coaching for pushing during descent of the fetus. After the birth, as the blockade wears off, the nurse monitors vital signs: BP, taken with the woman sitting, should be assessed for postural hypotension. Postural hypotension is a common problem during early recovery. Skin temperature of the legs should be checked because vasodilation recedes as the local anesthetic wears off; both legs should be equal in temperature. The client should not ambulate until full control has returned, which is usually in 4 to 6 hours.

Rare serious early reactions

Subarachnoid (total spinal) injection into the spinal fluid of the larger epidural dose may cause unconsciousness, apnea, bradycardia, or respiratory and cardiac arrest. Indications during test doses or early in the injection are *slurred speech* (notice that the anesthesiologist always asks the mother to talk during the injection), respiratory and pulse changes, and severe hypotension. Subarachnoid injection is an emergency, and cardiopulmonary resuscitation (CPR) is performed with ventilator support.

Accidental intravascular injection rarely occurs but may result at the time of injection or later as a result of migration of the catheter. There is a systemic reaction similar to that above, beginning as light-headedness and a metallic taste in the mouth.

Postdural puncture headache

Postdural puncture headache (PDPH) is not common after epidural administration. With use of the new pencil-point needles the incidence has diminished to approximately 0.8% (Benhamou, 1995). When it occurs, it often is related to poor technique; if the dura mater is punctured with a large-bore needle or the epidural catheter is withdrawn before any anesthetic is given, the loss of spinal fluid may cause a "spinal" headache. Related to stretching of the meninges, this headache may be severe and last as long as 1 week. Clients used to be kept in a supine or side-lying position for 6 to 24 hours after administration of a spinal anesthetic. The client with PDPH still may be instructed to follow the same regimen. Research, however, indicates that strict adherence to the flat position does not alter the incidence of headache (Albright et al, 1986).

Effective treatment is done by administration of an epidural blood patch (5 to 10 ml of the woman's blood inserted into the puncture site) to act as a plug to stop any more leakage (Figure 16-14). In addition, extra IV fluid (2000 to 3000 ml) and analgesics are given as needed to help the client until the intracranial fluid pressure returns to normal. Sometimes a tight abdominal binder is requested.

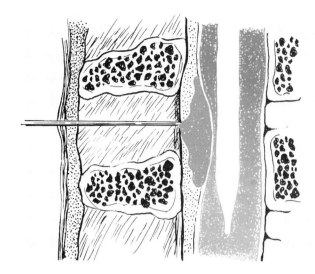

Figure 16-14   Epidural blood patch. (Modified from Bobak IM, Lowdermilk DL, Jensen MD: *Maternity nursing,* ed 4, 1995, Mosby.)

Other postpartum problems related to epidural anesthesia

Backache. This may result from multiple attempts with needles or hemorrhage into the intervertebral ligament. Other causes may be position during labor and birth plus pushing efforts. Reported rates vary widely, but the range for reported backaches in the first 6 months postpartum is 30 to 40% (Bader, 1993; Breen et al, 1994).

Shivering. Shivering or shaking can begin after birth. The cause is unknown. Epidural sufentanil or IV meperidine have been used to treat this response (Datta, 1995).

Hematoma. On rare occasions a *hematoma* may occur in the epidural space. It must be evacuated as soon as discovered. Because of this risk, if the mother has a bleeding disorder or platelet levels are below 150,000/mm³, epidural administration will not be done.

Infection. This is a possibility without absolute asepsis; if the client is already septic, epidural injections are not administered.

In rare instances a piece of the catheter may break off, usually when it is being removed. To avoid this problem the catheter is removed slowly by the anesthesiologist and then checked to see that it is intact. The nurse should *document removal of an intact catheter* on the nursing record.

Epidural Analgesia

Epidural analgesia is a positive development in pain management during labor. The epidural catheter is positioned in the same manner as for anesthesia, however, test doses are different and management and outcomes differ.

Analgesics are instilled into the epidural space and then diffused through the dura mater to the cerebrospinal fluid (CSF) to attach to the opiate receptors on the dorsal horn of the spinal cord (Nicholson, 1990). Morphine, fentanyl, and sufentanil are commonly used. Methadone, meperidine, or butorphanol are sometimes used. Ultra-low mixed doses begin with 10 mL of a mixture of 12.5 mg bupivacaine (0.125%) 1 to 2 μg/mL fentanyl and 16.5 μg epinephrine (1:600,000) in saline, given in two 5-mL increments (Youngstrom et al, 1996). Continuous, very low-dose infusion through the epidural catheter allows potent analgesic effects throughout the first stage of labor. To handle the pain of the second half of labor, many women need additional combined doses. Hourly monitoring of lower limb mobility and pain level is instituted. To ambulate safely, the woman should demonstrate (1) no orthostatic hypotension, (2) muscle strength in legs shown by being able to bend and straighten the knees, and (3) feeling in the plantar surface of the feet. She must be accompanied while ambulating and be assessed at regular intervals (Youngstrom et al, 1996).

Other units provide a bedside pump to administer small premeasured, self-regulated doses (Figure 16-15). **Patient-controlled epidural analgesia** (PCEA) has been shown to be safe and to reduce narcotic and local anesthetic doses by as much as 40 to 50% compared with women required to wait for their "top up" epidural dose to be given by the anesthesiologist after the pain returns (Nicholson, 1990). See Procedure 16-2.

Intrathecal Analgesia

Intrathecal analgesia is inserted directly into the spinal fluid (intrathecal or subarachnoid space) with the narrow gauge spinal needle (see Figure 16-13). This approach may be used either during active labor or as part of the epidural wash after cesarean birth. Pain relief lasts 4 to 7 hours during labor, with doses of 0.1 to 0.25 mg morphine (Manning, 1996). Fentanyl citrate 25 μg or sufentanil citrate 10 μg provide shorter acting analgesia with fewer side

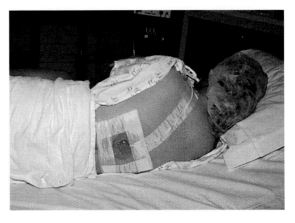

Figure 16-15   Woman with PCEA pump. (Courtesy Michael S. Clement, Mesa, Ariz.)

PROCEDURE 16-2
Patient-Controlled Analgesia

Purpose

Define role and responsibility of Registered Professional Nurse in administration of PCA or PCEA.

Anesthesiologist Responsibilities

- *PCEA:* Order hydration with IV fluids before epidural. Initiate epidural using test dose before therapeutic dose.
- *PCA and PCEA:* Specify medication, concentration, mode of delivery. Loading and incremental doses and lockout intervals. List parameters of timing on observations and when to intervene or call anesthesiologist.

RN Responsibilities

- Follow instructions for setup and management of PCA pump.
- Monitor vital signs:
  Before start of infusion, follow epidural routines. Monitor respiratory rate q15min × 1 hr, then q30min × 1 hr, then as ordered. For respiratory rate below 6/min stop PCA/PCEA and administer naloxone 0.08 mg IV push q3min until rate above 8/min. Notify anesthesiologist. Monitor contractions and FHR response q15min × 1 hr and then follow schedule for labor phase.
- Monitor pain level by observation and behavior. Record demand dosing and results.
- Monitor IV site if on PCA. Check PCEA catheter status and pump status at regular intervals.

OPTIONAL ACTIVITY

Write a sample nursing note correctly documenting the start of this procedure.

FHR, Fetal heart rate; *PCA,* patient-controlled analgesia; *PCEA,* patient-controlled epidural analgesia; *RN,* registered nurse.

effects. Only a single dose is used, and analgesia fades slowly during the second stage. Additional anesthesia such as local infiltration or pudendal infiltration must be used for the birth. Morphine applied locally to the spinal nerves in this way provides effective postoperative analgesia for 16 to 24 hours after surgery. See nursing interventions for assessments after this method.

Combined spinal-epidural technique

First, the larger gauge epidural needle is correctly placed. Then a smaller gauge spinal needle is inserted into the subarachnoid space until clear CSF drips out. The intrathecal narcotic dose is administered, and the spinal needle is withdrawn. Through the epidural needle the pliable epidural catheter is inserted, and then the second needle is withdrawn. The catheter is taped in place as is routine for an epidural (Datta, 1995). Continuous or intermittent (PCEA) infusion with mixtures such as sufentanil or fentanyl with bupivacaine can then begin. This approach allows low doses to be effective.

Side effects of epidural intrathecal opiates

Pruritus may occur in approximately 50% of clients, and the client should be observed for urticaria. Because nausea and vomiting accompany transition labor, the phase should be observed in relation to the timing of the medication. The physician may order an antiemetic, such as metoclopramide, transdermal scopolamine or perclorperizine, or may use naltrexone (Trexan).

Urinary retention is to be prevented for any laboring woman. Bladder distention and voiding frequency and amount should be monitored. A straight catheterization may be required. After the birth naloxone (Narcan) may be given if the woman is unable to void.

Delayed respiratory depression is a potential serious adverse side effect, especially with morphine; thus in the first 24 hours of monitoring of respiratory rates, use of an oxygen saturation monitor and nursing observation every hour is mandatory. Lethargy and a respiratory rate less than 6 to 8 breaths per minute should be noted and the narcotic antagonist given. Additional analgesics are not given without a specific order from the anesthesiologist (Nicholson, 1990). Diphenhydramine (Benadryl) po, naloxone IV or IM, or naltrexone po may be ordered after birth to relieve the symptoms of pruritus or respiratory depression.

Subarachnoid Spinal Block

Spinal anesthesia provides a subarachnoid block that erases motor tone and feeling below the block level. It is now used only for operative delivery. Because its technique is similar to that of a spinal tap, it may be performed by the obstetrician or nurse anesthetist. There are two types, saddle and spinal block; both are used less frequently today than epidural anesthesia (see Figure 16-13).

A low spinal is called a *saddle block* because the parts of the body that come in contact with a saddle are some of the parts anesthetized. Because a saddle block usually does not stop contractions, it can be administered during the second stage of labor and provides anesthesia from L5 to S5 for descent and delivery. If used for a forceps delivery visceral pain still may occur, depending on the dose. A modified saddle block provides anesthesia as high as T10 and complete pain relief during delivery for the perineum and contractions, but it does not anesthetize high enough for cesarean delivery.

The client is in a sitting position with the lower portion of her back rounded, feet supported, and forearms on her thighs or the over-bed table. Puncture into the dura mater is made at the L4 and L5 interspace with a long, small-gauge needle. CSF has been tapped when fluid drips back through the needle. *Hyperbaric solution* of the anesthetic (mixed with a glucose solution so it is heavier than CSF) is inserted, and the client is kept in a sitting position for 1 to 3 minutes to allow the anesthetic to settle downward in the CSF. The client is assisted by two persons to lie supine with her neck flexed on a pillow, and there should always be a lateral tilt to her lower back (with a small pillow or wedge) to prevent vena caval compression.

Spinal block

A cesarean birth performed with lower uterine incision requires anesthesia for at least 60 to 90 minutes. Sensory levels to T6 and T7 should be anesthetized. Because additional medication cannot be added if surgery takes longer than expected, concentrations of medication are chosen carefully for the duration of effect.

Spinal block for cesarean delivery is accomplished in the same way as saddle block, but the client may be placed in the side-lying position for needle insertion. Her lower back should be rounded. She must stay absolutely still during the injection. A higher volume of local anesthetic is inserted. Recovery is slower, and adverse reactions are more possible. A spinal anesthetic is administered just before surgery.

Adverse reactions. Adverse reactions are similar to those of epidural administration in some ways. Positioning in a lateral tilt prevents aortovenocaval compression. However, hypotension always occurs and is more severe than with an epidural injection. Epinephrine and a preload of IV fluids are administered to prevent lowered BP.

Allergic reaction to the medication or the occurrence of a high total spinal are rare. PDPH sometimes occur and are treated as already described. In rare instances the cord itself may be injured from too-deep or rough needle injection. In the recovery period, voiding may be a problem; most women have an indwelling catheter for 12 hours after cesarean delivery.

Nursing Responsibilities

Nursing interventions are similar to those for epidural after cesarean delivery. Return of sensation and postural hypotension are monitored, and position and fluids are managed to reduce the incidence of PDPH. The inability to void may continue into recovery; therefore the nurse monitors for bladder distention and bleeding.

GENERAL ANESTHESIA

In effective concentrations, general anesthetics cause unconsciousness by depression of the central nervous system. Uterine muscle becomes relaxed, which can be beneficial when hypertonic contractions are present but may precipitate hemorrhage during and after delivery. General anesthesia is used in smaller centers when an anesthesiologist is not available for epidural administration, when there is an emergency delivery and no time for another approach, and when regional anesthesia is contraindicated (e.g., for hemorrhage, infection, bleeding disorder, or a neurologic problem in the spinal area). General anesthesia places a maternity client at higher risk than does regional anesthesia because of the potential risk of aspiration of stomach contents during induction and recovery. In fact, aspiration and its consequences are one cause of maternal mortality.

General anesthetics are given by the IV route or by inhalation. In some countries, certain inhalants are used in low doses for labor analgesia. The mother uses a hand-held inhaler. When she is sleepy, the mask falls away from her face so that she does not receive significant doses. This method is not used in this country.

All principles of medication transfer across the placenta apply to general anesthesia. Because the anesthetic in the doses needed for surgery passes quickly into the fetal circulation and depresses the fetal respiratory center, the induction must be rapid. The time-to-birth interval is important. Investigators have shown a better neonatal outcome when induction-to-delivery is kept at less than 10 minutes. In addition, the time of uterine incision to the delivery of the infant is important. There are lower Apgar scores and more acidosis when there is an interval of more than 3 minutes (Datta, 1996).

Balanced Anesthesia

To prevent newborn depression, several agents in low doses are used. An IV dose of thiopental or ketamine is accompanied by a muscle relaxant and inhalation of anesthetic gas. *Nitrous oxide* has been used for more than 100 years. It provides rapid analgesia. With oxygen, it may be sufficient for vaginal delivery. The effect on the fetus is related to the length of analgesia. Within 15 minutes the equilibrium across the placenta is approximately 87%. With extended analgesia the infant may be depressed and hypoxic.

Therefore anesthetic administration for vaginal delivery must be timed as carefully as that for operative delivery.

Nitrous oxide has shown a teratogenic property in rat offspring when given during early gestation. Health professionals must be aware that there may be reproductive effects of chronic exposure to this gas.

Halogenated agents

Agents such as halothane, enflurane, and isoflurane have a smooth induction and stimulate less vomiting than other agents. Effective anesthesia occurs at low levels, and excretion and recovery are rapid. These agents have not replaced all others in obstetrics because of their relaxant effect on smooth muscles. Studies on bleeding after delivery, including that of Gilstrap et al (1987), conclude that women who received halogenated agents had significantly greater postpartum anemia as measured by reduced hemoglobin and hematocrit measurements and the need for transfusions. The nurse notes the type of anesthesia each client receives and observes for fundal firmness and amount of postanesthetic bleeding.

Ketamine

Ketamine induction is pleasant and rapid. Equilibrium in the fetal circulation occurs within minutes of IV injection. Deep analgesia may be obtained quickly, and recovery is rapid. For this reason it can be used just before difficult manipulation in a vaginal delivery. Ketamine also relaxes bronchial smooth muscle and is a good choice for clients with asthma. The risk of vomiting also is reduced. The cardiovascular stimulation of this medication raises the BP 10 to 15%, and uterine blood flow is increased. This drug is not used in hypertensive states, however it is often chosen when maternal hypotension is a factor or the fetus is distressed. During recovery the woman may have unpleasant dreams as she awakens and may be restless. If anesthesia has been deep, she should be watched for vomiting and aspiration during recovery.

Thiopental sodium

This is a short-acting barbiturate used for induction (in 30 seconds) but is not itself an analgesic. It must be used with a muscle relaxant, usually succinylcholine, and nitrous oxide or a halogenated anesthetic. An endotracheal tube is necessary. Hypotension will be evident and vena caval compression must be avoided by use of a lateral tilt position. Recovery is smooth, with little nausea and vomiting.

Prevention of Aspiration

For all general anesthesia, the woman is at risk because of vomiting and aspiration. These hazards lead to most of the deaths from general anesthesia. Aspiration of acidic contents of the stomach occurs if the woman vomits while her gag and cough reflexes are partially or completely anesthetized. The result is irritation to the lungs and possible respiratory arrest, cardiopulmonary changes, and death. In rare cases an inability to pass the endotracheal tube causes the woman to suffer from anoxia. In many of these cases the women were markedly obese.

The pregnant woman *always* is at risk for aspiration. Thus determination of the interval from the time of the last meal until general anesthesia is really unnecessary because all women in labor have slowed emptying of stomach contents. The woman who has fasted before elective cesarean has nearly the same stomach volume as the woman undergoing emergency cesarean (Datta, 1996). The woman who has received meperidine or another opioid analgesic is at much higher risk because her stomach emptying is markedly delayed by these drugs (see Drug Profile 16-3).

Most obstetric units now allow clear, nutritious fluids and ice chips during labor to provide energy and comfort and are addressing the problem of aspiration in a different way. Before operative delivery with general anesthesia and epidural anesthesia, the woman should receive a clear antacid such as sodium citrate (Bicitra or Alka-Seltzer Effervescent, two tablets in 30 ml water) just before induction. If the cesarean is scheduled, histamine blockers such as metoclopromide IV are effective. The goal is to raise the gastric pH above 2.5 (Box 16-2).

Cricoid pressure

The best protection from aspiration of stomach contents because of vomiting during induction is the use of **cricoid pressure** (Sellick maneuver) during tracheal intubation. A nurse may be asked to apply pressure to the cricoid cartilage, pressing it to the cervical vertebrae to close the esophagus during intubation (Figure 16-16). Pressure should be maintained or increased if the client begins to vomit. The anesthesiologist will direct the nurse's action. After the endotracheal tube is in place and the cuff inflated, the woman is protected from aspiration.

Recovery from General Anesthesia

After the birth, the infant is observed for signs of respiratory depression. The mother has no awareness of the birth or of the infant until she has recovered. Depending on the dose, the period of recovery may be 1 or 2 hours, with lingering drowsiness lasting as long as 8 hours.

After surgery the client continues to be observed for vomiting and is positioned to prevent aspiration. Her head and shoulders should be turned to the side and slightly elevated, and she requires close observation during waking. Recovery is gradual, depending in part on her body size and the dose received. Protection from injury is a priority because restlessness is typical during emergence. Because pain perception is distorted, clients may complain of pain unless intrathecal or epidural narcotics have been given. If not, intramuscular analgesics are given in one-half doses during immediate recovery because of the potential for

---

▌ *Box* **16-2**   **Steps to Decrease Risk of Pulmonary Aspiration during Induction of General Anesthesia**

1. Neutralize stomach contents by administering a clear antacid (e.g., sodium citrate 5 minutes before induction).
2. Preoxygenation: the effects of the physiologic changes of pregnancy on the respiratory system cause the woman in labor to desaturate faster than the nonpregnant client.
3. Use a rapid-acting barbiturate (thiopentone) and a depolarizing muscle relaxant (succinylcholine) to induce unconsciousness and facilitate tracheal intubation by muscle relaxation.
4. Immediately on administration of these drugs, apply cricoid pressure (Sellick maneuver) by a trained assistant.
5. Intubate the trachea and inflate the cuff to seal the airway.
6. Check to ensure that the endotracheal tube is properly positioned before releasing cricoid pressure.

From Douglas MJ: The case against more liberal food and fluid policy in labor, *Birth* 15(2):93, 1988.

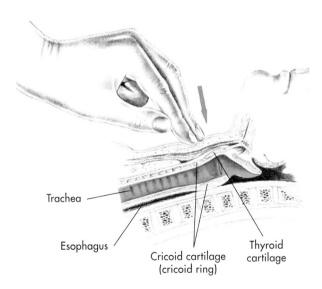

Figure 16-16   Technique of applying pressure on cricoid cartilage to occlude esophagus prevents pulmonary aspiration of gastric contents during anesthesia induction. (From Lowdermilk DL, Perry SE, Bobak IM: *Maternity and women's health care,* ed 6, St Louis, 1997, Mosby.)

Trachea

Esophagus

Cricoid cartilage (cricoid ring)

Thyroid cartilage

hypotension. Vital signs are monitored frequently. Smooth muscle may be relaxed; therefore postural hypotension is a possibility as is hemorrhage. Women may have difficulty voiding after general anesthetics and a Foley catheter remains in place for several hours.

TEST *Yourself* 16-4

a. List three reasons in favor of and three reasons against oral fluid intake during labor.
b. What is the best position to prevent aspiration should the client vomit?

General Nursing Responsibilities Related to Drug Use in Pregnancy

Because the nurse understands the effects of drugs, the care plan should include observation for and assessment of medication effects on clients along with teaching preventive care. The following steps can be taken to increase awareness and improve assessment and intervention in relation to perinatal drug use and effects. When these steps are taken, it should be possible to provide informed nursing support to any woman during pregnancy or recovery and to discover subtle signs of medication influence on the infant.

1. Include education about medications in antepartum and postpartum classes and for every lactating woman.
2. Explain the benefit-to-risk ratio for questionable medications.
3. Counsel all mothers about nonpharmacologic methods for alleviating minor discomforts of pregnancy and discomfort during labor and recovery.
4. Encourage women to take childbirth classes and support the educated mother in her attempts to cope with labor and delivery.
5. During the interview and assessment of the mother, include a record of any incidental nonprescription or prescription medications taken before labor.
6. Inform nursery nurses of transitional medications that might affect the newborn during recovery. Include timing and level of analgesia and anesthesia.
7. Increase your ability to assess the newborn for normal behavioral responses. Records must be more descriptive during the newborn period if long-term behavioral effects of drugs are to be evaluated.
   a. Note iatrogenic factors affecting responses.
   b. Be alert for delayed excretion, cumulative effects, and altered physiologic states when noting medication effects.

Key Points

- Pregnancy alters protein and tissue binding so that more of the drug may be free to seek receptor sites. Women note greater sensitivity to drugs as a result.
- Membranes permit transfer of most substances so that levels of the drug become equal on both sides of the placental barrier and, with some exceptions, also cross the blood-brain and blood-milk barriers.
- A woman's serum drug level during late labor and the time-dose interval are crucial in evaluating newborn signs of drug effects.
- Transfer through the blood-milk barrier is affected by the pH of milk, volume at each feeding, and metabolic breakdown in tissue or in the newborn's gastrointestinal tract. Only fractions of the maternal dose reach the newborn, compared with neonatal standard doses.
- Nurses should teach lactating women to space necessary drug intake so that the lowest level is in the milk just before a feeding.
- Fetal and neonatal drug effects must be evaluated by behavioral responses, Apgar scores, and vital signs.

- Induction of labor with oxytocics may be painful for a woman because the goal is to speed labor while the same pressure factors are required to dilate the cervix and cause fetal descent through the birth canal.
- Pain during parturition and after birth can be reduced with nonpharmacologic interventions. Support of the mother's choice of methods is a nursing intervention.
- PCA administered IV or by the epidural route results in less demand for analgesics and higher client satisfaction.
- Pain thresholds vary widely as do pain behaviors. Cultural differences are seen clearly in labor responses.
- Epidural anesthesia with local anesthetics or with addition of fentanyl is a widely used anesthesia for vaginal or cesarean birth.
- General anesthesia places the woman at risk of aspiration; therefore a clear antacid must be given before and cricoid pressure applied during intubation.
- Nurses should not withhold analgesia during recovery because pain interrupts mother-infant acquaintance.

Study Questions

16-1. Select the terms that apply to the following statements:
 a. Lipoprotein membrane between maternal and fetal circulation _____
 b. The fatty sheath of myelin around capillaries and nerves of the brain _____
 c. The limited amount of drug molecules that may attach to a specific type of protein in maternal circulation

 _____
 d. The measurable period in which half of a drug dose is metabolized and excreted _____
 e. Pain originating from smooth muscle and felt as dull and diffuse from these fibers _____
 f. Sharp and localized pain from these fibers _____

16-2. Pudendal block produces anesthesia for which parts of the body?
 a. Lower uterine segment and cervix
 b. Vagina and entire perineum
 c. Uterus, cervix, bladder, and rectum
 d. Parts affected by perineal nerve

16-3. Which types of drugs move more easily across membrane barriers?
 a. Hydrophilic, ionized drugs
 b. Low molecular weight, protein-bound drugs
 c. Lipophilic, partially ionized drugs
 d. Fat-soluble, nonionized drugs

16-4. If equilibrium of a medication is present in maternal and fetal circulations, which of the following is true:
 a. The drug accumulates in higher levels in the fetus than in the mother.
 b. An adverse effect will occur in the fetus.
 c. The fetus will be more affected by the drug than the mother.
 d. The ratio of free medication is the same on both sides of the placenta.

16-5. Which of the following situations would result in the highest level of drug in the newborn?
 a. Mrs. J., who has an infection, is being given ampicillin, 2 g, q6h, by piggyback IV. Her last dose was 4 hours before birth.
 b. Mrs. K., because of high BP, is receiving an IV with magnesium sulfate, 2 g/hr, by infusion pump.
 c. Mrs. L. received meperidine and promethazine IM 3 hours before birth.

16-6. Why is it safe to use oxytocin for induction when protocols for its use are strictly followed?
 a. There are several effective antagonists that may be administered.
 b. FHR do not respond to oxytocin.
 c. The drug follows a physiologic pattern even if too much is given.
 d. Rapid metabolism results in a short t$_{1/2}$.

16-7. After the first test dose of medication has been inserted into the epidural catheter, the client must be observed for which of the following?
 a. Allergic responses
 b. Hypertonic contractions
 c. Accidental injection into dural or intrathecal spaces
 d. Headache and nausea

16-8. After the therapeutic dose of an epidural anesthetic has been injected, one must observe for which of the following?
 a. A change in contraction rate and intensity
 b. Complaints of thirst and increased anxiety
 c. Vasodilation resulting in hypotension
 d. Increase in bloody show with possible rupture of membranes

Answer Key

16-1: *a*, Placental membrane; *b*, blood-brain barrier; *c*, bound drug; *d*, half-life; *e*, unmyelinated; *f*, myelinated. 16-2: b. 16-3: d. 16-4: d. 16-5: b. 16-6: d. 16-7: a, c. 16-8: c.

References

*Abboud TK: The neonatal neurobehavioral effects of mepivacaine for epidural anesthesia during labor, *Anesthesia* 63(9)A:449, 1985.

*Albright GA et al: *Anesthesia in obstetrics: maternal, fetal, and neonatal aspects,* ed 2, Boston, 1986, Butterworth.

Alderdice FA et al: A national study of labour and birth in water, *Mod Midwifery* 4(1):14, 1994.

American College of Obstetricians and Gynecologists: *Induction and augmentation of labor,* Technical Bulletin #157, Washington, DC, 1991, The College.

American College of Obstetricians and Gynecologists: *Obstetric analgesia and anesthesia,* Technical bulletin No 225, Washington, DC, 1996.

Anderson PO: Medication use while breastfeeding a neonate, *Neo Pharm Quarterly* 2(2):3, 1993.

Arkoosh VA: Labor analgesia, *Curr Opin Anaesth* 8:206, 1995.

Atkinson BD et al: Double blind comparison of intravenous stadol and fentanyl for analgesia during labor, *Am J Obstet Gynecol* 171(10):1994.

Bader AM: Neurologic complications of regional anesthesia in obstetrics, *Curr Rev Nurs Anesth* 16(4):27, 1993.

Beal MW: Acupuncture and related treatment modalities; II, applications to antepartal and intrapartal care, *J Nurse Midwifery* 37(4):260, 1990.

Belluomini J et al: Accupressure and obstetrics, *J Am Acad Nurse Pract* 6(10):490, 1994.

Benden J: TENS relief of discomfort, *Physiotherapy* 79(11):773, 1993.

Benhamou D: Complications of obstetric anesthesia, *Curr Opin Anaesth* 8:216, 1995.

Berlin M: Effects of drugs on the fetus, *Pediatr Rev* 12(9):282, 1991.

Bernat SH et al: Biofeedback-assisted relaxation to reduce stress in labor, *J Obstet Gynecol Neonatal Nurs* 21(4):295, 1992.

Blackburn ST, Loper DL: *Maternal, fetal and neonatal physiology,* Philadelphia, 1992, WB Saunders.

*Bodden C: *Relief of labor pain by acupressure,* master's thesis, Garden City, NY, 1986, Adelphi University.

*Brackbill Y et al: Obstetric meperidine usage and assessment of neonatal status, *Anesthesiology* 40:116, 1974.

Breen TW et al: Factors associated with back pain after childbirth, *Anesthesiology* 81:29, 1994.

Briggs GC, Freeman RK, Yaffee SJ: *Drugs in pregnancy and lactation,* ed 4, Baltimore, 1994, Williams & Wilkins.

Brodsky PL, Pelzar EM: Rationale for revision of oxytocin protocols, *J Obstet Gynecol Neonatal Nurs* 20:440, 1991.

*Cahill CA: Beta-endorphin levels during pregnancy and labor: a role in pain modulation? *Nurs Res* 38(4):200, 1989.

Caldwell LE, Rosen MA, Shnider SM: Subarachnoid morphine and fentanyl for labor analgesia, *Reg Anesth* 19(1):2, 1994.

Carter JH, Halpern SH: Anesthesia for cesarean section, *Curr Opinion Anaesth* 8:210, 1995.

Curry PD, Pacsoo C, Heap DG: Patient-controlled analgesia in obstetric anesthetic practice, *Pain* 57:125, 1994.

Datta S: *The obstetric anesthesia handbook,* St Louis, 1995, Mosby.

Datta S: Evolution of modern pain management. In Repke JT, ed: *Intrapartum Obstetrics,* New York, 1996, Churchill Livingstone.

Davies S: Pharmacology of obstetric anesthesia: part I, *Curr Rev Nurs Anesth* 17(1):22, 1994.

*Duchene P: Effects of biofeedback on childbirth pain, *J Pain Symptom Manage* 4(3):117, 1989.

Ferrante FM et al: Patient-controlled epidural analgesia: demand dosing, *Anesth Analg* 73:547, 1991.

Fields SA et al: Obstetric analgesia and anesthesia, *Prim Care* 20(3):705, 1994.

Fitzgerald M: Prescription and over-the-counter drug use during pregnancy, *J Am Acad Nurs Pract* 5(5):380, 1993.

*Gaston-Johannson F, Fridh G, Turner-Nowell K: Progression of labor pain in primiparas and multiparas, *Nurs Res* 37(2):86, 1988.

*Geden EA et al: Effects of music and imagery on physiologic and self-report of analogued labor pain, *Nurs Res* 38(1):37, 1989.

*Gift AG: Visual analog scales: measurement of subjective phenomena, *Nurs Res* 38(5):286, 1989.

*Gilstrap LC III et al: Effect of type of anesthesia on blood loss at cesarean section, *Obstet Gynecol* 69(3):328, 1987.

Gordon SC, Gaines SK, Hauber RP: Self-administered versus nurse-

administered epidural analgesia after cesarean section, *J Obstet Gynecol Neonatal Nurs* 23(2):99, 1994.

*Grim LC, Morey SH: Transcutaneous electrical nerve stimulation for relief of parturition pain; a clinical report, *Phys Ther* 65(3):337, 1985.

Jorgensen Dick MJ: Assessment and measurement of acute pain, *J Obstet Gynecol Neonatal Nurs* 24(9):843, 1995.

*Kuhnert BR et al: Meperidine and normeperidine levels following meperidine administration during labor; II. fetus and neonate, *Am J Obstet Gynecol* 33:909, 1979.

*Loeser J: Concepts of pain. In Stanton-Hicks M, Boss R, eds: *Chronic low back pain,* New York, 1982, Raven Press.

Manning J: Intrathecal narcotics: a new approach for labor analgesia, *J Obstet Gynecol Neonatal Nurs* 25(3):221, 1996.

*Melzack R et al: Severity of labor pain: influence of physical as well as psychologic variables, *Can Med Assoc J* 30(3):580, 1984.

*Moore ML: *Realities in childbearing,* Philadelphia, 1983, WB Saunders.

Nicholson JR: Nursing considerations for the parturient who has received epidural narcotics during labor and delivery, *J Perinat Neonat Nurs* 4(4):14, 1990.

Norris MC (ed): *Obstetric anesthesia,* Philadelphia, 1993, JB Lippincott.

Ohning BL: Neonatal pharmocodynamics—basic principles; I: drug delivery, *Neonatal Network* 14(2):7, 1995a.

Ohning BL: Neonatal pharmocodynamics—basic principles; II: drug action and elimination, *Neonatal Network* 14(2):15, 1995b.

*Olsson G, Parker G: A model approach to pain assessment, *Nurs* 87(5):52, 1987.

Patrick CH: Therapeutic drug monitoring in neonates, *Neonatal Network* 14(2):21, 1995.

*Rivera-Calimlim L: The significance of drugs in breast milk, *Clin Perinatol* 14(1):51, 1987.

Scott DA: Postoperative analgesia, *Anesthesiology* 83(4):727, 1995.

Settladge R: Drugs in pregnancy. In Mishell D, ed: *Management of common problems in obstetrics and gynecology,* ed 3, Cambridge, Mass, 1994, Blackwell Scientific Publishers.

Shyken JM, Petrie RH: The use of oxytocin, *Clin Perinatol* 22(4):907, 1996.

Simone C, Derewlany LO, Koren G: Drug transfer across the placenta, *Clin Perinatol* 21(3):463, 1994.

*Spielman FJ, Herbert WNP: Maternal cardiovascular effects of drugs that alter uterine contractility, *Obstet Gynecol Surv* 43(9):516, 1988.

Taylor T: Epidural anesthesia in maternity patients, *MCN Am J Matern Child Nurs* 18(2):86, 1993.

Telfeyan C, Santos AC: Pharmacology of local anesthetics during pregnancy, *Curr Opinion Anesth* 8:196, 1995.

Ward R, Mirkin B: Perinatal pharmacology. In Broady T et al, eds: *Human pharmacology,* ed 2, St Louis, 1994, Mosby.

Williams MC: Vacuum-assisted deliveries, *Clin Perinatol* 22(4):933, 1996.

Youngstrom PC, Baker SW, Miller JL: Epidurals redefined in analgesia and anesthesia: a distinction with a difference, *J Obstet Gynecol Neonatal Nurs* 25(4):350, 1996.

*Zimmer EZ, Divon MY, Vadasz A: Influence of meperidine on fetal movements and heart rate beat-to-beat variability in the active phase of labor, *Am J Perinatol* 5(3):197, 1988.

Student Resource Shelf

Lowe NK: The pain and discomfort of labor and birth, *J Obstet Gynecol Neonatal Nurs* 25(1):82, 1996.

An understanding of the multidimensional aspects of pain provides the basis for a woman-centered approach to holistic pain management.

Simkin P: Reducing pain and enhancing progress in labor: a guide to nonpharmacologic methods for maternity caregivers, *Birth* 22(9):3, 1995.

A review of numerous pain relief techniques that are simple and low cost and can be used by nurses and birth partners.

Stampone D: The history of obstetric anesthesia, *J Perinat Neonat Nurs* 4(1):1, 1990.

A review of the progress in pain management during labor and birth.

Weber SE: Cultural aspects of pain in childbearing women, *J Obstet Gynecol Neonatal Nurs* 21(1):67, 1996.

Clinical application of culturally sensitive care recognizes that expression of pain differs among women of various cultures.

*Classic reference.

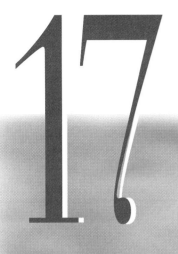

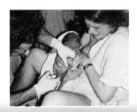

17. Immediate Recovery & Home Care

As soon as an infant is born, the processes that occurred during pregnancy begin to be reversed. This period of transition is known interchangeably as the recovery, the postpartum, postnatal, or postdelivery period, or the **puerperium**. It has also been described as the fourth trimester of pregnancy.

In addition to physical changes, the new mother and her family undergo emotional and psychologic adaptations as they adjust to new roles and responsibilities. Nursing care must be carefully planned to assess needs and ensure that the recovery period is successful.

PHYSICAL ADAPTATIONS

Uterus

Involution. Involution is the process whereby the pelvic reproductive organs, particularly the uterus, return to the approximate prepregnant size and position while the placental site of the endometrium heals. Failure to complete this process is referred to as **subinvolution**.

The decrease in uterine weight and size reflects a reduction not in the *number* of cells but rather a marked reduction in the *size* of the same cells, through the process of

389

catabolism. At delivery, the woman's uterus weighs approximately 1000 g (2.2 pounds); by the end of puerperium, it will have returned to its prepregnant weight of 60 g (2 ounces).

The position of the uterus also changes during puerperium, descending rapidly into the lower pelvic cavity. Immediately after delivery, the uterus lies midway between the symphysis pubis and the umbilicus. Within 12 hours of delivery it rises to the level of the umbilicus or slightly above it. On the first postpartum day, the uterus begins descent into the pelvic cavity at a rate of about 1 cm a day until the tenth day, when it may be palpated at or below the level of the symphysis pubis. Throughout the postpartum period the firm and contracted uterus should be found in the midline (Figure 17-1).

Along with uterine position, uterine *consistency* is the indicator of progressing involution. The strong, frequent myometrial contractions that control blood flow to the uterus cause it to become hard, and its consistency can be assessed by palpating the uterine fundus, which should feel firm and round. If the fundus is soft and not clearly defined in shape, the uterus is described as "boggy," an indication that contractions are inadequate, allowing blood loss to continue.

The endometrium also undergoes an involutional process. After the placenta is delivered, only the basal portion of the decidua remains. This separates into two layers; the more superficial layer necroses and sloughs off in the lochia. What remains regenerates into the new endometrium by about the sixteenth day. Healing of the placental site itself takes up to 6 weeks, as a lesion the size of a hand repairs itself through the regeneration of new tissue. This process prevents placental scarring. Otherwise, the inside lining of the uterus would be full of

scar tissue after a few pregnancies, making it unsuitable for further implantation.

Lochia. After delivery, decidual lining sloughs off as a vaginal discharge called **lochia.** This discharge contains blood, decidual tissue, epithelial cells from the vagina, mucus, bacteria, and on occasion, fragments of membranes and small clots. Its odor is fleshy but not offensive (as menstrual discharge can be).

- The first phase of lochia, when the discharge is red and bloody, is called *lochia rubra* (rubra meaning "red"). This phase lasts 1 to 3 days and initially may contain a few small blood clots.
- *Lochia serosa* occurs next, lasting 3 to 10 days. The discharge during this phase is described as a serosanguineous reddish pink-to-brown drainage.
- The third and final phase is called *lochia alba*, primarily because of the presence of leukocytes. It appears as a white or cream colored or almost clear discharge and resembles the leukorrhea of pregnancy; it lasts 10 to 14 days or even up to 3 weeks.

The color of lochia indicates the healing stage of the placental site (Table 17-1). Warning signs of abnormal flow are found later in this chapter.

Postpartum hemorrhage. Hemorrhage in the postpartum period is an emergency situation that requires careful assessment and prompt treatment. Early postpartum hemorrhage is caused by uterine atony, blood loss from lacerations, or hematomas. Whereas bleeding from a noncontracting uterus or a laceration is obvious, leakage of blood into tissue in a hematoma may go unnoticed. Even when a hematoma is recognized, blood loss is always more than estimated (Cunningham et al, 1993).

Excessive bleeding that continues or begins again 1 to 2 weeks after delivery is called *late* postpartum hemorrhage and is caused either by subinvolution or by retained placental fragments. (See Chapter 21 for a full discussion of bleeding during and after pregnancy.)

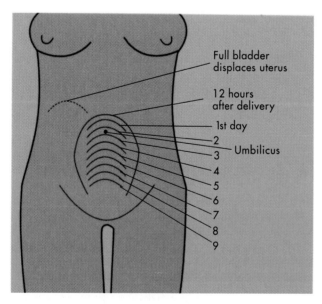

Figure 17-1   Postpartum descent of uterus into lower pelvis.

Table **17-1**	**Lochial Characteristics**		
	Rubra	**Serosa**	**Alba**
COLOR	Bright red; bloody	Pink-brown	Creamy white
CLOTS	Small clots	No clots	No clots
ODOR	Slightly "fleshy"	No odor	No odor or stale body odor
LENGTH	1-3 days	5-7 days	1-3 weeks

Uterine atony. Failure of the uterus to remain firmly contracted can lead to postpartum hemorrhage. Because uterine blood vessels and the uterine muscles are intertwined, a tourniquet action prevents bleeding or hemorrhage from the open blood vessels at the placental site when the uterus contracts. Factors that hinder uterine contractility include exhausted uterine muscle, over distention from multiple gestation or a large fetus, use of tocolytics, infection, lacerations of the cervix, or retained placenta.

A full bladder is a prominent cause of **uterine atony**. Because of changes in intraabdominal pressure after delivery and the considerable volume of intravenous (IV) fluids administered, the bladder becomes easily full and distended, pushing the uterus up and to the side (generally to the right), thus impeding contraction.

Cervix

Whereas the upper part of the uterus is firm, hard, and contracted after delivery, the lower uterine segment and cervix remain loose, thin, and stretched. The cervix may also appear edematous and bruised from the delivery and may have small tears or lacerations. It will allow entry of the entire hand for several hours, making manual examination of the uterus possible. By the first postpartum day, however, the cervix has sufficiently narrowed and regained its normal consistency to admit only two fingers. At the end of the first week it has narrowed considerably and begins to thicken to recreate a canal.

Involutional changes may continue for 3 to 4 months, but since the cervix has sustained trauma, the parous cervix will never again look like the nonparous cervix. The external os, which previously resembled a dimple, now resembles a slit, and any lacerations to the cervix during delivery may leave scar tissue.

Vaginal Canal

The vaginal canal, stretched to accommodate the delivery of the fetus and placenta, appears swollen and smooth after delivery. It gradually becomes smaller and firmer, although it never regains prepregnancy size. *Rugae* (vaginal folds) reappear by the third week, but secretions are diminished until ovulation begins again. This dryness is related to estrogen withdrawal. The woman may need lubrication to ease penetration during intercourse.

The external vaginal orifice or introitus appears jagged and irregular in shape after delivery and the *parous* (postdelivery) hymen has characteristic nodular skin tags at its edges. Trauma to vaginal tissue may occur as a result of delivery, particularly if it was very rapid or uncontrolled. Occasionally, a hematoma may develop as a result of descent and delivery. The usual places for the development of hematomas are the external vaginal orifice, vaginal wall at the ischial spines, and the episiotomy site. Any woman who complains of severe or excessive perineal pain or sensitivity should be carefully assessed for hematomas.

Perineum

After delivery, the muscles of the floor of the perineum are stretched, swollen, and often bruised. Even an intact perineum can be edematous, erythematous, and uncomfortable. If an episiotomy was performed or if lacerations occurred and were repaired, a scar on the perineum will be present, although it may not always be obvious.

Ovaries

The ovaries are inactive during the last two trimesters of pregnancy. Because of the drop in placental hormone level, ovaries gradually resume the prepregnancy cycle. (See Endocrine Funtion in this chapter for the discussion of ovulation and menstruation.)

Breasts

Already developed throughout pregnancy, the breasts respond to hormonal stimulus. For the first few days after delivery, both breast-feeding and non-breast-feeding women secrete **colostrum**, a creamy yellow precursor to milk, but the breasts remain soft and nontender. About 3 days postdelivery, in response to increased prolactin levels, breasts become firm and tender as milk supply is initiated. Breasts rapidly become distended, hard, and warm in response to increased blood flow and venous and lymphatic congestion. This development is called physiologic engorgement. Without the stimulus of suckling, engorgement lasts for about 24 to 48 hours and will resolve spontaneously, with the breasts receding to their prepregnant size.

Suckling by the infant stimulates on-going milk production (refer to Figure 17-12). The breast will remain firm, full, and somewhat tender until emptied by nursing. Nipples may be erect, flat, or inverted, and the areola remains more darkly pigmented and prominent. Leakage of colostrum may be noted. Further discussion of assessment of breasts and support measures for breast care is contained later in this chapter.

Cardiovascular Function

Volume adjustment

Some of the most dramatic changes in the puerperium occur in the cardiovascular system. During pregnancy, the blood volume increases by 30% to 50% over the prepregnancy volume. After delivery, however, there is no need for excess blood volume, and drastic shifts occur in body fluids. During vaginal birth and placental delivery, the woman loses approximately 500 ml of blood, with up to 1000 ml lost during cesarean birth. This loss depletes a portion of the additional fluid, but shifts in fluids that are redirected from the placenta compensate and increase the circulating volume. Without the extra blood vessels of the uterus and placenta, blood is returned to the central circulation. Vena caval compression from the large uterus is relieved, and blood from the pelvic region returns unimpeded to the general circulation, along with extravascular fluids that accumulated during pregnancy. Cardiac output (CO) increases anywhere from 25% to 80% depending on the type of delivery, with a resultant increase in stroke volume (SV) (Creasy and Resnick, 1994). This first critical adjustment may require special attention for the woman with cardiac problems (see Chapter 23).

Heart rate. During pregnancy, heart rate (HR) increases to 15 beats per min over the prepregnancy baseline and SV also increases, thus improving CO to effectively circulate a larger blood volume to the expanded uterine and placental vasculature ($SV \times HR = CO$). After delivery the body attempts to compensate for increased central venous load, slowing the HR to as low as 40 to 60 beats per min to control CO and prevent systemic overload and hypertension. Because this bradycardia is a normal postpartum adaptation, an *increase in pulse rate always signals a secondary cause,* such as hemorrhage, infection, thrombosis, anxiety, pain, or excitement related to the delivery, and this increase should be explored.

Blood pressure. In the immediate recovery period, blood pressure may decrease in response to anesthesia or blood loss, and although the delivery may have been uncomplicated, orthostatic hypotension may occur because of fluid shift and decreased intraabdominal pressure. It should return to normal within the first week after delivery, unless the woman experiences complications such as pregnancy-induced hypertension (PIH) (see Chapter 22).

Blood values

Hemoglobin and hematocrit. Because hemoglobin and hematocrit levels reflect actual loss of erythrocytes, as well as the percentage of formed cells to total volume, these values may fluctuate during the immediate postpartum period. During the first day, the fluid shift from extravascular tissues into the vascular compartment may depress the hematocrit level because of simple dilution. If levels have dropped on the first postpartum day, a repeat evaluation is obtained; this lower hematocrit may also reflect excessive blood loss.

During the initial period of postpartum diuresis, the increased volume of red blood cells (RBCs) that occurred in pregnancy will now become obvious because of the loss of extra body fluids. Hematocrit may rise in the first 3 to 7 days. RBCs gradually return to normal levels by 4 to 5 weeks, as old cells die out and fewer new ones form. Nonpregnant levels are reached by 5 to 8 weeks (Blackburn and Loper, 1992).

White blood cells. The normal adult white blood cell (WBC) count is between 5000 and 10,000/mm³. The count rises during late pregnancy and labor and can reach levels of 15,000 to 20,000/mm³. This count is within normal limits for pregnancy and immediate recovery. (Some experts state that levels 25,000 to 30,000/mm³ [Cunningham et al, 1993] or even up to 40,000/mm³ [Gleicher, 1992] are acceptable for the first 24 to 48 hours postpartum.) Levels fall quickly to normal levels in 4 to 7 days. Therefore, persistent elevation indicates infection (Blackburn and Loper, 1992).

Coagulation factors. Clotting factors increase near term and remain high in the immediate postpartum period. Platelet, fibrin, and fibrinogen levels are elevated during recovery. Their function is to protect against bleeding caused by delivery of the fetus and placenta, trauma, and possible postpartum hemorrhage, but they also contribute to formation of a thrombus if the woman is immobile or suffers additional trauma (see Chapter 22). All levels return to their previous normal ranges in 3 to 4 weeks (Table 17-2).

Respiratory Function

After delivery, with abdominal pressure decreased, the diaphragm descends to its normal position, permitting better lung expansion and ventilation, but the respiratory rate does not noticeably change. However, the respiratory system should be assessed regularly during the immediate recovery period. If the woman received inhalation or general anesthesia, extra precautions should be instituted to prevent stasis of secretions or aspiration of stomach contents if vomiting occurs. Lung sounds should be assessed by auscultation.

Excretory Function

Body water in the extravascular spaces and excess plasma volume from the pregnancy are rapidly eliminated. By the second postpartum day, diuresis and polyuria occur. Up to 3 L of urine are eliminated daily for a few days; this physiologic condition should be explained to the woman. Within a week, she will return to her prepregnancy voiding pattern.

Freed from the pressure of a pregnant uterus and possessing decreased muscle tone, the bladder increases its capacity dramatically, filling to 1000 or 1500 ml without discomfort. Retention of urine may result because of stretching of the perineal floor, with accompanying bruising and edema of the trigone and urethral meatus. During labor and delivery, the fetus places pressure on the bladder, particularly if it is full. Regional or general anesthesia may temporarily inhibit neural function, diminishing urinary sensations from the bladder. Urinary retention follows, putting the woman at risk for hemorrhage from a poorly contracting uterus. Stasis also predisposes to urinary tract infections.

Laboratory tests may be altered. Increased membrane permeability persists for the first week, thus proteinuria of up to 1+ may be seen. Although glucose is still easily

Table 17-2	**Postpartum Laboratory Values**	
	Normal	**Abnormal**
TEMPERATURE	97°-100.4° F (36.2°-39° C)	≥100.4° F (38° C) after first 24 hr
PULSE	50-80 bpm (may drop to 40 bpm)	Tachycardia because of hemorrhage, thrombosis, infection, dehydration, fever, medication, anxiety, excitement
RESPIRATION	16-24/min	↑ with respiratory difficulty
BLOOD PRESSURE	Pregnancy levels; orthostatic hypotension as a result of fluid shifts and lower intraabdominal pressure	↑ PIH, hypertension, delivery excitement ↓ because of hypovolemia from anesthesia or hemorrhage
RED BLOOD CELLS	3.75-5 million/mm³; gradual ↑ to prepregnancy levels	↓ because of hemorrhage or excess IV fluids
WHITE BLOOD CELLS	10,000-18,000/mm³	↓ 10,000/mm³ or ↑ 20,000/mm³ may indicate a problem
HEMOGLOBIN	11.5-14 g/dl	Blood loss of 500 ml decreases Hb 1-1.5 g/dl
HEMATOCRIT	32%-42%	Blood loss of 500 ml decreases Hct 3% to 4%
PLATELETS	↑ during recovery	↓ HELLP syndrome, lupus
FIBRIN	↑ during immediate recovery to normal by 3-5 days	↓ bleeding related to DIC
URINE		
Output	↑ 3 L/day	Concentrated urine
Glucose	↑ lactosuria	Check for diabetes, if glycosuria
Blood urea nitrogen	↑ because of catabolism	

Data from Blackburn and Loper, 1992.
DIC, Disseminated intravascular coagulation; *HELLP,* hemolysis, elevated liver enzymes, and low platelet count; *PIH,* pregnancy-induced hypertension.

passed into the urine, it is usually in the form of galactose and is not detected by conventional dipsticks. In addition, if the woman has been NPO through a prolonged labor and recovery, urinary ketones may be present. Also, as a result of catabolic changes taking place in the uterus, nitrogenous wastes are created and serum blood urea nitrogen (BUN) may be elevated.

Dilation of the ureters and renal pelves requires about 6 weeks to return to the prepregnancy condition. If there is urinary stasis, microorganisms can easily travel upward, causing kidney infection.

Gastrointestinal Function

Without placental hormones, the gastrointestinal (GI) tract begins to revert to its prepregnancy peristaltic and digestive activities. After being NPO or on clear fluids for most of labor and delivery, a woman is generally hungry or thirsty and wants to eat or drink. The type of analgesia

or anesthesia and the delivery route influence when the woman may have her first oral intake. Many units wait 1 hour to monitor recovery, then provide fluids as desired. No woman should be given oral fluids or food until she has recovered from general anesthesia. After initial adjustment, however, she may request extra portions of food. By discharge, most women have regained their appetite.

During pushing and the delivery of the fetal head, the straining and pressure on the lower bowel often cause the extrusion of internal hemorrhoids. After delivery, however, these reduce in size and can be manually reinserted into the rectum. Hemorrhoids present during the pregnancy also shrink. Surgical reduction after delivery is rarely necessary.

Most women do not have a bowel movement until a few days after delivery. The reasons are varied. The woman may have had diarrhea at the onset of labor and no solid food intake for up to 24 hours or more. In the postpartum period, constipation can occur as a result of decreased motility of the GI tract and decreased abdominal and perineal muscle tone, anesthesia, iron supplements, and even fear of having pain while defecating. The woman with an episiotomy or painful hemorrhoids may try to avoid straining and delay her first bowel movement. The speed with which her bowels become regulated will depend on her daily activities, diet (adequate roughage and fluids), activity (including exercises), and schedule. Stool softeners and mild laxatives may be ordered to facilitate emptying the bowel.

Gas buildup is a problem for many women after surgical birth because of anesthesia and intestinal manipulation during the procedure. Ambulation, progression of diet, antiflatulents, or exchange enemas generally make the woman more comfortable.

Integumentary Function

After delivery the skin changes caused by the pregnancy begin to recede. As the melanocyte-stimulating hormone that caused pigmentational changes is eliminated, melasma disappears, unless excessive pigmentation has occurred. Not all changes will completely disappear. *Striae gravidarum* (stretch marks) may fade to a silvery color in light skinned women, but they remain deeper than normal skin tone on darker skin. The linea nigra and the darkened areola fade, but in some women faint traces will persist. Palmar erythema caused by increased circulation and estrogenic influence also subsides. In a few months, hair and nail growth will return to prepregnancy patterns. Hair may appear to be falling out as the rapid growth of pregnancy ceases. Spider nevi also recede during the postpartum period and urticarial rashes disappear (see Chapter 9).

For the first postpartum week, it is common for the new mother to experience profuse afebrile diaphoresis, especially at night, as a mechanism to secrete excess accumulated fluids.

Musculoskeletal Function

Immediately after delivery, the woman may be fatigued or even exhausted. The labor position and pushing techniques may leave arms, neck, shoulders, and perineal muscles sore and aching.

Abdominal muscles

The uterine ligaments remain loose and relaxed, and the abdominal muscles have less tone because of having been stretched, resulting in the soft, flabby abdomen most women complain about in the first 6 to 8 weeks after delivery. Complete recovery is dependent on previous tone, genetic inheritance, and the kind of exercise begun in this period.

During pregnancy, labor, or delivery, overdistention of the uterus can lead to a separation of the vertical, central abdominal muscle group (the rectus abdominis muscles). This is called *diastasis recti abdominis* (*diastasis* means "separa-

tion"). If this occurs before or during delivery, pushing may become difficult or impossible because these muscles help push the infant through the birth canal. After delivery, such a separation decreases support for the abdomen, resulting in a pendulous abdomen and backache. In general, no particular treatment is indicated for this condition. Exercise may help, but restoration of the muscles may be prolonged.

Joints

Under the influence of relaxin, the pelvic joints, particularly the symphysis pubis, may separate slightly during labor and delivery, and as a result, some women feel pain and discomfort in this area. Eventually this pain, described as a "pinching," subsides. A few women have severe pain and difficulty in walking for a short time and need medical evaluation. Joints become stabilized by 6 to 8 weeks.

Endocrine Function

Placental hormones

Without the placenta, hormonal levels drop abruptly after delivery. Human chorionic gonadotropin (hCG), human placental lactogen (HPl), and human chorionic somatotropin (HCS) amounts fall within 24 hours, whereas estrogen and progesterone levels decrease more gradually. The lowest estrogen level between days 3 and 7 corresponds with the onset of lactation, and estrogen will remain low until days 19 through 21; the estrogen level will then slowly rise as a new follicle develops. Since prolactin inhibits follicular development, breast-feeding can suppress estrogen production. The progesterone level decreases markedly by 72 hours postdelivery and will not rise again until after the first ovulation.

Shivering. Many women experience transient trembling after delivery. Several theories concerning this shivering has been proposed: exhaustion from the strenuous activities of labor and delivery; the sudden decrease in intraabdominal pressure; the sudden and complete withdrawal of placental hormones; and a reaction to the small transfusions of fetal blood or amniotic fluid that may have entered maternal circulation during placental separation. The cool environment of labor rooms and room-temperature IV fluids are a leading cause of chilling. This trembling and chill are usually not associated with an elevation of temperature. Usually, this condition is relieved with warmed blankets, or epidural sufentanil or IV meperidine may be administered by an anesthesiologist (Datta, 1995).

Pituitary hormones

Follicle-stimulating hormone (FSH) and luteinizing hormone (LH) remain low for 10 to 12 days postpartum; LH does not rise until a follicle develops just before the first ovulation. FSH begins to increase by the third postpartum week. Serum prolactin rises throughout pregnancy and continues to be high after delivery, when production is taken over entirely by the anterior pituitary gland. Since the impetus for prolactin excretion is nipple stimulation, breast-feeding will maintain an elevated level, dependent upon the number of feedings given per day. Without the stimulus of breast-feeding, prolactin levels drop rapidly.

Stimulation of the breast during breast-feeding also induces the release of oxytocin, which causes the milk to be released from the breasts by the action known as the **let-down reflex.** At the same time, oxytocin causes strong contractions of the uterus, the "afterbirth pains."

Other endocrine functions

The thyroid and adrenal glands and the pancreas return to prepregnancy size and activity within a few weeks after birth. Because the antiinsulin factors of the placental hormones are gone, insulin is better used; insulin-dependent diabetics will need less insulin and will usually return to prepregnant requirements within 24 hours (see Chapter 24). Gestational diabetics will begin to stabilize serum glucose levels.

Return of ovulation and menses. The exact mechanism responsible for resumption of the menstrual cycle is not fully understood, and time of resumption is unique for each individual. Cycles can begin in lactating mothers as early as 8 weeks after delivery or as late as 18 months. Some nonlactating mothers (40%) may have their first menstrual period as early as 4 to 6 weeks after delivery, and 90% resume menses by 24 weeks (Creasy, 1994.)

Regardless of whether the woman is breast-feeding, the first cycle or two may be *anovulatory*—menstruation that occurs without the expulsion of a mature ovum—until follicles completely respond to pituitary stimulation. Ovulation in the breast-feeding mother may be further delayed because prolactin levels interfere with the development of the graafian follicle. Since the prolactin level is influenced by the strength of infant sucking, as well as the number and frequency of feedings, it is not predictable; therefore breast-feeding is unreliable as a method to control conception.

Immunologic Function

Infection

Recovering women are at special risk for wound infection and infections of the uterus, urinary tract, respiratory tract, or breast. However, because of early discharge, symptoms may first occur after the woman is at home. Thus it is crucial that the nurse recognize who is at higher risk and teach all women how to prevent and report symptoms of postpartum infections. Predisposing factors such as diabetes, chronic respiratory problems, anemia, malnutrition, substance abuse, or immunocompromised status alert the nurse, as do intrapartum events such as prolonged rupture of membranes, long labor or difficult delivery, multiple gestation, urinary catheterization, internal fetal or uterine

monitoring, episiotomy, lacerations, hematomas, or cesarean delivery.

Once the woman at risk is identified, a plan of care can be formulated to decrease additional risk. The woman must be taught to recognize early warning signs and seek medical intervention to prevent more serious complications. The most common adaptation is fever, but there are other more subtle symptoms as well. Lethargy, chills, anorexia, nausea and vomiting, myalgia, abdominal pain, cramping or tenderness, and foul-smelling lochia may be indicators.

Puerperal infection is the most common of postpartum infections (Clark, 1995). This term describes infections of the genital tract in the postpartum period, appearing before the tenth day after delivery. A new definition also includes fevers from infection within the first 24 hours of recovery (Clark, 1995). See Chapter 25 for a detailed description of postpartum infection.

An elevated temperature in the first 24 hours after delivery may be caused by dehydration, excitement, fatigue, chilling, and blood loss. The temperature may be as high as 38° C (100.4° F), which is considered within normal limits. If the temperature remains elevated after the first day, however, the cause must be found and treated. Infection should be considered, especially if there is a history of premature rupture of the membranes, hemorrhage, long or traumatic labor and delivery, or preexisting infection. A thorough assessment of the woman's condition and the chart history provide data about the source of the problem.

Fever related to breast engorgement. Most often, only a low-grade fever accompanies engorgement of the breasts. The infant is not separated from the mother when she has a fever, unless this is specifically directed by the physician. Because the infant and mother usually have the same bacterial and viral agents, nothing is usually gained by isolation (see isolation precautions in Chapter 25).

TEST *Yourself* 17-1

Fill in the normal findings in the first 24 hours after delivery.
   WBC count
   Lochial color and amount
   Temperature (oral)
   Appetite
   Fatigue level

PSYCHOSOCIAL ADJUSTMENTS

Attachment

The postpartum period is a time of transition from nonparenthood to parenthood (see Chapter 20 for further discussion). Parent-infant attachment that leads to parent-infant bonding depends in part on the infant's responsiveness to the parents. The infant's response reinforces the parental response and encourages them to continue interaction.

Bond formation is an outgrowth of reciprocal attachment stimulus-response and affectional ties that help form a coordinated, constructive social relationship. The nurse can only infer that bonding is progressing satisfactorily through observation of attachment behavior (i.e., behaviors that serve to maintain contact between the parent[s] and infant and demonstrate affection toward the infant) (Figure 17-2). Examples of this behavior include kissing the infant, fondling and cuddling it, and holding it "en face" (face to face) to maintain eye contact (see Figures 8-7 and 8-8).

Maternal development tasks

Rubin (1975a) delineated several stages or phases that the new mother goes through during recovery; these include **taking in, taking hold,** and **letting go.** After the delivery, the mother is exhausted and needs rest and sleep. During the first or second day, she will be *taking in* all the experiences of labor and delivery and may become introspective and contemplative She may ask many questions regarding the labor and delivery experience and worry about her condition and her infant. Her physical needs and deficits of nourishment, rest, and comfort must be met by a caring nursing staff; the new mother will then be able to care for the needs of her infant.

Taking hold describes the period when the mother attends to the infant's care needs, the role changes to come, and her own recovery needs. During this phase, the woman is usually eager to learn how to care for herself and her infant.

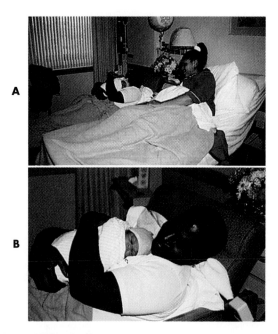

Figure 17-2   A, Getting acquainted in the labor-delivery and postrecovery (LDRP) room where mother and father have time with their new infant. **B,** Father may stay overnight in an LDRP setting. (Courtesy Marjorie Pyle, RNC, *Lifecircle.*)

During later recovery, the mother must also *let go* and view the infant as a separate person. Some women have difficulty accomplishing this task, and if it is not resolved, psychologic problems could ensue. Examples of problems include a mother who may have great difficulty letting others assist with care of the infant, or an overprotective mother may not allow herself to go out if a baby-sitter is needed. She is still attached to the child because she views the infant as an extension of herself. Because this behavior is not evident in the hospital stay, the clinic nurse or pediatric staff members may be able to identify this unresolved task.

Self-esteem needs

All people need *self-esteem*; it underlies personal satisfaction and effective functioning. It is the extent to which an individual believes herself or himself capable, worthy, successful, and significant. Self-esteem depends on maintenance of control over self and achievement of expectations. In adulthood, individual expectations are affected by demands from the common group, society, or culture and are experienced as roles. During pregnancy, these roles take on new meaning, and emphasis is placed on responsibilities toward the growing child. Studies show that women set for themselves psychologic tasks to carry out, especially during labor and delivery. In a study by Tribotti et al (1988), role performance was selected as a leading concern of women after birth. The congruence or lack of congruence between the idealized self and the actual self determines feelings of self-worth and self-esteem. Childbirth is a crisis event, an emotional milestone. The woman, already in a state of disequilibrium, is vulnerable to self-criticism and to anything that may be perceived as criticism from others.

In today's society, in which a great emphasis is placed on active participation in and control over life experiences, many couples desire the "ideal" childbirth experience. When a woman who planned birth without medication and with minimal assistance experiences a labor that deviates from the normal and then requires medication, anesthesia, or forceps or cesarean delivery, she often feels that she has failed. A woman who has planned for and expects to give birth in a controlled situation with her partner may feel disappointment, anger, sadness, guilt, and failure when she is unable to achieve this goal. As a result, she may feel some degree of shame and decreased self-esteem.

The husband or partner is undoubtedly the most important influence in the woman's self-satisfaction. His reactions to her performance greatly affect her self-esteem, and if she senses disappointment from him for any reason, she may feel less "successful."

Potential for mood changes

The first few days after delivery—even up to 10 or 14 days—could be considered a period of "normal" crisis and disequilibrium especially for the first-time mother (Rubin,

1977). It is a time of transition, readjustment, reappraisal of roles, added responsibility, excitement, fatigue, and recovery from pregnancy, labor and delivery. Relationships are strained. It rarely is a time of peace and tranquility, as the new family attempts to establish boundaries, functions, schedules, and roles.

The blues. Many new mothers (and even new fathers) experience mood swings know as "the blues," with episodes of unexpected crying, sensitivity, and sadness. Typically these start 3 to 7 days after delivery, are generally attributed to fatigue and hormonal shifts, and may last 1 to 2 weeks. Changes in mood coincide with the drop in the hormones estrogen and progesterone, which reach their lowest level during those days.

Postpartum depression. Beginning 2 weeks after delivery, more severe symptoms characterize postpartum depression. Some causes may include lack of sleep during the first month of recovery, demand of additional responsibilities, and discomforts of infection or pain. Several studies have examined the reasons for postpartum mood changes according to maternal responses. Some of the reasons given by mothers include worries about the infant, difficulties involving breast-feeding, homesickness, and pain, but many can give no reason for their depressed feelings.

The severest form of postpartum depression is postpartum psychosis or *puerperal psychosis*. This depression is characterized by acute psychotic behavior characteristic of affective, schizophrenic, or organic disorders. Professional help, not merely emotional support, comfort, and encouragement, is needed. When hospitalization is required, every attempt should be made to keep the mother-infant relationship intact while caring for both. This topic is discussed in greater detail in Chapter 26.

IMPACT OF EARLY DISCHARGE

Today, early discharge is a much-debated topic. Long hospitalization is not warranted for most women, but there is great concern that the new mother and infant are sent home before adequate assessment of needs and teaching is done. Early discharge limits the time the woman has to listen, to learn, and to practice self-care.

Ideally, discharge teaching is begun prenatally to introduce the woman to the process of labor, birth, recovery, and infant care and feeding. This is a perfect opportunity for education, since the woman is preparing for the birth experience and is not as stressed or rushed as she will be after delivery. With frequent visits to her health provider during the last month of pregnancy, the woman has the opportunity to ask for clarification and further information without the pressure of limited time. Teaching can be repeated and reinforced until it is clearly understood. This allows the woman to participate more fully in the birth experience and take more control over her own care and that of her infant.

After delivery, this teaching continues with the first postpartum check—reinforcing, expanding, and evaluating its effectiveness until the woman goes home. Because there are too many distractions in these first few hours after birth, the woman may not remember instructions and should receive written instructions. Use of videotapes may allow the woman to learn at her own pace and then review information with the nurse. Many units provide follow-up care by a telephone call during the next day to see how the parents are managing. Such follow-up care is especially appreciated by the patents (McGregor, 1996; Valaitis et al, 1996).

A follow-up home visit has also become more common. Maternal postpartum checks include the involution process and systemic stabilization, as well as prevention of infection and other complications. Parenting skills are also assessed and reinforced, and the infant's status is evaluated (Figure 17-3).

Nursing Responsibilities

Whether the woman has had a spontaneous vaginal delivery, assisted delivery, or a surgical delivery, certain aspects of care are universal. Specific needs of individual mothers with complications are discussed in later sections. Critical elements of care are listed in Box 17-1.

The woman in recovery is a person at risk; she is vulnerable in many ways. Physical stability must be ensured and a positive client-nurse relationship established so she can be assisted in her developmental tasks of parenting and maintaining self-esteem. Following the nursing process is a logical and organized way to approach planning and giving care to the woman in the early postpartum period. The following discussion of care by the nurse adheres to this format.

Box **17-1**	**Critical Elements: Maternity Care**

Universal precautions are considered an essential part of maternity nursing. Use latex gloves when there is contact with blood or other body fluids.

Obtain the client's consent before beginning a procedure or treatment, and explain findings after a procedure is completed.

Individualize care by determining the client's needs for nursing interventions.

Encourage and teach self-care during every contact with client.

Provide privacy, respecting cultural needs.

Support patient-infant and sibling-infant interaction during hospital stay.

Postpartum Visit Record
Maternal Assessment

MATRIA HEALTHCARE
OF NEW YORK, INC.

Date: _____ Time In: _____ Time Out: _____ Del. Date: _____ M.D. _____ Payor: _____

Patient Name: _____ DOB: _____ ID Number: _____

Infant Name: _____ ID Number: _____

Type of Delivery: ❑ Vag　❑ C/S Primary　❑ VBAC　❑ Multipara　❑ Primagravida

Number of Babies Delivered this Pregnancy: ❑ 1　❑ 2　❑ 3　❑ 4　❑ _____

Race/Ethnicity:　❑ White　❑ Black　❑ Asian　❑ Hispanic　❑ American Indian　❑ Other: _____

T - P - R - B/P	HEART	LUNGS	BREASTS
T: P: R: B/P: Wt:	❑ Regular rate & rhythm ❑ Denies chest pain ❑ Other _____	❑ Respiration regular ❑ Breath sounds clear in all fields ❑ Denies SOB ❑ Nailbeds and mucous membranes pink ❑ Other _____	❑ Soft ❑ Filling ❑ Tender ❑ Engorged Discharge: ❑ Colostrum ❑ Milk ❑ Other Support Bra: ❑ Y ❑ N Nipples: ❑ Erect ❑ Inverted ❑ Intact ❑ Cracked ❑ Red ❑ Bleeding Cleansing: ❑ Soap ❑ Water only Air drying: ❑ Usually ❑ Rarely ❑ Never Topical agent (type/frequency).

UTERUS		LOCHIA		PERINEUM
HEIGHT ❑ ___ F Above ❑ At Umbilicus ❑ ___ F Below ❑ Not Palpable CONSISTENCY ❑ Firm ❑ Boggy	POSITION ❑ Midline ❑ Right ❑ Left TENDERNESS ❑ Absent ❑ With touch ❑ Constant	No. pads/day: ____ Color ❑ Rubra ❑ Serosa ❑ Alba Clots ❑ Y ❑ N Frequency Size	Odor ❑ Fleshy ❑ Foul ❑ Absent Saturation ❑ Small ❑ Moderate ❑ Heavy	❑ Episiotomy ❑ Intact ❑ Edema ❑ Bruising ❑ Redness ❑ Hemorrhoids ❑ Gaping or not healing ❑ Laceration Cleansing appropriate ❑ Y ❑ N

INCISION		BLADDER	BOWEL HABITS	LOWER EXTREMITIES
❑ Tubal ❑ Vertical C/S ❑ Horizontal C/S ❑ Staples ❑ Removed ❑ Dry & Intact ❑ Redness ❑ Edema ❑ Pain ❑ Hematoma	❑ Absent ❑ Purulent ❑ Serosanguineous ❑ Foul odor ❑ Steri Strips ❑ Dehiscence	❑ Voiding ❑ Burning ❑ Frequency ❑ Incontinence ❑ Other _____	❑ Regular ❑ Constipated ❑ Diarrhea ❑ Passing Flatus ❑ On stool softener ❑ Other _____	R Calf: Homan's ❑ Positive ❑ Negative L Calf: Homan's ❑ Positive ❑ Negative Varicosities present: ❑ Y ❑ N

EDEMA		APPETITE	SLEEP	ACTIVITY	SUPPORT SOURCE
Absent ❑ Legs ❑ min ❑ mod ❑ pitting ❑ Feet ❑ min ❑ mod ❑ pitting	❑ Face ❑ min ❑ mod ❑ pitting ❑ Hands ❑ min ❑ mod ❑ pitting	❑ Normal/Regular ❑ Increased ❑ Decreased ❑ Absent ❑ Diet Supplement ❑ Special Diet	Amount of sleep/past 24 hrs. _____ Self-fatigue scale 1 - 2 - 3 - 4 - 5 None　　Exhausted	❑ BR & BRP ❑ Climbing stairs ❑ Resume routine activities ❑ Other _____	❑ Baby's father ❑ Maternal/Paternal family ❑ Friends/Neighbors ❑ Domestic help ❑ Other _____

ENVIRONMENT	PSYCHOLOGICAL	LABS COLLECTED
❑ Supplies are appropriately maintained and organized in the home. ❑ No apparent health/safety hazards. General hygiene: ❑ Adequate ❑ Inadequate	❑ Characteristics of appearance: behavior and verbalization appropriate to situation. ❑ Affect appropriate ❑ Other _____	❑ CBC ❑ H&H ❑ U/A ❑ Other _____

FAMILY ADAPTATION	MOTHER IDENTIFIED NEEDS
❑ Demonstrates adequate newborn care ❑ No evidence of inappropriate problem solving ❑ No verbalization of inability to cope with parenting or postpartum care ❑ Disorganized in caregiving activities ❑ Abusive situation	

SUMMARY	
❑ Assessment within normal limits	❑ Recommendations/Referrals

Nurse's Signature: _____ Date: _____

Figure 17-3 Postpartum Visit Record indicates some of the observations made during a home visit to a newly delivered mother. (Courtesy Matria Healthcare of New York, Inc, Home Care and Maternity Management Services.)

ASSESSMENT

The first hour after delivery does not end the recovery process. The critical phase of recovery continues throughout hospitalization and the weeks after discharge. During this time, accurate observations, nursing history, and physical assessment allow formulation of appropriate nursing diagnoses and an effective plan of care. A nurse who has been able to follow a woman through labor, birth, and immediate recovery will already know much of the information about the newly delivered woman. If the woman is transferred to a recovery setting, the nurse there must follow through with the steps to be mentioned.

Initial observations

First impressions of a woman provide the nurse with an overview of how she is recovering from childbirth. Two factors easily noted are her general appearance and the presence of pain. The woman's color reflects circulation and perfusion. Observe her for pallor, flushing, or cyanosis, and note general responsiveness. Is she extremely fatigued, unusually quiet, or very excitable or anxious? Does she look comfortable, or is she in distress?

An IV line may still be in place. Assess its patency and note the type of solution, any medication added, amount left in the bag, and the rate of flow. Also assess the insertion site for irritation or infiltration. If the woman has had a surgical delivery, a Foley catheter will be in place. In addition to physical findings, note whether the woman is alone or accompanied, and if so, by whom. Is support evident? Does the mother speak about the infant? Is she very concerned over her own welfare?

Physical assessment

Physical assessment is critical in this period. It may be performed in any order; the following is one suggested order of priority.

Vital signs. Take pulse, respiration, and blood pressure to assess normal blood volume and recovery. Temperature is taken to ensure that the woman is not dehydrated and to rule out infection.

Postpartum checks include vital signs every 15 minutes for 1 hour, then every 30 minutes in the second hour, then every 4 hours for 24 hours.

Uterus. For vaginal delivery, check the fundus for consistency, height, and position to ensure adequate uterine contraction and descent. Additionally, for cesarean delivery, check the dressing, including its condition, and check for the presence of bleeding.

Perianal area. Observe the perineal pad for amount and color of lochial discharge, noting unusual odor or presence of clots; check for intact sutures along the line of episiotomy, noting any bleeding, edema, ecchymosis, or pain; and observe the anus for repaired lacerations or hemorrhoids.

Bladder. Palpate for emptiness or fullness and distention. Observe whether a Foley catheter is in place.

Abdomen. Check for distention, softness or firmness, rigidity, and tenderness. Check also for the presence or absence of bowel sounds after general anesthesia or cesarean delivery.

Breasts. Ask the mother if she is planning to breast-feed. If so, ask is she has had an initial experience just after birth.

With initial physical assessment complete the nurse can determine whether the woman can be left comfortably and safely alone while the nurse completes data collection.

Nursing history

Depending on the institution, information can be obtained from a history taken on admission to labor and delivery, a chart review, or a second interview during the postpartum period. (Do not make the woman repeat basic information she has already provided). Necessary background data include the following:

- Type and time of delivery: estimated blood loss (EBL), length of labor, time from rupture of membranes (ROM) to birth
- Anesthesia and medications received during labor and delivery
- Present gravidity and parity; blood type and Rh factor
- Status of infant
- Chosen method of feeding the infant
- Significant past medical and surgical history
- Allergies, including medication, food, and environmental conditions
- Medications taken on a regular basis
- Diet, including medical, religious, or cultural limitations
- Social, occupational, and economic factors that may affect the woman's recovery and parenting
- General educational background for this experience, including childbirth preparation classes attended
- Home situations that will affect recovery and parenting, including whether she will have help with the infant or will need to climb stairs after a difficult or surgical delivery

Check the physician's orders regarding activity, diet, medications, IV infusion orders, and any special treatments or procedures (e.g., administration of rubella or Rh immune globulin injections). The antepartum chart usually contains laboratory data, including the woman's blood type and Rh factor, serologic tests, and rubella titer.

NURSING DIAGNOSES

The nurse identifies specific self-care needs or deficits appropriate to each postpartum woman and formulates nursing diagnoses that focus on the woman's problems. These diagnoses will be the basis for the plan of care that should reflect her physical, emotional, and developmental needs. Some nursing diagnoses are universal to every woman, regardless of the type of delivery. Although individual women may have different needs, the following are commonly recognized:

- Injury, risk for, related to bleeding from uterine atony, retained placental fragments, lacerations, or hematomas
- Infection, risk for (uterine, perineal, incisional, urinary), related to childbirth
- Pain, related to uterine contractions, incision, or breast engorgement
- Urinary retention, related to periurethral edema from delivery
- Constipation, related to anesthesia, diet, medication, or pain
- Knowledge deficit, regarding parenting, hygiene, and recovery processes related to prior experience
- Breast-feeding, effective; or breast-feeding, ineffective
- Fatigue, related to childbirth exertion
- Sleep pattern disturbance, related to hospital routine and need to care for new infant at home
- Role performance, altered, related to new parenting role
- Family processes, altered, related to addition of a new family mamber
- Sexuality patterns, altered, related to recovery from childbirth

In other instances the type of delivery or other special circumstances necessitate formulation of diagnoses related to specific needs. After a complicated birth or cesarean delivery, a woman may exhibit needs related to the following diagnoses:

- Altered tissue perfusion (phlebitis) related to immobility
- Situational low self-esteem related to childbirth difficulties
- Altered parenting related to disappointment, discomfort, or separation from infant
- Anxiety related to concern for self and infant

It is interesting to note that the nurse and client may focus on different problems. It saves time for the nurse and the new mother to discuss priorities. A study by Tribotti et al (1988) reports significant variations in concerns, which change day by day during recovery. The five nursing diagnoses recovering women most frequently select in the early period are as follows:

1. Alteration in comfort (pain)
2. Sleep pattern disturbance
3. Impaired physical mobility and activity intolerance
4. Alteration in bowel elimination
5. Anxiety

Women focus on their bodily changes at first. After cesarean birth, physical changes assume an even greater importance. By 25 to 72 hours after birth, women are concerned about altered sleep patterns and facing the future. By 73 to 96 hours after birth, many more diagnoses are selected by the participants (an average of nine diagnoses each).

EXPECTED OUTCOMES

Because of the brief hospital stay, the nurse will usually evaluate only short-term achievement. Therefore, outcomes must be possible and measurable within the time frame of initial recovery, with referral for problems that cannot be quickly resolved. It is reasonable to expect that the client will:

- Be free from injury and maintain normal involution pattern
- Exhibit no signs of infection during recovery
- Manage pain with or without medication
- Reestablish normal elimination patterns
- Demonstrate understanding of and ability to manage care of self and infant
- Express understanding of breast-feeding and demonstrate skills needed to successfully breast-feed her infant
- Report relief from fatigue and verbalize ways to improve sleep patterns at home
- Express comfort with new role and its impact on other roles
- Discuss ways to incorporate the new infant into the existing family structure
- Discuss plans for contraception (if chosen) and verbalize rationale for avoiding vaginal intercourse until healing occurs

NURSING INTERVENTION

During all recovery care, certain critical elements must be observed (Box 17-1), and adherence to these is assumed in good nursing practice. Each of the following topics restate the associated nursing diagnosis and expected outcome.

Potential for Hemorrhage

Uterine blood vessels are dilated and numerous. Hemostasis is effected by uterine contraction. Thus after the birth of the infant, uterine contraction is critical. The vaginal and perineal tissues are well supplied with blood vessels, and any birth trauma will precipitate excess bleeding. Hemorrhage is rapid loss of more than 10% of blood volume. (Hemorrhage is discussed in detail in Chapter 21.) Immediate nursing care includes observation for and interventions to prevent hemorrhage.

Nursing diagnosis: Injury, risk for, related to bleeding from uterine atony, retained placental fragments, lacerations, or hematomas.

Expected outcome: The client is free from injury and maintains a normal involution pattern.

Postpartum check. The postpartum "check" is first performed on the woman's admission to recovery, whether in a labor-delivery-recovery (LDR), labor-delivery-recovery and postrecovery (LDRP), or postpartum unit. During the first hour, uterine and lochial checks are performed every

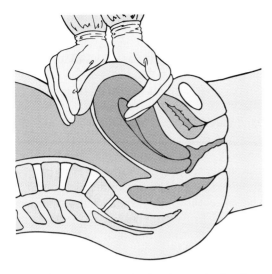

Figure 17-4   Palpating the fundus during the first hour after birth. The upper hand is cupped over the fundus; the lower hand dips in above the symphysis pubis and supports the uterus while it is gently massaged. (Redrawn from Bobak IM, Jensen MD: *Essentials of maternity nursing,* ed 3, St Louis, 1991, Mosby.)

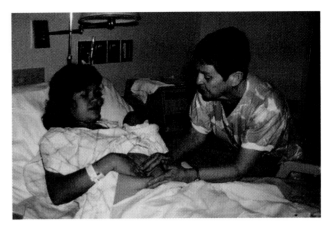

Figure 17-5   Demonstrating the fundal check. The woman should feel the fundus and learn to rub it at intervals in the first days. (Courtesy Marjorie Pyle, RNC, *Lifecircle.*)

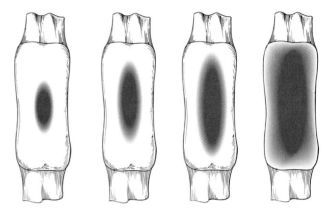

Figure 17-6   Differing amounts of lochia staining on peripads. (Redrawn from Bobak IM, Jensen MD: *Essentials of maternity nursing,* ed 3, St Louis, 1991, Mosby.)

15 minutes and then every 1 to 2 hours for the next 4 hours. If all signs show expected progress, reassessment is decreased to every 4 hours in the first 24 hours and then every 8 hours until the woman is discharged.

To remember priorities while performing postpartum assessments after uncomplicated vaginal deliveries, approach the check according to the following:

F—fundus
L—lochia
E—episiotomy
E—elimination
B—breasts

Fundal check. Palpate the abdomen to locate the *fundus* or top of the uterus by pressing in and down with the side of the palm (Figure 17-4). Describe the descent by measurements in *fingerbreadths* from the umbilicus (one fingerbreadth measures 1 cm)(refer to Figure 17-1).

After a surgical birth, palpation may be omitted when there is a vertical incision to avoid pressure on tissue and incision lines, depending on hospital protocol. If done, palpate gently, approaching from the sides to the midline.

The uterus should be *firm* in consistency, feeling like a grapefruit. A fundus that is hard to find or one that is soft or boggy signifies inadequate contraction, and hemorrhage could occur. If the fundus is firm at the midline and at the expected level and position, the nurse documents these data. If, however, the fundus is soft or boggy, gentle massage is applied by rotating the cupped hand over the fundus until it feels firm. Vigorous massage or kneading should be avoided because it may overstimulate the uterus and cause it to become more fatigued and thus decrease contractility. Note if the fundus becomes firm, and measure the amount of

blood on the pads after palpation since drainage and "old" clots pooled in the vagina may be expressed by palpation.

The fundus should be located *midline* in the abdomen. If it is felt on the side, assess the bladder for distention, which is the usual cause of a displaced uterus. After the bladder is emptied, the location and firmness are reassessed.

Discharge teaching. Explain fundal checks and why it is important for the fundus to be firm. Show the woman how to palpate the fundus, and teach her how to massage it to improve uterine contractility in the first few days (Figure 17-5). Emphasize that overmassaging should not be done because this may cause injury. Instruct the woman to call her health care provider if the uterus is not firm and there is increased lochia.

Lochia. Lochia is observed for amount, color, and consistency. It may be difficult to describe the amount objectively. The terms *scant, moderate,* and *heavy* are often defined subjectively (Luegenbiehl et al, 1991). A more standardized approach measures the size of the lochial stain or the weight of the pad. Absorbency of the pad will affect measurements; the type of pad used in each unit should be tested. AWHONN (1993) describes amounts of lochial flow as follows:

Scant— <2.5 cm stain on a perineal pad
Light— <10 cm stain
Moderate— <15 cm stain
Heavy—1 saturated pad in 1 hour
Excessive—1 saturated pad in 15 minutes

Figure 17-6 demonstrates lochial stain on a perineal pad with estimated stain amounts. If pads are measured by protocol, remember that 1 gm = 1 ml. A large saturated peripad holds 60 to 100 ml lochia. Blood loss is crucial to the recovering woman: for every 500 ml lost, the hemoglobin can drop 1 to 2 points. Be sure to check any bed pads under the woman and, when she is out of bed, ask her to save any pads to assess heavy flow. As the woman gets out of bed for the first time, it is common that a gush of lochia that has collected in the vagina will drain. Warn the woman before she stands, reassure her, and provide an extra disposable bed pad to catch the "drip" until she gets to the bathroom.

When the lochial flow is excessive or suddenly increases, check for a change in the client's activity level (e.g., excess straining, lifting, or walking). Check the fundus again for firmness and massage if necessary. If a fundal check and uterine massage do not produce a firm fundus, oxytocic agents may be indicated.

If the fundus is firm, bleeding is not the result of uterine atony. Constant trickling of oxygenated blood (brighter red) may mean arterial bleeding from an unrepaired laceration or a clotting defect. The physician or midwife should be notified for further assessment.

Discharge teaching. Describe the usual sequence of lochial changes. Instruct the woman of the warning signs: resumption of heavy bleeding after lochia serosa begins, clots passed in the lochia, or any unusual or unpleasant odor to the flow. Encourage her to avoid strenuous activity, especially lifting.

Oxytocic use during recovery. To stop excessive blood flow after birth, oxytocin doses of 10 to 20 units (U) may be given intramuscularly (IM) or in an IV solution of 1000

PROCEDURE 17-1
Fundal and Lochia Check

1. Assess that the woman has an empty bladder, and ask her when her pad was last changed.
2. Have the woman lie supine, if possible.
3. Put on nonsterile gloves.
4. Locate the fundus with the palm of the hand.
5. Cup the hand, and place lateral side of the hand slightly above fundus.
6. Place second hand above the symphysis pubis to support and stabilize the uterus during palpation.
7. Gently, but firmly, press into abdomen toward the spine and then slightly downward toward the perineum until a mass is felt in the palm of the hand. At the same time, note the degree of contraction.
8. Measure the number of fingerbreadths at which the fundus is felt below the umbilicus. In general, fingerbreadth measurement should correspond to the number of days after delivery.
9. With gloved hand, check perineal pad for color and amount of lochia.
10. Explain results to the woman, and encourage her to perform the check herself.
11. Offer perineal care, if needed, and provide a clean pad.

Perineal Care

1. Cleanse the perineum after voiding or defecating or after a fundal check with the aseptic solution, if used by protocol, or with plain warm tap water.

2. Cleanse from the front, moving toward the anus to prevent the spread of fecal organisms to the vaginal area.
3. Use soft wipes and a front-to-back single-tissue wiping technique.

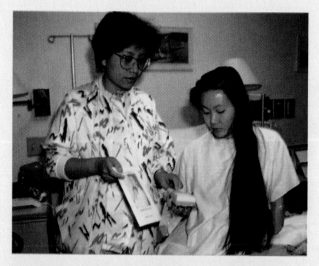

Figure 17-7   Teaching perineal care before the first time out of bed. (Courtesy Marjorie Pyle, RNC, *Lifecircle.*)

OPTIONAL ACTIVITY

Write a sample nursing note correctly documenting the performance of this procedure.

ml to run at 125 ml/hr. If the bag has less than 500 ml at the time recovery begins, a new bag of fluid with the oxytocic dose should be started to prevent too concentrated an infusion (see Drug Profile 16-1).

A side effect of oxytocin is an *antidiuretic effect*, since a partner hormone from the posterior pituitary is vasopressin, an antidiuretic hormone. Therefore during an infusion with oxytocin, the total fluid intake must be carefully watched and checked against output. It has been noted that doses over 20 U/1000 ml fluid in 8 hours can occasionally result in *oliguria*. When the solution is changed to an isotonic saline solution, diuresis immediately begins to occur. *Water intoxication* has also resulted if the dose is given in a prolonged infusion. Signs are elevated BP and headache.

Ergot derivatives. When there is frank hemorrhage uncontrolled by oxytocin, methylergonovine (Methergine) 0.2 mg may be given deep IM every 2 to 5 hours (sites should be rotated). The drug may also be given orally 0.2 to 0.4 mg once every 6 to 12 hours. Since the drug has a vasoconstrictive effect, it is administered only when the maternal blood pressure is within the normal range and there is no peripheral vascular disease.

Prostaglandin preparations. When postpartum bleeding is not controlled by other methods, carboprost tromethamine may be used. Side effects include severe hypertension, bronchospasm, flushing, tetanic contractions, GI upset, fever, joint and muscle pain, low abdominal pain, eye pain, or even shock (see Chapter 21 for more discussion).

Evaluation

- Is the fundus firm and at the appropriate level and position?
- Is the lochia normal in amount, color, and consistency?

Infection

Careful attention must be paid to clinical changes, since the usual diagnostics of fever and leukocytosis are altered in the postpartum period. Subjective symptoms such as complaints of pain, malaise, or chills should be reported to the physican for follow-up. When incisional discharge is present, always obtain a specimen for culture and sensitivity. Antibiotics should not be administered *until* the culture is obtained, but they may be given before the reports are received. Culture and sensitivity results are necessary for the definitive diagnosis of any infection.

Nursing diagnosis: Infection, risk for (uterine, perineal, or incisional), related to childbirth.

Expected outcome: The woman is free from infection.

Uterine infection. Delivery of the placenta leaves an open, raw decidual site. With a dilated cervix, there is risk of an ascending infection. Uterine infection impedes involution, predisposing the woman to hemorrhage. Palpate the abdomen for distention, rigidity, or tenderness. Note lochial odor. Normal lochia is described as "fleshy" or "musky." If there is unusual odor (unpleasant or foul), obtain a specimen for a culture and sensitivity test, check vital signs, and notify the physician for medical follow-up care.

Perineal infection. A perineum that has undergone the trauma of an episiotomy or a laceration is at risk for infection because of its proximity to fecal material and the potential growth medium the lochial bleeding provides. Once infected, the tissue allows pathogens to travel into the vagina and even to the uterus itself (see Chapter 25). Inspect the perineum for signs of infection. The acronynm **REEDA** describes findings (Box 17-2).

Abdominal incision. Following cesarean delivery, the abdominal incision is also assessed for REEDA. If infection occurs, warm soaks or irrigations with a peroxide and saline solution may be indicated, with frequent sterile dressing changes. Support of the woman during this time is vital: the treatment should be explained, and she needs help to cope with another interruption of the childbirth experience.

Discharge teaching. Beginning with the first perineal care (pericare) after birth, explain how to perform the correct technique (see Procedure 17-1). The woman should continue perineal care until the perineum heals and lochia ceases (see Figure 17-6). Emphasize that perineal pads should be applied and removed in a front-to-back direction. Reinforce that hand washing is necessary before and after pericare to prevent infection. Suggest that the woman inspect her perineum and episiotomy by means of a mirror (see discussion on incisional pain: episiotomy later in this chapter). A woman may feel uncomfortable handling her own genitalia because of personal or cultural factors.

Encourage the woman with a cesarean incision to inspect it and report any signs of infection. Also, instruct her to report fever or chills. The woman may want to keep a gauze pad over the incision to prevent irritation from clothing. Showering is allowed, but tub bathing is delayed because of the discomfort of getting into a tub. When the woman is able to negotiate the tub, warm water is soothing to the incision line.

 Box **17-2**

WARNING SIGNS

Perineal Infection

Redness inflammation around wound
Edema of surrounding tissues
Ecchymosis around area (includes evaluation for hematoma)
Discharge from wound
Approximation of skin surfaces

Evaluation

- Is lochial odor normal?
- Is the episiotomy or abdominal incision clean, dry, and intact?
- Is there any evidence of REEDA?
- Does the woman report severe pain at incision sites?
- In the first 24 hours, is the woman's temperature below 100.4° F?

Box 17-1

CLINICAL DECISION

If your client has a morning fever of 101.4° F 30 hours after birth, what assessments must take place before notifying the physician?

Pain

Any complaint of pain requires a nursing response. Because pain is subjective, the best assessment of the level of pain is obtained by asking for a description on a numerical scale, with the lowest number indicating absence of discomfort. Observe the woman's *pain behaviors* as well (see Chapter 16 and Figure 16-6). Location and kind of pain are determined—sharp, burning, throbbing, or aching. Precipitating factors are identified. Pain unrelieved by standard interventions usually indicates complications, and the physician is notified for follow-up.

Nursing diagnosis: Pain, related to uterine contractions, incision, or breast engorgement.

Expected outcome: The woman reports relief from pain.

Uterine contractions. Strong contractions of the involuting uterus are called *afterbirth pains.* Cramping is increased when the uterus has been overdistended, such as by a very large infant or a multiple pregnancy. The IV oxytocin used after delivery increases these contractions, as does breast-feeding, because sucking stimulates oxytocin release from the pituitary gland. Reassure the woman that uterine contractions are a normal part of recovery from childbirth and last for only a few days. She can lie prone with a small pillow or rolled towel under the middle of her abdomen. The cramping may worsen initially because of pressure on the uterus, but she should soon notice relief. A mild analgesic is often helpful in relieving this cramping, and it may be given before breast-feeding to decrease discomfort.

Incisional pain: episiotomy. Most women who have had an episiotomy or vaginal lacerations will experience some degree of pain during immediate recovery after the local anesthetic effect wears off. Assess any changes in the suture line by putting on a pair of gloves and using a light to inspect the perineum for REEDA. Observe also for hemorrhoids, anal fissures, or unrepaired surface vaginal tears. The external labia are carefully observed during the inspection. Note if touching the area elicits more pain.

Cold compresses are applied as soon after birth as possible and for the first 24 hours to prevent and decrease edema and to diminish local sensation. Commercial cold packs may be used, or an examination glove can be filled with crushed ice, tied shut, and wrapped in a paper washcloth. Never apply cold packs directly against skin without a barrier in between. Cold packs should be left in place only for about 20 minutes and removed for a period before reapplication. Sustained vasoconstriction from cold can cause tissue damage (see Chapter 15). Fortunately, the warmth of the perineal area melts the cold pack within the optimal 20 minutes.

After the first 24 hours, warm moist heat is offered by providing the woman with a sitz bath. She is taught to fill it with comfortable warm water, place it on the toilet seat, and sit in it, adding warm water to keep the desired temperature. Although some practitioners recommend cool sitz baths, most women find warmth more soothing. Topical analgesic creams or ointments provide some relief, but studies have found that plain warm compresses give as much, if not more, relief (Enkin, 1995).

Newer therapies involve the use of ultrasound and electromagnetic waves. Though these seem to show some promise, it is unsure whether the modality itself is what helps or the attention that the woman receives while receiving the treatment (Enkin, 1995).

Because analgesic use in the postpartum period is very common, there is generally a standing or routine order for medications such as Percocet or Darvocet. Newer approaches to pain management suggest that providing the new mother with a supply of nonprescription analgesics such as acetaminophen or ibuprofen is more effective than providing prescription analgesics. When the woman is more in control and the time needed for the nurse to respond is eliminated, the woman is better able to medicate herself as soon as she experiences pain. Studies show that this level of self-care results in higher patient satisfaction and less need for narcotic analgesia (Enkins, 1995; McGregor, 1996).

Pain: abdominal incision. The low, transverse "bikini" incision is usually less painful than a vertical incision because most movement does not pull on the muscles involved. However, skin and tissue trauma from the incision itself causes pain. In addition, a distended abdomen will cause pressure on suture lines and increase pain sensation. To rule out infection or bleeding as the cause for pain, the incision should always be reassessed before offering interventions.

The woman is taught to support the incision while moving and to *splint* by holding her hand or a pillow over the incision during deep breathing and coughing. If a binder is ordered, it should be applied when the woman is supine or in a low Fowler's position.

Pharmacologic management after cesarean birth has improved in the last few years. Long-acting epidural narcotic analgesia will last up to 24 hours. If this is not available, meperidine (Demerol) is given at doses of 75 to 100 mg, depending on body weight, and administered IM every 3 to 4 hours. Patient-controlled analgesia (PCA) is used in some centers (see Chapter 16). All PCA pumps have safety features to prevent accidental overdose, and a record is kept of the number of doses infused. The step down from PCA is to oxycodone (Percocet or Percodan) or propoxyphene (Darvocet) and then usually to oral acetaminophen or a prostaglandin inhibitor such as ibuprofen. By the third or fourth day, a woman should be for the most part free from pain, except for soreness on moving, and acetaminophen may keep her comfortable.

Discharge teaching. Encourage the new mother to use comfort measures such as relaxation techniques or lying prone on a pillow or towel. To decrease perineal pulling, suggest that the woman perform Kegel exercises as she sits or stands. Offer teaching about ordered analgesics and their relationship to breast-feeding. Teach the woman with an abdominal incision postoperative self-assessment: inspecting the wound for REEDA and noting any temperature elevation or localized, unresolving pain. Review dosages of ordered analgesics and their side effects.

Breast discomfort. Whether or not the woman is breast-feeding, she may experience discomfort on the third or fourth postpartum day. Therefore all women must know how to care for engorgement. Because women are discharged soon after delivering, engorgement may occur at home. Discussion related to breast pain in the lactating woman is found in the section on breast-feeding.

Discharge teaching. Show the nonlactating woman how to use ice packs to decrease fullness and pain, and emphasize that these packs should never be placed directly on the skin but should be wrapped in a washcloth to prevent tissue injury. The woman should avoid breast stimulation or expression of milk, manually or by pump. Although expression may seem to give relief initially, it actually stimulates milk production and causes the discomfort to last longer. The woman should be advised to wear a snug, well-fitting brassiere at all times until the engorgement subsides. If a woman asks for medication to "dry up" the milk, explain that such medications usually are not given and that the discomfort will decrease within 2 to 3 days.

Evaluation

- Does the woman report a decrease in pain?
- Is she able to explain and demonstrate comfort measures before discharge?
- Is she wearing a bra consistently?
- Can she demonstrate correct use of an ice pack?
- Can she explain the medication she will take at home, including the dose and its frequency and the medicine's side effects?

Elimination

A combination of factors—trauma from delivery, residual hormonal levels, anesthesia, and fluid shifts—influence both urinary and bowel elimination in the recovery period. Nursing care is planned to prevent or treat alterations in elimination since these also affect other systems.

Nursing diagnoses: Urinary retention, related to periurethral edema from delivery

Constipation, related to anesthesia, diet, medication, or pain

Expected outcome: The woman returns to normal elimination patterns

Urinary elimination. A record is kept on the first two voids after delivery. The first void should be within 4 to 8 hours after delivery and should be at least 200 cc. Voiding of less than 100 cc suggests overflow from a distended bladder. Palpate the lower abdomen for distention and discomfort, and if the woman is unable to void, increase fluid intake and ambulation. Running tap water, using a sitz bath to relieve edema and relax the sphincter, and applying warmth or ice to the suprapubic area are aids to urination. There may be a standing order for straight catheterization to relieve distention or check for residual urine after voiding. If this must be repeated, some protocols call for insertion of a Foley catheter attached to a closed drainage system.

There is a difference of opinion on how much urine can be safely drained out at one time without changing vital signs. Since the postpartum woman has been able to withstand increased intraabdominal pressures from a gravid uterus and a full bladder and has already experienced a sudden decrease in pressure with delivery, draining the bladder may not be traumatic. However, care should be taken to slowly drain the initial amount while assessing the patient for complications. The catheter may be clamped for a few minutes and then opened to drain the remaining urine.

Early specimens are always mixed with lochia. A clean-voided specimen must be obtained if there are any questions regarding urine color and clarity, if there is cloudiness or an unusual color, if the client becomes febrile, or if there are signs of dysuria or frequency. A specimen is sent for culture and sensitivity testing and the physician is notified for medical follow-up care. The only way to obtain a clear, sterile specimen is by straight catheterization.

Discharge teaching. Encourage the new mother to empty her bladder frequently and to keep track of the approximate amounts voided. Remind her to note any unusual color or odor and report it. Encourage her to increase fluid intake, and also instruct her to report dysuria or frequency as signs of urinary tract infection.

Evaluation

- Has the woman passed at least 200 cc with each void?
- Is her bladder nondistended after voiding?

- Does she report dysuria?
- Can she verbalize the need to maintain adequate fluid intake?
- Is she able to explain signs and symptoms that need to be reported?

Bowel elimination. The abdomen should be visually inspected for distention, palpated for firmness or rigidity, and auscultated for the presence of bowel sounds, especially after surgical delivery. The woman is asked if she is able to pass flatus rectally or if she feels the urge to defecate.

Encourage the woman to increase fluid intake, and recommend ambulation to enhance peristalsis. Stool softeners and laxatives are administered as ordered. If these measures fail, an enema or suppository may be needed.

Discharge teaching. Review the effect of fluid and dietary intake on bowel function with the new mother. Discuss foods that are high in fiber to assist with passing stool. If stool softeners are ordered, teach use, dosage and frequency, and side effects.

Evaluation

- Are bowel sounds present?
- Is the woman passing flatus and has she moved her bowels?
- Does she verbalize understanding of the need to increase fluids and fiber in her diet?
- Can she explain the use, dosage, and side effects of any stool softeners ordered?

Needs for Activity and Rest

The amount of energy expended during labor and birth leaves the new mother in great need of rest. Women often fall asleep during a quiet recovery. Others are so excited that they find it impossible to relax and sleep. After the initial period of elation and stimulation, encourage the woman to use relaxation techniques to calm herself. Although sleep may not seem very important to the new mother, she will become fatigued if she does not set regular times of rest. Fatigue adversely affects milk production, interferes with learning, can precipitate depression, and can lower her self-esteem (Atkinson and Baxley, 1994).

Nursing diagnoses: Fatigue, related to childbirth exertion

Sleep pattern disturbance, related to hospital routines and the need to care for new infant at home

Knowledge deficit, regarding safe resumption of exercise after childbirth

Expected outcomes: The woman reports improvements in fatigue levels.

The woman verbalizes ways to improve sleep patterns at home.

The woman verbalizes understanding of appropriate exercise patterns after discharge.

Care should be planned so that the new mother can rest while she is in the recovery unit. If the infant is staying in the mother's room, encourage the partner to help her rest. Discuss with her the ways she can get rest in the home situation by limiting visitors at first, encouraging helpers to do the noninfant care tasks, and disconnecting the telephone during feeding or nap times. She will miss sleep at night, so she should plan to nap when the infant does. The nurse can emphasize to the partner the importance of rest while encouraging him to assist with infant and mother care.

Exercise. When women were confined to bed for extended periods after delivery, many complications such as hypostatic pneumonia, thromboses, and pulmonary emboli occurred. For this reason, ambulation and exercise are encouraged soon after delivery.

Discharge teaching. Gentle isometric stretching exercises and Kegel exercises may begin after birth. Then the next few days, abdominal strengthening exercises, such as arm and leg lifts and flexing to touch the chin to the chest, start the process of returning the woman to her prepregnant condition. In the first 4 to 6 weeks after delivery, the new mother may gradually resume exercising in the same way she exercised during the prenatal period (ACOG, 1994; Artal and Buckenmayer, 1995). She should be cautioned not to exercise too strenuously at first but instead to pace her activities. Walking is one of the best exercises. Sit-ups are delayed for a few weeks. (Box 9-1 presents guidelines for exercise during the postpartum period, and Figure 17-8 demonstrates typical exercises to regain body contours.)

Evaluation

- Can the woman demonstrate isometric exercises before discharge?
- Does the woman verbalize understanding of the need to gradually resume exercise after discharge?
- Is the woman able to describe exercises to be avoided in the immediate postpartum period?

Immunologic Needs

Delivery of the fetus and placenta increases the chance of fetal blood entering maternal circulation. For the Rh negative mother with an Rh positive infant, this predisposes to the formation of antibodies that can endanger future pregnancies. Prevention of this isoimmunization is possible if Rh immunoglobulin (RhIG, RhoGAM) is administered within 72 hours after delivery. The Rh negative mother may have already received several doses during pregnancy at 28 and 34 weeks or if she underwent an invasive procedure such as amniocentesis, chorionic villus sampling, or if she suffered trauma (see Chapter 23).

Rh immunoglobulin. The Rh negative woman must be Coombs' negative to receive RhIG within 72 hours after birth. Both maternal and newborn blood types and Coombs' test results must be verified by the nurse before the dose is given (see Drug Profile 23-1).

Discharge teaching. Give the woman the card containing information about RhIG, including the dose given

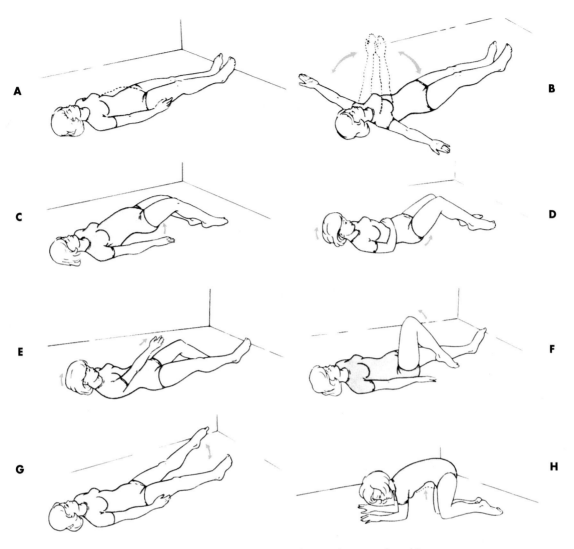

Figure 17-8   A to H, Postpartum exercises to regain muscle strength and improve posture.

and the date and time of administration. Explain to the woman the importance of notifying health care practitioners of her Rh status.

Rubella. If the woman has not had rubella infection and if her titre is negative (1:8 or less), she is a candidate for rubella vaccination. Assess the need for rubella vaccination before discharge (see Chapter 25).

Discharge teaching. Caution the mother to avoid becoming pregnant for at least 3 months after receiving this attenuated live virus. Since there is a very slight chance of a low grade viral infection being passed to another person, she should avoid contact with any nonimmune pregnant women. Rubella infection in early pregnancy may result in congenital birth defects (see Chapter 25).

Evaluation

- Does the woman who is Rh negative and Coombs' negative have an infant who is Rh positive and Coombs' negative? If so, has she received RhoGAM within 72 hours of delivery?

- Can she verbalize the need for RhoGAM in future pregnancies?
- Has the mother with a rubella titer of 1:8 or less received a rubella vaccine?
- Can she explain the need to avoid pregnancy for at least 3 months and to avoid contact with any pregnant nonimmune woman?

Sexuality and Contraception

The topic of sexual relations may have been introduced during pregnancy, but it must be discussed again as early as possible in the postpartum period, preferably with the mother's sex partner present. Before discharge, the woman's expectations and understanding of potential problems are assessed.

Nursing diagnoses: Sexuality patterns, altered, related to the need to recover from childbirth.

Knowledge deficit, regarding appropriate contraceptive methods for the postpartum period.

Expected outcomes: The woman and her partner express understanding of the reasons for delaying vaginal intercourse until after healing has occurred.

The woman verbalizes a choice of a contraceptive and explains its use.

To prevent hemorrhage and infection, sexual intercourse is usually restricted until the perineum and uterus have completely healed. Traditionally, healing was considered accomplished by 6 weeks, but it is probably adequate at 2 to 4 weeks. After that, intercourse may be resumed when desire and comfort dictate. Although new parents may be inhibited from intercourse because of pain from an episiotomy or laceration or fear of damaging them, discomfort from breast stimulation in the nursing mother, or abdominal tenderness after a cesarean delivery, teaching can alleviate anxiety and allow for comfortable resumption of sexual activity (refer to Chapters 8 and 9).

The nurse discusses methods of relieving discomfort during intercourse, such as the use of water-soluble lubricants or plain vegetable oil to decrease perineal trauma and vaginal dryness. The mother must be reassured that it is normal to experience strong contractions during orgasm. The nursing mother should be told that stimulation of full breasts may be uncomfortable, may cause some leaking, and will be less bothersome if "planned" after a feeding rather than before. The couple should be encouraged to try various positions that lessen pressure on the perineum, abdomen, and breasts.

The couple should also be encouraged to express their feelings about another pregnancy and what prevention is planned. Review facts about the return of menstruation and ovulation. The parents may be worried about another pregnancy but unsure of an appropriate method of family planning. Because birth control often is planned around the menstrual cycle, the woman should understand that she may not have her first menses for 4 to 8 weeks if she is not nursing, whereas breast-feeding mothers may have amenorrhea for as long as 4 to 18 months (AWHONN, 1993), therefore natural family planning may be unreliable at first (refer to Chapter 5).

Discharge teaching. Encourage the woman to freely express when she is ready to resume sexual activity. Explain that one way to determine the comfort level in coitus is to insert two fingers into her vagina and rotate gently. If there is minimal discomfort, she may feel better about initiating intercourse (AWHONN, 1993). Also remind her that she may need extra lubrication until hormones increase natural vaginal secretions.

Safe sex is always taught as essential, thus use of condoms with foam or gel should be encouraged. These are an especially useful method for the breast-feeding mother who should not use combined oral contraceptives that could affect prolactin levels in the first months of feeding and decrease milk supply. If a diaphragm is the method of choice, teach the woman that she will have to be refitted because the cervix and vagina are enlarged after delivery and her old diaphragm may not fit properly (see Chapter 5). Review natural family planning, but emphasize that since it involves menstruation and mucous secretions, it is not always possible to interpret the cycle until hormone levels have stabilized and several cycles have occurred.

Evaluation

- Does the woman verbalize the rationale for deferring coitus until healing has occurred? Does she state plans to discuss this with her partner?
- Can she discuss comfort measures to use during intercourse?
- Is she able to explain her choice of a contraceptive method?

SPECIAL NEEDS AFTER CESAREAN BIRTH

Although recovery from childbirth is the main factor in planning care for all postpartum women, the mother who has had a cesarean birth has special needs related to her surgery and will require additional nursing considerations. See the Care Path on Cesarean Birth for sequences of care.

The stress of childbirth is worsened when a woman is unprepared for a surgical procedure; often a woman will experience additional anxiety, pain, disappointment and frustration, and lowered self-esteem. She will need understanding, support, and encouragement to see surgical birth as an acceptable way to have an infant. If the birth was emergent or unexpected, she may have little memory of the details of the surgical birth and will need to be given details.

Nursing diagnoses: Injury, risk for, related to surgery and possible uterine bleeding.

Infection, risk for, related to abdominal incision, indwelling urinary catheter, and altered breathing patterns.

Pain, related to incision and uterine contractions.

Tissue perfusion, altered, related to immobility.

Self-esteem, situational low, related to childbirth difficulties.

Parenting, altered, related to discomfort and the recovery process.

Anxiety, related to concern for self and infant.

Expected outcomes: The woman is free from injury and maintains a normal involution pattern.

There is no wound or pulmonary or urinary infection.

Pain is relieved so that normal activity is quickly resumed.

Tissue perfusion is maintained without emboli formation.

Surgical birth does not interfere with self-esteem and parenting roles.

Anxiety for self and infant resolves.

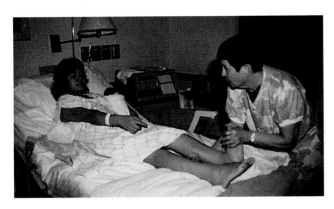

Figure 17-9   Checking Homans' sign for any woman who is not ambulatory in the first few hours. (Courtesy Marjorie Pyle, RNC, *Lifecircle*.)

Physical Recovery: Circulation

Because ambulation may be hindered by pain from abdominal surgery, the woman is at risk for circulatory complications. When muscular activity is decreased or absent, venous return is decreased and stasis may occur. When this is combined with increased viscosity from fluid losses and the temporary elevation in clotting factors in the immediate period, the woman is predisposed for the formation of phlebitis and thromboembolism (see Chapter 22).

Homans' sign. The initial assessment should note any history of or risk for blood clots. If complications require bed rest for even 1 to 2 days, preventive care should be initiated, which includes isometric exercises and active range of motion. Be alert for complaints of pain in the legs; examine extremities for warmth, redness, and swelling, and assess for Homans' sign (Figure 17-9). There may be a developing blood clot in the deeper veins of the calf if there is pain extending up the leg when the foot is flexed toward the shin. A positive Homan's sign must be reported for medical follow-up.

Obviously, the best prophylactic treatment plan calls for helping the woman walk as soon as possible. For the woman unable to ambulate soon after delivery, leg movement, isometric exercises, and turning are encouraged. Antiembolism stockings are applied to give support to the vein walls and thus aid blood flow. After cesarean or complicated delivery, the woman may enter the unit with a counterpressure mechanical pump. The pump, connected to bandages or plastic sleeves over thromboembolic disease (TED) stockings, provides intermittent inflation to apply the pressure needed to assist venous return. The nurse checks the settings, verifies the functioning of the system, and reassures the woman about the sensations she may experience.

Recovery from Anesthesia

Chapter 16 details the care of a person recovering from anesthesia. During the initial assessment, the type and

duration of anesthesia are noted. Some women will be groggy and confused on awakening from general anesthesia. There may have been a long labor before the decision for cesarean birth was made; fatigue will then be an important factor during recovery. When an epidural has been planned for and understood, women may have a very smooth recovery period. Other women feel heaviness in the legs after regional block anesthesia and have difficulty when first getting out of bed. The newly recovering woman should never get up alone and should sit on the side of the bed for a period of time to prevent orthostatic hypotension.

Respiratory needs. Discomfort from a surgical incision, especially a classic or vertical incision, and abdominal distention interfere with the mother's normal respiratory pattern. To prevent increased abdominal pressure, she often avoids deep breaths and coughing, which result in decreased tidal volume, decreased air exchange, and accumulation of bronchial secretions. This avoidance leads to complications of atelectasis and pneumonia.

As soon as possible, explain pulmonary exercises, assisting the woman to as high a Fowler's position as she can tolerate, and offer her a pillow to hold across her abdomen while she coughs. Gentle pressure supports the abdominal musculature, decreasing pain and relieving anxiety. "Ladder" breathing or "huffing" before coughing is useful, and an incentive spirometer should be ordered. These devices encourage deep breathing by having the woman use her breaths to make a ball or gauge move. The deeper the breath, the more the ball rises, and the woman can see results and work at her own pace, increasing respirations gradually as tolerated.

Pain medication is offered before beginning respiratory therapy, with the explanation that it will help the woman with the activity. After an IM injection, the wait is 15 minutes, and after oral analgesics, 30 minutes is allowed for adequate absorption and action. Auscultate the lung fields before and after treatment to assess patency and air flow.

Delayed peristalsis: gas pains. Intestinal peristalsis can be decreased by the action of anesthetics, analgesics, altered food intake, and a change in activity level. After a cesarean delivery, for example, it may take 24 hours for motility in the small intestine to resume and 3 to 5 days for complete function in the large intestine to return. Air and the breakdown of old materials in the colon produce flatulence and distention and thus increase pain and incisional discomfort because of distension.

Small sips of water and ice chips may be allowed until bowel sounds are heard, and then the ordered diet is advanced slowly. The woman avoids iced and carbonated drinks that may increase flatulence. Early and frequent ambulation is encouraged to stimulate normal peristalsis. If a medication such as simethicone is ordered prophylactically, the woman is instructed to chew the tablets thoroughly before swallowing. Gas

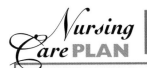

Nursing Care PLAN | *Recovery from Vaginal Birth*

CASE

Mary is an 18-year-old, G1, P 0000, who came to labor and delivery 2 weeks before her estimated date of birth. She reported rupture of membranes 4 hours before admission. After 22 hours of labor and a normal spontaneous vaginal delivery (NSD) of a 5 lb 10 oz, 37-week female infant, she was admitted to the recovery room with the following vital signs (VS): 99.8/80/22, BP 104/68. She had right medio-lateral episiotomy and third-degree laceration and complains of "pain in the bottom—a lot." Perineum is edematous, and reddened, with sutures intact.

Her social history includes being married to Leonard, age 20, a truck driver who is often out of town. Mary worked at a local fertilizer plant until her delivery and plans to return to work in 3 months. She states that she attended two childbirth preparation classes with a sister who also accompanied her to the hospital and stayed with her through delivery. Mary is eager to "try" to breast-feed her daughter.

Her nutritional history describes often eating out at fast-food restaurants, but as a result of prenatal guidance she has added more fruits and vegetables to her diet. While pregnant, she decreased smoking from two packs per day to one pack per day, and she reported drinking beer with co-workers after work a few nights a week.

Assessment

1. Obstetric, pregnancy, and delivery history
2. Vital signs and involutional status
3. Nutritional history and status
4. Pain level and medications ordered
5. Infant feeding plan: breast-feeding
6. Social history
7. Knowledge and developmental level: self-care, infant care, and feeding
8. Support systems

Nursing Diagnoses

1. Injury, risk for possible hemorrhage, related to blood loss secondary to uterine atony and third-degree laceration
2. Infection, risk for, related duration of ruptured membranes, impaired skin integrity, and invasive procedures during labor and delivery
3. Pain, related to episiotomy and third-degree lacerations, afterbirth pains, and breast discomfort
4. Altered elimination, risk for related to periurethral edema and NPO status during labor
5. Knowledge deficit, regarding postpartum recovery self-care, related to inexperience
6. Knowledge deficit, regarding infant care and feeding, related to inexperience as parents
7. Breast-feeding, ineffective, related to inexperience
8. Parenting, risk for altered, related to family structure and support and parental employment
9. Knowledge deficit, regarding sexual activity and contraception.

Expected Outcomes

The woman will be able to do the following:

1. Demonstrate normal involution, plus knowledge of subinvolution signs.
2. Show no signs of infection.
3. Report minimal discomfort, and know care for healing wound.
4. Urinate without difficulty, and evidence bowel sounds before discharge.
5. Discuss self-care needs during recovery, concerning nutrition, rest, activity, and reduction in smoking and drinking.
6. Demonstrate ability to feed the infant and give it safe care.
7. Demonstrate attachment and parenting behaviors.
8. Report adequate support system for self, husband, and infant; evaluate workplace and work schedule for maximum benefit for self and infant.
9. Discuss when sexual relations can be resumed and ways to increase comfort during sexual activity, and explain a contraceptive method.

Nursing Care PLAN | *Recovery from Vaginal Birth—cont'd*

▼

Nursing Interventions

1. Teach fundal checks, lochia assessment, and wound care. Follow routine focused assessments of vital signs, laboratory values, and recovery status.
   Demonstrate, explain, and encourage handwashing, correct disposal of peripads, and perineal care.
2. Assess for unusual pain.
   Encourage nonpharmacologic approaches to pain control, such as the use of ice packs for 24 hours, Sitz bath use after 24 hours, and perineal tightening exercises while sitting or standing.
   Teach analgesic dosage and side effects. Encourage rest periods.
3. Monitor urinary output and check for residual fullness after voiding.
   Assess bowel sound, flatus, and bowel function.
   Encourage adequate fluid and fiber intake.
   Administer stool softeners or laxatives as ordered, plus teach protocol for home use.
4. Review knowledge of self-care activities.
   Provide instruction on all aspects of self-care.
   Explain and encourage adequate nutrition, such as an increase in protein, vitamin C, and fluids for breast-feeding.
   Discuss effects of passive smoke, alcohol on breast-feeding infant.
5. Assess knowledge level about infant care, safety, feeding, and needs.
   Discuss developmental needs of the 37-week newborn.
   Discuss importance of using a car seat and returning for newborn checkup.
   Discuss the potential for jaundice because of gestational age.
   Describe situations that should be reported to health care provider.
6. Assess attachment and parenting behaviors.
   Discuss expectations of the parenting role and her support system.
   Encourage seeking help from family, friends, and community groups.
   Encourage Mary to include husband in parenting tasks.
7. Assist Mary with getting infant onto breast and teach her how to assess for sucking and swallowing.
   Discuss breast and nipple care and provide literature.
   Teach signs of engorgement and mastitis, and teach when to report problems.
   Refer to home care, lactation follow-up, and WIC.
8. Teach rationale for delaying sexual activity, and teach comfort measures.
   Discuss methods of contraception she may choose and encourage questions.

▼

Evaluation

1. Is involution progress appropriate for the day after birth?
2. Are episiotomy and laceration incisions clean, dry, and intact? Is she afebrile?
3. Does she report relief from pain and know at-home pain relief methods?
4. Is she urinating without difficulty? Does she have bowel sounds? Has she passed flatus or moved her bowels?
5. Is she performing pericare, assessing involution, and demonstrating self-care behaviors?
6. Can she give safe basic care to the infant? Does she have a car seat to take the infant home?
7. Do she and her partner demonstrate attachment and parenting behaviors?
8. Is she able to do initial breast-feeding? Does she have referrals and resources for feeding at home? Does she verbalize diet changes needed during breast-feeding?
9. Can she explain when to resume sexual activity? Has she chosen a contraceptive method, and can she describe how to use it?

---

pains generally occur on the third postoperative day. The woman is advised to lie on her right side and to turn frequently to facilitate passing gas. The nurse may place a rectal tube to decompress the lower bowel or administer a Harris flush (return-flow enema) as ordered. The use of analgesics that further slow peristalsis is discouraged.

Discharge teaching. Teach and assist the new mother with deep breathing and coughing exercises, and encourage her to continue them after discharge. Because of short hospital stays, respiratory complications may not become apparent until she is at home a few days. Teach her to report any congestion, productive sputum, dyspnea, or fever. Encourage her to elevate her legs at home when sitting and avoid crossing her legs while lying or sitting. Describe signs of phlebitis and emphasize the need to report any evidence of this to the physician.

Provide information on diet to maintain bowel elimination, especially the need for increased fluids and fiber. Review the correct use of simethicone.

Evaluation

- Is the status of the lochia and fundus appropriate for the postdelivery time?

- Are signs of REEDA absent from the abdominal incision?
- Does the woman understand how to manage splinting, position changes, and analgesics to reduce discomfort?
- Does she have clear breath sounds and understand the need for coughing and breathing exercises?
- Are elimination patterns reestablished?
- Are both partners able to verbalize understanding of reasons for surgery and outcomes?

Psychosocial Considerations after Cesarean Birth

To assess what the cesarean birth experience means to a new mother, the nurse can arrange a time to review the experience with her by using questions such as the following:

- What do you understand about what happened during surgery?
- Do you feel that you have unanswered questions?
- What could the nurses have done to make things easier for you?

Listen to the woman's feelings about her experience, and encourage her to recount her perceptions and express excitement, pride, sadness, regret, anger, or disappointment. There may be elements of the grieving process as she copes with the perceived loss of an active birthing experience. In the recovery period the nurse emphasizes the woman's individuality and ability as a new mother. As the woman talks about her cesarean delivery, the focus should be on achievement and the birth of her infant.

Postpartum "blues" may be seen more often after surgical delivery because of longer hospital stays. The nurse should be alert for signs of ineffective coping; refer the mother for counseling if coping mechanisms do not appear adequate.

Follow-up care by telephone or through home care visits is planned, and the new mother is given preparation for the fatigue and discomforts she may often feel at home and on her own with the new infant.

A father also needs to discuss his experience. The nurse offers understanding of the disappointment or even anger that he may feel and encourages him to communicate with his partner to foster mutual support. The nurse must emphasize the importance of his role as successful father, especially if the mother is unable to fully participate in infant care because of pain or limited mobility.

Complicated births often result in compromised infants who require special care in a neonatal intensive care unit (NICU). To the new parents, this results in additional stress caused by the interruption of the normal attachment process and a sense of loss because of fear for their infant's well-being. Encourage and assist them to visit the nursery to see, touch, and participate as much as possible in care of their infant (see Figure 17-19). If this is not possible, act as liaison between the parents and the

NICU nurses to relay information about the infant's condition and progress (see Chapter 29).

Discharge teaching. Emphasize that negative feelings about the birth experience are normal and acceptable, and encourage the mother to share them. Refer her to peer groups or individual counseling as indicated. Review with the couple the normal progression of postpartum "blues," and explain to the father that the mother's mood swings are most often not directed at him. Encourage opportunities for rest.

Evaluation

Because the hospital stay for birth is so brief, additional evaluation must be directed toward the preparation for going home, regardless of the method of birth.

- Can the woman demonstrate accurate self-assessment and care?
- Does she exhibit adequate confidence and competence in infant care?
- Are there needs for referral? Has she received follow-up literature and instructions in all areas of self-care, including family planning?
- Can she describe infant needs for nutrition, rest, sleep, activity, and safety?
- Have the parents obtained a car seat for going home?

Box 17-2

CLINICAL DECISION

Your client Susan (age 24, G1, P1, living in a small apartment) tells you that she is most troubled about two of the postpartum concerns you had not thought to discuss with her. She feels that social isolation and loneliness are her chief concerns after going home. How will you begin your conversation about these concerns, and what assistance might there be for her?

LEARNING INFANT FEEDING

Because breast-feeding is considered the best method of infant feeding, the nursing mother should receive encouragement, support, and assistance. The woman who chooses to bottle-feed also has many needs as she begins caring for and satisfying her infant (Figure 17-10). Regardless of the method, if there is an apparent lack of understanding about how to feed an infant, a new mother will become quickly frustrated if her infant does not respond to her efforts or is unsatisfied after a tense feeding time (Figure 17-11). The nurse assesses whether the mother is comfortable holding the infant, offering the breast or bottle, and bubbling the infant, and also whether she shows signs of attachment behaviors during feeding. The mother is encouraged to ask questions and express concerns while support and teaching is offered.

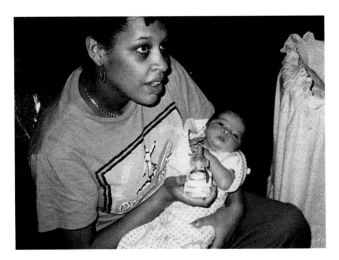

Figure 17-10 Bottle-feeding raises, many questions for new mothers. She will need assistance with her awkward position. (Courtesy Camille Bodden.)

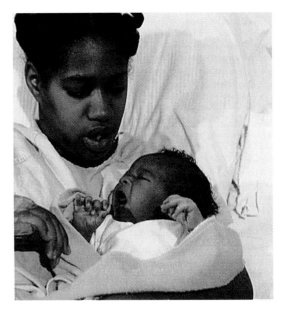

Figure 17-11 If the young mother is tense and the infant is crying, feeding times may seem a disaster. This situation requires intervention. (Courtesy Concept Media, Irvine, Calif.)

Lawrence (1994) emphasizes that, "The method chosen to feed a baby is but one item in a whole lifestyle of maternal-infant interaction," but since confidence about feeding her infant is essential to every mother, the nurse must be careful at this critical time not to appear judgmental if she does not wish to breast-feed or becomes frustrated with her infant's feeding. The new mother needs positive reinforcement for her ability to decide how she wishes to feed her child and to learn the best ways to do so. She also needs instruction and explanations about infant behavior so that she feels the infant "likes" her. If the infant does not meet her expectations and is sleepy at feeding time or slow to suck, the woman may feel anxious. There should never be "blame" assigned to the mother or the infant (Renfrew et al, 1990). Neither is a failure; there are simply needs to be met and problems to be solved.

Breast-feeding

Nutritional benefits of breast-feeding

Human milk provides all the nutrients necessary for the first 4 to 6 months of life and remains valuable up to and even beyond 2 years (Nicoll, 1995). Breast milk is "uniquely designed to meet the needs of human infants" (Lawrence, 1994). There is a low solute load, and it has more unsaturated fatty acids than cow's milk (Table 17-3). Proteins and fats are more easily digested, and carbohydrate content is appropriate for growth. When an infant is breast-fed, problems caused by poor sanitation, lack of refrigeration, ignorance, or illiteracy are avoided. Finally, for the infant, adequate protein intake is available even in a diet-deficient environment.

The composition of breast milk changes during the course of the feeding session. Initially the infant receives a large volume of lower caloric "foremilk." After the first few minutes, volume decreases as the milk becomes higher in fats and calories. It is this "hindmilk" that not only gives essential nutrients but also leaves the infant feeling full and satisfied.

Immunologic benefits

Human milk is a biochemically unique substance perfectly adapted to the infant's needs. Colostrum is available to the infant for the first 1 to 3 days of life. It contains antibodies consistent with maternal titers of antibodies, protecting against organisms such as *Staphylococcus, Salmonella,* poliovirus, influenza virus, *Bordetella pertussis, Escherichia coli* and others. Since the newborn has immature antibody response until about 6 weeks of age, without the full protection of the antibody system the infant is vulnerable. Secretory IgA found in colostrum binds with microorganisms while also protecting antibodies from being degraded by acids. Antibodies produced by the mother are specific to pathogens, sparing the infant's normal flora, and able to ward off disease without initiating an inflammatory response.

Other protective factors in colostrum include oligosaccharides, which intercept bacteria and help excrete them, and lactoferrin, which binds with iron to make it unavailable for pathogens that require it. Colostrum also contains interferon, known for its antiviral activity, and fibronectin, which activates phagocyte activity. Finally, immune cells (leukocytes, macrophages, and lymphocytes) attack pathogens, while hormones such as cortisol and other proteins work on mucosal lining to strengthen it against pathogenic invasion and permeability to other substances (Newman, 1995).

Cesarean Section

Focus	Discharge Outcomes	0 – 12 Hours
ASSESSMENT INTERVENTIONS	• Temperature <99.6 • Blood pressure $\geq \frac{90}{60}$ $\leq \frac{140}{90}$ • Pulse <100 • Voiding on own qs • Firm uterus • Moderate lochia rubra • Incision clean and intact • Passing flatus	• Vital signs per SOC • Cough, deep breathe, spirometer, splint incision • Assess vital signs, pain, level of consciousness, itching and nausea and vomiting as per the SOC for ordered method of pain management • Foley care as per the SOC for Foley catheter • Assess fundus and lochia as per SOC • Assess incision as per SOC • Assess bowel sounds as per SOC
DIAGNOSTIC TESTS	• Hgb > 8 grams • HCT > 24%	
MEDICATIONS/IV	• No IV • Able to take and retain PO medications • Pain relief obtained • RhoGAM given prn • Rubella vaccine given prn • Hepatitis status known	• IV per physician orders • Pain Management: ☐ PCA ☐ Morphine ☐ Other: ☐ • Antiemetic prn ☐ • Antipruritic prn • Determine need for RhoGAM • Review maternal rubella and hepatitis status
DIET	• Able to take and retain food and fluids	• Encourage PO fluids • First meal clear fluids as tolerated ☐ • (Other) Diet
CONSULTS	• Positive mother-infant interactions and parenting activities • All appropriate consults completed, and actions implemented as needed	• Monitor mother's delivery of care and refer prn • Ensure consults initiated: ☐ None needed ☐ Nutrition ☐ Home care ☐ Social work ☐ Lactation consultant ☐ Pain team ☐ (Other)
ACTIVITY/SAFETY	• Able to ambulate ad lib. • Security and safety of newborn maintained	• Assist first ambulation, then ambulate ad lib. • Review infant security with mother
PATIENT/FAMILY EDUCATION	• Successful completion of client education plan as per *Needs Assessment* • Receives written educational materials • Significant other involved in teaching and care	• Complete *Needs Assessment* with mother • Initiate teaching: ☐ Breast-feeding ☐ Expressing and storing breast milk ☐ Bottle feeding ☐ Mother care ☐ Infant care
DISCHARGE PLANNING	• Mother and infant discharged together • Home care referral prn • Receives prescriptions prn • Verbalizes understanding	• Assess Home Care/Discharge needs ☐ • Consider WIC ☐ • Assure circumcision permit prn • Inform mother of target discharge date and time

Courtesy Long Island Jewish Medical Center, New Hyde Park, NY.

ad lib., At pleasure; *CBC*, complete blood count; *HCT*, hematocrit; *Hgb*, hemoglobin; *IV*, intravenous, *PCA*, patient-controlled analgesia; *PO*, by mouth; *prn*, as needed; *qs*, quantity sufficient; *SOC*, standard of care; *WIC*, Women, Infants, and Children Food Supplementation Program.

13 - 24 Hours	25 Hours - Discharge	Initials

13 - 24 Hours

- Assess vital signs, pain, level of sedation, itching, and nausea and vomiting as per SOC for method of pain management
- Discontinue Foley catheter by 24 hours
- Measure first void after Foley catheter discontinued
- Catheterize if not voiding after 6 hours without Foley catheter
- Assess fundus and lochia as per SOC
- Assess incision as per SOC
- Assess bowel sounds as per SOC

☐ • Consider need for CBC

- IV per physician orders
- Pain management:
☐ PCA ☐ Morphine
☐ Oxycodone 2 tablets every 4 hours prn
☐ • Antiemetic prn   ☐ • Antipruritic prn
☐ • Acetaminophen 1 gram every 4 hours prn
☐ • Simethicone, milk of magnesia, bisacodyl

- Advance diet as tolerated
☐ Soft diet   ☐ Regular diet
☐ (Other)   Diet

- Continue to monitor mother's delivery of care and refer prn
☐ Nutrition
☐ Home care
☐ Social work
☐ Lactation consultant
☐ Pain team
☐ (Other)

- Encourage ambulation ad lib.

- Continue teaching as per *Needs Assessment*
- Continue involvement of significant other in care

Ensure birth certificate information obtained

25 Hours - Discharge

- Vital signs per SOC
- Assess pain as per SOC
- Assess fundus as per SOC
- Assess lochia as per SOC
- Assess incision as per SOC
- Assess bowel sounds as per SOC
- Assess continued ability to void on own

- CBC on day of discharge

- Discontinue IV after 24 hours
☐ • Oxycodone 2 tablets every 4 hours prn
☐ • Acetaminophen 1 gram every 4 hours prn

☐ • Rubella vaccine prn

- Advance diet as tolerated
☐ Soft diet   ☐ Regular diet
☐ (Other)   Diet

- Completion of consults

- Encourage ambulation ad lib.
- May shower after 24 hours

- Reinforce mother/infant care

- Complete discharge plan and instructions

Table 17-3	Contrast between Human and Cow's Milk Concentrations	
	Human	**Cow**
CALORIES	Higher	Lower
PROTEIN	Lower	Higher
FAT	Higher	Lower
CARBOHYDRATES	Higher	Lower
CALCIUM	Lower	Much higher
PHOSPHORUS	Lower	Higher
IRON	Low	Only trace
SODIUM	Lower	Higher
POTASSIUM	Lower	Higher
VITAMIN A	Higher	Lower

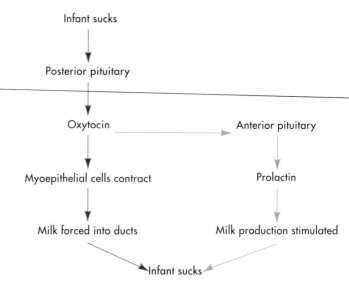

Figure 17-12 Let-down reflex is triggered by the infant's sucking.

In the absence of this protection, large molecules of protein can reach the intestinal tissues of the formula-fed infant and be absorbed into the circulation, producing an immune response that can predispose the infant to an allergy to cow's milk. In the breast-feeding infant, however, the intestine is coated with immunoglobulins from the colostrum. Human milk has low allergenicity and contains a factor that promotes growth of *Lactobacillus bifidus,* which produces lactic and acetic acids in the GI tract. These acids turn the stool acidic and provide additional protection against the growth of enteric infections. The formula-fed infant has a more alkaline stool that does not have the same protective effect. Because colostrum is rich in immunoglobulins, antiinflammatory agents, and immunologic modulators, there may be a relationship between breast-feeding and decreases in respiratory illnesses, especially those caused by respiratory syncytial virus (RSV), meningitis, and bacteremia. Colostrum may also be protective against chronic liver disease in later life (Cunningham et al, 1993) and against Crohn's disease and childhood cancers, such as leukemia, for infants nursed 4 months or more (Lawrence, 1994). Studies also indicate decreased incidence of otitis media, diarrhea (Dewey, 1995), insulin-dependent diabetes mellitus (Dermer, 1995), and even rheumatoid arthritis and inguinal hernia (Lawrence, 1994; Pisacane, 1995).

Another important benefit of breast milk involves its connection with sudden infant death syndrome (SIDS). Researchers point out that breast-feeding may be associated with a significantly lower incidence of SIDS (Renfrew et al, 1990; Lawrence, 1994).

Developmental benefits

Breast-feeding provides a unique bonding experience for mother and child. It stimulates most of the senses, and close body contact allows the infant to recognize its mother's smell and to feel and hear her heartbeat, as it did during gestation. Studies indicate this bonding may result in increased visual, oral, and intellectual development (Dermer, 1995). And because the sensory qualities of breast milk change with the mother's food intake, the infant is exposed to different odors, thus preparing it for the later introduction of other foods (Lawrence, 1994).

Physiologic benefits for the mother

Breast-feeding assists in the important process of involution. As the infant sucks, nipple stimulation triggers release of oxytocin from the posterior pituitary gland, causing the uterus to contract. When the infant nurses, the uterus contracts, blood vessels are constricted, the possibility of postpartum hemorrhage is reduced, and the descent of the uterus back into the pelvic cavity is enhanced (Figure 17-12).

The effect of breast-feeding on osteoporosis and breast, ovarian, and bone cancers is under study, with evidence showing a decreased risk in women who have breast-fed (Dermer, 1995; Renfrew, 1990). Weight reduction is also enhanced for the new mother. Breast-feeding requires the expenditure of a great deal of maternal energy to produce milk, thereby helping the mother lose weight and return to her prepregnancy weight sooner.

Psychologic benefits

Being a nursing mother often gives the woman "permission" to continue to take care of herself after pregnancy: she is able to plan and ask for help with meeting her needs for nutrition, rest, and time with the new infant. Mother-infant attachment is strengthened, since the mother is the primary caregiver and has to give full attention to the infant during feeding. Hormones also play a part, increasing feelings of well-being and interest in maternal behaviors (Lawrence, 1994).

Antenatal preparation. Most women who breast-feed have made the decision to do so before pregnancy or in its early stages (Enkin, 1995). Therefore the best time to begin teaching is in the antenatal period, along with teaching preparation for labor, birth, and postpartum. This is especially important because many women have limited exposure to correct breast-feeding facts and techniques in everyday life and may not receive them from their family. The popularity of bottle-feeding in recent decades has resulted in a lack of women experienced in the art of breast-feeding, and so mothers and grandmothers may not be able to share their personal knowledge with their daughters. Thus the nurse becomes the teacher, preparing the woman for a successful breast-feeding experience by giving correct information, strongly encouraging the decision, and clarifying misconceptions.

Physically, there is no preparation necessary during pregnancy, no need to "toughen" nipples by rubbing, rolling, or applying alcohol. In fact, these measures can irritate, injure, and dry the tissue, as well as cause increased contractions during the last trimester (see Chapter 9). Manual expression of colostrum is not necessary, but colostrum that does ooze from the nipples in the last trimester may be rubbed into the nipple as a lubricant. Soaps and other drying agents should be avoided. The mother should be taught that breast size and nipple size vary widely and usually are not important to breast-feeding. The woman should be reassured that milk supply depends not on breast mass but on the alveoli in the breast. Small, flat nipples are not a problem if the infant can latch on. To assess this, the woman can press the thumb and index finger into the breast behind the nipple. If the fingers can grasp the nipple, the infant will be able to do so too. Nipples that appear inverted often respond to pressure on the areola while the infant sucks. Only rarely do inverted nipples completely prevent lactation.

Some sources do recommend prenatal use of a nipple shell (a small dome that fits over the areola and presses in on it) or performing Hoffman's exercises (placing thumb and forefinger on opposite sides of the areola and gently pulling apart), but there is question if these techniques really improve nipple status (Enkin, 1995).

Initiation of Feeding

Breast-feeding should be initiated as soon as possible after delivery. After the placenta is delivered and the mother is comfortable, the infant can be put to the breast during the first period of reactivity (Lawrence, 1994) (see Figure 15-8). The infant may nurse enthusiastically or may just lick the nipple and not suck at all. However, this skin-to-skin contact is an intense experience for a woman and her child. There is a correlation between time of first feeding and the success and length of time of breast-feeding (Lawrence, 1995; Riordan and Auerback, 1993). Care should be taken so that the mother and infant do not become chilled. A radiant warmer, if available, can be placed over the delivery table or in the recovery area.

Positions for nursing

Common positions are the cross cradle, or "madonna hold," with the infant cradled in an arm; the "football hold," in which the mother's arm supports the infant's head and back and the infant's body and legs are to the side and behind the mother; and the side-lying position, with the mother and infant facing each other (Figure 17-13). Side lying may be the most comfortable position for

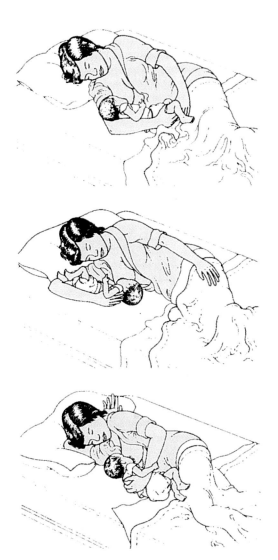

Figure 17-13 Three positions for nursing. Note infant's position in relation to mother. (From Fogel CI, Woods NF: *Health care of women,* St Louis, 1981, Mosby.)

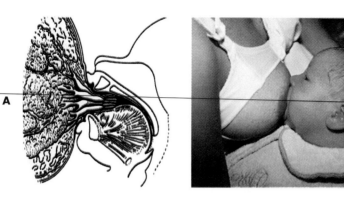

Figure 17-14 A, The position of the nipple should be above the infant's tongue and toward the hard palate. **B,** Football hold. Note correct widely flanged position of the infant's mouth so that nipple and areola are pulled forward into the mouth. (**A,** From *Clinical education aid: number 10,* Columbus, Ohio, Ross Laboratories. **B,** Courtesy Marjorie Pyle, RNC, *Lifecircle.*)

the woman who has had an episiotomy or a surgical birth, although many mothers prefer to sit upright to feed after cesarean delivery.

Regardless of position, the infant must be lined up with the mother's body "tummy to tummy" so that the head is directly in front of the breast and the nipple is within easy reach (Figure 17-14). Pillows can be used to support the mother's arm while she guides the infant's open mouth onto the breast. The mother supports her breast with four fingers under it and the thumb on top (C-hold or palmar grasp) or with the thumb and index finger above the areola and the other three fingers under (scissor hold).

Neither the infant's head nor the breast should be moved to the side, or the neck will be extended, hyperextended, or turned, interfering with swallowing and also creating traction on the nipple tissue. With correct positioning, the infant's open mouth is simply guided to and placed onto the breast for latching-on (Figure 17-14, *A*).

Latching-on. Latching-on, the ability of the infant to grasp breast tissue, is the single most important aspect of breast-feeding. It means that the infant will nurse from the breast and not suck on the nipple only, ensuring adequate milk ejection and preventing nipple trauma. The mother may express milk so that the infant can taste it by placing her thumbs on each side of the breast and moving firmly toward the nipple. The mother can utilize the infant's **rooting reflex** to interest the infant in the breast. When the infant approaches the breast with lips open, the mother moves the *infant to the breast* and "plants" the lower rim of the infant's mouth well below the nipple. Seen from below, the infant's jaw should be pressed against breast tissue, and from above, the nose also. In the process of latching-on, the infant draws nipple, areola and a good portion of breast into the mouth, forming a teat, with the nipple safely in the back of the mouth avoiding friction and directing the flow of milk to the back of the throat (Figure 17-15).

Sucking and swallowing. The **sucking reflex** is developed by week 34 of gestation. Because sucking involves

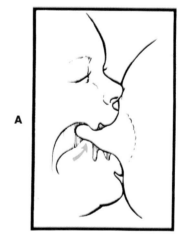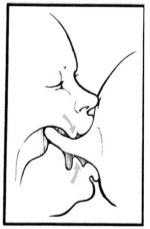

Figure 17-15 The sucking process. **A,** Tongue thrusts up and forward to grasp nipple. **B,** Gums compress the areola while the tongue moves backward to create a suction. (From Riordan J: *A practical guide to breast-feeding,* St Louis, 1987, Mosby.)

compression of the nipple and areola between the tongue and palate, the mouth must be opened wide and the tongue positioned over the lower gum. The mouth must cover the nipple and at least 1 inch of the areola as well. This amount of breast tissue must be within the mouth so that the lactiferous sinuses can be compressed (see Figure 17-15). It is essential to teach the mother that there is no milk in the nipple; if sucking does not involve the breast itself, no milk will be obtained.

Sucking should be quiet and rhythmic, quicker at first and deepening as the ejection of milk increases. Clicking or smacking noises or milk dribbling from the lips indicates attachment that must be corrected. Swallowing is seen in the infant's neck and is assessed after the first attempts at latching-on. Occasionally an infant may choke while trying to swallow a large amount of milk. The mother should simply remove the infant until it is calm, and then place it again on the breast.

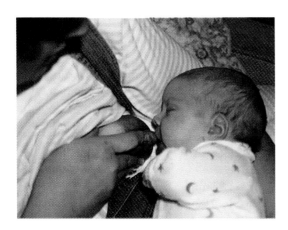

Figure 17-16   To take the infant off the breast, break the suction by inserting a finger into the infant's mouth. (Courtesy Marjorie Pyle, RNC, *Lifecircle*.)

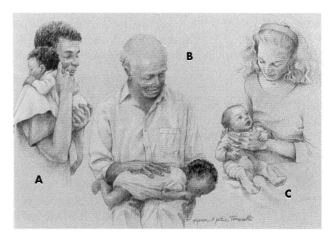

Figure 17-17   Once or twice during a feeding, the infant may need to be burped or bubbled by patting or rubbing the back for a minute. The three positions for burping the infant: **A,** Upright against the shoulder; **B,** Face down across the lap; **C,** Upright on the lap as the head and chest are supported with the hands. This is a good opportunity for the father or grandparents to provide nonnutritive cuddling and care. (Courtesy Childbirth Graphics, Waco, Texas.)

Timing of feedings. Hungry infants should be fed on demand, usually every 2 to 3 hours at first. This means that newborns have feedings 8 to 12 times a day. Hospital routines interfere with lactation when infants are brought to the mothers only every 4 hours. With the growth of mother-infant centered units, the infant is present to the mother all or most of the time, and she is taught to observe infant feeding cues and to respond by feeding the infant. When the infant is sleepy or seems disinterested at first, gentle stimulation, unwrapping, or talking may awaken the infant to eat. To feed well, breast-fed infants must be awake and interested, and it is often necessary to wake a sleepy infant to feed in the first few days.

Length of feeding sessions is no longer limited. Traditionally women were told to limit early feedings to 2 to 3 minutes on a side, building up time gradually. Because it may take at least 5 minutes of sucking to trigger the let-down reflex in first-time mothers, limiting the time is self-defeating. The nipples will not become sore if the infant is correctly positioned and therefore not "chewing" on the nipple. Instead the mother learns to recognize signs of satisfaction in the infant—slowing down in sucking and swallowing and finally falling asleep. When ready to take the infant off the breast, nipple pain is avoided by inserting the little finger into the infant's mouth to break the suction (Figure 17-16).

Bubbling. Bubbling, or burping, the infant should be performed before the feeding to eliminate air in the stomach that might displace milk or cause it to be spit up. Often the infant has been crying or sucking the fist, thus swallowing air. Because there is no air in breast milk, if the infant sucks correctly, less air is swallowed. Usually women find it easiest to bubble the infant halfway through the feeding, while changing sides, or when the infant appears to slow down (Figure 17-17). Small amounts of undigested milk may be regurgitated (spit up) with the bubble. This is different from vomiting partially digested milk.

Supplemental feedings

Early supplemental feedings with formula adversely affect the establishment of the mother's milk supply and may cause "nipple confusion," resulting in the infant's refusal to breast-feed. Therefore newborns should not be given supplemental feedings of glucose water or formula unless indicated by the medical condition of the mother or infant. In some states withholding supplementation for breast-feeding infants is mandated by state health policies. Mothers are strongly encouraged, especially in the initial establishment period of 2 to 3 weeks, to only breast-feed to ensure adequate milk supply. As a point of interest, it is noted that mothers who routinely supplement their infants with formula feedings are more likely to stop breast-feeding early or entirely (Lawrence, 1994). See Procedure 19-4 for early cup feeding when, for some reason, the mother cannot feed for one or two times.

Discharge gift packs that include formula may encourage formula supplementation. Therefore when a breast-feeding woman is going home, avoid sending mixed messages.

Variations for multiple births

A mother who breast-feeds twins can produce all the milk necessary for both infants. Two infants sucking provides a tremendous stimulus to the breasts, and milk production increases accordingly. The mother will need to increase her fluid and caloric intake and be particularly aware of her own nutritional needs. Twins can be fed at the same time or alternately (Figure 17-18). If fed together, the mother will need initial help in positioning the infants.

Breast-feeding twins can actually be easier to manage than bottlefeeding. Once a routine is established, nursing the two together can actually be simpler because both are satisfied at the same time. Breast-feeding also allows the mother to hold and cuddle one infant while feeding the other.

Breast-feeding after cesarean birth

Initially, breast-feeding may be more difficult after a cesarean delivery. If regional anesthesia was used, the mother should be able to nurse soon after delivery. Because general anesthesia can leave the mother and infant groggy, the nurse will need to help the mother get into a comfortable position and to wake the infant. Some women find it most comfortable to nurse in a side-lying

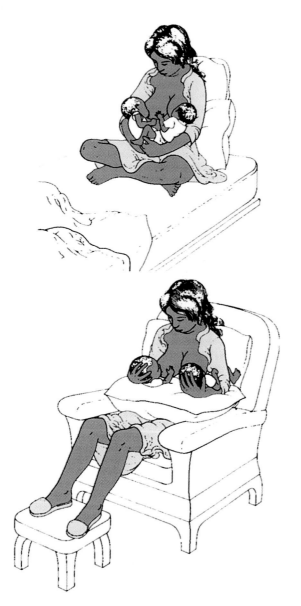

Figure 17-18 Positions for nursing twins. (From Fogel Cl, Woods NF: *Health care of women,* St Louis, 1981, Mosby.)

position, whereas others prefer using a football hold while sitting up in bed or a chair when allowed out of bed. This is especially true on the second and third postpartum days, when abdominal distention and gas pains occur. The woman may also need help switching the infant from one breast to the other. Leaving the bed rails up can give her something on which to hold as she turns over.

Common Problems

Discomfort: nipple pain. Prevention is the *key* element. Pain from sore or cracked nipples is not a normal or expected part of breast-feeding, nor is it related to length of time in early feedings. Rather it is caused by the infant's incorrect latching-on. If the infant only grasps the nipple or does not pull a sufficient amount of breast tissue into the mouth, then there will be pressure and friction on the nipple. With correct latching-on, the nipple is protected near the back of the infant's tongue. If soreness does occur, correctly repositioning the infant is effective in relieving it quickly. The infant should never be pulled from the breast; instead, the mother breaks suction by inserting a finger into the corner of the infant's mouth (see Figure 17-16).

Limiting time on the breast does not decrease damage to nipples and may in fact worsen it by inhibiting the let-down reflex, decreasing milk supply, and increasing the number of feedings demanded by the infant. Nipple creams and ointments are not recommended to treat sore nipples. These may clog ducts, predisposing to mastitis, and almost all contain some substance that should not be ingested by the infant. If a cream is ordered, probably vitamin A & D ointment is the most benign (Lawrence, 1994). Vitamin E should be avoided since the concentration exceeds recommended infant dosage (Riordan and Auerback, 1993).

Discharge teaching. Guide the new mother to recognize accurate latching-on and removal from the breast. Emphasize the need for on-demand feeding around the clock, at least 8 to 12 times in 24 hours. Show the mother how to assess her infant's sucking and swallowing and to recognize adequate intake by the infant's voiding and stooling patterns. Instruct her to report fewer than six wet diapers or less than three bowel movements a day.

Box **17-3**

CLINICAL DECISION

Ada S has been eager to prove that she is a good mother and has been breast-feeding her infant for long periods. Her nipples are now red and bleeding. Which strategies should be included in her plan of care and why?

Remind the mother to avoid soaps and other drying agents on her nipples, to avoid breast pads or change them when wet, and to expose her nipples to the air. She may also find relief with the heat from a hand-held hair dryer, set on the lowest setting and kept 6 to 8 inches away from the nipple. Using this for 2 to 3 minutes has been found to be helpful (Riordan and Auerback, 1993; Lawrence, 1994). If she requires analgesics, teach dosage, timing, and side effects.

Engorgement. The majority of women experience uncomfortable fullness on the second or third postpartum day. Breasts become full and heavy and pain may be mild or severe, with throbbing or aching extending to the lower edge of the rib cage and into the axillae. In devising a plan to decrease discomfort, the nurse must understand that this **engorgement** has two distinct parts: congestion caused by increased vascularity, and accumulation of milk.

The pain related to the first cause, vascular engorgement, can be decreased by providing support for the breasts and applying ice packs under the arms. Warm showers with gentle expression of milk may be helpful. Electric or hand pumping will not help and may actually traumatize breast tissue (Lawrence, 1994). The mother may also need analgesics to relieve pain.

The second cause, stasis of milk, occurs when an infant is unable to feed frequently, does not nurse long enough, or is not positioned to drain the breast adequately. Swelling may cause the nipple to recede into the areola, making it harder for the infant to grasp. Pressure from "back-up" hinders blood and lymph drainage, increasing vascular engorgement and compressing the milk ducts as well. Because intraductal pressure can damage milk-producing epithelial cells, it is essential that this pressure be relieved quickly.

The best treatment for engorgement is prevention (Lawrence, 1994: Enkin et al, 1995; Renfrew et al, 1990). If it does occur, encourage the mother to breast-feed as often as possible, around the clock. Warm soaks or showers, followed by expression of some milk before feeding, can relieve pressure behind the areola, softening it and making it and the nipple easier for the infant to grasp. If the mother is unsure of how well the infant is emptying the breast or if she still feels fullness after feeding, she may use a pump to express residual milk volume.

Some practitioners recommend the use of cabbage leaves as an adjunct therapy. Cool to cold raw cabbage leaves are placed on the breasts and left for 20 minutes or until wilted. Some studies show relief within 2 hours (Lawrence, 1994), whereas others question its efficacy (Enkin et al, 1995).

Mastitis. Mastitis may be either an inflammatory or infectious process related to poor drainage of the ducts and alveoli or to missed feedings once lactation is established. It can occur if organisms enter the breast through damaged nipples. The woman usually reports a temperature of 38.5° F or above, experiences chills and flu-like symptoms, and has a hot, red, swollen, sore portion of one breast.

In the presence of an infection, breast-feeding should *not* be discontinued. It is important to completely empty the breast; therefore the woman should either continue to nurse or, if that is too painful, temporarily use a pump.

Treatments include getting bed rest, increasing fluids, using ice or warmth for comfort, wearing a supportive bra, and possibly using analgesics. Antibiotics such dicloxacillin, penicillin, ampicillin, or erythromycin may be ordered and should be continued for 10 to 14 days (Lawrence, 1994; Enkin et al, 1995).

Plugged ducts. Unresolved engorgement may lead to clogged or blocked ducts. Plugged or clogged ducts are recognized as small, hard lumps throughout the breast and can be treated by changing the mother's and infant's position to facilitate drainage and by starting to nurse on the affected side. In addition, the mother can be taught to stroke the lump toward the nipple as she feeds. Also, undue pressure applied to the breast, as from a poorly fitting brassiere or from pressure of the infant's chin during nursing, can cause stasis in a duct. The water content of the milk there is absorbed by the tissue, leaving a thick viscous substance that irritates the tissue. Inflammation occurs as a response; this is *noninfective* mastitis.

Breast abscess. There is controversy about whether breast-feeding should continue when an abscess occurs. If it is located near the surface of the breast and away from the nipple, nursing is generally allowed (Riordan and Auerback, 1993), but if purulent drainage is present, breast-feeding may need to be interrupted until antibiotic therapy is underway. Pumping should be encouraged to empty the breast and maintain the milk supply (Renfrew et al, 1990; Lawrence, 1994).

Discharge teaching. Emphasis should be on unrestricted and uninterrupted breast-feeding. Since ductal problems, mastitis, and abscesses occur in the weeks after discharge, prepare the woman to recognize and report signs of complications. Teach her to avoid underwire bras, to be aware of the infant's pressure against her breast, and to assess for cracked or fissured nipples. Encourage adequate rest, nutrition, and fluids. Suggest warm showers to increase milk release, massage to relieve duct clogs, and manual expression to relieve engorgement. If she feels that her breasts are not being emptied with each feeding, the mother should express the milk manually or by a pump.

Antibiotic therapy should be reviewed, with emphasis on dose, timing, and side effects, as well as the need to continue for the entire 10 to 14 days as ordered. Analgesia is also discussed. Reassure that a breast infection will not harm the infant and that discontinuing breast-feeding can only worsen the condition.

Evaluation

- Does the infant latch-on, and can the mother remove the infant from the breast correctly?
- Does the mother express understanding of the need for frequent, unlimited feedings night and day?
- Is she able to describe ways to prevent and treat engorgement?
- Can she verbalize risk factors and signs and symptoms of mastitis? Does she understand the need to contact a physician for possible antibiotic or analgesic therapy?

TEST *Yourself* 17-2 _____

a. List two signs of breast fullness and breast engorgement. Are interventions different?

b. How do interventions differ between a woman who is breast-feeding and a woman who does not?

Contraindications to Breast-feeding

There are relatively few contraindications to breast-feeding. (See Chapter 25 for infections and breast-feeding precautions.) What then is a contraindication? Untreated tuberculosis, leukemia, drug abuse, and breast cancer diagnosed during lactation all prevent nursing the infant. There is much discussion about the mother with human immunodeficiency virus (HIV). In its 1992 statement, UNICEF advised against it (Riordan and Auerback, 1993), and many experts agree that the decision to breast-feed in the presence of HIV should be an individual one, based on risk versus benefit. If the infant is more at risk from illness or death from infection or malnutrition, such as in an area of extreme poverty, then more may be gained by breast-feeding. If, however, these risks are low, then the greater danger may be from the presence of HIV that can be transmitted via breast milk (Nicoll et al, 1995; Van de Perre, 1995; Lawrence, 1994; Lindberg, 1995).

Nutritional Considerations

Nutrition related to breast-feeding is discussed in detail in Chapter 10. Simply stated, the mother should increase her intake by 200 to 500 calories beyond her prepregnant amount. Less than adequate nutrition, however, does not appear to have any significant effect on the quality of milk production. The woman does not need to force fluids: drinking to simply satisfy thirst is accomplished by having something to drink each time she nurses.

There is no need to avoid or limit any foods. Although certain foods may change the odor and taste of the milk, these do not appear to have any adverse effects. Caffeine is generally tolerated in moderate amounts. Both passive smoke and smoking should be avoided during lactation (see Chapter 10).

Drugs and Breast-Feeding

Drug level in breast milk is dependent on many factors, including the drug's molecular size and solubility in lipids and water, its affinity to protein, the pH of the drug, and its diffusion rate. In addition, the infant's gestational age and status affect how a drug is transferred through the milk and is metabolized (see Chapter 16). When a woman must take a drug while lactating, careful timing of maternal doses may reduce drug concentrations in milk. Though there are differing opinions about when to administer the medication so that peak effects do not coincide with the full breast, the following are recommended on the basis that most milk is taken in the first 10 minutes on each breast.

1. Some authorities suggest giving oral doses at the beginning of a session. When absorption time to peak is about 20 to 40 minutes, most of the milk will have been taken before the medication crosses the blood-milk barrier.

2. Berlin (1981) suggests that all medications be given just after a feeding session.

3. IV and IM doses should be given just after a feeding session because medication reaches the minimum effective concentration more quickly than oral doses and will usually be metabolized and excreted before the next feeding. However, medications given by continuous IV infusions are more quickly concentrated in breast milk than medications given intermittently orally or IV because of higher sustained maternal serum levels. In certain cases, pumping and discarding the milk may be preferable until the high doses are discontinued.

4. If a medication is highly protein bound and given daily (such as digoxin or methadone) or is known to pass in larger amounts into breast milk, timing the dose after morning or late afternoon feeding allows at least 4 hours before the next feeding or formula may be substituted at the next feeding.

Safety principles. A number of authors recommend the following principles in regard to medication and lactation.

1. A medication should not be prescribed for a pregnant or lactating woman unless it is necessary for her health or the health of her infant. If medication is used, the most effective medication with the fewest side effects should be selected (Briggs, Freeman, Yaffee, 1994).

2. Drugs of low-molecular weight are passed into breast milk in low doses (at 1% to 2% of maternal dose), depending on frequency of dose and the amount and characteristics of the medication. Therefore the amount reaching the infant is very small. Drugs of large-molecular weight do not cross the barrier.

3. Even though certain drugs are found in milk, they may not be hazardous if metabolized in alveolar cells or destroyed in the infant's GI tract. (Exceptions are listed in Appendix 3A.)

4. A lactating woman should always discuss the drug with her physician before taking over-the-counter (OTC) drugs or prescribed medication.

Alcohol. Studies show that alcohol does pass into breast milk and levels rise quickly. Because an infant's liver is immature, alcohol is metabolized and excreted slowly. Alcohol also depresses sucking-induced prolactin and inhibits oxytocin release from the pituitary gland, decreasing milk production and the milk ejection reflex (Anderson, 1995; Schulte, 1995). Mothers should be encouraged to avoid alcohol completely, or to refrain from breast-feeding for 2 hours after ingesting an alcoholic drink. Milk containing alcohol should be pumped and discarded.

Special Problems

Jaundice

Approximately 50% of newborns develop visible jaundice, considered "normal" physiologic jaundice, during the first week of life (see Chapter 19). In most cases, jaundice will resolve with increased feedings, voidings, and stooling (Martinez et al, 1993).

Occasionally a condition known as breast milk jaundice occurs. Some breast milk has been found to actually inhibit the bilirubin-converting enzyme (glucuronyl transferase) and to also contain a progesterone metabolite, *pregnanediol,* that delays bilirubin synthesis. It is rarely seen before the end of the first week of life and must be differentiated from jaundice that is aggravated by poor breast-feeding technique. To rule out breast-feeding as the cause of jaundice, a physician may ask the mother to discontinue breast-feeding for 48 hours to allow the level to fall. In this case, the mother may continue to pump her breast to maintain supply. It is extremely rare that jaundice will be an indication to discontinue lactation (see Chapter 29 for discussion). Phototherapy may also be initiated.

In fact, some researchers believe that because of increased stooling, bilirubin levels actually drop more quickly in breast-fed infants than in those bottle-fed or supplemented with formula or water. If the infant receives adequate fluid by nursing, there is usually no need to interrupt breast-feeding (Lawrence, 1994).

Preterm infant

Breast-feeding for an infant weighing more than 1500 g is not only considered possible but is also recommended. Preterm and low-birth-weight infants need nutrition in the form of increased fats. Breast milk has the advantage of containing lipases, which are more available and better utilized by the preterm infant. Colostrum also plays a ben-

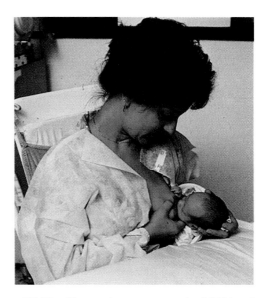

Figure 17-19   The mother may go to the NICU to feed a stabilized preterm infant. Note supporting the infant's chin to assist in sucking strength. (Courtesy Ross Laboratories, Columbus, Ohio.)

eficial role for the preterm infant by promoting growth of *Lactobacillus bifidus* in the GI tract, changing pH levels, and increasing lactic acid production (Hill, 1993).

If the infant's condition allows oral feeding, breast-feeding may actually be less stressful than bottle-feeding. Though sucking is slightly more difficult, the infant is able to control sucking, swallowing, and breathing. In addition, the close physical contact with the mother appears to calm the infant and decrease oxygen demands. All infants should be monitored carefully during feeding for any signs of hypoxia (Figure 17-19).

If the infant is not yet able to breast-feed, the nurse should teach the mother to massage her breasts before expressing milk and to use a handheld or electric breast pump (Figure 17-20). In this way, her milk supply will become established, and the expressed milk can be fed by tube or bottle to the infant. Expressing the mother's milk not only provides the infant with the best possible nutrition, but it can also be a source of comfort and bonding for the mother who has been physically separated from her child and feels helpless (see Chapter 29 for more discussion).

Infant with physical disabilities

When infants have a cleft lip or palate, Down syndrome, or other neuromuscular problems, breast-feeding is an important part of their protection against infection, as well as a means to promote bonding and developmental tasks. Depending on the severity of the disability, complete breast-feeding may be possible with or without assis-

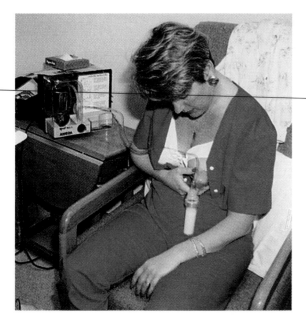

Figure 17-20 An electric breast pump is useful for working mothers and for alleviating breast fullness. (Courtesy Marjorie Pyle, RNC, *Lifecircle*.)

tive devices, or it may be necessary for the mother to express her milk and feed it to her infant by spoon, cup, or feeding tube. The nurse should make every effort to support the new mother in her decision to breast-feed and should offer any assistance to increase its feasibility.

The Impact of Health Care Professionals on Breast-Feeding

Though husbands, partners, mothers, and friends all influence a woman's decision of whether to breast-feed, the importance of physicians and nurses cannot be ignored (Losch et al, 1995). Physicians should introduce the topic of feeding choices early in pregnancy, offering teaching and guidance, and they should follow this up in the postpartum period by writing orders that support complete breast-feeding. Nurses play a special part in helping the mother be successful by sharing facts with a positive attitude and patience, thus helping the woman to master skills. The nurse should be careful to assist in ways that increase mastery, independence, and confidence (Renfrew et al, 1990).

Discharge Planning

Breast-feeding is usually only barely established during the 1 to 4 days that the mother and infant are in the hospital; during this time, the mother has the support of the hospital staff members and their assurance that her infant is doing well. When she goes home, however, she may be very much on her own and can easily lose confidence in her ability to feed her infant. Feelings of self-doubt may be fostered by relatives and friends who ask whether the infant is getting enough milk. "Not having enough milk" is a common reason mothers give for failure in breast-feeding.

An important part of the postpartum health team is the lactation consultant (LC), a certified specialist who acts as support and educator for patients, families, and staff. An LC may be available early to help initiate breast-feeding, and may follow up after discharge through telephone calls or return visits by the mothers for on-going assistance. In many areas, LCs have private practices.

In addition to the LC, the nurse takes on the role of teacher and support person and also refers the mother for assistance and women, infants, and children (WIC) food supplements as needed. Lactating women qualify for additional help and instruction through the WIC program, which has been very supportive of breast-feeding (see Chapter 10). In many areas, home care services are available to a mother when it has been determined that she needs follow-up care or is discharged early. Breast-feeding coordinators and clinicians may follow up with new mothers by telephone. Finally, the mother is encouraged to seek out other women who have breast-fed successfully. If a mother has no support in the home, she may contact La Leche League, an organization dedicated to promoting breast-feeding. By telephone and through local group meetings, support and advice are available to new mothers. To find a local group, a woman may write to La Leche League International, P.O. Box 1209, Franklin Park, IL 60131-8209; telephone (312) 455-7730.

HOME CARE

Self-care is a practical and real need. The nurse cannot possibly continue to monitor everything through the recovery phase but must instead teach the new mother to understand the processes of recovery and how to evaluate her successful progress (Box 17-3). Nursing follow-up after discharge must become the norm rather than the exception. The nurse will be called on to assess and to continue teaching after the new mother goes home. This may be achieved by telephone or in person, through classes and support groups. Innovative programs are being developed to compensate for shortened hospital stays, such as offering three home visits during the first week by an approved nurse if the woman is discharged within the first 24 hours after birth. In this way, the woman who chooses to go home early still receives professional assessment, planning, and care within the privacy and comfort of her home (see Figure 17-3).

Some hospitals use the expertise of perinatal nurses who alternate working in the home and hospital on a rotating basis. This nurse meets the woman on her first postpartum day, checks charts, receives physician orders, and plans to meet the woman at home. When making the home visit, the nurse is able to assess the situation and the needs of the mother and infant. The woman's response to both in-home visits and follow-up telephone calls is very positive because both give her opportunity to seek information, validate her experiences, and permit her to obtain help when she is at home alone without the constant support of hospital personnel and services (Williams and Cooper, 1993).

THE FAMILY AFTER BIRTH

Family processes always undergo alterations with the childbirth experience. Whether this infant is the first or is joining other siblings, changes in roles, routines, and priorities are a challenge to all family members. Understanding their concerns and encouraging participation in the restructuring of the family unit facilitate successful transition.

Fathers

Most fathers choose to be a vital part of the process during birth. With increased societal emphasis on shared parenting and the recognition of paternal bonding, many fathers are active in care giving and enjoy the closeness it brings (Figure 17-21). Providing cuddling, changing diapers, bathing, and singing to and playing with his infant are important parts of the paternal role (Figure 17-22).

Almost universally, hospitals have eliminated visiting restrictions for fathers. A father may provide much of the care of the infant in the woman's room and is also involved in discharge planning, since he is essential in early care at home (Figure 17-23).

Grandparents

The emotional and comforting support offered by grandparents during pregnancy and birth is finally being recog-

Box 17-3

TEACHING PLAN *for* HOME CARE

Postpartum Warning Signs to be Reported

FUNDUS
Soft, boggy in the first few days
Height higher than expected or deviated to right or left
Sharp pains in lower abdomen, tender to touch

LOCHIA
Bright red after more than 4 days or changing to red again after being pink
Clots passed after first few days
Increasing amount
Strong or strange odor
Constant trickling of blood
No lochia in first week

EPISIOTOMY
Red, bruised, swollen, oozing, or edges separating
Increased pain, unhelped by sitz bath or analgesics

ABDOMINAL INCISION
Reddened, bruised, swollen, oozing, or edges separating
Bleeding, warm to touch
Sharp pain, discomfort unrelieved by usual comfort measures

TEMPERATURE
Any increased temperature, sensation of chills, general aching
"Flulike" symptoms

URINATION
Decreased urine output or frequent voiding in small amounts
Pain or burning when urinating
Cloudy, strong, or foul-smelling urine
Lower abdominal or flank pain

BOWEL MOVEMENT
Constipation unrelieved by stool softener given by physician
No stool, diarrhea present

APPETITE
Decreased or no appetite, abdominal pain, gas pains

CIRCULATION
Any sharp pain or tenderness in legs or groin

BREASTS
Pain continues after initial engorgement
Redness, shiny skin, any red lines or spots
Lumps unrelieved by nursing
Cracked or sore nipples unrelieved by usual comfort measures

MOOD
Constant feelings of sadness, exhaustion, or anger
Disinterest in infant, self, or usual activities
Not able to return to normal activities of daily living
Not interested in seeing friends

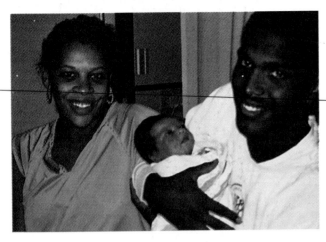

Figure 17-21 Early involvement of young fathers builds confidence. (Courtesy Camille Bodden.)

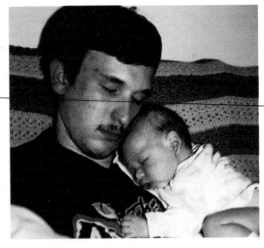

Figure 17-22 Father and son "tired out" together. (Courtesy Eric Schult.)

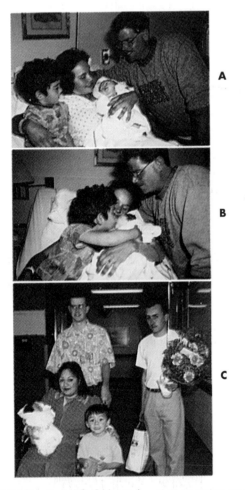

Figure 17-23 **A** and **B,** Sibling takes time to warm up to the new "intruder." **C,** Ready for going home. (Courtesy Marjorie Pyle, RNC, *Lifecircle.*)

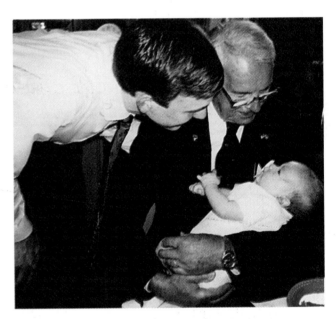

Figure 17-24 Three generations meet. Grandfather, grandson, and new great-grandson. (Courtesy Eric Schult.)

nized by health care personnel. Grandparents are allowed in some labor suites and are encouraged to visit the postpartum units because they are in a position to offer help and guidance as needed.

A special bond often develops between grandparent and grandchild. Special memories are formed as the grandparents do their best to spoil the child, often giving him or her things and time not available when their own children were young. It is as if they have been given a second chance at child rearing, with all the pleasures and joys and none of the responsibilities (Figure 17-24).

Despite all the joys and pleasures of having the grandparents around, conflicts can sometimes arise regarding

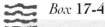

Box 17-4

TEACHING PLAN *for* HOME CARE

Caring for Siblings

BEFORE THE INFANT COMES
- Include the child in activities preparing for the event.
- Plan with the child where the child will stay during the mother's hospitalization. If staying with a neighbor or relative, he or she might stay the night as a "dry run" before the expected due date.
- Be aware that children can misinterpret; parents should be matter-of-fact and positive about the impending hospitalization.
- If the older child will be going into a new bed, make the transfer as early in pregnancy as possible.
- If possible, begin toilet training well in advance of the new infant's arrival. Otherwise, delay toilet training until the older child is accustomed to the new infant.
- Consider buying (and wrapping) inexpensive items and storing them for use when gift-laden visitors arrive for the newcomer.

WHEN THE INFANT ARRIVES
- Try to understand that the older child needs to express his continued dependency and need for attention. Gentle and frequent explanations of the positive aspects of "growing up" help prevent regressive behavior.

- When guests arrive with gifts for the infant, give the older child the tucked-away surprises at intervals and allow him or her to pull the wrappings from the infant's gifts, especially if the child is 2 or 3 years old.
- Consider giving the child a special gift when the infant is brought home from the hospital, specifying it as the newcomer's "thank you" for making everything ready for him or her.
- Remember that older children still need physical attention, including snuggling, rocking, and hugging. This extra assurance helps convince the child that love can be expanded to fit two or three or more children.
- Let the child "help" with the infant; this helps him or her feel important. However, do not overdo it to the point that he or she feels like "I'll never get to play again."
- Prevent any anger or hurt that might be displaced onto the infant.
- If there is a change in the expected plan for the newborn, deal with the older child's fears realistically. For example, if the infant is premature, try to have a picture taken to show to the older child.
- Take advantage of books that express the message of the problems the older child experiences in living with the new arrival.

Modified from Kappleman M: *What your child is all about*, New York, 1974, Reader's Digest Press.

child-rearing practices. If the new parents do not agree with each other in their views of child rearing, the grandparents may step in to offer advice, even when it is not desired. They may force their opinions on the inexperienced parents and evoke feelings of guilt if advice is refused. Therefore, ground rules for the raising of a child must be set down by the new parents so that conflict is reduced. Once the grandparents take over rearing tasks, it may be hard to reestablish the parents as the primary caregivers. Grandparents are a rich source of knowledge, but their knowledge must be made available without forcing the young parents to relinquish authority. This task must be worked out early within the family structure. When the new parent is an adolescent, the task is even more difficult (see Chapter 8).

Siblings

The arrival of a new addition to the family has a profound effect on the other members, including children (see Figure 17-23). The way in which the siblings are prepared before the birth may help to determine whether they will adjust to and accept the new infant (Box 17-4 and see Chapter 12). In labor-delivery-recovery and postrecovery settings, siblings visit freely.

Parents must realize that children often regress in their behavior after the infant's birth. The 4-year-old child may begin to wet in bed at night, and the 3-year-old child may want to suck at the breast with the new baby. These situations must be handled sensitively so the older child does not feel guilty because of the regressive behaviors. A special time with the child each day may restore confidence and security, and some lactating mothers have found that letting the toddler nurse allows him or her to realize that it is no "big" request and thus soon forgets about it. Each family has to work out its own way of handling sibling rivalry to suit the specific situation. Every child experiences feelings of rivalry when a new infant enters the family system.

Key Points

- The reproductive system returns to the prepregnancy state by reversing the unique developments that occur during pregnancy. The return of the uterus to its prepregnant state is called involution.
- Childbirth places stresses on the new mother and her entire family, and support networks may determine whether these stresses are easily resolved.
- Monitoring of involution, vital signs, pain, and infection is essential in the early postpartum period.
- Facilitating the mother's self-care and her care of the infant is the major goal of postpartum nursing care.
- Nursing responsibilities include assisting the woman in developmental tasks and in achieving beginning satisfaction in the parenting role.

- Support and teaching enable most women who choose breast-feeding to be successful, and they lessen the chances of problems or complications.
- Women who give birth by assisted or surgical methods may need more support to maintain self-esteem.
- Use of the nursing process assists the nurse in identifying focus areas for effective and appropriate care for the childbearing family.
- Discharge teaching must start either before delivery or with the first postpartum check, and it must be an integral part of all nursing care.

Study Questions

17-1. Select the terms that apply to the following statements:
   a. Through _____, the body returns to its prepregnant state.
   b. The fluids from the lining of the uterus are called _____.
   c. The beginning of outward interest in her infant and her surroundings occurs when a new mother starts _____.
   d. The _____ is the 6- to 8-week period of immediate recovery from birth.
   e. Intense discomfort in the incompletely emptied breasts is due to _____.
   f. Milk will not be ejected properly until the _____ reflex occurs.

17-2. Mrs. H is a 33 year-old gravida 3, para 1, who had a vaginal birth of a healthy, full-term baby girl 3 hours earlier. An IV solution of Ringer's lactate, with 20 units of Pitocin added, is infusing at 100 ml/hr. During initial postpartum check, you note that the pad is soaked and has multiple small clots. Choose the priority nursing intervention for Mrs. H:
   a. Giving and explaining perineal care and placing a new pad.
   b. Calling her physician to report lochia change.
   c. Performing a fundal check and ensuring the patency and flow rate of the IV solution.
   d. Taking no measures because this condition is common with multigravida women.

17-3. At 6 hours after birth, Mrs H's fundus is found to be one fingerbreadth above the umbilicus and deviated to the right. What is your assessment of this fundal status?
   a. Position is normal for this time in involutional process.
   b. Her body position is out of alignment.
   c. Position indicates a full bladder.
   d. Position indicates that there may be retained placental fragments.

17-4. Which of the following indicates the need for further assessment during the first 24 hours after a cesarean delivery?
   a. WBC count of 18,000/mm³
   b. Scant lochia rubra
   c. Thirst and fatigue
   d. Temperature of 100.4°

17-5. Vital signs are taken frequently during the immediate postpartum period because:
   a. The standing order indicates frequent checks.
   b. Early hemorrhage is best detected by changes in vital signs.
   c. Most recovery problems can be detected through assessment of vital signs.
   d. Vital signs may change rapidly throughout the immediate postpartum recovery period.

17-6. Which of the following lochial patterns should the mother report?

a. Bright red discharge with a small clot on the second recovery day

b. Serosanguineous discharge on the fourth day

c. No lochia on the third day

d. Yellowish white mucus on the fourteenth day

17-7. Kegel exercises are helpful in the recovery period because these will:

a. Tone up the upper thigh muscles.

b. Relieve lower back pain caused by the delivery position.

c. Relieve the pain of breast engorgement.

d. Strengthen the perineal muscles and promote healing of the episiotomy.

17-8. In addition to sufficient infant nursing, the woman should do which of the following to ensure adequate milk supply during lactation?

a. Avoid salty foods and eat balanced meals.

b. Drink at least 12 cups of fluid a day.

c. Drink at least 1 quart of fruit juice a day in addition to the required milk intake.

d. Increase vegetable and complex carbohydrate intake.

Answer Key

17-1: *a*, Involution; *b*, lochia; *c*, taking hold; *d*, puerperium; *e*, engorgement; *f*, let-down. 17-2: c. 17-3: c. 17-4: b. 17-5: d. 17-6: c. 17-7: d. 17-8: b.

References

American College of Obstetricians and Gynecologists: Recommendations on exercise in pregnancy and the postpartum period, *Am Fam Physician* 49(5):258, 1994.

Anderson PO: Alcohol and breastfeeding, *J Hum Lact* 11(4):321, 1995.

Artal R, Buckenmeyer PJ: Exercise during pregnancy and postpartum, *Contemp Ob Gyn* 40:62, 1995.

Association of Womens' Health, Obstetric and Neonatal Nurses (AWHONN) Maitson S, Smith JE: *Core curriculum for maternal-newborn nursing*, Philadelphia, 1993, WB Saunders.

Atkinson LS, Baxley EG: Postpartum fatigue: *Am Fam Physician* 50(1):113, 1994.

Beaudry M et al: Relation between infant feeding and infections during the first six months of life, *J Pediatr* 126(2):191, 1995.

*Berlin CM: Pharmacologic considerations of drug use in the lactating mother, *Obstet Gynecol* 58(suppl):5, 1981.

Berner LS: Early discharge rules for mothers and newborns: penny wise and 8 lbs/2 oz foolish, *J Womens Health* 4(5):479, 1995.

Bilyk PL: Teaching breastfeeding as a public committment, *Int J Childbirth Educ*, 11(2):34, 1996.

Blackburn ST, Loper DL: *Maternal, fetal and neonatal physiology*, Philadelphia, 1992, WB Saunders.

Boland M: Overview of perinatally transmitted HIV infection, *Nurs Clin North Am*, 31(1):155, 1996.

Briggs GC, Freeman RK, Yaffe SJ: *Drugs in pregnancy and lactation*, ed 3, Baltimore, 1994, Williams & Wilkins.

Brinton LA et al: Breastfeeding and breast cancer risk, *Cancer Causes Control* 6:199, 1995.

Buchko BL et al: Comfort measures in breastfeeding, primiparous women, *J Obstet Gynecol Neonatal Nurs* 23(1):46, 1994.

Burroughs MW: Should nursing mothers take ibuprofen? A response letter, *MCN AM J Matern Child Nurs* 23(1):122, 1996.

Clark RA: Infections in the postpartum period, *J Obstet Gynecol Neonatal Nurs* 24(6):542, 1995.

Creasy R, Resnick R: *Maternal-fetal medicine-principles and practice*, Philadelphia, 1994, WB Saunders.

Cunningham A, Jeliffe DB, Jeliffe EFP: Breastfeeding and health in the 1980's: a global epidemiological review, *J Pediatr* 118(5):659, 1991.

Cunningham FG et al: *William's obstetrics*, ed 19, Norwalk Town, Conn, 1993, Appleton & Lange.

Datta S: *The obstetric anesthesia handbook*, ed 2, St Louis, 1995, Mosby.

Dermer A: Overcoming medical and social barriers to breastfeeding, *Am Fam Physician* 51(4):755, 1995.

Dewey K et al: Differences in morbidity between breastfed and formula fed infants, *J Pediatr* 126(5 pt 1):697, 1995.

*Donovan B: *The cesarean birth experience*, Boston, 1977, Beacon Press.

Duncan B et al: Exclusive breastfeeding for at least 4 months protects against otitis media, *Pediatrics* 91(5):867, 1993.

Enkin M et al: *A guide to effective care in pregnancy and childbirth*, Oxford, 1995, Oxford University Press.

Freed GL et al: National assessment of physicians' breast-feeding knowledge, attitudes, training and experience, *JAMA* 273:472, 1995.

Gleicher N et al: *Principles & practice of medical therapy in pregnancy*, ed 2, Norwalk Town, Conn, 1992, Appleton & Lange.

Hamadeh G et al: Postpartum fever, *Am Fam Physician* 52(2):531, 1995.

Hill A, Roth I: The care and feeding of the low birth weight infant, *J Perinat Neonat Nurs* 6(4):56, 1993.

Hill PD, Humenick SS, West B: Concerns of breastfeeding mothers: the first six weeks postpartum, *J Perinatal Educ* 3(4):47, 1994.

Jensen D: LATCH: A breastfeeding charting system and documentation tool, *J Obstet Gynecol Neonatal Nurs* 23(1):27, 1994.

Kalkwarf HJ et al: Bone mineral loss during lactation and recovery after weaning, *Obstet Gynecol* 86(1):26, 1995.

Keppler AB: Postpartum care center: follow-up care in a hospital-based clinic, *J Obstet Gynecol Neonatal Nurs* 23(1):17, 1994.

Lawrence RA: *Breastfeeding: a guide for the medical profession*, ed 4, St Louis, 1994, Mosby.

Lawrence RA: The clinician's role in teaching proper infant feeding techniques, *J Pediatr* 126(6):S112, 1995.

Lethbridge DJ et al: Validation of the nursing diagnosis of ineffective breastfeeding, *J Obstet Gynecol Neonatal Nurs* 1:57, 1993.

Lin HH et al: Absence of infection in breastfed infants born to hepatitis C virus-infected mothers, *J Pediatr* 126(4): 589, 1995.

Lindberg CE: Perinatal transmission of HIV: how to counsel women, *MCN Am J Matern Child Nurs* 20(4):207, 1995.

Losch M et al: Impact of attitudes on maternal decisions regarding infant feeding, *J Pediatr* 126(4):507, 1995.

Luegenbiehl D et al: Standardized assessment of blood loss, *MCN Am J Matern Child Nurs* 15(4):241. 1991.

MacKendrich W, Caplan M: Necrotizing enterocolitis: new thoughts about pathogenesis and potential treatments, *Pediatr Clin North Am* 40(5):1047, 1993.

*Classic reference.

Martinez JC et al: Hyperbilirubinemia in the breast-fed newborn: a controlled trial of four interventions, *Pediatrics* 91(2): 470, 1993.

Mason T et al: Breastfeeding and the development of juvenile rheumatoid arthritis, *J Rhematol* 22(6):1166, 1995.

McGregor LA: Short, shorter, shortest: continuing to improve the hospital stay for mothers and newborns, *MCN Am J Matern Child Nurs* 21(4):191, 1996.

*Meier P, Anderson GC: Responses of small preterm infants to bottle-and breast-feeding, *Matern Child Nurs J* 12(1):97, 1987.

Miovech S et al: Major concerns of women after cesarean delivery, *J Obstet Gynecol Neonatal Nurs* 3(1):53, 1994.

Neifert M, Lawrence R, Seacot J: Nipple confusion: toward a formal definition, *J Pediatr* 126(suppl 6):125, 1994.

Nicoll A et al: Infant feeding policy and practice in the presence of HIV infection, *AIDS* 9(2):19, 1995.

Pheister D et al: Use of norplant contraceptive implants in the immediate postpartum period, *Am J Obstet Gynecol* 172(1 pt 1): 175, 1994.

Pisacane A et al: Breastfeeding and acute lower respiratory tract infections, *Acta Paediatr* 8:714, 1994.

Pisacane A et al: Breastfeeding and inguinal hernia, *J Pediatr* 127(1):109, 1995.

Renfrew M et al: *Bestfeeding: getting breastfeeding right for you,* Berkeley, Calif, 1990, Celestial Arts.

Riordan J, Auerbach KG: *Breastfeeding and human lactation,* Boston, 1993, Jones & Bartlett Publishers.

*Rubin RA: Maternal tasks in pregnancy, *Matern Child Nurs J* 4(3):143, 1975.

*Rubin RA: Maternity nursing stops too soon, *Am J Nurs* 10:1680, 1975.

*Rubin RA: Binding-in in the postpartum period, *Matern Child Nurs J* 6(2):67, 1977.

Schulte P: Minimizing alcohol exposure of the breastfeeding infant, *J Hum Lact* 11(4):317, 1995.

Seriven M et al: The importance of pubic pain following childbirth: a clinical study and ultrasonographic study of diastasis of the pubis symphysis, *Obstet Gynecol Surv* 50(9):634, 1995.

*Tribotti S et al: Nursing diagnoses for the postpartum woman, *J Obstet Gynecol Neonatal Nurs* 17(6):410, 1988.

Valaitis R et al: Meeting parents' postpartal needs with a telephone information line, *MCN Am J Matern Child Nurs* 21(2):90, 1996.

Van de Perre P: Postnatal transmission of human immunodeficiency virus type 1: the breastfeeding dilemma, *Am J Obstet Gynecol* 173(2):483, 1995.

Walker M: Fathers and breastfeeding, *J Obstet Gynecol Neonatal Nurs* 23(5):376, 1994.

Wang YS, Wu SY: The effect of exclusive breastfeeding on development and incidence of infection in infants, *J Hum Lact* 12(1):27, 1996.

Weinberg SH: An alternative to meet the needs of early discharge: the tender beginnings postpartum visit, *MCN Am J Matern Child Nurs* 19(6):339, 1994.

Wiessinger D: Watch your language, *J Hum Lact* 12(1):1, 1996.

Williams LR, Cooper MK: Nurse-managed postpartum home care, *J Obstet Gynecol Neonatal Nurs* 22(1):25, 1993.

 Student Resource Shelf

McGregor LA: Short, shorter, shortest: Improving the hospital stay for mothers and newborns. *MCN Am J Matern Child Nurs* 19(2):1166, 1994.

Compare these suggestions with what is occurring in your clinical setting.

Newman J: How breast milk protects newborns, *Sci Am* 273(6):76, 1995.

Review of all factors known to protect breast-fed infant.

Rubin RA

If possible, read all of Rubin's pioneer work on attachment and maternal tasks. See citations in preceding reference section.

Newborn Care

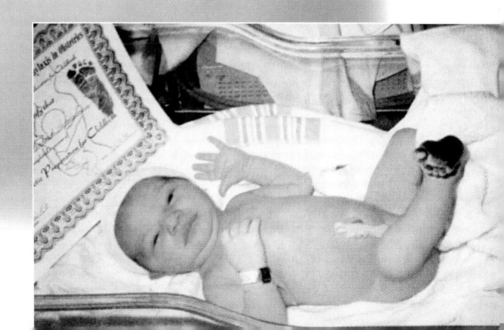

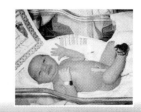

1.8 Newborn Physical Assessment

Learning Objectives

- Identify components of the neonatal health history and physical assessment.
- Determine the risk status of the neonate based on data from prenatal history and intrapartum progress.
- Describe major physiologic changes in the neonate's transition to extrauterine function.
- Distinguish between normal and abnormal structure and function for full-term neonates.
- Describe normal neonatal behavior patterns.
- Explain the purpose of gestational age assessment.
- Recognize physical characteristics of preterm, postterm, small-for-gestational age (SGA), and large-for-gestational age (LGA) infants.
- Determine gestational age using size, weight, and specific developmental characteristics.

Key Terms

Acrocyanosis
Caput Succedaneum
Cephalhematoma
Cold Stress
Desquamation
Developmental Reflexes
Epicanthal Folds
Erythema Toxicum
Gestational Age
  Assessment
Habituation
Hyperbilirubinemia
Macrocephaly
Microcephaly
Molding
Mongolian Spots
Nevi
Nonshivering
  Thermogenesis

Ortolani's Sign
Pallor
Petechiae
Physiologic Jaundice
Plethora
Polydactyly
Pseudomenstruation
Red Reflex
Regurgitation
Simian Line
Strabismus
Surfactant
Syndactyly
Temperature Gradient
Thermal Neutral
  Environment
Thrush
Vernix

$\mathcal{N}$ewborn infants are usually considered tiny and powerless, completely dependent on others for life. Although this is true for obtaining food and water, it is not true regarding basic life processes. Within 1 minute of birth, the normal newborn adapts from a dependent existence to an independent one, capable of oxygenation and carrying on life processes. Understanding and appreciating this transition are vital to the assessment of the newborn.

This chapter is organized by body systems and reviews techniques for assessing the normal transition to extrauterine function. For information on the at-risk infant and several of the problems mentioned here, refer to Chapters 28 and 29. The nurse frequently is the first health care provider who has contact with the neonate. In some birth settings it can be as long as 24 hours before a physician is required to examine a new infant. These first hours are crucial because multiple organ systems are making the transition from intrauterine to extrauterine functions. The nurse is required to have the skill to identify an infant who is having difficulty so that proper therapy can be implemented. The use of universal precautions with barriers such as gloves until the newborn has the first bath is important to protect both the nurse and client from communicable diseases.

Neonatal physical assessment is similar to adult assessment; that is, the same methods of data collection are used. An important focus is on assessment of growth and development. The objective of the assessment is to identify any alterations in health status that would make adjustment to extrauterine life difficult. A list of warning signs follows each system. These are assessment findings that necessitate interventions, discussed further in Chapter 29. Health history is a prelude to assessment; therefore the neonatal health history (Box 18-1) should be completed before beginning the physical examination. History of the pregnancy and birth

helps focus the assessment on specific risks that may be present.

Physical assessment is usually begun with the head, and then it proceeds downward. Infants are stimulated by physical assessment and may lose heat quickly when undressed. Therefore the order of the examination has been changed to minimize heat loss and to enlist the infant's cooperation. Attention is given to prenatal development; developmentally-related body systems are reviewed at the same time. In addition, the examiner notes differences in behaviors and vital signs during the early periods of reactivity.

Box 18-1 | **Neonatal Health History**

Date _____ Name of Infant _____

Sex _____ Time and date of delivery _____ Type _____

PRENATAL DATA

Maternal age _____ Blood type and Rh (Indirect Coombs') _____

EDC via dates _____ EDC via ultrasound _____

PREVIOUS OBSTETRIC HISTORY

Parity (explain all items) _____

Prior pregnancies: Date _____ Gestational age _____ Sex _____ Weight _____ Delivery _____

COMPLICATIONS OF THIS PREGNANCY

Preeclampsia _____ Hypertension _____ Diabetes (class) _____ Bleeding _____ Viral/bacterial infection _____

DRUG USE

Over the counter _____ Prescription _____

OTHER DRUGS

Alcohol _____ Cocaine _____ Heroin _____ Methadone _____ Other _____

FETAL TESTING AND RESULTS

AFP assay _____ Ultrasound _____ Amniocentesis _____ NST _____ BPS _____

INTRAPARTUM DATA

Onset of contractions _____ Rupture of membranes (ROM) When? _____

Any abnormalities? _____ Maternal vital signs _____ Any elevations? _____

Medications during labor: Anesthesia/analgesia _____ Time last administered _____

Length of stages of labor: First _____ Second _____

Fetal monitoring (external/internal) _____ Fetal distress? _____ Fetal pH? _____

IMMEDIATE CONDITION

Apgar score: 1 min _____ 5 min _____ 10 min _____

Any resuscitation? _____ Whiffs O$_2$ _____ Suction _____ Other _____

Spontaneous breathing established _____ Medications _____

OTHER OBSERVATIONS

Voided _____ Stool _____ Breast-fed _____ Bonding time _____

First Temperature _____ Eye prophylaxis with _____ Vitamin K IM? _____ Time _____

INITIAL ASSESSMENT

The nurse begins with a quick but thorough scan of the infant (Figure 18-1), looking for overt signs of difficulty for which immediate intervention is necessary. These manifest as abnormalities in vital signs, color, tone, movement, and size. The following seven questions provide a focus for the procedure.

Vital Signs

Are the vital signs—temperature, heart rate, respiration, and blood pressure—within normal limits?

Temperature

An axillary temperature can be taken with minimal disturbance by gently slipping the thermometer into the axillary space. Figure 19-8 illustrates the correct placement for an undressed infant. Rectal temperatures are not routinely taken because the vagus nerve is stimulated and there is risk of rectal perforation. No consensus has been reached on the use of infrared tympanic thermometers for newborns. The size of the newborn ear canal and the associated difficulty in positioning the thermometer in this small area makes accuracy of results uncertain. Some research indicates that the ear thermometer may be useful for initial newborn screenings but recommends that any decreases or elevations be verified with axillary temperatures (Weiss, Poelter, and Gocka, 1993). Other research recommends use of the tympanic measurement only after an infant is 3 months old (Wells et al, 1995). (Thermogenesis is discussed under metabolic control later in this chapter.) Normal ranges of axillary temperatures are 36.1° to 36.5° C (97.0° to 97.7° F). There are no widely accepted established normal ranges for tympanic thermometers.

Heart rate

An apical heart rate of 110 to 160 beats/min should be heard on the left side of the chest near the nipple on an awake newborn. Pulse rates may elevate to as high as 180 beats/min when the infant is crying and drop to as low as 80 beats/min when the newborn sleeps. The rate may be irregular for brief periods after crying. It is recommended that the apical pulse be taken for a full minute to assess for murmurs and irregularities. For alterations in heart sounds, see discussion of the cardiorespiratory system found later in this chapter.

Respiration

Because newborn respiratory rate is irregular, count for a full minute while looking at the upper abdomen. A range of 30 to 60 breaths/min is normal, with a possibility of brief (less than 5 to 15 seconds) periods of pause or apnea. Some otherwise healthy infants may show tachypnea (rate >60 breaths/min) during the first hour as excess lung fluid is absorbed. The examiner listens for the quality of breath sounds at each midaxillary line.

Blood pressure

Initial readings are taken on an arm and a leg with the Doppler device (Dinomap), and these are compared (see Figure 18-6, *B*). In the first 3 days, the range is from 75/45 to 50/30 mm Hg, with an average of 65/41 mm Hg. If there is a reading above or below these levels, further evaluation of blood volume is done. A marked difference between readings of arm and leg may indicate congenital heart disease and requires further evaluation.

Color

Does the infant's underlying color show a pinkish tone, with the exception of hands and feet?

Acrocyanosis (peripheral cyanosis) (Figure 18-2) is normal in the first 12 hours after birth. Later it may be a sign of difficulty controlling temperature or glucose. The rest of the body and mucous membranes should have a pink tone or be acyanotic. The examiner looks during feedings and crying to see whether the area around the infant's mouth becomes bluish (see Figure 18-6, *B*). Careful assessment is needed on newborns with highly pigmented skin.

Measurements

Are the infant's weight and length, as well as head and chest circumstances, consistent with the estimated gestational age?

The examiner needs an infant scale and paper barrier, a paper tape measure, and a growth chart. The head circumference is measured (Figure 18-3) from occiput to forehead, and the chest circumference is measured (Figure 18-4) at the level of the infant's nipples. Length is measured by a length board under the infant from tip of head to sole of foot. A very active infant can be positioned with the head touching the top of the crib and one leg gently extended. This distance can then be marked and measured.

Compare the infant's birth weight, length, and head circumference with the criteria in Table 18-1. These values can be plotted on a growth and development chart (see Figure 18-28) after gestational age assessment is completed. The normal range in weight is from 2500 to 4000 g. Measurements of length range from 44 to 55 cm. Head circumferences average from 33 to 35 cm, with chest circumferences always 1 to 2 cm less. If the chest is larger than the head, the infant should be closely observed for **microcephaly**. A head circumference less than the 10th percentile indicates microcephaly, which may be associated with congenital malformations and infection. A head circumference greater than the 90th percentile indicates **macrocephaly**, caused perhaps by hydrocephaly. Some infants whose par-

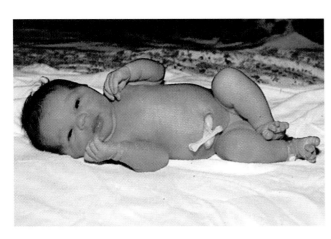

Figure 18-1 Healthy newborn. (Courtesy Marjorie Pyle, RNC, *Lifecircle*.)

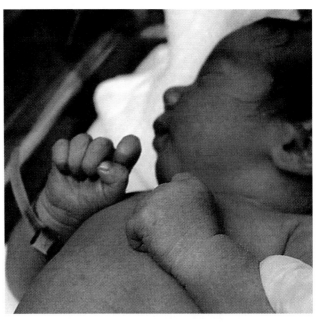

Figure 18-2 Acrocyanosis of hands in newborn. (From Seidel HM et al, eds: *Mosby's guide to physical examination,* ed 3, St Louis, 1995, Mosby.)

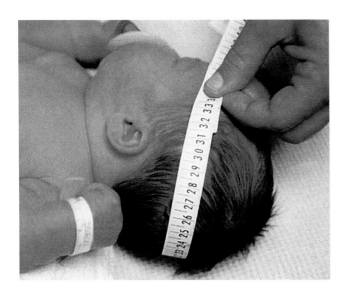

Figure 18-3 Appropriate placement of the measuring tape to obtain the head circumference. (From Seidel HM et al, eds: *Mosby's guide to physical examination,* ed 3, St Louis, 1995, Mosby.)

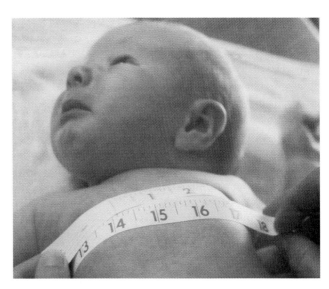

Figure 18-4 Measuring chest circumference. (Courtesy M Schult.)

Table **18-1** | **Normal Term Newborn Measurements**

Value	Normal Range	Variations
Weight	2500-4000 g	Average is 3400 g (7 lb).
Length	44-55 cm	Average is 50 cm (20 in); because molding of head can influence this value, remeasure before discharge.
Head circumference	32-37.5 cm, average 33-35 cm	Check molding of head.
Chest circumference	1-2 cm less than head circumference	Breast engorgement or molding of head can influence this ratio.
Axillary temperature	36.1°-36.5°C (97.0°-97.7°F)	Environmental temperature extremes, sepsis, and altered neurologic function can cause hypothermia or hyperthermia.
Respirations		
Rate	30-60 breaths/min	Respirations may be relatively tachypneic (rate over 60) during first hour but should not rise.
Quality	Easy, abdominal, without use of accessory muscles	Infant may have period of grunting, flaring, and retractions during first hour.
Apical pulse	110-160 beats/min	Rate of 100 to 120 beats/min is normal during sleep, but it should accelerate with stimulation; rate over 160 beats/min is common with increased activity and crying.
Blood pressure (*taken in arm and leg*)	**Systolic:** 50-75 mm Hg **Diastolic:** 30-45 mm Hg	Hypotension may mean low blood volume. Should be equal in upper and lower extremities.

Box **18-2** | **Periods of Neonatal Reactivity**

FIRST PHASE (AT 30-60 MIN AFTER BIRTH)
Active, alert
Eyes open, gazing
Active rooting, sucking
Vital signs labile: rapid irregular heart rate and respirations; may have rales, grunting, retractions, flaring nares
Activity labile: observe for tone, symmetric movement

FIRST SLEEP (AT 2-4 HR)
Quiet sleep, no interest in feeding
Stabilized vital signs
Onset of bowel sounds

SECOND REACTIVITY PERIOD (AT 4-10 HR)
Infant awake and alert
Rooting and sucking strong
Variable vital signs with mild cyanosis in extremities
Mottling, increased mucus
Passage of meconium and urine

Box **18-3**

WARNING SIGNS

Early Adaptation

- Axillary temperature <36.1° or >37.2° C (<97° or >99° F)
- Heart rate <110 or >160 beats/min (if asleep, may fall to 80 beats/min, or if active, may rise to 180 beats/min)
- Respiratory rate <30 or >60 breaths/min (if active, may rise transiently)
- Cyanosis other than acrocyanosis
- Jaundice
- Periods of apnea lasting >15 seconds
- Lack of movement and responsiveness
- Asymmetric position during flexion
- Hypotonic or hypertonic position
- Lack of interest in the environment
- Birth weight <5 pounds or >9 pounds
- Head circumference <5th percentile or >90 percentile
- Large or small for gestational age

ents are constitutionally large or small may exceed or fall short of these limits, but the measurements should not fall in widely divergent percentiles. For example, an infant whose weight and height fall within the 75th percentile should not have a head circumference in the 25th percentile. If the infant's head is greatly molded, the head and chest circumferences may be equal until the molding resolves. Remeasurement within 3 days is advised (Table 18-1).

Movement and Tone

Does the infant move all four extremities and return to a symmetric position of flexion?

Do all motions seem free and symmetrical in comparison with the other body parts?

Note especially birth injuries or anesthesia effects on muscle responses. A hypotonic infant may also have acidosis, hypoglycemia, hypothermia, or congenital problems (see Chapter 29).

Behavioral State

Is the cry vigorous and not high-pitched or shrill?

Does the infant seem interested in the environment? Is the transition from sleep to wake a smooth one?

Because the behavioral state will influence assessment, it is important to relate the infant's period of reactivity to these questions (Box 18-2) to the findings. If the answer is yes to all of the preceding seven, the infant will be in no immediate distress, and further evaluation can proceed.

CARDIORESPIRATORY SYSTEM

The respiratory and cardiovascular systems are considered together because of their obviously related functions, importance to survival, and proximity during assessment.

Normal Respiratory Transition

The first breath

There are several stimuli to breathing. During vaginal delivery, the infant's thorax is first compressed, then it rapidly reexpands, or recoils. This draws in a small amount of air. The comparative cold of the extrauterine environment, bright lights, noises, pressure on the infant's body, and sensation of weight from the addition of gravity all stimulate the newborn to take a deep gasping breath.

Mild hypercapnia, hypoxia, and acidosis normally accompany labor and delivery (see Chapter 14) and are chemical stimulants to the respiratory control centers in both adults and newborns. Studies show that animal fetuses that are warm and submerged will not breathe, despite this chemical stimulus, but will take a first breath

when they are exposed to the cooler environment. There are implications here for alternative birth practices that attempt to extend the intrauterine environment after birth. Several newborn deaths related to home underwater birth have been documented. These infants were submerged for up to 1 hour, with the parents thinking that the infant "enjoyed" the water (*Birth*, 1991).

Establishment of respiration

An adequate supply of **surfactant** is needed if normal respirations are to continue (see Chapter 7). In its absence, alveoli collapse with each exhalation, and there is no residual volume. With each breath the infant with inadequate surfactant must try to inflate lungs that are collapsed. The tremendously increased respiratory effort soon leads to respiratory failure. This is the basis of repiratory distress syndrome (RDS) (see Chapter 29).

Once respirations are established, the range will be between 30 and 60 breaths/min and will be irregular in rate, rhythm, and depth, with periods of apnea lasting up to 15 seconds. The face and trunk will have an acyanotic tone, although the extremities may still show a bluish color.

As the infant breathes, the partial pressure of oxygen (P_{O_2}) in the blood increases, whereas the partial pressure of carbon dioxide (P_{CO_2}) decreases. As acidosis resolves, blood pH approaches adult values. The pulmonary blood vessels, constricted in fetal life, dilate in response to the increased oxygen levels and allow a dramatic increase in blood flow to the newborn lungs. The results of normal transition occur as follows.

1. Surfactant production is maintained.
2. Residual volume is established.
3. Physiologic acid-base balance continues.
4. Blood flow to the lungs is increased.
5. Vital signs are within normal limits.
6. An oxygenated color is evident.

Normal Cardiovascular Transition

Transitional circulation

Fetal circulation (see Chapter 7) should be reviewed before transitional circulation is studied. Changes that occur during the transition from fetal to newborn circulation are closely linked to changes in the respiratory system. These changes are caused by the alterations in systemic and pulmonary pressures that result from the first deep breath and the establishment of respirations. Therefore, clamping the umbilical cord does not cause the reversal from fetal to adult circulation. Circulatory patterns will change from fetal to newborn even if the infant is born unattended and the cord is not clamped immediately after birth (see unexpected birth, Chapter 15). Figure 18-5 illustrates the following description of transitional circulation.

1. The infant's first breath raises the P_{O_2}, which causes the pulmonary arterial blood vessels to dilate and allows blood to flow freely to the lungs. Now the pulmonary blood pressure is decreased.
2. The *umbilical arteries* constrict in response to increased P_{O_2} levels, and the cord is cut.
3. Circulation through the *umbilical vein* ends.
4. As the *ductus venosus* closes, the systemic blood pressure rises.
5. These changes in pressure cause blood flow through the ductus arteriosus to reverse its direction, thus changing one of the right-to-left shunts. The ductus arteriosus then constricts (also in response to increased P_{O_2} levels), preventing blood flow through it by the end of the first day. It will later become the ligamentum arteriosum.
6. Because of increased blood flow to the lungs, there must be increased flow from the lungs through the pulmonary veins and to the left atrium.
7. The increased pressure of this blood against the *foramen ovale* forces it to close against the interatrial septum. This reverses the other right-to-left shunt. (The site of the old foramen ovale will later become the fossa ovalis.)
8. These allow blood to flow to the newborn lungs for gas exchange and return to the heart for distribution to the body. All fetal vessels, first functionally and then anatomically, adapt to adult circulation by atrophy (Table 18-2).

The rate of the neonatal heart will be relative to the fetal heart rate (FHR) but will gradually become slower. The rate continues to be irregular in rate and rhythm, but variability also decreases. The rate responds to stimuli as did the FHR. The results of normal transition are as follows:

1. Decrease in pulmonary blood pressure *with* resultant increase in pulmonary blood flow.
2. Closure of the foramen ovale.
3. Constriction of the ductus arteriosus.
4. End of flow through the umbilical vein.

Failure of this transition results in a life-threatening disorder—*persistent fetal circulation* (PFC) or *persistent pulmonary hypertension of the newborn* (PPHN)—which is reviewed in Chapter 29.

Assessment

Inspection. The infant is observed at rest and during activity. The examiner observes skin color and looks for symmetric expansion of the chest. The infant's color should be primarily acyanotic, but there may still be acrocyanosis. Bulging or asymmetry of the chest may indicate that air is trapped in the pleural space below (pneumothorax). The respiratory rate is counted by watching the lower portion of the chest and the abdomen rise and fall (watching the cord can be helpful) for a full minute, since the neonate's normal irregular pattern of respiration will cause the total to be inaccurate if the counting is discontinued before 60 seconds have elapsed. Although respirations range from 30 to 60 breaths/min (see Table 18-1), there may be changes according to state and period of reactivity. The quality of respiration is assessed by noting retractions or nasal flaring. *Retractions* are caused by use of accessory muscles of respiration and are seen as the inspiratory "pulling in" of the chest wall above and below the sternum (suprasternal and substernal retractions) and between and below the ribs (intercostal and subcostal retractions). Recognition of retractions as mild, moderate, or severe requires practice. When nasal flaring is present, the nares seem to dilate with each inspiration, indicating that the fluid that fills the lungs during fetal life has not yet been absorbed or that more serious difficulties in extrauterine adjustment may be present (see Figure 29-7).

Meconium staining of the skin, nails, and cord should be noted, since this indicates chronic fetal distress. Meconium stained amniotic fluid may be associated with respiratory distress if aspiration of fluid has occurred during labor. While assessing respiratory status, the examiner notes the number and spacing of the nipples and the presence of *gynecomastia*, or breast engorgement. A few infants may have extra nipple tissue (i.e., supernumerary nipples). The apical impulse, or *point of maximal impulse* (PMI) may also be seen.

Auscultation. The best place to listen to breath sounds is at the midaxillary line, but all lobes should be examined. An equal amount of air entry on each side of the chest should be heard. Scattered *rales* (sounds of moisture within the lungs) are considered normal during the first few hours of life, especially in the infant delivered by surgical intervention. There should be no stridor or noise during inspiration. *Grunting* is an abnormal expiratory sound heard as the infant forcibly exhales against a closed glottis to keep the alveoli from collapsing. It may be possible to hear this grunting without a stethoscope. Grunting is a warning of respiratory distress.

The examiner concentrates on the heart sounds, auscultating the entire cardiac region. One pattern is to begin at the apex, found on the infant at the PMI, the place where the pulse is best felt. The PMI is found just to the left of the midclavicular line at the fourth intercostal space. This point is higher in the infant than in the adult because the neonatal heart lies in a more horizontal position. The examiner works from the apex up to the left sternal border, then toward the base of the heart, then listens along the right sternal border, finally turning the infant over and listening between the scapulae.

If a rate of less than 110 is heard, stimulating the infant to cry should make the rate rise. Although neonatal heart rates have variability similar to FHR, obvious irregularities in the cardiac rhythm should not occur. Gestational age also influences heart rates (with faster rates earlier in gestation) because of the dominance of the sympathetic nervous system.

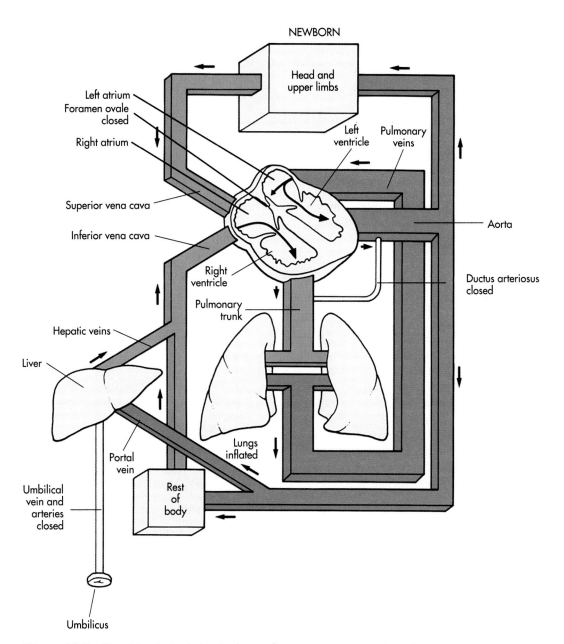

Figure 18-5   Transitional circulation in the newborn. (Courtesy G David Brown.)

Table **18-2**   **Anatomic Changes in the Fetal Structures after Birth**

Fetal Structures	Infant Structures	Range for Completion
Foramen ovale	Fossa ovalis	Several wk to 1 yr
Ductus arteriosus	Ligamentum arteriosum	Several wk to 1 yr
Ductus venosus	Ligamentum venosum of the liver	1-2 mo
Umbilical arteries	Lateral umbilical ligaments	2-3 mo
Umbilical vein	Ligamentum teres of the liver	2-3 mo

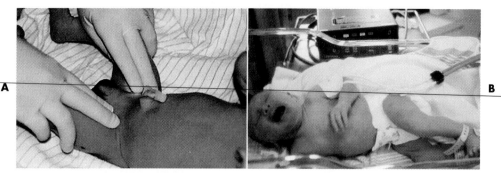

Figure 18-6   A, Palpating femoral pulses. **B,** Infant blood pressure is taken on each extremity. (**A,** Courtesy Marjorie Pyle, RNC, *Lifecircle.* **B,** Courtesy M Schult.)

The next focus is the quality of heart sounds and the presence of extra sounds. S_1 and S_2 are the first and second heart sounds. S_1 is heard when the atrioventricular valves (mitral and tricuspid) close, and S_2 occurs when the semilunar valves (aortic and pulmonary) close. The "lub-dub" sounds are S_1 and S_2, respectively. The time between S_1 and S_2 is *systole,* and the time between S_2 and S_1 is *diastole.*

In evaluating heart sounds, a separate and distinct S_1 and S_2 should be heard, usually with no extra sounds during systole or diastole. The sounds should be easy to hear (i.e., it should not seem as though the heart is far from the stethoscope). However, "closeness" of heart sounds to the chest wall is a parameter that can be assessed accurately only with experience. A good order to use when auscultating the heart is as follows.

1. Count the rate, noting its regularity and variability with the infant's activity.
2. Locate the place where the sounds are best heard in the chest.
3. Differentiate between S_1 and S_2.
4. Decide whether there are extra sounds.

Palpation. Brachial pulses are palpated at the antecubital space, and the femoral pulses are palpated bilaterally along the inguinal ligament halfway between the iliac crest and the symphysis pubis (Figure 18-6, *A*). Their relative rates and volumes should be equal.

Box **18-4**
WARNING SIGNS

Cardiorespiratory Problems

- Sustained heart rate <110 or >180 beats/min
- Respiratory rate <30 or >60 breaths/min
- Central cyanosis
- Difference in arm and leg blood pressure readings
- Apnea for more than 15 seconds
- Muffled heart sounds are heard, with PMI shifted to right
- Cardiac murmur
- Unequal breath sounds

Percussion. Percussion of the neonatal chest is not generally undertaken because any questions concerning the size and condition of organs are investigated by radiographic or ultrasonic examination.

TEST *Yourself* **18-1**

a. Recall the changes in fetal circulation shunts after birth.
b. Why should you count respirations for 1 full minute?
c. What is the significance of expiratory grunting heard in a 2-hour-old newborn?

METABOLIC CONTROL

Heat Transfer

The newborn enters an environment at least 20° to 25° F cooler than core body temperature. Unless the infant is protected against heat loss, core body temperature can drop 0.5° to 2° C (0.9° to 3.6° F) within 5 to 10 minutes of birth. Thermal receptors are present on the body surface, with many on the face. When triggered, the response is peripheral vasoconstriction. The head, 20% of the body surface, is wet at birth and difficult to dry completely. Because most of the heat loss is through evaporation and radiation, drying the infant is a priority. Use of radiant overhead warmers has significantly reduced initial heat loss. Incubators are also useful to control heat loss from convection.

The **temperature gradient** is the difference between the skin and the environment (external gradient) or between the core of the body and the skin (internal gradient). Temperature control in the newborn is influenced primarily by this temperature gradient.

When ambient temperature falls in the adult, increased metabolism raises internal or core temperature by means of involuntary high intensity, rhythmic shivering and by voluntary muscle activity. This muscle activity is *physical thermogenesis.* However, the newborn infant can use only **nonshivering thermogenesis.** Chapter 7 describes a special form of fat, brown adipose tissue (BAT), that is deposited during fetal life. Newborns produce body heat by increasing their metabolic rate and by metabolizing this tissue; they do not shiver. A decrease in ambient temperature stimulates production of norepinephrine, which increases brown fat metabolism. This response is impaired when an infant has hypoxia or if fat stores are already depleted. Certain drugs can also block this response. During BAT metabolism, oxygen is consumed and fatty acids and glycerol are produced. Newborns are vulnerable to heat loss despite these mechanisms because (1) there is a large skin surface to body weight ratio, which promotes a more rapid loss of heat from the core to the skin surface, and (2) the presence of substantial layers of subcutaneous fat as additional insulation depends on gestational age and birth weight.

Extremes of environmental temperature, therefore, will stress the infant. This may lead to *overheating,* which will cause an elevated body temperature, vasodilation with flushed skin, and tachypnea as the infant tries to dissipate the extra heat. For this reason, an infant should never be left unattended under a radiant warmer without a continuous *servomechanism* for temperature feedback. These devices monitor the skin temperature and change the heat output as needed to maintain the set temperature. More commonly, the environmental temperature will be too low and will initiate the adverse effects termed **cold stress.**

Cold stress

The infant responds to low environmental temperatures with peripheral vasoconstriction, which leads to increased anaerobic metabolism and acidosis. Initially, peripheral vasoconstriction will make the skin temperature drop while the core temperature is maintained. Later, core temperature will fall. (Neonatal cold stress is discussed in Chapter 29.) One goal of nursing care is maintaince of a **thermal neutral environment** is which heat production (measured as oxygen consumption) is minimal, yet core temperature is within the normal range. Infants cared for in such an environment need not expend extra energy or consume extra oxygen to maintain normal internal temperature. Although this may not make a tremendous difference to the healthy, full-term infant, the added stress can be disastrous for the sick infant.

Glucose and Calcium

Maintenance of adequate blood glucose levels is vital because of the brain's dependence on glucose for energy; lack of glucose may cause tremors, seizures, and permanent neurologic damage. Maintenance of serum calcium levels is also necessary for normal neuromuscular function; low calcium levels may cause tremors, tetany, and seizures. Abnormally increased calcium levels are rare in the neonate.

Glucose is needed for the increased energy demands that occur after delivery. The newborn infant must breathe and maintain body temperature. The infant's movements are also more vigorous than those that occur in utero. At birth, glucose levels are maintained by glycolysis of hepatic glycogen and gluconeogenesis. These prenatal stores will be the primary source of energy until feedings are well established.

The infusion of large amounts of glucose during labor may result in fetal hyperinsulinemia, with a postnatal rebound of hypoglycemia. For this reason, glucose is usually not infused during labor (Hazle, 1986). There may also be transient neonatal tachypnea, hyponatremia, and elevated bilirubin levels when fluid intake during labor has not been carefully regulated (Keppler, 1988). Therefore it is important that the nurse caring for a newborn be aware of the mother's intrapartum hydration status and the type and volume of any parenteral fluids she received.

Several factors influence neonatal calcium metabolism and increase the risk for hypocalcemia. At delivery, maternal calcium supplies end. Levels of hormones that control calcium metabolism are low at birth. In addition, the fetus that is stressed in utero is also at high risk for hypocalcemia (for treatment, see Chapter 29).

Results of a normal transition show serum glucose levels in the normal range of 50 to 100 mg/dl and total calcium in the normal range of 7 to 8 mg/dl. A difficult transition may manifest in several ways. Tremors are most commonly seen, but *lethargy, tachypnea, pallor,* and *cyanosis* are also common signs of hypoglycemia or hypocalcemia. It is important to anticipate metabolic imbalances in infants who are especially at risk: those who are small or large for gestational age, infants of diabetic mothers (IDM), and premature and postmature infants.

Box **18-1**
CLINICAL DECISION

After your assessment of a 3200 g full-term, 6-hour-old newborn boy, which of the following findings should be reported?
a. Heart rate of 140 beats/min during sleep, which rises to 160 beats/min when the infant cries
b. Pink with bluish color around mouth and in hands and feet when crying
c. Brachial pulses that feel much fuller in volume than femoral pulses, which are barely palpable

Box **18-5**
WARNING SIGNS

Poor Metabolic Control

- Infant is preterm, postterm, IDM, large for gestational age (LGA), small for gestational age (SGA)
- Temperature less than or above normal range
- Tremors, tachypnea, pallor, cyanosis
- Glucose <50 mg/dl
- Calcium <7 mg/dl

TEST *Yourself* 18-2

a. Describe how the neonate responds to a drop in ambient temperature.
b. What history and assessment data in the newborn are associated with hypoglycemia?

INTEGUMENTARY SYSTEM

The integumentary system is the next system to be evaluated. The information obtained from assessing this system is often related to the integrity of other systems (e.g., skin color provides information on the health of the cardiovacular and hematologic systems).

Normal Transition

At birth the skin and its structures are exposed to the dry, colder extrauterine environment. Any **vernix**—an unctuous substance made of sebum and desquamated epithelial cells—that remains is gradually absorbed. Therefore skin commonly becomes dry and may crack at the ankles and wrists. The term infant's skin will normally peel within 2 days of birth; peeling before that time is not normal. **Desquamation** (peeling) over the entire body is a classic sign seen in the postmature infant.

Cutis marmorata, which is a mottled or marbled appearance over the body, may be observed. It is caused by dilation of the small blood vessels, and is not an expected reaction to chilling (Figure 18-7, *A*). It usually is seen only during early infancy, but it may persist longer in infants with certain congenital problems. The *harlequin sign* is a phenomenon seen only in the newborn infant, most often in those of low birth weight. The infant who is lying on one side will become bright red over the dependent half of the body and very pale over the half that is superior. There is a definite line of demarcation between the two colors, which will reverse sides if the infant's position is reversed. This sign is benign and lasts a short while.

Pigmentation is genetically determined and influenced by the extrauterine environment. After birth, when the infant is exposed to light, the skin of African-American infants will continue to darken. About 90% of all infants of African-American, Asian, Latin American, or Native American origin will have **mongolian spots**, which result from the deep dermal infiltration of melanocytes. These flat, irregularly shaped, pigmented lesions are seen most commonly over the lumbosacral region. They vary in size (some may be quite large) and color (from gray-blue to blue-black). Though with age these lesions appear to fade, they actually become less obvious as the overlying skin loses its transparency. After age 4, these mongolian spots may seem to have disappeared (Figure 18-7, *B*).

The most common skin variation seen during the transition period is **erythema toxicum** (Figure 18-7, *C* and *D*), also known as newborn rash. The cause of this is not known, but its appearance has alarmed the mothers of many full-term infants. These pale yellow to white pustules and papules with reddened bases usually erupt first on the trunk but then may spread to the entire body, with the exception of the soles and palms. The lesions disappear spontaneously within hours to days after their appearance.

Many full-term infants are born with *milia,* or epidermal inclusion cysts (Figure 18-7, *E*). These small white or yellow papules are commonly found on the nose, chin, and forehead. When they appear on the palate or gums, these are called *Epstein's pearls.* Both types of skin variation disappear early in infancy. Sweat may be retained in small, noninflammatory vesicles called *miliaria.* These are also seen over the forehead, as well as on the neck and diaper area. Because this condition usually occurs in infants who live in a hot, humid environment, cooling and drying the infant will cause the vesicles to resolve.

Assessment

Inspection of the integumentary system takes place during the examination of other systems. It is presented at this point in the chapter to provide guidance for the balance of the examination.

The skin color is observed in natural light. If this is not possible, the examiner should recognize that fluorescent lights tends to alter true color. Skin thickens as gestational age increases; therefore the skin of the less mature infant is more transparent.

Skin pigmentation, which ranges from pale to dark brown, is assessed. Mucous membranes should have underlying pink tones, and no cyanotic changes should be seen with crying or activity. Acrocyanosis and mottling occur early but are abnormal if they persist. The examiner notes whether the infant is acyanotic or has **pallor** (pale or white underlying tone) or **plethora** (ruddy, purplish color). The skin of the forehead or abdomen is blanched by applying finger pressure momentarily and observing the return of color (capillary filling), which should be prompt. Capillary refilling is an indication of perfusion. The presence of jaundice is also noted.

It is important to examine the entire skin surface, including the neck and inguinal and axillary folds. At term, vernix caseosa is found only in these deep skin folds. Skin *turgor,* an indication of adequate intrauterine growth, is examined by gently pinching a fold of skin on the abdomen or thigh. If the skin fold does not appear elastic, turgor is poor. Any edema or extra folds of skin are also noted.

The quality and distribution of *hair* are important parts of both gestational age assessment and evaluation of the infant at risk for genetic disease. Unusual patterns and distributions of hair growth are associated with some genetic syndromes (e.g., Cornelia de Lange's syndrome). In addition, certain racial groups have heavier hair distribution at

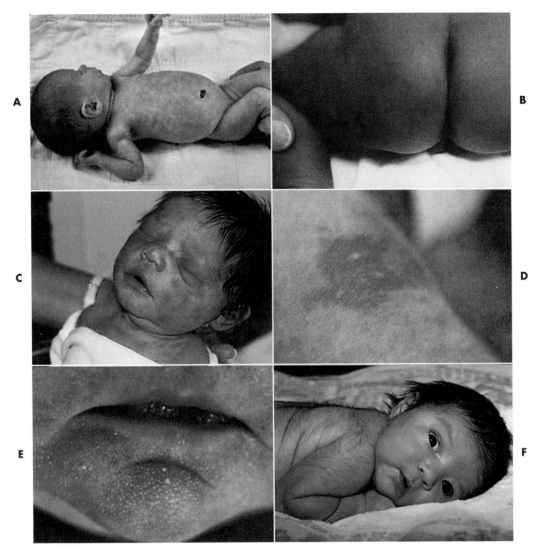

Figure 18-7   Skin characteristics of the newborn. **A,** Cutis marmorata—skin mottling. **B,** Mongolian spots. **C,** Newborn rash and swollen eyelids. **D,** Erythema toxicum. **E,** Milia. **F,** Hair distribution. (**A, D,** and **E,** Courtesy Mead Johnson; **B,** From Seidel HM et al, eds: *Mosby's guide to physical examination*, ed 3, St Louis, 1995, Mosby; **C** and **F,** Courtesy Marjorie Pyle, RNC, *Lifecircle*.)

birth (Figure 18-7, *F*). Lanugo is fine, downy hair that covers the back, shoulders, and forehead of a preterm infant and is present on the shoulders at term. Nail growth increases with gestation; nails will have grown to the end of the fingers at term and past the fingertips after term.

The examiner looks for birth marks, skin injuries, and meconium staining. He or she also gently *palpates* masses for consistency, tenderness, and return of color, noting whether a reddened lesion blanches with pressure, which indicates a vascular connection. Tiny red spots that do not blanch with pressure may be **petechiae,** or microhemorrhages within the skin, possibly caused by pressure during birth. Another cause of petechiae is thrombocytopenia, which can be life threatening, but it is also a sign of congenital infection. Oval reddened areas (forceps marks) may be observed on the cheeks of

infants whose delivery has been assisted with forceps. Use of vacuum extraction during delivery results in a chignon, a bruised, edematous area of the scalp. These marks gradually resolve.

Some integumentary structures are subject to prenatal stimulation by maternal hormones. One manifestation is secretion of a colostrumlike fluid ("witch's milk") by the breasts during the neonatal period, which is seen in both male and female infants. Other structures may also appear to mature early. Occasionally a tooth may erupt during fetal life and be seen at birth (natal teeth). It is almost always a prematurely erupted deciduous tooth rather than an extra, or supernumerary, one. An attempt is made to save the tooth, if possible. Before the infant is discharged, however, a loose tooth is removed to prevent possible aspiration.

Box 18-6   Neonatal Skin Lesions

NEVI (HEMANGIOMAS OR DEVELOPMENTAL VASCULAR ABNORMALITIES)

Flat (Telangiectatic) Hemangiomas

Salmon-pink color and easy to blanch; found at nape of neck, eyelids, and forehead; fade within 1 year

Nevus Flammeus (Port-Wine Stain)

Red to black in color; if found on face along trigeminal nerve tract, may be associated with cerebral vascular malformation

Raised and Giant (Cavernous) Hemangiomas

Bright red to reddish blue in color; tend to increase in size after birth; cavernous type may trap platelets, causing thrombocytopenia

PIGMENTED LESIONS

Mongolian Spots

Gray to blue; found on lumbosacral area in African-American, Asian, Latin American, and Native American infants; fade in first few years of life

Cafe-au-lait Spots

Small, brown patches; if more than six are present or any are larger than 4 by 6 cm, infant may have neurofibromatosis; with aging these may undergo precancerous changes

ERYTHEMA TOXICUM

Maculopapular rash that may include small pustulelike lesions containing sterile fluid and eosinophils (white cells indicative of an allergic response rather than infection); found on the trunk and face; fades within a few days

MILIA

Epidermal cysts containing keratogenous material; look like whiteheads found over the nose and chin; fade within a few days

MILIARIA

Retention of sweat in opened exocrine glands causing clear vesicles on the face, scalp, and perineum; resolves in a few days if environmental heat and humidity are not extreme

BULLAE

Blisters more than 1 cm in diameter

PUSTULES

Small lesions containing pus; may be signs of staphylococcal infection; must be differentiated from erythema toxicum

Box 18-7

WARNING SIGNS

Integumentary System Problems

- Long nails and desquamation indicating postmaturity
- Thin, translucent skin with abundant vernix and lanugo, indicating prematurity
- Pallor, possibly caused by hypothermia, anemia, sepsis, or shock
- Cyanosis, possibly caused by cardiorespiratory disease, hypoglycemia, polycythemia, sepsis, or hypothermia
- Petechiae, possibly caused by thrombocytopenia, sepsis, congenital infection, or pressure sustained during delivery
- Plethora, possibly caused by polycythemia
- Meconium staining, possibly caused by intrauterine asphyxia
- Abnormal hair distribution (unrelated to gestational age) or extra skin folds, possibly associated with genetic syndromes
- Poor skin turgor associated with intrauterine growth retardation and hypoglycemia
- Large (cavernous) hemangiomas, which may trap platelets within their borders and cause thrombocytopenia
- Bullae or pustules, possibly caused by syphilis or staphylococcal infection

Nevi are genetic changes in the skin. There are many types of nevi; some spontaneously disappear and others do not. Within each of these groups, there are two other subdivisions of nevi: *telangiectatic,* or flat, and *hemangiomatous,* or raised. Salmon patches are flat, pale pink, irregularly shaped lesions called "stork's bites" when found at the nape of the neck (Figure 18-8). About 50% of all white newborns have a simple hemangioma on the sacrum, the back of the neck, the face, or eyelids. These are small at birth, then they grow and eventually disappear. Although they fade with age, parents may express concern when these are first noticed. Nevus flammeus, or port-wine stain, is a serious disfigurement and found most often on the face; unfortunately, this does not disappear. Giant hemangiomas (strawberry marks) are larger and raised; these can be dangerous if they trap platelets and thereby lower the amount of circulating platelets (Figure 18-9).

Most skin lesions are harmless, although they usually are a source of concern to parents who naturally hope for the perfect infant. Parents need to know which of these will disappear spontaneously and which need treatment. Common skin lesions are described in Box 18-6.

GASTROINTESTINAL SYSTEM

Normal Transition

For the first 30 minutes after birth (first period of reactivity), the healthy, full-term infant will be alert and eager to suck—this is the ideal time to initiate breast-feeding. Newborn gastric capacity at term is about 10 to 20 ml. Although the stomach will not empty completely during the first few hours of life, this is not a concern because the breast-feeding infant will consume only a small amount of colostrum.

The suck-swallow mechanism that has been functioning prenatally further matures after birth to prevent aspiration. The result of this maturation is the rapid opening of the epiglottis during swallowing and its closing during respiration. The *cardiac sphincter* between the esophagus and stomach in the newborn infant is frequently less than fully functional; therefore **regurgitation**—reflux of gastric contents into the esophagus and upward into the pharynx—may occur, which increases the possibility of aspiration. This may occur especially during the second period of reactivity from about the second to sixth hour after delivery, when the infant demonstrates variability in several areas of adjustment to extrauterine life. It is also during this time that the infant may become "mucousy," having difficulty with mucous secretions. The infant may gag or choke, and it may be necessary to clear the airway by changing his or her position or by suctioning any secretions.

Bowel sounds can be heard as the first period of reactivity ends. Meconium is usually passed during the second period of reactivity, although it may occur in utero or at delivery.

There are several congenital defects that affect the gastrointestinal system. Early general assessment may detect if there is an *imperforate anus*. Upon feeding, an infant who lacks an intact esophagus would immediately begin to choke. (See Chapter 28 for full discussion of the *tracheoesophageal fistula* and atresias.)

Assessment

Inspection. The abdominal wall should be free of defects. The cord is observed for color and the amount of Wharton's jelly. Umbilical cord changes should be consistent with the infant's age in days; it will blacken and become dry within 2 to 3 days. An umbilical hernia may be present. This mass protrudes more when the infant cries and is seen more commonly in African-American infants. The abdominal girth is measured just above the umbilicus. The rectum should be patent, and meconium should be passed within 24 hours. Some meconium-filled loops of bowel may bulge through the abdominal wall until this occurs.

Auscultation. The examiner always auscultates for bowel sounds before palpating the abdomen because bowel motility can be affected by palpation. Bowel sounds should be present several hours after birth (see Box 18-2).

Palpation. Palpation of the newborn abdomen requires gentle firmness. It should be done at least 2 hours after a feeding. The entire abdomen is palpated in a systematic manner, noting masses. The liver should be evaluated for size by palpating from the right iliac crest up to the right costal margin, until the lower liver edge is felt to slip against the fingers; stop palpating 1 to 2 cm below the right costal margin (Figure 18-10). The spleen tip may be felt at the left costal margin.

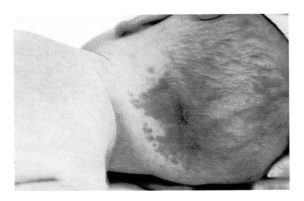

Figure 18-8　Nevus at nape of neck, "stork's bite" mark. (Courtesy Mead Johnson.)

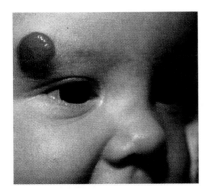

Figure 18-9　Giant hemangioma in infant. (From Habif TP: *Clinical dermatology*, ed 3, St Louis, 1996, Mosby.)

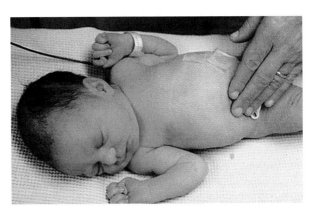

Figure 18-10　Positioning to examine infant's abdomen to palpate liver. (From Seidel HM et al, eds: *Mosby's guide to physical examination*, ed 3, St Louis, 1995, Mosby.)

Box 18-8

WARNING SIGNS

Gastrointestinal System Problems

- Obvious structural defects in the abdominal wall
- Single umbilical artery associated with congenital anomalies (especially renal)
- Meconium-stained or shriveled umbilical cord associated with intrauterine growth retardation or perinatal asphyxia
- Imperforate anus, which may be associated with a tracheoesophageal fistula or esophageal atresia
- Enlarged liver and spleen (hepatosplenomegaly) associated with congenital infections and hemolysis
- Flat or scaphoid abdomen, which may be associated with a diaphragmatic hernia (congenital defect in which abdominal contents are in the thorax)
- Failure to pass meconium stool within 24 hours
- History of polyhydramnios or oligohydramnios during pregnancy
- Masses anywhere in abdomen

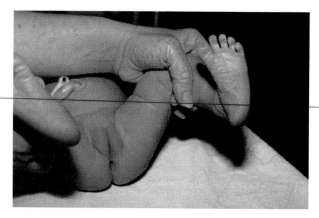

Figure 18-11   Full-term female genitalia. (Courtesy Marjorie Pyle, RNC, *Lifecircle*.)

There should be no masses, but the examiner may feel some loops of bowel. There may be *diastasis*, or separation of the rectus muscles, which feels like softness in the midline between the two bands of rectus muscles.

GENITOURINARY SYSTEM

Normal Transition

The removal of the placenta at birth ends the neonate's dependence on the maternal kidneys for renal function. The quality of renal function in the term infant is generally adequate for the infant's needs. However, the ability of the newborn kidney to adapt to stress is limited. This deficiency improves during the first week of life, and kidney function continues to mature to adult levels as infancy continues. During the neonatal period, urine composition changes from dilute (specific gravity 1.004 to 1.010) to more concentrated as renal function matures. By 2 months of age, the infant's urine has a strong odor and the specific gravity of adult urine.

The normal fetus responds to the stress of labor and delivery with secretion of catecholamines, which cause FHR accelerations and help mobilize hepatic glycogen for energy in the immediate neonatal period.

Assessment of kidneys and bladder

The quantity of amniotic fluid is the first prenatal clue that the kidneys are functioning. After birth the infant should void within the first 24 hours. The first voiding is easy to miss because newborn urine is quite dilute and may not be noticed in the excitement immediately after birth. Newborns then void frequently, wetting six to eight diapers

a day after the mother's milk is established. If measured, the normal infant's output of urine is 1 to 3 ml/kg of body weight per hour. The kidneys are palpated bimanually (using both hands). The examiner, supporting the infant's lumbar region from below, palpates the flank deeply to the spine just under the costal margin. This should not be attempted when the newborn has recently been fed.

Assessment of female genitalia

The examiner assesses the configuration of the labia and hymen and notes the placement of the urinary meatus and rectum and the length of the perineum, as well as the size of the clitoris and labia, which vary with gestational age.

In the full-term female infant, the labia almost completely cover the clitoris (Figure 18-11). There should be no fusion of the labia; hymenal tags (small tags of mucous membrane extending from the vagina) are not significant. **Pseudomenstruation**—a white mucous discharge, sometimes streaked with light pink blood—is often present and is the result of withdrawal of maternal hormones for a few days after birth. The labia may be edematous and darker than usual in response to birth pressure and maternal hormones.

Fused labia, clitoral hypertrophy, and placement of the urinary meatus anterior to the clitoris are signs of sexual ambiguity (see Chapter 27). In premature infants, there are widely spaced labia majora and a large clitoris. Bulging of the hymen may be caused by the pressure of fluid behind an imperforate hymen.

Assessment of male genitalia

The examiner inspects the penis for correct placement of the urinary meatus (Figure 18-12), which should always be at the tip of the penis. The scrotum is observed for color, size, and rugae (deep wrinkles), which vary with gestational age. The scrotum is larger and covered with rugae close to term. The color is dark because of the passive transfer of maternal hormones. After a breech delivery the infant may have bruising and edema of the genitalia, which resolves after several days, but gross

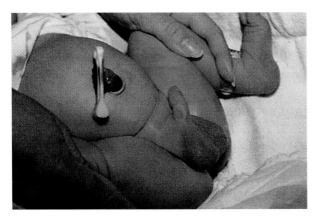

Figure 18-12 Full-term male genitalia. (Courtesy Marjorie Pyle, RNC, *Lifecircle*.)

Box **18-9**

WARNING SIGNS

Genitourinary System Problems

BOTH MALE AND FEMALE INFANTS
- Oligohydramnios
- Mass palpated in abdomen
- Defects of the abdominal wall
- Failure to void within 24 hours

FEMALE GENITALIA
- Clitoral hypertrophy
- Fused labia
- Abnormal placement of the urinary meatus

MALE GENITALIA
- Hypospadias (urinary meatus opening on ventral surface of penis)
- Epispadias (urinary meatus opening on dorsal surface of penis)
- Micropenis
- Bifid or split scrotum (not fused in midline)
- Scrotal masses
- Hydrocele (fluid within scrotal sac)

abnormalities should not occur. (See Figure 18-28 for gestational age assessment.)

The examiner palpates the testes by blocking the inguinal canal with one finger to prevent testicle retraction while gently palpating the scrotum with a thumb and forefinger. The fullness of the scrotal sac is noted. By 36 weeks each testis should have descended into the scrotum and is palpated separately. Each should be smooth, about 1 cm diameter, and freely movable. The testes may retract into the inguinal canal if the infant is cold. It is common for a male newborn to have a hydrocele, a collection of fluid surrounding the testicles in the scrotum. Transillumination will verify that this enlargement is not a mass. Most hydroceles resolve spontaneously.

Male infants have frequent erections, which may surprise new parents. Infants have been observed engaged in pelvic rocking. The possibility of infantile sexual reactions is disturbing to some. Cutaneous sensation, however, is the first sensory capability to develop.

TEST *Yourself* 18-3

> a. Why should you press on the groin to block the inguinal canal when palpating the scrotum?
> b. What is the significance of a whitish pink vaginal discharge in a newborn girl?
> c. What factors in an infant's birth history would make swollen genitalia an expected finding?

HEMATOLOGIC SYSTEM

Normal Transition

At birth the hematologic system is infused with oxygen. The relatively low oxygen tension of umbilical venous blood is replaced with the higher oxygen tension now supplied by the lungs via the pulmonary artery. Adjustment from a fetal to adult state of function occurs gradually. Observations focus on the ability of this system to carry oxygen, rid itself of its fetal hemoglobin load, and maintain normal coagulation.

Hemoglobin levels versus hematocrit values

The normal term infant has a blood volume of about 80 ml/kg of body weight. Hematocrit values will range from 45% to 65% if blood is drawn from a vein or artery; because of the normally sluggish peripheral circulation, it will be higher if a capillary sample is examined. Hemoglobin levels are about one third of the total hematocrit value; that is, an infant whose hematocrit value is 60% will have a hemoglobin level around 20 g/dl. Within the first few days, the red cell mass decreases from a prenatal 5 to 6 million/mm^3 to a more adult level of 4 to 5 million/mm^3. This extra red cell destruction contributes to the bilirubin load to be metabolized (Figure 18-13).

Blood volume is affected by birth technique. If the neonate is held above the level of the placenta before the cord is clamped, enough blood can flow back into the placenta from the infant to produce anemia. If the infant is held below the level of the placenta or if the cord is squeezed along its length toward the infant ("milked"), there will be enough extra blood transfused to cause *polycythemia*. Because each condition is dangerous, it is recommended that the infant be held level with the placenta until cord clamping is accomplished.

The function of hemoglobin is the same in fetal and adult life. Adequate growth and metabolism cannot pro-

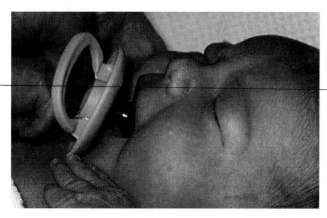

Figure 18-13 Plethora—ruddy color of newborn. (From Seidel HM et al, eds: *Mosby's guide to physical examination,* ed 3, St Louis, 1995, Mosby.)

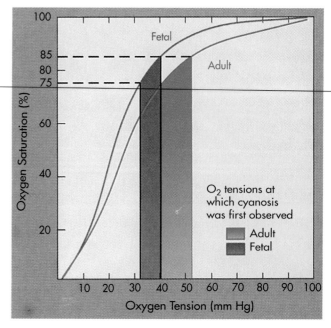

Figure 18-14 Hemoglobin-oxygen dissociation curve. (From Klaus M, Fanaroff AA: *Care of the high-risk neonate,* ed 3, Philadelphia, 1986, WB Saunders.)

ceed without a constant supply of oxygen. The infant's ability to sustain adequate oxygenation depends on the concentration of oxygen in the air, level of pulmonary maturity, adequate cardiac output, adequate volumes of blood and hemoglobin, and ability of the blood to carry and deliver oxygen to the tissues. The concentration of oxygen in the blood (Po_2) and the ability of the blood to carry oxygen (determined chiefly by the amount and type of hemoglobin) contribute to oxygen saturation. Normally 96% to 98% of hemoglobin is saturated with oxygen. During fetal life, oxygen is supplied via umbilical venous blood flow in a concentration far lower (Po_2 is 30 mm Hg) than that which is normal during extrauterine life. Thus fetal oxygen saturation must still be kept in the normal range, although less oxygen is available. The following adaptations have evolved in the human fetus to allow for this:

1. Total hemoglobin concentration is increased (15 to 20 g/dl in the fetus versus 11 to 13 g/dl in the adult).
2. Red cell mass is increased in the fetus to 5 to 6 million/mm³.
3. Fetal hemoglobin has a high hemoglobin-oxygen affinity (hemoglobin-oxygen binding). It will be several weeks before hemoglobin F (fetal) is replaced by hemoglobin A (adult) in the neonate.

The increased affinity of fetal hemoglobin for oxygen makes it harder to detect hypoxia by observing cyanosis in the neonate because a greater amount of hemoglobin is associated with oxygen at any Po_2. This concept is illustrated by the hemoglobin-oxygen dissociation curve (Figure 18-14).

Bilirubin

Bilirubin is produced when the heme portion of the hemoglobin molecule is catabolized. The destruction of 1 g of hemoglobin yields 35 mg of bilirubin. Bilirubin is produced in the reticuloendothelial system and is bound to albumin, a plasma protein, for transport to the liver. In the liver, two acceptor proteins remove the bilirubin from the circulation. The bilirubin at this point is *indirect,* also called unconjugated or fat soluble. When bilirubin is not conjugated, it is available for diffusion across cell membranes. Conjugation is a process by which fat-soluble, indirect bilirubin is converted to a water-soluble substance called *conjugated,* or *direct,* bilirubin. Bilirubin must be metabolized in the liver in this way to be excreted in the urine or feces (Figure 18-15). If the metabolic process is delayed, high levels of bilirubin, or **hyperbilirubinemia,** will produce jaundice or yellow discoloration of the skin and sclerae. More important, very high levels of indirect bilirubin in the brain will produce *kernicterus,* an abnormal toxic accumulation of bilirubin in the central nervous system tissues (see Chapter 29 for treatment).

Jaundice. Physiologic jaundice may develop because of several factors, including newborn polycythemia, accelerated destruction of fetal red blood cells, impaired conjugation of bilirubin, an immature liver in the newborn, cold stress, hypoglycemia, and increased reabsorption from an immature newborn intestine. The large hemoglobin load is one factor contributing to the frequency of physiologic jaundice because the maternal metabolism is no longer available. In utero, unconjugated bilirubin was easily carried across the lipid-rich cell membrane of the placental endothelium and trans-

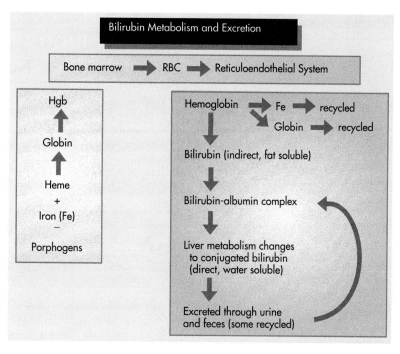

Figure 18-15   Bilirubin metabolism.

ported to the maternal liver for metabolism and secretion into bile, to be excreted via the mother's small and large intestines.

At birth, most infants, even those severely affected with intrauterine hemolytic disease, will not show jaundice. Jaundice does not become apparent until the serum bilirubin level rises above 5 mg/dl of blood and should not develop until the infant is more than 24 hours old (see Box 18-10). **Physiologic jaundice** should show falling levels before the end of the first week (see Chapter 19 for initial treatment). In certain cases, breastfeeding infants may have more persistent jaundice (see Chapter 17).

Coagulation

The newborn infant's bowel is sterile at birth and thus does not support the normal production of vitamin K until adequate food and bacteria are in the intestine. Because vitamin K will not be produced before adequate food intake has occurred, administration of vitamin K soon after delivery is an established way of correcting this lag in production. Most term neonates are deficient in factors II, VII, IX, and X. These deficiencies are even more prevalent in the premature infant. It may take weeks to several months for the neonate to develop adult levels of clotting factors. The normal newborn, however, has adequate platelets for hemostasis.

Small red spots that *do not blanch* with pressure are *petechiae* (microhemorrhages within the skin). Large

bruises (areas of ecchymosis) called *purpura* may also be present on the face of an infant whose cord was around the neck or on areas of pressure during the birth process (vertex or breech). These bruises may indicate thrombocytopenia (low platelet levels), which must be investigated.

Assessment

The examiner integrates assessment of the hematologic system with that of the skin, eyes, and GI and cardiorespiratory systems. In natural light the infant's skin tone is observed for pallor, *plethora* (ruddy color caused by a high hematocrit level), and jaundice. The examiner firmly presses the skin over the forehead, sternum, or calf and looks quickly for the first color in the pressed spot. Yellow indicates jaundice. In infants with brown skin, it may be necessary to look at the mucous membranes and sclera of the eye. Development of jaundice proceeds from head to foot in a cephalocaudal direction as bilirubin levels rise, although the sclera become yellow last. Though this examination provides some idea of the severity of the hyperbilirubinemia, a serum level should always be established for confirmation. (Box 18-10 shows normal laboratory values by newborn age.)

Palpation of the liver and spleen aids the assessment because enlargement of these organs often accompanies newborn hemolytic disease. The examiner also checks the maternal and neonatal blood types and indirect and direct Coombs' test results (see Chapter 23). (A full discussion of treatment is found in Chapter 29.)

| Box **18-10** | **Neonatal Laboratory Values** |

HEMOGLOBIN
13.5-21 g/dl

HEMATOCRIT
45%-65% (central)

RED BLOOD CELLS
4-6 million/mm³

WHITE BLOOD CELLS
10,000-30,000/mm³

PLATELETS
>100,000/mm³

TOTAL SERUM BILIRUBIN
First 24 hr: <5 mg/dl
Second 24 hr: <10 mg/dl
Third 24 hr: <12 mg/dl
  Decreases thereafter
  No jaundice after the first week

  Box **18-11**
WARNING SIGNS

Hematologic System Problems

- Pallor
- Plethora, hypoglycemia (associated with polycythemia)
- Jaundice
- Hepatosplenomegaly
- Petechiae or purpura, not over pressure area
- Thrombocytopenia

IMMUNOLOGIC SYSTEM

Normal Transition

Although developed prenatally, the immune system begins to function sluggishly at birth. The normal full-term newborn will experience exposure to and colonization with an endless number of organisms, but infection should not develop. Whether infection occurs is a function of the infant's own immunity, the presence of immunoglobulin A (IgA) and other immune factors found in breast milk, and the hand-washing diligence of the neonatal staff. Sepsis has been called the "great pretender" because its signs and symptoms are so varied in the neonate. Chapter 29 presents techniques for careful observation of signs of sepsis so that treatment may be started promptly. (See Chapter 7 for the immunoglobulins that may protect the infant.)

  Box **18-12**
WARNING SIGNS

Immunologic System Problems

- "Doesn't look right"
- Foul-smelling amniotic fluid
- Maternal fever during labor
- Pallor, cyanosis, lethargy, petechiae
- Respiratory distress
- Hypoglycemia
- Hypothermia

  Box **18-2**
CLINICAL DECISION

You observe that a 36-hour-old infant delivered by cesarean birth 26 hours after rupture of membranes is not feeding well. There is no change in temperature or stooling pattern from normal. What is the possible significance of this finding? What else should you check to add to the assessment data?

Assessment

The examiner observes the infant for pallor, cyanosis, jaundice, lethargy or irritability, and poor or shrill cry, with special attention given to an infant with the following risk factors:

1. Low birth weight
2. Prematurity regardless of birth weight
3. Birth more than 24 hours after rupture of membranes
4. Mother a known hepatitis B carrier or drug user or lacking in prenatal care

A complete blood cell count and a culture of blood and cerebrospinal fluid, and urine may be ordered for infants at risk for sepsis.

HEAD AND NECK

Examination of the head, ears, eyes, nose, and throat, as well as the special senses, will precede neurologic assessment because the condition of these structures is often a sign of the integrity of the neurologic system. Many anomalies of the head and neck are associated with neurologic dysfunction.

Assessment of the Head

The head is inspected from all sides for size, shape, and evidence of trauma. **Molding** may be present with vaginal or cesarean delivery (see Figure 18-17). If the fetus has been in the breech position, the vertex may be flattened and the occiput prominent.

The condition of the scalp and cranial bones is considered. If internal FHR monitoring or fetal blood sampling was performed during labor, lacerations of the scalp may be present. Occasionally an infant delivered by cesarean birth sustains a scalp laceration during incision of the uterus. The quality of the hair is also noted; premature infants have woolly hair, whereas the hair of full-term infants is soft and silky.

The examiner palpates the head from the frontal bone, following the suture line to the diamond-shaped anterior fontanelle, then along the coronal suture, and next along the sagittal suture to the triangle-shaped posterior fontanelle (Figures 18-16 and 18-17). The occiput is palpated, and the assessment continues laterally to the parietal bones until the entire skull has been examined. If there is molding, the suture lines may be overriding, or there may be only a small space between the cranial bones. Premature closure of one or more sutures (*craniosynostosis*) retards brain growth and causes the skull to develop an odd shape.

Fontanelles should feel soft and flat. The normal anterior fontanelle measures 2 by 3 cm and closes about 18 months after birth. The posterior fontanelle is much smaller and closes by the fourth month. Abnormally large fontanelles may be a sign of hydrocephaly, osteogenesis imperfecta, or congenital hypothyroidism. Unusually small fontanelles may also be normal, or they may be associated with microcephaly.

During birth the head is subjected to pressure from the forces of labor. The sutures and fontanelles provide space for movement of these bones during labor and delivery, causing temporary *molding* of the fetal head (Figure 18-18). If, however, the transitional stage of labor is excessively long, the pressure of the ischial spines on the fetal parietal bones may cause subperiosteal bleeding, or **cephalhematoma**. Pressure on the presenting part may cause it to become edematous. In a vertex presentation, this is seen as **caput succedaneum**, or edema of the scalp. Figure 18-19 compares cephalhematoma with caput succedaneum. Note that bleeding is *under* the periosteum in Figure 18-19, *B*.

Box 18-13
WARNING SIGNS

Head Problems

- Widely spaced suture lines or abnormally large fontanelles
- Abnormally small fontanelles or suture lines that do not override or have spaces
- Bulging fontanelles, a sign of increased intracranial pressure
- Depressed fontanelles, possibly associated with dehydration
- Large cephalhematoma, possibly associated with skull fracture, extreme molding, or intracranial bleeding
- Lacerations of the scalp with widely separated wound edges, which may need suturing
- Malformations of the head, face, or spine
- Abnormal head circumference (see general examination for warning signs)

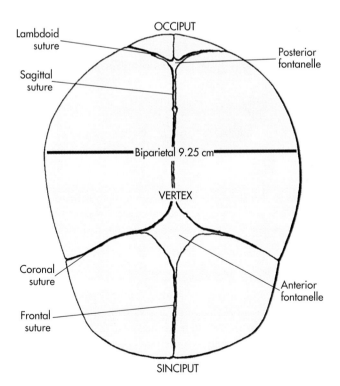

Figure 18-16   Anterior and posterior fontanelles. (From *Mechanisms of normal labor.* Courtesy Ross Laboratories, Columbus, Ohio.)

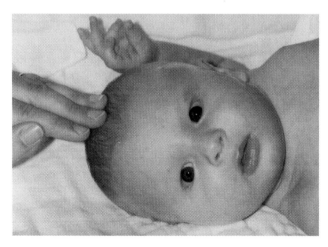

Figure 18-17   Palpating anterior fontanelle. (Courtesy of M Schult.)

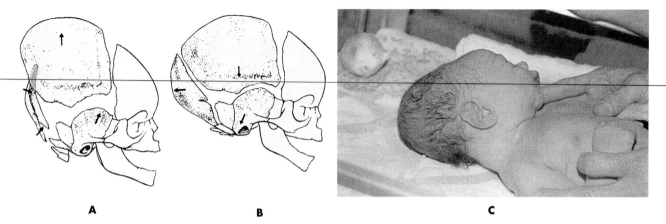

Figure 18-18   Molding during birth process causes **(A)** overlapping and movement of cranial bones and **(B)** reexpansion of cranium on third day with return to normal positions. **C,** Molding of head evident in newborn. (A and B, Courtesy Mead Johnson. **C,** Courtesy Marjorie Pyle, RNC, *Lifecircle.*)

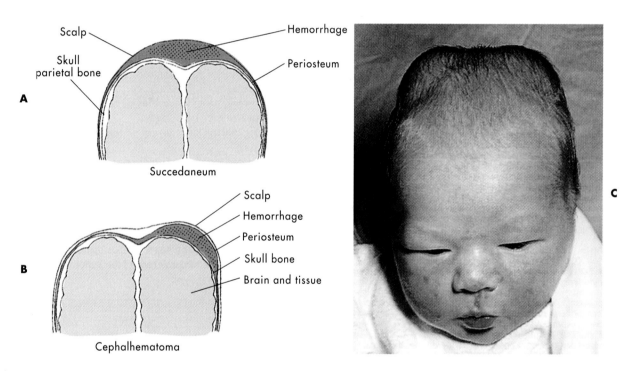

Figure 18-19   Note the differences between **A,** caput succedaneum, and **B** cephalhematoma. **C,** Bilateral cephalhematoma. (From Beischer AA, MacKay EV, eds: *Obstetrics and the newborn,* ed 3, Philadelphia, 1993, WB Saunders. Courtesy Harcourt-Brace Jovanovich Group.)

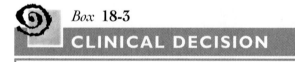

Box **18-3**

CLINICAL DECISION

Ann, a newborn, has a cephalhematoma over the right side of her head and swollen soft scalp over the occiput. Describe the differences between cephalhematoma and caput succedaneum.

Assessment of the eyes

The examiner observes for symmetry and size of the eyes, color of the sclera and iris, and the presence of exudate or any other deviations from normal. The eyes should be equal in size and symmetrically placed. The angle of slant from inner to outer canthus is noted (Figure 18-20, *A*). A mongolian slant is upward from inner to outer canthus; a downward slant from inner to outer canthus is an antimongolian slant. The sclera may be white to blue-white;

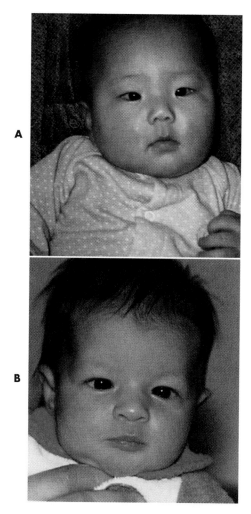

Figure 18-20 **A,** Epicanthal folds. **B,** Strabismus is normal in this week-old girl. (**A,** Courtesy S Ruhstaller; **B,** Courtesy R and B Silverman.)

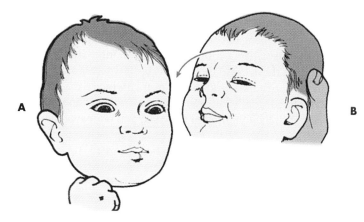

Figure 18-21 **A,** Sun-setting sign. **B,** Doll's eyes movement. (Courtesy Mead Johnson.)

subconjunctival hemorrhage can result from the pressure on the infant's face and head during delivery. The iris varies with heredity from dark or light slate blue to brown.

Brushfield's spots, speckling of the iris, **epicanthal folds** (a vertical fold of skin covering the inner canthus), and a slant up or down from the inner canthus to the outer are associated with trisomy 21 (Down syndrome).

Chemical conjunctivitis from eye prophylaxis may produce whitish exudate within the first 24 hours. Pressure during the birth may cause the eyelids to become edematous. When open, the lids should cover only the top part of the iris; drooping or ptosis is a sign of neuromuscular weakness.

The *sun-setting sign* (Figure 18-21, *A*) appears as a crescent of sclera over the iris and is caused by retraction of the upper lid; it is seen only with hydrocephalus. The examiner turns the infant's head from side to side and observes for *doll's eye movement,* a lag in eye movement when the head is turned (Figure 18-21, *B*); a slight lag in eye movement is normal in the newborn.

The examiner places the infant in the supine position and inspects the pupillary reflex by shining a light first into one eye and then into the other. Pupillary reflexes should be equal. The **red reflex,** a circular red area of light at the pupil, is noted. The red reflex should be equal and round. Inability to elicit this reflex indicates congenital cataract (opacity of the lens). The observation is commonly documented when checking pupils equal, round, reactive to light (PERRL).

Ocular movements are observed when the infant is alert. The examiner holds a light or red object 10 to 12 inches from the eyes and tries to get the infant to follow. The full-term infant should be able to follow a bright object or a face for 180 degrees horizontally and for 30 degrees vertically; however the eyes may not move smoothly and in unison because of immature muscular control. This is seen as crossing of the eyes, or **strabismus** (see Figure 18-20, *B*). The infant should blink in response to bright light (optical blink reflex) but will show habituation to this response.

Habituation is the newborn's ability to process stimuli and shut out overwhelming stimuli. After initial stimulation, the newborn's response to the same stimulus may diminish.

Newborn infants are relatively nearsighted and focus best on an object held at a distance of 10 to 12 inches. The newborn shows interest in highly contrasting patterns and in black and white patterns. This is why the human face, with its sharply contrasting features, holds the neonate's attention.

The bright lights and administration of eye prophylaxis in delivery room settings are deterrents to neonatal vision. In spite of normally decreased visual acuity, infants delivered in an environment where the lighting is dimmed will open their eyes and scan the area. When eye prophylaxis is delayed, the neonate will make eye-to-eye contact, an important part of early parent-infant interaction and bonding.

Assessment of the ears

The placement of the ears is noted by using a straight edge and visualizing a line between the inner and outer canthus of the eye and the pinna (Figure 18-22). The configuration, firmness, and degree of incurving of the pinna are observed; this is an important part of gestational age assessment. Examination of the canal and tympanic membrane soon after birth is not usually possible because vernix fills the canal. After vernix is absorbed, the membrane is visualized by pulling the ear lobe down and back. The membrane should appear light, pearly gray, and translucent. Often this examination is not included in the initial neonatal inspection.

Skin tags and preauricular sinuses may be innocuous, or they may be associated with renal malformations. Low-set or otherwise malformed ears are associated with chromosomal aberrations.

Hearing. Hearing may be impaired in the normal neonate if the external auditory canal is filled with amniotic fluid or vernix. This usually resolves within days.

The examiner observes the infant's startle reflex in response to loud noise and preference for high-pitched voices. The normal newborn will turn to the sound of the human voice and will show preference for the mother's voice. Refer to the Brazelton neonatal behavioral assessment found later in this chapter for a description of the infant's ability to habituate to repetitive, noisy stimuli.

Assessment of the nose

The examiner observes for gross abnormalities of the nose and face and for nasal patency by either closing the infant's mouth and noting slight nasal flaring as the infant breathes or by passing a soft catheter through both nares. The former of these methods is less traumatic. Air should easily enter through the nose. A small amount of clear or white nasal discharge may stimulate the sneeze reflex, which is not a sign of illness. Copious nasal discharge may be a sign of congenital syphilis, and difficulty with nasal breathing may be associated with *choanal atresia* (blocked posterior

nasal passages). Neonates are obligate nasal breathers—they will not breathe through the mouth if nasal passages are blocked. Therefore assessment of nasal patency is vital.

Assessment of the mouth

While the infant is quiet, the lips and mouth are inspected for external defects and symmetry. There should be no obvious defects. Mucous membranes should be moist and pink. All movements of the mouth should be symmetric; asymmetric facial movement may be caused by facial nerve palsy (commonly associated with forceps delivery). The examiner places a gloved finger near the mouth to note rooting, then places the finger in the infant's mouth to test sucking, and then runs the finger over the hard and soft palates (Figure 18-23, *A*) or uses a tongue blade to stimulate the gag reflex, which should be easily elicited. Sucking and rooting reflexes should be strong and coordinated with swallowing. Weak or absent root, suck, or

Box 18-14

WARNING SIGNS

Eye and Ear Problems

- Exudate that is copious or greenish yellow or that persists or appears after 24 hours of age, possibly caused by an infectious process
- Jaundice of the sclera caused by hyperbilirubinemia
- Ptosis (drooping of eyelid)
- Sun-setting sign
- Brushfield's spots, epicanthal folds, and mongolian slant associated with Down syndrome
- Antimongolian slant associated with chromosomal abnormalities
- Lack of optical blink reflex or failure to follow objects associated with blindness
- Failure to respond to loud noise or human voice or both
- Low-set or malformed ears

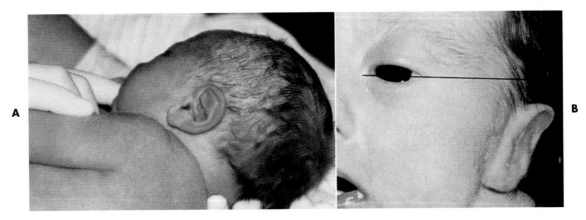

Figure 18-22 **A,** Normal ear placement. **B,** Down syndrome low-set ear. (**A,** Courtesy Marjorie Pyle, *Lifecircle.* **B,** Courtesy Mead Johnson.)

swallow reflexes may be associated with neonatal depression caused by maternal medication or perinatal asphyxia.

When the infant cries, the examiner notes the size of the tongue and its coordination with the soft palate and uvula during movement and observes for the presence of natal teeth. Figure 18-23, *B*, shows an infant's mouth with **thrush**. This *Candida albicans* infection in a newborn is often acquired intrapartally during a vaginal delivery and is treated with nystatin (Mycostatin).

Assessment of the neck

To properly visualize the anterior aspect of the normally short neonatal neck, the examiner extends it by placing one hand behind the neck and allowing the head to fall back slightly. The neck is inspected for skin tags, masses, and pits, and the posterior portion is observed for skin folds, the hairline, and the contour of the neck. The head should rotate freely during this process.

The examiner pulls the infant to a sitting position and looks for *head lag,* noting how well the infant can use the neck extensors and flexors to control the head in the upright position (Figure 18-24). Normal full-term newborns can temporarily support their heads in this position. This is the only time that the examiner does not support the infant's head.

The clavicles are palpated. Fractures may be sustained if a large infant has shoulder dystocia during delivery. The examiner may note a "crunchy" feeling (crepitus) or may actually feel the two ends of the broken bone. The sternocleidomastoid muscle is palpated and any masses are noted.

TEST *Yourself* 18-4 _____

a. PERRL means pupils _____, _____, and
   _____.
b. What do skin tags and sinuses near the ears signify?
c. What is molding and why does it occur?

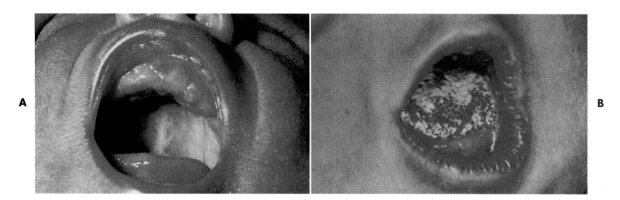

Figure 18-23 **A,** Normal mouth and palate. **B,** Mouth with thrush. (Courtesy Mead Johnson.)

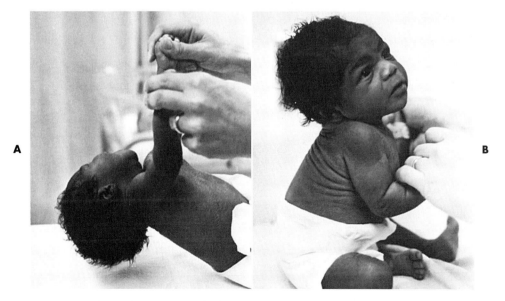

Figure 18-24 **A,** Pulling to sit. **B,** Sitting. Note head lag. (Courtesy Mary Olsen Johnson.)

Box 18-15

WARNING SIGNS

Nose, Mouth, and Neck Problems

NOSE
- Occluded nares
- Copious nasal discharge

MOUTH
- Cleft lip or palate or both
- Large or small mouth
- Thin upper lip and smooth philtrum (bow of lip)
- Weak or absent root, suck, swallow, or gag reflex
- Poorly coordinated suck and swallow
- Asymmetric facial movement or appearance
- Large tongue
- Natal teeth or other masses

NECK
- Masses, pits, or skin tags
- Abnormal hairline
- Head lag
- Crepitus or poor arm movement

NEUROMUSCULAR SYSTEM

Normal Transition

During intrauterine life the normally developing fetus exhibits voluntary and involuntary activities that increase in complexity and frequency with maturity. These prepare the infant for many behaviors vital for healthy extrauterine life. Chest wall movements encourage pulmonary development; rooting, sucking, and swallowing reflexes prepare for feeding; arm and leg movements keep limbs supple and promote symmetric muscular growth. Increasing muscle tone produces a posture of increased flexion as pregnancy advances. This flexion helps the newborn conserve body heat by exposing less body surface to the cooler environment. Although reflexes such as the Moro and grasp must have had a positive survival value for human beings' ancestors, these now have no critical use.

The normal intrauterine environment provides only minimal variations in temperature, tactile sensation, light, and sound. Labor and delivery bring wider extremes. The infant is quickly subjected to the colder temperature, firmer touch, brighter light, and louder sound of the extrauterine world. These sensations are functional because they provide the neonatal nervous system with necessary stimuli, as do rising carbon dioxide levels during the second stage of labor. Efforts can be made, however, for a gentler transition during the immediate neonatal period by shielding the newborn's eyes from harsh, direct lighting and by gently handling and speaking to the infant. A gentle delivery is especially important, since this is a time when pressure from maternal struc-

tures and assisting hands or instruments can injure delicate nerves, bones, and connective tissue.

The close relationship of the neurologic and musculoskeletal systems, both functionally and anatomically, allows simultaneous assessment. Normal structure and behaviors, both voluntary and involuntary, are indicators of normal fetal development and future neonatal function.

Overall assessment

Assessment of fetal neuromuscular status begins with the observation of heart rate variability and accelerations with movement. At birth, initial observations of the neonate's neurologic status are included in the Apgar score. The rest of the neurologic examination may be delayed for 24 hours to allow for recovery from birth and partial metabolism of any medications given to the mother. The examination is divided into three parts: general assessment; evaluation of motor function, developmental reflexes, and cranial nerve function; and behavioral assessment. This assessment is time-consuming and tiring for the infant. It might not be completed in one assessment; the demands in a busy unit may require an abbreviated examination.

Overall assessment should take place when the infant is quiet and neither too sleepy nor too hungry. The examiner should always remember to maintain warmth and to note especially the following:

1. Weight, height, and head and chest sizes (abnormal growth and development are associated with neurologic dysfunction)
2. Presence of any obvious congenital anomalies
3. Resting posture: position other than flexion (in a full-term infant) may be the result of the effect of maternal medications, sepsis, of congenital neuromuscular disease
4. Tremors (repetitive vibratory motions); may be caused by metabolic imbalance, neonatal drug withdrawal, or neurologic disorders
5. Abnormal eye movements or repetitive leg movements such as bicycling (leg movements in a cycling motion), tonic posturing, lip smacking, or rapid flexion-extension (clonic movements)
6. Level of responsiveness (see behavioral assessment)

Changes in neurologic status are often early markers for abnormalities of other systems; for example, lethargy is an important sign of sepsis and an abnormal quality of cry is a sign of some congenital syndromes.

Assessment of the back

The back is inspected for anomalies by placing the infant in a prone position and observing for birthmarks, hair distribution, dimples, or hair tufts anywhere along the spine (associated with spina bifida occulta). There should be no obvious defects (Figure 18-25).

The back is palpated by holding the infant under the chest in a prone position and lifting horizontally, allowing the spine to flex. The examiner stimulates the trunk incurvation reflex by firmly running a fingertip along the back from shoulder to hip just lateral to the spine and then running the fingers over the entire spine from neck to sacrum. Flexion of the pelvis to the stimulated side should occur. The examiner palpates for masses and absent vertebrae. Flexion and extension of the spine should be smooth and regular. (For defects of the back, see Chapter 28.)

Assessment of the extremities

With the newborn in a supine position, the extremities are observed for symmetry of movement and size, posture at rest, fractures, lacerations, bruising, or deficiencies in function. No evidence of trauma should be noted. The

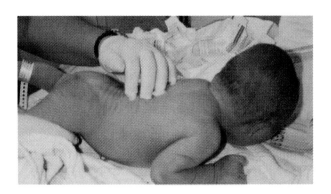

Figure 18-25   Inspection of back. (Courtesy M Schult.)

full-term infant should lie in a position of flexion (normal intrauterine posture) at rest.

The examiner inspects for number of digits, normal formation of the hands and feet, and condition of the nails. There should be no deformities. Fingernails should not be stained with meconium and at term should reach the ends of the fingertips. The degree and pattern of sole and palmar creases are noted. At term, creases are found over the entire sole. A single crease across the palm, the **simian line**, is associated with Down syndrome (see Chapter 28). An infant who has assumed the frank breech position in utero will lie with the hips flexed and with knees fully extended. These infants are at increased risk for *congenital dislocation of the hip.* The following characteristics indicate dislocation.

1. There is limited abduction of the affected hip.
2. The femur will appear shortened on the affected side.
3. The placement of thigh creases (gluteal folds) is unequal and deeper on the affected side.

Ortolani's sign is elicited during examination for detection of congenital hip dislocation. With the infant placed in the supine position, the examiner places the middle fingers on the outside of the femur (at the greater trochanter) and the thumb on the inside (at the lesser trochanter), flexing the infant's legs until the hips and knees are at right angles. The knees are abducted by pressing them toward the examining table. A click is heard and felt during this motion if the hip is dislocated (see Figure 18-26).

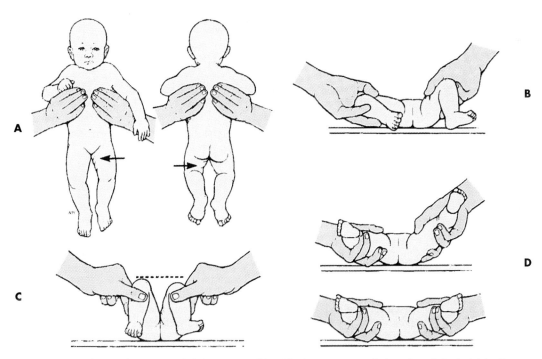

Figure 18-26   Signs of congenital dislocation of hip. **A,** Asymmetry of gluteal and thigh folds. **B,** Limited hip abduction, as seen in flexion. **C,** Apparent shortening of femur, as indicated by level of knees in flexion. **D,** Ortolani's click (if infant is younger than 4 weeks of age). (From Wong DL: *Whaley and Wong's essentials of pediatric nursing,* ed 5, St Louis, 1997, Mosby.)

Box **18-16**

WARNING SIGNS

Back and Extremity Problems

- Deformities of digits, including fusion (**syndactyly**) and an extra digit (**polydactyly**)
- Simian line associated with Down syndrome
- Lack of movement of limb, possibly from brachial nerve palsy caused by excessive traction and flexion of the neck during delivery (arm held adducted and internally rotated) or fracture
- Limited abduction and unequal femur length
- Asymmetric thigh creases or positive Ortolani's sign (clicks indicating congenital hip dislocation)
- Inability to have feet manually manipulated to midline position

If the feet seem to be abnormally positioned, an attempt is made to manipulate them gently into a neutral or midline position. This should be easy to do if the malposition has resulted from pressure in utero rather than from structural deformity. Further assessment is needed when feet cannot be manually manipulated to midline with ease, as *talipes equinovarus* (clubfeet) may exist.

Assessment of motor function

The infant's posture is observed for tone and movement on the basis of the head, back, and extremity examination results. Table 18-3 can be used as a guide.

Developmental reflexes. Assessment of neonatal reflexes should be performed with expectations appropriate for the infant's gestational age. Table 18-4 reviews assessment of **developmental reflexes**. The Moro reflex is elicited to evaluate whether there is any damage to the structure of the extremities and the function of the peripheral and central nervous systems. The Moro reflex should

---

Table **18-3** **Motor Function**

Observation	Normal Response	Abnormal Response	Causes
Resting posture	Flexion, even in sleep, for first 2-3 wk	Hypotonia* ("frog leg posture")	Hypoxia, prematurity, metabolic disturbances (e.g., hypoglycemia, hypothyroidism, hypermagnesemia), Down syndrome
Tone	Normal tone: some head lag; flexion at elbow and knee becomes extension when pulled to sitting	Hypertonia: infant moves "as a block"; no head lag, no elbow or knee extension when pulled to sitting. Hypotonia: excessive head lag	Hypoxia, intracranial bleeding, drug withdrawal
Symmetry†	No difference between two sides of body or upper and lower extremities	Tone increased or decreased from right to left or upper and lower parts of body	Hypoxia, intracranial bleeding, drug withdrawal, injuries to nerve plexus, fractures
Strength	Strong cry, spontaneous movements, resistance to painful or unnatural posture	Weak cry, lack of movement or response	Hypotonia, prematurity
Movement	Smooth when opening and closing hands, moving hand to mouth, kicking spontaneously	Seizure activity, tremors	Hypoxia, drug withdrawal
Fasciculations (fine tremors)	None noted	Fine tremors of fingers and toes at rest or during sleep, reduced spontaneous activity	Hypotonia
Spine Evidence of trauma to cervical area	Tonic neck reflex, symmetric Moro reflex, normal grasp	Lack of response unilaterally or bilaterally	Erb's palsy if unilateral, dislocation of cervical spine if bilateral, fractures
Lumbosacral disruption	Normal appearance and reflexes	Acute injury, bruising, mass in area, spinal shock, loss of knee and ankle reflexes	Congenital anomalies, traumatic breech delivery

*To demonstrate uncertain hypotonia, note position of head as infant is placed back on bed from sitting posture. As vertex of head touches bed, infant with normal muscle tone will flex head so weight of head is on occiput. Hypotonic infant will not be able to flex head.
†Head should be held in midline to avoid stimulating tonic neck reflex during evaluation of symmetry.

be brisk and complete bilaterally. The extremities should move symmetrically and return to the flexed position when movement ceases (see Table 18-4, *A*).

Cranial nerves. Observation of cranial nerve function is more detailed than observations made during other parts of the neurologic assessment; however, many parameters are assessed during these other parts of the physical examination. For instance, as the examiner looks for forceps marks, the mouth can be observed for symmetric movement because the same excessive pressure that damaged the skin can cause facial nerve palsy. Pupillary response and eye movements indicate functioning of optic and oculomotor nerves. Rooting and sucking reflexes test the trigeminal and facial nerves. Startle response to a loud noise indicates the health of the eighth nerve.

TEST *Yourself* 18-5 _____

a. What are the three parts of the neuromuscular examination? Why is Ortolani's sign elicited?
b. How can the rooting reflex be used to help the mother with breast-feeding?

Box 18-17

WARNING SIGNS

Neuromuscular Problems

- Low birth weight, short height, or small head size
- Hypertonia or hypotonia
- Lethargy, irritability, or abnormal cry
- Tremors
- Repetitive movements of the eyes or limbs
- Asymmetric development, movement, or strength
- Deformities of back or limbs
- Limited abduction and unequal femur length
- Asymmetric thigh creases or positive Ortolani's maneuver
- Poor or weak Moro reflex and grasp
- Absent or uncoordinated root, suck, and swallow
- Lack of self-quieting behaviors
- Failure to change behavioral states smoothly

Box 18-4

CLINICAL DECISION

What do you think of the following two findings? Is either a cause for concern and if so, why?
a. You note that a full-term infant assumes a resting posture of extension and feels "floppy."
b. You note an asymmetric Moro reflex after an especially long second stage of labor.

BRAZELTON NEONATAL BEHAVIORAL ASSESSMENT SCALE

Brazelton's research changed the way health care personnel think about a newborn infant's capabilities. Previously, neonates were thought to be passive receivers of environmental stimuli. It is now known that the normal full-term infant can influence the amount of stimuli intake and the caregivers' responses (Brazelton, 1984). The Brazelton scale consists of 28 items in 7 categories (Box 18-18). Use of the *Brazelton neonatal behavioral assessment scale (BNBAS)* as a research tool is limited to those who have completed an examiner's workshop training program. Nurses, however, can use items from this tool to assess the responses of infants and increase parental understanding of infant temperament and behavior patterns.

Neonates can attend to their surroundings (Figure 18-27) or sleep deeply, shutting out all distractions. Neonates can remain agitated and distressed or use self-quieting activities for consolation. Normal infants differ in these abilities, but the normal full-term infant should make the transition between states smoothly (Box 18-19).

Recognition of the infant's state is especially important to parents because it can cue them to the appropriateness of their parenting behaviors. For example, it is not appropriate to attempt to play with or wake up to feed an infant who has been sleeping deeply; to do so only creates in the parents a sense of failure. However, parents who recognize

Box 18-18 | **Brazelton Neonatal Behavioral Assessment Scale**

HABITUATION
Infant's ability to decrease response to external stimuli (bright light, rattle, bell, and tactile stimulation to the foot)

ORIENTATION
Infant's ability to attend to, focus on, and interact with animate and inanimate stimuli (auditory and visual)

MOTOR PERFORMANCE
Infant's ability to organize and control motor activity

RANGE OF STATE
State of consciousness during the entire examination period

REGULATION OF STATE
Infant's self-quieting abilities

AUTONOMIC REGULATION
Skin color

REFLEXES
Primary neonatal reflexes

Table 18-4   **Developmental Reflexes**

Technique	Normal Response	Abnormal Response
MORO REFLEX		
Use hand and forearm to support infant's head and back as upper body is lifted off the surface; supporting hand is dropped to simulate falling. Disappears: 4 months. (Photo A.)	Abduction and extension of arms and at least fingers three to five occurs, followed by adduction and flexion of upper extremities. Infant may startle and cry.	Asymmetry means hemiparesis, fractured humerus or clavicle, or brachial plexus injury. Sluggish responses are seen in premature and ill infants.
TONIC NECK REFLEX		
Position infant on back and turn head to side. Disappears: around 4 months. (Photo B.)	Arm and leg on same-side show extension and increased tone; arm and leg on opposite side flex and show decreased tone ("fencing position"). Response may vary.	Infant who is unable to break this posture soon after it is elicited exhibits abnormal obligatory response.
STEPPING REFLEX		
Hold infant upright and place one foot in contact with firm surface. (Photo C.)	Leg in contact with surface extends while other flexes. Infant then appears to take steps.	Hypertonic: both legs will be in extension. Hypotonic: will not extend legs.
BABINSKI'S REFLEX		
Stroke lateral aspect of infant's sole from heel to toe. Disappears: by 2 years.	Dorsiflexion of great toe with extension of other toes occurs.	Poor response may indicate neurologic dysfunction.
PLANTAR GRASP		
Press finger to infant's sole just below toes. Disappears: 10 months. (Photo D.)	Toes flex around examiner's finger.	Absence of reflex is seen in infants with hypotonia or spinal cord injuries.
PALMAR GRASP		
Place object in palm of infant's hand. (Photo E.)	Flexion of fingers with grasping of object occurs. Grasp is strong enough to lift infant from bed (see traction response).	Lack of grasp seen in infants with hypotonia or perinatal asphyxia.
TRACTION RESPONSE		
Place infant on back and firmly place one finger in each palm. After infant grasps examiner's fingers, pull up.	Infant grasps examiner's fingers and can be pulled to sitting position.	Lack of response indicates hypotonia.
ROOTING REFLEX		
When infant is awake, touch cheek. Disappears: 6 months. (Photo F.)	Infant turns head and mouth toward stimulus. Response may not be elicited in normal infants who have just been fed.	Response weak in infants with facial nerve palsy or central nervous system depression.
SUCK REFLEX		
When infant is awake, place clean finger or nipple in mouth.	Infant begins to suck.	Suck is weak or absent.
SWALLOW AND GAG REFLEX		
Observe infant during feeding.	Infant sucks and swallows fluid without distress or coughs or gags appropriately.	Drooling, lack of swallow, and lack of coordination are present between suck and swallow.

From Seidel HM et al, eds: *Mosby's guide to physical examination*, ed 3, St Louis, 1995, Mosby.

Table **18-4**   **Developmental Reflexes—cont'd**

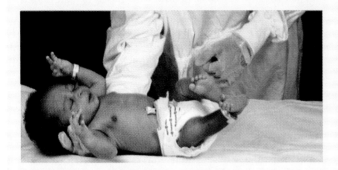

A, Moro reflex response.

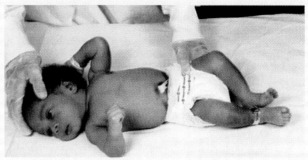

B, Tonic neck reflex.

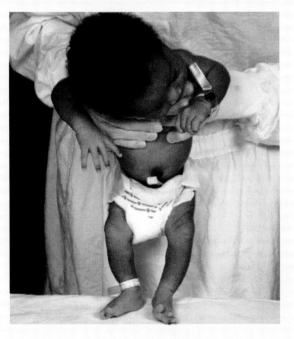

C, Stepping reflex.

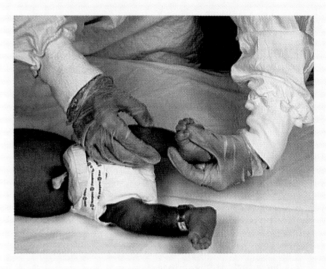

D, Plantar reflex.

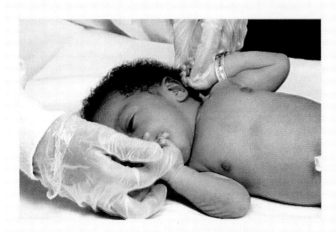

E, Palmar grasp.

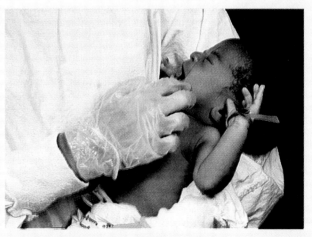

F, Rooting reflex.

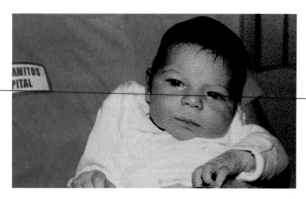

Figure 18-27 Quiet and alert. (Courtesy Marjorie Pyle, RNC, *Lifecircle.*)

■ *Box* 18-19   Neonatal States of Consciousness

SLEEP STATES

State I

Deep sleep: Regular breathing, eyes closed with no movements, no spontaneous activity except startles

State II

Light sleep: Irregular respirations, eyes closed with rapid eye movements, low activity level with sucking behaviors

AWAKE STATES

State III

Drowsy: Variable activity level, eyes open or closed with lids fluttering, dazed expression

State IV

Alert: Minimal motor activity, bright look with attention focused on source of stimulation, may appear dazed but easy to "break through" to infant

State V

Eyes open: Much motor activity, thrusting movements of extremities, reacting to stimuli with increasing activity or startles

State VI

Crying: High motor activity and intense crying, difficult to "break through" to infant

Modified from Brazelton TB: *Neonatal behavioral assessment scale,* ed 2, Philadelphia, 1984, JB Lippincott.

---

the alert state and initiate play during this time are more likely to be rewarded by responses. Parents can also be made aware that their infant's hand-to-mouth activity is a self-quieting, consoling behavior (Figure 20-10), not a bad habit to be eliminated. Fostering this kind of awareness will help new parents understand their newborn (see Chapter 20 for further discussion).

GESTATIONAL AGE ASSESSMENT

The gestational age of the newborn is calculated in weeks from the last menstrual period (LMP) (see Chapter 9). A more accurate fetal age is assessed by ultrasonic determination of biparietal diameter and crown-rump length. It is important to determine the actual maturity of each infant because complications of the neonatal period vary greatly with maturity; premature and postmature infants have the most difficulty adapting to extrauterine life.

Several attempts have been made to develop a system of **gestational age assessment** that is easy to perform, is replicable by many examiners, and has a high correlation with actual gestational age (Dodd, 1996; Ballard et al, 1991; Dubowitz et al, 1970; Lubchenco, 1970). Physical characteristics should be assessed soon after birth. With experience, a nurse may quickly determine the age of the infant.

Figure 18-28 illustrates the special observations needed for gestational age assessment. Circle the box on the tool that most closely represents the neuromuscular or physical maturity sign. Then use the charts in Figure 18-29 to evaluate the size of the infant in relation to gestational age.

Assessment of Physical Maturity

Skin. The examiner assesses the skin by first noting color, presence of peeling or cracking, and visible blood vessels. The *skin* thickens with maturity, causing peeling and making the blood vessels less visible. The amount and distribution of lanugo, which appears early in gestation and disappears as pregnancy progresses, are observed. Next, the *sole creases* are inspected (Figure 18-30); these increase in number and depth with gestational age.

Breast size. The *breast areolae* are palpated and their diameters measured. The areolae will barely be visible in the very immature infant and grow to 5 to 10 mm in diameter close to term.

Ear. The *pinnae* of the infant's ears curve in with increasing gestational age (see Figure 18-22). Cartilage formation also causes the pinnae to become stiffer and to recoil after being folded in the more mature infant.

Genitalia. Last, the *genitalia* are examined. In the male infant, testes descend through the inguinal canal as gestational age increases. As this occurs, the scrotum becomes larger and rugae (wrinkles) cover it (see Figure 18-12). In the mature female neonate, the labia majora cover the clitoris and labia minora. In the premature neonate, the labia minora may be prominent (see Figure 18-11).

Assessment of Neuromuscular Maturity

Neuromuscular assessment should be postponed for 24 hours to allow the infant to recover from the stress of birth. First the infant's *resting posture* is observed. The preterm infant lies in a position of extension, which becomes gradually more flexed with maturity. Next the

Name _____   Date/time of birth _____   Sex _____

Hospital No. _____   Date/time of exam _____   Birth weight _____

Race _____   Age when examined _____   Length _____

APGAR Score: 1 minute _____   5 minutes _____   10 minutes _____   Head cir. _____

Examiner _____

Neuromuscular Maturity

Neuromuscular Maturity Sign	Score							Record score here
	-1	0	1	2	3	4	5	
Posture								
Square window (wrist)	>90°	90°	60°	45°	30°	0°		
Arm recoil		180°	140°-180°	110°-140°	90°-110°	<90°		
Popliteal angle	180°	160°	140°	120°	100°	90°	<90°	
Scarf Sign								
Heel to ear								

Total neuromuscular maturity score

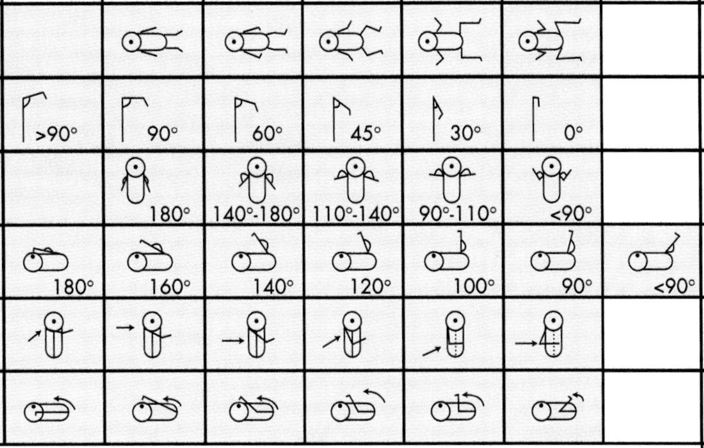

Score

Neuromuscular _____

Physical _____

Total _____

Maturity Rating

Score	Weeks
-10	20
-5	22
0	24
5	26
10	28
15	30
20	32
25	34
30	36
35	38
40	40
45	42
50	44

Gestational Age (weeks)

By dates _____

By ultrasound _____

By exam _____

Physical Maturity

Physical Maturity Sign	Score							Record score here
	-1	0	1	2	3	4	5	
Skin	sticky friable transparent	gelatinous red translucent	smooth pink visible veins	superficial peeling and rash, few veins	cracking pale areas rare veins	parchment deep cracking no vessels	leathery cracked wrinkled	
Lanugo	none	sparse	abundant	thinning	bald areas	mostly bald		
Plantar surface	heel toe 40-50 mm:-1 <40 mm:-2	>50 mm no crease	faint red marks	anterior transverse crease only	creases ant. 2/3	creases over entire sole		
Breast	imperceptible	barely perceptible	flat areola no bud	stippled areola 1-2 mm bud	raised areola 3-4 mm bud	full areola 5-10 mm bud		
Ear	lids fused loosely:-1 tightly:-2	lids open pinna flat stays folded	sl. curved pinna; soft; slow recoil	well-curved pinna; soft but ready recoil	formed & firm instant recoil	thick cartilage ear stiff		
Genitals male	scrotum flat, smooth	scrotum empty faint rugae	testes in upper canal rare rugae	testes descending few rugae	testes down good rugae	testes pendulous deep rugae		
Genitals female	clitoris prominent & labia flat	prominent clitoris & small labia minora	prominent clitoris & enlarging minora	majora & minora equally prominent	majora large minora small	majora cover clitoris & minora		

Total physical maturity score

Figure 18-28   Newborn maturity rating using Ballard tool, expanded to include extremely premature infants. Add points scored for neuromuscular maturity to those scored for physical maturity, then circle score and corresponding weeks of gestational age. (From Ballard JL et al: New Ballard Score: expanded to include extremely premature infants, *J Pediatr* 119[3]:417, 1991.)

angle of the square window is determined by flexing the hand onto the forearm and noting the angle at which resistance is felt (Figure 18-31). The angle decreases with increasing gestational age. The *degree of arm recoil* is assessed by first flexing the arms for 5 seconds and then pulling on hands to full extension, and then releasing the hands. The angle formed as the arms recoil also decreases with increasing gestational age. The *popliteal angle* is assessed by placing the infant on his or her back. The examiner extends one leg, taking care not to allow the

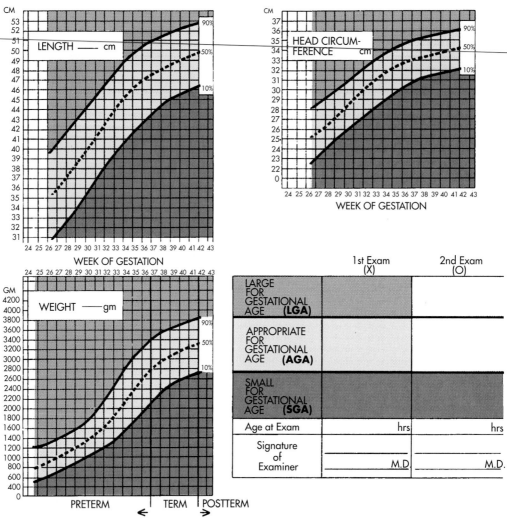

CLASSIFICATION OF NEWBORNS
Based on Maturity and Intrauterine Growth
Symbols: X - 1st Exam   O - 2nd Exam

Figure 18-29   Newborn classification. Plot gestational age against weight, height, and head circumference on appropriate graph. These should not be in widely divergent percentiles. If infant is AGA, weight will fall between 10th and 90th percentiles. Infant whose weight is below 10th percentile is SGA; infant whose weight is above 90th percentile is LGA. Problems associated with each are reviewed in Chapter 27. (*AGA*, Appropriately grown for gestational age; *LGA*, large for gestational age; *SGA*, small for gestational age.) (Courtesy Mead Johnson.)

buttocks to lift off the bed and noting the point at which resistance is met. The angle becomes more acute as gestation progresses. While the infant is on his or her back, the *scarf sign* is assessed by wrapping one arm across the infant's chest until resistance is met (Figure 18-32) and noting where the elbow lies in relation to the infant's midline. Finally, *heel-to-ear flexibility* is assessed by grasping the foot loosely, extending it toward the ear and letting go (allowing the back to rise up off the bed if necessary), and noting the point at which the foot slips out of grasp. The score for neuromuscular assessment is totaled in the same manner as for the physical characteristics.

Add the two scores together and find the corresponding gestational age (see Figure 18-28). After gesta-

tional age is determined, it is plotted against birth weight on the graph in Figure 18-29 and the infant is diagnosed as *small, appropriate,* or *large* for gestational age (*SGA, AGA,* or *LGA*), respectively.

Normally there is a positive relationship between gestational age and birth weight. This relationship, however, can be disturbed as a result of complications of pregnancy such as infection, diabetes, and hypertension. The weight of an infant who is AGA falls between the 10th and 90th percentile. SGA or LGA infants fall below and above these limits, respectively. The *interaction* of gestational age and birth weight greatly influences neonatal well-being (Figure 18-33). In addition, appropriateness of size and gestational age influences clinical decisions.

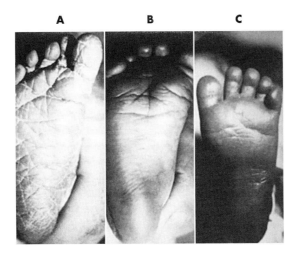

Figure 18-30 Plantar creases. Infant's sole becomes more creased with maturity. At 36 weeks there is only anterior transverse crease. By term, creases are found on entire sole. **A,** Postterm. **B,** Term. **C,** Preterm.

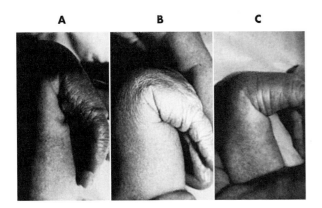

Figure 18-31 Square window. Flex the hand onto forearm and note the angle at which resistance is met. **A,** Postterm. **B,** Term. **C,** Preterm.

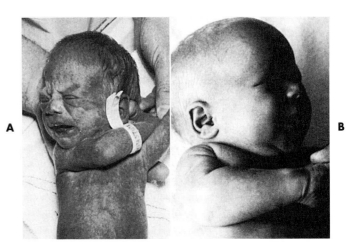

Figure 18-32 Scarf sign. Attempt to pull the arm across the upper chest until resistance is met. Note position of elbow in relation to midline. **A,** Preterm. **B,** Term. (**A,** Courtesy Kenneth Holt, MD; **B,** Courtesy John Young.)

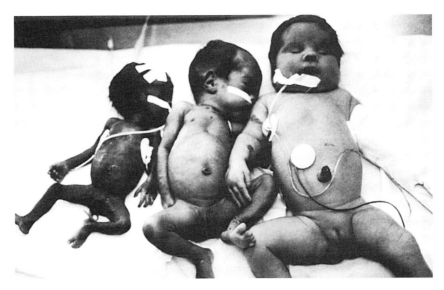

Figure 18-33 Three infants of same gestational age, weighing 600 g, 1400 g, and 2750 g, respectively, from left to right. (From Korones SB: *High-risk newborn infants: the basis for intensive nursing care,* ed 4, St Louis, 1986, Mosby.)

Determination of neonatal health may not be complete for 24 hours, when all three areas of assessment (history, physical examination, and gestational age) are completed. Box 18-20 summarizes complete neonatal physical assessment. Every infant should be completely evaluated soon after birth and then just before discharge.

Additional checks for skin color and cardiovascular, neuromuscular and temperature status are performed as necessary. The trend toward early discharge of postpartum mothers and their full-term infants has important implications for performing these examinations. Evaluation must be completed and plans for follow-up must be in place before discharge. This requires accurate assessment and comprehensive discharge planning within a very short time frame.

Box 18-20   Neonatal Physical Assessment

Date_____ Name of infant _____

Sex _____ Date and time of delivery _____ Age at exam _____

ADMISSION DATA

Time of admission_____ Placed in warmer? _____ Isolette_____ Servo temperature _____

Eye prophylaxis_____ Vitamin K _____ Time _____ Location _____

Time, type, and volume of first feeding _____

CORD BLOOD

Blood type and Rh _____ Direct Coombs' test _____ VDRL (serology) _____

Compare with maternal blood type _____

INITIAL PHYSICAL EXAMINATION

Date _____ Time _____ Age of infant _____

GENERAL FINDINGS

Vital Signs

Temperature _____ Pulse _____ Respirations _____ BP _____ Arm _____ Leg _____

Weight _____ Height _____ Head circumference _____ Chest circumference _____ Color _____

Activity _____ State _____ Cry _____

Skin

Color _____ Vernix caseosa _____ Hair distribution _____ Nails(length) _____

Lesions _____ Desquamation _____ Petechiae/ecchymosis/trauma _____

Turgor (evidence of subcutaneous loss) _____ Other _____

Head

Circumference _____ Shape _____ Fontanelles/sutures (size, placement, fullness) _____

Birth trauma: Forceps marks _____ Caput succedaneum _____ Cephalhematoma _____

Facial symmetry _____ Other _____

Ears

Position _____ Size _____ Cartilage formation _____ Other _____

Eyes

Position (slant, hypertelorism) _____ Size _____ Iris _____ Sclerae _____ Other _____

Nose

Patency _____ Flaring _____ Nasolabial folds _____ Other _____

Throat and mouth

Lips (color, formation) _____ Symmetric facial movement _____ Palate _____ Gums/teeth _____

Tongue (midline, gag) _____ Other _____

> *Box* **18-20**   **Neonatal Physical Assessment—cont'd**

Neck

Range of motion _____ Other _____

Chest

Circumference _____ Respiratory rate and quality (retractions/grunting) _____
Breath sounds _____ Thorax (symmetry of movement, anterior-posterior diameter, bulging _____
Breast tissue _____ Other _____

Cardiovascular

Color (cyanosis, pallor, plethora) _____ Heart rate _____
Unusual rhythm or murmurs _____
Location of PMI pulses: brachial/femoral _____ Capillary filling _____
Hematocrit (if done) _____ Other _____

Abdomen

Shape of umbilical cord/vessels (color, size, drainage) _____ Liver _____ Spleen _____
Kidneys _____ Anus (patency, location) _____ Other _____

Extremities and back

Spine _____ Upper extremities (digits, symmetry of size, movement, tone) _____
Lower extremities (digits, symmetry of size, movement, tone) _____
Gluteal and thigh creases _____ Ortolani's sign _____ Other _____

Genitalia

Female
Labia majora/labia minora/clitoris/vagina _____
Discharge _____ Edema/ecchymosis _____
Placement of urinary meatus _____ Patency and placement of anus _____ Other _____
Male
Penis (hypospadias or epispadias) _____ Scrotum _____ Testes _____
Patency and placement of anus _____ Other _____

Neurologic and behavioral

Reflexes

Moro _____	Tonic neck _____
Neck righting _____	Stepping _____
Babinski _____	Palmar grasp _____
Traction response _____	Plantar grasp _____
Rooting _____	Sucking _____
Swallowing _____	Other _____

Behavioral

State _____	Visual following _____
Auditory following _____	Consolation _____
Hand-to-mouth activity _____	

Tremors
Description (location, type) _____
Stimulus related_____

ASSESSMENT OF GESTATIONAL AGE

Via dates _____ Via ultrasound _____ Via examination: initial _____ After 24 hours _____
Classification
Preterm   Term   Postterm

SGA
AGA
LGA

Box **18-5**

CLINICAL DECISION

Your assessment of infant boy Roger reveals the following characteristics. Using gestational age assessment and Figures 18-29 to 18-32, determine the total score for this infant and his age in weeks. If the infant weighed 2040 g at birth, is he SGA, AGA, or LGA? Plot weight against gestational age on the graph in Figure 18-28.

NEUROLOGIC CHARACTERISTICS

Posture: all extremities flexed
Square window: 30 degrees
Arm recoil: 90 degrees

Popliteal angle: 90 degrees
Scarf sign: elbow will not reach midline
Heel to ear: lower leg at right angle to trunk

PHYSICAL CHARACTERISTICS

Skin: cracking, pale, few veins
Lanugo: mostly gone
Sole creases: two thirds of sole
Breast: full areola, 5-mm bud
Ear: well formed and firm
Genitalia: good rugae, testes descended

Key Points

- The purposes of assessment are to identify those infants experiencing a difficult transition to extrauterine life and to aid bonding between family and newborn; therefore at least one assessment in the presence of the family is advised.
- Each neonate should be fully assessed at birth and before discharge. If the infant is born at home or dis-

charged early, assessment at 24 to 48 hours is recommended.
- Nurses caring for newborn infants should be proficient in neonatal assessment and necessary urgent interventions.
- Directions concerning communication of information obtained from assessment must be clear.

Study Questions

18-1. Select the terms that apply to the following statements:
  a. Skin that is dry and peeling just after birth is _____.
  b. An unusual line crossing the center of the palm of the hand is _____.
  c. Enlarged breast tissue caused by maternal hormones in male or female infants at birth is _____.
  d. Early bluish tone on hands and feet of newborn is _____.
  e. Color of an infant who is anemic is _____.
  f. Color of an infant whose hematocrit value is over 65% is _____.
  g. Actions taken internally and externally to protect the infant from chilling are _____.
18-2. A father is concerned because his infant's hands and feet are deep blue. How would you respond to his concern?
  a. "The baby must have a low blood oxygen level. I'll get the oxygen right away!"
  b. "Don't worry about that now; we'll ask the pediatrician about it later."
  c. "It's normal. Once the baby's peripheral circulation is established, her extremities will become pink."
  d. "As long as she's moving, her color doesn't really matter."
18-3. A male infant, born at 40 weeks, weighs 2040 g. His status is:
  a. LGA
  b. SGA
  c. AGA
18-4. Match the cardiac sounds with the appropriate events.
  a. S$_1$ 1. Systole
  b. S$_2$ 2. Diastole
  c. S$_1$ to S$_2$ 3. Closure of atrioventricular valves
  d. S$_2$ to S$_1$ 4. Closure of semilunar valves

18-5. Match the stage with the numbered manifestations.

a. First period of reactivity   1. Meconium passage

b. First sleep   2. Labile vital signs

c. Second period of reactivity   3. Active and alert

                                               4. Onset of bowel sounds

                                               5. Increased mucous secretions

18-6. When assessing the skin, you note that a 16-hour-old infant is jaundiced "in face and chest." You conclude:

a. This is a normal developmental event and not a concern.

b. There must be a maternal-infant blood incompatibility.

c. The jaundice must have begun in utero.

d. This is *not* normal and must be investigated.

18-7. After a forceps-assisted delivery, one of the following is an *unlikely* possibility.

a. Facial nerve palsy

b. Bruising of cheeks

c. Cephalhematoma

d. Puffy eyelids

Answer Key

18-1: *a,* Desquamation; *b,* simian; *c,* gynecomastia; *d,* acrocyanosis; *e,* pallor; *f,* plethoric; *g,* thermoregulation. **18-2:** *c.* **18-3:** SGA. **18-4:** *a,* 3; *b,* 4; *c,* 1; *d,* 2. **18-5:** *a,* 2, 3; *b,* 4; *c,* 1, 5. **18-6:** *d.* **18-7:** *d.*

References

Ballard JL et al: New Ballard Score: expanded to include extremely premature infants, *J Pediatr* 119(3):417, 1991.

*Brazelton TB: *Neonatal behavior assessment scale,* ed 2, Philadelphia, 1984, JB Lippincott.

Dodd V: Gestational age assessment, *Neonatal Network* 15:27, 1996.

*Dubowitz LMS et al: Clinical assessment of gestational age in the newborn infant, *J Pediatr* 77:1, 1970.

*Hazle NR: Hydration in labor: is routine hydration necessary? *J Nurse Midwifery* 31:171, 1986.

*Keppler AB: The use of intravenous fluids during labor, *Birth* 15(2):75, 1988.

*Lubchenco LO: Assessment of gestational age and development at birth, *Pediatr Clin North Am* 17:125, 1970.

News, *Birth* 18:2, 1991.

Taeusch HW: Initial evaluation: history and physical examination of the newborn. In Taeusch HW et al, eds: *Schaffer and Avery's diseases of the newborn,* ed 6, Philadelphia, 1991, WB Saunders.

*Classic reference.

Weiss ME, Poelter D, Gocka I: Infrared tympanic thermometry for neonatal temperature assessment, *J Obstet Gynecol Neonatal Nurs* 23:798, 1993.

Wells N et al: Does tympanic temperature measure up? *MCN Am J Matern Child Nurs* 20:95, 1995.

 Student Resource Shelf

Brazelton Training Center
1295 Boyleston St., Suite 320
Boston, MA 02215
(617) 355-4959

A 2-day intensive training in using the BNBAS.

Seidel HM et al: *Mosby's guide to physical examination,* ed 3, St Louis, 1995, Mosby.

An excellent general introduction to the skills needed for physical examination. It is extensively illustrated with interpretation of findings; however, the focus is not specifically on assessment of the newborn.

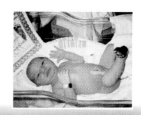

19

Early Care *of the* Normal Newborn

The nurse supports and assesses the normal newborn's body system adjustment in the transition period that begins after birth. In some birth settings it can be as long as 24 hours before a physician is required to examine a newborn. These first hours after birth are crucial because multiple organ systems are making the transition from intrauterine to extrauterine functions. Nurses must be skilled enough to identify an infant who is having difficulty so that proper therapy can be instituted. They also need to remember to protect themselves and their clients from communicable diseases by using universal precautions with barriers such as gloves until the normal newborn has the first bath. Following the bath, gloves should still be worn for diaper changes, injections, blood work, and any other situations that might involve exposure to blood or body fluids.

Psychosocial support given during the early neonatal period coincides with the "maternal sensitive period" (Klaus and Kennell, 1982), during which infant-parent attachment begins. An environment that allows this process is vital in facilitating attachment. Families vary in their ability to recover from interruptions during this period. Although controversy continues regarding the importance of the maternal sensitive period, every attempt should be made to keep interruptions to a minimum. Assessment of infant-family interaction and parental knowledge regarding infant care must be performed before an individualized health education plan can be written.

IMMEDIATE CARE OF THE NEWBORN

Care given immediately after birth should be limited to measures necessary to support neonatal life, provide for identification of the neonate, and promote infant-parent attachment. All other interventions, such as eye prophylaxis, vitamin K administration, and extended physical examination, should be postponed until the parents and infant have become acquainted.

The setting for the birth may vary, but materials needed for care during the immediate period do not. The following supplies are needed:

- A radiant warmer with oxygen supply
- Warmed blankets or towels
- Materials for identification (i.e., footprint ink pad and sheet, name bands)
- Suction apparatus including bulb syringe and wall suction with modified DeLee tray and catheters (size 8 and 10 French) and Ambu bag.
- Stethoscope with neonatal bell and diaphragm
- Plastic cord clamp (sterile)
- Documentation forms

All materials may be placed on a cart or shelf for easy access but need not be visible. The radiant warmer should be turned on when a birth is imminent.

Assessment of Transition

Apgar score

In 1952 Virginia Apgar, an anesthesiologist, designed a tool for evaluating newborn infants. The **Apgar score** provides a quick assessment of an infant's immediate adjustment to birth, tells when an infant needs help, and indicates whether interventions have been successful. The score has limitations but is used in virtually all birth settings in this country. An assessment of five characteristics of adjustment is performed between 55 and 60 seconds after birth (the 1-minute score) and again at 5 minutes after birth (the 5-minute score). If problems continue, a 10-minute Apgar score is recorded as well (Table 19-1).

Low gestational age appears to invalidate the significance of Apgar scoring because prematurity affects the heart rate (higher), respiratory rate (more irregular), muscle tone (more flaccid), and reflex responses (less responsive). Nevertheless, the Apgar scoring method has led to significant changes in the ways newborns are supported in the crucial first few minutes. Five parameters are examined by an "independent" person, usually the nurse. Apgar scores should not be assigned by the person who delivers the infant because the score may be higher than warranted (Jepson et al, 1991). Scoring begins 55 seconds after birth, but of course one should not wait to begin assistance if it is obvious the newborn is having a difficult first few seconds of transition. (See resuscitation methods in Chapter 29.)

Five parameters are examined and scored (see Table 19-1) as follows:

1. *Heart rate* (HR): Listen to the apical heart rate or palpate the pulsations of the umbilical cord. Do not count for a full minute; with experience you will know a dangerously slow HR almost instantly. Count 6 seconds, and multiply by 10.

Table **19-1**   **Apgar Newborn Scoring System***

Acronym	Sign	Score		
		0	1	2
A — Appearance	Heart rate	Not detectable	Below 100	At or above 100
P — Pulse	Respiratory effort	Absent	Weak cry, hyperventilates	Good strong cry
G — Grimace	Muscle tone	Flaccid, limp	Some flexion of extremities	Well flexed
A — Attitude (tone)	Reflex irritability	No response	Grimace, some motion	Cough, sneeze, or cry
R — Respirations	Color	Blue, pale	Body, pink; extremities, blue (acrocyanosis)	Completely pink undertone

*If the child is not light skinned, alternative tests for color are applied, such as color of mucous membranes of mouth and conjunctiva, color of lips, palms, hands, and soles of feet.

2. *Respiratory effort:* You may count the respiratory rate by watching the infant's chest rise and fall, but it is best to assess air entry by auscultation. The normal neonate's irregular pattern of respiration may make it difficult to recognize weak, irregular respiratory effort. Observation for central cyanosis will help; the infant who has a pink tongue and mucous membranes has adequate oxygenation.

3. *Muscle tone:* Observe the position of the infant at rest. The full-term infant who is not distressed will be well flexed at the elbows and hips. Attempts to straighten the extremities will be met with some but not rigid resistance, and the extremities will recoil to their original flexion when released.

4. *Reflex irritability:* Observe the infant's reaction to suctioning or to stimulation of the sole of the foot. Either action should elicit a cry or at least a grimace. In practice the infant who has an HR above 100 beats/min, well-established respirations, good muscle tone, and pink or acrocyanotic color does not have to be stimulated to assess reflex irritability; any irritating stimuli, such as drying with a towel, will cause a cry, a grimace, or some motion. Assess the response to a catheter in the infant who is being resuscitated; crying, grimacing, and even pushing away tubes are signs of success.

5. *Color:* Observe the infant's peripheral (skin) and central (tongue and mucous membranes) color. Most infants are cyanotic for a short time after birth as drastic alterations in fetal circulation take place. The bluish color, termed **acrocyanosis**, may persist in the extremities. The face and trunk of the infant should show oxygenated color (pink undertone) after only a few respirations. Because brown-skinned newborns may look "ashy" rather than cyanotic, the mucous membranes of the lips, mouth, and tongue are assessed for central cyanosis.

In the normal infant, the Apgar score often is 8 or 9 at 1 minute and 9 or 10 at 5 minutes (Figure 19-1). The lower the score the more acidotic the infant usually is; in addition, infants with lower scores have worsening cardiorespiratory function (see the discussion on asphyxia in Chapter 29). By 5 minutes of age, scores should improve markedly. A falling score or a 5-minute score below 7 indicates that neonatal intensive care must be instituted. (See Chapter 29 for care.)

The score's sensitivity is inadequate to predict acidosis because when the newborn is in trouble, the adrenal hormones *(catecholamines)* may be elevated. These substances increase respiratory and heart rates and reflex responses in an effort to compensate for the acidosis. Thus it is apparent that if catecholamines were elevated, the score result would improve. Yet the low pH, indicating metabolic acidosis, may be similar. In general, if the cord pH is above 7.24, the 1-minute score will be above 8. If the cord pH is 7.0 to 7.23, the score will be between 4 and 7. When pH is below 7, the infant is seriously acidotic, and

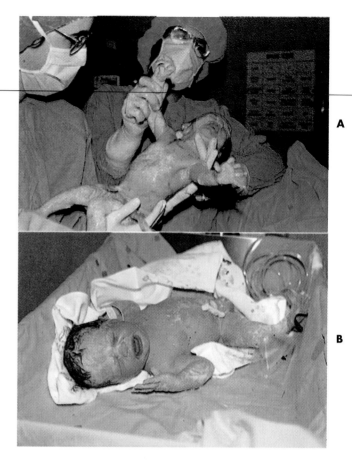

Figure 19-1   A, Note color and activity just after birth. **B,** Observe color of lips and mucous membranes on newborns rather than color of extremities. (Courtesy Marjorie Pyle, RNC, *Lifecircle.*)

the Apgar score will reflect a rating of 1 to 3 (Apgar et al, 1958; Letko, 1996).

All nurses in this area of care are required to have preparation by the Neonatal Resuscitation Program (NRP).

Nursing Responsibilities

NURSING DIAGNOSES

Early nursing diagnoses that guide newborn care are as follows:

- Ineffective thermoregulation related to limited ability to adjust to environmental temperature
- Potential for aspiration or ineffective airway clearance related to oropharyngeal mucus
- Potential for altered parenting related to attachment, preventing abduction
- Risk of altered protection related to low production of immune factors; potential of low vitamin K resulting in increased bleeding rates
- Altered nutrition: less than required related to delayed sucking, limited intake, or potential hypoglycemia

EXPECTED OUTCOMES

- Core temperature is maintained with help of environmental control methods.
- Infant will establish respirations and maintain oxygenated color.
- Infant will be safe from abduction or injury.
- Infant will be free of infection and any untoward bleeding.
- Adequate fluid and nutritional intake prevents hypoglycemia and dehydration.

NURSING INTERVENTION

Maintenance of respiration

Maintenance of a patent airway for respiration is a priority. As the infant's head is delivered, secretions are squeezed out of the mouth and nose by the pressure of the birth canal. The infant's airway may be occluded by respiratory secretions, mucus, and blood from the maternal birth canal or amniotic fluid mixed with meconium and vernix. There is increased risk of secretion aspiration in infants delivered in a posterior position. To prevent aspiration the mouth and then the nose can be suctioned with a bulb syringe before the rest of the infant is delivered and the first breath is taken.

After the body is born, the infant is placed in a 15-degree, head-dependent, side-lying position to promote drainage of secretions. The infant is positioned either on the mother's abdomen or under a radiant warmer (Figure 19-2). Care is taken in positioning not to extend the infant's neck too far because overextension can cause compression of the soft trachea.

The oral airway is cleared first inasmuch as suctioning the nose stimulates a gasp that could cause aspiration of blood and mucus. In cases of infection (amnionitis), gastric aspirate may be required as well. A sterile DeLee trap is used to suction the infant's stomach. At one time the strength of suction was controlled by the nurse using a plastic mouthpiece of the trap as a straw, but because of universal precautions against blood-borne pathogens, the mouthpiece must be connected to low mechanical suction. Oversuction must be avoided. If the infant is breathing, has equal bilateral breath sounds, has an HR in the normal range, and is pink to acrocyanotic, suctioning is stopped (Figure 19-3). The infant will complete airway clearance by coughing and also by absorption of residual fluid in lungs. This early suctioning is especially important in cases of suspected meconium aspiration or maternal serum hepatitis or HIV infection (MacDonald, 1990).

The following signs indicate that the airway has become clear:

- An irregular respiratory rate of 40 to 60 breaths/min with periods of apnea lasting as long as 15 seconds

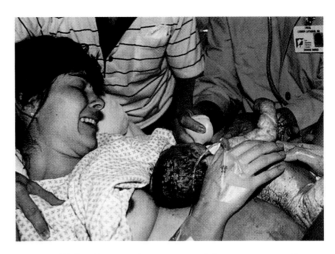

Figure 19-2 Skin-to-skin contact while suctioning is done allows the mother the opportunity to "claim" her newborn. (Courtesy Marjorie Pyle, RNC, *Lifecircle.*)

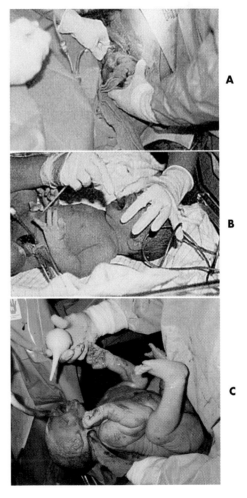

Figure 19-3 **A,** Suctioning on the perineum with tubing attached to low suction at the wall. **B,** Suction of oropharynx with straight catheter. **C,** Suctioning with bulb syringe before first breath. (**A** and **B,** Courtesy Marjorie Pyle, RNC, *Lifecircle.* **C,** Courtesy M Schult.)

- Symmetric rise and fall of the chest and abdomen with each breath
- Absent or minimal nasal flaring, grunting, or retractions
- Pink mucous membranes and tongue (absence of central cyanosis)
- Spontaneous activity with good muscle tone (a reliable sign of adequate oxygenation)

Maintenance of circulation

A patent airway and adequate air exchange are indicated by an apical HR of 110 to 160 beats/min that is easily heard on the left side of the chest near the nipple and by the absence of central cyanosis. Infants who cannot maintain *a*irway, *b*reathing, and *c*irculation (ABCs) are at high risk and include those with low Apgar scores or other problems that interrupt this process.

Cord clamping. The cord stops pulsating soon after the first breaths reverse fetal circulation. Because it becomes limp it does not need to be cut immediately. A reason for clamping and then cutting just after delivery is that it facilitates care in the warmer away from the mother. If, however, she is to hold the infant on her abdomen for a period of time, the cord may be clamped and cut later. The possibility of transfusion of blood back into the placenta by gravity flow is another reason for clamping and cutting the cord just after delivery. For the same reason the newborn should not be held for a long period below the perineum; this position could transfuse extra blood into the newborn and cause a high hematocrit level (**plethora**) with associated jaundice (see Chapter 29).

Two metal hemostats are used to clamp the umbilical cord at delivery, and the cord is cut between them. The cord is examined for the presence of two arteries and one vein before the plastic clamp is applied. Any variation from these findings is noted at once, and a thorough assessment of the infant is warranted because this congenital defect may indicate that others are present. A sterile plastic or metal clamp is applied 2 cm from the skin. The clamp is not placed closer to the skin because if an intravenous (IV) infusion is needed for an ill infant, catheterization of the vessels in a cord that is too short is difficult.

Maintenance of warmth

Thermoregulation is easily overlooked in the busy atmosphere of the birthing room. If the infant's core temperature is not maintained, the transition to extrauterine life can be compromised (Thomas, 1994).

Four mechanisms cause heat loss. The first way in which an infant begins to lose heat is by **evaporation** of amniotic fluid and secretions. Drying with warmed towels or blankets not only removes these fluids but also provides tactile stimulation, which encourages continued respiration. Some units use large soft paper towels for first drying.

Heat loss by **conduction** to colder surfaces is controlled by placing the infant on the mother's abdomen or on a prewarmed bed and covering the infant with pre-

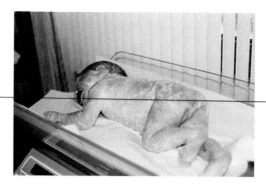

Figure 19-4   Birth weight obtained quickly to prevent chilling. Note large amount of vernix on infant. (Courtesy Marjorie Pyle, RNC, *Lifecircle.*)

warmed blankets. Heat loss by **radiation** to colder air masses is controlled by placing the infant under a radiant heat source or on the mother's abdomen. Because much body heat is lost through radiation from the head, covering the head with a warmed cap has been used (see later discussion on temperature control). There are thermal receptors on the face and body as well. Heat loss by **convection** is difficult to control because it necessitates limitation of air conditioning and other sources of air currents. The best way to control convective loss is to limit the number of persons attending the delivery and keep the environmental temperature as warm as possible (Figure 19-4).

Many nursing actions are available to prevent heat loss. The least heat loss occurs when the infant is dried promptly, the cord is clamped, and the infant is placed in a warmed incubator. Because this procedure does not allow for bonding, other methods have developed. The use of an overhead radiant warmer is standard care in birthing room and delivery room. Skin-to-skin maternal contact is also a way to warm the infant whose body is dry and head is covered. Greer (1988) compared use of an insulated bonnet, a stockinette cap, and no head covering in a birth setting where a radiant warmer was used. Her results showed that the stockinette cap was the least useful in maintaining heat, perhaps because the wet hair transmitted moisture to the cap, and evaporation continued. Mean rectal heat loss was between 0.65° and 1.2°F in each case with use of the same radiant overhead warmer. Her conclusion was that when a radiant heater was used, a stockinette cap should not be used. More research needs to be done to validate these findings. Currently, a stockinette cap is used in most settings.

In one setting, newborns were persistently cold under the overhead radiant warmer. It took some investigation to realize that the ceiling air-conditioning vent delivered cold air at an angle to disperse the warm air. Clear plastic food wrap was then placed over the sides and top of the open crib to shield the newborn's body until engineering services could adapt the vent flow.

Some suggestions for nursing care to prevent heat loss immediately after birth include the following:

1. Birth rooms should be warmer than are most rooms. Doors should be shut and personnel limited to reduce convection.
2. Radiant warmer hoods may be placed above the newborn and mother while the initial bonding period occurs; however, the mother may become too warm.
3. The infant should be dried well with warmed, large, soft paper towels and then cocoon-wrapped in one or two warmed blankets and placed by the mother's side or on her abdomen.
4. The head should be dried as much as possible. An insulated bonnet or blanket loosely covering the scalp will reduce loss from evaporation and convection.
5. Oxygen should be administered by a tube (not mask) held close to the newborn's nose only for as long as needed. Oxygen is cold and will trigger the many receptors on the face.

Initiation of infant-parent attachment

Assisting the new family in the acquaintance process is an important part of maternal-infant nursing care. The bonding process begins before birth (see Chapter 8). Ideally, the nurse facilitates the following measures to encourage further bonding:

1. Skin-to-skin and eye-to-eye contact
2. Privacy and comfort for both parents
3. Initial breast-feeding if desired

The first hour of life is an ideal time for initial infant-parent interaction because the infant is quiet and alert (first period of reactivity) and may be eager to nurse or at least may make an attempt to nurse.

Skin-to-skin contact is promoted by encouraging the mother to hold the infant. In some settings the infant is immediately placed on the mother's abdomen after birth. (An overhead radiant warmer should be used if there is concern about thermal environment.) Christensson et al (1995) found that infants who were placed in skin-to-skin contact with their mothers during the first 90 minutes after birth had significantly less crying and had higher temperatures than infants placed in cots near the mother.

Infants who are breast-fed during the first hour of life are more likely to continue breast-feeding longer (Klaus and Kennell, 1982; Klaus, 1995). During this period the nurse observes for signs of positive interaction, keeping in mind individual variations in behavior. This behavior includes hesitant touching that progresses to more confident touching, *en face* contact, expressions of approval, comparing newborn with other family members, and calling the newborn by name. Research has shown (Prodromidis, 1995) that rooming-in and the associated increased maternal-infant contact promotes attachment. The mothers in this study who had rooming-in watched less television, talked on the phone less, and had more

intimate face-head touching and talking to the infant than mothers with minimal contact with their infants.

Identification

Identification (ID) of each newborn infant always takes place in the immediate neonatal period before the mother and infant are separated. The identification system may vary from agency to agency. One common practice is to place prints of the newborn's soles and the mother's right index finger on the "footprint sheet" (Figure 19-5). This document also contains other information such as the date and time of birth; mother and infant's hospital numbers: infant's sex, race, weight, and length; and the signature of the person by whom it was completed (Figure 19-6).

Many parents enjoy receiving a copy of this form. Hospitals may use only ID bands today because newborn footprints have not been as useful as expected in later identification. A set of name bands with preprinted matching identification numbers also is affixed to the infant's wrist or ankle and the mother's wrist. If mother and infant are separated at any time, the matching preprinted numbers are used to verify the infant's identity on discharge (Figure 19-7).

These methods of identification are not foolproof, however; prints are often smudged and unreadable, and bands can fall off. When an infant's identification is questioned, blood and tissue typing or other genetic markers are used for confirmation.

Preventing abduction

Infant abduction from hospitals has happened, especially where there is rooming-in. According to the National Center for Missing and Exploited Children (NCMEC), each year 12 to 18 infants are abducted. The typical case involves an "unknown," almost always female of child-bearing age abductor who impersonates a nurse, hospital employee, volunteer, or relative to gain access to an infant. She may have recently lost an infant or learned she was unable to conceive. NCMEC guidelines explain that "Because there is generally easier access to a patient's room than to the newborn nursery and a newborn infant spends increasingly more time with mother rather than in the traditional nursery setting, most abductors take the infant directly from the mother's arms" (*Birth*, 1992.)

Without frightening the mother, the nurse must provide the following specific precautions:

1. Do not leave the infant alone in the room, even to use the restroom.
2. Be alert for unidentified visitors, especially those who inquire about hospital routines. Every hospital employee should wear an ID displayed on the uniform.
3. Check ID bands when the infant is returned to or brought from the nursery.
4. Transport infants one at a time and always in a bassinet, never carried.
5. Have parents designate names of visitors and include this information in infant's chart (Rabin and Lincoln, 1994).

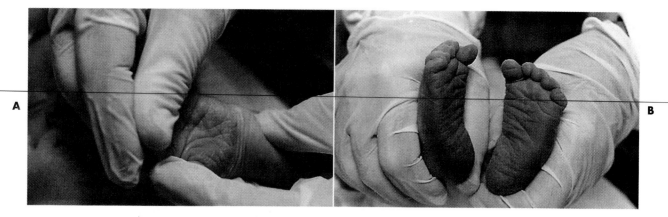

Figure 19-5 Check normal creases on hand (**A**) and sole (**B**) when doing footprints. (From Seidel HM et al: *Mosby's guide to physical examination,* ed 3, St Louis, 1995, Mosby.)

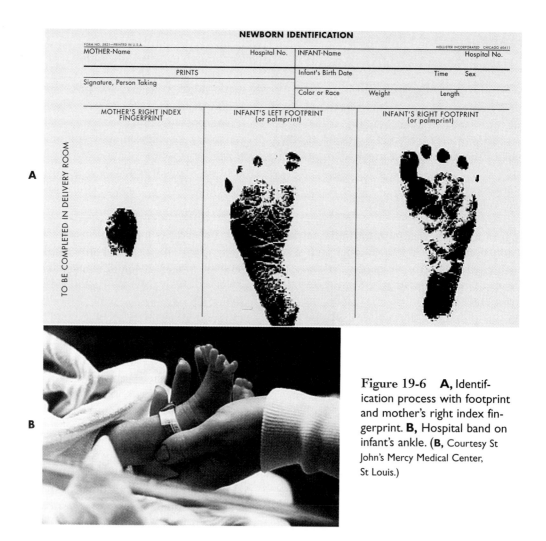

Figure 19-6 A, Identification process with footprint and mother's right index fingerprint. **B,** Hospital band on infant's ankle. (**B,** Courtesy St John's Mercy Medical Center, St Louis.)

Several hospitals have instituted bands with beeper alarms that are activated if the newborn is illegally carried out of the maternity unit. These beepers are removed at the discharge hour in the mother's presence. If the mother is discharged before the infant, she keeps her ID bracelet and shows it when the infant is discharged.

If an infant is abducted the agency security and local law enforcement authorities should be notified at once and the NCMEC called at 1-800-843-5678 (1-800-THE LOST) for technical advice on handling the situation. Of all infant abductions from hospitals approximately 95% are located and safely returned within 2 weeks (Rabin and

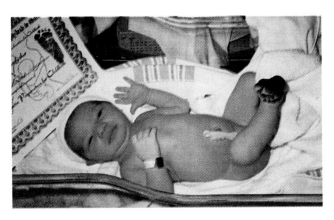

Figure 19-7   Footprinted and banded, this healthy newborn is ready to meet the world. Note cap for warmth. (Courtesy BL Silverman.)

Lincoln, 1994). But clearly prevention of this traumatic event is a priority nursing activity.

Vital signs

Pulse. An infant with a pulse in the normal range (110-160 beats/min) with an underlying pink skin tone and mucous membranes should have sufficient oxygen, which the nurse usually can check at a glance. Cyanosis will develop if oxygen falls below 50 mm Hg pressure. (The normal range is above 70 to 80 mm Hg.) Cyanosis first appears around the mouth (circumoral) and then spreads to the face and trunk before appearing in extremities. A newborn may turn "dusky," with a grayish undertone to the skin. Periods of apnea may occur in some seemingly normal newborns. If this occurs for longer than 15 seconds, the infant should be quickly stimulated to see if the color "pinks up." Oxygen and suction equipment are placed in each nursery but not in each mother's room.

Blood pressure. Newborn blood pressure (BP) may be taken initially in an upper and lower extremity to compare pressures, which should be equal (see Table 18-1) (Axton et al, 1995). The average BP is 68/41 mm Hg on admission to the nursery. Pressures are higher just after birth, then stabilize within the week. Often, BPs are not taken in normal full-term infants (see Figure 18-6, *B*).

An infant who becomes pale during sleep or an infant with **pallor** may have a lower blood volume. Hematocrit levels will indicate anemia and low blood volume. A *plethoric* (ruddy) infant may have a higher BP and may become more jaundiced than normal because of an increased blood volume.

Respirations. Nasal passages should be clear, which is indicated by adequate air exchange. There should be no respiratory effort, nasal flaring, or retractions. Respirations are observed by watching the diaphragmatic line between the chest and abdomen. After the initial period the rate averages 30 to 60 breaths per minute, with irregularities in rhythm and depth. The nurse listens for abnormal sounds.

Rales indicate amniotic fluid still in the lungs. **Stridor** indicates inspiratory constriction of the larynx perhaps caused by too vigorous suctioning. **Grunting,** substernal and subcostal retractions on expiration, and nasal flaring are classic signs of respiratory distress. **Periodic breathing** is a more irregular rate and rhythm accompanied by periods of apnea of 5 to 15 seconds. A newborn with repeated episodes of periodic breathing should be followed up because of a related risk of sudden infant death syndrome (SIDS) (see Chapter 20).

Temperature. Monitoring of the infant's temperature continues, usually on a schedule of every 1 to 2 hours in the first 4 hours of life. Axillary or inguinal sites are preferable to rectal (Figure 19-8). The normal range for an infant's axillary temperature is 97.0° to 97.7° F (36.1°-36.5° C). Rectal temperatures are not done because these may not measure an accurate core temperature; deeper insertion increases the possibility of trauma to rectal mucosa and stimulation of the vagus nerve, which can cause bradycardia. Tympanic thermometers are increasingly being used in pediatrics, but their use in newborns is still not universally accepted (Weiss, Poelter, Gocka, 1993; Wells et al, 1995).

Located lateral to the femoral artery, the femoral inguinal site has many advantages over the rectal or axillary. There is no brown adipose tissue here as in the axillary site, the tissues come together more firmly, and the thermometer registers accurately within 5 minutes. In a recent series of studies, it has been shown that there is little difference between axillary and rectal temperature in the newborn. The mean differences range from 0.2° F by axillary and rectal sites and 0.8° F for inguinal and rectal sites. Axillary temperature took longer to reach maximum temperature (11 minutes) but rose only 0.1° F after 5 to 6 minutes (Bliss-Holtz, 1989). On the basis of these findings, a 5-minute limit for temperature taken in the axillary or inguinal site with a glass and mercury thermometer is adequate. The site should be noted and the fact acknowledged that inguinal temperatures average 0.2° F lower than axillary and 0.8° F lower than rectal temperatures. With an electronic thermometer the time of register is significantly shorter.

The infant usually is maintained under an overhead warmer until axillary temperature approaches 97.8° or 98.0° F. If the infant's temperature is higher, the nurse investigates the environmental temperature first and then checks dehydration. Often, feeding the infant will bring the temperature down to the normal range. Signs of infection should be considered as well (see Chapter 18). A persistent low temperature should be investigated; one cause could be hypoglycemia. In addition, environmental temperature and sources of convection should be checked.

Hypoglycemia and early feeding

In birthing rooms and in labor, delivery, and recovery rooms, the infant is put to the mother's breast as soon as she is ready. Then after approximately 1 hour, the sleep phase begins, and the infant is fed again on awakening.

Routines of feeding every 4 hours were adhered to when one or two nurses had a nursery population or 10 to 20 infants to feed. With rooming-in the mother keeps a record of feeding times on infant demand and records intake and output (see the discussion of nutrition later in this chapter). The system involves the parents immediately, promotes bonding, and allows staff members to assess for problems before early discharge.

Testing for hypoglycemia. Tests for whole blood glucose and calcium levels are performed on any infant who is small for gestational age (SGA) or large for gestational age (LGA), an infant of a diabetic mother (IDM), or an

infant who was stressed during labor and delivery. Some of the signs of a hypoglycemic infant are hypothermia, tremors, high-pitched cry, cyanosis, and respiratory distress. Venous blood is obtained from the lateral sides of the heel (see Procedure 29-2).

Pain associated with the heelstick procedure was investigated by Campos (1994). She compared the comforting measures of rocking and pacifiers with no behavioral intervention and found that newborns who were either rocked or given pacifiers had significantly less crying than those with no intervention. Pacifiers reduced HR more than rocking or no intervention and produced a sleep state, while the rocking intervention was associated with the alert state. Treloar (1994) measured transcutaneous oxygen tension levels in newborns following heelsticks. She found that infants who were given pacifiers during this procedure had significantly higher oxygen levels than those who did not. She concluded that nonnutritive sucking, which decreases crying, may alleviate crying-induced oxygen decreases in healthy newborns. Clearly, both interventions produced a beneficial response in the newborn and are worth incorporating into the care of the newborn during a heelstick procedure.

Any newborn who seems slow in transition in color, temperature, or neurologic state may be tested at the nurse's discretion. In this case testing follows a schedule of 30 to 60 minutes after birth, then every hour for 4 hours, and then every 4 hours for 24 hours. Capillary blood sampling (see Procedure 29-2) to monitor blood glucose is done in the nursery using the agency-approved method. Normal blood glucose range in the newborn is 50 to 100 mg/dl. A reading below 35 to 45 mg indicates a need for glucose water or formula by mouth and careful continued assessment because untreated hypoglycemia in the newborn can lead to permanent central nervous system (CNS) damage or death.

Infants with *hypocalcemia* exhibit signs similar to those seen with hypoglycemia. Blood levels are measured by means of a sample sent to the laboratory. Hypoglycemia or hypocalcemia will delay an infant's discharge. Care is discussed in Chapter 29.

TEST *Yourself* 19-1 _____

a. What is the schedule for testing a 10-lb newborn infant for hypoglycemia? Would you report a finding of 60 mg/dl?
b. What additional information should you collect to evaluate an infant whose glucose capillary level is below 45 mg/dl?

Eye prophylaxis

Eye prophylaxis is mandated within 1 hour of birth in the United States to prevent **ophthalmia neonatorum**. The newborn may become infected with microorganisms during

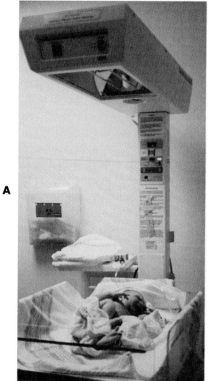

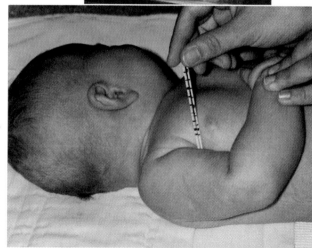

Figure 19-8 A, Newborn under overhead warmer. **B,** Taking axillary temperature. (Courtesy M Schult.)

the descent through the vaginal canal at birth. Because 4 million women each year report symptoms of *Chlamydia trachomatis* and 2 million cases of gonorrhea are diagnosed each year (Hammerschlag et al, 1991), universal prophylaxis effective for both infections is now standard practice (Hess, 1993) (Procedure 19-1).

Silver nitrate 1% is still used in some places, but antibiotic ointments are standard in the United States because these ointments are effective against both infections (Drug Profile 19-1). Untreated infections and inadequately treated infections result in classic signs—swollen, bruised-looking eyelids with yellow exudate—that can result in corneal damage and blindness if left untreated (see Figure 25-3).

Eye prophylaxis is delayed until after bonding has been initiated because the irritation can disrupt initial infant-parent eye contact. However, within 1 hour of birth the nurse should administer the medication. Improper technique is thought to be responsible for many cases of inadequately treated ophthalmia neonatorum.

Before discharge, parents should be taught about the difference between the chemical conjunctivitis caused by treatment and the inflammation from inadequately treated infectious conjunctivitis. Chemical conjunctivitis causes some edema and inflammation that will subside within 48 hours. Inadequately treated infectious conjunctivitis will progress with increasing amounts of exudate, and parents

should contact a pediatrician so the infant can receive repeat treatment before complications occur.

TEST *Yourself* 19-2 _____

Why is erythromycin ointment recommended instead of silver nitrate for newborn eye prophylaxis?

Vitamin K

Hemorrhagic disease of the newborn (HDNB) is a result of a deficiency of prothrombin and other clotting factors. Vitamin K-dependent factors are low in the newborn. The vitamin is produced in the bowel by means of bacterial flora that are initially low in newborns and continue to be so in those infants who are breast-fed. Infants who are breast-fed exclusively have different bacterial colonization (Faucher and Jackson, 1992).

A routine procedure is to administer 1 mg of vitamin K within 6 hours of birth (Drug Profile 19-2). Vitamin K may cross the placenta, and some settings have used it for a woman in the last week of pregnancy when preterm birth is expected. In the United States parenteral vitamin K is routinely given to newborns (Procedure 19-2) although other countries give oral vitamin K_1, 1 mg, or

PROCEDURE 19-1

Eye Prophylaxis

1. Within 1 hour of birth, wash infant's face with mild soap (e.g., Aveeno, diluted Hibiclens) and water to remove maternal blood and body fluids and to reduce the risk of hepatitis B virus (HBV) and human immunodeficiency virus (HIV) transmission via mucous membrane (Ross and Dickason, 1992).
2. Dry the face.
3. Place forefinger on ridge of eyebrow and thumb on cheekbone, and spread eyelid to expose subconjunctival sac.
4. Place a 1- to 2-cm ribbon of antibiotic into each conjunctival sac and gently close the eyelid. Wait for 1 minute, and wipe off excess ointment from the eyelid. In some settings, two drops of silver nitrate 1% are used, then the eye is flushed with saline after 1 minute (Figure 19-9).

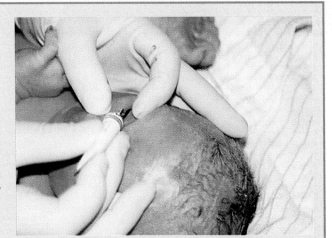

Figure 19-9 Eye prophylaxis. Instillation of 1-cm ophthalmic erythromycin ointment into subconjunctival sac for prevention of chlamydia and gonorrhea. Note that the nurse is wearing gloves. (Courtesy Marjorie Pyle, RNC, *Lifecircle*.)

OPTIONAL ACTIVITY

Write a sample nursing note correctly documenting the performance of this procedure.

Box **19-1**

DRUG PROFILE

Antibiotic Ointments Used in Eye Prophylaxis

Erythromycin ophthalmic ointment 0.5% (Ilotycin)
  Available in single-dose tube
Tetracycline ophthalmic ointment 1%
Chlortetracycline ophthalmic ointment 1%
  (Achromycin ophthalmic 1%)
  Available in single-dose tube

ACTION

Bacteriostatic, bactericidal, inhibits protein synthesis. Effective against *Chlamydia* and gonorrhea.

DOSAGE

Instill 1- to 2-cm ribbon of ointment into subconjunctival sac. Wait 1 minute, then wipe excess off lid.

SIDE EFFECTS AND ADVERSE EFFECTS

Chemical conjunctivitis in approximately 20% lasting 24 to 48 hours.

NURSING CONSIDERATIONS

Must be used within 1 hour of birth.
Inadequate instillation may result in inflammation with organisms beginning 3 days after administration. Inform mother to observe and report. Be sure to wash maternal blood off face and eyes before manipulating eyelids. Wear gloves. Observe for hypersensitivity.

 Box **19-2**

DRUG PROFILE

Vitamin K (phytonadione, AquaMEPHYTON, Konakion)

ACTION

Vitamin essential in the coagulation cycle

DOSAGE

Instill 0.5 to 1 mg by IM injection any time during the first 6 hours of life. Administer IM into the midanterior thigh (vastus lateralis muscle), using a tuberculin syringe and 25-gauge, 5/8-inch needle.

ADVERSE REACTIONS

Sweating, flushing, erythema, pain, edema or hematoma at injection site (rare)

NURSING CONSIDERATIONS

Observe for signs of poor blood clotting such as oozing from cord or petechiae or postcircumcision bleeding.

EVALUATION

- Did infant maintain a stable temperature in an open crib?
- Were infant's vital signs within normal range?
- Do parents position and handle infant safely?
- Were all medications administered and laboratory tests completed?
- Did infant get established with feedings?

vitamin K_2, 5 mg. Research comparing the two methods has not been definitive (Faucher and Jackson, 1992).

Hepatitis prophylaxis

The Centers for Disease Control (CDC) recommend HBV vaccination to begin for all newborns within 48 hours of birth (CDC, 1991). When the mother is HBV positive, her infant is also given hepatitis B immunoglobulin (HBIG) within 12 hours of birth (see Chapter 25 and Table 19-5).

Positioning

In 1992 the American Academy of Pediatrics recommended that healthy infants be placed to sleep on their backs or sides. This recommendation was based on several decades of research on sudden infant death syndrome (SIDS) that indicated that prone sleeping position was associated with a risk of SIDS. In 1994 a coalition of professional organizations, including the U.S. Public Health Service, sponsored the "Back to Sleep" campaign to promote back and side sleeping positions for infants. Nurses should inform parents about these recommendations and demonstrate safe positions in the hospital setting (Dwyer et al, 1995; Havens and Zink, 1994).

DAILY CARE OF THE NEWBORN

Nursing responsibilities include preparing the parent for care of the newborn. With short hospital stays this instruction must include written material and videotaped programs. Whenever the nurse is with the client, some instruction should take place. When the newborn is at the bedside, instruction is facilitated. At a minimum the mother should know the use of the bulb syringe, bathing, cord care, circumcision and perineal care, nutrition and elimination requirements, infant behavior, and characteristics and signs of illness. There is much a new parent must learn; with the current early discharges much of this knowledge must be gained at home. The nurse, however, should maximize the limited time with the new parents to equip them with the knowledge and resources they will need to feel confident at home.

PROCEDURE 19-2
Vitamin K Injection

1. The infant should be bathed before the skin is punctured to prevent tracking HBV or HIV into the tissues. An alternate choice is to use chlorhexidine (Hibiclens) solution for cleansing the site (Ross and Dickason, 1992). Alcohol is ineffective against these viruses unless the alcohol is allowed to dry on the skin for 1 minute (MacDonald, 1990).
2. Select site by measuring distance from the greater trochanter to knee. Inject in center of the midanterior portion of the thigh (vastus lateralis muscle).
3. Prevent movement by pressing on knee with lower palm while grasping muscle with thumb and forefinger of other hand.
4. The IM injection is administered with a 1-ml syringe with a 25–gauge ⅝-inch needle (Figure 19-10). Observe for signs of bleeding from the site.

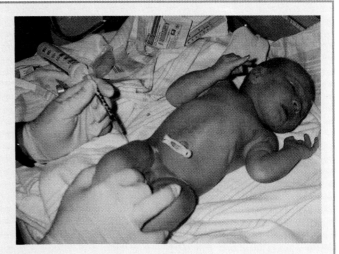

Figure 19-10   Vitamin K injection into midanterior lateral thigh. (Courtesy M Schult.)

OPTIONAL ACTIVITY

Write a sample nursing note correctly documenting the performance of this procedure.

Hygiene

The infant does not have protective skin flora at birth and is exposed to a variety of infectious agents. Abrasions from forceps or fetal scalp electrode and the wound on the tip of the umbilical stump can provide entry points for such agents. The newborn has passive immunity from the mother, but this immunity will not protect against all organisms. Acquired agents such as HIV may be transmitted to the infant or to medical staff personnel from the mother's blood and fluids on the newborn's skin. Therefore all supplies used in care of newborns must be medically clean and not interchanged with other infant's supplies. Universal precautions require the use of gloves until the newborn has been bathed and for contact with secretions or blood when drawing capillary samples.

Recommendations for skin care during the neonatal period have changed. Previously, dry care was advised; the infant was washed only as necessary for the first days to preserve the protective function of the vernix caseosa. However, the possible presence of HIV in maternal body fluids has led to the complete bathing of neonates soon after birth, with careful attention to stabilization of body temperature. Sponge baths are used thereafter to keep the cord dry until it detaches. At birth and after the cord falls off, infants may be immersed in water and usually express pleasure at being in water again.

First bath

The first bath has assumed new importance because of universal precautions. Because of rising numbers of women with HIV and HBV, use "infant universal precautions" to protect the newborn as much as possible from the maternal virus that may be transmitted during the birth process (MacDonald, 1990). Removing birth blood and fluids from the infant's skin is the first line of defense in the postbirth period. This should be done before eye medications (less than 1 hour) or parenteral medication (as long as 6 hours) after birth. If the complete bath must be delayed because of unstable body temperature, then only the face is washed before eye medication is instilled. By 6 hours the temperature should have stabilized enough to wash the infant under an overhead radiant warmer (Penny-McGillivray, 1996) (Procedure 19-3).

Bathing at home.   Until the cord detaches, a sponge bath is given. The sequence is the same as the complete bath; hair washing is done last (Figure 19-11). Parents should be instructed to use a small amount of an unperfumed, mild soap. The room in which the bath is given should be warm, without drafts. All bathing articles and the infant's change of clothes should be available before bathing begins. Parents should be shown how to safely handle the infant during the bath (Figure 19-12). Any safe receptacle may be used for a tub. If the kitchen sink is used, it first must be scrubbed. Place a soft towel on the bottom of the sink or use a "bath

PROCEDURE 19-3

First Bath

Nurse Protection: Waterproof gown and gloves.

1. *Preparation:* Determine that axillary temperature is above 97.8° F (36.5° C). Under radiant warmer set at 36.5° C. Place disposable pad under newborn.
2. *Equipment:* Plastic disposable bath basin, warm water (access to running water adjacent to warmer is helpful), gauze squares, disposable washcloth or sponge. (Some units save chlorhexidine [Hibiclens] sponges with soft plastic brushes for the hair wash; others use small combs.) Two warm blankets: one for a towel (or use large, soft paper toweling), one for a wrap.
3. *Soap:* Ideal is chlorhexidine diluted to 4 to 5%. Alternative choice is a mild soap that does not change skin pH.
4. *Face:* Wash face with soap and water; infant will not open eyes. Rinse once. Lingering antiseptic may be beneficial. In some studies dilute chlorhexidine was not rinsed with no untoward effect (Cowan et al, 1979).
5. *Body:* With some small amount of friction, soap entire body, paying attention to creases where blood may linger.

6. *Rinse:* You may immerse infant in warm water (some have suggested a small shower head) or liberally squeeze water from sponge onto infant. In any case, rinse water should be clean (do not put soapy cloth or sponge into the water). Lift infant out of water onto towel and dry thoroughly.
7. *Wrap:* Wrap the body in a cocoon wrap.
8. *Hair:* With sponge or gauze squares, soap hair, scrubbing firmly to remove all blood and mucus from hair. Rinse and dry hair as much as possible.
9. *Rewarming:* Infant may remain under the radiant warmer for as long as 1 hour. In this case, unwrap body and attach servomechanism temperature probe. Infant, completely dressed, may also be placed into a crib with a stockinette cap and double blanket. Temperature should be rechecked 1 hour after the bath.

The skilled nurse can complete the bath in a short period while protecting the infant from chilling.

OPTIONAL ACTIVITY

Write a sample nursing note correctly documenting the performance of this procedure.

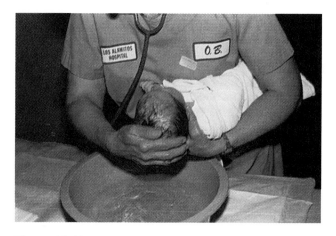

Figure 19-11 In daily care, wash hair after bath to prevent heat loss from wet scalp. (Courtesy Marjorie Pyle, RNC, *Lifecircle*.)

raft," a sponge pad that supports the newborn. Some parents use a commercially obtained tub, but its usefulness is brief because the infant grows so fast. Water must be tested for temperature and the infant protected against chilling.

The tub bath can be a time for sociability. Many parents find the evening bath relaxes the infant before sleep. This routine carries through effectively for the older infant. The father may be more available to help, and this can be a special time for him and the infant.

Cord care. After the first bath the cord stump and clamp may be painted with a bacteriostatic agent such as alcohol or Triple Dye (a mix of brilliant green, proflavine, hemisulfate, and crystal violet), which colors the cord and adjacent skin dark purple. Daily care in the nursery involves application of Triple Dye or alcohol (protocol varies) and folding the diaper under the cord stump to prevent wetting from urine.

The plastic clamp is removed when the cord appears shriveled and drier, usually on the second day (Figure 19-13). In cases of early discharge the cord clamp may be kept on until the cord falls off; it does no harm. The mother should be told that there may be a small oozing site where the stump separated. She should be instructed to keep the stump clean and continue to swab alcohol over it after each diaper change. Diapers should be fastened below the cord to allow air-drying. Contact with a wet or soiled diaper will slow the cord's drying process and increase the chance of infection. The cord usually will fall off after approximately 10 to 14 days. If it remains soft and red or begins to have a foul odor, the infant should be checked by the primary care provider. **Omphalitis** is an infection of the umbilical cord that begins with these color and odor changes, is potentially dangerous, and can lead to septicemia.

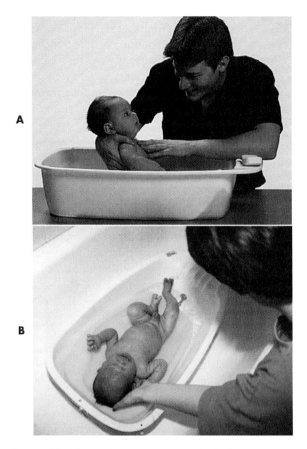

Figure 19-12   **A,** Bathing newborn. **B,** Bathing using sponge mat for safety. (**A,** Courtesy Ross Laboratories, Columbus, Ohio; **B,** Courtesy M Schult.)

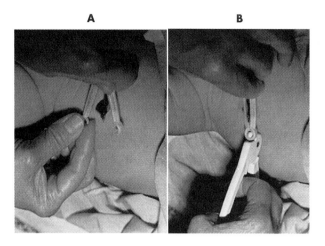

Figure 19-13   Plastic cord clamp is removed when cord is dry. (Courtesy Marjorie Pyle, RNC, *Lifecircle.*)

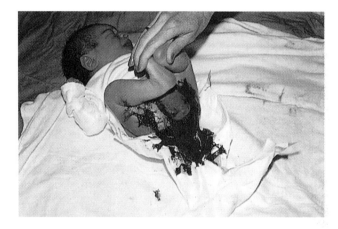

Figure 19-14   Meconium is black and sticky with a consistency like peanut butter. (Courtesy Marjorie Pyle, RNC, *Lifecircle.*)

Elimination

Meconium usually is passed within the first 24 hours after birth and is characteristically dark greenish black in color (Figure 19-14). As feeding is established, meconium stools gradually are replaced by stools that are greenish brown (transitional stool). Gradual change in the color and consistency of the stool varies with the type of feeding (breastfeeding or bottle-feeding). A breast-fed infant may pass four or more variable stools in 24 hours but also may have as little as one stool in 3 days. The stool may be looser and more pasty than that of bottle-fed infants and will reflect changes in the mother's diet. As long as stool is not hard and has a characteristic consistency and color, a variable pattern is acceptable. Bottle-fed infants have stools that are firmer and stronger smelling. Constipation and diarrhea usually occur with other signs such as fever, vomiting, and anorexia.

Most infants void within the first 12 hours and will wet six to eight diapers a day. Actual urine output varies with intake. Parents should understand the connection between intake and output (i.e., that more concentrated urine means that the infant needs more fluids).

Perineal Hygiene

Cloth or paper diapers may be used. Both types have advantages and disadvantages and parents should become acquainted with the differences so they can make an informed decision. They need to be aware that the ultraabsorbent diapers are so effective that it is often difficult to determine if the infant has actually urinated. The environmental impact of continued use of disposable diapers is of concern to many parents and health care providers.

Diaper changes should be done with each feeding and as necessary. The perineal area should be cleaned from front to back, using a wash cloth with plain water or a commercial cleansing wipe. Parents of female infants need explicit instructions on the importance of perineal hygiene to decrease the incidence of urinary tract infections. A soap that removes normal skin flora should not be used. Although smegma may be gently washed off, it has a protective function and can remain. The use of plastic diaper covers that prevent air circulation should be avoided. If cloth diapers are used, "breathable covers" are satisfactory. To protect from irritation, plain petroleum jelly (from a tube) may be applied after the skin is dry. If a rash develops, a zinc oxide ointment is recommended.

Circumcision

Circumcision is a surgical procedure that involves separating and excising the **prepuce** from the glans penis; it allows exposure of the glans for easier cleaning. The current rate in the United States is approximately 50%; circumcision is the most commonly performed operation on both male infants and adults today (Gelbaum, 1992).

Circumcision issues

Opponents of routine neonatal circumcision note that they are advocates of choice; the newborn has no choice. They state that it is a human rights issue. According to the National Organization of Circumcision Information Resource Center, "There is perinatal encoding of the brain with violence, excruciating pain, interruption of maternal-infant bonding, betrayal of infant trust, and denial of the right to a sexually intact body by genitalia mutilation, as well as the right to individual religious freedom to choose" (Milos and Macris, 1992). Proponents cite religious beliefs, hygiene, and possible decreases in infection (Table 19-2).

How can the parents decide? For some the decision is made before birth. For others the decision is made for them because a number of insurance companies and public hospitals have stopped paying for or performing newborn circumcisions, even by request, as a cost-cutting measure (Poland, 1990).

In 1989 the American Academy of Pediatrics changed its position and now supports routine circumcision because increased data suggested some medical benefits. Urologists have contributed data that indicate approximately 10% of men will require later circumcision for various reasons. In addition, uncircumcised men have developed penile cancer at rates two times that of circumcised men. Yet penile cancer is rare. Studies of urinary tract and sexually transmitted infection rates have shown conflicting results. One report (Gelbaum, 1992) states that there is an increased incidence of HIV in the uncircumcised man, perhaps because the virus can linger behind the foreskin. Human papillomavirus has been implicated in increased rates of cervical cancer in the sexual partners of infected men who are uncircumcised.

Concerns. Risks of the procedure are approximately 0.25% for any complication. Most are minor and result from lack of skill of the physician. Serious complications are rare and involve bleeding in unrecognized cases of hemophilia, infection, or surgical trauma (Gelbaum, 1992). Since 1948 there have been only three recorded circumcision-related deaths of newborns (American Academy of Pediatrics, 1989).

Contraindications. A sick, premature, or poorly adjusting infant should not be considered for circumcision. Boys with **hypospadias**, an opening of the meatus on the underside of the penis, may need the foreskin for future repair of the defect and should not be circumcised at birth. A boy with a small penis also should not be circumcised.

Penis care. Parents who do not want their son to be circumcised need to know how to give penile care and teach their son penile self-care later. Knowledge of the development of the foreskin and glans helps this process. As the foreskin begins to develop, it grows from the base of the

---

Table **19-2**	**Reasons to Proceed with or to Avoid Neonatal Circumcision**
Reasons to Perform Neonatal Circumcision	**Reasons not to Perform Neonatal Circumcision**
HEALTH	
Penile cancer more common if not done	Rates of penile cancer extremely low
Cervical cancer more common in female partners if men have human papillomavirus (HPV)	Conflicting evidence; admit some HPV involvement but advocate other ways to treat
Facilitates better hygiene	Removes natural protection of sensitive glans
May decrease urinary tract infections and balanitis	Minor infections are treatable
Less traumatic if procedure done early	Infants feel and remember pain; encode trauma, upset; breaks trust
RELIGION AND CULTURE	
Religious requirement or custom for Arabs, Jews, and many Christians	Should allow child to choose
Boy will develop sexual and cultural identity with father if circumcised	Some state it reduces sexual pleasure

Data from American Academy of Pediatrics, 1989; Gelbaum, 1992; Poland, 1990.

glans toward the tip. It is composed of inner and outer layers of skin, which adhere to the glans and protect the end of the penis. Small areas of separation begin to develop during the third trimester of pregnancy. Total separation of these layers is necessary before the foreskin can be completely retracted from the penis, usually by 3 to 4 years of age.

Parents are concerned about **smegma**, which is a harmless sterile material formed by the normal sloughing of the epithelial cells as the prepuce gradually separates from the glans. The uncircumcised penis is cared for as is the rest of the body. Only the exposed surface should be cleaned until gradual separation of the foreskin from the glans is completed. The foreskin should not be forcibly retracted to cleanse the underlying surface. **Paraphimosis**, a condition in which the foreskin cannot be replaced, will cause pain and edema. Medical help must be sought.

The question of circumcision should be discussed with parents during the prenatal period. If this has not been done, the nurse will need to take the time to listen and provide information so they can make a decision. Parents who choose to have their son circumcised need to know about the procedure, which usually is performed in the hospital on the second day. With early discharge, circumcision may take place later.

Cultural considerations. Circumcision has been practiced in many cultures throughout history, often as a coming-of-age ritual. Arabs, Jews, and many Christians base the practice of circumcision on religious principles. North and South American Indians, African groups, Australian aborigines, and many Pacific Islanders use circumcision as well (Gelbaum, 1992). Most families from the Orient and parts of Europe do not. The rates in Europe, England, and Scandinavia are approximately 1%.

For the Jewish male infant a ritual circumcision known as a *briss* occurs on the eighth day of life to celebrate their covenant between God and the Jewish people (see Cultural Awareness box). Women, including the infant's mother, have traditionally been banned from the room. In recent times, however, all adult family members and guests are included. There is special attention and love directed to the mother during this time.

The ceremony is performed by a *mohel*, a person trained in both the religious and surgical aspects of briss. Some mohels require the **bilirubin** level to be no higher than 8 mg before they will perform the circumcision. If the infant is still in the hospital, the ceremony can be arranged there. The actual ceremony is quite short, with the principal honor being given to the *sondek* (godfather), who holds the infant during the procedure. The infant is swaddled in clean, white garments. Afterward the infant is placed in his father's arms and given sweet wine on clean gauze.

Methods of circumcision

To prevent possible vomiting the infant is not fed for 1 hour before circumcision. Hunger may add to his discom-

CULTURAL AWARENESS

I remember the day of my son's briss. It was hot and sunny, and 50 well-wishers were crammed into my small house. I chose to remain in the next room, and as I handed him over to my best friend, I thought of the meaning of this 5000-year-old ritual. I wished that it did not involve pain for my baby, but I embraced it as a physical, visual acceptance of the covenant and the beginning of Adam's life as a Jewish boy and man. Our family grew closer on that day, both to each other and to our heritage.

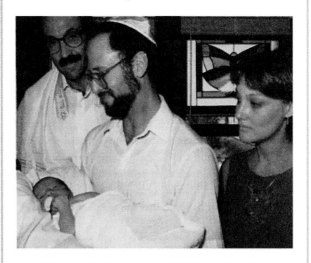

fort and irritability. A molded plastic "circ board" is used as a restraint when the procedure is done in the hospital (Figure 19-15). The plastibel method uses a plastic ring placed between the glans and prepuce and secured with a suture. The prepuce is then removed, and the plastibel remains in place until it falls of spontaneously in approximately 8 days (Figure 19-16).

The Gomco method uses a bell-shaped apparatus that is fitted over the glans. A ring is then placed over the prepuce and tightened for 3 to 5 minutes. The prepuce is then excised. Gauze coated with petroleum jelly is wound around the penis. This gauze usually falls off within a day. Although little attention has been paid to neonatal pain during any procedures, it is increasingly unacceptable to circumcise an infant without the use of anesthesia. Use of pacifiers and audiotapes of music and maternal heart beats during painful procedures has led to reduced crying but may not reduce pain during circumcisions and heel sticks. Marchette et al (1991) found significant elevations in HR and systolic BP, with reductions in transcutaneous oxygen values, during the invasive steps of the procedure. These changes indicate pain response, and it seems important to use local anesthesia during circumcision. Practitioners may use either a topical or local anesthetic to block pain impulses via the dorsal penile nerve. Even with the use of anesthesia, the infant may

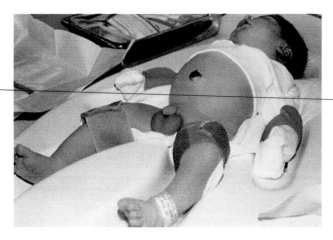

Figure 19-15   "Circ board" restrains infant during circumcision. (Courtesy Marjorie Pyle, RNC, *Lifecircle*.)

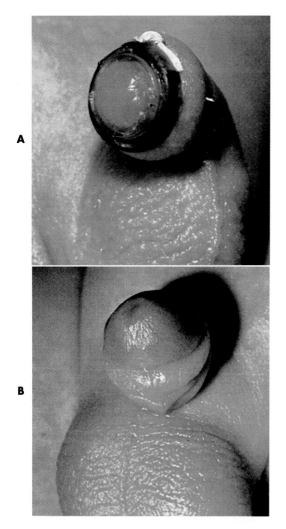

Figure 19-16   Circumcision using Hollister plastibel. **A,** Suture around rim of plastibel controls bleeding. **B,** Plastic rim and suture drop off in 7 to 10 days. (Courtesy Hollister, Inc, Chicago.)

be irritable or lethargic for several hours after the procedure. Comfort measures include cuddling and offering feeding, which may be taken eagerly or rejected (Phillips, 1995).

Aftercare. Circumcision care involves keeping the exposed glans covered with gauze squares on which sterile ointment has been placed. This protects the area from abrasion, excessive bleeding, and infection. Routine cleaning may begin after approximately 4 to 5 days with use of a soft cloth and omitting soap. Cleansing should be done with every diaper change, and diapers should be applied loosely. The caregiver observes for early complications such as bleeding, infection, or difficulty voiding. Complications that may occur later include meatitis (inflammation of the meatus), adhesions of the remnants of the foreskin to the glans, or meatal stenosis caused by meatitis. See Box 19-1, Teaching Plan for Home Care.

Nutritional Needs

In the past the well neonate was not fed until 4 to 12 hours after birth to allow for adjustment to extrauterine life. Now early feedings are standard for the well full-term infant for the following reasons (see Chapter 17):

- During the first period of reactivity, the neonate is alert and eager to feed, making this an ideal time to start breast-feeding or bottle-feeding.
- Early feedings stimulate early passage of meconium, which reduces enterohepatic circulation and potential bilirubin level elevations.
- Early ingestion of colostrum coats the gastrointestinal tract with secretory immunoglobulin E (IgE) and other immune factors, which may offer protection against gastroenteritis.
- Early feedings help the infant's gastrointestinal tract to colonize with "friendly" organisms, allowing less opportunity for pathogens to proliferate. These organisms are necessary for vitamin K production in the intestine.
- Early feedings may lessen the chance of hypoglycemia because the act of feeding stimulates glucagon secretion and therefore glycolysis.

Feeding is a complex system that involves several components. Examination of each of these is crucial in determining whether the neonate is feeding successfully.

Neurologic component

Eating involves a chain of responses that are reflexive in nature. Recall that the *rooting reflex* is elicited by touching the cheek, which causes the infant to turn toward the stimulus. This survival maneuver allows the infant to seek food. Swallowing is an automatic mechanism that helps propel food into the stomach. The *gag reflex* protects the trachea by preventing aspiration. Coordination among sucking, swallowing, and breathing are necessary for successful feeding and should be present by approximately week 34 of gestation. All infants, whether breast-fed or bottle-fed, used

Box 19-1

TEACHING PLAN *for* HOME CARE

Circumcision

1. Keep area clean by using plain water *only* around area, not on sore area.
   - Petroleum jelly gauze around penis may detach or be taken off within 12 to 24 hours. Use a big dab of petroleum jelly on a 4-inch sterile gauze square and place over penis to protect it against rubbing against diaper.
   - If the plastibel method was used, expect the plastic ring to detach when the scab is dry. Use petroleum jelly as described previously.
2. The normal healing process will look like the following:
   - Slightly swollen under the head of the penis, which should be pinkish red for several days. If head of penis is bluish, check amount of swelling and **call** health care provider.
   - There may be a watery pink-yellow oozing substance but no bright red bleeding.
   - A small blood clot may form underneath the head of the penis.
3. **Call** health care provider if any of the following happen:
   - Active bleeding: apply pressure with a sterile gauze for 5 minutes. If it does not stop, **call** health care provider and keep applying pressure.
   - Infant does not urinate after he is at home. If more than 12 to 18 hours, **call** health care provider, and check swelling of penis.
   - Infection will show redness and swelling after the first few days. Look for any pus or fever, and **call** health care provider if present.
   - **Call** health care provider if infant is not eating or sleeping well.

to be offered a "test feeding" of sterile water to check suck, swallow, and gag reflexes. Now water is not offered to breast-feeding infants before first feeds. Feeding also is part of the assessment for congenital anomalies. Infants with tracheoesophageal fistula and esophageal atresia will choke and become cyanotic when first fed.

Nutritional component

Breast milk or formula provide the major source of calories during the first 6 months. The energy requirement for a healthy infant is 115 kcal/kg/day during this period. Fluid requirements vary with the age of the infant and range from 80 to 160 ml/kg/day (Table 19-3). The calories to fluid ratio of formula and breast milk is the correct one to achieve needed fluid intake (20 kcal/30 ml). During the first day of life the infant will need 80 ml/kg/day. This increases to 100 to 110 ml/kg/day on the second and third days of life and to 150 ml/kg/day by the end of the first week. Adequate intake will ensure that the young infant gains approximately 30 g daily. It should be kept in mind that normal infants will lose as much as 10% of birth weight during the first week because of limited intake, loss of extracellular fluid, and passage of urine and meconium. Parents should be informed that this is an expected loss and should be regained by 2 weeks if the newborn is feeding adequately.

TEST *Yourself* 19-3 _____

Jon weighed 3900 g at birth. On the basis of his weight, what are his 24-hour caloric needs and fluid needs?

Expected weight gain. The average weight gain is 7 kg in the first year. Half of that, 3.5 kg, is gained in the first 4 months. After the first week, this means that the neonate will gain at a rate of 5 to 6 ounces a week, doubling the birth weight by 4 months. At approximately 5 months the rate of growth slows, and the infant becomes ready for the gradual introduction of other foods (Table 19-4).

Interactional component

Satisfactory feeding not only affects the relationship between parent and infant; it depends on the quality of interaction between parent and infant. The parent should have the ability to focus attention on the infant during the feeding, read cues accurately, and respond to these cues appropriately. This is a learned skill and parents may express surprise that cues vary from one child to the next. Nurses have an important role in helping parents achieve a satisfactory relationship with their infant.

Feeding meets several basic human needs. It satisfies the infant's craving for oral satisfaction and gives an infant a sense of security and love while providing parents with positive feedback about their ability to nurture a child. (See development of the senses in Chapter 20 for the value feeding time has in infant development.)

These factors should be kept in mind when assessing the infant's ability to feed. The nurse observes the following:
- Coordination of root, suck, and swallow reflexes
- Quantity of intake sufficient for growth
- Adequate output in stool and urine
- Elastic skin turgor
- Feeding experience pleasurable for infant and parent

Table 19-3 | **Recommended Dietary Allowances for Infants during the First Year of Life**

	0-6 Mo	6-12 Mo
WEIGHT	6 kg (13 lb)	9 kg (20 lb)
HEIGHT	60 cm (24 in)	71 cm (28 in)
KILOCALORIES	kg × 115	kg × 108
PROTEIN, G	(kg × 2.2)13	(kg × 2.0)14
FAT-SOLUBLE VITAMINS		
Vitamin A, μ RE	375	375
Vitamin D, μg	7.5	10
Vitamin E, mg TE	3	4
WATER-SOLUBLE VITAMINS		
Ascorbic acid, mg	30	35
Folate, μg	25	35
Niacin, mg NE	5	6
Riboflavin, mg	0.4	0.5
Thiamin, mg	0.3	0.4
Vitamin B_6, mg	0.3	0.6
Vitamin B_{12}, μg	0.3	0.5
MINERALS		
Calcium, mg	400	600
Phosphorus, mg	300	500
Iodine, μg	40	50
Iron, mg	6	10
Magnesium, mg	40	60
Zinc, mg	5	5

Modified from *Recommended daily dietary allowances*, 10, Washington, DC, 1989, National Academy of Sciences.
NE, Niacin equivalents; *RE*, retinol equivalents; *TE*, α-tocopherol equivalents.

Nursing responsibilities

Nursing responsibilities in establishing feeding include evaluating the mother's knowledge within the brief hospitalization period. Because extended families may not be readily available to support the new mother, literature and resources for support become critical in most situations (see Chapter 17).

Breast-fed infant. An infant who is to be breast-fed is given a first try just after birth or during the first recovery hour if the condition is stable. The infant should be breast-fed again during the second period of reactivity. Advantages of this early feeding are seen in establishing early attachment; stimulation of maternal oxytocin secretion occurs as well. The infant should be fed on demand, that is, when crying from hunger. The intervals between feedings vary from 2 to 3 hours. At first, not all infants will demand feeding. Some infants may be sleepy. Variations exist because of different methods of birth and use of analgesics and anesthetics. For this reason close observation and assessment of output are important. An infant may have to be coaxed to breast-feed the first few days.

Successful breast-feeding depends on the mother's desire and is influenced by her level of understanding and her support persons in the home (Figure 19-17; see also Chapter 17 for techniques and maternal support; see Box 19-2 for advantages of breast milk). Most mothers who are new at breast-feeding are concerned about adequate intake. Frequent feeding is the best way to establish lactation. Signs of satisfaction include a content infant after feeding who shows a weight gain of approximately 25 to 30 g/day in the first few months. There will be an average of six to eight wet diapers a day with elastic skin turgor and soft or pasty stools. There may be frequent stools or stools every other day, depending on the maternal diet.

Table 19-4 | **Developmental Milestones and Suggested Infant Feeding Guidelines: Birth to 5 Months**

	0-2 Wk	2 Wks–2 Mo	2 Mo	3 Mo
Breast milk/formula				
Volume per feeding	2–3 oz	3–5 oz	5 oz	6–6.5 oz
Number of feedings (per day)	6–8	5–6	5–6	4–5
Average total	20 oz	28 oz	30 oz	32–34 oz
Recommended calories (115 kcal/kg)	403	483–598	598	656
Total calories	440	560	600	660–680

During the first 2 months of life, infants display the following oral and muscular development related to feeding: rooting, sucking, and swallowing. During the third month, the extrusion reflex diminishes and sucking becomes voluntary. Therefore liquid is the appropriate food texture.

During months 4 and 5, the infant learns to put hands to mouth and develops a grasp. By the sixth month, chewing begins and the lips can be put more accurately to the rim of a cup. Food texture will continue to include liquids but baby soft foods can be added.

From Bronner YL, Paige DM: Current concepts in infant nutrition, *J Nurs Midwifery* 37 (suppl 2):475, 1992.

The mother who eats a balanced diet with adequate fluid intake will produce milk in adequate quantities for her infant's growth. If she does not drink enough fluids, the quantity of milk will be *reduced* while the quality stays stable. (See discussion on maternal nutrition in Chapter 17.)

Mothers often ask about offering water supplements. Initially water through a rubber nipple may result in "nipple confusion" for the infant because the sucking action is different. Later, especially in hot weather, water may be given between feedings but must be boiled, cooled, and placed in a clean bottle (Procedure 19-4).

Box 19-1

CLINICAL DECISION

Mrs. Jones wants to breast-feed exclusively but is afraid she won't have enough milk. Nutrition counseling should include which three principles? She should be able to state that her infant is eating satisfactorily if which three events are occurring?

Bottle-fed infant. Bottle-feeding allows fathers and siblings to participate in feeding. Some mothers feel that they have more freedom when feeding responsibilities are shared. Infants usually require less frequent feeds because of the slower digestion of the larger milk curd. Demand feeding should be encouraged. Initially the infant may need to feed every 2 to 3 hours, but as the infant matures, feedings may be further apart.

Although many brands of formula are available, mothers tend to buy the brand that was given in the hospital. The formula companies provide free samples to hospitals for this reason (Novak, 1988). All formula companies in the United States must follow strict regulations and are attempting to make their products as similar to breast milk as possible. Parents should be told that cow milk (any type) is not to be added to the infant's diet until after 1 year of age. Cow milk curd is not well digested unless the milk is boiled. Thus fresh whole milk is not advised. In addition, skim milk has a low fat content, and to gain sufficient calories would require too much fluid volume.

Infant formulas are available in several forms, which influence the ease of preparation.
- Powdered formula is mixed with boiled water in specific quantities to yield full-strength formula.
- 13 ounces of concentrated formula when mixed with 13 ounces of boiled water yields 26 ounces of full-strength formula.
- Ready-to-use formula in 32-ounce cans is convenient but expensive.

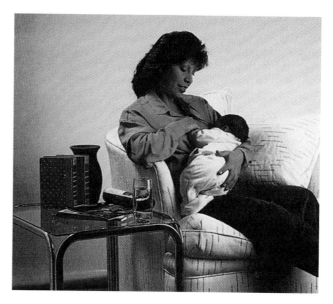

Figure 19-17   Breast-feeding. (Courtesy Ross Laboratories, Columbus, Ohio.)

Box 19-2   Advantages of Human Milk versus Cow Milk

- Contains adequate (not excessive) protein; has greater quantities of certain amino acids, including cystine and taurine
- Contains more lactalbumin (produces easily digested curds) than casein (produces large, hard curds)
- Contains more lactose, which in the gut stimulates growth of microorganisms, which synthesize some B vitamins and produce organic acids that may retard growth of harmful bacteria
- Contains more monounsaturated fatty acids, which enhance absorption of fat and calcium
- Contains adequate (not excessive) minerals with exception of fluoride (low in both)
- Amounts of iron and zinc are low but more readily absorbed
- Contains less calcium and phosphorus but a more favorable ratio of the minerals, which prevents excessive calcium excretion
- Contains adequate amounts of vitamins A, B complex, and E; vitamin C content depends on maternal intake; vitamin D is low but more readily absorbed (vitamins C, D, and E are low in cow milk, but vitamin K is higher)
- Contains growth modulators that modify growth or maturation
- Offers several immunologic benefits: contains various immunoglobulins (Ig), especially IgA; macrophages; granulocytes; T-cell and B-cell lymphocytes; and other factors that inhibit bacterial growth
- Has laxative effect
- Is economical, readily available, and sanitary
- Has psychologic benefits of close bond between infant and mother during feeding

From Wong DL: *Whaley and Wong's essentials of pediatric nursing*, ed 5, St Louis, 1997, Mosby.

PROCEDURE 19-4
Cup Feeding of the Preterm or Term Infant

Purpose

An alternative method of feeding when the mother is not available to breast-feed, an infant needs supplements because of low blood sugar, or an infant tires easily while breast-fed or has uncoordinated suck and swallow patterns.

Rationale

Requires little energy expenditure, stimulates tongue and jaw movements and production of saliva and lingual lipase (aids in milk digestion). Infant paces intake in time and quantity. Infant does not become confused with rubber nipple verses breast nipple. Reduces need for nasal or oral feeding tubes.

1. Position infant in upright sitting position, wrapped securely. Place cloth under chin.
2. Tip cup slightly so milk is just touching lips. Do not pour in mouth. Infant will sip. Ideally, infant's tongue will extend under the bottom of the tipped cup.
3. Leave cup in position during feeding because infant will pause at intervals. Let infant determine rate of feeding.
4. Bubble infant at appropriate intervals.

Only breast- and cup-feed. Do not bottle feed.

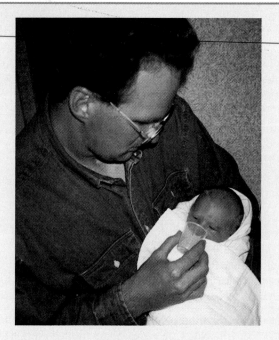

Figure 19-18   Cup feeding. (Courtesy M Schult.)

Lang S: Cup-feeding: an alternative method, *Midwives Chronicle* 107(1276):171, 1994.

• 4-ounce feeders like those used in the hospital are available but expensive.

Some health care professionals want parents to sterilize the bottles and nipples. Others believe that washing with hot, sudsy water and a hot-water rinse is enough. In either case the water used to mix the formula should be boiled before using.

Instruction on the later addition of solids. The most desirable diet for infants up to 6 months of age is breast milk. Bottle-feeding with commercially prepared formula is an acceptable substitute. Since 1984 the American Academy of Pediatrics (Broussard, 1984) has recommended that supplemental food not be introduced before 4 to 6 months of age. Anticipatory guidance is required in explaining this because parents have cultural habits and backgrounds that will influence their choices of food. Parents need to know that there is a time for introduction of solids. The infant's weight, activity, and appetite are factors to consider in this decision. Signals of the infant's readiness include the following:

• Has doubled birth weight
• Demands breast-feeding more than 8 to 10 times in a 24-hour period
• Drinks more than a quart of formula a day
• Often seems hungry

Parents need to know that adding solids does not initially increase the infant's nutrition; rather the infant is experimenting with the texture and taste of new foods and probably will not consume much. Introducing new foods one at a time and at weekly intervals allows for identification of allergies. Solids are introduced at the beginning of a meal when the child is hungriest and may be thinned with formula and fed by spoon. Solids should not be mixed in the bottle of formula. Sucking thickened liquid can cause choking and also will deprive the infant of learning spoon feeding. At first the infant may push the food away and appear dissatisfied. The *extrusion reflex,* the tongue thrusting of sucking, makes the infant appear to be spitting out the food. Feedings, although messy, should be enjoyable for both parents and child. Recommendations for the introduction of solid food are as follows:

1. From birth to 1 year of age, breast milk or formula is the food of choice. Whole, nonmodified cow milk is introduced only after 1 year of age, which allows for maturation of the gastrointestinal tract.
2. Between the ages of 4 and 6 months, continue with breast milk or formula. Begin introducing solids in the following order: rice cereal (offered first because it is least allergenic and also supplies dietary iron), fruits, barley and oatmeal, and prepared vegetables and meats (with applesauce-like texture). Commercial baby foods free of added sugar and salt or home-blended food can be used.

Weaning. An infant can be successfully weaned once grasping with both hands, reaching, and sitting well are accomplished. Infants often lose interest in breast-feeding after 7 to 8 months; others will continue longer. The mother who is breast-feeding can wean directly to a cup. A bottle-fed baby often will hold on to the night bottle until well into the second or even third year. The infant gets satisfaction from sucking, and it will do no harm if only a small amount of juice or milk is given. Diluting the drink with water may hasten the weaning. Parents should be cautioned *never* to allow an infant to fall asleep while drinking anything, even water, from a nursing bottle. This causes a pattern of tooth decay called "nursing bottle mouth," which can be severe enough to necessitate extraction of the affected teeth.

To begin weaning the infant, the mother should put a small amount of milk in a sturdy shallow cup. Training cups are available that have two handles, covers, spouts, and rounded bottoms to cope with the inevitable spills. Each infant differs in adjustment to drinking from a cup. The amount of milk consumed may decrease until the infant gets used to drinking from a cup. Water or juice can be offered from a bottle to give the infant intake during transition.

Supplements

Vitamins and minerals. Parents often are concerned about vitamin and mineral supplements. Supplements of individual vitamins rarely are used for infants, however, with the exception of vitamin K at birth to prevent hemorrhagic disease of the newborn and vitamin E to prevent hemolytic anemia in premature infants. It is common for the pediatric health care provider to prescribe selected multivitamin preparations (Tri-Vi-Flor or Poly-Vi-Sol) but probably unnecessary. Full-term infants normally are born with iron supplies adequate for the first 4 months of life. Breast milk, although relatively deficient in iron, provides adequate supplies because the breast milk iron is more easily digested. Bottle-feeding with iron-supplemented formulas sometimes increases iron deficiency because the harder stool can cause microhemorrhages.

Fluoride supplements. Fluoride is incorporated in structures of the dental enamel that forms during the early months of life before teething occurs. Fluoride supplementation is recommended by the American Academy of Pediatrics Committee on Nutrition (1992) if the local water supply is not fluoridated. The addition of fluoride to the diet can cause a 50 to 70% decrease in dental caries.

EVALUATION OF NEWBORN TRANSITION

A complete assessment includes review of the prenatal, intrapartal, and neonatal history. A complete physical examination should have been performed within the first 24 hours after delivery. Examining the infant in the parents' presence just before discharge gives them the opportunity to ask questions pertaining to the infant's status and the opportunity for the examiner to observe early parent-infant interaction. Several deviations become evident in the first day, whereas others do not manifest until after several days. (See Chapter 18 for warning signs.)

The physician will evaluate the newborn's condition and sign a discharge release. When mother and child are discharged early (less than 24 hours after delivery), it is necessary to perform another physical examination during an early home visit and to have newborn follow-up examination at 1 or 2 weeks of life.

Screening for Potential Problems

Metabolic screening tests provide for early diagnosis and treatment of *inborn errors of metabolism* (IEM), which can prevent or lessen the severity of potential handicaps. In the United States metabolic study programs use the filter paper spot technique. Capillary blood specimens from a heel stick are obtained (Figure 19-19). Blood samples are placed on the filter paper to fill and saturate each circle. The samples are analyzed for levels of enzymes, metabolites, and other substances. If these are not within normal limits, further testing is necessary.

Phenylketonuria (PKU) is an inherited autosomal recessive disorder caused by the absence of phenylalanine hydroxylase, an enzyme necessary for the conversion of the essential amino acid phenylalanine to tyrosine. Tyrosine is needed for the synthesis of hormones, skin, and hair pigment, and its absence leads to brain damage. This is why PKU is seen more frequently in fair-haired (or lightly pigmented) persons. Because maternal metabolism of fetal phenylalanine occurs in utero, clinical signs will not be seen immediately in the neonate. The screening test must be performed after the newborn has consumed enough milk that contains phenylalanine (either breast milk or formula) to produce levels high enough for detection. Newborns who are discharged early need to be retested by the primary care provider. Once the diagnosis is established, diet therapy that restricts phenylalanine intake is begun. During infancy, Lofenalac formula is recommended.

Primary congenital hypothyroidism is a defect in which the thyroid gland does not produce adequate thyroxine (T_4). If left untreated, severe brain damage may result. Clinical signs include hypotonia, widely spaced fontanelles, a large tongue that may cause feeding difficulties, and prolonged jaundice. Treatment consists of thyroid hormone replacement therapy.

Congenital galactosemia is a hereditary disorder of galactose metabolism. Signs that occur after the infant begins feeding include lethargy, hypotonia, and diarrhea. Treatment is elimination of galactose from the diet for 6 to 8 years. During infancy, lactose-free formulas such as Nutramigen or Prosobee are recommended. Hemoglobinopathies such as *sickle cell anemia* and *glucose-6-phosphate dehydrogenase deficiency* are tested for as well (see Chapter 23).

A

NEWBORN SCREENING BLOOD COLLECTION FORM

0 0 6 8 9 4 9 1

☐ * Tests within Acceptable Limits

☐ SEE ATTACHED REPORT

Lab I.D. 06894912

DOH USE ONLY--DO NOT WRITE IN THIS AREA

Infant's Last Name | First Initial | 1 ☐ Male 2 ☐ Female | Multiple Birth A B C Other ☐ ☐ ☐ ☐ | Ethnicity/Race 1 ☐ Wht. 3 ☐ Hisp. 2 ☐ Blk. 4 ☐ Asian 5 ☐ OTHER | ☐ Special Handling

Date of Birth Mo. Day Yr. | Birth Weight Grams | Date of Specimen Mo. Day Yr.

Specimen Collected: 1 ☐ Less than 24 hrs. of age 2 ☐ More than 24 hrs. of age | 1 ☐ Initial Specimen 2 ☐ Repeat Specimen

Infant's Medical Record No. | ☐ Premature ☐ Transfused ____ Date | Mother's Social Security No. | Mother's age

Hospital PFI Code | Hospital of Birth? 1 ☐ Yes 2 ☐ No | ☐ Homebirth | Physician License No. | Mother's Name Last First

Hospital Name | Physician's Name

City | Address | Zip

Zip | Tel. ( )

DO NOT USE ADDRESSOGRAPH | Tel. ( ) | County of Residence:

*Tested For: Phenylalanine, Leucine, Methionine, Galactose-1P Uridyl Transferase, Sickle Hemoglobin (SS), Thyroxine.

SATURATE ALL CIRCLES COMPLETELY See reverse side for instructions

B

BLOOD COLLECTION FORM
(INSTRUCTIONS)

With ballpoint pen, print all information requested on form, including current address information.

1. See diagram for puncture site. Avoid previous puncture sites or curvature of the heel.
2. Place infant's limb in a position to increase venous pressure.
3. Warm heel for 3 minutes.
4. Cleanse puncture site with 70% alcohol.
5. Wipe dry with sterile gauze.
6. Make puncture using sterile lancet with tip not longer than 2.44 mm.
7. Wipe away first drop of blood with dry sterile gauze.
8. Allow second, larger drop of blood to form.
9. Gently apply filter paper to large drop of blood. Allow blood to soak through and completely fill preprinted circle. Apply blood to one side of filter paper only. (Either side may be chosen for procedure.) **Do not use capillary tubes for specimen collection.**
10. Fill circle with **single** application to drop of blood. Do not layer successive drops of blood.
11. Fill all five circles.
12. **Allow blood spots to thoroughly air dry for at least 4 hours** on a flat, nonabsorptive surface, away from direct heat and sunlight. Avoid touching or smearing blood spots. Never superimpose one filter paper on another before thoroughly drying. Do not refrigerate.
13. When placing more than one specimen in an envelope, alternate forms so that blood spots on adjacent forms are not in contact.
14. Mail completed collection forms to the testing laboratory within 24 hours of collection.
15. Specimens identified as **special handling** must be thoroughly dry and then individually sealed in a plastic bag. The outside of the plastic bag must be labeled as requiring **special handling.**

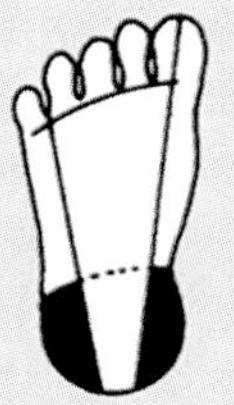

Preferred puncture site is indicated by shaded areas on heel.

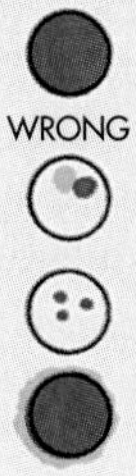

Figure 19-19 **A,** Metabolic screening form. **B,** Blood collection form instructions. Note that circles must be completely saturated with blood to ensure identification of metabolic disorders. (Courtesy Newborn Screening Program, Wadsworth Center for Laboratories and Research, New York State Department of Health, Albany, NY.)

Congenital lactose intolerance

A deficiency of the enzyme lactase (needed for the digestion of lactose), becomes evident in early infancy but is not life-threatening. Diagnosis is based on a history of diarrhea, abdominal pain, distention, and flatus after ingestion of milk containing lactose. Clinitest tablets are used to test the stool for malabsorbed sugar (reducing substances). Elimination of milk products and their gradual reintroduction while observing for return of symptoms is the easiest way to confirm the diagnosis. Treatment includes elimination of cow milk products and substitution of a soy-based formula such as Isomil, Prosobee, or Lactofree. Dairy products that have been fermented such as yogurt can be consumed safely. Lactose-reduced milk (Lactaid) also may be used by 1 year of age, and the child is observed for any digestive difficulties as milk products are slowly reintroduced. (See Chapter 28 for groups with genes for lactose intolerance.)

Other rare inborn errors of metabolism

There are a number of rare IEM. In general, if there is failure to thrive, unusual stools, or difficulty digesting feedings the infant should be screened for an IEM. In many cases these metabolic problems can be treated with strict diet modifications. Figure 19-19 indicates the usual genetic conditions included on the initial testing.

Human immunodeficiency virus

The final blot on the test paper may be reserved for HIV maternal antibody testing. Currently some states perform *blind testing* of newborns, that is, without identification of the individual. Only the state and hospital are listed, and reports are sent back to notify these agencies of the rate of HIV-positive mothers in their units. Newborns of HIV-positive women will show the presence of maternal antibodies in their blood, but only approximately 25% of these will actually be HIV infected. No permit is obtained from the mother because there is no individual identification. (See Chapter 25 for the current status of the infant of an HIV-positive woman).

Bilirubin level

Hyperbilirubinemia occurs when the normal pathways of bilirubin metabolism and excretion are impeded. This may occur when the mother and infant blood types are incompatible (see Chapter 23). Cord blood is used to determine the infant's blood type and Rh factor, and to perform the direct Coombs' test, which detects antibodies on the neonatal erythrocytes. When an infant is found to be jaundiced (regardless of the reason), serum bilirubin levels are determined from a capillary heel stick sample. Various treatments are available (see Chapter 29). The infant's discharge will be delayed until this problem has resolved.

Venereal Disease Research Laboratory

The Venereal Disease Research Laboratory (VDRL) is a serologic screen for congenital syphilis. This screening has been mandated by law in the United States as one of the cord blood tests (see Chapter 25). As a cost-saving measure, many hospitals currently save cord blood to examine only if the blood test result of a woman who has recently given birth is positive. Table 19-5 summarizes common test for newborns.

 Box **19-2**

CLINICAL DECISION

When cord blood reports return from the laboratory, you note the following:
Blood type A+, Coombs' test negative (mother is O+)
Hemoglobin 20 g/dl, hematocrit 68%, VDRL negative
Which finding is reportable?
On the discharge day (day 3) the newborn looks jaundiced. Why was the newborn more likely to become jaundiced at this time?

EARLY DISCHARGE PLANNING

Parenting is both a learned and an instinctive behavior. Even for experienced parents, the first time caring for an infant is a time of turmoil and decreased confidence. The perinatal nurse will find that most couples need education to reduce knowledge deficits related to infant care. Taking the time to provide the family with more knowledge about their infant will increase their confidence and ability to care comfortably for their newborn. Box 19-3 includes common questions asked by new parents.

The best time for teaching varies with experience and prenatal preparation. The nurse must assess the parents' readiness to learn and the knowledge base and support systems available once the mother and infant are discharged.

Objectives for Parent Education

1. Parents describe a positive support system and adequate housing.
2. Basic needs of the newborn infant are described.
3. Parents state signs of difficulty in nutritional intake and know how to seek help.
4. Parents evaluate home environment for hazards, infections, and temperature control and plan to childproof the home against accidents (including use of car seat).
5. Parents state source of primary care planned for their infant.
6. Parents state recommendations for immunizations and schedule of visits.
7. Parents describe when to notify health care provider regarding alterations in infant status, and they consistently follow up as necessary.
8. Parents start the attachment-bonding process, giving indication that this will continue to develop.
9. Parents can demonstrate safe sleeping positions for infant.

Planning for bringing the newborn home begins well before birth as families gather the materials necessary for their newborn's care, begin to educate themselves about parenthood, and anticipate lifestyle changes. Still, there is much to be done after the birth. Traditionally, new mothers and infants remained in the hospital for at least 3 days after birth, allowing time for assessment of parent needs and appropriate teaching. However, mothers and newborns may now leave as soon as 12 to 24 hours after birth with home care follow-up. (Several states have enacted rules requiring insurance companies to pay for at least 48 hours of care after vaginal birth. Forced early discharge is a critical issue). Families who *choose* early discharge may feel that the healthy new infant is safer and more comfortable at home (see Box 1-1). They may be concerned about finances, or their insurance company will not pay for more days. In either case it is vital that these families have a solid support system at home and that provisions are made for assessment of both mother and newborn on the third postpartum day. The mother is evaluated as described in Chapter 17. Neonatal adjustment is assessed in the same manner as described in Chapter 18, with special attention to the presence of cardiorespiratory difficulty or jaundice, the quality of

Table **19-5**   **Diagnostic Tests for Newborn Infants**

Laboratory Tests	Normal Results	Comments
CORD BLOOD		
Blood type	A, B, AB, O	Potential for incompatibility, especially if infant is type A or B with a type O mother.
Rh factor	Negative or positive	Potential for incompatibility if mother is type Rh negative and infant is Rh positive.
Direct Coombs' test	Negative	Detects sensitized red blood cells. Does not define blocking agent.
Bilirubin	1.0-1.8 mg/dl	Elevated level at birth indicates that fetal hemolysis is present.
Serology-Antibody Titers*		
Syphilis	Negative	If mother has been treated during pregnancy, newborn titers may still be positive but should decrease by 3 months.
IgM	Negative	If present, indicates maternal infection during pregnancy with transfer of IgM antibodies to fetus. Specific antibody titers of mother and infant are compared to rule out infections such as TORCH (see Chapter 27).
IgG	Negative	Formed in infant in response to antigen and does not cross placenta. If found, indicates that infant responded to maternal infection.
HEEL-STICK CAPILLARY BLOOD		
Glucose	45-90 mg/dl	If Dextrostix below 45 mg/dl, take venous sample for laboratory analysis. Infants of diabetic mothers, infants <5 lb or >8 lb, preterm infants, and stressed infants need additional testing.
Hematocrit	40%-65%	<40% anemia, >65% polycythemia
Bilirubin	At 3-4 days normal elevation of 4-6 mg/dl and may reach 12 mg/dl	For infant with levels elevated above normal, expect q12h tests, extra oral fluids. Infant may receive phototherapy if above 10-14 mg/dl.
Thyroid Screening		
T_4 level	Less than 6 µmg/dl at 3 days is abnormally low	Done on all infants at 2-3 days; especially important for those with wide-open suture lines, large fontanelles, thickened tongues.
TSH on suspected hypothyroid	TSH level >20 µmU/dl at 3 days is diagnostic of hypothyroidism	Signs of thyroid deficiency developed by first week.
Inborn Errors of Metabolism		
PKU	Blood levels of 4 mg or more by 48 hr indicate problem	PKU needs to be repeated by pediatrician if infant discharged early, before adequate milk intake.
Leucine, Methionine		
Histidinemia		Ferric chloride reaction turns urine blue-green.
Glucose-6-phosphate dehydrogenase	Elevated indirect bilirubin level in infant affected by maternal drug	Consult list of drugs causing hemolysis that may excrete in breast milk and affect infant.
Sickle cell trait/disease	Absent	Usually no initial problems. Watch for reduced oxygen tension.

Ig, Immunoglobulin; *PKU,* phenylketonuria; *TORCH,* Toxoplasmosis, rubella, cytomegalovirus, and herpes simplex; *TSH,* thyroid-stimulating hormone.
*These tests may be done selectively as ordered.

Table 19-5   **Diagnostic Tests for Newborn Infants~cont'd**

Laboratory Tests	Normal Results	Comments
MECONIUM*		
Cystic fibrosis	No elevated albumin in meconium	Test strip changes to deep blue if positive. Sweat test done to measure sodium and chloride concentrations of collected sweat.
PERIPHERAL CULTURES*		
Cord, anorectal, ear canal, nasopharyngeal	Negative	Use varies. Done especially if mother had premature rupture of membranes or if nursery epidemic occurs.
Any lesion		
URINE*		
Urinalysis	1.004-1.018 specific	Urobilinogen associated with jaundice in infant.
Possible culture	gravity. Uric acid crystals; no protein or red blood cells	

Box 19-3   **Common Questions Parents Ask Concerning Infant Care**

HYGIENE
How often should an infant be bathed?
When can I give my newborn a tub bath?
How do I care for the diaper area?
How do I care for his circumcision?

FEEDING
What is the best diet for an infant in the first year of life?

Breast-feeding
What kind of diet should I follow while breast-feeding?
How long should I let my infant nurse? How often?
Should I offer my infant extra water?
Does my infant need extra formula?
How should I hold my infant when nursing?
How do I burp my infant?
Should I let my infant use a pacifier?
When should I start offering solids?
When should I start weaning?

Bottle-feeding
What type of formula should I use?
How do I sterilize bottles, caps, and nipples?
How much should my infant be fed? How often?
Should I offer extra water?
How do I burp my infant?
Should I let my infant use a pacifier?
When should I start offering solids?

TEMPERATURE
How do I know if my infant is too hot or cold?
How should I dress my infant when going outdoors?
How warm or cool should I keep the house?
Is extra humidity necessary?

SAFETY
How do I choose a car seat, stroller, crib, or infant carrier?
How do I childproof my house?
I have a pet; is that safe for my infant?

SLEEP NEEDS
What are the normal patterns of sleep for an infant in the first year?
How can I help my infant go to sleep?
What do I do if my infant has colic?

HEALTH MAINTENANCE
When do I bring my infant back for a check-up?
When will my infant be immunized? Are there risks?
How will I know if my infant is sick?
How do I take my infant's temperature?
How can I keep my infant from getting sick?
When should I call my doctor or nurse practitioner?

Postpartum-Newborn Visit Record
Newborn Assessment

MATRIA HEALTHCARE OF NEW YORK, INC.

Infant Name:_____ ❑ Female ❑ Male DOB:_____ ID Number:_____

MD:_____ MD Address:_____

Mother Name:_____ SS#:_____ ID Number:_____

ECD:_____ DOB:_____ NB Age:_____ Date of Visit:_____ Payor:_____

Type of Visit: ❑ Home ❑ Telephone ❑ Well Visit ❑ Complication:_____

Race/Ethnicity: ❑ White ❑ Black ❑ Asian ❑ Hispanic ❑ American Indian ❑ Other:_____

VITAL SIGNS	HEAD, NECK, CHEST		
Temp._____ ❑ Rate regular ❑ Rate irregular Resp. ❑ Normal ❑ Other_____	❑ Normal ❑ Caput ❑ Bruising ❑ Molding	Fontanelle ❑ Soft ❑ Full ❑ Bulging ❑ Depressed ❑ Flat	Eyes: (right) ❑ Normal ❑ Edema ❑ Discharge (left) ❑ Normal ❑ Edema ❑ Discharge Ears: ❑ Symmetrical ❑ Normal ❑ Discharge Mouth: ❑ Lips and palate intact ❑ Teeth ❑ Mucous membranes pink/moist Nose: ❑ Normal ❑ Congestion ❑ Flaring Nares Neck: ❑ Full ROM Clavicles:❑ Bilat equal mvmnt

WEIGHT	SKIN COLOR/CONDITION	ABDOMEN/GENITALIA
Birth _____ Today _____	❑ Pink ❑ Pale ❑ Mottled ❑ Jaundice ❑ No ❑ Acrocyanosis ❑ Dusky ❑ Warm ❑ Lanugo ❑ Birthmark ❑ Good Turgor ❑ Dry/Cracked ❑ Cool ❑ Sclera ❑ Peeling ❑ Head (3 MG/DI) ❑ Rash ❑ Head & Chest (9 MG/DI) ❑ Lesions ❑ Head & umbilicus (12 MG/DI) ❑ Smooth ❑ Head & abdomen (15 MG/DI) ❑ Petechiae ❑ Head to feet (18 MG/DI)	Abdomen: ❑ Normal ❑ Distended ❑ Bowel sounds present Umbilical Cord: ❑ Normal ❑ Oozing Male genitalia: ❑ Urethral opening at tip of penis Testes: ❑ Right ↓ ❑ Left ↓ ❑ Right ↑ ❑ Left ↑ ❑ Normal Female: ❑ Labia normal ❑ Vaginal tag ❑ Discharge

CIRCUMCISION	UMBILICAL CORD	ELIMINATION	MUSCULOSKELETAL
❑ Yes ❑ No ❑ Intact, healing ❑ Redness ❑ Bleeding ❑ Draining ❑ Other	❑ Umbilical cord dry ❑ Umbilical cord moist ❑ Umbilical cord foul smell ❑ Cord care performed ❑ Cord clamp present ❑ Cord clamp removed ❑ Other:	Stools: # in last 24 hrs. Meconium passed ❑ Y ❑ N Color: Consistency:_____ Urine: # wet diapers in last 24 hrs._____ Color:	Spine: ❑ Straight ❑ Curved ❑ Dimple ❑ Hair at base Hip: ❑ Ortolani's Sign ❑ Neg. ❑ Pos. Hands/Arms: ❑ Normal ❑ Extra digit ❑ Webbed digit ❑ Fingernails present ❑ Abnormal shape/deformity Legs/Feet: ❑ Normal ❑ Extra digit ❑ Webbed digit ❑ Toenails present ❑ Abnormal shape/deformity ❑ Stepping reflex present

LABS DRAWN	BEHAVIOR PATTERNS	NEUROMUSCULAR
❑ Metabolic screen form #_____ Date:_____ Time:_____ Date mailed:_____ ❑ Bilirubin Results:_____ ❑ MD notified ❑ Other_____ Maternal blood type:_____	❑ Alert at intervals ❑ Responds to auditory stimuli ❑ Awakens regularly for feeding ❑ Sleeps for____hrs. at a time ❑ Lethargic ❑ Fussy, irritable or jittery ❑ Able to be consoled by care giver ❑ Self-consoling behaviors noted Cry: ❑ Normal ❑ High pitched ❑ Weak ❑ Excess	Muscle tone: ❑ Normal ❑ Other:_____ ❑ Symmetrical strength and movement in all extremities ❑ Adequate neck control ❑ Head lag not > 45° Reflexes: ❑ Suck ❑ Blink ❑ Moro ❑ Rooting ❑ Tonic neck Babinski: ❑ Positive ❑ Negative Grasp: ❑ Toes ❑ Hand

NUTRITION	FAMILY ADJUSTMENT	BABY IDENTIFIED NEEDS
❑ Breast ❑ Bottle ❑ Breast with supplement Formula_____oz. feeding Min. breast_____ Frequency of feedings_____ Feeding observed ❑ Yes ❑ No Proper latch on breast ❑ Yes ❑ No Coordinated suck/swallow ❑ Yes ❑ No Baby satisfied after feeding ❑ Yes ❑ No Emisis ❑ Yes ❑ No Amount:_____	Eye-to-eye contact ❑ Yes ❑ No Holding close ❑ Yes ❑ No Interest in care ❑ Yes ❑ No Verbal interaction ❑ Yes ❑ No Husband/significant other accepting of infant and participates in care ❑ Yes ❑ No Siblings adjusting to baby ❑ Yes ❑ No Other:	

MEDICATIONS			
Name	Dose	Route	Frequency

❑ Assessment within normal limits
❑ Recommendations/Referrals

Nurse's Signature:_____ Date:_____

Figure 19-20   Postpartum-newborn visit record. (Courtesy Matria Healthcare of New York.)

skin turgor, feeding and elimination patterns, and parental attachment (see the Care Path for newborns). Figure 19-20 illustrates the activities of the nurse at a home visit.

Because of time constraints, teaching must be efficient and effective. Some suggestions are the following:

1. Begin classes in the prenatal period, reviewing infant care, growth, and development.
2. Perform predischarge infant assessments while the parents are present so that teaching can be included.
3. Give written information in the parent's language to reinforce verbal instructions.
4. Follow up with telephone contact from nursery staff member or other designated provider.

Extended Stay

Unfortunately, some families have to extend the hospital stay because of maternal or neonatal illness. Prematurity, sepsis, and congenital anomalies are the most common reasons for extended hospitalization of neonates. These conditions and the effects on family interaction are discussed in Chapter 29. Assessment of parental needs should be completed before the infant is discharged and each plan individualized according to the parent's knowledge base. Nursing interventions reflect common concerns parents express about infant care and safety.

Referrals

If at any time before or during the discharge process a question arises about the abilities of the parents to care for the newborn, the family should be referred to an appropriate community agency. Usually this is done by the primary nurse with help from social services. Referral forms should be made out in advance so that early contact can be made with the family.

The women, infants, and children (WIC) program is a program of the federal government that provides pregnant and lactating women and their children with adequate nutrition. Essential foods are supplied to those who qualify. Ideally referrals to WIC are made prenatally but can also be made after birth (Dobson, 1994).

It is recommended that the following families and infants have referrals to social service and home care agencies made at or before discharge:

1. Maternal problems
- Medical disorders
  - 16 years old or younger at time of delivery
  - Birth at less than 28 weeks' gestation
  - Birth at home or en route to the hospital
  - No prenatal care or came for less than four visits
2. Infant problems
  - Multiple gestation
  - Weight less than 2001 g at birth
- Major congenital anomaly
- Inherited metabolic disease
- Discharged to home from the neonatal intensive care unit (NICU)

The infant and mother are ready for discharge when the health care giver has completed the newborn physical assessment (Figure 18-20) and necessary parental teaching, and the parents sign the identification form for their child (Figure 19-21). See Box 19-4 for an example of a discharge summary sheet given to the parents for future referral.

Evaluation

Questions that may elicit evaluation data on parental and newborn readiness for discharge include the following:

1. Is the infant within normal parameters of vital signs, bilirubin, gestational age, and behavior?
2. Have feeding behaviors been established? Are there feeding problems that need referral? Do parents know whom to call if help is needed?
3. Have parents read handouts and asked questions? (Were handouts available in their primary language?)
4. Have all laboratory tests been performed? Does the parent know when to obtain results and when to see a pediatrician or nurse clinician?
5. Do parents know the signs of illness and when to report problems?
6. Do parents indicate they have a car seat and understand safety guidelines, including safe positioning?
7. Do parents indicate a support system, or do there seem to be problems with attachment, bonding, or support?

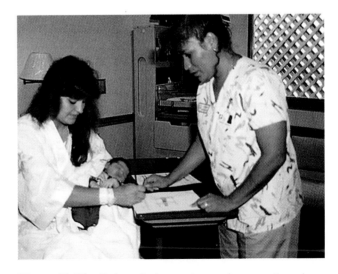

Figure 19-21 Before discharge, the mother examines the identification form and signs it. It is witnessed by the nurse. *(Courtesy Marjorie Pyle, RNC, Lifecircle.)*

Care | *Newborn Care*
PATH

Category	0 - 12 Hours
PHYSICAL ASSESSMENT	
1. The neonate will maintain:	
• Airway	Respiratory rate 30-60 bpm with apnea < 15 sec Bilateral breath sounds; wet rales normal/increased for cesarean section only
• Circulation	Apical rate 110-160/min with slight murmur BP equal in upper and lower extremities Syst. 50-75 Diast. 30-45 Skin color pink with acrocyanosis Bilateral femoral pulses
• Thermoregulation	Initial temperature:
2. Neonate will demonstrate norms related to:	
• Umbilical cord	Bluish-white color Three vessels (two arteries, one vein) Cord clamp in place
• Measurements	Weight: 2500 g-4000 g Length: 44-55 cm Head circumference: 32-37.5 cm (allow for molding) Chest: 1-2 cm less than head
• Reflexes	Expect: Early reflexes diminished by type of birth, anesthesia, or sleep
• Hemorrhagic disease of newborn	Neonate does not have colonizing bacteria in colon for synthesis of fat-soluble vitamin K Decreased prothombin levels
• Eye condition	Chemical conjunctivitis from erythromycin ointment Eyelids may be puffy from birth pressure
3. Newborn will initiate:	
• Nutritional intake	Tolerates initial breast-feeding, then on demand Initial bottle feed only 15-30 ml, water or formula (per hospital policy)
• Elimination	First void/stool may occur during birth, check record

BP, Blood pressure; *HBV,* hepatitis B virus; *IDM,* infant of a diabetic mother; *IM,* intramuscularly; *LGA,* large for gestational age; *PDA,* patent ductus arteriosus; *PKU,* phenylketonuria; *prn,* as necessary; *SGA,* small for gestational age; *WIC,* Women, Infants, and Children Supplementary Food Program.

12 - 24 Hours	Interventions	Initials
Respiratory rate 30-60 bpm with apnea < 15 sec, in lower range when asleep Bilateral breath sounds Wet rales decreasing	Suction nose/mouth with bulb syringe immediately and prn Place neonate in head-dependent, side-lying position Assess breath sounds Continue to monitor respiration q1h × 4 then q4h (per policy) Record findings, report significant changes	
Murmur may still be present if PDA has not closed Stable apical rate and BP Acrocyanosis disappears (now related to chilling or hypoglycemia)	Continue to monitor apical rate q1h × 4 (or per policy); skin color, femoral pulses, prn condition Record findings, report significant changes	
Expect same temperature range	Place in radiant warmer for 1-2 hr with thermistor attached until temperature stable > 97° F. Recheck ax temperature q4h. Postpone initial bath if temperature low. After bath, recheck temperature. Double wrap, and place in crib. Teach mother to maintain warmth of infant.	
Drying, no redness, drainage, foul odor Clamp remains in place	Provide cord care Assess cord for three vessels Teach parents cord care	
By 24 hrs, head circumference may change if significant molding or caput Cephalhematoma may form in the early period depending on birth pressures Edema/bruising over scalp if ventouse method used for delivery All reflexes should be elicited	Remove clamp before neonate's discharge Weigh on balanced scale Measure head and chest with correct landmarks Report/record significant variations Observe for cephalhematoma, caput Observe for bleeding after circumcision Assess and document findings Administer vitamin K before 6hr after birth.	
Edema and inflammation begin to subside by 24 hr Improved ability to focus eyes	Administer erythromycin ophthalmic 1-in ribbon of ointment within 1 hr postbirth (after eye contact with parents); wait 1 min before removing excess Teach parents need for prophylaxis, and side effects to report Observe reaction. Document medication time.	
Breast-feed on demand at least q3-4h Bottle-feed on demand at least q3-4h	Assess readiness to feed and tolerance of volume; record Support breast-feeding techniques, refer to lactation specialist if problems. Discuss normal feeding requirements, bottle-feeding preparation, and refrigeration	
Will void and pass meconium stool	Assess voids/color of stools q4h. Record per protocol. Report no stool in 24 hr, distention.	

Continued.

Newborn Care~cont'd

Category	0 - 12 Hours
SCREENING/MEDICATIONS	
1. Laboratory tests	Cord blood for type, Rh, Coombs' test Glucose by heelstick, if LGA, SGA, IDM, or prn signs of hypoglycemia
2. Medications	Vitamin K 0.5 mg IM by 6 hr after birth. Hepatitis B immunoglobulin per order and HBV vaccine within 12 hrs of birth if mother is HBV positive.
PARENT-INFANT ATTACHMENT	
• Parent will demonstrate positive interaction with newborn	Parent-infant en face position noted Investigates physical characteristics Infant opens eyes in dim light
DISCHARGE PLANNING/ HOME CARE	
• Parents are prepared for care of infant at home	Discuss discharge plans with parents Teach at every contact of mother/infant

---

Box 19-4   Discharge Summary Sheet

Name_____

Date of birth _____   Date of discharge _____

Birth weight_____   Weight at discharge _____   Length _____

Suggested diet _____

_____

Medications _____

Activity _____

_____

Community referral/resources _____

_____

Poison control No. _____   Hospital No. _____

Private physician No. _____   Clinic No. _____

Return visit: Date _____   Time _____

                       Place _____   Phone _____

Special instructions:

1. Continue applying alcohol to the cord with each diaper change.
2. Sponge bathe your newborn every day until the cord falls off. Then a tub bath may be given when the cord is completely healed.
3. Buckle the infant in infant seat with infant facing rear of car.

Other instructions:

_____

_____

A copy is made so that parents can use this as a reference guide after discharge.

12 - 24 Hours	Interventions	Initials
Blood type reported, should be Coombs' test negative Glucose level > 50 mg/dL Bilirubin < 5 mg/dL Give appointment in 48 hr for PKU and other genetic screening if early discharge	Evaluate ABO incompatibility in relation to jaundice. Report Coombs' test (check maternal status) Glucose and water or formula by bottle for hypoglycemia. Lavage if poor sucking.	
Touches infant, uses en face postion Continues attachment behaviors Names infant Careful to meet infant needs	Assess parent/infant interaction Incorporate siblings and grandparents Assess knowledge of newborn behaviors	
Knowledge of newborn care Assess level of comfort in doing tasks Determine need for home care/follow up	Assess social support and knowledge base Teach basic infant care needs Review use of bulb syringe, positioning, warmth, sleep/wake cycles, voiding/stooling Give written instructions and emergency telephone numbers. Make out referrals. Be sure mother has car seat for trip home, plus initial supplies. WIC referral	

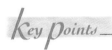

Key Points

- Monitoring infant transition is critical and guided by Apgar scoring.
- Vital signs must be monitored frequently during the first 4 hours of life.
- The nurse's role in assessment of the newborn is based on knowledge of growth and development. The nurse is responsible for detecting variations from normal and reporting findings to the appropriate person.
- Protection from heat loss and infection are primary nursing responsibilities in the transitional period.
- Nurses have a major role in prevention of infant abduction from hospital settings.
- Medications for the newborn must be given within the specific periods after skin cleansing to prevent infection.
- There is controversy about the value of circumcision. Nurses need to be prepared to discuss pros and cons of circumcision with parents.

- Education for care of the infant can be accomplished with demonstrations, literature, and audiovisual materials. Teaching related to all aspects of newborn care should be covered before discharge.
- Documentation of client's levels of understanding should be included in nursing care plans and discharge notes.
- Nutritional needs begin soon after birth. When transition is troubled, the infant should be assessed for hypoglycemia.
- Some tests for metabolic screening may need repetition if the infant is discharged early.
- A referral for home care should be made whenever problems with the mother or newborn are identified in the immediate newborn period.

Study Questions

19-1. Select the terms that apply to the following statements:
   a. Noisy breath on inspiration _____.
   b. Sign of respiratory distress _____.
   c. Black, sticky first stools _____.
   d. White, cheesy material secreted at female and male genitalia _____.
   e. Red, ruddy tone to skin other than high hematocrit _____.
   f. Bluish tone to hands and feet in first few hours after birth _____.
   g. Reason nurses check environment with infant's temperature _____.

19-2. Mary is delivered at term by normal spontaneous delivery (NSD) to a 28-year-old woman after an uneventful pregnancy, labor, and delivery. No maternal analgesia or anesthesia were used. She coughs several times, and you observe moderate amounts of white mucus expelled from her mouth and nose. Her apical heart rate for 6 seconds is 12. You note that she is moving her arms and legs vigorously and that for the first minute she is pink, but her hands and feet are blue. Select the points for each of the five items of the Apgar score at 1 minute.
   a. Heart rate 2; respirations 2; tone 2; reflexes 2; color 1, = 9
   b. Heart rate 0; respirations 2; tone 2; reflexes 0; color 0, = 4
   c. Heart rate 1; respirations 2; tone 2; reflexes 1; color 2, = 8
   d. Looks like 6 or 7.

19-3. At 5 minutes of age, the Mary's Apgar score is unchanged. What should you do?
   a. Chart the Apgar score, and continue to observe her.
   b. Start positive pressure ventilation with 80% oxygen via bag and mask.
   c. Move the infant from the warmer to footprint her and put on the identification band.
   d. Obtain another Apgar score.

19-4. Which mechanism of heat loss is prevented by the following methods of temperature control in the delivery area:
   a. Place the infant on warmed surfaces only
   b. Dry the infant thoroughly
   c. Place the infant under a radiant warmer if the infant is not placed on the mother's abdomen
   d. Minimize air-conditioning currents and movement of people

19-5. A pulse rate of 110/min in a deeply asleep term infant most probably indicates:
   a. A normal response for this phase of sleep.
   b. A heart problem to be evaluated.
   c. Bigeminal pulse deficit.
   d. Dehydration.

19-6. Robert is circumcised the morning of discharge. Which statement is inaccurate regarding immediate postcircumcision care?
   a. Check for bleeding from site for the first 12 hours.
   b. Clean penile area thoroughly with each diaper change.
   c. Use petroleum jelly as lubricant to prevent diaper irritation.
   d. Observe for and chart voiding before discharge.

19-7. Which of the following mothers must receive a referral for home care?
   a. Primipara with a 4000 g full-term male infant and adequate support systems
   b. Mother of twins with two siblings at home
   c. Mother of 2400 g female infant who had elevated bilirubin level at 3 days of age and discharged on the fourth day
   d. Diabetic mother of 3300 g full-term female infant

Answer Key

19-1: a. Stridor; b. grunting; c. meconium; d. smegma; e. plethora; f. acrocyanosis; g. thermoregulation. 19-2: a. 19-3: a. 19-4: a. Conduction; b. evaporation; c. radiation; d. convection. 19-5: a. 19-6: b. 19-7: b, c, d.

References

*American Academy of Pediatrics: Report of the task force on circumcision, *Pediatrics* 84(4):388, 1989.

American Academy of Pediatrics, Committee on Nutrition: Follow up on weaning formulas, *Pediatrics* 89:1105, 1992.

*Apgar V et al: Evaluation of the newborn infant—second report, *JAMA* 168:1985, 1958.

Axton SE et al: Comparison of brachial and calf blood pressures in infants, *Ped Nurs* 21(4):323, 1995.

Beachy P, Deacon J: Preventing neonatal kidnapping, *J Obstet Gynecol Neonatal Nurs* 20(1):12, 1992.

*Bliss-Holtz J: Comparison of rectal, axillary and inguinal temperatures in full-term infants, *Nurs Res* 38(2):85, 1989.

Bronner YL, Paige DM: Current concepts in infant nutrition, *J Nurse Midwifery* 37(suppl 2):59, 1992.

*Broussard A: Anticipatory guidance: adding solids to an infant's diet, *J Obstet Gynecol Neonatal Nurs* 13(6):239, 1984.

Burgess AW et al: Infant abductors, *J Psychosocial Nurs* 33(9):30, 1995.

Campos RG: Rocking and pacifiers: two comforting interventions for heelstick pain, *Res Nurs Health* 17:321, 1994.

Centers for Disease Control (CDC), Immunization Practice Advisory Committee: Hepatitis B virus: a comprehensive strategy for eliminating transmission in the US through universal childhood vaccination, *MMWR* 1-25, Nov 22, 1991.

Christensson K et al: Separation distress call in the human neonate in the absence of maternal body contact, *Acta Paediatr* 84:468, 1995.

Clinical Guide Lines: Measles, mumps, rubella, *Nurs Practitioner* 21(10):88, 1996.

*Cowen J et al: Absorption of chlorhexidine from intact skin of newborn infants, *Arch Dis Child* 54:379, 1979.

Dobson B: A WIC primer, *J Hum Lactation* 10(3):199, 1994.

Doherty LB et al: Detection of phenylketonuria in the very early newborn blood specimen, *Pediatrics* 87(2):240, 1991.

Dwyer T et al: The contribution of changes in the prevalence of prone sleeping position to decline in sudden infant death syndrome in Tasmania, *JAMA* 273:783, 1995.

Editorial: Birth news, *Birth* 19(1):45, 1992.

Faucher MA, Jackson G: Pharmaceutical preparations: a review of drugs commonly used during the neonatal period, *J Nurse Midwifery* 37(suppl 2):74, 1992.

Gilbaum I: Circumcision, *J Nurse Midwifery* 37(suppl 2):97, 1992.

*Greer PS: Head coverings for newborns under radiant warmers, *J Obstet Gynecol Neonatal Nurs* 17(4):265, 1988.

Hammerschlag MR et al: Efficacy of neonatal ocular prophylaxis for the prevention of chlamydial and gonococcal conjunctivitis, *N Engl J Med* 320(12):769, 1991.

Havens DH, Zink RL: The "back to sleep" campaign, *J Pediatr Health Care* 8:240, 1994.

*Herzog LW: Urinary tract infections and circumcision, *Am J Dis Child* 143(3):348, 1989.

Hess DL: Chlamydia in the neonate, *Neonatal network* 12(3):9, 1993.

Isenberg SJ et al: A controlled trial of povidone-iodine as prophylaxis against ophthalmia neonatorum, *N Engl J Med* 332:562, 1995.

Jepson HA et al: The Apgar score: evolution, limitations, and scoring guidelines, *Birth* 18(2):83, 1991.

*Kemper D et al: Jaundice, terminating breast-feeding, and the vulnerable child, *Pediatrics* 84(5):773, 1989.

*Klaus M, Kennell J: *Parent-infant bonding*, St Louis, 1982, Mosby.

Klaus MH: Commentary: the early hours and days of life: an opportune time, *Birth* 22(4):201, 1995.

L'Archeuesque CL, Goldstein-Lohman H: Ritual circumcision: educating the parents, *Ped Nurs* 22(3):228, 1996.

Larsen GL et al: Postneonatal circumcision—population profile, *Pediatrics* 85(5):808, 1990.

Lawrence R: *Breastfeeding*, ed 4, St Louis, 1994, Mosby.

Letko MD: Understanding the Apgar score, *J Obstet Gynecol Neonatal Nurs* 25(4):299, 1996.

MacDonald M: Infection control considerations for management of the newborn in the delivery room, *Pediatr AIDS HIV Infect: Fetus to Adoles* 1(1):16, 1990.

Marchette L et al: Pain reduction interventions during neonatal circumcision, *Nurs Res* 40(4):241, 1991.

*Marecki MA: Chlamydial trachomatis: a developing perinatal problem, *J Perinat Neonat Nurs* 1(4):1, 1988.

Milos MF, Macris D: Circumcision, *J Nurse Midwifery* 37(suppl 2):87, 1992.

Morbidity and Mortality Weekly Report: Guidelines for immunization, *MMWR* 45(RR-12):1, 1996.

*Newborn screening for sickle cell disease and other hemoglobinopathies, *Pediatrics* 83(suppl 5), 1989.

*Novak J: Formula for profit, *Common Cause* Mar/Apr: 18, 1988.

*O'Brien C et al: Effect of bathing with 4% chlorhexidine gluconate solution on neonatal bacterial colonization, *J Hosp Infect* 5(suppl A):141, 1984.

*O'Neill J et al: Percutaneous absorption potential of chlorhexidine in neonates, *Curr Ther Res* 31(3):485, 1982.

Penny-McGillivray T: A newborn's first bath: when? *J Obstet Gynecol Neonatal Nurs* 25(6): 481, 1996.

Phillips P: Neonatal pain management: a call to action, *Ped Nurs* 21(2):195, 1995.

Poland RL: The question of routine neonatal circumcision, *N Engl J Med* 322(18):1312, 1990.

Prodromidis M et al: Mothers touching newborns: a comparison of rooming-in versus minimal contact, *Birth* 22(4):196, 1995.

Rabin JB, Lincoln J: Preventing infant abductions from health care facilities, *Neonatal Network* 13(8):61, 1994.

Ross T, Dickason EJ: Nursing alert: vertical transmission of HIV and HBV, *MCN Am J Matern Child Nurs* 17(4):192, 1992.

Ryan CA, Finer NN: Changing attitudes and practices regarding local analgesia for newborn circumcision, *Pediatrics* 94:230, 1994.

Schoen EJ: The status of circumcision of newborns, *N Engl J Med* 322(18):1308, 1990.

Schoen EJ: Urologists and circumcision of newborns, *Urology* 40(2):99, 1992.

Sutton MB, et al: Baby bottoms and environmental conundrums—disposable diapers and the pediatrician, *Pediatrics* 88(2):386, 1991.

Thomas K: Thermoregulation in neonates, *Neonatal network* 13(2):15, 1994.

Treloar DM: The effects of nonnutritive sucking on oxygenation in healthy, crying full-term infants, *Appl Nurs Res* 7(2):52, 1994.

Weiss ME, Poelter D, Gocka I: Infrared tympanic thermometry for neonatal temperature assessment, *J Obstet Gynecol Neonatal Nurs* 23:798, 1993.

Wells N et al: Does tympanic temperature measure up? *MCN Am J Matern Child Nurs* 20:95, 1995.

Wiswell TE et al: *Staphylococcus aureus* colonization after neonatal circumcision in relation to device used, *J Pediatr* 119(2):302, 1991.

*Classic reference.

 ## Student Resource Shelf

Darby MK, Loughead JL: Neonatal nutritional requirements and formula composition: a review, *J Obstet Gynecol Neonatal Nurs* 25(3):209, 1996.

Review of requirements and sources of formulas.

J Nurse Midwifery 37(suppl 2), 1992.

Entire issue devoted to infant care issues: infant nutrition, assessment, circumcision, and drug use.

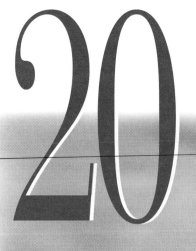

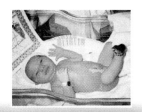

20 Home Care *of* *the* Young Infant

Learning Objectives

- Identify the process of initial attachment, and relate parent-infant interactions to the various infant temperaments.
- Compare normal growth and development milestones, while recognizing the unique responses of a particular infant.
- Discuss the infant cues to learning, as well as the process of and need for stimulation.
- Identify the essentials for basic home care of the infant.
- Describe the steps in the home health visit, the need for follow-up care, and the need for referral to various health care agencies.
- Describe immunizations recommended during the first year, including timing and potential adverse reactions.
- Review measures necessary for the infant's safety in the environment.
- Describe anticipatory guidance for parents to ensure health maintenance during infancy.
- Know adoption and foster care guidelines.

Key Terms

Acquaintance
Attachment
Bond Formation
Claiming Cues
Colic
Continuity
Cradle Cap
Diaper Rash
En Face Position
Gaze Aversion
Goodness-of-Fit
Infant Cues
Infant Stimulation
Parental Role Cues
Reye's Syndrome
Rhythmic Neonatal Functions
Self-Consolation
Temperament

$\mathcal{C}$oming home with a newborn infant is an experience requiring the total attention of the parents. Everything is new, and the infant's needs are largely unknown. Growing into the role of new parent will take approximately 1 to 3 months; adaptation includes being comfortable with reading the infant's cues to hunger, distress, and pain or anger and with being able to satisfy the infant's needs. Small successes breed greater confidence, and confidence is essential. Parents must have support while their confidence grows.

Anticipatory guidance about the growth and development of the infant's abilities and needs should focus on the way parents will be able to recognize needs and manage care. The nurse's role during this time has always included guiding and teaching. However, there have been major changes in health care delivery that require more intense preparation. In the past, new mothers stayed several days in the hospital after delivery, allowing the postpartum staff more time to assess the mother-infant dyad and to teach parents the basics of child care. Today, under insurance strictures and the increase in managed care, new mothers and infants may be discharged 12 to 48 hours after vaginal birth and 3 to 4 days after cesarean birth. These changes reduce the amount of postpartum teaching in the hospital and necessitate careful identification of the mother and infant who require home care follow-up.

Some insurance groups and managed care organizations will pay for new mothers to have one or more visits from a home care nurse; others will cover payments for these visits only if specific problems have been identified. These problems usually involve mothers who are very young, have a chronic illness (such as diabetes or hypertension), or have a history of substance abuse or domestic violence; infants who have congenital birth defects or are identified as poor feeders in the hospital; or an assessed problem in mother-infant attachment. It is easy to see how many of these problems can be missed by a postpartum staff that only has 12 to 48 hours for assessment. For this reason, nurses in physicians' offices, clinics, and emergency departments should be alert to the need for home care referrals after the initial hospital discharge (Hardy-Havens and Hannan, 1996).

The nurse in the postpartum or nursery area usually provides immediate help and anticipatory guidance. The home care nurse's role is to follow up on helping the parents make adjustments at home. There are many areas of childcare and postpartum self-care that may necessitate nursing intervention. Though all mothers and all infants will not have adjustment problems, it is helpful to have a comprehensive teaching tool to identify possible areas of concern that require follow-up. A sample teaching pathway during a home visit appears in Figure 20-1. Though the focus of this chapter is on home care of the infant, the nurse giving comprehensive care will recognize that the mother and infant continue to affect each other even after delivery, therefore maternal responses to infant behavior become an important part of any newborn assessment (see Chapter 17).

ATTACHMENT AFTER BIRTH

In pregnancy, achievement of the motherhood self-image is built first on prenatal attachment to the "fantasy" infant. After birth, the parents must reconcile this image with the "real" infant. In addition to the physical separation of birth, there is a psychologic process of separating from the unity and oneness of pregnancy and forming a new relationship with the child in the outside world (Rubin, 1977). Many factors influence how well this attachment proceeds, including maternal parity and previous parenting experiences, parental attitudes toward the infant, socioeconomic status, and the condition of the mother and infant. Parent-child bonding is a process that involves the steps of *acquaintance, attachment,* and *bond formation* (see Chapter 8).

Acquaintance

During pregnancy, an infant's health can be inferred only from secondary sources such as fetal monitors or ultrasound. After delivery, however, the parents can observe the newborn directly and are hungry for affirmation of the infant's well-being.

The parents have a strong urge for visual, then tactile, observations. The visual contact helps the mother psychologically relocate her infant as existing outside of herself. If the infant is healthy, she touches him, beginning with a light fingertip inquiry, tracing contours, counting fingers and toes, and feeling the texture of hair and skin, moving toward the center of the body. This process of **acquaintance** will be repeated over and over in the early days until the mother's discoveries are confirmed and stabilized for recognition (Rubin, 1984).

With these discoveries, each facet of the newborn's appearance or behavior will be bound into the parents' selves and family system by the process of claiming. This is one of the early tasks of parenthood. New parents often claim that the infant's features "look like" his or hers or grandmother's or another family member's. This linking is a way of claiming the newborn and incorporating him into the family system.

At the same time, the new mother is examining the "fit" of this new relationship. As she examines her infant's body with her fingertips (Figure 20-2; see also Figure 8-7), she looks for cues from the infant. Fingertip touch causes the newborn to turn toward the touch and to contract the muscle tissues around it. The infant finds touch pleasurable. When the lips are touched, the infant produces a "kiss" or "smile," or when the palm is stroked, the infant grasps the finger. Sometimes, the touch is not as pleasurable to the infant; when the brow is stroked, he may grimace, thus causing the mother to withdraw and resume exploration elsewhere. Through the repeated experience of "reading" the infant's cues, the new parents gain a sense of both infant predictability and competence in their ability.

Attachment

After recognizing and claiming the infant as their own, the parents begin to form bonds with the infant; these bonds occur through time and will ensure commitment to the infant's care. Both parents enter this process; perhaps it takes more time for the father if he must be out of the home for much of the day. (Parenting leave helps to allow this early attachment time.)

Studies show that a predictable group of reciprocal interactions takes place to foster and reinforce **attachment**. Each interaction between the mother or father and the newborn elicits a response in the other that is satisfying to both. For example, the infant cries, triggering soothing and comforting behaviors by the parent that satisfy the infant;

Newborn Educational Assessment and Teaching Pathway

MATRIA HEALTHCARE OF NEW YORK, INC.

Patient Name: _____   Patient ID# _____

SS#: _____ Date:_____/_____/_____

Baby's Name: _____

Circle Y or N for Yes or No
✓ = Objective met
* = Needs reinforcement
N/A = ~~Not Applicable~~
Int = Initials

Assessment & Teaching	Prior Inst.	Expected Outcome	Outcome		
			Status	Date	Int

KNOWLEDGE NEEDS RELATED TO NEWBORN CARE
A. Bathing   C. Cord Care
B. Skin Care   D. Nail Care
E. Clothing
F. Diapering
    * elimination patterns   * genitalia care
    * diaper rash   * circumcision care
G. Use of thermometer   I. Positioning
H. Use of the bulb syringe
	Y N
	
	Y N
		At the completion of the nursing visitit the mother is able to verbalize or demonstrate appropriate and safe newborn care.
		
		Environmental temperature and baby's clothing appropriate for thermoregulation.			

ALTERATION IN INFANT NUTRITION
A. Breastfeeding   * positions
    * supplements   * scheduled vs. demand
    * pumping and storage   * introduction to solid foods
B. Bottlefeeding   * frequency and amount
    * cleaning bottles   * introduction to solid foods
	Y N	At the completion of the nursing visit the mother expresses a comfort level with feeding method chosen and is able to express or demonstrate the appropriate feeding technique.			

KNOWLEDGE NEEDS REGARDING INFANT SAFETY A. Car seat usage C. Emergency measures B. Choking/CPR	Y N	At the time of the nursing visit the mother is able to state safety measures for her newborn and available resources.			

POTENTIAL FOR INFECTION, FLUID, AND WEIGHT LOSS (COMPLICATIONS)
Mother is instructed to call physician if infant has:
A. Fever
B. Persistent vomiting
C. Persistent diarrhea
D. No interest in eating
E. Excessive drowsiness
F. Jaundice (yellowing of the skin)
G. Excessive crying or unusual irritability
H. Foul odor or purulent drainage from cord or circumcision
FOLLOW-UP VISITS
A. Growth and Development
B. Immunizations
		1. At the time of the nursing visit the baby does not have a fever and the mother is able to describe signs of infection.
		2. Newborn's weight is stable or increasing.
		3. Feedings are well tolerated with no:
		   *vomiting *choking
		   *large spit-up (amount of regurgitation)
		4. The mother is able to express signs of dehydration.
		5. The mother is able to express when to call the health care provider for problems and concerns.
		6. The mother verbalizes understanding of hyperbilirubinemia (if applicable)
		7. The mother is able to state the importance of follow-up visits to the physician for assessments and health of her infant.			

❑ Newborn Discharge Summary included in Postpartum Teaching Pathway

Referral made: ❑ Yes ❑ No By whom?_____

Follow up with Health Care Provider: ❑ Yes ❑ No Whom?_____ Notified at: _____

Discharge Instructions Given: ❑ Verbal ❑ Written ❑ None

Discharge Reason: ❑ Therapy Completed   ❑ Admitted to Hospital   ❑ Patient Refused
                   ❑ Physician Request   ❑ Unsafe for Home Care   ❑ Other_____

Summary of Care and Services Provided:
   ❑ Maternal Assessment   ❑ Other Home Care Therapy   ❑ Breast Pump Rental   ❑ Other Labwork Drawn
   ❑ Newborn Assessment   ❑ Self-Care Instruction   ❑ Infant Immunization Schedule ❑ IV Therapy
   ❑ Phototherapy Dates:____to____ ❑ Baby Care Instruction   ❑ PKU   ❑ Antepartum Visit

Patient Status and Achievement of Goals - Verbalized Understanding Of:
❑ Environmental safety   ❑ When to call physician   ❑ Self-Care   ❑ Infant Care

Postpartum Appt: ❑ Scheduled ❑ Agrees to Schedule   Well Baby Visit: ❑ Scheduled ❑ Agrees to Schedule

Written Physician/Health Care Provider Notification - Copy of: ❑ This Form ❑ Visit Record:

❑ Faxed:___/___/___ ❑ Mailed:___/___/___ ❑ Given:___/___/___   to Maternal Health Care Provider:_____

❑ Faxed:___/___/___ ❑ Mailed:___/___/___ ❑ Given:___/___/___   to Infant Health Care Provider:_____
                                                                                                  Date

Figure 20-1   Newborn Educational Assessment and Teaching Pathway. (Courtesy Matria Healthcare of New York, Comprehensive obstetrical home care and maternity management.)

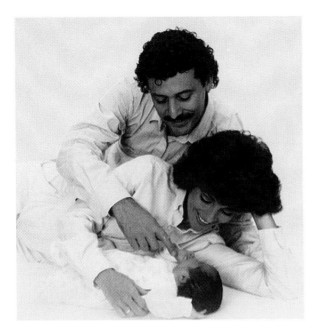

Figure 20-2 Fingertip exploration. (Courtesy Marjorie Pyle, RNC, *Lifecircle*.)

the infant then becomes quiet, thus satisfying the parent and enhancing self-esteem and confidence in care-giving skills (Figure 20-3). Attachment, now synonymous with "bonding," is defined as a slowly developing, continual, reciprocal affectionate tie that occurs over time (Gay, 1981). (See Chapter 8 for prenatal attachment.)

In early studies on attachment, Klaus and Kennell (1982) identified touch, vocalization, eye contact, odor, heat, hormonal and antibody exchange, entrainment, and time giving as major components involved in early attachment (Figure 20-4). By *touch,* the new mother gains knowledge of her infant's responses and a kinesthetic sense of his texture, temperature, moisture, and contours. Maternal touch helps the infant define body boundaries and will contribute to his sense of self-worth in the months to come. The mother touches the infant first with her fingertips, then progresses to massages with palm contact. The mother positions the infant for eye-to-eye contact, which helps establish the infant's identity and provide positive feedback to his parents; this is called *reciprocal interaction.*

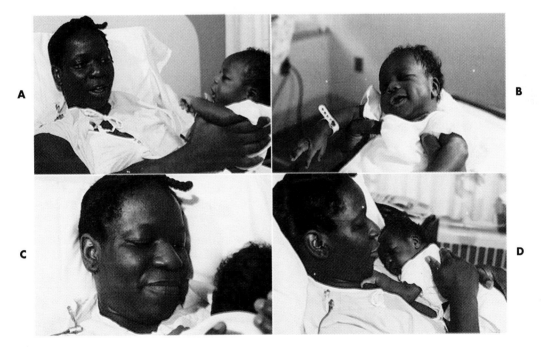

Figure 20-3 **A,** Early acquaintance process proceeding well. **B,** The mother first holds the infant away to look at her. **C,** The mother then brings her infant close, noticing details. **D,** Finally, she cuddles her up close. The nurse should wait and allow the natural sequence of bonding to occur rather than urging the mother to immediately cuddle the infant. (Courtesy Concept Media, Irvine, Calif.)

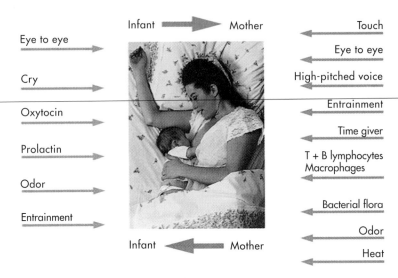

Figure 20-4 Mother-to-infant and infant-to-mother interactions can occur simultaneously in the first days of life. (Modified from Klaus MH, Kennell JH: *Parent-infant bonding,* ed 2, St Louis, 1982, Mosby. Courtesy Ross Laboratories, Columbus, Ohio.)

Eye contact

For new mothers, the need to look into the infant's eyes is nearly universal. Comments like "Open your eyes and then I'll know that you're real" are common. Parents often hold infants upright in the **en face position** (face-to-face) in an attempt to look into the infant's eyes. This eye contact strongly evokes parental feelings (Figure 20-5).

Pitch of voice

Infants are more responsive to and comfortable with high-pitched voices, enhancing the probability that the speaker will continue to speak in this range. Because of vibrations in the inner ear, the infant may cry when approached by a person with a deep, loud voice.

Cry

Crying brings an immediate reaction from the caregiver to soothe the infant or look for the cause of distress. The ability to interpret the cry and comfort the infant will enhance the parent's self-esteem; inability to provide comfort leads to feelings of failure. Thus it is difficult for parents to care for an infant with colic or withdrawal from drugs.

Odor

The olfactory sense also helps the process of identification and attachment. Studies have indicated that by approximately 5 days of age, breast-fed infants can discriminate between the breast pads of their own mother and those of others. Many mothers report that each of their infants had his or her own scent.

Heat

In times past, a mother provided heat for her infant by wrapping him and placing him close against her body.

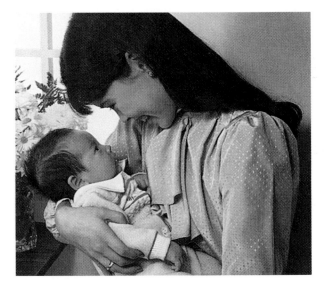

Figure 20-5 Mother-infant reciprocal interaction. (Courtesy Ross Laboratories, Columbus, Ohio.)

This method is less important in many cultures because of central heat, but using a front infant carrier does bring comfort to the infant.

Entrainment

Entrainment is the synchronization of the infant's movement to the patterns and rhythms of the mother's speech. When there is a change in the speech pattern, such as a pause or an accented syllable, subtle changes in the infant's behavior are noted.

Time giver

The rhythm of the mother's speech is only a part of entrainment. The intricate pattern of response of the

Box 20-1 | **Clues to Difficulty in Parent-Infant Bond Formation**

The nurse will be alerted to potential problems in mother-infant bond formation if:
- The mother is young or immature.
- The mother must struggle against a nonsupportive or isolated environment.
- The mother is beset by stress-causing situations (e.g., poor environmental conditions, serious illness in the family, severe disappointment, or rapid and repeated pregnancies) in addition to the birth of the new infant.
- The mother is separated from her infant for a prolonged period after birth (e.g., prematurity, maternal illness).

The nurse will strongly suspect that there is a problem in parent-infant attachment if:
- The parent expresses inappropriate feelings (e.g., anger, frustration, or helplessness) in response to the infant's crying.
- The parent fails to express anything about the infant that she or he likes (i.e., the parent has not found in the infant a claiming clue—a physical or psychologic attribute valued in self).
- The parent expresses unresolved feelings over a "dream" child (e.g., disappointment over the sex of the infant).
- The parent expresses mostly negative feelings about the infant (e.g., disgust over messy diapers or a perception that the infant is too demanding).
- The parent expresses expectations of the infant far beyond the infant's developmental stage.
- The parent fails to exhibit close, gentle, physical contact with the infant (e.g., holds infant away from body, plays roughly, or avoids eye contact and the en face position).

fetus to its mother's sleep-wake cycle and hormonal patterns are thrown out of equilibrium by birth. As a result, the mother becomes a "time giver" for the infant after he is born; in other words, she causes the formation of **rhythmic neonatal functions** (Klaus and Kennell, 1982). An example of this is the frequency with which the mother holds the infant in the alert state (which reinforces the infant). In this state, he is awake and ready to respond to her cues (which is reinforcing to the mother). The mother's steady routine of holding the infant when she wants him awake and of quieting when she wishes him to sleep helps establish predictable sleeping and waking patterns.

Hormonal stimulation

The infant's breast-feeding or stimulation of the breast by licking or touch induces the release of the maternal hormones oxytocin and prolactin. Although this interaction does not occur with a formula-fed infant, every mother gives her infant her antibodies prenatally and gives her bacterial flora postnatally (see Figure 20-4).

Therefore in many ways the infant's responsiveness reinforces the parents and encourages them to continue interaction. The result is a stable bond between the infant and parents that will endure and that will not be extinguished despite separations. **Bond formation** is an outgrowth of reciprocal attachment-stimulus response and affectional ties that form a coordinated, constructive social relationship. It is possible to only infer that bonding is progressing satisfactorily through observation of attachment behavior (i.e., behaviors that serve to maintain contact with and demonstrate affection toward the infant) (Figure 20-6). See Box 20-1 for clues to difficulty in parent-infant bonding formation.

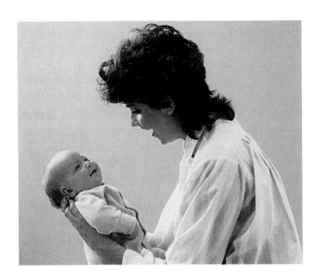

Figure 20-6   Social smile. (Courtesy Ross Laboratories, Columbus, Ohio.)

INFANT TEMPERAMENT AND PARENTAL RESPONSES

Differences in children amaze and puzzle parents. One child will be easy to raise, whereas the next will be difficult. In any effort to explain behavior, parents will point out how different a child is from themselves and other children and will search for **claiming cues**—is she like my own mother or my sister? Does she react like this because of some way I am treating her?

These claiming cues are observed in the immediate postnatal period, when the parents begin to explore and touch the infant with fingertips. Parents will describe characteristics that the infant shares with other family members, as well as remark on unique features. (This initial reaction is important, even if the infant is stillborn. [Kodadek, 1986].)

The *degree of consolidation cues* is observed during the first 2 months, when the parent talks to the infant in endearing terms and infant response is observed. Parents are still uncertain and often seek guidance and reassurance that they are perceiving their infant's responses correctly.

Growth in **parental role cues** is observed after the second month, as parents adjust to their infant and become comfortable with infant care. If positive cues are not observed, further evaluation must be done to diagnose potential or real alteration in role. Early intervention to support and teach parents will usually bring long-term positive changes.

Meaning of Temperament

Today, it is fairly clear that **temperament** is distinctly identifiable early in infancy, although its impact on behavior may not be seen until early childhood. Chess and Thomas (1985) defined temperament as "the general nature or characteristic mood of the individual determining the general way a person behaves." Others have defined temperament as the behavioral style, the "how" of behavior, which includes such things as degree of approach behavior, activity level, degree of persistence in performing activities, and mood characteristics (positive or negative) (Coffman, Levitt, Guacci-Franco, 1995). Chess and Thomas describe nine aspects of temperament:

- Activity level—the proportion of active and inactive periods
- Rhythmicity—the predictability versus the unpredictability of biologic functions
- Adaptability—the response to change imposed by situations or others
- Approach or withdrawal—initial response to new people or situations
- Sensory threshold—amount of stimulus (touch, sound) needed to produce a response
- Intensity of reaction—the level of response
- Quality of mood—amount of joyful, playful, or friendly behavior
- Distractibility—how easily ongoing behavior can be diverted
- Persistence—the length of time engaged in a difficult activity

When parents need help in understanding their infant, temperament must be recognized. The infant's and parents' temperaments determine the **goodness-of-fit**, or how well the infant integrates into the family (see Chapter 2). If the infant easily meets the parents' expectations, the transition is easy. Medoff-Cooper et al (1995) state that "achieving a goodness-of-fit between a parent's expectation and the child's behavioral style is a critical element of a positive parent-child relationship."

Dissimilarity often leads parents to label the child as "difficult," requiring much more energy and patience than they expected. The nurse noting comments such as, "Where did this baby come from?" can inquire about the parents' expectations versus the reality of the infant's patterns of behavior. For instance, parents become distressed when an infant develops colic and may confuse colic with a difficult temperament (see colic, later in this chapter).

A number of tools have been developed to identify infant temperament (Medoff-Cooper, 1995; Carey and McDevitt, 1978). The *Infant Temperament Questionnaire* (ITQ) (Carey and McDevitt, 1978) may be used to assess parents' perception of their infant between 4 and 8 months of age. Today, there are many questionnaires based on this ITQ. The ITQ assumes that temperament is a stable characteristic. When the answers are scored, the child is placed into one of the following behavioral groups: (1) easy, (2) slow to warm up, (3) difficult, (4) intermediate high difficulty, and (5) intermediate low difficulty. The ITQ appears to be a useful tool in acquainting parents with their infant. Because there are more than 90 questions, Box 20-2 shows only a sample of the questions that may be asked for each of the nine categories they define.

1. The *easy* child is characterized by a positive rhythmic mood, and has a low to moderate intensity of reaction. This child is adaptable and predictable in most circumstances, as long as expectations are consistent.

2. In the *slow-to-warm-up* child, response is less apparent. This infant responds with tentative withdrawal and slower adaptability, lower intensity, and a mildly negative mood when stimulated. This child gradually adapts to new situations as long as the parent is patient, relaxed, and does not force the child to demonstrate specific expected behaviors. As the child grows, limits for behavior should be set with leeway given for individual differences.

3. The *difficult* child may be unpredictable, extremely active, and intense and may tend to withdraw in situations and have a negative mood. The parents must help this child by clearly setting limits, which requires patience and a consistent set of parental behaviors.

   The parents may be upset or disappointed with the difficult child's reactions and must be reassured that their own parenting skills are not at fault. The child will need gentle and repeated negative and positive reinforcement. Rules should be simple and few, and specific outlets should be planned for this energetic child.

4. Finally, the *intermediate* child is one who is a mix of these three sets of characteristics and may be of intermediate high difficulty or intermediate low difficulty.

Infants display distinct individuality in temperament in the first weeks of life. In addition, studies show that maternal postpartum depression will negatively influence infant temperament (Beck, 1996). Responsiveness to stimulation is directly related to infant temperament. For instance, Korner (1990) has shown a significant relation-

| *Box* **20-2** | **Sample Items by Category from the Revised Infant Temperament Questionnaire*** |

ACTIVITY

The infant moves about much (many kicks, grabs, or squirms) during diapering and dressing.

The infant plays actively with parents (much movement of arms, legs, and body).

RHYTHMICITY

The infant wants and takes milk feedings at about the same times (within 1 hour) from day to day.

The infant's bowel movements come at different times (over 1 hour difference from day to day).

APPROACH OR WITHDRAWAL

The infant immediately accepts any change in place or position of feeding or the person giving it.

For the first few minutes in a new place or situation (new store or home), the infant is fretful.

ADAPTABILITY

The infant objects to being bathed in a different place or by a different person (after 3 months), even after two or three tries.

The infant accepts regular procedures (hair brushing, face washing) any time without protest.

INTENSITY

The infant reacts strongly to foods, whether positively (smacks lips, laughs, or squeals) or negatively (cries).

The infant reacts mildly to meeting familiar people (quiet smiles or no response).

MOOD

The infant is pleasant (smiles or laughs) when first arriving in unfamiliar places (friend's house or store).

PERSISTENCE

The infant amuses self for 30 minutes or more in crib or playpen (looking at mobile or playing with toy).

The infant watches other children playing for under 1 minute and then looks elsewhere.

DISTRACTABILITY

The infant stops play and watches when someone walks by.

The infant continues to cry despite several minutes of soothing.

THRESHOLD

The infant reacts to even a gentle touch (startle, wriggle, laugh, or cry).

The infant reacts to a disliked food even when it is mixed with a preferred one.

*The mother rates each of the following items on a scale of 1 to 6: 1—almost never; 6—almost always. Revised in 1977 by WB Carey and SC McDevitt. The entire instrument is available for $10. Send to WB Carey, MD, 319 West Front Street, Media, PA 19063.

ship between neonatal activity and responses with later activity levels and temperament between ages 4 and 8 years. The ability to persist in tasks is elicited in the *Dimensions of Mastery Questionnaire* (DMQ) designed for use with an older infant. The DMQ assesses the parents' perceptions of the infant's skill mastery in four areas: persistence, mastery pleasure, independent mastery, and competence (Morrow and Camp, 1996). Even in an infant younger than 7 months, the parents can be encouraged to promote infant learning and skill accomplishment by following the principles listed in Box 20-3.

Self-Discovery

Think about the temperaments expressed in your siblings and parents. Are there clashes in temperament? How does your family work these out? ~

SIGNIFICANCE OF GROWTH AND DEVELOPMENT

The idea of successful growth and development involving completion of tasks across the life cycle was introduced by Erikson and is accepted today as a standard. Parents must realize that the infant's behavior is an attempt to master these tasks. Without an understanding of this need, parents may respond in a way that hinders this attainment by acting in more controlling ways and not allowing free exploration (see Box 20-3).

The first few months of life establish the groundwork for the ability to love and trust. Because the infant may sleep for a majority of the day, parents often believe the infant is not learning from them or the environment. In reality, the new infant is responding intensely, especially to the emotional tone of the caregivers. The extent to which the infant interacts with the environment has only begun to be appreciated. Instructing parents about the newborn's visual, auditory, and cognitive abilities helps them begin appropriate stimulation for intellectual, social, and emotional growth. They may also learn to prevent adverse stimulation.

Recognizing that successful growth and development are important, the nurse who is able to assess the infant's progress may be able to identify developmental delays and suggest early interventions to overcome lags (Collin, 1995). A number of studies with premature infants have found that appropriate stimulation may allow these infants to catch up in terms of growth and development. Studies also show that there are significant differences between infants whose mothers use appropriate stimulation and understand infant cues and those whose mothers

| Box 20-3 | Ways to Promote Infant Learning and Mastery Motivation |

- Encourage unobtrusive assistance during play.
- Share pleasure in accomplishments with infant.
- Do not give immediate assistance during tasks.
- Do not interrupt infant during tasks.
- Let infant initiate activities.
- Limit controlling feedback during play.
- Provide auditory and visually responsive toys.
- Provide early kinesthetic stimulation (picking up or rocking).

From Morrow JD, Camp BW: Mastery motivation and temperament of 7-month-old infants, *Pediatric Nursing* 22(3):215, 1996.

do not (Mahler, Pine, and Berman, 1975). The nurse who understands the importance of parental input can strongly encourage and guide parents in positive interaction with their infant.

Biophysical maturation may be assessed by examining the infant's ability to control gross and fine motor movements, as well as the responses to sound, color, and light. The infant is observed for motor tone, social interaction, growth, and sleep patterns. If these assessments are within the normal ranges, the infant is thought to be developing well.

Cognitive growth is assessed by observing the infant's curiosity and interest in the environment. The infant who reaches monthly milestones in a timely manner shows the ability to manipulate and interact with the environment. Tests of infant intelligence also exist (Fagan and Detterman, 1992).

Verbal growth is assessed by observing the infant's attempts at vocalization. Note the quality of voice and communication with parents and others, the increasing depth of comprehension, and the ability to communicate in verbal and nonverbal ways.

First Task: Development of Trust

Infants are the center of their own worlds They are preoccupied with their own needs and experience the outside world only as it meets their needs. It is as if the infant believes that there is a magical connection to the mother. A need is expressed, and someone answers it; this is their first understanding of relationship.

Positive, comforting early encounters with the repetition, **continuity**, and routine of the parenting experience are the infant's building blocks for developing an internal framework of trust. With *continuity* and *repetition*, perceptions are organized into the earliest memories. Feeding is probably the most significant activity, because of its frequency and

routine of physical gratification; it is organized into memories of satisfaction and pleasure. Sensations in the infant's mouth and stomach experienced while feeding are of such intense gratification that these become the unconscious essence of satisfaction throughout the rest of life.

The child is also stimulated and gratified through cuddling and simple play. The child responds and begins to subtly "understand" the personal warmth the mother transmits through her body and tender gestures. As needs are met, the infant is able to direct increased amounts of attention toward the outer world.

Without parents who gratify and stimulate, the young infant concentrates only on unmet inner needs, particularly the demands of hunger and touching. The infant who is left for long periods without personal contact or is left to cry when food or other forms of attention are needed learns not to expect satisfaction of these needs (i.e., learns to *mistrust*.) As a result, the infant may develop primarily in a self-absorbed way and exclude the outside world. Thus *spoiling* is not an issue in this early period. Rather, parents are taught to promptly and consistently meet the infant's needs in as comforting a way as possible. When parents understand the importance of their actions on future development, most are eager to interact in these ways.

Perception of feeling

While developing a relationship with the mother, the infant is learning how the mother feels. Initially, the infant will reflect on and remember only the mother's feeling tone, but later, as the ability to perceive and remember develops, the infant will remember particular things about their relationship. If a child has a mother who can provide the necessary emotional atmosphere, the early impressions are warmth, tenderness, comfort, and as a result, the "satisfying" milk from the mother. If, however, the mother is unable to provide a healthy emotional tone, early impressions are isolation, frustration, coldness, and as a result, "undesirable" milk from the mother. Even food can be given in such a way as to make it seem bitter; thus feeding is not a nurturing experience. Even at a very early stage, inadequate mothering can greatly affect the child's development because the impressions developed at this stage are carried for the rest of the child's life. Because early fundamental feelings are essential to personality makeup, adults who have had an unsatisfying infancy may not have met their first task and are thus unable to move on to accomplish later tasks. As a result, some children continue to act in "babyish" ways until they reach adolescence. In adolescence they rebel or overreact and may become destructive in their desire to be independent. As adults they can be dependent and cling to friends, spouses, or parents as they seek someone who will consistently meet emotional needs. This is one example of why it is necessary for infants to have positive relationships. If trust is not established early, further development is impeded.

Development of the Senses

The sensory system parallels other systems in that it is initially uncontrolled and unrefined and requires physical maturation and experience to develop. Thus although the infant receives sensory input readily, the ability to interpret this input accompanies maturation.

Touch and motion perception

Motion and touch are perhaps the most important perceptions to the infant. Although tactile sensation has not been studied in depth, research has shown that the fetus in utero responds to manipulation of the mother's abdomen by squirming away. After birth, skin conveys sensations from patting, stroking, cuddling, carrying, and diapering. Touch creates quiet states and decreases tension. For instance, an infant will move around in a crib against the crib wall before relaxing and falling asleep. Infants wrapped snugly tend to sleep more soundly and be less fretful.

Response to stroking and the rooting reflex is increased over the first 5 days of life. Skin-to-skin stroking is extremely soothing for an adult, and many parents are now stroking infants lightly, though they use the misleading term *infant massage* to describe this activity. Infant stroking is a widely used relaxation therapy in other countries (e.g., in India a baby is rubbed with oil several times a day). Strokes should move from central to distal regions from head to toe. When stroking the head, move from the forehead to the occiput. Stroking is used with premature infants because it promotes more regular respirations and reduces periods of apnea (Field et al, 1988).

Most children and adults respond with satisfaction to hugging and loving touches. (When a child does not respond positively, inquire further into early tactile experiences.) Field's 1995 research indicates that both healthy infants and those with medical conditions respond positively to light massage therapy. They exhibit lower anxiety and stress hormones and have an improved clinical course. Field suggests that grandparent volunteers and parents be taught these massage techniques to improve their own wellness and provide this cost-effective treatment for the child.

Vestibular sensitivity reflects body posture, balance, and the sense of falling. The canals of the inner ear are functional at birth but must develop further afterward. Vestibular sense is integrated with visual perception slowly; the infant is unaware of heights from only visual perception. Even up to 3 years of age, children will climb and jump with no real idea of how far they are above a surface.

The awareness of motion is already acute at birth, having been present in utero. Infants respond with pleasure to rhythmic rocking motions and to tactile sensations of warmth, closeness, and snugness (see Cultural Awareness box). An infant's consolability often relates to body position (e.g., an infant becomes more alert and quiet when held upright). Infants enjoy being rocked, riding in cars or strollers, or swinging. One sign of neglect may be a child rocking himself or moving rhythmically and restlessly in the crib.

CULTURAL AWARENESS

The mothering pattern of the Kikuyu tribe of central Kenya stands out as strikingly different from many American styles. Infants are almost never put down, whether for sleep or any other reason. They are continuously carried, usually tied on their mothers' backs, and therefore are rarely deprived of physical contact with their mothers.

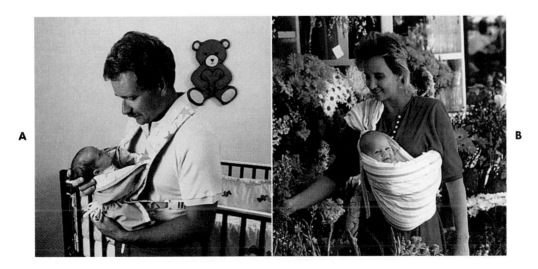

Figure 20-7   **A,** Father with Snugli carrier. **B,** Mother with sling carrier. (**A,** Courtesy Ross Laboratories, Columbus, Ohio; **B,** Courtesy Marjorie Pyle, RNC, *Lifecircle*.)

Recognizing the value of body contact gained from observation of cultures that use infant carriers, many American parents are now using such carriers for young infants. The infant sleeps well and seems to find pleasure being close to the parent's body in this way (Figure 20-7). Nurses must reinforce the importance of early kinesthetic stimulation for the infant through being picked up, rocked, and carried through space. The hospitalized infant also needs this movement (Morrow and Camp, 1996).

Hearing and verbalization

At around 6 months of gestation, the fetus begins to move in rhythm with maternal speech. Response to music while in utero has been noted; infants are soothed by quiet music and become more active with noisy music. Preterm infants are soothed by the effects of music and the mother's voice.

At birth the auditory canal is shorter in the infant than in the adult, and higher tones are tolerated more easily than those of lower frequency (resonance). The closer the infant is to the sound, the easier discrimination will be. Little reaction occurs below the level of normal speaking voices (50 to 60 decibels). Infants tend to like sounds around the higher range of the human voice and are sensitive to rhythmic and continuous sound. Infants like to listen to sentences uttered with exaggerated variation in pitch.

Auditory responses in infancy are as follows:

4 to 5 weeks—Occasional turning of eyes in direction of sound origin

4 months—Consistent turning of head toward site of sound; widening of eyes; quiet, listening attitude (audio-visual link important)

6 months—Turning toward sound; recognizing it below eye level first, then above eye level

Groundwork for verbal ability begins to be developed long before words are spoken. Ruben (1994) states that the cooing, babbling and crying are "protospeech," essential for developing language. Infants who have sensory deprivation from hearing loss show abnormal changes in their prespeech sounds. Many observers believe that infants whose mothers often talk to them tend to begin using words and sentences earlier than infants who are not so exposed (Table 20-1). *Thus the quality of linguistic exposure during the first few years of life will be a determinant of the child's linguistic ability* (Ruben, 1994). The ability to listen and to discriminate among sounds is an important task to be undertaken in the second half of the first year. Language comprehension precedes verbalization, and by 9 to 12 months the infant should be responding to simple commands such as "no." It is well known that an infant raised in a bilingual or trilingual setting will respond with the appropriate language to each speaker.

A verbal deficit should alert the parents to a possible physical problem. For instance, infants with hearing deficits often do not vocalize early. In fact, the Surgeon

Table **20-1**	**Normal Speech Development**
Age	**Speech**
1 month	Throaty sounds
2 months	Vowel sounds ("eh"), coos
3 months	Babbles, initial vowels ("ah")
4 months	Guttural sounds ("guh, goo"), some consonants
6 months	Imitates sounds, vocalize to toys ("m-m-m"); babbling intensifies
9-12 months	Language comprehension, understands "no"
	Begins articulation of short words ("mama, dada")

General warns that if an infant is not verbalizing "Mama" and "Papa" by 1 year, there may be a hearing problem. Infants should be evaluated at each well-baby visit for hearing deficiencies, which may develop from even minor head trauma, otitis media, and other infections.

Smell and taste

The sensation of smell is demonstrated by placing an alcohol swab under the newborn's nose and eliciting a startle reflex and a turn away from the smell. Facial expressions of rejection are similar to those of adults. The infant quickly becomes more sensitive to smell, and by the fifth day of life, a less potent smell elicits the same response. By the end of the first week, the infant can distinguish between the mother and a stranger by smell. The classic study on this ability was done by McFarlane (1975) with infants at 6, 8, and 10 days of age. When presented with a breast pad, these infants showed a consistent preference for the breast pad used by their own mother.

Research shows that the infant can discriminate tastes. Infants especially savor fluid that has been sweetened; the infant sucks harder and consumes more sweet fluid. When a sour and bitter taste is presented, facial expressions of rejection are similar to those of children and adults (Haith, 1986).

Sight

The visual ability of the fetus at 16 weeks is demonstrated by a startle reflex when strong light is shone on the mother's abdomen. All neurologic development for visual perception is functional before birth, but a number of studies indicate that the visual system experiences marked growth and development during the first 6 months (Box 20-4). At birth the infant's visual skill is an important factor in parent-infant attachment because it allows the infant to find, concentrate on, and prefer the human face to all other stimuli. Eyes can fixate on one object for a specific time and are especially attracted to contrasting pat-

Box 20-4   Early Visual Awareness

NEWBORN
Perceives changes in light intensity and movement
Blinks protectively
Follows bright object to midline if 6 to 8 inches from eyes

5 TO 6 WEEKS
Fixes gaze on object that is 12 to 24 inches away from eyes
Shows interest in bright colors, black and white patterns, faces

6 TO 12 WEEKS
Follows increasingly well objects that are 12 to 24 inches away from eyes

3 TO 5 MONTHS
Possesses rapidly developing visual and tactile links (see-touch-grasp)
Begins to inspect hands
Focuses increasingly on distance

Data from Holt K: *Developmental pediatrics,* London, 1977, Butterworths.

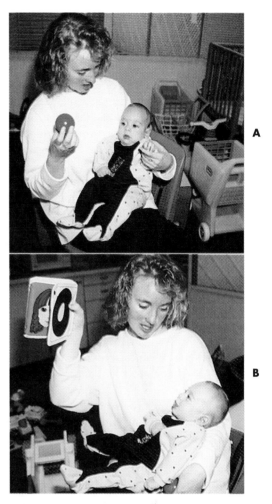

Figure 20-8   Presenting a red ball (**A**) and black and white diagrams (**B**) for infant interest. (Courtesy Marjorie Pyle, RNC, *Lifecircle.*)

terns. Initially the best focal point is approximately 10 to 12 inches away; this is the distance between faces when the infant is being held in the traditional feeding position. The infant can coordinate both eyes to move together and track a moving object for a short arc. The eyes can be oriented to an area to find an object (Figure 20-8). Changes in looking occur by about 2 months. Infants then detect changes in structure in pictures (e.g., faces with a frown instead of a smile or a box with a piece missing), indicating that perhaps structure is being recognized (Haith, 1986). Infants appear to enjoy primary colors, black and white contrasts, and colored mobiles that move (Figure 20-9).

Infant Stimulation Programs

It is now accepted and written into state regulations that early stimulation be provided for high-risk infants (Collin, 1995). The parents of normal newborns have concerns about how soon their infants should receive extra stimulation. This question never arose in the past; in extended families infants were always with some family member, and practices of child rearing were very different. Today, the infant may be with a baby-sitter or in day care or may have only a single parent with whom to interact.

There are activities parents may perform to stimulate an infant, but there must be a balance. Anxious, usually well-educated parents may misguidedly never give their infant a chance to build a routine or to relax because they insist on presenting multiple stimuli. On the other hand, as Horowitz (1990) indicates, it may be the parent's inability to *modulate*

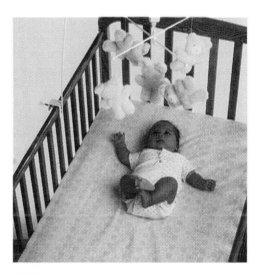

Figure 20-9   Crib mobiles keep the infant interested. (Courtesy Ross Laboratories, Columbus, Ohio.)

infant state (i.e., to console or calm a tired, crying infant) that predicts the possibility of future child abuse. The person who cannot deal with a crying infant may, in frustration, hit or hurt the infant. A more subtle abuse may be psychosocial, such as not allowing the infant or child to develop in a way that fits her unique temperament. Therefore nursing interventions can focus on teaching parents what to look for in infant states and responses, when to provide stimulation, and how to console the crying infant so as to alter the tension in an upset state.

Most of the work in **infant stimulation** studies has been done with preterm infants, but findings can be useful for parents of normal full-term infants. The goals for parent learning of **infant cues** have been spelled out in a number of early intervention programs. These goals include the following (Rauh et al, 1990).

1. Helping the parent focus on the infant's ways of responding by pointing out positive infant cues and the best interaction periods
2. Encouraging the parent to recognize signs of fatigue, exhaustion, overload, and hunger in the infant
3. Teaching parents when to stimulate, when to comfort, when to decrease stimulation, and how to encourage sleep
4. Teaching parents the progression of growth and development so they can note and enjoy the infant's rapid progress

Box **20-1**

CLINICAL DECISION

Andy's father did not know what to "say to a baby." He was a serious businessman who had had no prior experience with infants. He stated that he "felt silly" talking with an infant who could not respond. How could he be encouraged to vocalize with his infant?

Cues to infant responses

The kinds of visual cue the infant gives are related to time, attention, and gaze. In the early weeks, a newborn cannot maintain looking or gazing for more than a short period. As eye muscle control improves, the infant will scan and, if interested, focus, looking at an object for a longer period. By 2 months, **gaze aversion**, turning away from a person or object, signals that an infant needs a break from interaction. Brazelton (1978) made it clear that the infant has a drive to learn, seeks external satisfaction, and only "turns off" attention, as a defense, when it is too much, too fast, or when fatigue sets in. Adults respond in similar ways.

Infants learn best in the quiet alert state. If an infant becomes hyperalert and wide-eyed, almost staring during extended stimulation, she may be *overstimulated* and unable to break away. Encourage the parent to break eye contact to allow the infant to quiet down. Persistent stimulation (often by siblings) may cause the infant to turn away or stiffen with the palms outstretched. Stiffening and pulling away indicate that the infant wants a change. Body language is the infant's way of communicating.

On the other hand, early positive signs of an infant's enjoyment are lip pursing or sucking, leaning toward an object, or cuddling into the person holding her. Breathing and pulse become slower when the infant is interested (Haith, 1986). Families can learn to read their infant's messages easily after these messages are pointed out.

Self-consolation may be observed during evaluation with the *Brazelton Neonatal Assessment Scale* (see Chapter 18). During the assessment, it is a good time to point out these responses and encourage the parents to become aware of the infant's behavior. One pleasurable activity that decreases tension is sucking; infants need at least 120 minutes of sucking each day. If an infant takes formula or breast milk rapidly, nonnutritive sucking may supplement sucking time. The infant may quickly find a finger or thumb (Figure 20-10), or a pacifier may be used as a self-quieting tool for the infant. Help parents feel more accepting toward this behavior by using parallel examples in adults' self-consoling behaviors, such as chewing gum or eating when upset. Sucking must be done in an emotionally positive atmosphere. Thus propping a bottle should be avoided because it denies the gratification of interaction.

The Mother's Assessment of the Behavior of Her Infant (MABI) scale is a tool that may be used to help a mother become aware of her infant's patterns (Field et al, 1978). The scale is keyed to the Brazelton Assessment Scale. It was found using the MABI scale with lower socioeconomic-status teenage mothers of premature infants was useful and appeared to significantly increase their interaction with their infants. It is suggested that early use of the Brazelton scale at the bedside and the MABI may be a cost-effective way of affecting mother-infant interaction (Box 20-5).

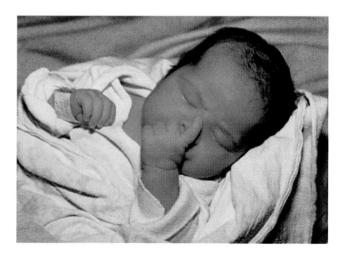

Figure 20-10 Hand-to-mouth consolation. (Courtesy Marjorie Pyle, RNC, *Lifecircle*.)

Box 20-5	MABI Questionnaire for Mothers, Modified from Brazelton Neonatal Assessment Scale*

Directions to the mother: Because a mother knows her baby better than anyone else, we would like you to give your impressions of your baby by circling answers to these questions. Before answering, you might want to watch your baby for a while and try playing some of the games with him or her. For example, before answering question 9, we ask you to shake a rattle to the side of your baby's face to see if he or she turns to look at the rattle. We have discovered that newborn babies can do many interesting things, which you will probably discover in your baby too.

1. *(Predominant state)* When you play with your baby he or she is often:
   - ☐ Sleepy (1-2, 2-3)
   - ☐ Alert (3-4, 4-5)
   - ☐ Upset (5-6)

2. *(Descriptive paragraph)* How would you describe your baby?
   - ☐ Fairly attractive (1)
   - ☐ Quite attractive (2)
   - ☐ Very attractive (3)

3. *(Descriptive paragraph)* How much do you have to stimulate your baby to get her to look at you?
   - ☐ Not very much (1)
   - ☐ A fair amount (2)
   - ☐ A lot (3)

4. *(Descriptive paragraph)* When your baby is upset, what does he or she do to quiet him- or herself?
   - ☐ Brings his or her hand to his or her mouth (1)
   - ☐ Sucks with nothing in his or her mouth (2)
   - ☐ Looks at you (3)

5. *(#9)* Try talking to your baby, holding your face about 1 foot away from his or her face, and then slowly move your face to one side and then to the other as you continue talking. When you do this, your baby:
   - ☐ Doesn't look at you (1-2)
   - ☐ Becomes quiet and looks at you (3-4)
   - ☐ Follows your face to each side with his or her head and eyes (5-7)
   - ☐ Follows your face with his or her head and eyes, up and down and to each side (8-9)

6. *(#7)* Now try the same thing, only move your face without talking. When you do this, your baby:
   - ☐ Doesn't look at you (1-2)
   - ☐ Becomes quiet (3-4)
   - ☐ Follows your face with his or her head and eyes (5-7)
   - ☐ Follows your face with his or her head and eyes, up and down and to each side (8-9)

7. *(#8)* Try talking to your baby from one side of his or her head and then from the other. When you do this, he or she:
   - ☐ Has no reaction or blinks (1-2)
   - ☐ Becomes quiet (3-4)
   - ☐ Turns his or her eyes and head to your voice once or twice (5-7)
   - ☐ Turns his or her eyes and head to your voice more than twice (8-9)

8. *(#5)* Now try holding a colorful toy or some shiny object in front of your baby's face and then move it slowly to each side of his or her head and then up and down in front of the face. When you do this he or she:
   - ☐ Doesn't look at the toy (1-2)
   - ☐ Becomes quiet and looks at the toy (3-4)
   - ☐ Follows the toy you are moving with his or her head and eyes (5-7)
   - ☐ Follows the toy you are moving with his or her head and eyes, up and down and to each side (8-9)

9. *(#6)* Try shaking a rattle on one side of your baby's head and then on the other side. When you do this, he or she:
   - ☐ Has no reaction or no blinks (1-2)
   - ☐ Becomes quiet (3-4)
   - ☐ Turns his or her eyes and head to the rattle once or twice (5-7)
   - ☐ Turns his or her eyes and head to the rattle more than twice (8-9)

10. *(#10)* When you did the preceding activities with your baby, he or she usually:
    - ☐ Paid little attention to you or the toy (1-2)
    - ☐ Had short periods of watching you or the toy (3-4)
    - ☐ Watched you or the toy for a fairly long time (5-7)
    - ☐ Paid attention most of the time (8-9)

11. *(#11)* How does your baby feel when you handle or hold him or her?
    - ☐ Limp like a rag doll (1-2)
    - ☐ Limp some of the time (3-4)
    - ☐ Relaxed but firm (5-6)
    - ☐ Very tense (7-9)

12. *(#12)* When your baby moves his or her arms, the movements are:
    - ☐ Jerky most of the time (1-2)
    - ☐ Jerky some of the time (3-4)
    - ☐ Smooth some of the time (5-7)
    - ☐ Smooth most of the time (8-9)

Modified from Field TM: University of Miami Medical Center, Mailman Center for Child Development, Miami, FL 33152. By permission of the author and *Infant Behavior and Development* 1:156, 1978.

*Note how questions parallel Brazelton items and scoring. The number of the Brazelton items that corresponds to the MABI item is placed in parentheses before the question; the corresponding Brazelton rating is placed in parentheses after each MABI rating.

Continued.

| *Box* 20-5 | **MABI Questionnaire for Mothers, Modified from Brazelton Neonatal Assessment Scale—cont'd** |

13. *(#14) When you pick up your baby and hold him or her in a rocking position, he or she:*
- ☐ Often swings his or her arms and kicks his or her legs and squirms (1-2)
- ☐ Is like a sack of meal in your arms (3-4)
- ☐ Relaxes and nestles his or her head in the crook of your arms (5-7)
- ☐ Moves his or her face toward you and reaches his or her hands out to grab your clothing (8-9)

14. *(#16) When your baby is crying very hard:*
- ☐ Nothing seems to quiet him or her
- ☐ Only a pacifier will quiet him or her (2)
- ☐ Holding and rocking will quiet him or her (3-6)
- ☐ Talking to him or her and holding your hand on the stomach quiets him or her (7-9)

15. *(#17) How would you describe your baby most of the time?*
- ☐ Very sleepy
- ☐ Awake a lot of the time and quiet
- ☐ Crying occasionally but easily quieted
- ☐ Crying a lot and difficult to quiet

16. *(#19) Please circle those activities that upset your baby:*
- ☐ Changing diaper (1-2)
- ☐ Undressing or dressing (3-4)
- ☐ Putting him or her back in the bassinet (5-7)
- ☐ Lying him or her on the stomach (8-9)

17. *(#20) How active is your baby?*
- ☐ Not very active
- ☐ Somewhat active
- ☐ Quite active
- ☐ Very active

18. *(#21) How often does your baby tremble when he or she is warmly dressed?*
- ☐ Not very often (1-2)
- ☐ Occasionally (3-4)
- ☐ Fairly often (5-6)
- ☐ Very often (7-9)

19. *(#23) How would you describe your baby's color changes?*
- ☐ Rarely changes color
- ☐ Changes to blue around the mouth when uncovered and to red when crying, but only for a minute (3-4)
- ☐ Changes color when uncovered or crying but changes back to his or her natural color when covered up or comfortable (5-6)
- ☐ Seems to get blue or red very often but will get his or her natural color back after being held for a while (7-9)

20. *(#24) How often and how quickly do your baby's moods change?*
- ☐ Sleeps most of the time and hardly ever cries (1-2)
- ☐ Is quiet much of the time (3-4)
- ☐ Goes back and forth from being quiet to crying fairly often (5-6)
- ☐ Often changes from being sleepy or quiet to crying and then back again—changes mood often and very quickly (7-9)

21. *(#25) When your baby is crying, how successful is he or she at self-quieting activities:*
- ☐ Cannot quiet self (1-2)
- ☐ Makes several attempts to quiet self but is usually unsuccessful (3-4)
- ☐ Has many brief successes at quieting self (5-6)
- ☐ Often quiets self for long periods (7-9)

22. *(#26) How would you describe your baby's hand-to-mouth activity?*
- ☐ Makes no attempt to bring hands to his or her mouth (1-2)
- ☐ Often brings hands next to his or her mouth (3-5)
- ☐ Sometimes puts fist or fingers in his or her mouth (6-7)
- ☐ Sometimes sucks on fist or fingers for as long as seconds at a time (8-9)

23. *(#23) How many times has your baby looked like he or she was smiling at you?*

Parental interventions for stimulation

Parents do not always instinctively know how to positively stimulate their infant. The nurse can offer teaching to help parents understand and promote early infant learning:

1. Explain the normal development of the senses and the relation of sleep states to responses. Infants respond best in the quiet alert state.
2. Assess the abilities of each infant before demonstrating how an infant responds. There is much variation in newborn and infant responses. Use the differences to introduce the topic of the uniqueness of each child.
3. Place the infant in a position that will promote eye-to-eye contact. Use mobiles over the infant's seat or crib.
   - Make mobiles out of cardboard with colors of dark and light contrast and medium intensity.
   - Use black and white contrast in stripes and checkerboards, as well as smiley faces.
   - Make the mobile light enough to respond to air movement.
   - Place the mobile low enough so the older infant can touch it, preferably with the feet.
4. Add auditory stimulation when possible.
   - Use soft, rhythmic sounds (singing, music boxes) but regulate the loudness (decibels).
   - Talk in higher tones, with variations in pitch.
   - Read stories, even to a young infant.
5. Promote tactile stimulation by encouraging skin-to-skin contact.
   - Learn infant stroking techniques.
   - Provide toys that have different textures.
   - Use a soft crib bumper.

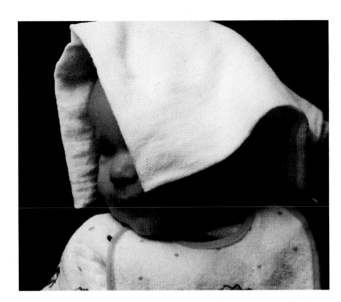

Figure 20-11   Teach parents how to play games with the infant. (Courtesy E Schult.)

- Carry the infant in a soft body carrier on the front of the parent; backpacks are appropriate only for older infants.
6. Since an infant learns through exploration and play, creative play should be fostered (Figure 20-11).
- Several books on games to play with infants are available for parents. These games were often passed on naturally to new parents in extended families but may have been forgotten in the generation of nuclear families.

HEALTH MAINTENANCE IN THE FIRST YEAR

Health maintenance is important because it allows the normal processes of growth and development to occur. In a positive setting, the infant is protected from the hazards of the environment. The infant whose physical and psychologic health is maintained is better prepared to live in an increasingly challenging world. Nursing care includes teaching parents about hazards to the infant. A young infant is vulnerable to temperature extremes, environmental hazards, and choking.

Automobile Safety

Motor vehicle accidents are the leading cause of mortality and mobidity for children in the United States. Automobile safety laws in most states require the use of a car restraint system for infants and children through 4 years of age. As a result, many hospital policies require the use of a car seat before allowing the newborn infant to be discharged. Civic groups often sponsor a car seat lending program for a small deposit, which is reimbursed when the seat is returned. Ideally, the hospital provides manage-

ment of the program so that seats are available and demonstrated before leaving the hospital. The nurse must teach and reinforce the importance of using a car seat. One study on child safety seat compliance (Wolf et al, 1995) recommends that education on hospital policy regarding child safety seats be offered in the prenatal and childbirth preparation classes, since the current brief postpartum stay does not allow adequate time for this important topic.

When an infant restraint system is always used, the chances of serious injury or death during an accident are greatly reduced. Holding an infant in one's lap is *unsafe* and underestimates the collision force that will throw the infant around inside the vehicle and may also throw him out. Seat restraints have the following purposes:

1. Helps absorb and dissipate the shock of the accident and minimize its impact
2. Holds the infant in place during travel
3. Regulates the infant's behavior, which allows parents to drive safely

Two types of restraints are available: the nonconvertible type, which is used for newborns and young infants (faces toward the rear of the car in a reclined position); and the convertible type, which is intended for children through the toddler years (faces backward for infants and forward for older children). Car seats are secured with the auto restraint belt on the rear seat of the car. Since the introduction of air bags, placement of car seats on the front seat is less safe. All car seats must meet the following Federal Motor Vehicle Safety Standards criteria: (1) seats are tested for front-end collision at 30 mph, (2) harnesses must have buckles that require adult strength to open, and (3) the device must have directions clearly displayed. Safety depends on correct installation of the seat within the car. These safety issues should be addressed before the infant is born. Parents should be asked the following questions:

1. How do you plan to take your infant home?
2. Do you know where to rent or buy a car seat?
3. Do you recognize the features that make a safe car seat?

Giving this guidance to parents before they purchase a car seat is the responsibility of the health care provider (Figure 20-12). Never leave an infant unattended in a car seat, even if the infant is well-secured. Heat and cold are intensified with the windows shut and are potentially lethal. In addition, an unattended child could be abducted through kidnapping or car theft.

Eliminating Household Hazards

Safety is an important topic that is a priority on any initial home care visit. There are several injury prevention surveys that help parents and health care professionals focus on areas that need attention. A copy of a safety teaching guide can be left with the parents to serve as a reminder for areas that necessitate change. The home care nurse will follow-up during the next visit. Though some of these

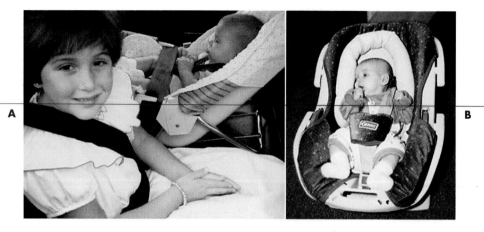

Figure 20-12 **A,** Federally approved infant car seat. Note placement in middle of back seat. **B,** Infant seat placed on the floor for safety. (**A,** From Wong DL: *Whaley & Wong's essentials of pediatric nursing,* ed 5, St Louis, 1997, Mosby. **B,** Courtesy Marjorie Pyle, RNC, *Lifecircle.*)

topics are not relevant for a newborn, parents need encouragement to start preparing early for the time when the infant becomes more mobile and is exposed to dangers in the home.

Temperature control

Infants are frequently overheated and overdressed. When an infant is dressed in a shirt, diaper, and sleeper, the temperature of the room may be kept as low as 70° F, which is comfortable for most adults. Add extra layers if the temperature drops further. Where houses are heated, avoid overheating, and avoid a dry atmosphere by placing a bowl of water near the source of heat or using a cold spray humidifier (must be cleaned daily). Parents should be cautioned against extremes in temperature and may need to monitor air conditioning. Care must be taken to keep the infant well-hydrated, especially during spells of extreme heat and humidity and when no air conditioning is available.

Show parents how to dress the infant appropriately for the weather, using as many layers of clothing as they themselves need. Always *cover the head, hands, and feet* when going out in cold or windy weather. A hat is advisable during the summer months to protect the infant from the heat of the sun. To prevent burning, use sunscreen (with a skin protection factor [SPF] of +15 or more) on infants exposed to sunlight, even on those who are heavily pigmented.

Pets

Pets may respond to infants with jealousy, regression, withdrawal, or hostility (Bahr, 1981). There are several guidelines to prepare the pet for the infant's arrival:
1. Discipline the pet not to enter the infant's room.
2. Never allow the pet to sleep in the empty crib.
3. Bring home a blanket used by the infant and let the pet smell it while giving the pet extra attention. Once the infant is brought home, allow the pet to smell the infant to establish her identity.
4. Keep the pet's immunizations current.

Accidents

Fifty percent of all children will require medical attention for injuries sustained in an accident. The greatest dangers to the helpless infant are burns, drowning, suffocation, and falls. Parents are responsible for the child's safety but may not know how to provide an environment that is both safe and stimulating. Teach the parents these specific guidelines:
1. Check the temperature of hot water; regulate the water heater to less than 140° F. When running water for the bath, turn on the cold water first and then add hot. Never leave the infant alone in the bath for any reason; even a few inches of water can cause an infant to drown. Place the infant in the bath after the water is drawn and the faucets are turned off.
2. Provide full supervision for an infant at all times. If the infant must be left out of sight (parents do need to use the bathroom), the only safe places for a small infant are the crib, playpen, or a sturdy infant seat placed on the floor with the restraint buckled (see Figure 20-12, *B*). Never leave an infant on an open surface without sides or a strap attached, and never leave an infant unsecured in a carriage, stroller, or high chair.
3. Keep plastic bags, telephone cords, soft pillows, heavy blankets, small objects, and balloons away from the infant.
4. Keep pins and other sharp objects out of reach.
5. Keep the infant away from the stove and other hot surfaces, such as wood stoves, fireplaces, and space heaters.
6. Be aware that other children may present a danger to an infant by rough handling or poking with sharp objects or toys.

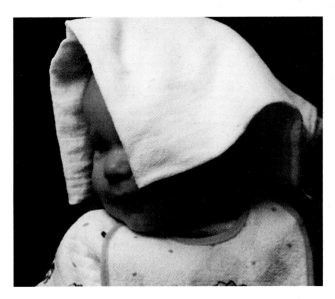

Figure 20-11   Teach parents how to play games with the infant. (Courtesy E Schult.)

- Carry the infant in a soft body carrier on the front of the parent; backpacks are appropriate only for older infants.
6. Since an infant learns through exploration and play, creative play should be fostered (Figure 20-11).
  - Several books on games to play with infants are available for parents. These games were often passed on naturally to new parents in extended families but may have been forgotten in the generation of nuclear families.

HEALTH MAINTENANCE IN THE FIRST YEAR

Health maintenance is important because it allows the normal processes of growth and development to occur. In a positive setting, the infant is protected from the hazards of the environment. The infant whose physical and psychologic health is maintained is better prepared to live in an increasingly challenging world. Nursing care includes teaching parents about hazards to the infant. A young infant is vulnerable to temperature extremes, environmental hazards, and choking.

Automobile Safety

Motor vehicle accidents are the leading cause of mortality and mobidity for children in the United States. Automobile safety laws in most states require the use of a car restraint system for infants and children through 4 years of age. As a result, many hospital policies require the use of a car seat before allowing the newborn infant to be discharged. Civic groups often sponsor a car seat lending program for a small deposit, which is reimbursed when the seat is returned. Ideally, the hospital provides manage-

ment of the program so that seats are available and demonstrated before leaving the hospital. The nurse must teach and reinforce the importance of using a car seat. One study on child safety seat compliance (Wolf et al, 1995) recommends that education on hospital policy regarding child safety seats be offered in the prenatal and childbirth preparation classes, since the current brief postpartum stay does not allow adequate time for this important topic.

When an infant restraint system is always used, the chances of serious injury or death during an accident are greatly reduced. Holding an infant in one's lap is *unsafe* and underestimates the collision force that will throw the infant around inside the vehicle and may also throw him out. Seat restraints have the following purposes:
1. Helps absorb and dissipate the shock of the accident and minimize its impact
2. Holds the infant in place during travel
3. Regulates the infant's behavior, which allows parents to drive safely

Two types of restraints are available: the nonconvertible type, which is used for newborns and young infants (faces toward the rear of the car in a reclined position); and the convertible type, which is intended for children through the toddler years (faces backward for infants and forward for older children). Car seats are secured with the auto restraint belt on the rear seat of the car. Since the introduction of air bags, placement of car seats on the front seat is less safe. All car seats must meet the following Federal Motor Vehicle Safety Standards criteria: (1) seats are tested for front-end collision at 30 mph, (2) harnesses must have buckles that require adult strength to open, and (3) the device must have directions clearly displayed. Safety depends on correct installation of the seat within the car. These safety issues should be addressed before the infant is born. Parents should be asked the following questions:
1. How do you plan to take your infant home?
2. Do you know where to rent or buy a car seat?
3. Do you recognize the features that make a safe car seat?

Giving this guidance to parents before they purchase a car seat is the responsibility of the health care provider (Figure 20-12). Never leave an infant unattended in a car seat, even if the infant is well-secured. Heat and cold are intensified with the windows shut and are potentially lethal. In addition, an unattended child could be abducted through kidnapping or car theft.

Eliminating Household Hazards

Safety is an important topic that is a priority on any initial home care visit. There are several injury prevention surveys that help parents and health care professionals focus on areas that need attention. A copy of a safety teaching guide can be left with the parents to serve as a reminder for areas that necessitate change. The home care nurse will follow-up during the next visit. Though some of these

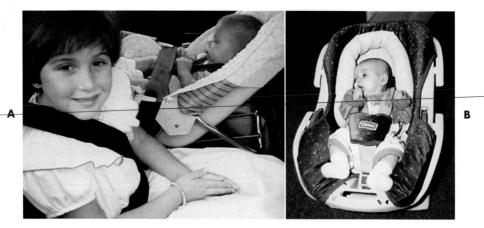

Figure 20-12   A, Federally approved infant car seat. Note placement in middle of back seat. **B,** Infant seat placed on the floor for safety. (**A,** From Wong DL: *Whaley & Wong's essentials of pediatric nursing,* ed 5, St Louis, 1997, Mosby. **B,** Courtesy Marjorie Pyle, RNC, *Lifecircle.*)

topics are not relevant for a newborn, parents need encouragement to start preparing early for the time when the infant becomes more mobile and is exposed to dangers in the home.

Temperature control

Infants are frequently overheated and overdressed. When an infant is dressed in a shirt, diaper, and sleeper, the temperature of the room may be kept as low as 70° F, which is comfortable for most adults. Add extra layers if the temperature drops further. Where houses are heated, avoid overheating, and avoid a dry atmosphere by placing a bowl of water near the source of heat or using a cold spray humidifier (must be cleaned daily). Parents should be cautioned against extremes in temperature and may need to monitor air conditioning. Care must be taken to keep the infant well-hydrated, especially during spells of extreme heat and humidity and when no air conditioning is available.

Show parents how to dress the infant appropriately for the weather, using as many layers of clothing as they themselves need. Always *cover the head, hands, and feet* when going out in cold or windy weather. A hat is advisable during the summer months to protect the infant from the heat of the sun. To prevent burning, use sunscreen (with a skin protection factor [SPF] of +15 or more) on infants exposed to sunlight, even on those who are heavily pigmented.

Pets

Pets may respond to infants with jealousy, regression, withdrawal, or hostility (Bahr, 1981). There are several guidelines to prepare the pet for the infant's arrival:
1. Discipline the pet not to enter the infant's room.
2. Never allow the pet to sleep in the empty crib.
3. Bring home a blanket used by the infant and let the pet smell it while giving the pet extra attention. Once the

infant is brought home, allow the pet to smell the infant to establish her identity.
4. Keep the pet's immunizations current.

Accidents

Fifty percent of all children will require medical attention for injuries sustained in an accident. The greatest dangers to the helpless infant are burns, drowning, suffocation, and falls. Parents are responsible for the child's safety but may not know how to provide an environment that is both safe and stimulating. Teach the parents these specific guidelines:
1. Check the temperature of hot water; regulate the water heater to less than 140° F. When running water for the bath, turn on the cold water first and then add hot. Never leave the infant alone in the bath for any reason; even a few inches of water can cause an infant to drown. Place the infant in the bath after the water is drawn and the faucets are turned off.
2. Provide full supervision for an infant at all times. If the infant must be left out of sight (parents do need to use the bathroom), the only safe places for a small infant are the crib, playpen, or a sturdy infant seat placed on the floor with the restraint buckled (see Figure 20-12, *B*). Never leave an infant on an open surface without sides or a strap attached, and never leave an infant unsecured in a carriage, stroller, or high chair.
3. Keep plastic bags, telephone cords, soft pillows, heavy blankets, small objects, and balloons away from the infant.
4. Keep pins and other sharp objects out of reach.
5. Keep the infant away from the stove and other hot surfaces, such as wood stoves, fireplaces, and space heaters.
6. Be aware that other children may present a danger to an infant by rough handling or poking with sharp objects or toys.

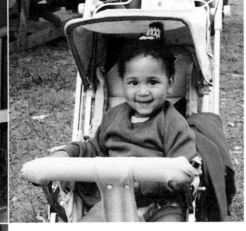

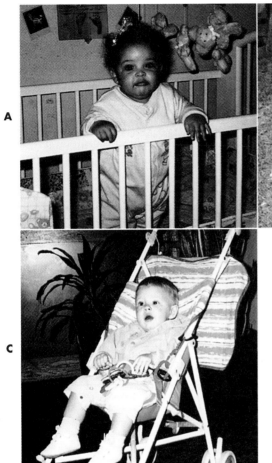

Figure 20-13   Safety features for cribs and strollers. **A,** Note the narrow crib slats to prevent injury. Mattress height needs to be adjusted as the infant grows. **B,** This stroller will adjust to a growing infant and saves money in the long run. **C,** A portable stroller is less expensive but not usable for as many months. The infant's back is always flexed in this stroller. (**A, B,** Courtesy Camille Bodden; **C,** Courtesy Marjorie Pyle, RNC, *Lifecircle.*)

Furnishings and equipment

Since there are so many new infant furnishings on the market, parents must be cautious. Standards are set by the United States Consumer Product Safety Commission for infant furnishings, and these should be used as a guide when making a purchase. A copy of *Guide to Baby Products* (Jones and Freitag, 1994) should be in each postpartum unit for reference. This guide is especially important for parents who receive or borrow used equipment. Be aware that infants need both comfort and safety. Figure 20-13 illustrates safety features for cribs and strollers.

Toys

Toy safety, a potential hazard area, is an important consideration. The first toys for an infant are often gifts not chosen by parents. The ability to select toys appropriate for age, interest, and play value is a skill (Box 20-6). The long-range usefulness of a toy lies in its play value, safety, and ability to capture the child's interest and imagination. Instructions should be read carefully until understood. Be aware that toys can be dangerous if they are not related to the age level of the child. Observe especially for any sharp edges and loosened parts. Finally, safe disposal is necessary if the toy is no longer usable.

Box 20-6   **Age-Appropriate Toys**

NEWBORN TO 4 MONTHS
Toys that are visual, auditory, and tactile
Something suspended over crib, such as a hanging mobile that is colorful with contrasting geometric designs and faces
Stuffed toys that are soft, cuddly, and washable
Bath toys such as sponges or squeeze toys
Music box
Safety mirror to see their own image
Soft and firm chewable "teethers"
Crib gym with items to hold, push, and pull

Choking

Choking is a leading cause of accidental death in infants under 1 year of age. Prevention of choking includes teaching parents not to force-feed their infant and to choose age-appropriate foods. Snack foods should not be left within reach of a cruising infant. Toys must be checked for small, loose parts. Prenatal classes are the best place to begin this instruction (Figure 20-14).

Additionally, instruct the parent *never to prop* the feeding bottle, since aspiration may occur with choking if the feeding is taken too fast.

Airway obstructions usually occur while an infant is eating or playing. Before intervening, parents must determine that the airway is actually obstructed. The child's respirations will become increasingly difficult, coughing will be frequent and ineffective and have a high-pitched crowing quality, and the infant will become cyanotic or pale. Every parent should know how to help a child (or adult) who is choking (Figure 20-15). The following standards for infants up to 1 year of age are from the American Heart Association (Bloom, 1994).

- Do *not* sweep mouth or pharynx with a finger.
- Support the head and neck with one hand, place the infant face downward, with head lower than trunk over your forearm and supported on your thigh.

- Deliver five back blows forcefully between the shoulder blades with the heel of the hand (Figure 20-16, *A*).
- While supporting the head, sandwich the infant between the hands and turn the infant on the back, head lower than trunk.
- Deliver five chest thrusts in the midline, one finger-breadth below the nipple line, in the same manner as external chest compressions (Figure 20-16, *B*).
- Open airway with head-tilt or chin-lift maneuver.
- If infant is not breathing, attempt one ventilation, and then turn infant over and repeat the back blows and chest thrusts until the foreign body is expelled or the infant becomes unconscious.
- Once the infant does lose consciousness, cardiopulmonary resuscitation (CPR) should be started (see Procedure 20-1).

TEST *Yourself* 20-1 _____

A 2-month-old infant who has inhaled a small object is coughing and pale. Describe the necessary actions the parent should take.

Preventing Illness

Communication must flow in both directions for illness prevention education to be effective. Parents must be armed with specific information that will allow them to accurately determine whether intervention is needed for their infant. Learning warning signs will increase their confidence and decrease anxiety.

Warning signs of illness in a newborn are found in Box 20-7 and should be taught to the new parents. A printed copy is sent home with each family.

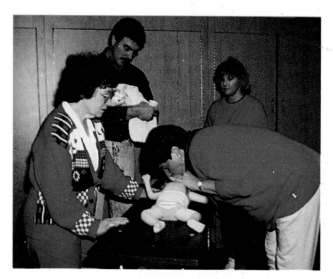

Figure 20-14 Parents learn mouth-to-mouth resuscitation in class. (Courtesy Marjorie Pyle, RNC, *Lifecircle*.)

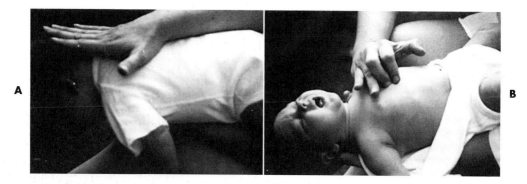

Figure 20-15 Modified Heimlich technique for a choking infant. **A,** Four back blows with palm of hand between scapulae. **B,** Four chest thrusts by placing two fingers below nipple line and pressing down ¹/₂ inch. (Courtesy P.O Roberson.)

PROCEDURE 20-1
Infant CPR

Observe color; tap or gently shake shoulders.
Yell for help; if alone, perform CPR for 1 minute before calling for help again.

Turn infant to back, supporting head and neck.
Place on firm, flat surface.
Clear airway, as required (see text).
Tilt head back gently to "sniffing" or neutral position; use head-tilt or chin-life maneuver (Figure 20-16, *A*).
Do not hyperextend neck.

Assess for evidence of breathing
Observe for chest movement
Listen for exhaled air, and feel for exhaled air flow.

Breathe for infant (Figure 20-16, *B*)
Take a breath.
Open mouth wide and place over mouth and nose of infant to create seal.

Note: Repeat the word *ho* as you gently puff the volume of air *in your* cheeks into infant. *Do not* force air.

Infant's chest should rise slightly with each puff; keep fingers on chest wall to sense air entry.
Give two slow breaths (1 to 1.5 sec/breath), pausing to inhale between breaths.
Check pulse of brachial artery (Figure 20-16, *C*) while maintaining head tilt.

If pulse is present, initiate rescue breathing. Continue until spontaneous breathing resumes at rate of every 3 seconds or 20 times/min.
If pulse is not present, initiate chest compressions and coordinate with breathing.

Chest compressions
Maintain head tilt. With other hand, position fingers for chest compressions.
Place index finger of hand farthest from infant's head just under imaginary line drawn between nipples (Figure 20-16, *D*). Move index finger to a position one finger-breadth below this intersection.
Using two or three fingers, compress sternum to depth of 1/2 to 1 inch (see Procedure 29-1 for newborns).
Release pressure without moving fingers from the position.
Repeat at a rate of at least 100 times/min, with 5 compressions in 3 seconds or less.
Perform 20 cycles of 5 compressions and 1 ventilation. (If possible, compressions are accompanied by positive-pressure ventilation at a rate of 40 to 60 /min. After cycles, check the brachial pulse to determine presence of pulse.
Discontinue compressions if spontaneous heart rate reaches or exceeds 80 beats/min.

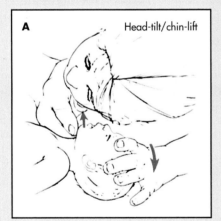

A Head-tilt/chin-lift

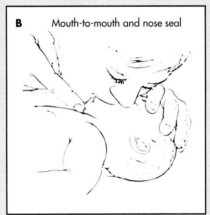

B Mouth-to-mouth and nose seal

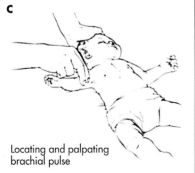

C Locating and palpating brachial pulse

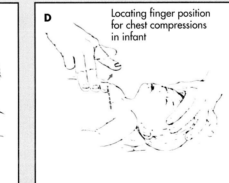

D Locating finger position for chest compressions in infant

Figure 20-16 A to D, Procedures for cardiopulmonary resuscitation. (From Guidelines for Cardiopulmonary Resuscitation [CPR] and Emergency Cardiac Care [ECC]: *JAMA* 286[16]:2171, 1992.)

OPTIONAL ACTIVITY

Write a sample nursing note correctly documenting the performance of this procedure.

Box 20-7

WARNING SIGNS

Illness in an Infant

CALL THE PRIMARY HEALTH CARE
PROVIDER* WHEN THE FOLLOWING OCCUR:

The eyes, umbilical cord, or circumcision site is red or swollen.

The infant appears lethargic or sleeps a lot.

The infant does not cry normally.

The infant is not eating well or frequently vomits feedings.

The infant does not move all extremities well.

The infant's skin seems yellow, even in sunlight.

The infant's stools are watery and frequent.

The infant has a stuffy nose and seems to have difficulty breathing (i.e., breathing is shallow, rapid, and regular more than 60 breaths a minute).

The infant has an axillary temperature over 99° F.

You notice anything unusual or have a vague, uneasy feeling that all is not well.

*This list may be given to parents upon discharge from hospital or by a home health nurse.

Immunizations

All children should be immunized against childhood infectious diseases. These diseases took a terrible toll in the days before immunizations became safe and standardized. It is a tragedy that still occurs, not only in many underdeveloped countries but in some populations within the United States as well. Children who have not been immunized die or are damaged by these preventable diseases. Cost should not be a deterrent—free immunizations are available at Department of Health Clinics—and immigration status is not questioned. Table 20-2 lists immunizations and guidelines for administration. However, schedules may vary with each health care provider.

The actions, adverse effects, contraindications, and implications for the vaccines administered must be known (see Appendix 3B). Since many vaccines are made from live attenuated viruses, there is a slight risk that multiplication of the virus may cause a reaction. Although universal vaccination seems ideal, it may create problems for some infants. The benefit-to-risk ratio should be considered for any infant with allergic or medical problems. Immunization is postponed if the child has an acute, infectious, febrile illness, since any reactions to the vaccine could be confused with disease symptoms. Children with immunologic deficiencies are not routinely vaccinated. Children

Table 20-2 Immunization Recommendations during Infancy

Disease/Type of Vaccine	Timing	Possible Side Effects
DIPHTHERIA Toxoid (inactivated toxin)	At 2, 4, 6, and 15 to 18 months, then at 4 to 6 years	Erythema, induration, tenderness, mild to moderate fever, vomiting, malaise
PERTUSSIS Killed vaccine	At 2, 4, 6, and 15 to 18 months; not administered over 6 years of age	Same as for diphtheria, plus central nervous system effects: local swelling, excessive tiredness, rare convulsions, encephalopathy
TETANUS Toxoid	At 2, 4, 6, and 15 to 18 months; 4 to 6 years and 11 to 12 years	Fever, local soreness and swelling
MEASLES (Rubeola, 10-day measles) Live attenuated virus	Usually at 15 months, either alone or with measles, mumps and rubella (MMR) and repeated at 4 to 6 years or 11 to 12 years	Rash, fever about 10 days after immunization (both rare)
MUMPS Live attenuated virus	At 15 months with MMR	Mild fever 7 to 14 days after vaccine
RUBELLA (German measles, 3-day measles) Live attenuated virus	Administered at 15 months with MMR	Rash, joint pain, lymphadenopathy (all rare)

Modified from American Academy of Pediatrics: *Report of Committee on Infectious Diseases*, ed 22, Elk Grove, Ill, 1991, The Academy, and from MMWR: *Guidelines for immunizations*, 45(RR-12):1, 1996.

with malignancies (such as leukemia or lymphoma) who are receiving corticosteroids or radiation therapy or who have altered immune systems (such as those who are human immunodeficiency virus [HIV] positive) should not be immunized with live attenuated virus. Rapid multiplication of the virus in these children can cause severe illness.

Recently, with some publicized negative reactions to the pertussis vaccine, parents have been hesitant to have their infants receive the diphtheria-pertussis-tetanus (DPT) vaccine. It is true that many more children die or suffer damage from pertussis (whooping cough) than from the vaccine. However, a neurologic history should be obtained before the administration of the pertussis vaccine because of certain adverse neurologic reactions. If there is any history of neurologic disorders, the pertussis vaccine should be omitted, but diphtheria and tetanus vaccines should be given on schedule.

In 1995 The American Academy of Pediatrics Committee on Infectious Diseases recommended the vaccination against varicella (chicken pox). Each year about 3.5 million children contract this usually benign disease. About 90 people die annually from complications, usually because of **Reye's syndrome** (a severe neurologic disorder) or encephalitis. A single subcutaneous (SC) dose of the vaccine is recommended for children 12 months to 12 years, and two doses 4 to 8 weeks apart is advised for children 13 years and older (Farrington, 1995). The vaccine may be administered at the same time as the measles, mumps, rubella (MMR) vaccine, with separate syringes and sites. Salicylates should be avoided for 6 weeks following vaccination to reduce the chance of developing Reye's syndrome.

Because of fear of adverse reactions, some parents are delaying their child's immunizations until school entrance or are refusing to immunize them at all. As a result, there is an increase in the incidence of preventable diseases in preschoolers. Providing adequate information is essential to correct misconceptions about immunizations.

Table **20-2**	**Immunization Recommendations during Infancy—cont'd**	
Disease/Type of Vaccine	**Timing**	**Possible Side Effects**
POLIO Live attenuated virus (TOPV), containing three different viruses; use killed vaccine (inactivated poliomyelitis vaccine [IPV] and Salk) for immuno-compromised patients	Trivalent oral polio vaccine (TOPV) administered at 2, 4 and 10 months and again at 4 to 6 years	No reaction; not administered to infant with human immunodeficiency virus (HIV)
INFLUENZA (HIB) Haemophilus influenza type B conjugate vaccine anti-Haemophilus influenzae serum	At 2 to 4 months; begin at 1 to 3 months if infant in day care	Slight fever
HEPATITIS B Vaccine for infants of hepatitis B negative women Infants of women who are hepatitis B positive or status unknown receive the vaccine, plus Hepatitis B immunoglobulin	Within 48 hours of birth or at 1 to 2 months; second dose 1 month later; third dose before age 18 months Within 12 hours of birth	Pain at intramuscular (IM) site, possible fever Report all adverse immunization effects to VAERS 1-800-822-7967
TUBERCULOSIS (TB) Limited immunity: BCG (Bacille Calmette-Guérin vaccine) Screening is done with tine test	If high risk, testing to be done every year starting at 12 months; if low risk, testing should be done at 12-15 months Should precede or be given simultaneously with measles vaccine because measles can give a false-positive TB test result	False negative can be produced if child exposed to childhood diseases within 4 weeks of TB testing; false positive reports if child has received BCG vaccine
VARICELLA (Chicken pox) Live attenuated vaccine (Varivax)	Single dose for children 12 months to 12 years; two doses 4 to 8 weeks apart for children over 13 years	Pain at site, fever, generalized rash

TEST *Yourself* 20-2 _____

Which infants should not receive immunizations on the regular schedule?

Health Problems during Infancy

Fever

A fever in an infant is frightening to the parents. They should be taught that fever is a normal response to a viral or bacterial infection. Fever is defined as a rectal temperature above 100.4° F (38° C) or an axillary temperature above 99° F (37.2° C). Tympanic (ear canal) measurements may not be as accurate for young infants (see Chapter 19) (Weiss, Poelter, Gocka, 1993). Normal body temperature rises during the day and peaks between 6 and 10 PM, then it drops to its lowest point between 2 and 4 AM. Febrile patterns follow the same cycle. With an illness, many infants will "spike" high fevers, going quickly from a relatively normal temperature to a very high one. Observations of spontaneous activity are often more reliable indicators of the severity of illness than fever (see Box 20-7). However, fever should not be ignored. The primary health care provider should be notified if the following are present:

- The infant is irritable, difficult to awaken, has difficulty breathing, or holds his head and neck stiffly.
- The infant appears dehydrated.
- The axillary temperature is greater than 99° F.

Interventions for treating a fever are as follows:

1. Monitor axillary temperature at least twice a day (morning and night) to account for diurnal variations. Hold the infant securely so the thermometer remains in place for at least 3 minutes. An inguinal temperature may also be taken (see Chapter 19).
2. Monitor temperature more often during the first day of the illness and if the infant feels warm, is irritable, shivers, or is flushed.
3. Reduce the infant's activity to conserve energy.
4. Dress the infant lightly.
5. Increase fluid intake.
6. Sponge bathe with tepid water if the temperature is greater than 103° F, and recheck the temperature after the bath. Never add alcohol to the bath since this dries the skin and may lower the temperature so rapidly that shivering occurs.
7. Parents should know how to calculate the appropriate dosage of acetaminophen for their infant's age and weight; if they are not sure, they should call the health care provider. (Never give aspirin, because it has been associated with Reye's syndrome.)

Common colds

Symptoms usually include cough, nasal congestion, and possibly anorexia and fever. Colds are viral illnesses and require no antibiotic therapy; thus all treatment is for symptomatic relief. To prevent colds, attempt to keep the infant out of crowds and away from visitors who are sick. This may be difficult for the working mother, especially if she uses a day care facility. Frequent hand washing with antibacterial soap before handling the infant is essential. Older siblings should also be encouraged to follow this practice. The following interventions help ease the discomfort of the infant with a cold:

- Use a cool mist vaporizer to increase the moisture to the infant's mucous membranes. Clean the vaporizer daily according to directions.
- Show parents how to use a bulb syringe to relieve nasal congestion, especially before feeding and sleeping.
- Increase intake of clear fluids.
- Contact the primary health care provider for advice about medications that may ease symptoms.

If the infant looks sick, has a temperature over 101° F (38.5° C), has a bad cough or a congested chest, is refusing liquids or vomiting, has diarrhea, or is pulling at his ears, then the problem may be more serious than a simple cold. Infants with these symptoms should be examined promptly.

Vomiting and diarrhea

Vomiting should be distinguished from spitting up. Spitting up or regurgitation is expelling a small amount of liquid when the infant burps or is handled actively after feeding. Vomiting is not always associated with these activities, and the amount of fluid expelled is greater. It can be caused by factors such as overeating, food allergies, pyloric stenosis, or gastroenteritis, or it can be indicative of altered maternal-infant attachment. *Diarrhea* is an increase in the fluidity, frequency, and volume of stool and can be caused by certain foods, excessive sugar or fluid intake, infections or allergies, or inability to digest milk. Dehydration is a serious complication of both diarrhea and vomiting. Assessment of the infant with these problems should include the following:

- A description of the onset, duration, and frequency of diarrhea
- Consistency, amount, and color of the diarrhea or vomitus
- Approximate oral intake within last 24 hours
- Signs of dehydration—weight loss, sunken fontanelle, dry eyes and mucous membranes, decrease in number of wet diapers

When diarrhea or vomiting occur, the following should be done:

- Stop all milk intake and encourage clear fluids in small amounts.
- The younger infant must be seen by the health care provider and then may be given an electrolyte formula such as Pedialyte, Vivonex, or sometimes Gatorade for 24 hours. After this the infant may then be slowly restarted on breast-feeding or formula.

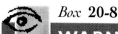

Box 20-8
WARNING SIGNS

Diarrhea and Vomiting

- Vomiting and fever
- Persistent vomiting or diarrhea with dehydration and sunken fontanelle
- Blood or bile in the vomitus or stool
- Vomiting with abdominal distention, localized tenderness or pain, or palpable abdominal mass
- Vomiting with visible peristalsis or projectile vomiting
- Vomiting and a history or suspicion of ingestion of a drug or poison

Refer infant to the health care provider if any of the warning signs in Box 20-8 are present.

Constipation

A constipated infant has hard, dry, infrequent stools. Constipation may occur when the infant is switched from formula or breast milk to cow's milk; fluid intake may fall during the weaning process. Great effort is required to pass the stool, producing anal irritation or a fistula and pain. Other causes of constipation include insufficient sugar in the formula, low fluid intake, starvation, prolonged vomiting spells, intestinal constriction, chronic disease, fissures, and severe diaper rash. Constipation can also be a sign of Hirschsprung's disease or hypothyroidism.

Some older infants can withhold stool and will do so if having a bowel movement causes pain. In toddlers, the pressure of early toilet training and the toddler's striving for control over bodily functions can cause the same result. Constipation should be discussed with the primary care provider, who may advise changes in diet. Infants should not be given laxatives or enemas. However, sometimes a small amount of Karo syrup mixed into formula or water is effective.

Skin problems

The epidermis and the immune system of the infant are immature, which increases susceptibility to irritation and infection. Thus the addition of any irritating agent may cause the skin to become inflamed and lose its protective quality. There are many types of skin lesions, some of which may be treated with prescription medication. Parents need to know how to relieve symptoms of skin irritation to increase an infant's comfort.

Contact dermatitis. In assessing skin conditions, the first step is to identify and eliminate environmental factors that could cause irritation, such as laundry soaps and detergent and wool clothing. Symptomatic relief can be achieved by giving a tepid bath or by applying cool lotions to relieve itching and pain from chafing. Apply cornstarch to areas that are not weeping wounds, taking care not to scatter the powder. Do not use baby powder or scented talcs since these substances may act as further irritants.

Cradle cap. A common infant condition is seborrheic dermatitis, resulting in yellowish oily scales on the scalp. Seborrhea of the face is frequently seen as well. Instruct parents to rub a small amount of baby or mineral oil into the scalp before shampooing. This softens the scales, and a fine-tooth comb can be used to remove the loose scales. Stubborn cases may require the use of an antidandruff shampoo and an application of 0.5% hydrocortisone cream to the face. Do not attempt to remove all scales after the first treatment. It is safer to try several applications over a few days or to leave the mineral oil on overnight than to try to loosen all the scales at once. Explain to the parents the need to avoid picking or scratching at crusty scales to prevent secondary infection.

Diaper rash. Perhaps the most frequent skin problem is diaper dermatitis, seen as reddened, excoriated skin of the perineum. Washing routines for cloth diapers should be reviewed; changing detergents or fabric softeners may be all that is needed. Cloth diapers should be double rinsed in a solution of sodium borate (Borax). Occasionally, the parent may need to switch to disposable diapers for a time. For some infants, the irritant may be plastic waterproof pants or paper diapers with plastic covers.

Diaper rash may also occur with a change in diet that alters what is excreted in the stool or urine. Teething may increase acidity of urine and stool. Finally, frequent liquid stool leaves the skin irritated. Whatever the cause of the rash, the diaper area should be washed with mild soap and water at each diaper change, then dried gently and exposed to air. A thick coat of petroleum jelly or an ointment containing zinc oxide (Desitin) can be applied preventively before a rash begins or to protect against further exposure of raw skin to the elements of urine and stool.

Candida **infection.** This requires special treatment. *Candida albicans*, or monilia infection, is acquired from the mother and may be present in the mouth or the diaper area. The rash has defined, scalloped edges and a wet, oozing look. White lesions that seem like curdled milk will appear in the mouth (see Figure 18-23). Nystatin is the treatment of choice and can be obtained only by prescription.

Heat rash. Some infants develop miliaria rubra when they are too warm; reddened papules appear on face, neck, trunk, and diaper areas. Reducing the environmental temperature by cooling the infant with a tepid bath or changing to lighter clothing will improve the rash. Cornstarch can be applied sparingly in the creases around the neck and in the axilla to absorb perspiration.

Newborn sleep cycles

Infants have unique cycles of sleep and wakefulness. Some infants sleep through any noise, whereas others wake and cry more frequently. By 10 days of age, the infant should be more in tune with the parents' sleep and wake cycles and should begin to establish a consistent pattern of sleep. During the first few weeks of life, infants may sleep up to 5 hours at a time and awaken for feeding and social time. However, some infants spend a considerable block of time awake. Until 2 to 3 months of age, the infant will require about 18 to 20 hours of sleep daily. By 4 months of age, 95% of all infants sleep through the night (about 8 hours), but during growth spurts, the infant may awaken for a feeding in the night. By 1 year of age, about 12 hours of sleep plus two nap times are needed. Routines should be set to establish good sleeping habits, although the age at which parents can anticipate an uninterrupted night's sleep varies.

Sleep disturbance. Parents need to be assured that each infant establishes a sleep pattern of his own, related in part to maturing of the neurologic system. Thus the infant cannot be "blamed" for waking during the night. It will be easier to establish settled patterns if specific routines are followed at bedtime. When the infant and the family's sleep schedules conflict, the parents become distressed, uncertain, and exhausted.

Research on night sleeping in infants (Anders et al, 1992) suggests that by age 3 months, infants who are put awake into the crib at bedtime and allowed to fall asleep on their own are more likely to return to sleep on their own after awakenings later in the night. In contrast, infants who are put into the crib already asleep at the beginning of the night are significantly more likely to be removed from the crib following a subsequent nighttime awakening. Infants allowed to develop self-soothing behaviors before falling asleep, such as holding a favorite blanket or using a pacifier, seem to continue these measures when they wake during the night and do not require parental intervention. Anders et al add that this is a complex research issue and parental attachment, expectation, and interventions, as well as culture, play a role in nighttime sleep regulation.

Adair et al (1992) tested a primary care intervention to prevent night waking in infants. It was based on findings that suggest parents contribute inadvertently to night waking when they rock, hold, or feed their infant to promote sleep. Such behavior establishes a learned association between parental presence and falling asleep. Adair's intervention consists of giving parents information about sleep-onset associations, having them keep a sleep chart for their infant, and discussing sleep with their pediatrician. By age 9 months, the intervention-infants were reported to experience 36% less night waking than those in the control group.

Guidelines for parents with sleep-related questions should include the following:

- When an infant is not synchronized with day and night schedules, keep him awake rather than encouraging extra sleep during the day.
- When an infant is a trained night feeder, make night feeding brief and boring. Do not use solids at bedtime because extra calories do not encourage sleep. Give the last feeding at 10 to 11 PM and not in the bed.

- *Do not prop the bottle* or let infants suck on bottles while falling asleep. This leads to "bottle mouth," tooth decay, and to inner ear infections (Von Burg, Sanders, Weddell, 1995). Use a pacifier or an alternative.
- When an infant is a night crier, it is often because the parent reinforces this behavior with extra attention. Soothe the infant as quickly as possible, and leave the room.
- Place the infant in bed before he is asleep, so the last waking memory is of the crib and comfort toy or blanket and not the parent. Avoid changing diapers at night when possible.
- When an infant is a fearful night crier and suffers from separation anxiety (beginning at about 6 months), give the infant a security object. Leave the door open and a nightlight on in the room.
- Position infant on back or side (refer to the section on sudden infant death syndrome [SIDS] later in this chapter) for the first several months of life. Later when the SIDS risk is over (6 to 8 months), the infant may assume any position. Most infants, in fact, have a preferred sleep position after they are able to turn themselves.

Many parents feel comfortable bringing the infant who has night wakefulness into their own bed, believing that this will increase the child's comfort and security. In many ethnic groups, sleep in a family bed is a normal arrangement.

Crying and fussiness

An infant's cry is his only means of communication, as well as a method of releasing tension. Most newborns cry intermittently for about 2 hours out of every 24. There are differences between cries of hunger, discomfort, boredom, and fatigue, and parents become able to distinguish the cry's meaning to meet the infant's needs. Crying seems to be a channel for the infant's energies, a time to let off steam, or an exercise period. Parents may become discouraged if their actions do not influence the infant's

Box **20-2**

CLINICAL DECISION

Andy was born at 37 weeks but weighed 6 pounds, so he was sent home after a 2-day recovery in the hospital. Mary decided to bottle feed him. At first, his sucking was irregular; he would often pause to rest. Mary felt he "wasn't hungry" and tended to remove the bottle before he was satisfied. "Oh, you're done?" she'd ask. "Well, time to go to sleep." She would put Andy down and leave the room. Within 10 minutes, he was crying again. This frustrating pattern developed early in the first month. Using the baseline data about feeling tone, sleep patterns, and feeding satisfaction, what interventions by the home care nurse might help Mary and her infant develop better continuity?

crying, and the infant who cries inconsolably is a real challenge to parents and health care providers.

Colic

Infants who cry for sustained periods during the first 3 months may have **colic**. They appear very distressed after feeding, draw their legs up to the abdomen, and scream. The pattern varies, but infants with colic may cry for 4 or more hours. These crying episodes are more likely to occur during the evening and late night, since the infant is influenced by the fatigue, tension, and busyness of the parent at the end of the day. Parents become extremely anxious over an inconsolable infant, and this leads to frustration, reduced confidence, and even anger at the infant, which may increase the infant's distress.

Wessel et al's (1954) widely accepted definition of an infant with colic is "one who, otherwise healthy and well-fed, has paroxysms of irritability, fussing, or crying lasting more than 3 hours a day and occurring on more than 3 days in any one week." Another definition of colic is "excessive crying in infancy with multiple causes" (Treem, 1994). Although the infant regulates the volume of the feed, he may still appear frantically hungry immediately after a feeding; a pacifier may be used to satisfy sucking needs.

There has been a wide range of explanations for colic. Many believe that allergy to cow's milk or the breast-feeding mother's diet contributes to colic. One study (Hill et al, 1995) showed that a low allergen diet for the infant and nursing mother reduced colic by 39%. Often the first impulse is to change formula; the average number of formula changes during the span of colic is 3.5 (Treem, 1994). Before making such changes, other explanations must be explored, including maternal tension, inappropriate parental responses, and infant hunger and boredom.

Metcalf et al (1994) compared the use of simethicone (taken to control intestinal gas in adults) and a placebo to treat colicky infants. Though both produced perceived improvement, simethicone was no more effective than the placebo in the treatment of infant colic. Treem (1994) reported that in some infants there is changed intestinal motility that responds to a fiber-supplemented soy protein formula. Methylcellulose (Citrucel) and extract of barley malt (Maltsupex) have been used with some benefit. The hormone *motilin*, which increases motor activity of the gut is present in higher levels in infants with colic than in those without it, suggesting a biologic predisposition to colic because of more intestinal cramping and abdominal distention. Finally, a number of infants have gastroesophageal reflux resulting in esophagitis. This irritation of the esophagus leads to excessive crying, spitting, and vomiting, and the period of distress extends beyond the expected 10 to 12 weeks.

To treat colic, first determine that no functional or organic disorder exists that is causing the infant's distress. A complete nursing history should be obtained and should include inquiries about maternal drug intake, both legal and illegal; infants of mothers who use cocaine or crack are extremely irritable and may be inconsolable.

Then, recommend an infant behavior diary for 4 to 7 days to track crying, stooling, and feeding times and results. The process of keeping this journal helps the parent approach colic in a more objective manner. The intent is to detect whether the infant belongs in a group of infants who cry even more than those with the expected colic pattern. These infants are more likely to have a cow's milk allergy or some other organic cause of irritability, and they need further medical assessment. Many different interventions have been tried: snugly wrapping the infant or walking her, or using gentle motion, touch and soothing words. Parents can try placing the infant in a front-pack carrier that allows free movement of the parent's hands, taking the infant for a ride in the car, playing music or making rhythmic sounds, using a mechanical infant swing, and even running the vacuum to provide a steady noise. Most important, urge the parents to seek help from friends and relatives to satisfy their need for "time out." Encourage parents to try various methods of quieting the infant and not to get excited if these do not work. Box 20-9 lists the parental counseling that has been shown to be effective for infant colic. If parents are able to relax, taking constructive steps, the infant's tension will diminish.

Brazelton (1976) found that as parents become worn out, infants cry even more. Crying diaries show the following results:

1. The more frantic the maneuvers a parent institutes, the more the infant cries.
2. The crying begins to decrease by 7 weeks, and by 10 weeks, it is just about gone.

 Box **20-9**   **Parent Instruction When Colic Occurs**

Try to never let your infant cry.
In attempting to discover why your infant is crying, consider these possibilities:
    The infant is hungry and wants to be fed.
    The infant wants to suck, although she is not hungry.
    The infant wants to be held.
    The infant is bored and wants stimulation.
    The infant is tired and wants to sleep.
If the crying continues for more than 5 minutes with one response, try another.
Decide on your own in what order to explore the above possibilities.
Don't be concerned about overfeeding your infant. This will not happen.
Don't be concerned about spoiling your infant. This also will not happen.

From Taubman G: Clinical trial of the treatment of colic by modification of parent-infant interaction, *Pediatr* 74:998, 1994.

3. By 12 weeks, the time of day formerly used for crying becomes the infant's most sociable period.

Follow-up studies on some of these colicky infants show that they often grow up to be very intelligent, which may be of some encouragement to distraught parents. In 1970, an organization called Mothers Anonymous (now Parents Anonymous) was formed. Although known by different names in various locations (e.g., Parental Stress Hotline, COPE, CALM), it is a helpful resource for parents who have crying infants.

Parents' fatigue and frustration levels may be a cause of subsequent abuse of the infant. An irrational idea emerges that the crying is the infant's deliberate attempt to irritate the parent. Interventions are important *before* this irrational idea becomes fixed. Unfortunately, in families where abuse is seen, there may not be a support network of people who are knowledgeable about infant growth and development. Often there is a repeated cycle of abuse (see Chapter 27).

Less Common Problems of Infancy

Sudden infant death syndrome prevention

SIDS is defined by the Centers for Disease Control as the sudden unexpected death of an apparently healthy infant, which remains unexplained after a death scene investigation, case report, and autopsy. In 1989 there were over 5,000 SIDS deaths in the United States. Table 20-3 summarizes the epidemiologic information known about SIDS. There does not seem to be one underlying cause of SIDS, but instead there is a subtle abnormality present from birth that increases the infant's risk of SIDS (Freed et al, 1994). Research shows the presence of some common factors associated with SIDS. It is necessary for health care professionals to share this information with parents so they can act responsibly.

"**Back to sleep.**" Based on a wide variety of international studies, the 1992 recommendation by the American Academy of Pediatrics Task Force Statement called "Infant Positioning and SIDS" advises placing healthy infants on the side or back for sleep. There has been a national campaign to publicize this recommendation, and all health care professionals are encouraged to promote its adoption in their practice and anticipatory guidance with parents. Acceptance of this new recommended positioning has been slow (Rainey and Lawless, 1994; Carolan et al, 1995). Lerner (1993) notes the importance of nurses as role models for parents since they are the ones who demonstrate infant position in hospitals and answer parents' questions about sleep. Positioning just after feeding is a common concern. Careful burping after each feeding is recommended, and placing the infant in a side-lying position for the first 30 minutes after a feeding is usually sufficient to prevent aspiration should regurgitation or vomiting occur.

Table 20-3	**Epidemiology of Sudden Infant Death Syndrome**
Factors	**Occurrence**
Incidence	1.4:100 live births
Peak age	2 to 4 months: 90% of cases occur by 6 months, but they may occur for up to 1 year
Sex	More males affected
Time of death	During sleep
Time of year	Increased in winter; peak January
Race	Native and African-American have higher incidence, followed by Caucasian
Socioeconomic status	Increased in lower socioeconomic groups

Birth status	Higher incidence in:
	    Preterm or low-birth-weight infants
	    Multiple births: although rare, simultaneous death in twins has been seen
	    Infants with central nervous system disturbance and respiratory disorders
	    Less in firstborn, more in subsequent siblings

Sleep habits	Prone position Use of polystyrene-filled pillow Overheating
Feeding habits	Lower in breast-fed infants
Siblings of SIDS victims	May have greater incidence
Maternal status	Younger age Smoker during pregnancy and infant exposed to passive smoke Addicted to drugs: heroin, methadone, and possibly cocaine

(From Wong DL: *Whaley and Wong's essentials of pediatric nursing*, ed 5, St Louis, 1997, Mosby.)

Passive smoke. Another factor now strongly associated with SIDS is the infant's exposure (including prenatal exposure) to passive smoke. Several research studies (Klonoff-Cohen, 1995; Mitchell, 1993) indicate that infants spending considerable amounts of time in homes where there is a smoker, particularly if it is the mother, have a higher rate of SIDS. Again, nurses have a responsibility to share this information with parents. It may not be welcomed by the parents, particularly if they are smokers, but it may give them the encouragement they need to stop smoking, or it might protect the infant from relatives who smoke. Parents should also be informed that passive smoke inhalation by infants is associated with a higher incidence of respiratory diseases and ear infections (Freed et al, 1995).

Caregivers are also alerted to the possibility of SIDS by episodes of apnea and gastrointestinal reflux in the infant with a history of bradycardia, premature delivery, and maternal drug use. The parent may report a sudden episode of apnea or respiratory difficulty associated with a change in skin color—pallor or cyanosis—and a change in muscle tone. When this episode occurs, the infant should be examined in a SIDS prevention center and should be followed with continuous home apnea monitoring. Regardless of the initiating cause of SIDS, the majority of SIDS victims die during an acute asphyxial event. Thus if the onset of apnea can be discovered and the infant is stimulated or resuscitation is begun, the potential for survival is increased. The highest risk of SIDS occurs before the infant is 8 months old, then the factors that place the infant at risk seem to diminish by 1 year of life.

Nonorganic failure to thrive

This term refers to an alteration in growth and development that cannot not be attributed only to a disease or systemic cause but also includes psychosocial factors. It is not apparent in the very young infant, but it slowly becomes obvious as the infant fails to gain weight and demonstrates development lags. The home care nurse is in an ideal position to assess the home environment and the parent-child interaction and to plan strategies for intervention before the problem develops. Klein (1990) encourages this role for the home care nurse and emphasizes the nurse's ongoing relationship with the family as a vital part of the intervention.

SEPARATION FROM THE BIRTH MOTHER

Some infants do not become a part of the families into which they were born but instead are placed in adoptive or foster homes. The reasons for this are as widespread and varied as the situations and personalities of the families themselves. Some parents recognize that because of their personal or financial circumstances, they cannot care for an infant or raise a child at this point in their lives. Other parents, because of social pressures, drug addiction, or mental illness, surrender or abandon children, or some may even have a child removed from their homes by protective agencies, either temporarily or permanently. For parents to recognize that they are unable to care for a child requires great courage. Depending on circumstances, there may also be a great deal of anger or sadness.

Infant's Needs

Infants who are placed into adoptive or foster home placement may remain in the hospital nursery longer than other infants. The staff must plan to supply the missing personal attention, warmth, comfort and stimulation that an enthusiastic and loving parent would normally provide. Although all their physical needs may be met, these infants have great need for psychologic stimulation from tender and playful handling. Studies have shown that infants in institutions without personal contact, given adequate food and comfortable but unstimulating surroundings, may become retarded in their physical and psychologic development, and in extreme cases, they may even die (Bowlby, 1965).

Nurses' Needs

Nurses become attached to an infant left for several weeks in the hospital, suffering feelings of separation, loss, and grief when the infant is taken away. These feelings are painful, but they are normal signs of attachment and separation, indicating that the infant has had a relationship that approximates a normal experience. Nurses need support to continue to involve themselves with each new infant waiting for placement.

Adoption

Adoption is the legal process by which the state gives full responsibility for the child to suitable parents, with the child becoming an actual legal member of the family. After a child is adopted, the adoptive parents are entirely responsible for the child's life. Adoption assures the child of having continuing family relationships throughout life, relationships that can begin as soon as the infant leaves the hospital, sometimes within 1 or 2 weeks after birth. Adoption requires that the child's biologic mother voluntarily surrender her legal rights to the child or that a court terminate her rights, usually on the basis of abandonment. After a period in foster care or adoptive placement (usually a total of 1 year), an adoption is legally finalized in the courts. In most states, a new birth certificate is issued showing the adoptive parents as the only parents. At this point, there should be complete protection against removal of the child from the adoptive home because of claims to the child made by another party.

The putative father's rights

There have been challenges to parental rights, and the legal scene is changing. In many states, the putative biologic father (unwed to the mother) must register his relationship to the infant within 30 days of the child's birth. Many states have established a birth-father registry. Currently, all states require that the putative father be informed before an adoption may be finalized (Ratterman, 1994). Some fathers want to raise the child, either alone or with their extended family. Others decide to marry or live with the birth mother and raise the child with her. The birth father may not want to raise the child but may still desire to know where the child will be placed and to have visitation rights, as well as provide medical and genetic background information (Horowitz, 1995).

Cross-cultural considerations

Challenges based on cross-cultural considerations are currently highly charged. The loss of a child's cultural heritage is deemed a tragedy by ethnic groups. The Indian Child Welfare Act (1978) won the fight to allow Native American tribal groups to have significant input on placement of a child with as little as $1/64$ Native American ancestry. Currently, some provisions of the Multiethnic Placement Act (1994) have been superceded by the Adoption Promotion and Stability Act (HR 3286) of 1996, which allows certain tax credits for adoptive parents and reduces barriers to interracial adoption. There are usually people interested in adopting infants, but older children, sibling groups, and special-needs children are often on long waiting lists for a permanent home.

Open adoption

Open adoption occurs when the birth and adoptive parents agree before the adoption that they will all play a part in raising the child. This approach to adoption is relatively new, and outcomes are slowly becoming understood (Gross, 1993). One study of 583 open adoptions found that 90% of the families were highly satisfied with the arrangement and would adopt this way again (Berry 1991).

It is important to understand that openness in adoption is better represented as a continuum rather than as an either/or proposition. Openness can range from the sending of cards to a third party on a yearly basis to an ongoing relationship between the birth and adoptive families that includes regular visitation. Levels of satisfaction with openness depend on such factors as the degree of openness, age of the children, number of siblings, and the conditions that led to the child's adoption.

International adoption

International adoptions are becoming a more frequently used avenue for couples to acquire a young infant. There is a great variation in the cost, the time it takes to complete the adoption, and the satisfaction with international adoption. Online AdoptINFO is a current source for domestic and international agencies involved.

Foster Care

Other infants leave the hospital's nursery for foster homes. If the birth mother chooses not to surrender her rights to the child and remains at least somewhat interested in the child so abandonment cannot be proven (even though the birth mother may be unable to care for the child herself), the child is placed in a foster home. Often, foster care is used for children who could be adopted but for whom adoptive homes are difficult to find because the children are older, have medical problems, or are members of sibling groups that should not be separated.

Foster care, in theory, is temporary placement with the goal of stabilizing the birth parent's situation or of finding adoptive parents. The child is placed with a family that is given primary responsibility for the child's care. Legal responsibility for the child is assigned to a state agency or a state-licensed private agency. Foster homes are usually administered directly through these agencies. Foster parents are paid a monthly rate through the agency to cover the child's expenses. A social worker is assigned to evaluate each home. A social worker works with the birth parent to resolve the uncertainty of the child's status in one of three ways.

1. The child is returned to the birth mother. This gradual process may begin with weekly supervised visits, followed by unsupervised visits in the birth parent's home, and finally a full return to the birth parent.

2. As the birth parent tries to follow arrangements with the agency, often mandated by a family court judge (such as attending counseling or drug rehabilitation sessions or parenting support groups), it may become apparent that the parent is unable or unwilling to make the changes required in order to ensure the child's return into the home. The parent may then voluntarily surrender rights to the child. This is generally a formal procedure that must take place with a lawyer and a witness, either in or out of court. Unfortunately, there are a number of problems today related to an overwhelming number of placements (often related to drug-using parents) and a shortage of supervising personnel.

3. The birth parents' rights are involuntarily terminated. This may occur because of abandonment, mental illness or retardation, abuse, or neglect. This proceeding is final and must take place in a family court.

Kinship care

Another arrangement gaining popularity in some states is *kinship foster care*. A family member of the birth parent will become the legal foster patent and receive the financial support accorded by this role. This serves to keep the family tie and, theoretically, the child will be better off because she is still with the family and can be returned to the birth parents when they are able to assume this responsibility. Kinship foster care has its own set of critics and crusaders, but it certainly has some special issues that must be addressed if the kinship foster care home is to be permanent. In some states, this growing trend has become extremely expensive, and a debate has begun regarding the state's responsibility to support children who reside with kin. In a state like New York, where 45% of children freed for adoption reside in kinship foster care homes, the argument is made that families should take care of their own without being paid; the state cannot afford to care for all these children (NYSDSS, 1994). However, loss of state funding may financially strain kinship homes to the point that they return children to foster care with strangers.

In theory, when children are placed in foster care, their birth parents should be given the support they need to eventually reunite the family. This approach is often referred to as *family preservation.* It values the family unit and encourages birth parents to raise their own children. Yet in recent years, situations have occurred where children are in foster care for years, awaiting birth parent rehabilitation that does not happen. There are important policy discussions weighing the rights of the birth parents and the rights of the child as the number of children in foster care escalates.

The distinction, then, between a child who can be placed for adoption and a child who is placed in a foster home for extended care is a legal one. The adopted child must first be *free for adoption,* which means that there is no parental claim to the child. Birth parents may voluntarily surrender their rights to the child by signing affidavits stating that this is their wish. Birth parents can also be sued in court and have their rights to children severed. The judicial systems of many states have historically favored the *blood bond* over the *psychologic bond* that the child has with the family with whom he lives, but this appears to be changing. Complete abandonment of the child by birth parents is one reason why the courts usually sever parental rights. If the birth parent's rights remain intact while the child lives with a foster family, many psychologically damaging conflicts can cause problems for the child.

Foster parents' needs. Many foster parents find it difficult to commit themselves totally to the child because of the possibility that he will be removed from their home and returned to the birth parents. The child may not understand the situation and may be confused by having two sets of parents (one set which the child knows as his "real" parents but who, in fact, are hardly known); later the child may be in conflict because he does not know where his identity and allegiance really lie. The foster care situation is difficult from the foster parents' viewpoint because legal uncertainties make them insecure in their feelings of love for their foster children. Many foster parents who commit themselves fully to children placed in their care suffer agonizing loss when the child is removed from their home, especially if the child is being returned to birth parents whom the foster parents feel remain "unfit." Even for the child who remains in the foster home, deep emotional conflicts can arise around matters such as visits from the birth parents. Foster parents must be unusually strong to be able to reach out to the child and explain the very mixed feelings involved in this situation. An ideal arrangement is to have foster parents and biologic parents all working together for eventual return to the biologic parents.

Finally, the birth parents are also frequently in conflict over the situation, torn between guilt over not being able to care for their child and their sense of inadequacy for being unable to do so. Unresolved grief may continue over an extended period.

The trend in the legislative and judicial systems is to give the children and foster parents more rights. Children, even infants, are being assigned their own lawyers to protect their rights and to guarantee that the best possible living situation is available to them in terms of their psychologic and physical development. Every state has its own laws concerning foster care, but as an example of progressive legislation, New York has given the preference for adoption to foster parents who have had a child in their home for 1 or more years. This is a step protecting the psychologic bonds—the delicate, fragile feelings of relationship—between the foster child and parents. Foster care must be restructured legally to guarantee that the "psychologic" parents of the foster child will have the fullest possible opportunity to develop normal family relationships and, most important, that the child will have an opportunity to feel that he is a secure and wanted member of a family.

Many states now also have subsidized adoption for foster parents who cannot afford to adopt a child who has been their foster child. This means that the state will provide adoption subsidy payments to such a family. These payments are usually subject to an annual review of the parents' income, but they may continue in cases of special needs children.

Compared with other forms of child care, foster care is the best way devised by our society of taking care of the child who cannot be brought up by the birth parents. In a foster home, a child relates to a complete family and can form close relationships on an individual basis. Even in the present legal situation, it is possible for a child to enter a foster home immediately after birth and to remain as a member of the family throughout childhood and adolescence, although this usually does not happen. The infant who enters a foster home will be able to relate to a parent with whom he can form the comforting, satisfying, and stimulating relationship that every infant needs in order to go on to more mature levels of psychologic development.

Key Points

■ Early discharge of mothers and newborns has shifted the location of a nurse's anticipatory guidance and teaching to home and clinic settings.

■ An understanding of child development can help parents enjoy and appreciate their infants.

■ Infant temperaments vary and are a significant factor in parental attachment and family interactions.

■ Instruction on maintaining temperature, avoiding household hazards, and resuscitating an infant is important content to include in parental teaching.

■ Immunizations play a vital role in keeping children and communities healthy.

■ Parents can be taught to manage problems with sleep and colic.

■ Avoiding both the prone sleeping position and exposure to passive cigarette smoke can decrease the incidence of SIDS in infants.

■ There are legal and psychosocial aspects to adoption and foster care that involve the nursing role.

Study Questions

20-1. Select the terms that apply to the following statements:
   a. A new infant who integrates well into the family has _____.
   b. A child who responds with tentative withdrawal and slower adaptability is _____.
   c. The general nature or characteristic mood of the individual is _____.
   d. For an infant, sucking a thumb is a way of _____.
   e. The infant cue of looking away when fatigued is _____.
   f. The condition that can result from allowing an infant to fall asleep while nursing from a bottle is
      _____.
   g. Sustained periods of crying during the first 3 months is _____.
   h. An infant placed with a grandmother for temporary care is receiving _____.

20-2. Which of the following behaviors is not present in a normal newborn infant by 1 week of age?
   a. The infant will be able to recognize the parents by sight.
   b. Habituation is used to block out stimuli.
   c. Loud noise will produce a startle response.
   d. The infant will distinguish between his mother and another by smell.

20-3. Parents question the nurse about newborn crying. The most helpful answer would be:
   a. "Infants cry to express frustration with their parents."
   b. "Crying only indicates a need for attention."
   c. "Newborns cry to release tension or ask for help."
   d. "This is their way of communication with bigger people."

20-4. Mary asks about whether her infant can "see." Choose the most appropriate answer the nurse could give.
   a. "A baby can follow a red ball or light like adults can."
   b. "Eye muscles are weak, so your baby cannot gaze more than a few minutes."
   c. "A baby will focus on objects about four to ten inches away, such as your face."
   d. "At first she probably sees only black and white objects."

20-5. During a home visit, the mother states that she can't afford fancy toys for her 2-week-old infant. Which intervention would be appropriate for the nurse?
   a. Ask her to think of safe toys that she can construct.
   b. Agree with the mother that new infants do not need toys.
   c. Encourage the mother to find sources of used, safe toys.
   d. Assess if she may be unable to provide other necessary items of care.

Answer Key

References

Accident facts: 1991 edition, Chicago, 1991, National Safety Council.

Adair R et al: Reducing night waking in infancy: a primary care intervention, *Pediatr* 89(4):585, 1992.

American Academy of Pediatrics: *Report of committee on infectious diseases*, ed 22, Elk Grove, Ill, 1991, The Academy.

Anders et al: Sleeping through the night: a developmental perspective, *Pediatr* 90(4):554, 1992.

*Anderson C: Integration of the Brazelton Neonatal Behavioral Assessment Scale into routine nursing care, *Issues Compr Pediatr Nurs* 9:341, 1986.

*Bahr J: Canine and feline rivalry, *Pediatr Nurs* 1(4):18, 1981.

Beck C: A meta-analysis of relationships between post partum depression and infant temperament, *Nursing Res* 45(4):225, 1996.

Berry M: The effects of open adoption on biological and adoptive parents and the children: the arguments and the evidence, *Child Welfare* 70(6):637, 1991.

*Betelheim B: *A good enough parent: a book on child-rearing*, New York, 1987, Alfred Knopf, Inc.

Blandon T, Deschner J: Biological mothers' grief: the postadoption experience in open versus confidential adoptions, *Child Welfare* 69(6):525, 1990.

Bloom RS, Cropley CC: *Textbook of neonatal resuscitation*, Dallas, 1995, American Heart Association.

*Bowlby J: *Child care and the growth of love*, Baltimore, 1965, Penguin Books.

*Brazelton TB: *Doctor and child*, Boston, 1976, Delacourt Press.

*Carey WB, McDevitt SC: Revision of the infant temperament questionnaire, *Pediatr* 61(5):735, 1978.

Carolan et al: Infant sleep position and the sudden infant death syndrome, *Clinical Pediatr* 34(8):402, 1995.

*Chess S, Thomas A: Temperament differences: a critical concept in child health care, *Pediatr Nurs* 21(2):167, 1985.

Collin RM: Nurses in early intervention, *Pediatr Nurs* 21(6):529, 1995.

Donaher-Wagner BM, Braun DH: Infant cardiopulmonary resuscitation for expectant and new parents, *MCN Am J Matern Child Nurs* 17(1):27, 1992.

Fagan JF, Detterman DK: The Fagan test of infant intelligence, *J Appl Devel Psychol* 13:173, 1992.

Farrington EA: Varicella zoster vaccine (Varivax), *Pediatr Nurs* 21(4):358, 1995.

*Field TM et al: The mother's assessment of the behavior of her infant, *Infant Behav Develop* 1:156, 1978.

*Field TM et al: Tactile/kinesthetic stimulation effects on preterm neonates, *Pediatrics* 77(5):654, 1988.

Field TM: Massage therapy for infants and children, *Developmental Behavior Pediat* 16(2):105, 1995.

Freed GE et al: Sudden infant death syndrome: prevention and an understanding of selected clinical issues, *Pediatr Clin North Am* 41(5): 967, 1994.

Fuller BF: Acoustic discrimination of three types of infant cries, *Nurs Res* 40(3):156, 1991.

*Funke J, Irbe MI: An instrument to assess the quality of maternity behavior, *J Obstet Gynecol Neonatal Nurs* 7(5):19, 1978.

*Gay J: A conceptual framework of bonding, *J Obstet Gynecol Neonatal Nurs* 10(6):440, 1981.

Gross H: Open adoption: A research based literature review and new data, *Child Welfare* 72(3):269, 1993.

*Haith M et al: Sensory and perceptual processes in early infancy, *Pediatr* 109(1):158, 1986.

Hardy-Havens DM, Hannon C: Legislation to mandate maternal and newborn length of stay, *J Pediatr Health Care* 10(3):141, 1996.

Hill DJ et al: A low allergen diet is a significant intervention in infantile colic: results of a community-based study, *J Allergy Clin Immunol* 96(6):886, 1995.

Horowitz FD: Targeting infant stimulation efforts, *Clin Perinatol* 17(1):185, 1990.

Horowitz R: *Adoption laws: answers to the most-asked questions*, Rockville, Md, 1995, National Adoption Information Clearinghouse.

*Klaus M, Kennell J: *Parent-infant bonding*, St Louis, 1982, Mosby.

Klein MJA: The home health nurse clinician's role in the prevention of nonorganic failure to thrive, *J Pediatr Nurs* 5(2):129, 1990.

Klonoff-Cohen HS et al: The effect of passive smoking and tobacco exposure through breast milk on sudden infant death syndrome, *JAMA* 273(10):795, 1995.

*Kodadek MP: Parenting the newborn, *NAACOG Update Series* 5(10):1, 1986.

Koepke JE et al: Becoming parents: feelings of adoptive mothers, *Pediatr Nurs* 17(4):333, 1991.

Korner, AF: Infant stimulation: issues of theory and research, *Clin Perinatol* 17(1)176, 1990.

Lerner H: Sleep position of infants: applying research to practice, *MCN Am J Matern Child Nurs* 18(5):275, 1993.

Lewis-Abney K, Smith ER: Managing fever of unknown source in infants and children, *J Pediatr Health Care* 10:135, 1996.

*Mahler M, Pine F, Berman A: *The psychological birth of the human infant*, New York, 1975, Basic Books.

*McFarlane A: Olefaction in the development of social preferences in the human neonate, *Ciba Foundation Symposium* 33:103, 1975.

Medoff-Cooper B: Infant temperament: implications for parenting from birth through 1 year, *J Pediatr Nurs* 10(3):141, 1995.

Melvin N: Children's temperament: intervention for parents, *J Pediatr Nurs* 10(3):152, 1995.

Metcalf TJ: Simethicone in the treatment of infant colic: a randomized placebo-controlled, multicenter study, *Pediatrics* 94(1):29, 1994.

Mitchell EA et al: Smoking and the sudden infant death syndrome, *Pediatrics* 91(5):893, 1993.

Morbidity and Mortality Weekly Report (MMWR): *Guidelines for immunizations*, 45(RR-12):1, 1996.

Morrow JD, Camp BW: Mastery motivation and temperament of 7-month-old infants. *Pediatr Nurs* 22(3):211, 1996.

New York State Department of Social Services (NYSDSS) and Community Development Office of Family and Children Services (Performance Monitoring and Evaluation Unit): *1994 Monitoring and analysis profiles with selected trend data: 1990-1994*, New York, 1994, The Department.

Rainey DY, Lawless MR: Infant positioning and SIDS, *Clin Pediatr* 33(6):323, 1994.

Ratterman D: *Adoption and the rights of putative fathers*,Washington, DC, 1993, American Bar Association Center on Children and the Law.

Rauh VA et al: The mother-infant transaction program, *Clin Perinatol* 17(1):91, 1990.

Rosenberg EB: *The adoption life cycle*, New York, 1992, The Free Press.

Ruben RJ: Communicative disorders: the first year of life, *Pediatr Clin North Am* 42(5):1047, 1994.

*Rubin RA: Binding-in in the postpartum period, *Matern Child Nurs* 6(2):67, 1977.

*Rubin RA: *Maternal identity and the maternal experience*, New York, 1984, Springer.

Standley JM, Moore RS: Therapeutic effects of music and mother's voice on premature infants, *Pediatr Nurs* 21(6):509, 1995.

Treem WR: Infant colic: a pediatric gastroenterologist's perspective, *Pediatr Clin North Am* 41(5):1139, 1994.

Unti SM: The critical first year of life: history, physical examination and general developmental assessment, *Pediatr Clin North Am* 41(5):859, 1994.

Von Burg MM, Sanders BJ, Weddell JA: Baby bottle tooth decay: a concern for all mothers, *Pediatr Nurs* 21(6):515, 1995.

Wegman ME: Annual summary of vital statistics: 1991, *Pediatrics* 90:835, 1992.

Weiss ME, Poelter D, Gocka I: Infrared tympanic thermometry for neonatal temperature assessment, *J Obstet Gynecol Neonatal Nurs* 23:798, 1993.

*Wessel MA et al: Paroxysmal fussiness in infancy, sometimes called "colic," *Pediatrics* 14:421, 1954.

Wolf D et al: Promoting hospital discharge of infants in safety seats, *J Community Health* 20(4):345, 1995.

Parent Resources

Brazelton, TB: *Touchpoints: your child's emotional and behavioral development*, Reading, Mass, 1992, Addison-Wesley.
The well-known Cambridge pediatrician's guide to children's psychosocial development. Organized by developmental stage with special section on infant and child issues such as allergies, bedwetting, sleep, crying, toilet-training, and illness.

*Classic reference.

Caplan T: *The first twelve months of life,* New York, 1995, Bantam Books.
 This guide to child development is organized by months and has general
 information on changes at each stage. Great photographs and growth
 charts.

Eisenberg A, Morkoff HE, Hathaway SE: *What to expect the first year,* New
 York, 1989, Workman Publishing.
 *This guide to growth and development and parenting issues is organized
 by months. A sequel has similar information on toddlers.*

Jones S, Freitag W: *Guide to baby products,* ed 4, New York, 1994,
 Consumer Reports Books.
 *Covers everything from furniture to food, plus a number of toys and
 health and safety devices.*

Spock B, Rothenberg MB: *Dr. Spock's baby and child care,* ed 6, New York,
 1992, Pocket Books.
 *This classic child care manual includes practical, reassuring advice
 about a wide variety of child care issues, with an emphasis on fostering
 parental confidence that begins with its well-known first sentence, "You
 know more than you think you do."*

Adoption Resources

AdoptINFO: Web site with research, opinion, and policy documents
 related to issues for adoptive families
http://www.cyfc.umn.edu/AdoptINFO.htp

Adoptive Families: Bimonthly journal available by writing to the following address:
Adoptive Families of America, Inc.
3333 Highway 100 North
Minneapolis, MN 55422
1-800-372-3300

The National Adoption Information Clearinghouse (NAIC)
5640 Nicholson Lane, Suite 300
Rockville, MD 20852
(301) 231-6512

*Spaulding for Children: National Resource Center for Special Needs
 Adoption*
16250 Northland Drive, Suite 120
Southfield, MI 48075
(810) 442-7080

Student Resource Shelf

Coffman S, Levitt MJ, Guacci-Franco N: Infant-mother attachment: relationships to maternal responsiveness and infant temperament, *J
 Pediatr Nurs* 10(1):9, 1995.
 *Study explores relationships among maternal responsiveness, infant tem-
 perament, and infant-mother attachment. Implications of findings are
 discussed.*

Lobar SL, Phillips S: The couple choosing private infant adoption,
 Pediatr Nurs 20(2):141, 1994.
 *Nurses can assist couples choosing private adoption by learning about
 the process and supporting the couple before and after they receive their
 infant.*

Five

Pregnancy *at* Risk

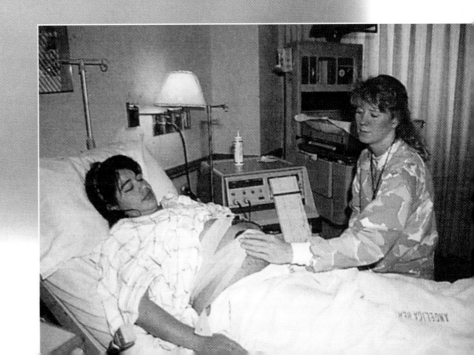

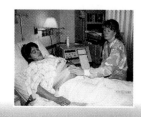

21

Reproductive System Problems *during* Pregnancy, Birth, *&* Recovery

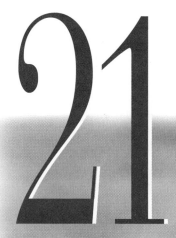

Learning Objectives

- Apply the steps of the nursing process to planning care for a woman with complications of the reproductive system.
- Correlate risk factors for preterm labor or premature rupture of membranes with physiology of pregnancy.
- Given a selected client situation, plan preterm labor prevention strategies.
- Correlate the changes of multiple pregnancy with the increased discomforts, risks, and interventions.
- Describe current rules and regulations that govern elective abortion.
- Summarize methods of psychosocial support for a woman when pregnancy is interrupted by spontaneous or elective abortion and by fetal death.
- Associate reproductive anatomy with causes of bleeding during pregnancy and the birth process.
- Compare and contrast signs and symptoms for each life-threatening cause of obstetric hemorrhage, and relate them to intervention choices.

Key Terms

Abruptio Placentae
Diovular Twins
Ectopic Pregnancy
Hemorrhage
Hydatidiform Mole
Hypovolemia
Incompetent Cervix
Induced Abortion
Intrauterine Fetal Death (IUFD)
Lacerations
Monovular Twins
Oligohydramnios

Placenta Accreta
Placenta Previa
Polyhydramnios
Premature Rupture of Membranes (PROM)
Preterm Labor (PTL)
Spontaneous Abortion
Tocolytics
Trophoblastic Disease
Uterine Atony
Vasa Previa

The complications of pregnancy that cause high risk for the woman and infant are presented in the last third of this text. Approximately 85% of all pregnancies that progress to the expected birth date are normal and without problems. When problems do occur, extreme anxiety and fear for the safety of the woman and her infant often occur. Figure 21-1 illustrates the varied "things that can go wrong" as documented in the maternal and infant health portion of the birth certificate. Throughout the following chapters it should be kept in mind that preventive care and interventions that support

maternal and fetal health and survival are the goals of all maternal and newborn interventions.

The reproductive system is complex and, if disturbed, can place a woman at risk for loss of her fetus or rarely her own life. This chapter will focus on the reproductive problems related to preterm labor and multiple pregnancy; abnormal functions such as polyhydramnios or oligohydramnios, hydatidiform mole, and ectopic implantation, which have underlying pathologic conditions; loss of the pregnancy before viability (abortion) or after viability (intrauterine fetal death [IUFD]); and abnormal placental

36a. MEDICAL RISK FACTORS FOR THIS PREGNANCY
(Check all that apply)

Anemia (Hct. <30/Hgb. <10)...................... ☐
Cardiac disease.. ☐
Acute or chronic lung disease.................... ☐
Diabetes.. ☐
Genital herpes... ☐
Hydramnios/Oligohydramnios.................... ☐
Hemoglobinopathy..................................... ☐
Hypertension, chronic................................ ☐
Hypertension, pregnancy-associated.......... ☐
Eclampsia.. ☐
Incompetent cervix.................................... ☐
Previous infant 4000+ grams...................... ☐
Previous preterm or small-for-gestational-age
   infant.. ☐
Renal disease... ☐
Rh sensitization... ☐
Uterine bleeding.. ☐
None.. ☐
Other_____ ☐
          (Specify)

30b. OTHER RISK FACTORS FOR THIS PREGNANCY
(Complete all items)

Tobacco use during pregnancy.................. Yes ☐ No ☐
   Average number cigarettes per day_____
Alcohol use during pregnancy.................. Yes ☐ No ☐
   Average number drinks per week_____
Weight gained during pregnancy_____ lbs.

39. OBSTETRIC PROCEDURES
(Check all that apply)

Amniocentesis.. ☐
Electronic fetal monitoring......................... ☐
Induction of labor...................................... ☐
Stimulation of labor................................... ☐
Tocolysis.. ☐
Ultrasound... ☐
None.. ☐
Other_____ ☐
          (Specify)

40. COMPLICATIONS OF LABOR AND/OR DELIVERY
(Check all that apply)

Febrile (>100°F or 38°C.)........................... ☐
Meconium, moderate/heavy........................ ☐
Premature rupture of membranes (>12 hours)........... ☐
Abruptio placentae.................................... ☐
Placenta previa... ☐
Other excessive bleeding........................... ☐
Seizures during labor.................................. ☐
Precipitous labor (<3 hours)...................... ☐
Prolonged labor (>20 hours)...................... ☐
Dysfunctional labor.................................... ☐
Breech/Malpresentation............................. ☐
Cephalopelvic disproportion...................... ☐
Cord prolapse.. ☐
Anesthetic complications........................... ☐
Fetal distress.. ☐
None.. ☐
Other_____ ☐
          (Specify)

41. METHOD OF DELIVERY *(Check all that apply)*

Vaginal... ☐
Vaginal birth after previous C-section........ ☐
Primary C-section...................................... ☐
Repeat C-section.. ☐
Forceps.. ☐
Vacuum.. ☐

40. ABNORMAL CONDITIONS OF THE NEWBORN
(Check all that apply)

Anemia (Hct. <39/Hgb. <13)...................... ☐
Birth injury... ☐
Fetal alcohol syndrome.............................. ☐
Hyaline membrane disease/RDS................. ☐
Meconium aspiration syndrome.................. ☐
Assisted ventilation < 30 min..................... ☐
Assisted ventilation ≥ 30 min..................... ☐
Seizures.. ☐
None.. ☐
Other_____ ☐
          (Specify)

43. CONGENITAL ANOMALIES OF CHILD
(Check all that apply)

Anencephalus... ☐
Spina bifida/Meningocele........................... ☐
Hydrocephalus... ☐
Microcephalus.. ☐
Other central nervous system anomalies
   *(Specify)*_____ ☐

Heart malformations.................................. ☐
Other circulatory/respiratory anomalies
   *(Specify)*_____ ☐

Rectal atresia/stenosis............................... ☐
Tracheo-esophageal fistula/Esophageal atresia...... ☐
Omphalocele/Gastroschisis........................ ☐
Other gastrointestinal anomalies
   *(Specify)*_____ ☐

Malformed genitalia................................... ☐
Renal agenesis... ☐
Other urogenital anomalies........................
   *(Specify)*_____ ☐

Cleft lip/palate.. ☐
Polydactyly/Syndactyly/Adactyly............... ☐
Club foot.. ☐
Diaphragmatic hernia................................. ☐
Other musculoskeletal/integumental anomalies
   *(Specify)*_____ ☐

Down's syndrome....................................... ☐
Other chromosomal anomalies
   *(Specify)*_____ ☐

None.. ☐
Other_____ ☐
          (Specify)

Figure 21-1 Maternal and infant health categories from the revision of the U.S. Standard Certificate of Live Birth.

function that underlies major bleeding problems during the perinatal period.

PRETERM BIRTH

Birth after 20 weeks and before 37 completed weeks of gestation will result in various degrees of immaturity in the newborn. The less mature the infant, the greater the risk of respiratory distress, intraventricular hemorrhage, necrotizing enterocolitis and neurologic deficits, and the risk of neonatal death. Thus the clinical management goal is to prevent or arrest premature labor long enough to allow the fetus to reach the best level of maturity, which is hopefully more than 36 weeks of development. After this gestational age, serious complications occur less frequently. Chapter 29 defines prematurity and low birth weight in more detail. Here the focus will be on the process of premature labor and preventive measures.

PRETERM LABOR

Preterm birth is preceded either by **premature rupture of membranes** (PROM) with or without signs of labor or only by signs of early labor. There may also be a structural defect leading to early dilation without labor or membrane rupture. Without intervention an **incompetent cervix** will result in the birth of a nonviable infant between 16 and 20 weeks of gestation.

Management will vary depending on gestational age, the maternal status, and the potential causes. Many interventions are controversial, have not proven to be effective, or have only limited effectiveness (Enkin et al, 1995).

To reduce the incidence of prematurity a number of factors must be considered, including high-risk socioeconomic or physical factors that require improved preventive interventions. Home monitoring of **preterm labor** (PTL) coupled with nursing management and support is a growing field. Every nurse needs to know the sequence of PTL and the recommended interventions.

Risk

An emphasis on reducing the U.S. PTL rate has not been as successful as programs in other developed countries because of the fragmentation of health care here. In fact, in spite of many early intervention programs, the rate has risen from 8.9% in 1980 to above 10% in 1995 (ACOG, 1995). It is expected that the rate will remain above 10% in 2000. Multiple pregnancies account for 10% of premature births.

For many women the cause may be unknown, and for them preterm birth is unpreventable. In other cases, the causes are treatable if the potential for preterm birth can be recognized early enough. Factors that are related to PTL are listed in Box 21-1.

In general, those who have preterm birth fall into one of the following categories:

- Almost one third of preterm births are related to maternal medical complications such as pregnancy-induced hypertension, cardiac disease, or insulin-dependent diabetes (see Chapters 22 and 23), and obstetric complications such as placenta previa, cervical incompetence, and multiple births.

- Another one third results from rupture of membranes (ROM) before term, leading to labor.
- Among one third of women, labor begins with no apparent reason. These last two may have an underlying cause of genitourinary infection (Iams, Johnson, and Parker 1994).

Women who give birth prematurely more frequently have urinary, vaginal, or amniotic fluid infection and may develop postpartum endometritis. Neonatal pneumonia develops more frequently in the infants of women with perinatal infections.

Research has shown that microbial colonization and resultant inflammation cause disruption of the decidua and membranes and a release of prostaglandins. Some vaginal flora also produce enzymes that increase the concentration of *arachidonic acid* (a precursor of prostaglandins). Microorganisms and host white blood cells produce a variety of *proteolytic enzymes*, substances that break down protein (Queenan and Hobbins, 1996). In addition, microorganisms may break down the mucous plug and facilitate the entrance of vaginal and cervical bacteria into the uterus. Figure 21-2 shows the relationship of potential causes of PTL.

The microorganisms detected in the first trimester and associated with increased risk of preterm birth are *Trichomonas vaginalis, Ureaplasma urealyticum, Myco-*

Box 21-1   Preterm Labor Risk Factors

SOCIAL HISTORY

Maternal age < 17 or > 40
Weight/height below standard
Prepregnancy weight < 50 kg
 Poor weight gain by 22 wks
Poor nutrition
Poverty
No or late prenatal care
Minority ethnic population
Heavy work, long commute
DES exposure in utero
Substance abuse
 Cocaine use
 Alcohol, smoking

HISTORY OF MEDICAL PROBLEMS

Pyelonephritis
Cone biopsy
Uterine anomaly or fibroids
Insulin-dependent diabetes

HISTORY OF PRETERM LABORS

Prior premature ROM
Prior preterm birth

PROBLEMS WITH PRESENT PREGNANCY

Genitourinary Infection

Bacteriuria, STDs

Bleeding Problems

Bleeding after 12 wks
 Placenta previa
 Placental separation
More than two spontaneous or elective abortions
Mid-trimester loss of pregnancy
 Incompetent cervix

Changed Uterine Volume

Oligohydramnios/polyhydramnios
Multiple pregnancy

Hypertension

Protein in urine >1+, more than 300 mg/L in 24 hr

Changed Status of Fetus or Cervix

Early fetal distress, intrauterine growth retardation
Premature ROM
 Early dilation of internal os
 Uterus irritable

DES, Diethylstilbestrol; *ROM,* rupture of membranes; *STD,* sexually transmitted disease.

plasma hominis, and *Bacterioides spp.* (Ergarter, 1996). In the second half of pregnancy *Gardnerella vaginalis, Chlamydia trachomatis,* group B *streptococcus,* and aerobic and anaerobic microorganisms that cause bacterial vaginosis (BV) may precipitate early labor.

Analysis of preventive strategies shows that antibiotic treatment during the first trimester may prevent later preterm birth (see Chapter 4). There may need to be retreatment. Metronidazole and intravaginal or oral clindamycin seem the most promising (McDonald et al, 1994).

Signs

The diagnosis of PTL usually is made when the following criteria are present (Beringer and Niebyl, 1990):
- Gestational age of 20 to 37 weeks
- Four uterine contractions in 20 minutes or eight or more in 60 minutes and ROM
- Intact membranes with clinical effacement of 50% or more and dilation of more than 2 cm

Beginning after weeks 20 to 28, normal uterine activity includes low-intensity contractions of less than 15 mm Hg pressure, which gradually increase in frequency and intensity until term when there should be fewer than four an hour by the external tocotransducer (the woman may not sense these mild contractions). Normal diurnal activity occurs with two periods of more frequent contractions and two quiet periods between 4 and 11 AM and 2 and 10 PM. This *diurnal* (twice a day) pattern is absent when preterm uterine activity is irritable (Figure 21-3).

Preterm uterine irritability may begin as early as 24 weeks. These low-amplitude, high-frequency (LAHF) waves are an early warning sign. This hyperactivity is evidenced as erratic but frequent mild, wavelike contractions. If the rate increases before 28 weeks to more than eight to ten an hour, the intensity may exceed 15 mm Hg (Figure 21-4). Without intervention, contractions will become organized and more intense, resulting in premature birth (Eganhouse and Burnside, 1992).

Through home uterine monitoring it has been shown that there is a sudden increase in numbers of contractions an hour in the 24-hour period before overt signs of PTL. This sudden increase is one of the only clear signs that can be observed. If a woman can learn to detect this increased activity, she can receive intervention *before* significant cervical dilation occurs.

Fetal fibronectin

A protein normally found in fetal membranes and the decidua may be found in the cervicovaginal fluid before the twentieth week but rarely after. The presence of *fibronectin* in the second half of pregnancy is now closely

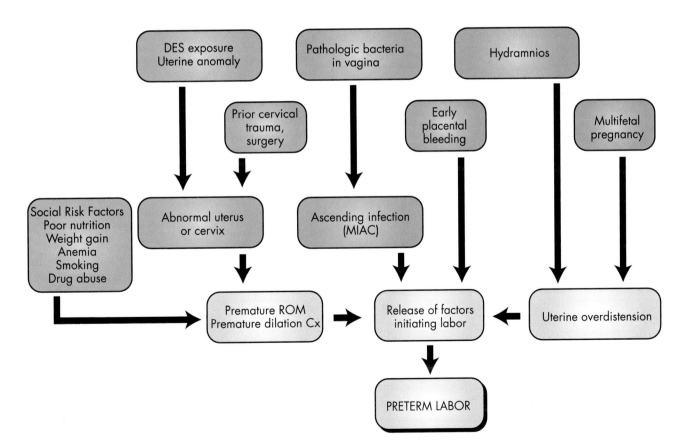

Figure 21-2   Factors affecting the onset of preterm labor.

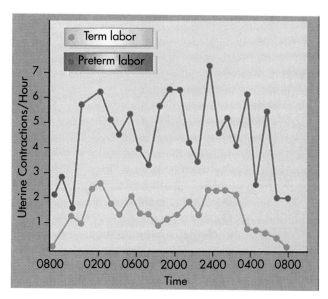

Figure 21-3 Comparison of contraction rates in 24 hours in normal pregnancies (*red*) and those with uterine irritability (*blue*). (Modified from Schwenzor TH, Schumann R, Halberstadt F: The importance of 24 hour cardiotocographic monitoring during tocolytic therapy. In Jung H, Lambert G, eds: *Beta-mimetic drugs in obstetrics and perinatology,* New York, 1982, Thieme-Stratton.)

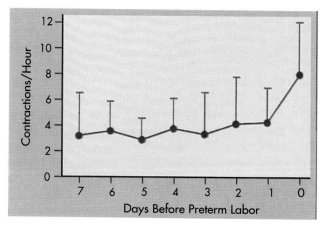

Figure 21-4 Frequency of contractions during the last 7 days before preterm labor. (From Katz M, Newman RB, Gill PJ: Assessment of uterine activity in ambulatory patients at high risk of preterm labor and delivery, *Am J Obstet Gynecol* 154:44, 1986.)

associated with pathologic changes at points where fetal and maternal tissues meet. This is a diagnostic marker for potential PTL with approximately a 93% sensitivity (Iams et al, 1995). There is a bedside test kit (Adeza Biomedical, Sunnyvale CA) to make the assay, which may come into wider use.

Transvaginal ultrasonography of the cervix

To narrow the group that needs therapy for PTL, Timor-Tritsch et al (1996) suggest that an image of the internal cervical os obtained by transvaginal ultrasound will confirm that dilation is truly beginning. This test added to fetal fibronectin assay may show which women need therapy and which cases are "false alarms."

Premature rupture of membranes

Membranes may rupture without subsequent organized labor contractions, or contractions may begin without membrane rupture. When membranes rupture before onset of full-term labor it is called *premature rupture of membranes* (PROM). When the rupture occurs before onset of PTL it is called *premature PROM* (PPROM). Causes are most likely to be related to infection of the genitourinary tract, as discussed earlier. Membrane rupture may be just a small leak or may be evidenced by a gush of fluid. A small leak may seal, and pregnancy may continue. The longer that leaking continues after rupture, the more likely there is to be ascending infection and chorioamnionitis.

Some women can recognize contractions; others talk of "feeling something change." Because the subtle signs of

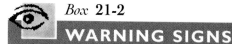

Box 21-2
WARNING SIGNS

Subtle Signs of Preterm Labor

Menstrual-like abdominal aching or cramps
General sense that something is wrong
Rhythmic dull backache or pelvic ache
Heavy feeling of pressure in the pelvis
Increase or change in vaginal discharge (more mucus that is watery or blood-tinged)
Intermittent uterine cramping, more than four every 20 minutes or eight an hour, often not sensed as painful
Intestinal cramping with or without diarrhea
Urinary frequency, perhaps with urgency
Change in fetal movement patterns

PTL may be missed, women should be taught the warning signs and the importance of reporting any changes promptly (Box 21-2).

Clinical Management

Some approaches have been attempted to standardize early detection of the potential for PTL. Women in the risk categories are observed more frequently and are instructed in self-monitoring of contractions.

Upon admission for reported labor or PROM, the woman is observed in the labor unit while a decision is made about labor status. Remember, the earlier she comes for diagnosis, the more likely it is that interventions will be effective.

Uterine cramping is monitored externally. A careful speculum examination is performed to assess cervical dilation and to note the presence of bulging membranes or the presence of amniotic fluid in the vagina. If membranes are leaking, a positive nitrazine test of the vaginal fluid will show a more alkaline pH (> 7) than urine, marked by a change to blue color. Amniotic fluid spread on a glass slide will show a fern pattern as it dries. This *ferning* is caused by crystallization of sodium chloride. A careful digital examination may follow the speculum examination, and a modified Bishop score is determined (see Chapter 13). Thereafter vaginal examinations are kept to a minimum to prevent the risk of transmitting infection from the lower vaginal canal into the cervical os.

Protocols for premature ruptured membranes

Vaginal cultures are taken for *Neisseria gonorrhea, Chlamydia trachomatis,* and group B *streptococcus* (GBS) to determine if there is *microbial invasion of the amniotic cavity* (MIAC). Prophylactic antibiotics are started, usually with ampicillin IV, with doses given until the results of the cultures are returned, and then broad-spectrum antibiotics, such as gentamicin, clindamycin, or erythromycin, are added if there is infection. Urinalysis and urine culture will indicate a urinary infection. Treatment with antibiotics has prolonged the pregnancy safely with a reduction in chorioamnionitis and adverse effects of prematurity (Queenan and Hobbins, 1996; Ergarter et al, 1996).

A baseline complete blood count is done. Nonstress testing is done (a nonreactive response and tachycardia are associated with MIAC), and ultrasound evaluation will indicate the amount of remaining amniotic fluid, with the biophysical profile. Some centers do routine amniocentesis to rule out MIAC and determine fetal lung maturity.

Decisions for preterm management are difficult. First, the woman should be transferred to a center where there is a neonatal intensive care unit (NICU). If the leaking continues, labor usually follows within the week, and the woman should remain in the hospital. Tocolysis is not done. If the leaking stops, she may be cared for at home with modified activity and evaluated every 2 weeks to determine fetal status.

If membranes rupture before full-term labor, but the fetus is mature enough (> 37 weeks), labor will be allowed to continue or will be induced. Usually only a short period, less than 12 hours, is allowed for observation before inducing labor. Observations must include ascertaining development of ascending infection by following maternal vital signs and fetal heart recordings.

Protocols for preterm labor

Assessment for PTL includes evaluating risk factors and subtle signs. If a woman is sent home after evaluation, careful documentation of the assessment is crucial to prevent risk of liability later should she deliver unexpectedly and fault the hospital personnel for sending her home.

The woman always is monitored for at least 1 hour in the labor area until a decision is made regarding potential outcome. Because a woman may be dehydrated, immediate intravenous (IV) hydration with 500 ml in 1 hour (Beringer and Niebyl, 1990) is a common practice. A more rapid fluid intake is not advised in the event tocolytic agents are to be used because fluid retention with pulmonary edema may occur with beta-mimetic drugs. During this hour the woman maintains a side-lying position and is monitored. The goal is to relax the uterine muscle with these interventions. If contractions stop, she may remain in the area for a few more hours. Care is individualized based on gestational age.

If contractions do not improve, and the cervix is less than 3- to 4-cm dilated, tocolytic therapy will be instituted if the risk of prolonging the pregnancy is less than the risk of the early delivery. Tocolysis is not used in cases of fetal distress or anomaly, ROM, and maternal disease such as severe hypertension, hemorrhage, or infection.

Tocolytic agents

Tocolytics belong to a class of drugs that inhibit contractions by affecting smooth muscle action. Analyses of tocolytic effectiveness show that these drugs will delay labor at least 24 to 48 hours and sometimes up to several weeks, but there are many failures (Drug Profile 21-1). In cases of possible infection, the addition of antibiotic therapy has improved effectiveness (Reece et al, 1995; McGregor, 1994).

Ritodrine (Yutopar) and *terbutaline* (Brethine) are commonly used. Terbutaline was initially used for asthma to relax bronchioles and has fewer side effects than does ritodrine, although terbutaline is in the same category of beta-mimetics. Currently, studies show that ritodrine is more effective than terbutaline, although terbutaline continues to be used. (Major actions are illustrated in Figure 21-5). Beta$_1$ receptors are found in the heart, small intestine, and adipose tissue; beta$_2$ receptors are in the uterus, blood vessels, bronchioles, and liver (Reece et al, 1995). Side effects are an exaggeration of physiologic effects. There is always an elevated heart rate, increase in cardiac output (pounding heart), and narrowing of coronary arteries, which for some may lead to ischemia and chest pain. A small number of women develop pulmonary edema with IV administration. The client complains of nervousness, headache, and palpitations and may have nausea and vomiting. Thus these drugs have significant effects on the maternal system and must be administered with caution and monitored carefully. Tolerance to the drug develops quickly and probably explains why these drugs are not as effective for long-term tocolysis.

Nifedipine, a calcium channel blocker used for hypertension, has been found useful because it relaxes smooth muscle. Results are comparable with the beta-mimetics, but administration and maintenance are simpler, a 10-mg capsule is given sublingually to be absorbed slowly or may be bitten to increase speed of absorption. Then additional

Box 21-1

DRUG PROFILE

Tocolytic Drugs

Drug/Dose/Route	Maternal/Fetal Effects	Monitoring
BETA-ADRENERGIC AGONISTS		

Ritodrine (Yutopar)

Dosage: IV bolus 0.25 mg, then 0.05-0.10 mg/min IV. Increments of .05 mg/min q20min to maximum of 0.35 mg/min. Decrease for 24 hr in same steps until lowest effective dose, then phase in po dose of 5-10 mg q4hr. First dose po 30 min before d/c IV dose. Stabilize before sending home on po doses.

Action: Beta-adrenergic receptor stimulant relaxes smooth muscle of uterus, respiratory tract; $t_{1/2}$ is 6-9 min at first, then 2-3 hr. Tolerance develops quickly.

Precautions: Hypovolemia, bleeding, hypertension, thyroid dysfunction, cardiac disease of any kind, diabetes, migraines, significant chronic fetal distress, infection. Discontinue drug 6 hr before birth.

Maternal

Effects are dose-related, and dose is titrated by woman's response; screen ECG before starting dose. *CV:* tachycardia, arrhythmias, chest pain, increased systolic and decreased diastolic pressure. *CNS:* tremors, headache, malaise, anxiousness, weakness. *GI:* nausea, vomiting, bloated feeling, diarrhea, constipation. *Metabolic:* hyperglycemia, hypokalemia, metabolic acidosis. *Other:* erythema, sweating, chills, hyperventilation.

Fetal/Newborn

Only with severe maternal effects: tachycardia, acidosis, hypoxia. Check newborn for these effects and paralytic ileus, hypotension, and hypoglycemia at birth.

Vital signs: BP q5min until stable, then q15min during IV route, then q4hr until stable. Pulse, respirations q1hr. Notify physician if pulse >130. Auscultate chest for rales and rhonchi. Daily weight. Urine for ketones. Blood for electrolytes, glucose. Give antiemetic, ice chips at first. Maintain quiet, restful environment with side-lying or Fowler's position. Reassure for anxiety. Teach to self-monitor contractions and fetal movements at home. Often use home monitoring.

Terbutaline (Brethine)

Dosage: 0.25 mg SC q20-60min until contractions stop. May be delivered SC by terbutaline pump or IV. Then 2.5-5 mg po q4hr for 48 hr. Maintenance dose is 5 mg q6hr.

Action: Acts on beta$_2$-receptor in smooth muscle of uterus, bronchi, $t_{1/2}$ is 3.7 hr. Also used with fetal distress to reduce hypertonic contractions and increase placental blood flow.

Precautions: Not used for diabetes, cardiac, asthma, severe PIH, thyroid conditions. Risk of pulmonary edema with IV fluid related to colloid osmotic pressure (COP), especially with betamethasone use.

Maternal

CV: increases systolic, decreases diastolic pressures related to peripheral vascular resistance; increases heart rate CO, SV; pounding heart, flushing, palpitations. *CNS:* tremors, nervousness, headache. *GI:* nausea, vomiting. *Metabolic:* glucose metabolism altered, hypokalemia, ketonuria.

Fetal/Newborn

Tachycardia; monitor glucose, heart rate.

Screen baseline glucose status; follow urinary ketones and serum glucose levels during treatment and electrolytes and serial hematocrit values. Screen baseline ECG; follow maternal-fetal vital signs closely; strict I&O. Monitor pulse for rate exceeding 120 bpm.

MAGNESIUM

Magnesium Sulfate

Dosage: Loading dose, 4-6 g of 10% solution for 20 min. Then 2 to 4 g/hr until contractions stop. Then po with 1 g tab magnesium oxide: q2-4hr for 24 hr. Many physicians use magnesium sulfate after terbutaline or ritodrine in lower doses with good effect.

Maternal

CV: Vasodilation with hypotension. *CNS:* depressed deep tendon reflexes, depressed respirations, muscle weakness, paralytic ileus, confusion. *Other:* sweating, flushing, hypothermia, oliguria.

Fetal heart tone and contractions. If unsuccessful, discontinue infusion 2 hr before expected delivery of infant to decrease adverse effects.

bid, Twice daily; *BP,* blood pressure; *CO,* cardiac output; *CNS,* central nervous system; *CV,* cardiovascular; *d/c,* discontinue; *ECG,* electrocardiogram; *EENT,* eyes, ears, nose, and throat; *FDA,* Food and Drug Administration; *GI,* gastrointestinal; *I & O,* intake and output; *po,* by mouth; *qid,* four times daily; *SC,* subcutaneous; *SV,* stroke volume; $t_{1/2}$, half-life.

Box 21-1

DRUG PROFILE

Tocolytic Drugs — Cont'd

Drug/Dose/Route	Maternal/Fetal Effects	Monitoring
MAGNESIUM — cont'd **Magnesium Sulfate — cont'd** *Action:* Competes with calcium entry into muscle, thus affecting contraction intensity. Short $t_{1/2}$; difficult to obtain therapeutic level. Toxic level may occur if renal function is poor. *Precautions:* Renal impairment, hypotension, myocardial damage.	**Fetal/Newborn** Hypermagnesemia, lethargy, hypotonia, possible magnesium toxicity, and neuromuscular and respiratory depression.	Antidote is calcium gluconate. Because excreted unchanged in urine, check output < 30ml/hr. Check respiratory rate > 14/min; check deep tendon reflexes (Box 22-4). Check Mg levels q6hr for therapeutic range of 4-7 mEq/L.
CALCIUM CHANNEL BLOCKERS **Nifedipine (Adalat, Procardia)** *Dosage:* Sublingual for quick onset using gelatin capsule. Repeat 10 mg q20min x 3. Then po 10-20 mg q4-6h. Chew and swallow with water. Reduce dosage after 3 days to two times a day (bid) for 5 days. *Action:* Inhibits calcium flow in muscle tissue, relaxes smooth muscle; extra benefit if woman has hypertension. $t_{1/2}$ is 2-3 hr. *Precautions:* Hypersensitivity, increases effects of beta-blockers; with other beta-blockers, may cause cardiac failure, hypotension. Caution: not FDA approved as yet for this purpose.	**Maternal** *CV:* palpitations, hypotension, peripheral edema. *CNS:* headache, weakness, dizziness, transient facial flushing, disturbed sleep. *EENT:* nasal congestion, dyspnea, cough, wheezing, blurred vision. *GI:* nausea, heartburn, diarrhea, abdominal cramps. *Other:* muscle cramps, joint pain, fever, chills. **Fetal/Newborn** Tachycardia.	Fetal heart tones and contractions. Maternal vital signs. When on bed rest use left lateral position. Obtain laboratory data: electrolyte levels. Monitor blood status.
ANTIPROSTAGLANDINS **Indomethacin** *Dose:* Rectal suppository 50-100 mg, then 25 mg po q6hr until contractions cease, or 50 mg po, then 25 mg po q4hr for 24 hr. Observe contractions and repeat for another 24 hr if recurs. Sometimes used with ritodrine. Usually not used after 35 weeks to avoid potential of ductus arteriosus closure. *Action:* Prostaglandin inhibition. Decreases effects of prostaglandin, thus relaxing smooth muscle. $t_{1/2}$, 2-3 hr. Transferred across placenta. Neonatal $t_{1/2}$ is 11-15 hr and longer if immature. *Contraindications:* Woman with any bleeding potential or peptic ulcer (because of slight anticoagulant effect).	**Maternal** Few effects, no change in heart rate or BP; nausea, heartburn, and vomiting occur; rare postpartum hemorrhage. **Fetal/Newborn** Potential of premature closure of ductus arteriosus—used for this purpose in neonate. Persistent pulmonary hypertension in neonate is rare possibility. Oligohydramnios—inhibits voiding and thus volume of amniotic fluid. Used as therapy when polyhydramnios occurs. Potential for hyperbilirubinemia if indomethacin displaces bilirubin from binding sites.	In small doses, few side effects. Observe contraction patterns for dizziness, drowsiness. Avoid alcohol, salicylates. Observe for change in bleeding pattern postpartum. Fetal assessment by serial ultrasound to determine amniotic fluid levels and any change in ductus arteriosus. Because drug levels reach equilibrium within 5-6 hr observe infant in neonatal period for prolonged excretion. D/C indomethacin 24 hr before labor if not halted by drug.

doses are given, up to four in the first hour, to stop contractions. Maintenance dose is held to 20 mg every 4 to 6 hours. Because it is a potent vasodilator, the mother may experience dizziness, flushing, and headache. Magnesium sulfate and nifedipine are not given together; profound hypotension may result.

A frequently used IV agent is *magnesium sulfate.* Effective as a neuromuscular blocking agent in cases of hypertension during pregnancy, it relaxes smooth muscle by affecting the flow of calcium out of the muscle cell. Magnesium sulfate is a familiar drug in labor and birth and has fewer side effects than do other tocolytic agents. Initial doses are given IV with a loading dose of 4 to 6 g and infusion 1 to 2 g an hour until contractions cease. Oral magnesium is rarely used for maintenance, however, a comparison of side effects of magnesium oxide and terbutaline is shown in Figure 21-6. A complete description of magnesium sulfate monitoring is found in Chapter 22 and in Drug Profile 21-1.

Because prostaglandins are involved in initiating labor (Chapter 13), antiprostaglandins have been used; currently *indomethacin* is used, but only for short periods (24-48 hr). Indomethacin is not considered for maintenance therapy because of adverse effects on the fetus. Inhibition of voiding and closure of the ductus arteriosus can occur, and, like acetylsalicylic acid (ASA), indomethacin inhibits platelet function and prolongs bleeding time.

The newest agent, *Atosiban,* is an oxytocin antagonist. The drug is administered either IV or SC and has an apparent lack of maternal or fetal side effects (Repke et al, 1996; Shubert, 1995).

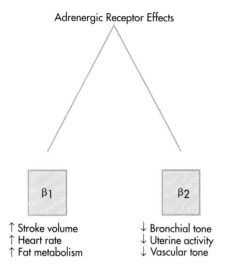

Figure 21-5   Adrenergic receptor effects. Beta$_1$ and beta$_2$ receptor effects often overlap. Search is for drug that has more specific beta$_2$ effects.

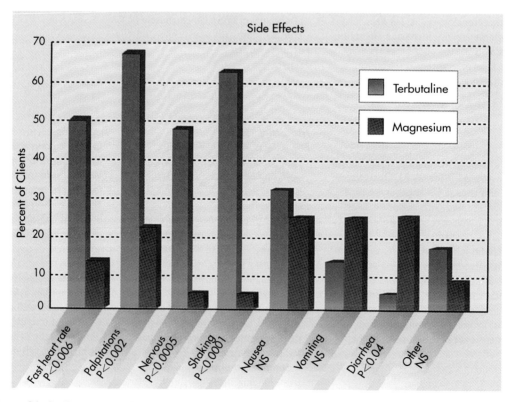

Figure 21-6   Percentage of clients reporting side effects with oral terbutaline and oral magnesium oxide. (Redrawn from Ridgeway LE et al: A prospective randomized comparison of oral terbutaline and magnesium oxide for the maintenance of tocolysis, *Am J Obstet Gynecol* 163:879, 1990.)

Box 21-1
CLINICAL DECISION

Lisa is receiving IV magnesium sulfate (2 g/hr) because of PTL. She complains of a heavy feeling in her limbs and of feeling too warm. What assessments must be done, and what would you expect to find? (See Drug Profile 21-1.)

Stimulation of lung maturity. When preterm birth between 28 and 34 weeks is threatened, the woman is usually given betamethasone IM to stimulate production of fetal lung maturity by increasing production of pulmonary surfactant (see Chapter 29). Glucocorticoids such as betamethasone work to prevent respiratory distress and also reduce the incidence of intraventricular hemorrhage and necrotizing enterocolitis in the young preterm infant (ACOG, 1994). For the greatest effect, doses must precede birth by 24 to 48 hours. Effects last as long as a week, and the dose may be repeated if needed (Drug Profile 21-2).

Thyrotropin-releasing hormone (TRH) may also be administered to the mother in PTL (at least 24 hours before birth) to reduce the incidence of respiratory distress and other complications of prematurity. TRH accelerates lung maturity, with an additive effect with glucocorticoids, producing *surfactant,* the necessary substance in the lung that enables oxygen transfer across the mucous membrane (Ballard et al, 1992). In several clinical trials, reduced chronic lung disease after 36 weeks of age was found in preterm infants when the mother received the full course of TRH (Ballard et al, 1992; Knight et al, 1994). This substance is given by IV intermittent infusion of four doses in 24 hours. The woman is continuously monitored for blood pressure (BP) and heart rate (HR) every 10 minutes, beginning 10 minutes before the 30-minute infusion and ending 10 minutes after it is over. Side effects may be temporary breast enlargement, headaches, increased HR, nausea, light headedness, feeling of warmth, and less commonly, anxiety, sweating, urge to void, and chest pressure. In rare instances, there may be convulsions. Informed consent is required.

Treatment for cervical incompetence

By 16 weeks the pressure of the gestational sac may be sufficient to slowly dilate the cervix. Because of prior trauma, diethylstilbestrol (DES) exposure in utero, or unknown factors, the cervix dilates painlessly. The condition is recognized only by vaginal examination or PROM. If noted before 4-cm dilation or PROM, treatment is possible. A suture is placed at the upper end of the cervix, encircling the cervix. This *cerclage* is removed before labor in some cases. If future pregnancies are desired, the suture may be left in place, and cesarean section may be done to conserve integrity of the cervix. Once the suture is in place, bed rest is needed to allow adjustment. If no contractions are noted, modified daily activity can be resumed.

Box 21-2
DRUG PROFILE

Betamethasone (Celestone)

ACTION

Used in cases of PTL to stimulate maturity of fetal lungs Given if fetus is between 24 and 34 weeks to lessen chance of RDS. Steroid action with onset 10 minutes with IM route

DOSAGE AND ROUTE

12 mg IM 24 to 48 hours before preterm delivery. Repeat once 12 to 24 hours after first injection, or 6 mg IM q12hr × 4. Inject deep into large-muscle mass with 21-gauge needle. Avoid deltoid site.

SIDE EFFECTS AND ADVERSE EFFECTS

Sometimes not used in presence of overt infection of genitourinary tract. Contraindicated for woman taking phenytoin (decreases action) or indomethacin (increases side effects).

PTL, Preterm labor; *RDS,* respiratory distress syndrome.

$\mathcal{N}$ursing $\mathcal{R}$esponsibilities

ASSESSMENT

A collaborative effort is required to determine if PTL is indeed present or advancing (see discussion of clinical management). All the assessment activities are performed by the nurse, physician, or midwife.

NURSING DIAGNOSES

PTL may require extended therapy at home or in the hospital. (See the discussion of problems with bedrest in the following section.) Women in PTL may have the following nursing diagnoses:

- Sleep pattern disturbance related to frequency of medication, contractions, reduced activity, or monitoring
- Anxiety related to outcome of PTL and side effects of medication
- Self-esteem disturbance related to feeling she may have caused onset of PTL
- Risk for ascending infection related to membranes rupturing or subclinical vaginal infection

EXPECTED OUTCOMES

The following are examples of expected outcomes that may apply to PTL clients:

- Obtains adequate sleep and rest using side-lying position
- Maintains adequate fluid intake, nutrition, and excretion if on modified bedrest
- Copes with limitations or lifestyle as a result of medication or rest requirements
- Understands and complies with self-monitoring and medication regimen
- Labor and infection inhibited because of treatments

NURSING INTERVENTION

Nursing interventions are crucial in effective prevention programs. In fact, nurses have been credited for much of the positive results of prevention programs. A pattern of care that is producing results includes the following (Eganhouse and Burnside, 1992):

- Instruction about early signs and preventive care for all pregnant clients before the twentieth week (Box 21-3)
- Identification of those at risk for PTL
- Instruction on self-monitoring of contractions twice a day from weeks 20 to 36 for women at high risk
- A 24-hour hot line to a nurse in the labor unit, clinic, or prevention program; staff education so that uniform responses are made to clients' telephone calls

- Frequently scheduled visits to evaluate clients at high risk
- Telephone contact with high-risk clients between visits
- Home uterine monitoring with regular home visits for those who have had one episode of PTL

Women need instruction regarding premature labor signs, and each pregnant woman should be given an illustrated handout that teaches self-monitoring of contractions. If she develops symptoms of PTL, she is instructed to do the following:

- Empty her bladder.
- Drink three to four cups of juice and water.
- Palpate for contractions, and record times.
- Rest in a side-lying position for 30 minutes, then gradually resume activity if contractions diminish.
- Notify health care provider if symptoms persist.

Care during tocolytic therapy

Once tocolysis has been chosen, care will depend on the agent. Box 21-2 lists doses, side effects, and monitoring requirements. Beta-mimetic agents and magnesium sulfate demand closer initial monitoring than do calcium channel blockers of antiprostaglandins because of cardiovascular and renal effects. Ritodrine and magnesium sulfate are begun with an IV bolus dose, and then are titrated to the woman's responses. Once contractions have stopped, oral doses may be started but should always overlap the IV doses to maintain the minimum effective

---

 Box **21-3**

TEACHING PLAN *for* HOME CARE

Prevention of Preterm Labor

REST PERIODS

Lie down on your left side for 1 hour twice a day. The physician may prescribe more rest if needed.

FLUID INTAKE

Make sure to drink eight to ten cups of fluid each day. If you are having increased contractions, drink three to four cups within the first hour.

STRENUOUS ACTIVITY

Do not perform any strenuous activity, including jogging, running, tennis, long walks, heavy lifting, or frequent trips up and down stairs. Do not do heavy cleaning, scrubbing floors, changing curtains, or moving furniture. Discuss long trips by car with your physician or midwife.

EMPLOYMENT

You may have to decrease, stop, or modify your work pattern.

SEXUAL ACTIVITY

You may have to limit or stop vaginal intercourse depending on the cause of PTL. If after vaginal intercourse, you have a marked increase in contractions, report this to the physician.

BREAST PREPARATION

Avoid breast massage, nipple stimulation, and preparation for breast-feeding until 2 weeks before your due date.

CHILDBIRTH CLASSES

Attend childbirth education class unless your physician or midwife has prescribed bed rest. Avoid the physical exercises taught for childbirth preparation, but practice breathing techniques.

STRESS REDUCTION

Discuss stressful or anxiety-producing situations with your support person, physician, or midwife. Seek appropriate helpers.

Modified from Johnson FF: Assessment and education to prevent preterm labor, *MCN Am J Matern Child Nurs* 14(3):158, 1989.

concentration of the drug (see Chapter 16). Drug and electrolyte levels must be followed during this period. Before going home on maintenance therapy, each woman should have written instructions for medication times with side effects noted and directions for notification of her primary care person.

Home care management. A woman can manage her treatment regimen at home. She learns how to palpate and record contractions. First she lies on her side, and with fingertips of both hands placed over the fundal area, she counts and records any sensation of hardening of the uterus; feeling of tightness; cramping; back, thigh, or hip pain; or any regular or irregular intermittent sensation. She must notify her nurse or physician if the number of allowed contractions in an hour (her threshold) is exceeded.

Electronic monitoring is helpful in identifying uterine activity, especially for those who routinely "miss" palpating their own contractions. Twice a day, she should void and then assume a comfortable semireclining position (Figure 21-7). She places the tocotransducer over the uterine fundus and records for 1 hour (and whenever unusual uterine activity occurs). The recorder stores information, and when the session is over, she sends the data via telephone modem to the nurse specialist or physician for analysis. The nurse will call back if there is needed action for threatened labor.

Most agencies that supply home monitors are accessible for 24-hour support and consultation. Although researchers are not in agreement about the efficacy of monitoring itself in preventing PTL and delivery, many do agree it is a positive benefit to have a nurse available to the client on a consistent basis for explanations, support, and treatment management (Iams, 1995).

Candidates for this program include women who have multiple pregnancies, prior episodes of PTL, previously delivered preterm infants, and those with risk factors known to increase the incidence of PTL.

Home therapy by terbutaline pump

If uterine activity is not successfully decreased with oral tocolytics, continuous subcutaneous terbutaline infusion by portable pump is available for home use. Figure 21-8 illustrates the pump size. Medication can be delivered at a continuous *basal rate*, with additional doses given every 3 to 4 hours (*scheduled bolus*), or, if uterine activity increases, the woman may be instructed to administer an additional prn dose (*demand bolus*).

The role of the nurse in teaching, assisting, and supporting the woman throughout this therapy is essential as the woman learns to use the equipment and to insert a subcutaneous needle. Follow-up visits are needed to clarify or reteach, and daily telephone consultations assist her to manage therapy at home.

Problems connected with in-home monitoring are cost and the ability of the woman to comply with the testing schedule. Women most in need of in-home monitoring are often those who are most affected by these factors; thus in-home monitoring or tocolytic therapy by pump currently is not used by all who need it. However, compared with the cost of extended hospitalization, home management is a reasonable approach. Figure 21-9 indicates the multiple decisions that are made in cases of PTL.

Psychosocial effects of preterm labor

There is interesting research into the body image differences between women who have preterm birth and those who carry pregnancy to term (Richardson, 1996). Those with PTL seem to have more lasting distress about body changes in the first half of pregnancy and to worry more about coping. They appeared to be ready to release the infant early and to feel the infant was ready to be born despite the infant's small size.

A woman being treated for PTL often feels powerless, and she should be encouraged in decision making in other aspects of her life. Family coping and support during this time are important.

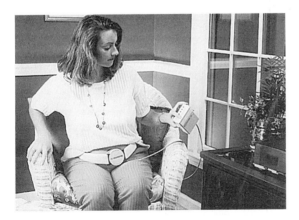

Figure 21-7 Home monitoring with Healthdyne contraction monitor. (Courtesy Matria Health Care, Marietta, Ga.)

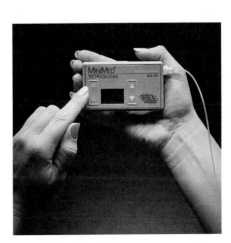

Figure 21-8 Terbutaline pump. (Courtesy MiniMed Technologies.)

Decision TREE | *Preterm Labor*

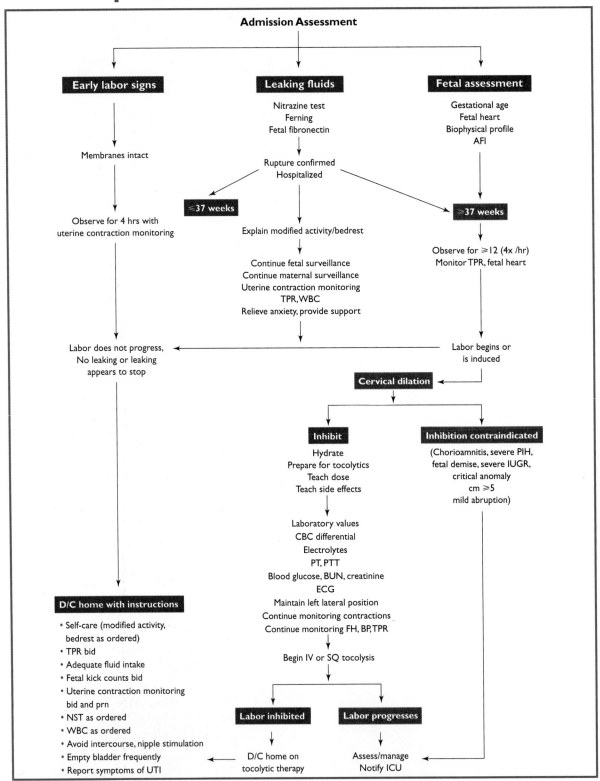

Admission Assessment

Early labor signs

Membranes intact

Observe for 4 hrs with
uterine contraction monitoring

Leaking fluids

Nitrazine test
Ferning
Fetal fibronectin

Rupture confirmed
Hospitalized

≤37 weeks

Explain modified activity/bedrest

Continue fetal surveillance
Continue maternal surveillance
Uterine contraction monitoring
TPR, WBC
Relieve anxiety, provide support

Fetal assessment

Gestational age
Fetal heart
Biophysical profile
AFI

≥37 weeks

Observe for ≥12 (4x /hr)
Monitor TPR, fetal heart

Labor does not progress,
No leaking or leaking
appears to stop

Labor begins or
is induced

Cervical dilation

Inhibit

Hydrate
Prepare for tocolytics
Teach dose
Teach side effects

Laboratory values
CBC differential
Electrolytes
PT, PTT
Blood glucose, BUN, creatinine
ECG
Maintain left lateral position
Continue monitoring contractions
Continue monitoring FH, BP, TPR

Begin IV or SQ tocolysis

Inhibition contraindicated

(Chorioamnitis, severe PIH,
fetal demise, severe IUGR,
critical anomaly
cm ≥5
mild abruption)

D/C home with instructions

• Self-care (modified activity,
  bedrest as ordered)
• TPR bid
• Adequate fluid intake
• Fetal kick counts bid
• Uterine contraction monitoring
  bid and prn
• NST as ordered
• WBC as ordered
• Avoid intercourse, nipple stimulation
• Empty bladder frequently
• Report symptoms of UTI

Labor inhibited

D/C home on
tocolytic therapy

Labor progresses

Assess/manage
Notify ICU

Figure 21-9 Decision tree for preterm labor. *AFI,* Amniotic fluid index; *bid,* twice a day; *BP,* blood pressure; *BUN,* blood urea nitrogen; *cbc,* complete blood count; *DIC,* disseminated intravascular coagulation; *ECG,* electocardiogram; *ICU,* intensive care; *IV,* intravenous; *NST,* nonstress test; *prn,* as necessary; *PT,* prothrombin time; *PTT,* partial thromboplastin time; *SQ,* subcutaneous; *TPR,* temperature; *UTI,* urinary tract infection.

When preterm birth becomes likely, maternal transport to a tertiary center must be arranged if a local NICU is unavailable. Distance from home will intensify feelings of loneliness and depression. Interventions to help the woman remain hopeful and interested in her environment are important. Primary nursing care can be an important factor in the continued support for this client. If the infant is premature, anxiety about outcome is a crucial factor. (The support for parents of a premature infant is outlined in Chapter 29.)

EVALUATION

The following questions may be asked to evaluate expected outcomes for PTL care:

- Were sleep and rest patterns maintained satisfactorily?
- Did the woman cope adequately with changes in lifestyle?
- Did her increased understanding of the PTL process prevent loss of self-esteem?
- Was infection controlled?
- Was labor delayed long enough to allow maturation of fetal lungs?

TEST *Yourself* 21-1

> a. Why is early detection of an irritable uterus so important?
>
> b. List the early warning signs of PTL.

MULTIPLE PREGNANCY

The occurence of twins, triplets, or quadruplets had a stable rate until ovulation-inducing agents and assisted-reproduction technologies were introduced (see Chapter 6). Now the twin rate approximates 1 in 43 births, and the triplet rate 1 in 1340 births (Luke, 1994). Without the assisted fertility technologies, the triplet rate would stay at 1 in 10,000 births (Ventura, 1996).

There are differences in twinning depending on when after fertilization the embryo divided. Figure 21-10 shows the possible embryologic origin of multiple pregnancies. The *monovular* (monozygotic, identical) rate accounts for one third of twins. This monovular rate is not affected by maternal age, race, or parity. Incidence is 3 to 4 per 1000 births worldwide, a fairly steady rate in every area.

The tendency for *diovular* (dizygotic, fraternal) twinning, when two ovum are released and fertilized at the same time, is inherited in certain families across the ethnic spectrum and is more common in African-American women and less common in Asian-American women.

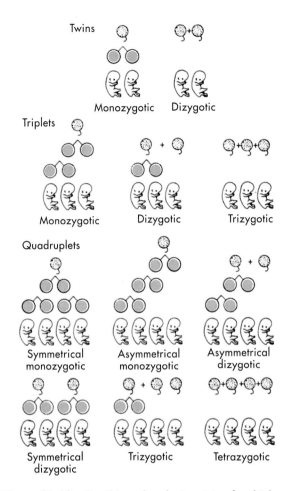

Figure 21-10 Possible embryologic origin of multiple pregnancies. (From Hafez ESE: Physiology of multiple pregnancy, *J Reprod Med* 12:88, 1974.)

Types

Monovular twins (monozygous) are the result of a single fertilized ovum that has divided into two before implantation. This process of "twoing," or twinning, may occur from 2 to 7 days after fertilization. The time of division affects whether the fetuses have separate amnions and chorions, but there always is a single placenta when separation has occurred early; later separation may result in two placentas (Figure 21-11, *B-D*). Placentas must be saved for complete examination.

Because a single ovum has been fertilized by a single sperm, each of the blastocysts develops into an individual with similar intelligence, physical characteristics, and gender. Identical twins are interesting to study from psychosocial and biologic aspects because both individuals have the same genetic makeup.

Diovular twins, or fraternal twins, stem from two ova released at the same time, either from a single ovary or one from each ovary. The placentas may fuse together or develop separately (Figure 21-11, *A*). Each embryo has an individual chorion and amnion. Fraternal twins may look so much alike that they are thought to be identical, or they

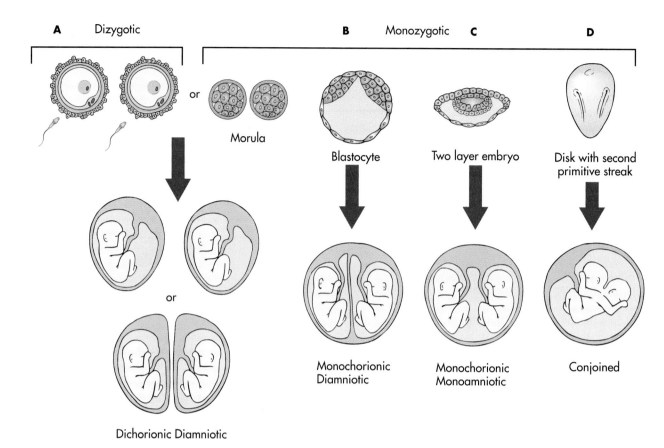

Figure 21-11 A, Formation of dizygotic twins; fertilization of two ova, two implantations, two placentas, two chorions, and two amnions. **B to D,** Formation of monozygotic twins. **B,** One fertilization: blastomeres separate, resulting in two implantations, two placentas, and two sets of membranes. **C,** One blastomere with two inner cell masses, one fused placenta, one chorion, and separate amnions. **D,** Later separation of inner cell masses, with fused placenta and single amnion and chorion. (From Whaley LF: *Understanding inherited disorders,* St Louis, 1974, Mosby.)

may be as different in size, coloring, personality, and ability as other brothers and sisters in a family.

Triplets and *quadruplets* may be diovular or monovular, but single-ovum pregnancies are less frequent. There may be mixed groups, with a set of monovular infants and one or two diovular infants.

Quintuplets and *sextuplets* are rarely the product of single-ovum pregnancies. In most cases two or three distinct placentas or masses of two or three have fused together. These pregnancies are linked to ovulation stimulants (see Chapter 6). A multifetal reduction of one or more of the embryos is done in some centers to improve the outcome for the remaining ones. With careful consideration for informed choice, and with ultrasound guidance, the embryo(s) to be aborted are approached through the maternal abdomen. Injection of potassium chloride into the intrathoracic space is done. The embryos remain in situ or may be expelled (Berkowitz et al, 1996). In fact, in multifetal pregnancies, it is not unusual for a woman to spontaneously lose one or more and still complete the pregnancy.

Conjoined twins are caused by the failure of the fertilized ovum to separate completely. If the embryonic disk divides after 13 days, it will remain united at one or more connections. The thorax, abdomen, and umbilical cord are common fusion sites. Sometimes surgery is possible when all organs are fully formed and function independently (Beischer and MacKay, 1993).

Tests for twin type

Blood factors are identical in monovular twins as are chemical substances such as haptoglobins and gamma globulins.

Footprints and fingerprints are nearly the same. Skin grafts from one identical twin always will be accepted by the other twin. "Ear prints," however, can assist in differentiating identical twins because ear formations are distinctive from birth onward. Often an identical twin appears to be a mirror image of the other (e.g., the whorl of hair on the crown of the head is on the opposite side) (Figure 21-12).

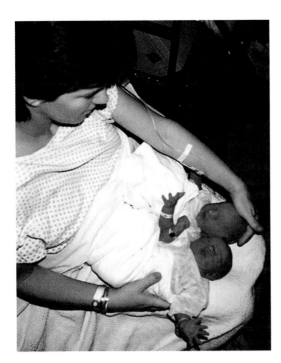

Figure 21-12 New twins meet their mother. (Courtesy James Suddath.)

Placental structure is studied for relationships of the chorion and amnion. The examiner searches for one or two chorionic membranes. (Monochorionic membrane indicates a monovular twinning.)

Risk

A multiple pregnancy carries a higher risk of perinatal morbidity and mortality because preterm birth occurs much more frequently compared with single births. Perinatal mortality for twins is 3 to 11 times higher than for single infants (Hollenbach and Hickok, 1990). The greater the number of fetuses, the higher the rate of premature birth and poor survival. Therefore medical intervention attempts to achieve the best possible outcome by maintaining the pregnancy as long as possible. The goal of treatment is to maintain a healthy pregnancy to at least 34 weeks' gestation.

Twins may differ considerably in weight. Especially in fraternal girl-boy pairs, girls often weigh less than the boy at birth. Sometimes one infant has dominated because of better placement of its placenta. The smaller infant is called the *discordant twin* and may have severe intrauterine growth retardation (IUGR) and postnatal problems.

Signs

Twins often came as a surprise in the past when confirmation depended only on palpation and auscultation of fetal heartbeat. Today, diagnosis occurs by ultrasonographic examination at 8 to 10 weeks (see Figure 11-2). Occasionally, if more than two fetuses are present, diagnosis may be complicated by overlapping outlines. At times, there is one more infant than predicted.

Although most multiple pregnancies follow a normal course, delivery comes early. The length of gestation from the onset of the last menses to birth is approximately 22 days less than in a single birth, averaging 37 weeks. Pregnancy proceeds normally during the first trimester, when the embryos are small, with the exception that blood volume increases to a higher level. Maternal alpha-fetoprotein levels are elevated.

An early problem may be increased nausea and vomiting. Because of increased levels of placental hormones, the mother may experience more frequent hot flashes and sweating. The major physiologic problems are caused by pressure of the overlarge uterus on the surrounding organs and by anemia and fatigue.

Pressure effects

The uterus causes pressure on the ureters, bladder, intestines, vena cava, and renal vasculature, and later on the diaphragm. Increased pressure from more than one fetus may lead to varicose veins of the rectal, saphenous, or vulvar veins. In addition, many women experience marked dependent edema in the lower portion of their legs. Constipation and digestive problems may be accentuated during the second and third trimesters. Pressure on the ureters may favor urinary stasis and infection. Pressure effects in each case are relieved by the side-lying position when the mother rests. Finally, during the day she may have to wear a maternity corset to provide some support for the abdomen.

 Box **21-2**

CLINICAL DECISION

Jenny visits the clinic at 16 weeks. She has had nausea, fatigue, and urinary frequency longer in this pregnancy than the last one. In addition, she is worried about her rapid weight gain. All the signs of pregnancy are present, and physical examination shows that her fundus is 2 cm below the umbilicus.
a. Is this finding appropriate for estimated gestational age?
b. What anticipatory guidance should she receive if twin gestation is diagnosed?

Clinical Management

Anemia and nutrition

Maternal anemia may be prevented by a diet rich in iron and the addition of supplemental iron and folic acid. The iron requirement is increased for a multiple pregnancy; iron needs are 60 to 80 mg/day. In addition to the normal (2000 to 2800 calories) requirements of pregnancy, an additional 300 calories per fetus is recommended. Because the woman usually can tolerate only small meals because of increased pressure on the stomach, she may have difficulty achieving that goal.

Bed rest

Rest for the woman carrying more than one fetus has been considered an important factor in preventing preterm delivery. Although bed rest is still prescribed in 20% of all pregnancies to treat conditions such as PTL, multiple pregnancies, hypertension, spontaneous bleeding, or abortion, there is little evidence that it is effective (Goldenberg et al, 1994; Enkin et al, 1995). There is evidence that bed rest is harmful, contributing to major effects of venous stasis, constipation, muscle atrophy, glucose intolerance, calcium loss from bones, and numerous other changes (Maloni, 1993). Therefore currently modified activity may be prescribed rather than bed rest. Certainly, during the third trimester, she will need the semi-Fowler's position for sleep and should always assume the side-lying position when in bed.

Monitoring

Because of the higher incidence of PTL, a multiple pregnancy is monitored closely. Home uterine monitoring may be prescribed. Contraction monitoring for preterm irritability is important because the overdistended uterus may begin significant contractions sooner than expected.

During labor, fetal monitors with dual capability are desirable. A spiral electrode may have to be placed on the first infant and an external ultrasound transducer on the second infant. Both may also be monitored externally by newer technology: the monitor strip of one machine shows two fetal heart rates (FHRs), and two tracings are provided by which to read the rates. Monitoring of the FHRs should continue during the birth process because there is as much as a 30-minute delay in the birth of the second twin.

Altered labor process

Uterine overdistension with resultant ineffective contractions is a problem during labor. Abnormal presentation of one fetus may cause special hazards to the second. The first infant may have a vertex presentation, but the second often is in a transverse or breech position, with the attendant problems of difficult delivery and possible prolapse of the cord. Cesarean birth under regional anesthesia is planned when there is any question of fetal positions. General anesthesia is not used because the infants would be exposed too long a time and become depressed.

Preparation for a multiple delivery requires a multidisciplinary approach. Neonatologists, nurses, and the anesthesiologist and obstetrician must coordinate activities. Resuscitation equipment for several infants must be available, and if necessary, the NICU must be ready to receive the infants. Each cord is tagged at the maternal side, and each infant is identified in order of birth. After delivery, the placentas are examined to aid in the diagnosis of zygosity.

High risk for hemorrhage. Because of the enlarged placental site, the internal os may be completely or partially covered. The warning signs of bleeding before labor should be noted carefully. During delivery a lower uterine or a cervical tear is not uncommon. After delivery the woman may have postpartum hemorrhage because of uterine atony and the large placental site.

Recovery and planning home care

Parents who expect the arrival of more than one infant have time to prepare psychologically and financially to receive them. The birth of more than one infant often rallies the whole family to help. Extended hospitalization for preterm infants is costly, however. Every possible referral to supportive agencies may be needed.

Because multiple births occur more often in women who have had children, it is important to prepare older siblings for the newborns (Figure 21-13). Most parents find that it makes no difference whether the infants are fraternal or identical in the first year. One infant may be behind the other in developmental tasks, however, and the parents may suffer undue anxiety. The nurse can assist in helping the parent recognize the uniqueness of each infant.

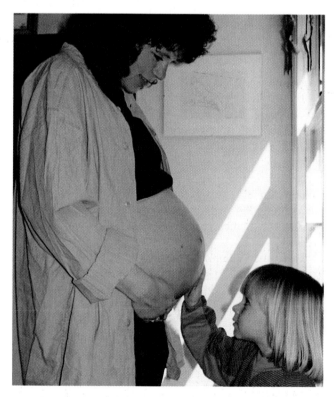

Figure 21-13 Siblings need special attention when twins are coming to "take up the space." (From Lowdermilk DL: *Maternity and women's health care,* ed 6, St Louis, 1997, Mosby.)

TEST *Yourself* 21-2 _____

a. List the expected maternal discomforts from pressure effects during a twin pregnancy.

b. What are the modifications of diet for a woman with multiple pregnancy?

c. What are the basic reasons bed rest is being challenged as a therapy for reproductive problems?

ECTOPIC PREGNANCY

An **ectopic pregnancy** is one that is "out of place." The fertilized ovum implants in the fallopian tube (95% to 98%) and rarely can implant on the ovary or be attached to the broad ligament and intestine. Cell growth proceeds at the same phenomenal rate of speed whether the blastocyst implants in the fallopian tube, ovary, cervix, interstitial area of the fundus, or in the peritoneal area (Figure 21-14). The rapidly developing embryo and placental tissue usually begin to show specific pressure effects by 10 weeks of gestation, and by 12 weeks, all overt signs are evident. As the placenta and embryo grow in the abnormal location, blood vessels proliferate, and when the pressure is too intense, the tube will rupture.

Risk

Ectopic implantation occurs in 2% of all pregnancies (ACOG, 1989). The number may be considerably higher for women of low socioeconomic status, however, and is associated with general lack of prenatal care and chronic tubal infection. Since 1982, ectopic pregnancy has become the second leading cause of maternal mortality from hemorrhage. Two thirds of the deaths are related to misdiagnosis or delayed diagnosis. Early diagnosis with ultrasound and β-hCG will result in a lower morbidity and mortality (Carson and Buster, 1993), but the woman must come for diagnosis for this to be true. Because signs are

subtle at first, the pregnancy often continues until the potential for rupture is present.

The following conditions contribute to the development of an ectopic pregnancy:

- Adhesions in the fallopian tubes from infections (salpingitis) usually caused by pelvic inflammatory disease (PID) especially from sexually transmitted diseases (STDs). The incidence of ectopic pregnancy is slightly increased in those who use intrauterine contraceptive devices (IUDs) and in those who have had infections after previous pregnancies.
- Scars with adhesions from prior pelvic surgery
- Low levels of estrogen and progesterone, causing a delay in transport of the fertilized ovum
- Ovum migrating to the opposite tube, approximately one in four have the corpus luteum on the opposite ovary
- Use of ovulation induction agents such as human menopausal gonadotropin (hMG)
- Presence of uterine benign muscle tumors (fibroids)

The incidence of recurrent ectopic with future pregnancies is increased when the contributing conditions still are present or when one tube has been damaged and removed.

Signs

All signs of early pregnancy are present: amenorrhea, breast tenderness, and nausea. β-hCG levels, indicating the presence of placental tissue, are usually lower and do not rise as rapidly as levels do for normal pregnancy. Signs and symptoms may be confusing and may lead to a delay in seeking a diagnosis (Table 21-1).

Before rupture, signs are related to increasing pressure or hidden bleeding. Pressure in the tube increases fairly rapidly, and by 10 weeks the woman will feel pelvic discomfort, beginning with dull aching and cramping and increasing to sharp stabbing pain in the lower portion of the abdomen. She may have referred shoulder pain (Figure 21-15) because a slow leak of blood in the peritoneal cavity causes irritation to the phrenic nerve, or pain may be referred to other parts of the body. If the ectopic pregnancy ruptures, an episode of severe pain occurs, and the woman may show rapid signs of hypovolemic shock from blood loss into the peritoneum.

Depending on the site, bleeding may be visible or internal and begins as a slow leak. Blood may collect in the peritoneal cavity in the cul-de-sac behind the vagina and anterior to the rectum.

The woman feels pressure and the need to defecate; the "bathroom sign" includes feeling faint when pressing down to evacuate the bowels. An abdominal examination elicits pain over the tube or ovary. The abdomen may be rigid and tender. During vaginal examination, if the cervix is moved, severe pain may occur. If there has been extensive bleeding, Cullen's sign shows a bluish tinge to the umbilicus.

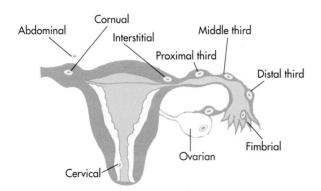

Figure 21-14 Ectopic sites of implantation. (From Breen JL: A 21-year survey of 654 ectopic pregnancies, *Am J Obstet Gynecol* 106:1004, 1970.)

Table 21-1	Signs and Symptoms of Tubal Implantation*

Signs and Symptoms	Comments
BLEEDING	
Painless, periodic vaginal spotting may resemble a light menstrual period.	Client may not notify physician. Bleeding may be caused by breakdown of decidual tissue after death of embryo in tube.
Hidden bleeding into peritoneum ("slow leak") causes symptoms of lower abdominal pressure (dark unclotted blood collects in cul-de-sac).	Hidden bleeding is caused by slow separation of placenta.
Sudden massive bleeding associated with rupture of tubal site causes woman to go into hypovolemic shock.	Bleeding usually is preceded by pain.
ANEMIA	
Fatigue and pale mucous membranes (out of proportion to observed blood loss) occur.	Hemoglobin and hematocrit levels fall slowly, especially with hidden slow bleeding.
ABDOMINAL PAIN	
Feeling of fullness in lower part of abdomen or backache and mild abdominal aching occur.	3 to 5 weeks after the woman misses the first period, symptoms begin, gradually increasing in intensity. (See Figure 21-14 for sites.)
Pain my be referred and occur at time of usual menstrual period.	
Pain may be excruciating during vaginal examination when cervix is moved.	Vaginal examination often brings first clue.
Intense, "tearing" pain may occur at time of rupture of tube.	Pain may still masquerade as appendicitis (see Figure 21-15).
SYNCOPE	
Light-headedness and fainting have been observed is 35% to 50% of ectopic pregnancies. It is called the *bathroom sign* because fainting often occurs while straining to defecate.	Bathroom sign is a response to feeling of fullness and pressure in rectal area. Cause is pressure of growing embryo or collection of blood in cul-de-sac or pressure on nerves of the perineal area.
EARLY SYMPTOMS OF PREGNANCY	
There will be breast tenderness, nausea for approximately 50%, a positive pregnancy test result, and uterus enlarged to approximately an 8-week size.	As long as corpus luteum is functioning, effects of pregnancy hormones will be experienced.

*Early diagnosis and intervention will prevent more serious signs.

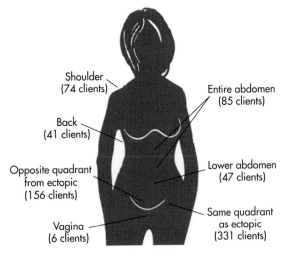

Figure 21-15 Sites of referred pain from ectopic pregnancies. (From Breen JL: A 21-year survey of 654 ectopic pregnancies, *Am J Obstet Gynecol* 106:1004, 1970.)

Shoulder (74 clients)
Entire abdomen (85 clients)
Back (41 clients)
Opposite quadrant from ectopic (156 clients)
Lower abdomen (47 clients)
Vagina (6 clients)
Same quadrant as ectopic (331 clients)

TEST *Yourself* 21-3

a. Which early signs of pregnancy are missing when there is an ectopic pregnancy?
b. Why is it not possible for an ectopic tubal pregnancy to develop beyond 14 weeks?

Clinical Management

The clinical problem is confirmed by the following tests:
- Pelvic examination for masses and cervical signs of pregnancy
- Ultrasound to verify placement of gestational sac in an unruptured tubal or intraabdominal pregnancy; transvaginal sonography is most accurate
- Culdoscopy or culdocentesis to extract old blood from the cul-de-sac or to view the site with fiberoptic light

Laboratory tests reveal low hemoglobin and rising leukocyte counts. The red blood cell count may be low, and the sedimentation rate is elevated. The serum-hCG level is followed every 48 hours if there is any question and although rising, has a lower level than in normal pregnancy. One study reports a 95% predictive diagnostic success with ultrasound and hCG levels. If used early enough, these tests may reduce the chance of rupture (Carson and Buster, 1993).

Treatment is to remove the ectopic pregnancy, stop the bleeding, and, when possible, repair the tubal damage. A tuboplasty may be performed to save the tube, or the tube may have to be removed because scar tissue here would raise the risk of a future ectopic pregnancy. *Methotrexate,* a folic acid antagonist that inhibits cell division, has been used as an adjunct to surgery (Queenan and Hobbins, 1996).

If further pregnancies are not desired, *salpingectomy,* which is the excision and removal of the entire tube, may be done. When a woman desires to have a future pregnancy, the tube is not removed; instead newer conservative treatments are performed by laparoscopy. Depending on the gestational size and tubal damage, one of the following techniques is used:

- Ampullary salpingotomy (incision into the tube) under laparoscopy by which products of conception are removed by gentle suction
- Resection of isthmic section, or at cornua, removing damaged narrow portion of tube (less commonly done)
- Medical treatment of the early ectopic pregnancy managed by use of chemotherapy; methotrexate and leucovorin calcium injected into gestational sac; follow-up more extensive with this method

When conservative treatment is used, adverse effects can include a persistent ectopic pregnancy, that is, a failure to disrupt placental growth. hCG levels remain elevated and pain persists; 5% of clients require a second surgical procedure or further instillation of methotrexate (Stock, 1991). There is no guarantee of future fertility, and tuboplasty has led to occasions for lawsuits. Documention is critical, and often, as evidence, photographs are taken of the tubal damage and the repair technique.

When the woman is admitted, vital signs and blood loss are observed and recorded frequently. If emergency surgery is required, preparation may be done in the emergency or operating room. A urine sample is obtained from the Foley catheter inserted before surgery. The blood must be typed and cross-matched. IV fluids through a large-bore catheter are continued throughout this initial period. After return from the recovery room, the woman will consume nothing by mouth until bowel sounds are heard. Paralytic ileus is a possibility because of the proximity of the bowel. Ambulation is encouraged to promote movement of flatus, and bowel sounds are monitored. Recovery depends on the degree of blood loss and the complexity of the surgery. When there has been significant blood loss, the client is observed for signs and symptoms of infection and anemia. If rupture occurs, she will be given prophylactic antibiotics during recovery. All Rh-negative women receive Rh immunoglobulin to prevent sensitization.

Nursing Considerations

The nurse initiates discussion of recovery and future pregnancies and teaches the use of contraception and the method most suitable to use for at least three menstrual cycles. The woman is encouraged to allow time for recovery. Finally, she should know the signs of ectopic implantation because there is a greater risk of recurrence if one tube has been removed.

Box **21-3**

CLINICAL DECISION

Ann is in emergency admission with abdominal pain and suspected ectopic pregnancy of 10 weeks' gestation.
a. What is the first care priority?
b. List questions you could ask during assessment.

GESTATIONAL TROPHOBLASTIC DISEASE: MOLAR PREGNANCY

In some instances the placental chorionic villi undergo abnormal degenerative changes in which the trophoblastic epithelium proliferates to form grapelike cysts (Figure 21-16). These cysts eventually completely fill the uterus. Only a calcified embryo may be left, or there may be no embryo. This change is termed **hydatidiform mole**, or molar pregnancy. It also may be called **trophoblastic disease**. There are several types. The *complete mole* has only the paternal chromosome present—the sperm chromosomes have duplicated or two sperm entered the ovum. In this case there is no embryonic tissue or membrane, only swollen, cystic villi. Choriocarcinoma may develop in 20% of the cases (ACOG, 1993).

A *partial mole* has some normally formed villi. There is only focal hyperplasia of tissue and a calcified or macerated embryo. The chromosome pattern is 69—the 23 female chromosomes plus 46 paternal chromosomes that have duplicated, or rarely there is fertilization by two sperm. hCG titers are lower with a partial mole, and levels return to normal more quickly after removal. A partial mole less often becomes malignant (5% to 10% of clients).

Risk

This abnormal condition occurs in 1 in 1200 to 1500 conceptions (ACOG, 1993). Some other parts of the world, particularly Southeast Asia, India, and Mexico, report an inci-

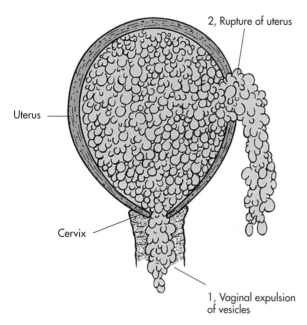

Figure 21-16 Uterine view with hydatidiform mole, *1*, Evacuation of mole through cervix. *2*, Rupture of uterus and spillage of mole into peritoneal cavity (rare). (From Lowdermilk DL: *Maternity and women's health care*, ed 6, St Louis, 1997, Mosby.)

dence as high as 1 in 200. A relationship may exist between low protein intake or low socioeconomic status and its occurrence. The cause is unknown; however, contributing factors may include malnutrition, chromosomal abnormalities, and hormonal imbalance. It has been seen more frequently after use of clomiphene to induce ovulation.

Malignant changes may take several forms. *Invasive mole* invades the myometrium but does not metastasize; chemotherapy is used. *Gestational choriocarcinoma* can metastasize quickly and to all organs; chemotherapy is used. *Placental site trophoblastic tumors* are rare and not sensitive to chemotherapy; hysterectomy is used.

Signs

A gestation with a complete mole will demonstrate an abnormally rapid growing uterus and signs of threatened abortion. Bright red or brownish vaginal bleeding may occur in the first trimester, with vaginal discharge of clear vesicles. Symptoms of hypertension often are present before 20 weeks. Nausea and vomiting may be much more severe than normal.

Laboratory tests reveal hCG levels completely out of the normal range; levels may be 1 to 2 million IU, compared with hCG levels of less than 300,000 IU in a normal pregnancy. Although hCG levels may be normally elevated in multiple gestation, these abnormal levels continue to rise after day 100 of pregnancy. Other laboratory values

show reduced hematocrit and lower estriol, pregnanediol, and 17-ketosteroid levels. Because of elevated triiodothyronine (T_3) and thyroxine (T_4) levels, maternal pulse may be faster (Queenan and Hobbins, 1996), and other signs of hyperthyroidism such as sweating and intolerance to heat will be present.

The problem is confirmed by use of ultrasound, which reveals the absence of fetal growth. Multiple diffuse echoes are seen. The ovaries may have theca luteal cysts.

Clinical Management

Medical treatment is to remove the molar tissue by dilation and suction curettage (D&C). Depending on the length of gestation, type of mole, bleeding, or other adverse signs the woman will be scheduled for immediate evacuation of the uterus. The client is prepared for surgery while blood loss is monitored. Respiratory distress may occur during or after evacuation of the mole related to embolus, congestive heart failure, or hypertension. The woman must be carefully observed in a special care setting during recovery from anesthesia (ACOG, 1993.)

Each client is followed to determine if malignant cells have developed. Serial β-hCG determinations are done 48 hours after surgery and then every 1 to 2 weeks until normal levels return and then every 1 to 2 months for the rest of the year. Because almost all malignancies develop within the first 6 months, a return to a normal level of β-hCG indicates lack of metastases. Future pregnancies should be delayed until the year ends.

Nursing Considerations

The nurse should assess level of anxiety and determine the level of understanding regarding the diagnosis and immediate treatment. After surgery it is important that the woman become knowledgeable about self-care in the follow-up period. She must not skip weekly laboratory evaluations. The woman's fears for herself may be well founded, depending on the outcome of the treatment; therefore she should not be reassured lightly.

Recurrence is possible, therefore the woman should be instructed about early signs, including vaginal bleeding, hypertension, aggravated nausea, and rapid uterine enlargement. She should wait at least a year before becoming pregnant again. This means that selection and use of an effective method of delaying pregnancy are important.

Because the variation in uterine growth is so strange and the prognosis so variable, the woman may suffer from lack of self-esteem and fear for herself. She may ask, "Why me?" The nurse can be a supportive contact person for her during follow-up care in the clinic and if chemotherapy is advised.

Continuity of care, teaching, and support needed when a molar pregnancy is confirmed may be a significant nursing role. The woman's involvement in her care and, consequently, the outcomes may be largely determined by successful nursing interventions. The woman's future may be determined by her own compliance with diagnostic testing and treatment.

ABNORMAL AMNIOTIC FLUID VOLUME

Polyhydramnios or **oligohydramnios** exist when the normal volumes of amniotic fluid are not maintained. These volumes average as follows:

- 16 weeks: 200ml
- 28 weeks: 1000 ml
- 36 weeks: 800 ml
- After 40 weeks: declines 8% a week

When an infant is postmature, there may only be 400 ml of amniotic fluid.

Fluid volume is maintained by means of various mechanisms that change in ratio as pregnancy progresses (see Chapter 7). After 20 weeks, significant amounts of fetal urine are added to the volume of fluid. Fetal swallowing removes fluid at a rate of 15 to 20 ml/hr at term; because fluid is reabsorbed across membranes, the balance should be precise. Even a small variation either way will lead to too much or too little fluid (Blackburn and Loper, 1992).

The amniotic fluid index (AFI) is determined by ultrasound measurements of pockets of amniotic fluid (see Chapter 11). If ultrasound examination reveals a cramped fetal position and few pockets of fluid (< 1 to 2 cm), or if the biophysical profile shows poor fetal breathing expansion, a diagnosis of oligohydramnios is made (Peppert and Donnefeld, 1991).

Oligohydramnios

A long list of congenital anomalies will produce oligohydramnios (< 500 ml at term or < 50% of expected amount at a specific week of development). In cases of defects in renal and gastrointestinal systems in which urine is not excreted or swallowing is affected, imbalance occurs quickly. Maternal hypertension, vasoconstriction, and IUGR will affect volume. PROM is always considered (see earlier discussion of preterm labor).

Amniotic fluid is necessary for lung development. If diminished fluid volume occurs, lungs may be poorly functioning. Severe oligohydramnios that occurs early may be life threatening because the fetus cannot move freely or exercise the lungs with fetal breathing. *Pulmonary hypoplasia* may be lethal in the fetus. Furthermore, diminished fluid occurs normally with increasing gestational age, and it is expected that the postmature infant may have fetal distress from compression of the cord related to lower volumes of fluid. Finally, certain drugs such as the prostaglandin inhibitors indomethacin and ibuprofen have been shown to diminish fluid (Beringer and Niebyl, 1990).

As labor approaches, if oligohydramnios is acute or related to earlier rupture of membranes that did not result in PTL, the first line of treatment is to expand maternal blood volume by a rapid IV infusion of 1000 ml lactated Ringer's solution. Amnioinfusion may be attempted during labor (see Chapter 14). In any case if the pockets of fluid are less than 2 cm, a cesarean section is planned because it is believed that the fetus cannot withstand the pressures of labor without the cushioning effect of adequate amniotic fluid (Queenan and Hobbins, 1996).

Polyhydramnios or Hydramnios

Polyhydramnios or hydramnios is the presence of an abnormally large amount of amniotic fluid (> 2000 ml) usually seen by the third trimester. The condition may occur for no known cause. Congenital malformation of the gastrointestinal tract that inhibits swallowing, defects of the central nervous system, and, rarely, multiple gestation are associated factors. Hydramnios is also associated with severe diabetes mellitus.

The uterus enlarges more rapidly than normal in the second half of pregnancy, and the pressure symptoms felt by the mother may be severe. An amniocentesis may be one way to relieve pressure, but a definite risk is connected to repeated tapping of the amniotic sac, therefore it is used primarily in acute cases. As a further complication, when membranes rupture before or during labor, the risk of a prolapsed cord is much greater. Management includes bed rest, sedation, hydration, high protein diet, and parenteral infusion of albumin (Queenan and Hobbins, 1996). Indomethacin has been used to reduce fetal voiding (see Drug Profile 21-1).

PREGNANCY LOSS BEFORE VIABILITY

A pregnancy may be terminated by **spontaneous abortion** (i.e, a miscarriage) or by **induced abortion** for elective or therapeutic medical reasons. Abortions are further divided into early abortions, which take place before the sixteenth week of gestation, and late abortions, which occur between the sixteenth and twentieth weeks of gestation. To be classified as an abortion or *previable,* the fetus must weigh less than 500 g and have a crown-rump (CR) length of less than 16.5 cm. The *age of viability* is considered to be the beginning of the twentieth week. Although few of the 20- to 25-week-old infants are able to survive, even with intensive support, these infants are counted as potentially viable for vital statistics.

Spontaneous Abortion

There are several types of spontaneous, involuntary abortion. The following descriptions are based on the woman's signs and are listed in order of severity:

1. *Threatened:* Slight bleeding with mild uterine cramping and backache. The cervix is closed.
2. *Inevitable:* Moderate to severe bleeding with uterine cramping similar to labor contractions. The cervical os is dilating.
3. *Incomplete:* Heavy bleeding with severe uterine cramping, with some tissue already partially out of uterus in the vagina.
4. *Complete:* Products of conception are totally passed. There remains slight bleeding with mild to moderate uterine cramping.
5. *Missed:* Slight bleeding with no uterine cramping and closed os. Embryo or fetus dies but is retained. Pregnancy growth ceases.
6. *Habitual:* Any of the above repeated in three consecutive pregnancies, usually after 16 weeks.

Risk

It is estimated that 15% of all conceptions are lost spontaneously, many so early that the woman is hardly aware of it. More than half of these spontaneous abortions are caused by fetoplacental defects, such as genetic defects or implantation abnormalities. Other causes are maternal problems such as poor nutrition, low hormone levels, severe diabetes, infections, uterine structure (e.g., fibroids or incompetent cervix), and, rarely, severe trauma such as an automobile accident or abuse. Some evidence indicates that emotional shock results in abortion through an elevation in maternal epinephrine, which then leads to vasoconstriction and necrosis of the decidua basalis.

Signs

Cramping or spotting that leads to frank bleeding is the major sign of spontaneous abortion. Membranes may rupture at this time.

A spontaneous abortion may become septic, with signs of fever, odorous bleeding, and a tender uterus. The later in the gestation the abortion occurs, the more bleeding there may be.

A threatened abortion may reverse itself or progress to an inevitable abortion. After cervical dilation is established and progressing, no therapy to prevent loss will work. The products of conception will be expelled completely or incompletely.

Complete abortion occurs when all parts of the conception pass out of the uterus. This may happen in the home, and the woman reports a delayed menses with much heavier flow at the next menses, or tissue is passed as large clots. The recovery period is one of normal involution, and most women do not need therapy. In cases in which an inevitable abortion has been completed at home and the products of conception are not seen by the health care provider, the woman may be observed, undergo blood tests, and receive follow-up care in a clinic or private office within 2 days.

Incomplete abortion is accompanied by heavy bleeding as fragments of the conceptus are expelled. Bleeding does not stop, and most women seek medical help. (The nurse should be aware that an incomplete abortion may be the result of an incompetent procedure performed by a non-licensed person.) The woman is seen by a physician or midwife to determine her status; if incomplete, the client is prepared for a dilation and evacuation (D & E). Oxytocin and antibiotics are given postoperatively. Depending on the client's condition, she may then be discharged the same day.

Missed abortion is diagnosed when the uterus fails to grow, and the signs of pregnancy begin to diminish. Although a fetal heartbeat may have been obtained at an earlier prenatal visit, ultrasound examination is needed to confirm the absence of fetal movement and heartbeat. Because placental function may continue for some weeks after fetal death, tests such as that for hCG may be misleading. Retention of a missed abortion is treated like a later **intrauterine fetal death** (IUFD) (see discussion on nursing interventions).

Habitual abortion may be caused by genetic, structural, immunologic, or hormonal problems. The search for cause may take time. Most commonly, for unknown reasons, the cervix loses its muscular integrity and begins dilation in the second trimester. This condition is called *cervical incompetence.*

Clinical management

Treatment of threatened abortion consists of limiting activities for 24 to 48 hours and observing the result. Controlled studies have failed to prove that bed rest, progesterone, or sedatives have any effect on the outcome of a threatened abortion (Enkin et al, 1995). Some centers are treating the woman with corticosteroids and with low doses of acetylsalicylic acid (ASA) to act as an antiprostaglandin. If the bleeding can be stopped, it will do so within 48 hours. The woman may be asked to avoid stress, intercourse, fatigue, and extended activity until the pregnancy seems to be progressing satisfactorily.

It is important to realize that a spontaneous abortion often occurs because something is not going well with the fetus. Thus a woman who has a rocky beginning may in fact have a fetus with a structural or genetic defect, or hormonal support may be deficient.

The clinical problem is confirmed by history, pelvic examination, and ultrasound to determine the presence of a gestational sac as early as 6 weeks. Laboratory values may show a decrease in hemoglobin (< 10.5 g/dl) with bleeding and an increase in white blood cell count if infection is present. Serial ultrasound examination may document lack of fetal growth if there is a question about missed abortion.

Treatment for *missed abortion* before 12 weeks includes baseline blood studies and ultrasound evaluation of location and size of the gestational site. Prostaglandin E_2

(Prepidel gel), is placed at the cervix 6 hours before a D & E (Queenan and Hobbins, 1996).

After 13 weeks, there usually is a period of 2 weeks of waiting for spontanous labor to begin. If labor does not begin spontaneously, then it is induced with vaginal prostaglandin E$_2$, oxytocin infusion or both.

Induced Abortion

In 1973 the U.S. Supreme Court (*Roe v. Wade*) ruled that elective abortions could follow these guidelines:
1. During the first 12 weeks the state could not bar a woman from obtaining an abortion by a licensed physician.
2. Between 12 and 20 weeks the state could regulate the performance of an abortion to protect the woman's health.
3. After 20 weeks the state could regulate and prohibit abortion except those deemed necessary to protect the woman's health or life.

The state may impose safeguards for the fetus. Most state laws have "conscience clauses" that allow a physician, nurse, or other hospital personnel to refuse to assist in abortion without fear of reprisal if it conflicts with their ethical or religious principles.

Abortion is an issue of intense debate in the United States. The trends in rules and regulations are following the Supreme court decisions of 1986, 1989, 1990, and 1991. There will be yet more challenges as individual states and groups of citizens seek through legal recourse to change the way abortions are allowed or restricted. In many states challenges have resulted in laws that restrict the times (only first trimester), the reasons (only rape, incest, fetal anomaly, or if life or health of mother threatened), and the notification or permission requirements before an abortion. Finally, the issues of who may counsel women, who may do an abortion, and who pays the bill are subjects of a bitter battle. The result is that accessibility becomes more limited for indigent women who would have to continue the pregnancy, whereas more affluent women continue to have access to services. Thus the balance between those who can and those who cannot obtain abortions remains proportionately the same as before 1973. The nurse will want to update knowledge of any change in this controversial choice, especially for individual states. (See Chapter 30 for legal issues arising from or surrounding elective abortion.)

Induced abortion may be the woman's choice for many reasons, including the following:
- Inability to care for or support a child
- Desire not to be pregnant
- Interference with current or long-range life goals
- Rape or incest
- Emotional problems, mental incompetence, or both

Medically advised abortion may be recommended for maternal disorders such as heart disease, cancer, sickle cell disease, neurologic disorders, or psychiatric disorders. Fetal disorders, such as those discovered by amniocentesis include chromosome disorders, severe structural defects, and gene defects, may lead a woman to choose to terminate the pregnancy (see Chapter 28).

Risk of induced abortion

Approximately 1.3 million abortions are performed in the United States each year, a rate that has continued at almost the same level since 1981. Compared with the maternal mortality risk of 7.8 per 100,000 live births, the mortality rate for induced abortion is less than 0.5 per 100,000. Most abortions today are done for white, unmarried women under 25 years of age. Teenagers less than 19 years of age account for 20% of the cases (Spitz, 1996). The proportion of second-trimester abortions has decreased sharply since knowledge of abortion methods has become more widely known. The development of the D & E procedure for later, safer abortions has reduced the frequency of transabdominal methods; 98% of abortions are done by D & E (Ventura et al, 1996).

Efforts continue to find safer abortifacients. The introduction of RU 486 may change all these statistics in the future (see Chapter 5) (Donaldson, Briggs, McMaster, 1994).

Follow-up care on the effects of repeated abortions on fertility and birth complications is important. Hemorrhage is the most common problem after abortion, contributing to the maternal mortality rate.

Asherman's syndrome. With repeated and frequent abortions, a condition known as *Asherman's syndrome* may exist. Although this syndrome may be caused by other problems such as hormonal imbalance, repeated surgery by D & C will affect the endometrium. In Asherman's syndrome the endometrium does not build up an adequate lining during the proliferative period of the cycle because of adhesions, usually from infections. No shedding or menstruation occurs, and occasionally the inner uterine tissue may adhere. Repeated abortions have also been linked to the incidence of PTL (Queenan and Hobbins, 1996).

Clinical management

Pregnancy is confirmed by a positive pregnancy test result and a pelvic examination to estimate gestational size. If size is questioned, ultrasound may be used. A low-lying placenta and fibroids, which would affect the safety of the procedure, also may be identified by ultrasound. Laboratory tests are performed to determine Rh factor, blood type, and hemoglobin and hematocrit levels. A health history is taken to assess special needs and risks. Counseling is offered to determine knowledge of alternative options and to ensure that abortion is the woman's choice.

Methods

D & E is the method of choice for an early termination of pregnancy of 7 to 8 weeks' gestation. The cervix must be dilated enough to allow the passage of instruments. Dilation is the most difficult part of the procedure because it must proceed slowly and may be met with considerable resistance, especially in the nullipara.

D & C may be performed until the end of the first trimester. Instead of a suction device, a spoon-shaped instrument is used to scrape the lining out of the uterus. Dilation of the cervix is achieved as in a suction evacuation. A D & C usually is not performed after the first trimester because the uterine lining becomes thinner and could be penetrated (Figure 21-17).

Transabdominal prostaglandin F$_2$ (PGF$_2$) may be used to induce labor in a second trimester abortion. An amniocentesis needle is inserted through the abdominal wall into amniotic fluid, and 20 to 40 mg PGF$_2$ is inserted. Labor begins within 1 to 2 hours or up to 24 hours later. Labor contractions follow the usual pattern of mild to increasingly strong intensity until the fetus is delivered, usually when the cervix is 4- to 5-cm dilated. The placental tissue must be checked to see if it is intact. Side effects may be diarrhea, nausea and vomiting, and appropriate medication is administered. Alternatively, PGF$_2$ may be given IM every 2 to 3 hours until contractions are well established (Queenan and Hobbins, 1996).

Transabdominal instillation of hypertonic saline or urea is performed by inserting an amniocentesis needle and withdrawing 200 ml of amniotic fluid and replacing it with 20% saline or a urea solution. Contractions begin within 8 to 12 hours and may last 48 hours before the fetus is delivered. To shorten the waiting period, oxytocin infusion may be used. Side effects may be significant, especially if saline is inadvertently drawn into the maternal circulation. For this reason, saline abortions are performed much less frequently today.

For an abortion after 12 weeks, a missed abortion, or IUFD a vaginal suppository of *prostaglandin E$_2$ (PGE$_2$)* is the most convenient method with the fewest side effects (see Drug Profile 16-2). For an abortifacient to work, the cervix must become dilated. To speed this process, dried seaweed that absorbs water has been used in the form of a rod, a *Laminaria* inserted into the cervical canal 10 to 24 hours before induction. The substance swells three to four times its original size, and painless cervical dilation takes place. The Lamisi is removed, and a 20 mg PGE$_2$ suppository is inserted into the posterior vaginal canal and repeated every 3 to 5 hours until delivery. Birth of the fetus should take place within 24 hours. Oxytocin may be used to shorten the time for a more advanced pregnancy (see discussion of intrauterine fetal death).

Nursing Responsibilities

Few nurses using this text will work with women seeking induced abortion in the first trimester because most are

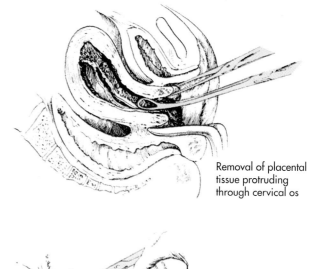

Removal of placental tissue protruding through cervical os

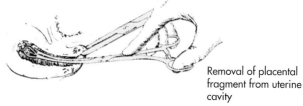

Removal of placental fragment from uterine cavity

Figure 21-17　Use of ring forceps to remove placental tissue. (From Willson JR: *Management of obstetric difficulties,* ed 6, St Louis, 1961, Mosby.)

seen in specialized clinics. All nurses, however, need to examine their own positions on these issues. Often, too, a nurse's counsel is informally sought in the community.

When the woman is debating whether to have an abortion, the nurse gives her information about the procedure. If she decides to proceed with the pregnancy, she should be informed about available resources. The woman should have a supportive environment while she deals with the issues and results of her decision. Many young women in their teens have not had an opportunity to develop their own values and to differentiate themselves from other people. This may be the first time some have had to make a decision about their own bodies.

Choice of attitudes. Nurses must develop an understanding of their own attitudes toward pregnancy termination to effectively counsel a woman seeking abortion. The confusion resulting from ambivalent feelings or incompletely understood ideas interferes with a therapeutic approach to such clients.

Burchell (1979) identified five possible positions on abortion and effectively discussed professional questions, attitudes, and approaches to it. He noted that legal changes do not usually affect deeply held attitudes, which he described as follows:

1. The first position allows no indication for abortion. Carried to its extreme, an ectopic pregnancy could not be removed, nor could a client with pelvic cancer be treated until the infant was born.
2. The second position holds that no direct abortion is accepted, but if necessary, an indirect abortion sec-

ondary to a life-saving procedure may be performed. It appears that most persons against elective abortion hold this position.

3. The third position allows medical indications to govern whether an abortion is necessary. This position promotes therapeutic abortions. The indications, however, became so vague that restrictions were almost negligible if the client could afford to obtain different medical opinions. The physician became the one who governed the choice of instituting an abortion.

4. The fourth position supports direct abortion based on the judgment of the physician and client. The reasons may be social, economic, or medical, but it is a fairly joint decision. The physician, however, may refuse to perform the procedure.

5. The fifth position allows the client to be the sole deciding agent (i.e., abortion on request, based on the woman's judgment alone). This last position has no restrictions, and although she may be counseled otherwise, the woman has the responsibility of the final decision.

Most people in the United States agree that abortion should not be used as a method of contraception. Therefore professional nurses involved in health education can help a woman to prevent future conception when pregnancy is unwelcome. Nurses who have gained a degree of empathy with a woman going through an unwanted pregnancy can begin to comprehend the aspects of her choice.

Self-Discovery

Consider the five positions of abortion discussed in light of your own ethical, moral, and religious convictions. For an imaginary early pregnancy in your current life situation, can you identify your position? How would you counsel another person? What considerations would you want to know about in the situation? ∼

NURSING DIAGNOSES

The following diagnosis may apply to those with spontaneous abortions or with induced abortions:

- Ineffective individual coping or dysfunctional grieving related to unresolved feelings about loss of pregnancy or choosing elective abortion
- Spiritual distress or grieving related to conflicts in choices or reasons for loss
- Potential for infection related to procedure, presence of concurrent vaginal infection
- Potential for injury related to being Rh-negative and isoimmunization possibility
- Knowledge deficit: methods, outcomes, or use of family planning in recovery period related to inexperience, anxiety

EXPECTED OUTCOMES

- Verbalizes to at least one person her feelings about pregnancy termination; finds support from significant others
- Seeks spiritual help as needed; experiences nondysfunctional grieving
- Describes method of preventing pregnancy she will use regularly
- If Rh-negative, receives Rh immunoglobulin
- Recovery proceeds without infection or undue bleeding

NURSING INTERVENTION

Recovery care for early abortion. After an elective abortion the woman is taught to look for symptoms of infection such as a change in vaginal discharge, uterine cramping, nausea, vomiting, or chills. She should call the clinic or physician if these signs occur. An oxytocic agent and an antibiotic will be prescribed. After a gestation of 59 days, all Rh-negative, Coombs' negative women will receive Rh immunoglobulin to prevent isoimmunization. The nurse explores with the woman the reasons she became pregnant, counsels and teaches her about contraceptive methods that may be more acceptable to her, and, finally, acknowledges the client's statements about the pregnancy in relation to her religious beliefs. She may wish to have the conceptus baptized, for instance. It may be important for her to talk with a chaplain or clergyperson.

The prevailing mood for a woman who has chosen to terminate an early pregnancy is relief. A period of grieving may still follow, and the nurse can prepare the woman for such an event. The importance of good counseling cannot be overemphasized. It is critical to prevent long-term adverse effects of the abortion process. The goal is to prevent *recidivism,* or repeated elective abortions (Mueller, 1991).

Care for abortion in the second trimester. Today a woman seeking second-trimester abortion has a set of psychosocial problems with which to cope. In some cases this decision is based on a fetal anomaly established after many tests, which included a waiting period for results. For others, denial of the pregnancy or financial considerations caused the delay. In any case these women need nursing assessment, support, and guidance (Mueller, 1991).

The nurse establishes communication to elicit the woman's reasons for seeking the procedure and completes required tests and assessments, depending on the week of pregnancy and the situation. The client usually is in the labor area for this procedure (see discussion of IUFD therapy).

Care at the bedside involves monitoring and treating the side effects of PGE_2 administration, which are nausea, vomiting, and diarrhea. Scopolamine, promethazine (Phenergan), diphenoxylate (Lomotil), and acetaminophen

(Tylenol) may be used. For more severe pain of contractions, maternal comfort can be achieved with adequate doses of morphine or meperidine (Demerol) because fetal depression need not be considered. In cases of IUFD an epidural anesthetic is offered.

The woman must go through the process of labor, although often with a shortened second stage because of the size of the fetus. (See also support techniques of labor care in Chapter 13.) Recovery follows a usual pattern, with lochia and lactation. The standard postpartum recovery instructions are given. It should be emphasized to a family member that if the woman has had previous unresolved losses and shows symptoms of extended denial or anger or delayed grieving, she may need to be referred to a counselor.

TEST *Yourself* 21-4 _____

a. Describe interventions for threatened abortion.
b. Compare and contrast the use of PGE$_2$ for induction (see Drug Profile 16-2) and second-trimester abortion.

EVALUATION

Depending on the reason for pregnancy loss, its conclusion may bring great relief or great sadness. The nurse refers to data and expected outcomes while asking evaluative questions such as the following:

- Is there support for her in the home situation?
- Does she talk of managing care in the recovery period?
- Is she aware of which family planning method to use?
- Does she know self-care for involution?
- Was pregnancy terminated without infection or hemorrhage?
- Has she received Rh immunoglobulin, if indicated?

Loss after Viability: Intrauterine Fetal Death

After the age of viability (20 weeks) a fetus that dies in the uterus or during the process of birth is an IUFD. *Stillbirth* is another term used to define the status of a fetus that does not breathe, exhibit a heartbeat, or show pulsation of the umbilical cord or movement of voluntary muscles at birth. Fifty percent of the perinatal mortality rate is related to IUFD. The causes are numerous. Maternal conditions that result in loss of placental functioning, including abruptio placentae, severe hypertension, or an aging placenta, lead to fetal hypoxia and acidosis. Chronic maternal conditions such as severe Rh sensitization, sickle cell disease, or diabetes mellitus may make an intrauterine environment incompatible with life. Unusual events such as trauma or uterine rupture may lead to death. Fetal conditions include genetic conditions not supportive of life,

IUGR, prolapse of the cord, nuchal cord, true knot in the cord, chronic fetal distress that worsens during labor, and many unknown reasons.

Clinical management

The only warning signs are changes in fetal movement patterns (see Chapter 11). Once fetal death has been diagnosed before labor begins, treatment involves waiting as long as 2 weeks for spontaneous labor to begin. Coagulation problems such as disseminated intravascular coagulation (DIC) may develop if a dead fetus is retained longer than 3 to 4 weeks. Laboratory evaluation of coagulation levels helps to monitor early changes that lead to DIC (see Chapter 22).

If labor does not occur naturally, it will be stimulated with oxytocin infusion, vaginal prostaglandin gel, or both in the same methods as midtrimester abortion. If the placenta is still functioning, progesterone inhibits oxytocin, and several attempts may be needed to deliver the fetus. Physicians are hesitant to subject the woman to surgery for a nonviable infant (Queenan and Hobbins, 1996).

Nursing considerations

Especially in cases of IUFD or an anomalous fetus, the behavior of the health care team during labor and birth and during recovery sets the tone and model for a woman's grieving (Mueller, 1991). Avoidance, lack of empathy, and inability to initiate discussions retard a woman's grieving process (see Chapter 26). Therefore it is the nurse's responsibility to initiate discussion and to show empathy but not to give false reassurance. Time to explore the woman's feelings and responses is required. For instance, in cases of IUFD, autopsy may be desired and useful to gain information about causes. The physician introduces the topic of autopsy with the rationale that at least the woman and her family will know there was no evident contributing cause. It may be helpful in the grieving process to know there are no known avoidable reasons for death. The woman should be encouraged to express her feelings and fears to reduce anxiety about the autopsy. The cause will be sought because such knowledge is needed to prevent possible future fetal deaths, and because the woman and her family need to know to assuage guilt. The grieving process is aided by understanding (see Chapter 26 for perinatal grief).

The nurse may suggest clergy support and baptism of the nonviable fetus, depending on the woman's beliefs.

HEMORRHAGE IN OBSTETRICS

During pregnancy the blood supply to the uterus increases enormously to provide for placental circulation. The myometrium is supplied mainly from the uterine and ovarian arteries, and these arteries enter the uterine

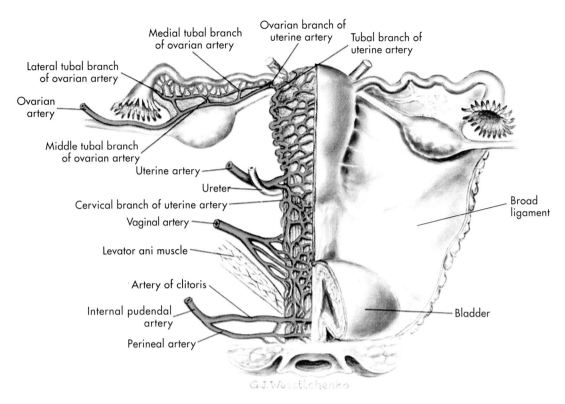

Figure 21-18   Blood supply to uterus and surrounding structures. Note how vessels enter at every level. (From Bobak IM, Jensen MD: *Essentials of maternity nursing: the nurse and the childbearing family,* ed 2, St Louis, 1987, Mosby.)

muscle, coiling and looping to allow for the stretching of the growing uterus (Figure 21-18). Pathways into the myometrium at every level of the uterus from the cervix to the fundus allow the uterine muscle to act as an elastic web that controls blood flow by constricting vessels that pass through it as the uterus contracts and allow normal flow as the uterus relaxes. For *hemostasis* the myometrium must function to close off blood vessels.

This unusual action of the uterus does not provide hemostasis in cases such as low implantation or ectopic pregnancy in which the placental blood supply is not under the control of uterine contraction. In other cases the placenta is correctly implanted in the body of the uterus, and bleeding may occur because of separation of part of the placenta. Until delivery and uterine contraction, hemorrhage may be rapid. Remember that 500 ml/min circulate through the placenta in the last part of pregnancy. Without hemostasis, this amount can be lost from the placenta during each minute. When uncontrolled, the result is hypovolemic shock from hemorrhage. Hemorrhage affects 7% to 8% of pregnancies. Of these, 1% are related to placental location, 1.5% to placental separation, and the rest to all other causes during birth and recovery. Today with careful monitoring, morbidity and mortality may be reduced to a low rate (Zahn and Yeomans, 1991; see also discussion of trauma in Chapter 23). However, hemorrhage accounts for 30% of maternal deaths (Ritter and deShazo, 1994).

Hemorrhage is rapid loss of blood of more than 1% of body weight or 10% of blood volume. This is calculated as follows: 1 ml of blood is equivalent to 1 g of body weight. In a woman weighing 50 kg (110 pounds) or 50,000 g, 1% of body weight is 500 g or 500 ml. Rapid blood loss of more than 500 ml can cause inadequate tissue perfusion, deprivation of glucose and oxygen in tissue, and build-up of waste products.

Most healthy persons tolerate gradual loss of 500 ml of blood with replacement of oral fluids (e.g., when donating a pint of blood). Hypovolemic shock begins if bleeding progresses to 1.5 to 2 L. Fortunately, normal pregnant women are protected against **hypovolemia** by the excess plasma and red blood cells already present by 14 weeks. With the exception of small women, women who bleed steadily during the antepartum period, or women with severe preeclampsia with reduced blood volume, signs of hypovolemia do not become clearly evident until 30% to 35% of volume is lost. By then, tachycardia and recognizable signs may be present, but the shock is more advanced than it would appear. Body responses are initiated to maintain tissue perfusion; intricate processes for hemostasis and reflex vasoconstriction begin (Table 21-2). Often the only initial signs in the woman are pallor, cold wet skin, and oliguria, all related to vasoconstriction. There may be expressions of anxiety, restlessness, and "air hunger" (feeling short of breath). Whether or not overt blood is observed, these early warnings of hypovolemia should always be noted.

Table **21-2** **Hypovolemic Shock**		
Physiologic Changes	Client Symptoms	Interventions
CARDIAC AND CIRCULATORY STATUS		
Decreased venous pressure, cardiac output, pulse pressure, arterial pressure	Client feels weak, anxious, dizzy and may feel rapid heartbeat.	Record vital signs; if necessary, take apical pulse. Support blood volume with plasma expanders, whole blood, and an isotonic solution. Military anti-shock trousers (MAST) may be used.
Peripheral vasoconstriction: to protect vital organs, adrenal medulla is stimulated to produce catecholamines, adding to vasoconstriction	Client feels cold; peripheral tissues are pale. Nails blanch slowly; client feels restless, anxious, fearful.	Keep client warm; check skin color, turgor, mucous membrane moisture, temperature. Reassure client. Record expressed statements, observations.
RESPIRATORY STATUS		
Tachypnea Respiratory center stimulated by hypoxia	Client complains of "air hunger" (shortness of breath)	Note rate, rhythm, depth of respirations. Administer oxygen by mask. Place client in side-lying position or in left-lateral tilt with legs at 45°-angle to hips.
GASTROINTESTINAL STATUS		
Fluid shift from interstitial tissues and intestinal tract to vascular compartment (takes several hours)	Sensation of thirst increases.	Drop in hematocrit observed after shift. Draw blood for serial hemoglobin and hematocrit determinations. Allow nothing by mouth if returning to operating room or delivery room for correction of bleeding.
Decreased parasympathetic activity plus reduced gastrointestinal motility, secretions	Nausea may occur.	Nasogastric tube may be inserted.
RENAL STATUS		
Conservation of fluids and salts stimulated by vasoconstriction of renal arterioles (needs 70 mm Hg pressure to effectively filtrate blood)	Client may have no sensation of need to void.	Observe closely for oliguria (lower limit of normal 30 ml/hr). Record hourly output, and specific gravity from Foley catheter.

General treatment follows these guidelines:

1. Replacement of fluid to restore adequate blood volume
2. Repair or removal of causes of bleeding
3. Support of body systems during treatment

Protocols for Management of Hemorrhage

The management of hemorrhage in obstetrics is a complex subject. The following is a summary of steps that are taken in collaborative care among physician, midwife, nurse, and anesthesiologist (Lowe, 1990; Zahn and Yeomans, 1991) (see discussion of trauma in Chapter 23).

1. Estimate the actual blood loss, relate it to the prehemorrhage blood volume, and make a comparison.

(Remember that small women and those with severe preeclampsia have lower than average volumes). Guessing by observation of the blood is not accurate, as indicated by the saying, "Twice of what the doctor estimates. . . ." When blood is on the floor or in the pads or sheets, the only accurate way to determine the amount of blood loss is to weigh pads, sheets, or sponges or to measure collected blood or clots. (A saturated perineal pad can absorb approximately 60 to 100 ml). In the emergency situation, no one can stop to do this, but later it may be useful.

2. Find the source of the bleeding and correct the cause. This complex and possibly time-consuming task is the physician's primary responsibility. The anesthesiologist and nurse assist in supporting the woman while this

process proceeds. Laboratory determinations are required for clotting time, platelet counts, prothrombin time (PT), partial thromboplastin time (PTT), and thrombin time (TT), which are important to direct the blood replacement and to detect DIC, which can lead to massive hemorrhage (see Chapter 22).

3. Support blood volume and body functions until hemorrhage ceases and functions normalize. Remember that vital signs do not change at first because of the compensatory mechanisms of vasoconstriction and fluid shift to the central circulation. Unfortunately for the fetus, the uterus is not a vital organ therefore as blood flow shifts centrally, fetal distress occurs. Fetal tachycardia occurs and late decelerations reflecting fetal hypoxia will be observed on the monitor strip.

It is important to correct hypovolemia, if possible, before the signs of shock appear. This potential risk underlies the sometimes large amounts of IV fluids administered during a cesarean operation. Protecting the BP will allow oxygen pressures to remain high enough for maternal and fetal tissues. If hypovolemia progresses to the second stage of blood loss, after approximately 30% to 35% of the volume is lost, preload falls, cardiac output falls, pulse rises, and BP (reflecting afterload) drops, sometimes dramatically. Tissues become hypoxic. If uncorrected, this leads to metabolic acidosis with damage to the tissues, platelet consumption, and then vasodilation reversing the protective vasoconstriction. Blood may pool in the peripheral circulation, causing further hypoxemia.

Volume expansion

Blood volume is supported in the following several ways (Santoso, Lin, Miller, 1995):

1. *Crystalloids* that are useful in expanding volume are normal saline (0.9%) and lactated Ringer's solution. The ratio is two to three times the estimated blood loss. Too great a volume of these fluids without albumin will lower the colloid osmotic pressure (COP), which regulates movement of fluid across body membranes. A lowered COP contributes to accumulation of interstitial fluid and pulmonary edema. Units of *albumin,* either 5% or 25%, may be given in these cases. (After cesarean birth, significant edema sometimes may be noted, especially in the lower extremities, when all else appears normal. The nurse can check the volume of fluids received in the operative period as part of the assessment of this situation).

2. *Packed red blood cells* (PRBC) may be given to increase oxygen delivery. Later the hematocrit level will be checked; women do best if it is maintained above 28% (Lowe, 1990).

3. If bleeding continues and the clotting system appears to be affected, *platelets* may be given to maintain counts above 80,000/mm³. *Cryoprecipitate* contains

---

| **Box 21-4** | **Autologous Transfusion** |

- The third trimester is an appropriate time for the woman who anticipates operative delivery to donate her own blood, which can be stored and used if needed. Blood volume is quickly replaced in this trimester. Such an arrangement eliminates the small risk accompanying blood transfusions and is an expensive process (Etchason et al, 1995).
- Intraoperative blood salvage (IBS) can be done, capturing the client's own blood in a canister, transporting to the blood bank where RBCs are washed, and returning to the client. Current machines can process a unit of blood in 3 minutes (Santoso, Lin, Miller, 1995).

---

clotting factors and fibrinogen, and *fresh frozen plasma* contains clotting factors and albumin.

Unless the hematocrit level falls drastically, whole blood is avoided because of the slight risk of serum-induced viral infections. (See Box 21-4 for an alternate choice of *autologous transfusion.*) When there is the facility to reinfuse the client's own blood, an *autotransfusion* may be done when massive amounts of blood have been lost (Santoso, Lin, Miller, 1995).

IV access must be maintained with a large-bore catheter (16 to 17 gauge). A second IV line will be started, and occasionally a *blood pump* attachment will be used to push in the fluids at a faster rate. Remember, if bleeding is arterial or from many sites around the placenta, the blood loss may be rapid. (During pregnancy, 500 to 600 ml of blood circulates through the placenta per minute.)

Stabilization

After the first emergency stage of intervention is over and the client is stabilized, a Foley catheter, if not already in place, will be inserted, and output will be evaluated by means of a bag with hourly volume markings. Infusions should maintain an output of 30 to 50 ml/hr and a hematocrit level of more than 30% (Zahn and Yeomans, 1991). (A falling hematocrit in the absence of bleeding may indicate crystalloid overhydration.) If volume is difficult to correct, a central venous line may be placed using the neck (external jugular) or antecubital fossa (brachial) route, because fluid overload and pulmonary edema are significant possibilities. Central access must be carefully considered when there is a clotting deficiency inasmuch as localized bleeding can be dangerous.

Oxygen by mask or nasal cannula should be started at the first indication. A pulse oximetry monitor may be used to monitor oxygen saturation. The woman must be kept warm. Rapid infusion of room temperature IV fluid can cause extreme chilling and a fall in core temperature. A *blood warmer* attachment may be used to avoid this problem.

Reversing hypovolemia takes a coordinated team effort and is an obstetric emergency. With today's current technology and a competent team, the woman almost always will survive the ordeal and recover well.

Placenta Previa

Placenta previa occurs when the placenta is attached in the lower uterine segment rather than in the body of the uterus. Because a thin decidual layer is located here, the placenta develops over a larger surface and may cover the internal os as follows (Figure 21-19):

- *Complete:* entirely covering the internal os
- *Partial:* covering a portion of the os
- *Marginal:* within 2 cm but not covering the os
- *Low-lying:* within 2 to 5 cm of the os

Toward the last part of pregnancy the lower uterine segment contracts and relaxes, and the cervix slowly effaces. With this movement, when the placenta is covering or lying partially across the internal cervical os, it pulls away from the placenta. Villi are torn from the walls exposing the uterine sinuses of the placental site. The earlier the bleeding begins, the more serious the type of previa. The cause is implantation in the lower uterine segment (LUS). Predisposing factors include uterine scarring from prior surgery such as uterine curettage or cesarean delivery, multiple gestation with a large placental site, infection with endometritis, and a previous episode of low implantation. Women with problems of infertility, with multiple pregnancies, and older multiparas account for many of the cases (Gonik and Brobrowski, 1996).

Risk

Lower uterine attachment requiring treatment occurs in 0.5% (1 in 200) of pregnancies and is a cause of perinatal mortality related to prematurity. Because blood is lost during an extended period, sometimes the fetus may be affected by maternal anemia. However, the highest risk to the fetus is preterm birth. With effective treatment, maternal mortality is low.

Signs

There may have been spotting in the first trimester. An ultrasound should have been done and the poor placental location identified. However, Enkin et al (1995) state that 90% of these early diagnosed cases are found in the last trimester to have "moved up" on the uterine wall and be normally placed. This is because the LUS develops further as pregnancy progresses.

If placental previa persists, the classic sign by 28 weeks is *intermittent, painless vaginal bleeding*. Bright red bleeding may begin slowly as spotting or come in intermittent gushes. Continuous bleeding is more common in the third trimester. Bleeding is not related to activity level, and the uterus is relaxed and nontender. Placental location prevents movement of the fetus into the pelvic canal. The head remains high, or fetal position may be transverse, oblique, or breech. Bleeding may not begin until the time of labor with grades 1 (low-lying) and 2 (marginal), and the cause may be confused with premature separation of the placenta.

Clinical management

The clinical problem is confirmed by ultrasound to view placental position. If bleeding is significant, the woman must be hospitalized and placed on a regimen of modified bed rest. There is a chance of dislodging more of the placenta if a vigorous pelvic examination is performed. Therefore, after the first speculum examination, no vaginal examinations are done, unless the woman is in the delivery room and ready for birth. If the cervix is even partially dilated, the placental tissue may be visualized at the cervical os.

Laboratory tests are ordered every 12 hours for hemoglobin and hematocrit levels. Blood type and match will be determined; two units will be kept on call. If the woman is Rh negative, the Kleinhauer-Betke test for pres-

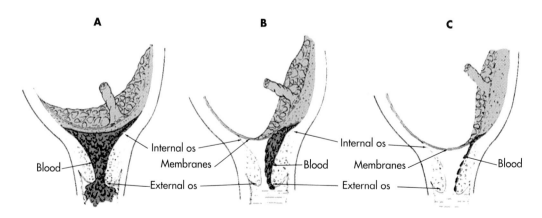

Figure 21-19   Types of placenta previa. **A,** Total, or complete, placenta previa. **B,** Partial placenta previa. **C,** Marginal placenta previa. (From Lowdermilk DL: *Maternity and women's health care,* ed 6, St Louis, 1997, Mosby.)

ence of fetal cells in the maternal circulation is done and the woman will be given Rh immunoglobulin to prevent sensitization (see Drug Profile 23-1).

After diagnosis is made of the degree of placental growth over the os, fetal age is determined. FHR and activity will be monitored at regular intervals. The amount of bleeding and the woman's response will be weighed against the age of the fetus. A recommendation for continuing the pregnancy and for the type of birth is made. When the risk to either mother or child seems greater than the risk associated with birth, the infant will be delivered. The result of this waiting and watching is increased anxiety.

Vaginal delivery may be possible if the head is well down in the birth canal; the head may act as a pressure tourniquet in this case. If the placenta partially (grade 3) or completely (grade 4) covers the os, bleeding begins earlier, and a cesarean delivery always will be required. Eighty percent of women with placenta previa require operative delivery. Surgery must be performed with care, especially if the placenta is lying over the anterior part of the lower uterine wall, because it is possible to cut blood vessels and cause more bleeding.

After delivery the placenta must be examined carefully. Fragments may adhere to the placental site, leading to infection. Hemorrhage may occur because the LUS does not have the same muscle strength in contraction to shut off the bleeding.

Premature Placental Separation: Abruptio Placentae

Premature separation of the normally implanted placenta is known as **abruptio placentae** or retroplacental hemorrhage. Separation occurs in many degrees (Box 21-5) and may occur at any stage of pregnancy (Enkin et al, 1995). Premature separation occurs most often after 20 to 24 weeks and often just before or at the time of labor. Severity is classified by grades 0 to 3, or as mild, moderate, or severe, depending on the location and amount of bleeding (Figure 21-20). Separation may be as follows:
- *Marginal* or *apparent*: separation at the edge of the placenta, with bleeding seen at the vagina
- *Central* or *concealed*: separation occurring in the center of the placenta so that no bleeding is observable

> ### Box 21-5   Degrees of Abruptio Placentae
>
> **MILD**
> No or slight external bleeding; less than 250 ml
> Placenta showing infarcted areas of less than one sixth of placenta
> Vague lower abdominal backache, slight uterine tenderness
>
> **MODERATE**
> Retroplacental or vaginal bleeding of less than 1000 ml, separation of less than two thirds of placenta, cramping and mild abdominal aching to more severe pain, fetal heart tone present but may show irregularities, DIC may occur
>
> **SEVERE**
> More than two thirds of placenta separated; uterus du bois (woodlike), uterine tenderness, rigidity, or severe pain, Couvelaire uterus (bruising of uterine muscle); FHTs showing severe distress or FHTs absent
> Entire separation; maternal shock, fetal death; severe pain; DIC coagulation

DIC, Disseminated intravascular coagulation; *FHT,* fetal heart tone.

PLACENTAL ABNORMALITIES

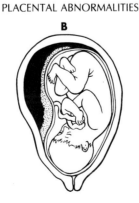 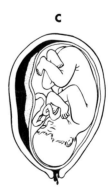

Figure 21-20   Classification of abruptio placentae. **A,** Marginal with apparent bleeding; **B,** central or concealed (many degrees of severity); **C,** complete, bleeding is retroplacental and also vaginal, but large volume makes uterus tense and painful. (From Gilbert ES, Harmon JS: *High risk pregnancy & delivery,* St Louis, 1993, Mosby.)

Table **21-3**	**Comparison of Placenta Previa and Abruptio Placentae**
Placenta Previa	**Abruptio Placentae**
No underlying chronic disease	Associated with hypertension, diabetes, and kidney diseases
Warning signs of spotting hemorrhage always externally visible	Usually no warning signs
	Hemorrhage may be internal or externally visible
No pain	Pain may be present in varying degrees
Occurs rarely during labor but is unrelated to labor	Usually occurs in labor
FHTs and movement usually present and unaffected	FHTs reflecting uteroplacental insufficiency
Placenta in lower uterine segment	Placental attachment in normal locations
Soft uterus	Uterus tender to woodlike

FHTs, Fetal heart tones; *LUS,* lower uterine segment.

- *Missed* or *combined:* various portions of placenta separate, bleeding is trapped in the uterus or is visible at the vagina

Differentiating types of placental separation is difficult, and often it may be confused with placenta previa. Differences between the conditions are listed in Table 21-3. The cause varies, but any condition that contributes to vascular changes at the placental level contributes to separation. In some cases the vessels may necrose, and infarcts (dead tissue) occur, which may split from the decidua. If the infarct is thought of as a stroke in the placental vessels, it is easier to relate the possible precursors. Pregnancy induced or chronic hypertension is present in 50% of the cases, and multiparas older than 35 years are more often affected (Beischer and MacKay, 1993). In addition, severe diabetes and renal disease with vascular changes are associated with separation (Queenan and Hobbins, 1996). Chronic smoking and cocaine use also contributes 5% to the rate. Mechanical factors may be responsible in some cases, including trauma from automobile accidents (5% to 10%). Sudden release of a large amount of amniotic fluid, rapid descent of an infant with an unusually short cord, or precipitate labor placenta may contribute. In many clients, however, there is no clear cause.

Risk

Between 0.5% and 1.5% of all pregnancies have premature separation of some grade; most are minor. If separation begins at home and if there is a delay in obtaining assistance, maternal mortality is approximately 6% when moderate to severe separation occurs. Separation accounts for more than 15% of perinatal deaths and, although perinatal mortality has decreased, the fetal death rate still is 20% to 40% (Saftlas, 1991).

Signs

Signs of separation often occur as labor begins. If the woman is at home, the first sign may be vaginal bleed-ing. Fetal movements may become hyperactive and then cease. If membranes break, meconium staining may be observed. Pain will occur in many degrees; persistent escalating pain indicates concealed bleeding with an enlarging clot (Box 21-6).

When blood loss is significant, signs of shock will be present. If the woman is in labor in a hospital setting, the monitor strip will show uteroplacental insufficiency (UPI) with baseline changes and reduced variability. Tonus will rise, and contraction patterns will change. In addition, if bleeding is concealed, erratic hypertonic contractions, uterine tension, and severe pain will be present. There may be bruising of the uterine muscles (Couvelaire uterus), resulting in poor hemostasis after birth. Fetal condition deteriorates rapidly, and emergency surgical intervention must be instituted.

Laboratory tests show a decrease in complete blood cell count values, and coagulation factors may change. In the case of severe abruptio placentae, 10% to 30% of women develop DIC (see Chapter 22).

Clinical management

Treatment is determined by the amount of separation and blood loss compared with fetal age and status. For grade 0 (mild) with concealed or overt blood loss of less than 250 ml, conservative treatment of bed rest, sedatives, and close observation is continued until the fetus is 37 weeks of age. In cases of moderate blood loss, when 250 to 1000 ml have been lost but less than one half of the placenta is affected, cesarean delivery will be performed after stabilization of maternal and fetal perfusion. Severe cases that affect more than two thirds of the placenta often result in fetal death in utero. The woman has a rigid abdomen and pain, and her condition is serious. A cesarean delivery is done as soon as she is stabilized enough to undergo anesthesia. This condition may cause an intermingling of maternal and fetal blood; therefore Rh-negative women receive Rh immunoglobulin.

Box 21-6

WARNING SIGNS

Abruption

Vaginal bleeding
Uterine tenderness or severe pain
Back pain
Fetal distress (late decelerations, decreased variability)
Change in contractions:
    Rising baseline tonus
    Hypertonic, frequent

Vasa Previa

A rare but serious defect in the structure of the umbilical cord may lead to fetal bleeding and death during labor. In **vasa previa** the umbilical vessels leave the placenta surrounded only by the amnion and chorion and enter the umbilical cord a few inches away from the placenta. These vessels, unprotected by Wharton's jelly, are vulnerable to compression and rupture during labor, especially after ROM. Therefore any bleeding beginning during labor should be tested by Kleihauer-Betke test for the presence of fetal cells, in case the blood is of fetal origin. An emergency cesarean is done to rescue the infant from further blood loss.

Uterine Rupture

Rupture is not common. It is almost always related to separation of a prior uterine scar. If the placenta is attached where the scar is located, it is more likely to invade into the myometrium causing placenta accreta or to be associated with rupture. Classical incisions are more likely to rupture, and for these cases, vaginal birth after cesarean (VBAC) is not usually permitted.

Risk

Uterine rupture results in serious maternal morbidity and mortality and carries a high risk, 22%, of maternal deaths from hemorrhage (Ritter and deShazo, 1994). Depending on when and where it occurs—at home or in the delivery unit—the blood loss can be significant, usually concealed, and into the peritoneum.

Signs

Signs of uterine rupture include a change in station of the presenting part during labor, with the fetal body rising up in the abdomen, or a change in contour of the abdomen. Abnormal fetal tracings signal distress. Approximately 18% of women have pain that may be confused with abruptio placentae. With upper or miduterine

rupture, there may be tearing pain, collapse, and shock. The fetus usually dies.

With rupture of the LUS, which is less vascular, signs may be less dramatic. Fetal distress, with aching or pain in the lower abdomen, will be evident. Labor contractions change or cease at the same time. In these less dramatic cases, the tear in the lower uterine wall may be seen only after birth, when exploration of the cause of bleeding occurs.

Clinical management

Ultrasound evaluation may quickly establish the presence of blood in the peritoneum and a shift in fetal position. Maternal signs of hypovolemia rapidly progress, and emergency cesarean section must be carried out as soon as possible.

Hysterectomy (removal of the uterus) or repair of the rupture must be chosen. If repair is possible, the woman is not allowed to labor in a subsequent pregnancy but is scheduled for an early cesarean birth when fetal lungs show maturity (approximately week 36).

Hemorrhage Related to Birth Method

Common factors that raise the risk for hemorrhage include a history of previous hemorrhage, underlying medical problems such as hypertension, preeclampsia, reduced platelets, anemias, and infection. Bleeding happens more often with a nullipara than a multipara unless she has had more than four births, a *grand multipara.* Finally, any woman with a long labor and a prolonged second stage is at risk for bleeding. Fatigue of the muscle from these causes and overstretching of the uterine muscles related to multiple pregnancy increases risk (Table 21-4).

Risks with vaginal birth

Vaginal birth adds risks related to forceps or vacuum extraction, prolonged third stage, mediolateral or midline episiotomy, and lacerations of the birth canal. Bleeding averages 500 ml at birth, including the first few hours of recovery (Combs, Murphy, Laros, 1991).

Risks with cesarean birth

The main cause is general anesthesia, which quickly exerts a vasodilating effect. Bleeding with cesarean birth averages 900 to 1100 ml and may total much more as risk factors are added. A classic surgical incision adds to blood loss as well. Any woman having an emergency cesarean section is at high risk because of factors leading to surgery—preeclampsia, uterine dystocia, second-stage arrest, and amnionitis. Therefore staff members must always be prepared for additional blood loss. Lowe (1991) estimates that 7% to 8% of women will exceed the average blood loss for vaginal and cesarean birth.

Table 21-4	**Risk Factors for Hemorrhage**

Vaginal Birth	Cesarean Birth
CAUSES IN DESCENDING ORDER OF OCCURRENCE*	

• Prolonged third stage
   Placenta accreta in some degree, manual extraction of
   placenta
	General anesthesia
	Amnionitis

• Preeclampsia: low platelets and blood volume, and effects of magnesuim sulfate	Preeclampsia
• Mediolateral episiotomy	Protracted active labor
• Previous postpartum hemorrhage	Prolonged second stage
• Twins or more than two fetuses	
• Prolonged second stage	
• Soft tissue lacerations	
• Oxytocin-augmented labor	
• Asian or Hispanic ethnicity	Being Asian or Hispanic
• Forceps/vacuum extraction	Classic uterine incision
• Midline episiotomy	
• Nulliparity (not multiparity unless > 4)	

Data from Combs CA, Murphy EL, Laros RK Jr: Factors associated with hemorrhage, *Obstet Gynecol Surv* 46:362, 1991.
*For women who bled during labor or birth and whose hematocrit dropped 10 points or more from admission or who received a transfusion.

Hemorrhage After Birth

There may be hemorrhage as a result of uterine atony, trauma, or subinvolution with infection. Hemorrhage is described as early or primary in the first 24 hours or as late or secondary if heavy bleeding with clot formation occurs after 24 hours and for as long as 2 weeks. Causes may be factors that inhibit uterine contractions, trauma, or infection and subinvolution.

The placental site is a raw wound with numerous blood vessels that spill blood if ineffective uterine contractions are evident. If the uterus stays firmly contracted, blood loss follows the normal pattern. If reduced tone begins again after initial contraction, the newly formed clots on the surface of the placental site will be loosened, and fresh bleeding will begin.

Uterine Atony

Uterine atony is the most frequent cause of early bleeding. Reasons for poor contractility of the muscle are numerous (Box 21-7). Common reasons are a long, exhausting labor or uterine inertia with excessive oxytocin stimulation. Foremost is the effect of a distended bladder on the uterus. The bladder and anterior lower portion of the uterus are attached by fascia. When the bladder becomes distended, the uterus must be pulled up with it and thus is unable to maintain contraction. With the fundal check, the uterus is found to be soft and located to the right side, at or above the umbilicus. Signs may not be evident until fundal pressure is applied and clots are expressed. Clots may collect in the

Box 21-7	**Risk Factors for Uterine Atony**

Multiparity
Overdistended uterus, twins, polyhydramnios
Placenta previa or abruptio placentae
Fibroids causing asymmetric contraction
Long, exhausting labor
Prolonged second stage
Oxytocin stimulation during labor
General fatigue, anemia, and preeclampsia
Distension of bladder
Too vigorous massage of fundus
Precipitate labor

vagina and not become evident until the client changes position or stands up.

Placenta accreta

A rare cause of bleeding is **placenta accreta**, an anomaly in which the placental trophoblastic tissue entered the myometrium when the placenta was formed. When placental separation after birth is expected, parts adhere to the wall and prevent uterine contracture. This is an emergency, and in some cases requires a hysterectomy to save the life of the woman.

Lacerations

Lacerations of the birth canal may occur with large infants, when breech or other dystocias are present or when forceps are used. The vagina and cervix are inspected after the birth to detect tears that need to be sutured. Continuous bright red bleeding with a contracted uterus indicates a laceration in the birth passage. The laceration may be in the lower uterine segment, and bleeding then is retroperitoneal and unobserved until signs of hypovolemia begin. Periurethral lacerations may accompany the birth of a large infant. Perineal lacerations are evident to the physician or midwife and may occur especially with precipitous or uncontrolled final moments of the descent phase of birth. See Box 15-4 for the description of each type of laceration.

Hematoma

A hematoma is a collection of blood within tissue. During birth certain vessels may be torn, with bleeding into tissues of the upper part of the vagina, around the perineum, or into the labia. Blood loss usually is underestimated and hidden. Pain often out of proportion to the size of the hematoma occurs. In most cases the hematoma is visible as a swelling within the vagina, at the labia, or in the rectal area. The pain may be severe and felt in the entire perirectal area. The woman may have fever, chills, and thigh pain, and on occasion, if left undiscovered, leg edema. Treatment is to make an incision to allow trapped blood to escape from the hematoma. Sometimes a pressure gauze pack is inserted for 12 hours. Then the incision is sutured, and antibiotics are given. An ice compress applied intermittently is an important early treatment of a perineal hematoma.

Subinvolution

Hemorrhage may occur later as a result of poor involution of the uterus related to infection or retained placental fragments or membranes. The woman should be given instructions regarding the expected changes in lochia. When bright red bleeding or clotting begins again, she should contact the physician at once because the amount may vary from a normal menstrual flow to volumes that precipitate shock.

Box 21-4
CLINICAL DECISION

a. An hour after birth a primipara develops a bright red steady trickle of blood from the vagina. List the sequence the nurse should follow in assessment. What initial steps are taken?
b. When Mary first gets out of bed to void, a huge gush of clotted blood runs down her leg and onto the floor. Identify the steps in assessment and priorities for immediate care.

Clinical management. Treatment of inadequate uterine contraction is to strengthen muscle tone with oxytocic agents (see Chapter 16).
- *Oxytocin,* 20 U, may be given in IV fluids. (Oxytocin also has an antidiuretic action and delays diuresis if more than the usual dosage is administered.)
- *Methergine,* 0.2 mg, may be injected IM if the client is not hypertensive.
- *PGF$_2$,* 0.25 mg, may be directly injected into uterine muscle or given IM.
- *PGE$_2$,* 20 mg suppository, may be inserted into the uterine cavity.

If oxytocics do not cause muscle contraction, bimanual compression of the hypotonic uterus may be done. Wearing a sterile glove, the physician compresses the placental site with the right fist while grasping the fundus and exerting downward pressure. This pressure should be released for 1 minute every 5 minutes.

The bladder is the first area that must be checked if bleeding develops in the recovery area. There is a standing order for straight catheterization to keep the bladder empty; assessment of bladder status is a nursing priority.

Severe bleeding from rupture, lower uterine lacerations, and cervical or perineal lacerations will require surgical repair.

Nursing Responsibilities

The potential for antepartal bleeding must be considered in all care. Because placental perfusion may diminish and fetal distress may occur, monitoring of the fetus always accompanies a risk of bleeding. Placenta previa may seem to subside, but at any time may recur with painless, silent bleeding. Women with risk factors for hemorrhage need frequent monitoring of vital signs and intake and output. Documentation is critical because events may transpire so quickly.

ASSESSMENT

The nurse ascertains risk factors in the woman's history, compares current vital signs and laboratory reports with the last prenatal visit, and assesses for signs and symptoms of blood loss. On admission, if there is heavy bleeding, status is monitored with assessment of amount on pads by visual comparison with a standard chart or by weighing the pads (pad count). Vital signs are monitored frequently if there is bleeding and every 4 hours when it subsides. Clients with a diagnosis of placenta previa that is more severe than grade 2 may not leave the hospital. Exceptions may be made if the woman lives nearby and has home help, easy transportation, and understands her self-care regimen completely. Bleeding related to abruption or rupture is a crisis, and assessment is a collaborative event in the labor area.

NURSING DIAGNOSES

The following nursing diagnoses that apply to the type and time of occurrence of bleeding in pregnancy are selected:

- Impaired maternal or fetal gas exchange related to maternal hypovolemia and decreased placental perfusion
- Risk for infection related to anemia, surgical procedures, and blood loss
- Pain related to uterine rupture, placental abruption, surgical or traumatic events
- Severe anxiety and fear for self and infant related to unknown diagnosis and potential for fetal injury and prematurity
- Potential for altered parenting or individual coping with delayed attachment with a potentially ill, preterm infant
- Knowledge deficit related to multiple rapid tests and interventions

EXPECTED OUTCOMES

Some outcomes that may be selected for clients with placenta previa, abruption, and birth-related bleeding are as follows:

- Improvement of maintenance of blood volume and tissue perfusion is evidenced by hematocrit, platelet, and white blood cell levels, normal FHR; maternal vital signs; and urine output
- Pain is managed with relief
- Client expresses feelings about self and fetal risk; seeks support; states understanding of purpose of interventions and treatments
- Postpartum recovery follows normal parameters
- Speaks of fetus or newborn with hope and plans

NURSING INTERVENTION

For *placenta previa* the regimen may be prolonged bed rest of 5 to 10 weeks. The woman is advised to change positions; sitting up in a chair may be as restful as lying in bed. Even though bleeding is not aggravated by activity, bed rest appears to lessen the bleeding potential. However, all the body changes that accompany bed rest, including reduced muscle tone, constipation, fatigue, and calcium loss, become a problem. The activity of walking to the bathroom is decided with the physician, depending on the grade of previa. To prevent calcium loss, the woman stands to bear weight several times a day. Isometric exercises and simple upper body and lower leg exercises must be done several times daily to retain muscle mass. The woman must work toward maintaining normal body functions (Maloni, 1993).

Fluid and food intake are encouraged. Because iron tablets are constipating, iron-bearing foods and roughage are preferred to maintain stooling. No enemas are to be given. For an active person who feels well, bed rest is distressing. A woman on bed rest needs a full understanding of the care plan to gain her compliance. The plan should be clear so that those involved in her care do not insist on different regimens. A primary nurse should follow the woman's progress and initiate discussion about coping and family needs. The nurse refers the woman to social service and discusses plans with the family early in the hospitalization. An extended stay is costly both before birth and later for the premature infant. Because most families do not have adequate financial coverage, anxiety about financial matters will be always present.

The nurse ensures that the woman has a relationship with several staff members so she does not feel isolated; works to provide diversion, including books, handwork, and television; and checks often on her mental state. Depression often occurs during prolonged bed rest.

After birth, the nurse carefully observes the woman who has placental previa for hemorrhage from the larger placental site where muscles do not constrict as completely as in the fundus.

Mild placental separation is treated like placenta previa; there is bed rest and watchful waiting. Depending on the degree of separation, fetal age and well-being, and the woman's status, she may be sent home or kept under observation.

Conservative treatment of moderate separation includes watchful monitoring, analgesics, and evaluation of the degree of abruption by ultrasound examination. If the infant is mature enough, cesarean delivery is planned.

Severe separation is always an emergency; the client goes to surgery from the emergency or labor room. Until the placenta is removed, there is no hemostasis.

Remember the general risk diagnoses even during an emergency. The plan of treatment must be fully explained to the client and her partner. The nurse works with them to modify their escalating level of anxiety. When the woman has recovered, she should be encouraged to review what has happened so that she may understand and recover equilibrium. The nurse should enlist the family's support, keeping them informed. Because this problem may be a real threat to the woman's self esteem, she should be encouraged to express her beliefs about why this has happened. When she is in early grieving, observe for signs that she has support from significant others.

Box **21-5**

CLINICAL DECISION

Sally comes to the unit with moderate vaginal bleeding at 36 weeks' gestation. Immediate physical assessment should include FHTs and activity, visualization of type and volume of blood on pad or at vagina, and which other actions?

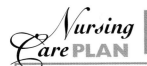

Birth-Related Hemorrhage

CASE

Joan, para 2012, had an extended second stage after a long first stage of labor. Membranes had been ruptured 16 hours before birth, and rectal temperature was 100° F. Because of lack of descent, a cesarean delivery occurred, with general anesthesia. During surgery, blood loss was 3000 ml. She received 2 U of PRBC and 6000 ml of crystalloids during surgery. She has now been transferred to the recovery area.

Assessment

1. Current IV fluids, rate, and replacement orders
   - Output per Foley catheter compared with amount of intake and oxytocin dosage
   - Status of lochia, wound drainage, abdominal dressing, fundus
   - Vital signs, chest sounds, color of mucous membranes and nail beds
   - Level of consciousness and pain sensation
2. Laboratory assessments of complete blood count, PT, PTT, fibrinogen, and platelets
3. Joan's knowledge of why and what happened

Nursing Diagnoses

1. Risk for poor tissue perfusion related to loss of blood and rapid replacement of crystalloids
2. Risk for infection related to blood loss, extended ROM, and surgical procedure plus anesthesia
3. Pain related to fatigue, surgical procedure, and potential inflammation of tissues
4. Anxiety for self and infant related to complicated labor, potential newborn infection

Expected Outcomes

1. Balanced fluid status is evidenced by hematocrit level above 28%, urine output of 30 to 50 ml/hr or more, lack of generalized edema
2. Tissue perfusion maintained as evidenced by pulse oximetry reading showing Po_2, Pco_2 within normal limits
3. White blood cell count, vital signs, incision status remain within normal limits for recovery.
4. Pain is managed, with relief; client gains adequate rest.
5. States understanding of reasons for surgery. Speaks of newborn with hope and anticipation of going home.

Nursing Interventions

1. Maintain warmth with extra blankets. Place all infusions on IV pumps.
2. Monitor vital signs.
   - Maintain pulse oximetry to assess oxygenation.
   - Evaluate lung sounds. Position in low semi-Fowler's position turned slightly to one side. Observe for vomiting.
3. Check total oxytocin dose to prevent antidiuretic action. Hourly output compared with intake until active diuresis occurs.
4. Observe for signs of infection. Administer antibiotics. Follow laboratory reports.
5. Monitor need for analgesic. Administer before severe pain returns. Assess if pain seems more severe than usual.
6. Include partner in discussion of progress. Orient family to reasons for surgery, responses to hemorrhage. Assure woman when signs of recovery are apparent. Inform her of newborn status.

Evaluation

1. Did diuresis begin and hematocrit level remain above 28%? Did bleeding follow normal recovery patterns?
2. Was infection avoided or counteracted?
3. Did fatigue levels diminish? Was pain managed?
4. Did she understand the events through which she just passed? Does she recognize the need for surgical interventions?
5. Has she seen and begun attachment to the infant?
6. Is the infant's condition stable?

For *postbirth hemorrhage* the initial nursing role includes monitoring and detection of developing problems. Remember, signs of shock, evidenced by an increase in pulse and a decrease in BP, are late results of hemorrhage. In an emergency, the nurse supports blood volume by increasing flow rates of infusing fluids or by beginning an infusion with a large-bore intracatheter. Oxytocic agents are administered as ordered. The woman may be placed in a position that allows elevation of knees and lower legs to 45° or military antishock trousers (MAST) may be applied (see Table 21-2). Hemorrhage may be rapid, and a team approach is essential.

If bleeding is local and the source is determined, initial application of an ice pack to the perineum may be effective. Most commonly, the condition can be corrected in the delivery area, and the client returns to the recovery area with blood volume restored. Hematocrit and hemoglobin levels may be low, but transfusions are used only if necessary. Laboratory values are monitored at least every 12 hours during recovery.

The hemorrhaging woman will be anxious and requires explanations of the management and expected outcomes. It is important to explain the rationale for treatment and give her as much information as she desires about the techniques being used to stop the bleeding.

The woman is at special risk for infection and usually is given prophylactic antibiotics. She should be taught the signs of lingering infection and subinvolution.

Box 21-6

CLINICAL DECISION

The client in labor says that she does not feel well. She is chilly, breathless, and pale. You see no vaginal bleeding. List the assessment steps and early interventions you can do while notifying the physician.

EVALUATION

Questions similar to the following may be asked to form an evaluation of outcomes of care for a woman with bleeding from the reproductive tract:

- Did the woman realize why treatments and interventions were performed?
- Did both mother and infant receive adequate perfusion during the bleeding episode?
- Did fluid volume replacement result in output within the normal range?
- Did supportive staff and family members assist her in coping with anxiety?
- Does she understand the signs of infection, changes in lochia, and self-care in the recovery period?
- Are referrals needed for home care or assistance?

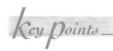

Key Points

- Approximately 85% of all pregnancies are completed normally without problems, but complications of the reproductive system may be life threatening for the mother or fetus.
- PTL remains a leading cause of morbidity and neonatal mortality. Every nurse should be knowledgeable about signs, symptoms, and recommended interventions.
- Some risk factors for PTL are amenable to prevention, especially smoking, infection, stress, and drug abuse.
- Multiple gestation places extra stress on the woman from pressure effects, nutritional demands, and labor complications. Early monitoring is mandatory.
- Signs of ectopic pregnancy are confusing. Early diagnosis and intervention prevent morbidity. The embryo is lost and fertility may be altered.
- The age of viability is the dividing point in pregnancy loss. Early abortions have many serious implications.

Second-trimester abortions cause significantly greater maternal risk.
- There is a choice of attitude toward elective abortion, and nurses have the responsibility of becoming self-aware and cognizant of state rules and regulations.
- Hemorrhage in obstetrics is a risk because of the greater vascular supply to tissues during pregnancy.
- Pregnant women are protected against effects of moderate blood loss, but when hemorrhage exceeds 30% to 35% of blood volume, sudden signs of severe shock will occur.
- Risk factors for hemorrhage can be estimated, which facilitates the implementation of preventive watchful care.
- Nursing monitoring during labor and recovery will identify early warnings of hemorrhage.
- Care is collaborative when hemorrhage occurs. Documentation is essential because events transpire rapidly.

Study Questions

21-1. Select the terms that apply to the following statements:
   a. Abnormal site for implantation of embryo _____
   b. Too much amniotic fluid for gestational age _____
   c. Lack of maternal chromosomes results in "empty ovum" _____
   d. Precursor of uterine cancer _____
   e. Untreated result of an irritable uterus _____
   f. Two embryos from one fertilized ovum _____
   g. Agents that inhibit uterine contractions _____

21-2. Jenny is pregnant with twins. She complains of being warm and sweating at 28 weeks. To further evaluate these findings you should first ask her about which of the following?
   a. Her weight gain pattern
   b. Her usual activity and rest pattern
   c. Any allergies or changes in environment
   d. Signs of infection

21-3. During the last trimester of a twin gestation, it would be most important to teach self-monitoring of which of the following?
   a. Fatigue levels and interrupted sleep patterns
   b. Patterns of edema in lower extremities
   c. Heartburn and inability to take full meals
   d. Changes in mild contraction patterns

21-4. After two warnings of impending labor, Sue calls to say that she is having abdominal aching, diarrhea, and increased watery vaginal mucus. Which instructions should be given over the phone?
   a. "Drink several glasses of water, void, and rest on your left side for 30 minutes."
   b. "Take an acetaminophen tablet and a glass of water. Try to sleep."
   c. "Come in to see us in the labor unit as soon as you can, and drink two glasses of water as you get ready."
   d. "Rest in a side-lying position and call again in an hour because you tend to have these feelings off and on."

21-5. A woman would be at highest risk for premature labor if her history includes which of the following?
   a. Is working full time at a mildly active job
   b. Has gained 40 pounds by week 35 of gestation
   c. Was treated for a bladder infection and is now reinfected
   d. Is a vegetarian having difficulty getting enough iron in her diet

21-6. A woman in her first trimester of pregnancy calls, wondering if she is miscarrying. During a telephone assessment, which question is not pertinent?
   a. "What is the amount of bleeding and uterine cramping?"
   b. "Do you know the time fetal movements stopped?"
   c. "Was a pregnancy test done, and when?"
   d. "Do you know the exact length of pregnancy?"

21-7. Nursing assessment of a woman admitted for an inevitable abortion at 18 weeks includes which of the following?
   a. Determination of fetal heart sounds or movement
   b. Evaluation of bleeding and frequent vital signs
   c. Evaluation of character of the contractions
   d. Measurement of height of fundus and noting time since membranes ruptured

21-8. Anna was admitted at 6 AM because of a painless bleeding episode during the night. She is 26 weeks pregnant and is frightened. Before the physician arrives to examine her, how can you help to limit her complications?
   a. Perform a vaginal examination to determine bleeding site; place her in Trendelenburg's position.
   b. Reassure her that this pregnancy may turn out normally, and explain admission process.
   c. Maintain bed rest, and monitor vital signs and bleeding.
   d. Encourage bed rest, urge oral fluids, and ask companion to stay.

Answer Key

21-1. *a*, Ectopic pregnancy; *b*, polyhydramnios; *c*, hydatidiform mole; *d*, trophoblastic disease; *e*, preterm birth; *f*, monovular twins; *g*, tocolytics. 21-2. *a*; 21-3. *d*; 21-4. *c*; 21-5. *c*; 21-6. *b*; 21-7. *b*; 21-8. *c*.

References

*American College of Obstetricians & Gynecologists (ACOG): *Multiple gestation,* Technical bulletin 131, Washington, DC, 1989, The College.

ACOG: *Management of gestational trophoblastic disease,* Technical bulletin 178, Washington, DC, 1993, The College.

ACOG: *Antenatal corticosteroid therapy for fetal maturation,* Committee Opinion 147, Washington, DC, 1994, The College.

ACOG: *Preterm labor,* Technical bulletin 206, Washington, DC, 1995, The College.

ACOG: *Vaginitis,* Technical bulletin 221, Washington, DC, 1996, The College.

Ballard RA et al: Respiratory disease in very-low-birthweight infants after prenatal thyrotropin-releasing hormone and glucocorticoid, *Lancet* 339:510, 1992.

Barnhart K: Prompt diagnosis of ectopic pregnancy in a ED setting, *Obstet Gynecol* 84(11):1010, 1994.

Beischer NA, MacKay EV, eds: *Obstetrics and the newborn,* ed 3, Philadelphia, 1993, WB Saunders.

Beringer RE, Niebyl JR: The safety and efficacy of tocolytic agents for the treatment of preterm labor, *Obstet Gynecol Rev* 45(7):415, 1990.

Berkowitz RL et al: The current status of multifetal pregnancy reduction, *Am J Obstet Gynecol,* 174(4):1265, 1996.

Blackburn ST, Loper DL: *Maternal, fetal and neonatal physiology,* Philadelphia, 1992, WB Saunders.

*Burchell RC: Professional perspectives on abortion, *J Obstet Gynecol Neonatal Nurs* 3(6):25, 1979.

Carson S, Buster JE: Ectopic pregnancy, *N Engl J Med* 329:1174, 1993.

Combs CA, Murphy EL, Laros RK Jr: Factors associated with hemorrhage, *Obstet Gynecol Surv* 46:362, 1991.

Cowan M: Home care of the pregnant woman using terbutaline, *MCN Am J Matern Child Nurs* 18(1):99, 1993.

Donaldson J, Briggs J, McMaster D: RU 486: an alternative to surgical abortion, *J Obstet Gynecol Neonatal Nurs* 23(7):555, 1994.

Eganhouse DJ: Fetal monitoring of twin gestation, *J Obstet Gynecol Neonatal Nurs* 21(1):17, 1992.

Eganhouse DJ, Burnside SM: Nursing assessment and responsibilities in monitoring the preterm pregnancy, *J Obstet Gynecol Neonatal Nurs* 21(5):355, 1992.

Enkin M et al: *A guide to effective care during pregnancy & childbirth,* Cambridge, Mass, 1995, Oxford University Press.

Ergarter C et al: Antibiotic treatment in preterm premature rupture of membranes and neonatal morbidity: a metaanalysis, *Am J Obstet Gynecol* 174(2):589, 1996.

Etchason J et al: The cost effectiveness of preoperative autologous blood donations, *N Engl J Med* 332:719, 1995.

Gilbert ES, Harmon JS: *High risk pregnancy & delivery,* St Louis, 1993, Mosby.

*Gill SA, ed: Twin pregnancy, *Clin Perinatol* 15(1):162, 1988.

Goldenberg RL et al: Bed rest in pregnancy, *Obstet Gynecol* 84(1):131, 1994.

Gonik B, Bobrowski RA, eds: *Medical complications in labor and delivery,* Cambridge Mass, 1996, Blackwell Science.

Gordon MC, Iams JD: Magnesium sulfate, *Clin Obstet Gynecol* 38(4):706, 1995.

Harrison LK, Naylor KL: The laws that affect abortion in the United States and their impact on women's health, *Nurs Pract* 16(12):53, 1991.

Hausknecht RU: Methotrexate and misoprostol to terminate early pregnancy, *N Engl J Med* 333:537, 1995.

Heuston WJ et al: The effectiveness of preterm-birth prevention educational programs for high-risk women: a meta-analysis, *Obstet Gynecol* 86(4, part 2):705, 1995.

Hollenbach KA, Hickok K: Epidemiology and diagnosis of twin gestation, *Clin Obstet Gynecol* 33:3, 1990.

Iams JD, Johnson FF, Parker M: A prospective evaluation of the signs and symptoms of preterm labor, *Obstet Gynecol* 84(2):227, 1994.

Iams JD: Current status of home uterine activity monitoring, *Clin Obstet Gynecol* 38(4):771, 1995.

Iams JD et al: Fetal fibronectin improves accuracy of diagnosis of preterm labor, *Am J Obstet Gynecol* 173(1):141, 1995.

Jones JM, Sbarra AJ, Cetrulo CL: Antepartum management of twin gestation, *Clin Obstet Gynecol* 33:32, 1990.

King T: Clinical management of premature rupture of membranes. *J Nurse Midwifery* 39(suppl 2):81, 1994.

Knight DB et al: A randomized controlled trial for antepartum thyrotropin-releasing hormone and betamethasone in prevention of respiratory disease in preterm infants, *Am J Obstet Gynecol* 171(1):11, 1994.

Lowe TW: Hypovolemia during hemorrhage, *Clin Obstet Gynecol* 33(3):454, 1990.

Luke B: The changing pattern of multiple births in the United States: Maternal and infant characteristics, 1973 and 1990, *Obstet Gynecol* 84(1):101, 1994.

McDonald HM et al: Changes in vaginal flora during pregnancy and association with preterm birth, *J Infect Dis* 170:724, 1994.

McGregor JA et al: Prevention of premature birth by screening and treatment for common genital tract infections: results of a prospective controlled evaluation, *Am J Obstet Gynecol* 173(3):157, 1995.

*Mehta I, Young ID: Recurrence risks of common complications of pregnancy: a review, *Obstet Gynecol Surv* 42(4):218, 1987.

Mercer BM, Ramsey RD, Sibai BM: Prenatal screening for group B *Streptococcus,* *Am J Obstet Gynecol* 173(1):842, 1995.

Mittendorf R et al: Reducing the frequency of low birth weight in the United States, *Obstet Gynecol* 83(6):1057, 1994.

Mueller L: Second-trimester termination of pregnancy: nursing care, *J Obstet Gynecol Neonatal Nurs* 20(4):284, 1991.

Peppert JF, Donnenfeld AE: Oligohydramnios: a review, *Obstet Gynecol Rev* 46(6):325, 1991.

Peterson DF: Preterm labor: update on assessment and management, *J Emerg Nurs* 20(5):373, 1994.

Queenan JT, Hobbins JC: *Protocols for high risk pregnancy,* ed 3, Cambridge, Mass, 1996, Blackwell Science.

Ray D, Dyson D: Calcium channel blockers, *Clin Obstet Gynecol* 38(4):713, 1995.

Reece EA et al: *Handbook of medicine of the fetus and mother,* Philadelphia, 1995, JB Lippincott.

Repke JT et al, eds: *Intrapartum Obstetrics,* New York, 1996, Churchill Livingstone.

Richardon P: Body experience differences of women with preterm labor, *Maternal Child Nurs J* 24(1):5, 1996.

Ritter DC, deShazo RD: Peripartum complications, *Postgrad Med* 95(2):178, 1994.

Saftlas AF et al: National trends in the incidence of abruptio placentae, 1979-1987, *Obstet Gynecol* 78(6):1081, 1991.

Sala DJ, Moise KJ: The treatment of preterm labor using a portable subcutaneous terbutaline pump, *J Obstet Gynecol Neonatal Nurs* 19(2):108, 1990.

Santoso JY, Lin DW, Miller DS: Transfusion medicine in obstetrics and gynecology, *Obstet Gynecol Surv,* 50(6):470-481, 1995.

Shubert PJ: Atosiban, *Clin Obstet Gynecol* 38(4):722, 1995.

Spitz AM et al: Pregnancy, abortion and birth rates among US adolescents, *JAMA* 275:989, 1996.

Stock A: Ectopic pregnancy, *Clin Obstet Gynecol* 33(3):448, 1991.

Timor-Tritsch IE et al: Can a "snapshot" sagittal view by transvaginal ultrasonography predict active preterm labor? *Am J Obstet Gynecol* 174:990, 1996.

Vaccine side effects, adverse reactions, contraindications and precautions, *MMWR* 45(RR-12):1, 1996.

Ventura SJ et al: Final natality statistics: 1994, *Monthly Vital Statistics Report,* 44(11s):1, June 1996.

Wheeler DG: Preterm birth prevention, *J Nurse Midwifery* 39(suppl 2):66, 1994.

Zabielski MT: Recognition of maternal identity in preterm and fullterm mothers, *Maternal Child Nurs J* 22(1):2, 1994.

Zahn CM, Yeomans ER: Postpartum hemorrhage: placenta accreta, uterine inversion and puerperal hematomas, *Clin Obstet Gynecol* 33(3):422, 1991.

*Classic reference.

Student Resource Shelf

Eganhouse DJ: A nursing model for a community hospital preterm birth prevention program, *J Obstet Gynecol Neonatal Nurs* 23(9):756, 1994.
  A demonstration of a planned approach for nursing interventions to prevent preterm labor.
Harrison LK, Naylor KL: The laws that affect abortion in the United States and their impact on women's health, *Nurs Pract* 16(12):53, 1991.
  Review of Supreme Court rulings since 1973 with analysis of how they affect women's choices.

Maloni JA: Bed rest during pregnancy: implications for nursing, *J Obstet Gynecol Neonatal Nurs* 22(5):422, 1993.
  Details the adverse effects of bed rest on the physiology of the pregnant woman.
Nolan TE, Gallup DG: Massive transfusion: a current review, *Obstet Gynecol Surv* 46(5):289, 1991.
  Concise review of uses of blood components when massive hemorrhage occurs. Clarifies tests and reasons for using different blood fractions.

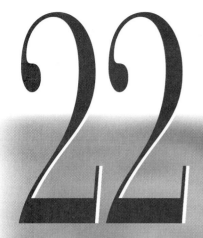

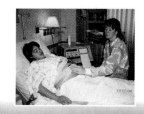

22 Hypertensive, Embolic, & Immune Problems *during* Pregnancy

Learning Objectives

- Apply steps of the nursing process to planning care for a pregnant woman with hypertensive, embolic, or immunologic complications.
- State strategies for identification and treatment of pregnancy-induced hypertension.
- Contrast normal hemodynamic changes of pregnancy with alterations caused by severe preeclampsia and pulmonary edema.
- Describe the various subtle signs of antiphospholipid syndrome and lupus erythematosus.
- Compare events of embolic disorders with normal increases in clotting activity during pregnancy.
- Identify health care instructions for a woman with pregnancy-induced hypertension, thromboembolic problems, and lupus erythematosus.

Key Terms

Adult Respiratory Distress Syndrome (ARDS)
Amnesia
Amniotic Fluid Embolism
Antiphospholipid Syndrome (APS)
Colloid Osmotic Pressure (COP)
Disseminated Intravascular Coagulation (DIC)
Eclampsia
Gestational Hypertension
HELLP Syndrome
Hemoconcentration
Papilledema
Photosensitivity
Platelet Aggregation
Preeclampsia
Pregnancy-Induced Hypertension (PIH)
Pulmonary Embolism
Scotoma
Thrombocytopenia
Thrombophlebitis

HYPERTENSIVE DISORDERS OF PREGNANCY

Approximately 23 million persons in the United States have hypertension, and many are not receiving treatment. Because a woman may seek health care for the first time as an adult when she becomes pregnant, if she is discovered to be hypertensive it is important to differentiate between chronic hypertension and **pregnancy-induced hypertension** (PIH). The reported incidence of *all* hypertensive disorders of pregnancy is 6% to 8% (ACOG, 1996). Hypertensive disease is responsible for 15% of maternal

deaths in the United States (Berg et al, 1996). Maternal hypertension greatly affects fetal well-being primarily because of placental insufficiency and potential premature birth.

Hypertension observed during pregnancy is divided into two categories:

1. Chronic hypertension, which predates the pregnancy or continues beyond 42 days postpartum
2. PIH, with onset of signs after the twentieth week of gestation and resolution before 42 days after birth (ACOG, 1996).

PIH is hypertension that first appears during pregnancy, usually after 20 weeks of gestation. It is a multi-organ disease process with several manifestations.

- **Preeclampsia** includes renal involvement and classic signs of hypertension, edema, and proteinuria. Classification of pregnancy-induced hypertensive states is shown in Box 22-1.
- **Eclampsia** occurs when cerebral involvement leads to seizures or coma.
- **HELLP syndrome** occurs when, in addition to hypertension, there are pathologic changes in the liver, platelets, and erythrocytes.

TEST *Yourself* **22-1** _____

Before going any further, recall the cardiovascular stresses experienced during pregnancy (see Chapter 9).
a. Vascular changes
b. Cardiac output changes
c. Pulse and blood pressure (BP) changes

Preeclampsia

The Greek word *eklampnis*, meaning "shining forth, or sudden development," refers to the sudden onset of the characteristic convulsion that distinguishes preeclampsia from eclampsia. Preeclampsia has a slow onset and is usually detected after the twentieth week of gestation when a slowly rising blood pressure (BP) is accompanied by renal involve-ment; preeclampsia is shown by signs of increasingly severe edema, proteinuria, or both. However, the processes that initiate preeclampsia *begin with implantation* and early placental development and may be detected by 8 to 12 weeks of gestation by the methods listed in the following pages.

Although the etiology for preeclampsia is unknown, for some women there may be genetic predisposition to an altered angiotensin response because of the *angiotensinogen T 235* gene. Women with this gene are 20 times more likely to develop preeclampsia than women without it (Ward et al, 1993). In addition, the renin-angiotensin-aldosterone system (RAAS) is altered from normal pregnancy functions. Renin and angiotensin I and angiotensin II are elevated during normal pregnancy. Angiotensin II stimulates release of aldosterone, which promotes the retention of sodium by the kidney so that there is an increase in plasma volume and extracellular volume. Together with renin, these substances act to maintain BP, fluid volume, and sodium balance. With preeclampsia, the levels of all the factors of the RAAS are significantly lower.

Finally, the reduced peripheral resistance in normal pregnancy allows increased perfusion to placenta and kidney and increased blood volume. Preeclampsia results when factors affecting the peripheral resistance do not allow the normal vasodilation of pregnancy.

Studies have also pinpointed prostaglandin *imbalance* as a primary factor in the increased vasoconstriction of preeclampsia. The first of these prostaglandins is *thromboxane* A_2 (TXA_2), a powerful vasoconstrictor that *stimu-*

▌ *Box* **22-1**   **Classification of Hypertensive States during Pregnancy**

I: PREGNANCY-INDUCED HYPERTENSION (PIH)
Preeclampsia: Hypertension with renal involvement, edema, and proteinuria.
Mild preeclampsia
BP > 140/90 mm Hg after 20 weeks' gestation or > 30/15 mm Hg elevation from the early or prepregnant baseline
Increase in mean arterial pressure (MAP) to more than 105 mm Hg
Mild edema, evidenced by weight gain > 2 lb/week
Proteinuria > 100 mg/L or +1
Severe preeclampsia or eclampsia
Oliguria; increasing proteinuria > 5 g in 24 hr or 3-4+; generalized edema; hypertension > 160/110 mm Hg scotoma; epigastric pain or onset of seizures or coma (no prior history of neurologic pathology)
HELLP syndrome
Hypertension with liver involvement, hemolysis, elevated liver enzymes, and low platelet count (< 100,000 μL)

II: PREEXISTING HYPERTENSION, CHRONIC
With or without renal disease
BP > 140/90 mm Hg before 20 weeks' gestation, persists more than 6 weeks after birth; pressures may rise to high levels
Gestational hypertension
Elevated BP occurring for the first time during pregnancy after 20 weeks but without proteinuria or edema
Usually resolves within 6 weeks of birth
Warns of future hypertension

III: CHRONIC HYPERTENSION WITH SUPERIMPOSED PREECLAMPSIA OR ECLAMPSIA

lates **platelet aggregation** (clumping that often causes thrombosis). Thromboxane is important in the normal processes of hemostasis.

The second important prostaglandin is *prostacyclin* (PGI$_2$), a potent *vasodilator* and an *inhibitor* of platelet aggregation. PGI$_2$ is produced in the blood vessel epithelium and in the renal cortex and should be present in higher amounts during pregnancy than in a nonpregnant state. It contributes to the general vasodilation that is normal during pregnancy. When an imbalance between thromboxane and prostacyclin develops, however, there is *progressive vasoconstriction* in the blood vessels instead of normal vasodilation, leading to hypertension and reduced circulation to the placenta and throughout the cardiovascular system. This imbalance appears to underlie PIH (Reece et al, 1995).

What is not known is the exact cause of the imbalance between these two prostaglandins. It is thought that a defect in placental development is involved wherein the muscular walls of the placental vessels *do not adequately dilate* to accommodate the normally rapid increase in placental blood volume. The pathophysiology is related to a defect in trophoblastic cells, which erode the spiral arteries of the placental bed (see Chapter 7). (This early development is necessary for uteroplacental circulation to *increase*.) As a result, the fragile blood vessel walls are progressively injured by the increased pressure of blood flow through constricted vessels. Platelets and fibrin are deposited and begin intrinsic processes that will inhibit normal prostacyclin. Secretion of TXA$_2$ occurs in increasing ratios and fosters further vasoconstriction.

This theory can partially explain the vasoconstriction that is seen in placental vessels and that leads to intrauterine growth retardation (IUGR), abruptio placentae, and a higher risk of fetal death during the pregnancies of hypertensive women (Tomada, 1996). In the *early phase,* there is gradually developing general vasoconstriction, but initially there is a normal plasma volume. Unless the woman is diagnosed early and responds to treatment, the disease process worsens. A *late phase* develops in which there is escalating hypertension, proteinuria, and a *reduced* plasma volume with **hemoconcentration**. Without intervention, the disease may progress to convulsions and coma (eclampsia). The only cure for preeclampsia is the birth of the infant. Thus a clinical decision must often be made concerning the benefit-risk issues of delivery of a very preterm infant versus worsening maternal disease. Delivery of the fetus and placenta mark the beginning of recovery from preeclampsia.

Risk related to pregnancy-induced hypertension

Preeclampsia is most likely to develop during pregnancy in those women who already have hypertension or diabetes or are obese, and in those who have a family history of hypertension or other complications of pregnancy such as multiple pregnancy, hydramnios, or hydatidiform mole. The risk for nulliparas, especially those younger than 14 or older than 35, is three times that of women in the middle young adult years (ACOG, 1996). The association of preeclampsia with poverty and protein malnutrition is recognized but not really explained. Although African-American women have a two to three times higher rate of chronic hypertension than do European-American women, the incidence of preeclampsia is similar between groups of women who do not have chronic hypertension (MMWR, 1995). The current incidence is 32 out of every 1000 births (Ventura, 1996). Women with chronic hypertension or renal disease have a high risk of superimposed preeclampsia, and certain women with the angiotensinogen gene T 235 have a 20 times greater risk of pregnancy-induced hypertension (see risk factors summarized in Box 22-2).

Because recognition and treatment of early preeclampsia have improved, the incidence of eclampsia has diminished during the last 20 years to less than 1 per every 2000 births (Saftlas, 1990). Although the incidence of eclampsia has been reduced with prenatal care, women with prenatal care may still have seizures if their health care providers delay administration of magnesium sulfate, the drug of choice for prevention of seizures (Perinatal Trial Service, 1995). Eclampsia also occurs in women who are chronically hypertensive but develop superimposed preeclampsia and in women with the hemolysis, elevated liver enzymes, and low platelet count (HELLP) variation of PIH.

Predicting pregnancy-induced hypertension. Doppler flow-velocity waveform measurement of the uteroplacental circulation or in the umbilical cord can demonstrate if there are pathologic changes in the placental circulation (see Chapter 11). *Lack of vasodilation* may be detected as early as 8 to 12 weeks, long before any evident signs appear (Tomada, 1996). However, Doppler flow studies are costly and not widely available. Tomada's research used the mean arterial pressure (MAP) and body mass index (BMI) (Chapter 10) at the first visit before the twelfth gestational week. If the MAP was more than 80 mm Hg, the BMI was over 23.6, and there was a family history of chronic hyper-

---

Box 22-2	**Risk Factors for Preeclampsia**

Nullipara
Age: Nullipara younger than 20 or over 35 to 40
Prior family history of pregnancy-induced hypertension (PIH)
Chronic hypertension, renal disease
Prior superimposed preeclampsia (70% recurrence)
Antiphospholipid syndrome, lupus erythematosus
Obstetric complications: hydatidiform mole, fetal hydrops
Multiple gestation
Angiotensinogen gene T 235
Diabetes, especially with vascular changes

From ACOG, 1996; Ferris, 1996.

tension or PIH, the woman was 3.7 to 4.2 times more likely to develop PIH. Thus women at risk could be selected for early intervention.

Signs

In PIH, the normal cardiovascular adjustments of pregnancy are altered in the following ways.

- Generalized vasospasm results in BPs rising above 140/90 mm Hg or a reading of 30/15 mm Hg over baseline. MAP rises above 105 mm Hg.
- Systemic vascular resistance is increased, including pulmonary vascular resistance.
- Cardiac output is *lower* than normal.
- Blood volume becomes *lower* than normal *as the disease progresses.*
- As a result, hematocrit readings related to the changes in blood volume rise, and there is hemoconcentration.

- Platelet counts may fall below 150,000/mm³.
- **Colloid osmotic pressure** (COP) is lowered, contributing to generalized edema and potentially to pulmonary edema.

Classic signs of hypertension, edema, and proteinuria are discussed in the following pages. See Figure 22-1 for the sequences in development of signs and symptoms of PIH.

Hypertension. In an adult, hypertension is a lasting elevation of BP to a level greater than 140/90 mm Hg. This arbitrary figure was based on a normal average BP of 110/75 and equals a 30/15 elevation. Because younger women may have a lower baseline, a change of more than 30 systolic and 15 diastolic points above the nonpregnant normal baseline reading may indicate hypertension during pregnancy. Young women usually enter pregnancy with a lower baseline reading, which should fall even further in the first trimester (by at least 5 systolic and 10 diastolic

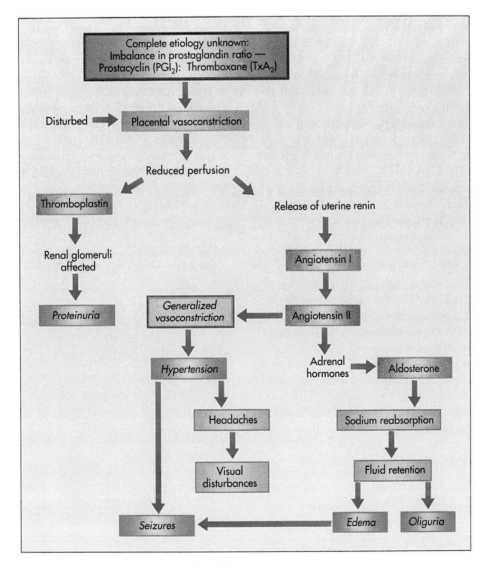

Figure 22-1   Cycle of responses in pregnancy-induced hypertension. (Data from Walsh SW: Preeclampsia: an imbalance in placental prostacyclin and thromboxane production, *Am J Obstet Gynecol* 150:335, 1985.)

points), so that the normal baseline before 20 weeks' gestation would be 103 (±11) systolic / 56 (±10) diastolic. Readings then gradually rise to reach levels at term of 110 (±12) / 69 (±9) (Ferris, 1996). (These changes are a result of normal vasodilation and the decreased systemic vascular resistance of pregnancy).

It may be that those women who will develop preeclampsia symptoms after the twentieth week of pregnancy do not show this significant first trimester drop in pressure. They demonstrate higher baselines early in pregnancy. However, Ferris (1996) also states that one third of chronically hypertensive women demonstrate what appears to be a normal reading in the second trimester. Remember, *a diastolic pressure above 80 in a young woman should always be investigated.*

Mean arterial pressure. MAP is a significant reading that identifies a rising diastolic pressure. A reading of 120/80 mm Hg equals a MAP of 93 mm Hg (the diastolic reading plus a third of the pulse pressure). Current studies show that a MAP of more than 90 in the *second trimester* warns of—but does not absolutely predict—a higher risk of preeclampsia and fetal growth retardation, related to reduced placental circulation (Ferris, 1996). A MAP of 105 mm Hg in the last trimester indicates PIH. The second and third trimester readings should be compared with the woman's earliest baseline (see Chapter 9).

Assessing blood pressure readings. Technically, BP elevation must be observed at two readings taken at least 6 hours apart. However, the woman cannot be kept in a clinic for this period of time. Therefore readings should be taken several times during each prenatal visit, allowing a 10-minute rest period after exercise, excitement, anxiety, or pain.

Readings taken in different positions are not comparable (Roberts, 1994). Therefore, the same position should be used and the position should be recorded. BPs are highest when the woman is supine or standing and lowest when in the lateral recumbent position. Using this position, the BP cuff should be on the upper arm (Working Group, 1990). The sitting position is best during ambulatory care; the arm should be supported at the level of the heart and the same arm used for each reading (Roberts, 1994).

The trend of the readings is observed. For example, a woman who normally has a BP of 100/65 mm Hg would demonstrate potential preeclamptic hypertension if her pressure increased to 130/80 or 135/85 mm Hg. The diastolic pressure is more significant because it reflects the cardiac resting phase. Since pregnant women have a lower diastolic reading, *both* Korotkoff's phase 4 (muffled) and phase 5 (disappeared) sounds should be recorded (Sibai et al, 1993; Working Group, 1990). The low fifth phase is thought to better indicate intraarterial pressure (ACOG, 1996).

Edema. Edema is a common occurrence during pregnancy. Moderate edema, especially in the lower extremities (dependent edema), is seen in 80% of normal pregnancies (Reece et al, 1995). Normal edema is related to the increase

TEST *Yourself* 22-2

Amy, a 17-year-old pregnant woman, comes to the clinic at 24 weeks' gestation with a BP of 128/78 mm Hg. What information does the nurse need to determine the significance of this reading? What is the MAP of this reading?

in femoral venous pressure caused by obstruction of the enlarging uterus and to the effects of gravity when the woman is in the upright position. Resting in bed in a lateral recumbent position relieves the collection of fluid in the interstitial spaces and causes diuresis to occur. Such physiologic edema develops *smoothly and slowly.*

The difference between normal *dependent edema* and abnormal *generalized edema* is important. With increasing kidney involvement and vasoconstriction, intravascular fluid may move into both the intracellular and interstitial spaces and is seen in the face, hands, and abdomen, unrelated to body position. In PIH, there may be *early-onset* or *late-onset* edema. The characteristic appearance is with *sudden onset* and a rapid weight gain of *more than 2 pounds per week.* In severe states, the woman often gains 5 or more pounds in a week.

Pitting edema is a sign of increasing generalized edema and can be demonstrated during assessment of the lower legs (Figure 22-2). When the examiner presses on the client's ankle or pretibial area for 15 seconds, pitting edema is present if the finger pad leaves an indentation in the tissue. Assessment of the degree of edema is summarized in Box 22-3.

Renal changes and proteinuria. Renal involvement is produced by vasoconstriction and edema of the endothelial cells so that glomeruli look enlarged and bloodless; a lesion called *glomerular capillary endotheliosis* develops. Fibrin is deposited, and the function of the glomeruli is affected.

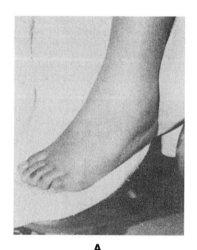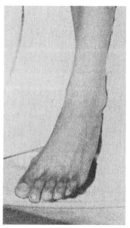

A   **B**

Figure 22-2   A, Marked pedal edema. **B,** Same foot and ankle after recovery from PIH.

Poor renal function allows protein to be spilled into the urine and leads to a decreased serum albumin level.

Renal ischemia and proteinuria of varying amounts correlate with the severity of renal involvement. Thus spilling of protein of 1+ or more (> 300 mg/L in 24 hours) is considered a sign of renal abnormality and requires treatment. The degree of proteinuria is more accurately determined by a 24-hour urine collection. A level of 3 to 5 g/L in 24 hours is considered very serious. The cycle worsens as protein is spilled into the urine; as the plasma COP decreases more fluid moves into the intracellular, spaces, including the brain, liver, and kidneys. Although proteinuria may be first recognized from results of a urine test strip, a clean-voided midstream specimen must be obtained to eliminate secretions from the vagina that could distort findings.

Because of the reduced flow to the kidneys, serum levels of blood urea nitrogen (BUN), uric acid, and creatinine become elevated. Sodium conservation is triggered, and urine output is further decreased (Blackburn and Loper, 1992). Sodium retention increases the woman's sensitivity to angiotensin II, reinforcing the pathologic cycle (see Figure 22-1 and Table 22-1).

For many years, retained sodium was considered the major cause of preeclampsia, and women were put on

---

Box 22-3	**Assessment of Edema**

- Minimal edema of lower extremities: +1
- Marked edema of lower extremities: +2
- Edema of lower extremities, face, and hands: +3
- Generalized massive edema, including the abdomen and face: +4

Table 22-1	**Signs and Symptoms of Preeclampsia and Eclampsia**

Mild	Severe
WEIGHT GAIN: EDEMA	
More than 1-2 lb/wk begins	Edema above waist in abdomen, fingers, face, extremities
No visible edema	Weight gain may be more than 5 lb/wk
HYPERTENSION	
30/15 mm Hg rise over baseline reading	Systolic pressure 160 mm Hg or greater; diastolic, 110 mm Hg
Increase in MAP ≥ 105	or greater
Feels some lethargy, fatigue	If preexisting hypertension, BP may be very high
May complain of headaches	Complains of lasting frontal headache unrelieved by analgesics
	Cerebral and visual disturbances, ringing in ears, fainting episodes
	Possible grand mal convulsion in sleep
	May experience amnesia up to 48 hours before convulsion
	Epigastric girdling pain, related to edema or hemorrhage in liver capsule (hemolysis, elevated liver enzymes, and low platelet count [HELLP])
	Hyperactive reflexes (clonus)
RENAL CHANGES	
Just a trace of proteinuria	Increased proteinuria +3, +4; 5 g/24 hr
Insignificant change in output	Oliguria: 500 to 600 ml or less in 24 hr (or > 30 ml for 2 hr)
	Begins as dark, scanty urine and progresses to severe oliguria, sometimes anuria
BLOOD CHANGES	
Some increase in plasma volume; not as much as normal.	Hct elevated because of hemoconcentration; plasma volume lowered
Platelets normal	Lower platelets <150,000/μL
Uric acid begins rising	Uric acid above 6 mg/dl, rising BUN level
CHANGES IN EYE	
Some retinal arteriolar spasm	Edema: papilledema, ischemia of retina

BUN, Blood urea nitrogen; *HELLP,* hemolysis, elevated liver enzymes, and low platelet count; *MAP,* mean arterial pressure.

rigid low-sodium diets. Now this regimen is considered to be *hazardous* to the mother because a low-sodium diet actually *stimulates* renin-angiotensin II output, whereas a less restricted sodium diet (2 g per day) and modified bed rest inhibit renin output (Ferris, 1996).

Signs of severe preeclampsia

If a woman's BP continues to rise in spite of interventions, severe preeclampsia is diagnosed when one or more of the following criteria appear (Dekker and Sibai, 1991; Ferris, 1996):

- Systolic BP >160 mm Hg or a diastolic BP >110 mm Hg on two occasions at least 6 hours apart when the client has maintained bed rest
- Proteinuria level of at least 5 g/24 hr or +3 or +4 by semiquantitative analysis with Tes-Tape or Clinistix
- Persistent temporal or occipital headache
- Hyperreflexia (Box 22-4)
- Cerebral or visual disturbances
- Epigastric pain
- Oliguria of less than 500 to 600 mL in 24 hours (25 mL/hr) (ACOG, 1996)

Abruptio placentae, disseminated intravascular coagulation (DIC), thrombocytopenia, pulmonary edema, congestive heart failure, cerebral hemorrhage, liver necrosis, or renal failure may also develop in a woman with severe preeclampsia.

A seemingly unrelated late sign in preeclampsia is right upper quadrant pain or tenderness. *Epigastric pain* is a result of severe edema of the liver capsule or hemorrhage into or necrosis of the liver. Because epigastric pain may be confused with symptoms of gastric illness, careful assessment is necessary.

Oliguria. Dark concentrated urine results from water and sodium retention with reduced renal output. Normal urine output of greater than 30 to 50 ml/hr is reduced and may lead to *oliguria* (<500 to 600 ml/24 hours) or to *anuria*, a lack of urine production. Oliguria is a late sign of severe PIH.

Other signs. **Thrombocytopenia** (platelet count <150,000/μL) occurs in 30% to 50% of women with severe preeclampsia. (See HELLP syndrome found later in this chapter for further discussion.)

Plasma volume reduction decreases renal perfusion and increases the risk of hypovolemic shock should hemorrhage occur.

Box 22-4   Deep Tendon Reflex Assessment Scale

- No response (abnormal): 0
- Diminished response (low normal): +1
- Average response (normal): +2
- Brisker than average response (high normal): +3
- Hyperactive (jerky or clonic) response: +4

Hyperreflexia develops as the brain tissue becomes more irritable because of vasoconstriction and edema. Reflexes become increasingly hyperactive (see Box 22-4). Deep tendon reflexes are assessed regularly during therapy. Hyperactive (jerky or clonic) responses of +3 to +4 indicate the potential for a seizure.

Amnesia occurs in the 48 hours before a seizure. The woman may appear vague and confused and will have no memory of recent events.

Scotomas are visual changes related to retinoarterial spasm and edema of the optic disk, which may include temporary loss of vision in one part of the eye (Figure 22-3). Spots, rings, or blurred vision accompanied by headache and aggravated by bright lights are also signals of severe vasoconstriction in the eyegrounds. Partial lower retinal detachment may occur in 10% of eclampsia cases and in 1% of preeclampsia cases (Seidman, Seir, Ben-Rafael, 1991). The scotoma resolves spontaneously in most cases, within 2 weeks of the birth.

Blindness is a rare symptom of eclampsia, caused either by thrombosis or detachment of the retina or by cortical involvement with hypodense areas in the occipital lobes. This event is also reversible as vasospasm and edema diminish with treatment. A scan by computed tomography (CT) can be diagnostic.

Eclampsia

Severe preeclampsia becomes *eclampsia* when grand mal seizures or coma occurs. The eclamptic convulsion is a result of cerebral edema and vasoconstriction and is an acute emergency that can result in hypoxia, acidosis, cerebral hemorrhage, or physical injury. Seizures can occur at any time after 20 weeks' gestation, before labor, during labor and birth, or within 14 days after birth (Miles et al, 1990). *Early-onset* seizures are those occurring before 48 hours after birth; *late-onset* seizures are those beginning after 48 hours postbirth until 14 days after birth. The HELLP syndrome is associated with 30% to 50% of late-onset cases.

Risk

Hypertension is one of the first three causes of maternal death. Forty percent of the deaths related to hypertensive causes during pregnancy are the result of eclampsia (Berg, et al, 1996). (See Figure 1-5 for comparison of mortality rates in the last two decades.) Those with early antepartal eclampsia before 28 weeks' gestation have the highest risk of maternal and fetal morbidity and mortality. Women with chronic hypertension combined with preeclampsia more often fall into this category.

Signs of eclampsia

The plasma COP decreases, and more fluid moves into the intracellular spaces, including the brain, liver, lungs, and kidneys. The cycle worsens as protein is spilled into the urine. Because of these fluid shifts out of the vascular compartment, there will be hemoconcentration.

Warning signs that a convulsion may occur are amnesia, epigastric pain, hyperreflexia, or clonus. Convulsions may occur during sleep, and unlike some types of seizures, they are not specifically triggered by light or noise. Eclamptic convulsions often begin with facial twitching. During the *tonic phase*, the woman arches her back, and muscles contract and stiffen. Her jaw closes tightly, sometimes injuring her tongue. Thoracic muscles contract tightly, and breathing stops temporarily. After 15 to 20 seconds, the *clonic phase* begins, during which the woman thrashes about; muscles alternately contract and relax. Cyanosis, sometimes apnea, continues through this phase, and incontinence of urine or feces may occur. A coma usually follows, which leads to another convulsion if it is not treated.

Hypoxia and acidosis may be present in both the woman and fetus for several hours after a seizure. Measures are taken to control BP, seizures, and hypoxia. Delivery should be postponed if possible until seizures are controlled and the woman is responsive.

The birth of the infant is the only *cure* for preeclampsia or eclampsia. Recovery begins with onset of *diuresis of greater than 100 ml/per hour for more than 2 hours*, but there remains a risk of seizure until proteinuria and BPs return to more normal readings.

HELLP Syndrome

A form of PIH occurs with little warning and often no "regular signs." **HELLP** stands for **H**emolysis, **E**levated **L**iver enzymes, and **L**ow **P**latelet count. This syndrome, which was first described in 1982, occurs in every geographic area. BPs may not be severely elevated and edema may not be noted, but proteinuria will be present and epigastric pain indicating liver involvement occurs in 90% of cases. A woman may seek help from an internist or the emergency department for the symptom of right upper quadrant pain. Because the diagnosis may be missed until a seizure occurs, it is important to look carefully at platelet counts and at liver enzyme levels, which may rise very high (Figure 22-4). Table 22-2 compares laboratory values found in preeclampsia, HELLP, and DIC states.

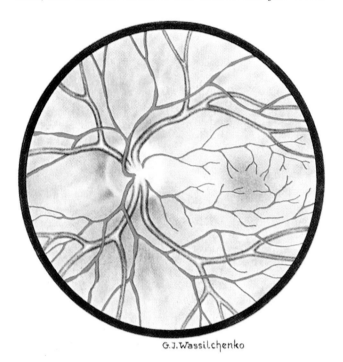

Figure 22-3 Funduscopic evidence of severe pregnancy-induced hypertension: arteriospasm, edema, hemorrhages, arteriovenous nicking, and exudates. (From Bobak IM: *Maternity and gynecologic care: the nurse and the family,* ed 5, St Louis, 1993, Mosby.)

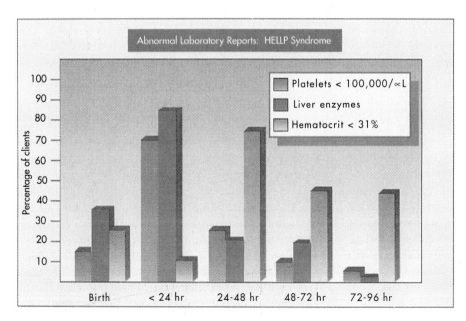

Figure 22-4 Liver enzyme levels. Percentage of clients with HELLP whose postpartum laboratory reports showed abnormal findings. Abnormalities tend to peak before 72 hours after birth—usually LDH/g > peak AST/g ALT. (Data from Catanzarite V: HELLP syndrome and its complications, *Contemp Ob Gyn* 36[12]:13, 1991.)

Table 22-2	**Comparison of Laboratory Values: Pregnancy-Induced Hypertension, HELLP, and Disseminated Intravascular Coagulation (Third Trimester)**			
Value	Normal	PIH (severe)	HELLP	DIC
Hb (g/dl)	11.5-13	Same	< 11 g/dl	Hemolysis
Hct	32%-40%	Elevated	< 32%	
Burr cell (schistocyte)	Absent	Possibly some	Possibly some	Present
Bilirubin				Elevated
PT (sec)	10.2-13.8	Slightly shorter	Same as PIH	Prolonged
PTT (sec)	40-60	Slightly shorter	Same as PIH	Prolonged
Platelets (per/μL)	200,000-400,000	< 150,000	As low as 30,000	< 150,000
Fibrinogen (mg/dl)	300-600	Same	Elevated	Decreased
Clotting time (min)	6-12	Same	Same	Varies
FSP	Absent	Absent	Usually absent	Always present
Creatinine (mg/dl)	0.4-1.3	Higher	Higher	Unchanged
BUN	< 11	> BUN	> BUN	Unchanged
Uric acid (mg/dl)	< 6	> 6	> 6	Unchanged
LDH (IU/dl)	Slight increase over nonpregnancy levels: 84-220	Same	> 500	Unchanged
Proteinuria	Negative	2+ to 4+	1+ to 4+	Negative
Serum albumin	Down 15%	Decreased		

BUN, Blood urea nitrogen; *FSP*, fibrin split products; *Hb*, hemoglobin; *Hct*, hematocrit; *LDH*, lactic dehydrogenase; *PT*, prothrombin time; *PTT*, partial thromboplastin time.

Risk

The HELLP syndrome may occur anytime after 28 weeks' gestation but it occurs more often just after birth, usually within 72 to 96 hours (Catanzarite, 1991). The rate of incidence is between 4% and 12% among women with PIH. There is a perinatal mortality rate as high as 37%. Until clear signs of improvement occur, the woman is at risk for **adult respiratory distress syndrome** (ARDS), seizures, liver hematoma, hepatic failure, renal failure, and death. Acute fatty liver of pregnancy may be confused with this syndrome. HELLP is managed in the same way as PIH.

Signs

Edema of the extremities often does not occur, and the first presenting sign is *right upper quadrant pain*. The differential diagnosis of HELLP depends on recognizing this as a variation of PIH. Laboratory studies of liver function and platelets will clarify diagnosis. Liver enzymes are greatly elevated in the classic ratios of LDH (lactic dehydrogenase) *higher than* >AST (aspartate aminotransferase [SGOT]) *higher than* >ALT (alanine aminotransferase [SGPT]). In severe cases, platelet levels fall lower than 50,000/mm³ (class I) or may be below 100,000/mm³ (class II). Platelets will be transfused if levels fall below 20,000/mm³ because of the danger of hemorrhage from many sites (see DIC).

Hematocrit (Hct) levels fall because of the micro-hemolytic process. A blood smear on a slide will show fractured, broken red blood cells (RBCs) that have been torn by forceful passage through tightly constricted vessels. These broken RBCs are called schistocytes, or *burr cells*. Once the RBCs are fractured, burr cells are removed from the system, causing an elevated serum bilirubin value (see Table 22-2). Clients with elevated serum bilirubin values are very ill and may have sudden seizures. Until platelet counts and liver enzymes return to normal, danger is present. The client developing HELLP may or may not have observable edema. There will be proteinuria and moderate hypertension.

CHRONIC HYPERTENSION

Chronic hypertension is always a secondary sign of a primary problem that may stem from other problems, such as renal disease, chronic stress, or lupus erythematosus (LE). Chronic hypertension exists when BP is greater than 140/90 mm Hg before pregnancy or before the twentieth week of gestation and persists more than 6 weeks after the birth. In this case, hypertension is not associated with pregnancy, but it may be aggravated by it. During pregnancy, some women develop mild hypertension *without* edema or proteinuria. This mild hypertension may be a "warning sign" for the development of hypertension later in life (formerly termed mild or **gestational hypertension**). Other women come to the pregnancy with an elevated pressure. If a woman has had untreated or poorly controlled chronic hypertension for several years, she may show signs of hypertensive vascular disease. Vascular changes such as arteriosclerosis, retinal hemorrhage, or renal disease may be present. Pregnancy is especially stressful for these women.

Risk

Women with preexisting hypertension are considered to have 10 times the risk for superimposed PIH (ACOG, 1996) and are monitored with close supervision throughout pregnancy. Extreme increases in systolic pressure may occur; thus the risk of cerebral vascular accident (CVA) is increased. There is also a higher incidence of developing adult-onset diabetes in this chronically hypertensive group (see Chapter 24 for the link between hypertension and diabetes).

Signs

Differential diagnosis is obtained by several tests. An ophthalmologic examination may reveal varying degrees of vascular sclerosis, hemorrhage, of **papilledema** (engorgement and swelling of the optic disk) (see Figure 22-3). Plasma urea nitrogen levels over 20 mg/dl and creatinine levels of more than 1 mg/dl indicate a chronic underlying renal problem. Systolic BP may soar above 160 mm Hg. Placental injury from such an elevated pressure leads to infarcts, with resulting poor circulation to the fetus causing growth restriction in the fetus. Finally, the damaged placenta may separate prematurely (abruptio placentae).

During pregnancy a woman with chronic hypertension continues her usual antihypertensive medication unless it has an adverse effect on the fetus. She may need to be hospitalized to gain control of the hypertension. See Drug Profile 22-2 for antihypertensives that are safe for use during pregnancy and during a hypertensive crisis. Each newborn infant must be evaluated for residual drug effects.

Chronic Hypertension with Superimposed Preeclampsia

Some form of preeclampsia develops in about 15 to 30% of women with chronic hypertension. Those with moderate to severe hypertension before pregnancy are in the most danger; the disease develops and moves to a crisis more rapidly than in other women. Increased risks of severe renal failure, abruptio placentae, and stillbirth are found in this group. Finally, preeclampsia tends to recur in about 30 to 40% of these women in a subsequent pregnancy.

Signs

In addition to a rise in systolic and diastolic BP over the usual readings, any of the classic signs of headache, fatigue, generalized edema, oliguria, and proteinuria indicate the onset of PIH. Hospitalization for careful monitoring and antihypertensive treatment to maintain a diastolic BP below 100 mm Hg is the only safe way to care for these women. Multiple nursing problems can arise during care of a woman who has severe hypertension with superimposed preeclampsia. Assessment often reveals alterations in many body systems. There may be self-care deficits, and the nurse should explore whether there were problems with medication compliance.

T E S T *Yourself* 22-3

a. Distinguish between the types of PIH in relation to signs and onset.
b. Compare signs of preeclampsia with signs related to chronic hypertension.

Clinical Management of Pregnancy-Induced Hypertension

Preventive therapy

Two preventive therapies are recommended for PIH. *Calcium* supplements during pregnancy can inhibit preterm birth and are now recommended for reducing the risk of preeclampsia (Bucher et al, 1996). Low zinc or magnesium levels also have been linked with the development of PIH, but there is no current recommendation for supplements.

Calcium supplementation. When calcium supplements are used, there has been a threefold reduction in preeclampsia in angiotensin-sensitive women (Ferris, 1996; ACOG, 1996). The rationale is that calcium may reduce vascular and uterine muscle tone; thus it is therapeutic for both hypertension and preterm labor (see Chapter 21). Daily doses of 2 g for pregnant adolescents and 1.5 g for adult pregnant women are recommended, in addition to the 1200 mg (1.2 g) that should be obtained in the diet (Bucher et al, 1996). Because of renal changes, women should also be observed for hypercalciuria and renal stones. Calcium carbonate offers the best absorption: Tums and Os-Cal are readily available over the counter (see Chapter 10).

Low-dose aspirin. *Aspirin* has been used since the mid-1980s for cardiovascular and thrombotic disease because of its antiprostaglandin effect, reducing platelet aggregation and inactivating TXA_2. Larger aspirin doses (1 to 2 g/24 hr) actively inhibit the clotting mechanism. Women have been warned against using these larger doses of aspirin because of potential fetal effects, maternal bleeding, and prolonged gestation and labor (Dekker and Sibai, 1993). However, *low-dose aspirin* (60 to 75 mg/24 hr) has been extensively studied for use in preventing PIH. The antiprostaglandin action of aspirin in these low doses appears to promote vasodilation and to slightly prolong pregnancy but has no effect on fetal bleeding or maternal clotting mechanisms. However, a slightly higher rate of abruptio placentae is noted in those receiving low-dose aspirin (Sibai, Caritas, Thom, 1993). Therefore, with the woman's informed consent, this low-dose therapy is currently used for women at risk of PIH (initial systolic pressures of 120 to 134 mm Hg, history of hypertension, PIH with last pregnancy, or multiple pregnancy) and not for every normotensive pregnant woman (ACOG, 1996).

Anticonvulsants: magnesium sulfate. In the United States, *magnesium sulfate* is the treatment of choice for PIH and the prevention of eclamptic convulsions. The magnesium ion provides a neuromuscular blockade at the myoneural junction by reducing acetylcholine release. Its parasympathetic effects on the vessel walls and on the flow of intracellular calcium cause peripheral vasodilation. Although there is only a small effect on the BP level, some reduction in smooth muscle tone increases blood flow to the placenta and in the brain. Because the frequency and intensity of labor contractions are decreased, it is also frequently used to block preterm labor (Gordon and Iams, 1995) (see Chapter 21).

Magnesium ion is excreted by the kidneys. Thus when there is generalized vasoconstriction and reduced urine output, *cumulative* doses may develop. These toxic doses result in hypotonia, loss of deep tendon reflexes, respiratory failure, and cardiac arrest. Dosage is planned to maintain a level between 4 and 7 mEq/dL (Box 22-5). Magnesium illustrates the small *window of effective concentration* (see Chapter 16) and the ease with which toxic levels may be reached.

Regulation of magnesium levels must be exact and is best achieved by intravenous (IV) infusion and by monitoring serum levels. Serum magnesium levels are drawn before the dose is ordered and at regular intervals. The *antidote* is kept at the bedside: 1 g (10 mL) of a 10% calcium gluconate solution, to be given by IV bolus over 2 minutes. Administration of a diuretic will also hasten magnesium excretion. If toxic levels occur, respiratory support may need to be provided with oxygen and, as necessary, with endotracheal intubation and cardiac monitoring.

At regular intervals, three standard observations are made and documented:

1. Determine the presence of the knee-jerk reflex response. Deep tendon reflexes are lost if magnesium levels rise above 10 mEq/dl (see Box 22-5).
2. Respiratory rate must remain above 12 breaths per minute (ACOG, 1996).
3. Urine output should exceed 25 ml/per hour through an indwelling catheter (ACOG, 1996).

Administration. The usual route is by continuous IV infusion (Drug Profile 22-1). First, a loading dose of 4 to 6 g in 250 ml D$_5$W is given as a bolus over 20 minutes. Then, 2 per hour is continuously infused by pump. The drug should be continued for at least 24 to 48 hours after

---

Box 22-5   **Magnesium Levels**

Normal: 1.8-2.5 mEq/dl
Therapeutic: 4.0-7.0 mEq/dl
Hyporeflexia, slurred speech, nausea, somnolence, double vision: 9.0-12.0 mEq/dl
Respiratory distress: > 12.0 mEq/dl
Cardiac arrest: > 15.0 mEq/dl
Antidote
10% calcium gluconate 10 mL IV over 2-3 min as a bolus

Box 22-1

DRUG PROFILE

Parenteral Magnesium Sulfate

ACTION
Blocks release of acetylcholine at neuromuscular junction, thus decreasing neuromuscular irritability, including vasomotor and uterine irritability. Causes slight peripheral vasodilation, reduces edema in the brain, and increases perfusion to brain and placenta. Not used in kidney impairment because it is excreted unchanged from kidney. Cumulative doses may occur if output is too low.

DOSAGE AND ROUTE
IV by infusion pump: Loading dose is 4 to 6 g in 250 D$_5$W or Ringer's lactate over 15 to 20 minutes.
Maintenance dose: To keep in therapeutic range must be 2 g/hr, regulated by titrating with client's responses of reflexes, output, respirations, and magnesium levels.

ANTIDOTE
10% calcium gluconate 10 mL; keep syringe and ampule at bedside.

SIDE EFFECTS AND ADVERSE EFFECTS
Sweating, warmth, flushing, and heavy feeling in limbs. May become lethargic and confused, with depressed reflexes and respirations. Nausea and vomiting.
Fetal effects: Decreased beat-to-beat variability and potential for tachycardia. Monitor newborn for magnesium levels, hypotonia, and hyporeflexia.

PRECAUTIONS
More difficult to obtain therapeutic levels in preterm labor than in PIH because kidney involvement in PIH reduces excretion. Monitor for respiratory rate under 12 breaths/min, urine output under 25 ml/hr, and depressed reflexes, and perform neurologic check every 4 hours. Assess for changes of headache, visual disturbances, and epigastric pain. Continue seizure precautions for PIH. Monitor contractions and fetal heart tones in both preterm labor and PIH.

birth or until a specified period after the diuresis of 100 mL/per hour has begun. (Diuresis indicates a reversal of the vasoconstrictive effects of PIH).

In settings where an IV pump is not available, the intramuscular (IM) route may be used. IM injections of a 50% solution into the gluteus medius are painful and rarely ordered in this country. (Sometimes 1 ml of 1% procaine is added to the solution if the client has no allergies.) The loading dose is 5 g (50% solution) in the right and left dorsogluteal areas and then 3 to 5 g every 4 hours depending on client response. There is a lag of 90 to 120 minutes before plasma levels are effective. This drug must be administered by Z-track injection, using a sufficiently long needle to place the solution well into the body of the muscle because a subcutaneous injection would cause edema and pain and possibly result in an abscess.

Effect on fetus and newborn. Magnesium crosses the placenta and may result in temporary loss of fetal heart variability. Cord blood levels will reflect magnesium levels of the mother. Thus if the woman had been on continuous infusion before the infant was born, the newborn may demonstrate signs of hypotonia, lethargy, and low Apgar scores related to reflexes and respirations. Magnesium is slowly excreted, and within 3 to 4 days the newborn should recover.

New studies indicate that magnesium has a significant benefit in *reducing the risk* of cerebral palsy and intraventricular hemorrhage in premature infants (Nelson and Grether, 1995). This is a valuable side effect to maternal treatment.

Phenytoin. When a seizure is imminent, *phenytoin* may be used, although studies suggest that magnesium sulfate is superior in preventing a convulsion (Gordon and Iams, 1995; Perinatal Trial Service, 1995). One regimen recommends a dose of 1 g by IV infusion over 20 min, diluted to give 10 to 12 mg/ml, and then a dose of 100 mg every 6 hours for 24 hours. The only side effects are transient burning at the IV site, mild euphoria, dizziness, nystagmus, and a mild decrease in BP (Miles et al, 1990; Perinatal Trial Service, 1995). The newborn may have transient hypotonia.

Antihypertensives. Opinions differ on the use of antihypertensives for the treatment of preeclampsia, since the mechanism of action must not affect fetal perfusion. The usual approach is to delay their introduction unless the diastolic BP rises above 110 mm Hg or the systolic BP, above 180 mm Hg (ACOG, 1996).

Hydralazine (Apresoline). Hydralazine is safe in pregnancy because it acts directly to relax arteriolar smooth muscle. A decrease in peripheral resistance brings about a reflex increase in cardiac output and better perfusion of the placenta. To maintain adequate blood flow to the placenta, the diastolic BP should not drop *below* 90 to 100 mm Hg after it has been elevated above this level.

Although the drug has no direct action on the heart, it may cause reflex tachycardia, increased stroke volume, and cardiac output to occur. Side effects include flushing, headache, dizziness, and cardiac irregularities. Given IV as a 5- to 10-mg bolus as often as every 20 minutes, doses should not exceed 40 mg/day (Drug Profile 22-2). Because antihypertensive drugs must be titrated with BP responses, IV use always includes fetal and maternal continuous monitoring.

Labetalol. In a hypertensive emergency, Labetalol 20 mg may be given IV every 10 minutes to a maximum of 300 mg, either as a bolus or continuous infusion. After the BP is stabilized, the woman's condition may be controlled with oral doses of this mixed alpha- and beta-blocker.

Nifedipine. A calcium channel blocker acts as an antihypertensive by relaxing smooth vascular muscle and also inhibiting uterine contractions (see Drug Profile 21-1). Nifedipine is used successfully during the second half of pregnancy to treat chronic hypertension (10 to 20 mg three times a day after meals) and may be used in an acute hypertensive episode. In an acute episode, the dose is one 5- to 10-mg capsule, bitten into and retained sublingually. The dose may be repeated every 30 minutes to a total of 180 mg per every 24 hours (Gonik and Bobrowski, 1996).

Nursing Responsibilities

Chronic hypertension

Multiple nursing problems may arise in the care of a woman with chronic hypertension. Assessment often reveals alterations in many body systems, as well as knowledge and self-care deficits. Problems with compliance must also be explored. Chronic hypertension is often related to life stress, obesity, smoking, and poor nutrition.

Any woman with preexisting hypertension is encouraged to have *preconception* counseling. A full assessment of her condition can be done, and the potentially harmful effects of antihypertensive drugs can be discussed. After rigorous testing, the woman will be classified as either high or low risk for pregnancy. If high risk, she will be hospitalized as necessary during the pregnancy for regulation of her pressures to keep the diastolic BP between 90 and 100 mm Hg. If low risk, she may be followed on an outpatient basis (see home care management). She will be seen every 2 weeks in outpatient follow-up until 28 weeks and then weekly until the time of labor.

The woman should be on a 2 g sodium diet and receive calcium supplementation and nutritional counseling. The high-risk woman also receives fetal evaluation as early as 28 weeks. Daily fetal movement counts and a regular biophysical profile (BPP) are used to determine fetal status. Antihypertensive medication is chosen for maternal and fetal safety. Diuretics are not routinely used, but may be necessary in severe hypertension. Early warning signs of

Box **22-2**

DRUG PROFILE

Acute Antihypertensive Therapy

Drug	Action	Dose	Maximum Dose	Adverse Reaction	Time to Effect
Hydralazine	Direct vasodilator	Initial: 5 mg IVP Repeat: 5-10 mg q20min	40 mg	Tachycardia, nausea, headache	20 min
Labetalol	Alpha-1 and beta blocker	Initial: 20 mg IVP Repeat: 40-80 mg q10min	300 mg	Postural hypotension	10 min
Nifedipine	Calcium channel blocker	Initial: 10 mg SL Repeat: 10 mg SL 30 min after initial dose	180 mg/day	Hypotension when given with $MgSO_4$	10-20 min
Nitroglycerin	Venous dilator at low dose	Initial: 5 µg/min, continuous infusion	Undetermined	Methemoglobinemia at > 7 µg/kg/min	3-5 min
	Arterial dilator at high dose	Increase: Double dose q3-5min			
Nitroprusside	Venous dilator	Initial: 0.25 µg/kg/min Increase: 0.25 µg/kg/min q5min	10 µg/kg/min	Cyanide toxicity, methemoglobinemia	1-5 min

IVP, Intravenous push; *SL,* sublingual. From Gonik B, Bobrowski RA: *Medical complications in labor and delivery,* Cambridge, Mass, 1996, Blackwell

superimposed PIH are taught to the client. Laboratory testing includes testing the values of 24-hour urinary protein and sodium, serum creatinine, uric acid, creatinine clearance, and Hct (Reece, 1995).

If the chronic hypertensive woman remains free of PIH and maintains a stable BP, she has a normal chance of a healthy outcome to the pregnancy. Those who develop superimposed PIH are at very high risk for fetal demise and maternal morbidity.

Pregnancy-induced hypertension. Because the development of PIH during pregnancy is gradual, much has been written about early detection. However, PIH is difficult to predict. Refer to the section on predicting PIH and note that a family or personal history of hypertension, combined with an increased BMI, a higher than normal hematocrit level, and a less than expected fall in diastolic BP in the first half of pregnancy, should alert the caregiver to a potential for PIH. The woman should understand the importance of following rest, diet, and fluid instructions. Cigarette smoking must be strongly discouraged because it promotes vasoconstriction.

ASSESSMENT

Admission BP is compared with the earliest available baseline pressure, and the MAP is calculated. Urinalysis indicates the severity of proteinuria. Assess for reflex response and edema, plus any of the warning signs of progressive PIH.

Often the woman with preeclampsia manifests several of the overt signs. More subtle changes will be established by laboratory evaluations in cases of chronic renal disease, HELLP, and LE-induced hypertension.

NURSING DIAGNOSES

Mild pregnancy-induced hypertension

- Knowledge deficit, related to preventive care, stress reduction, and smoking
- Knowledge deficit, related to self-care measures and treatment modalities
- Alteration in nutritional and fluid requirements, related to hypertension during pregnancy
- Alteration in activity level, related to hypertensive requirements
- Anxiety, related to potential for maternal and fetal morbidity

Severe pregnancy-induced hypertension

Additional nursing diagnoses will be needed as the status changes:

- Altered tissue perfusion related to generalized vaso-spasm; potential for reduced fetal perfusion and growth restriction
- Altered fluid volume in vascular compartment related to shift to interstitial tissue or renal involvement
- High risk for injury caused by seizures, acidosis, hypoxia, and potential for thrombosis
- Fear related to risk of maternal or fetal compromise

EXPECTED OUTCOMES

- Verbalizes self-care activity to reduce risk of preterm labor or increasing BP
- Alters nutrition, fluid intake, and smoking to prescribed levels
- Adjusts activities of daily living to prescribed level of activity
- Able to verbalize feelings of apprehension relative to current status and future outcomes

Severe pregnancy-induced hypertension

- Maternal or fetal injury does not occur; perfusion to vital organs and fetus is maintained.
- Biophysical parameters remain stable.
- Safety related to adequate oxygenation and airway clearance is maintained.
- Woman and family know reasons for interventions.

NURSING INTERVENTION

Prenatal care for early preeclampsia or mild chronic hypertension involves assessment to detect early signs of worsening hypertension. Clinic care includes instruction in self-care related to symptoms, weight, diet, and calcium intake. The nurse should telephone any client who skips an appointment and should question her regarding signs of PIH, or a home visit should promptly be scheduled if a client does not return to a clinic after showing signs of preeclampsia. Conservative management involves modified bed rest in the lateral position to promote renal excretion. The woman may be placed on low-dose aspirin and may be given calcium supplements.

Provide the client with a weight guideline and involve her in identifying signs of problems; compare daily weights with previous measurements. Nutrition assessment may determine if the client's weight is related to intake or edema. It is difficult to gain more than 2 pounds per week through nutrition alone. Nutritional guidelines include a high protein diet of 60 to 70 g per day and increased fluid intake up to 3000 mL per day. The client should use a nutritional analysis to detect deficiencies in the diet (Chapter 10). Calcium intake through the diet should meet the 1200 gm requirement, and an additional 1.5 to 2 g of oral calcium will be recommended. The *warning signals* found in Box 22-6, which are noted as part of the assessment process at each prenatal visit, should be taught to every client.

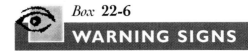

Box 22-6

WARNING SIGNS

Pregnancy-Induced Hypertension

- Visual disturbances (blurred vision or spots before eyes)
- Dizziness
- Persistent frontal or occipital headache
- Edema in face, hands, or legs on arising from sleep
- Changes in urine color and consistency and a reduction in volume
- Nausea, vomiting, or right upper quadrant epigastric pain
- Decreased or absent fetal movements
- Signs and symptoms of preterm labor (see Chapter 21)

Home care management. Increasingly, clients with mild gestational hypertension or PIH are being managed at home. In a number of trial cases, the outcomes have been similar to those for hospitalization, but it is easier and less costly for the woman to stay at home (Helewa et al, 1993; Barton, Stanziano, Sibai, 1994). To be considered for home care, the client must be willing to follow the care guidelines and to transmit results to the physician or nurse clinician.

- Electronic BP measurements 2 to 4 times daily, using same arm and position
- Daily morning weight
- Daily fetal movement count; biweekly or weekly clinic visits for uterine and nonstress fetal monitoring after 28 to 32 weeks
- Daily urine dipstick for protein on first voided midstream urine, and weekly 24-hour urine sample for protein (Simpson, 1995)

There may be home visits and daily phone contact by the home care provider to assess compliance, review signs and symptoms, and observe for escalation of PIH. (See Chapter 21 for home monitoring of fetal heart and contractions.)

The issue of bed rest. As discussed in Chapter 21, bed rest during pregnancy has both risks and benefits. Periods of modified bed rest in a lateral position are often recommended in mild hypertension. Complete bed rest is currently questioned because of its potential side effects. Maloni (1993) summarizes these as muscle atrophy, failure to gain weight at recommended rates, and general cardiovascular deconditioning. There is also increased risk of thromboembolic problems, bone demineralization, and calcium depletion. In addition, separation from the family results in isolation and depressed feelings (Maloni, 1993); there is increased stress on the family and postpartum recovery is prolonged (Goldberg et al, 1994).

By following these home care instructions and by assessing at frequent prenatal visits, it may be possible to prevent the woman's condition from progressing to the more severe phase. If her condition does not resolve and PIH signs continue or worsen, hospitalization will be necessary.

Care for severe pregnancy-induced hypertension. When a hypertensive crisis occurs, the entire health team works together rapidly to manage the life-threatening aspects of illness. Upon admission of a woman with severe PIH, physical assessment will detect degrees of edema, proteinuria, and deep tendon reflex status. Query the client regarding visual changes, headache, fatigue, and apprehension. Note the woman's level of consciousness and her recall of past events, and also query family members about changes noted in the last few days. Levels of consciousness should be regularly assessed because the client can slip into a coma without a convulsion. A rapidly rising BP, decreasing urinary output, and increasing amounts of albumin in the urine are alarming signs of deterioration. Vital signs should be assessed by monitors, and the MAP requires careful watching by this means. If no electronic BP monitor is available, check BP every 15 minutes and temperature, pulse, and respirations every hour. Continuous monitoring of uterine contractions and fetal heart rate is performed to detect late decelerations, changes in baseline variability, and other signs of distress.

Intake and output. A Foley catheter will be inserted, attached to a urimeter for measurement of hourly output. Protein levels are also checked every hour. All IVs are regulated by an IV pump. To avoid overload, the volume of solutions with antibiotics or antihypertensives and main-line IV fluid volume are added together for a *total volume of 125 ml per hour.*

When laboratory reports indicate hypovolemia, a one-time bolus of 250 to 500 ml isotonic fluid infused rapidly may relieve the hypovolemia and increase urine output. Precautions must be followed carefully, and the BP, pulse, respiratory rate, and breath sounds are assessed frequently in case pulmonary edema is precipitated.

Magnesium sulfate is initiated, and the client may receive additional anticonvulsants or antihypertensives. Hourly assessments of reflexes, respirations, and output give an indication of whether the serum concentration is in the therapeutic range. The physician is notified of adverse responses. Potassium depletion is also checked. Magnesium sulfate will be continued for 24 to 48 hours after birth, until diuresis begins. In the postdelivery period, ergot medications (ergotamine, methylergonovine [Methergine]) are contraindicated because these act as vasoconstrictors.

Protection from hazards. This is important because the woman may have a convulsion during sleep. Pad the sides of the bed rails. During a seizure the chance of biting the tongue is possible. If there is an opportunity, an airway should be inserted; both the airway and a padded tongue blade are kept at the bedside. Suction and oxygen must also be available in the room.

If the woman is not already in the left-lateral position when the convulsion occurs, she should be positioned promptly to promote circulation to the placenta and to provide for drainage of oral mucus. The airway must be suctioned to clear away mucus. If not already in place, oxygen is begun by mask. Fetal status is monitored closely.

The woman's status is frequently assessed for circulatory or renal failure and for signs of cerebral hemorrhage. She is also observed for signs of abruptio placentae, as evidenced by uterine rigidity, decreased fetal heart rate, and, at times, vaginal bleeding. The possibility of DIC exists (see later discussion). *Labor may begin during a convulsion.* In these cases, it usually progresses rapidly to a precipitate delivery, often with excessive bleeding.

Hemodynamic monitoring. In some cases, *central venous pressure* (CVP) measurements are needed to measure pressures on the right side of the heart, *preload* (see Figure 23-1). In serious cases, the use of a triple pulmonary artery catheter (PAC) or quadruple lumen line (Swan-Ganz catheter) is recommended to continuously measure CVP and *pulmonary artery* (PA) pressures. *Pulmonary capillary wedge pressures* (PCWP) and *cardiac output* (CO) may also be measured to ascertain cardiac function. Systolic BP indicates the *afterload* (see Table 23-1). Because the client requires intensive care, a one-to-one nursing ratio is mandatory (ACOG, 1996). (See discussions on pulmonary edema, DIC, and stroke as additional complications found later in this chapter.)

 Box **22-1**

CLINICAL DECISION

Ms. Jones is hospitalized for severe preeclampsia. Magnesium sulfate is begun. Four hours after the loading dose, her assessment shows the following: tendon reflexes +2, BP 150/100 mm Hg, fetal heart rate 144 beats/min, respirations 10 breaths/min, and urine output 40 ml in the last 2 hours. Choose the appropriate initial action(s).

Family support. The family will be very anxious about the client. The woman with threatened seizures will not remember events from before the convulsion or for several hours after. Her family will be frightened and will need a careful explanation of what is happening. It is critical to reduce anxiety and anger in the family so that they will feel that every possible measure is being taken. Therefore bedside visits are important; encourage the family to talk with the woman so that she is also comforted.

Recovery. The time of birth will depend on the woman's condition and the presence of fetal distress. Emergency cesarean delivery may be instituted. Recovery may be very rapid, with the BP returning to moderate levels within 48 hours. The mother is cared for in the labor recovery area or in an intensive care unit until she is out of danger. After the birth, severely affected clients are not out of danger until at least 2 hours of diuresis take place (>100 ml per hour), showing that the edema and vasoconstriction in the brain and kidney have begun to improve (see Nursing Care Plan).

EVALUATION

- Was she able to follow prescriptions for activities of daily living (ADL), diet, and rest?
- Did personal and community resources allow her to cope with limitations?
- Did she verbalize understanding of instructions for self-care and recovery care and report findings to health care personnel?
- Were maternal and fetal perfusion maintained with good outcomes?
- Were client and family members kept informed of progress and clinical management decisions?

RESEARCH

PURPOSE OF STUDY
To determine if maternal hypertension is related to pregnancy complications among African-American and other women in the United States.

REVIEW OF LITERATURE
Hypertension is a common complication of pregnancy and a major cause of maternal-fetal morbidity and mortality. The etiology of maternal hypertension is unknown. Some studies cite a higher incidence among African-Americans than among any other ethnic group. Hypertension during pregnancy is associated with intrauterine growth retardation, preterm delivery, and antepartum hemorrhage.

FINDINGS AND IMPLICATIONS FOR PRACTICE
Medical records from a national hospital discharge data bank were surveyed, and findings indicated that the rates of pregnancy-induced hypertension (PIH) did not vary significantly by ethnicity. Higher rates of PIH were identified in those women who had a history of prepregnancy hypertension. Age was also a significant factor, with higher PIH rates among women aged 15 to 19 years and 40 to 49 years.
Prepregnancy screening is essential to identify women at risk for PIH. Prenatal management and education interventions may decrease the risk of intrapartal complications

Samadi A, Mayberry R: Maternal hypertension and associated pregnancy complications among African-Americans and other women in the United States, *Obstet Gynecol* 87(4):557, 1996.

DISSEMINATED INTRAVASCULAR COAGULATION

The coagulation system involves factors that assist in blood clotting and those that affect breakdown, or *lysis*, of a clot. **Disseminated intravascular coagulation** (DIC) is a condition in which the coagulation sequence is activated by injury to the epithelium, or by bacterial particles or other foreign material. Events related to pregnancy that may trigger DIC are sepsis, intrauterine fetal death, hemorrhage, and partial abruptio placentae with a retained clot, amniotic fluid embolism, and preeclampsia. DIC may develop as a chronic low-level condition, or it may cause life-threatening hemorrhage and organ damage (Figure 22-5). Other terms sometimes used to describe this condition include *consumptive coagulopathy* and *defibrination syndrome*.

The pregnant woman is already in a hypercoagulable state during the later part of pregnancy. Should any of the above conditions exist, additional microemboli occur in the small vessels. The intrinsic and extrinsic pathways are activated. The intrinsic factors exist within the vascular system and respond to vessel damage. The extrinsic factors are within body tissue and respond to tissue trauma (Gilbert and Harmon, 1993). Through multiple steps and factors, the clotting cascade begins. Fibrinogen is released and converted into fibrin in the extrinsic pathway. Calcium is key in the process of converting prothrombin to thrombin as clots form. Platelets play an important role in hemostasis. As platelets *aggregate* (clump and adhere to exposed and damaged epithelium), the clot enlarges. Platelets are consumed and their levels fall.

The blood vessels also secrete various substances needed for coagulation and anticoagulation. These anticoagulation factors include plasminogen, which is integrated into the fibrin mass and is converted to plasmin. Plasmin will then produce *fibrinolysis* (clot breakdown). A number of other substances work together to dissolve the clots. Especially important are fibrin degradation products (FDPs) and fibrin split products (FSPs), which are produced to reduce platelet aggregation (Perry and Martin, 1992). FSPs have anticoagulation effects and exacerbate bleeding.

The DIC process begins with a trigger cause and may exist as a low-level chronic condition for a period of time, or it may escalate suddenly. Signs begin when the liver cannot compensate for the increased consumption of clotting factors. Therefore fibrin and platelet consumption occur at the same time as rapid fibrolysis, which further depletes coagulation factors.

Preeclampsia carries a major risk of triggering DIC because of microinjuries to the epithelium of blood vessels in the placenta related to the processes discussed earlier. Investigators note that fibrin and platelet thrombi have been found in numerous organs of preeclamptic patients, including liver, brain, adrenals, lungs, heart, spleen, and kidneys (Perry and Martin, 1992). This multiorgan effect is

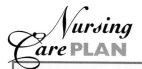

Nursing Care PLAN | *Pregnancy-Induced Hypertension*

CASE

Karen, age 16, single, para 0000, first visited the clinic at 24 weeks' gestation; she had a BP 120/76 mm Hg and her weight was 115 pounds. She was counseled on nutrition, given instructions to take calcium 2 g PO two times a day and a list of warning signs, and she was asked to return in 2 weeks. However, she made the next visit at 32 weeks; she stated that she had skipped coming because of headaches and feeling tired and "blue." Her weight gain in the last 8 weeks has been 17 pounds; currently she has BP 138/94 mm Hg, 2+ edema, and 2+ proteinuria.

Social History: Her family support is moderate, with no support from the father of the child. She seems unaffected by the diagnosis and is resistant to being admitted to the labor area for intensive monitoring and treatment.

Assessment

1. Single adolescent primigravida with unknown onset of hypertension. MAP is 108.
2. Weight gain of more than 2 pounds per week.
3. Complains of headaches, fatigue, and "down" mood.
4. Verbalizes no need for assistance; appears frightened of hospitalization.
5. Demonstrates lack of knowledge of condition and the implications of it.

Nursing Diagnoses

1. Fluid volume excess, edema related to sodium and water retention
2. Injury, risk for, related to seizure activity, hypoxia, fetal distress
3. Fear, related to potential for injury to self and fetus and to unknown hospitalization events
4. Knowledge deficit, related to signs, interventions for PIH, self-care
5. Potential noncompliance with therapies, related to developmental age, anxiety

Expected Outcomes

1. Returns to weight gain at normal pace with control of BP by therapy.
2. Suffers no injury resulting from central nervous system involvement.
3. Verbalizes fears to primary nurse or physician regarding complications and treatments.
4. States signs and symptoms that indicate need for interventions.
5. Actively participates in decisions about treatments and follows therapy guidelines.

Nursing Interventions

1. Monitor daily weight, vital signs, and fetal responses every 4 hours. Monitor intake and output. Assess location and degree of edema. Monitor urine for proteinuria every 4 hours. Maintain modified bed rest in side-lying position.
2. Monitor for neurologic changes, and assess level of consciousness every 4 to 8 hours. Administer magnesium sulfate as ordered, and monitor magnesium levels by respirations, output, and reflexes. Institute seizure precautions as per order.
3. Acknowledge validity of Karen's feelings; assign a primary nurse to establish rapport. Provide emotional support, and involve family members in increasing support.
4. Provide Karen with accurate information about treatments and procedures. Involve her in self-care activities to gain a measure of control over events.
5. Discuss with Karen and family the decisions that must be made; give choices where possible. Arrange for counseling if necessary or requested.

Evaluation

1. Did weight gain return to normal pattern? Did vital signs return to normal ranges?
2. Were neurologic changes (including seizures) experienced?
3. Did Karen verbalize feelings of fear for herself and infant? Did supplying support and information help reduce fears?
4. Did she state acceptance of therapies necessary to control PIH?
5. Did she actively participate in care?
6. Was the fetus developing normally for gestational age?

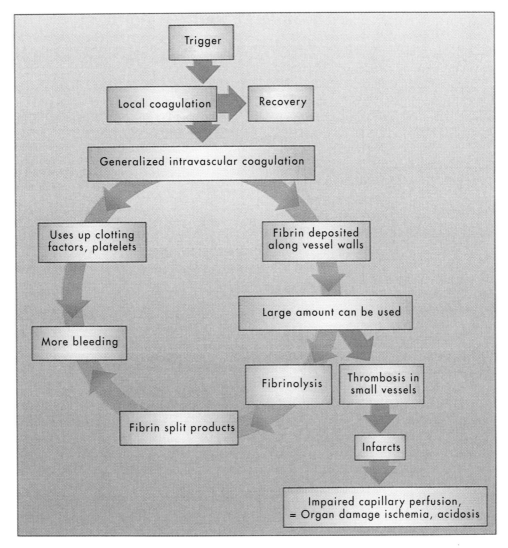

Figure 22-5 Mechanisms of disseminated intravascular coagulation can escalate into a vicious cycle.

 Box **22-7**

WARNING SIGNS

Disseminated Intravascular Coagulation

- Oozing at venipuncture site, or mucous membranes of mouth or nose
- Hematoma enlarging or wound drainage increasing
- Bruising under BP cuff
- Hematuria or oliguria or both, related to renal infarcts or microemboli
- Pain at site of organ infarcts from emboli
- Adult respiratory distress syndrome (ARDS) from thrombosis in lung capillaries
- Acute fatty liver of pregnancy (AFLP) with liver failure

observed in preeclampsia in response to endothelial injury in the placenta related to severe vasospasm. The microemboli may cause ischemia in these organs, causing a reduction in fibrinogen and platelets and an increase in FSPs.

Signs

The chief characteristic of DIC is that its signs vary widely. DIC may first be identified when a tube of blood fails to clot or *oozing* occurs at a venipuncture site or *bruising* occurs after a BP cuff has been used. There may be multiple petechiae, ecchymosis, and purpura. There may be bleeding into the gastrointestinal tract, vagina, and all mucous membranes, as well as the presence of hematuria. If DIC begins during or after the birth, hemorrhage may be difficult to control (Box 22-7).

Laboratory evaluation will reveal fractured (broken) RBCs called *Burr's cells*, or schistocytes, which result from RBCs passing through vasoconstricted vessels. These broken cells are removed from the circulation. There will be elevated FSPs, increased partial thromboplastin time (PTT) and prothrombin time (PT), and decreased fibrinogen levels. (See Table 22-2, which compares variations found in PIH, DIC, and HELLP syndrome). If blood coagulation is questioned, the following screening tests are performed: bleeding time, clotting time, PT (factors II, V, VII, X), and PTT (all factors except VII and XIII) (Ives, 1996).

Clinical management

Because the major effect of DIC in pregnancy is uncontrolled bleeding, the source of hemorrhage must be assessed for possible repair. The following priorities must be followed.

- Correct trigger cause if possible.
- Maintain central blood volume.
- Replace deficiencies (see Chapter 21).
- Support body system functions.

When DIC is diagnosed, it is possible that the fetus must be delivered, depending on the stage of the pregnancy. This cannot be done until the threat of hemorrhage is reversed by factor replacement with platelets, by plasma exchange with fresh frozen plasma, and by packed RBCs (see hemorrhage in Chapter 21). Low-dose heparin is sometimes given to reverse the hypercoagulability (Clark et al, 1994). Supportive care includes all interventions for impending shock—cardiac and fetal monitoring, careful regulation of intake and output, hemodynamic monitoring, warmth, and correction of the cause.

Nursing responsibilities

The nurse should be aware of risk factors for DIC and alert to presenting signs. Carefully following lab reports may give an early warning of a changing condition. When overt signs begin, there is a high risk for fetal or maternal demise, and the client must have intensive care with one-to-one nursing. Fetal perfusion is important and is promoted by a side-lying position and oxygen by mask. Administer blood products. Observe for hypervolemia, maintaining strict hourly intake and output. Monitor breath sounds for pulmonary edema and perform all preeclampsia checks. Invasive hemodynamic monitoring may be instituted.

Bruising may be aggravated by skin pressure during turning or during activities. The BP cuff should be quickly inflated to only 20 mm Hg above expected systolic pressure. Observe for bruising under cuff. Check for skin breakdown, and avoid using a harsh toothbrush on potentially bleeding gums. Finally, support the family during this time of intense concern about the client and her infant. With aggressive support, recovery takes 2 to 7 days as the liver returns to normal function.

Box **22-2**

CLINICAL DECISION

Mary had a lengthy labor, which included amnionitis and finally a cesarean delivery. She returned to the recovery room with a Foley catheter in place, O_2 by nasal catheter, and IV fluids with oxytocin. On her admission, urine was clear. An hour later, you note hematuria and, in checking her skin under the BP cuff, you find bruising. Including further assessment, what actions should you now take?

THROMBOEMBOLIC DISEASE: ANTIPHOSPHOLIPID SYNDROME

Autoimmune antibodies were first described only 40 years ago. **Antiphospholipid syndrome** (APS) and its partner, *lupus anticoagulant* (LA), are related to recurrent spontaneous abortion, IUGR, and severe PIH. This is an abnormal immune response. Normally, antibodies are formed against "nonself" foreign proteins by means of B and T lymphocytes. When activated, B cells produce an antibody substance that will bind to a specific antigen to form an *immune complex*. This complex is then eliminated from the body by means of a substance called *complement* (Figure 22-6).

In the APS syndrome, immune complexes, after interacting with complement proteins, are *not* eliminated but instead are deposited in body tissue and cause additional antibody production against the cells in those tissues.

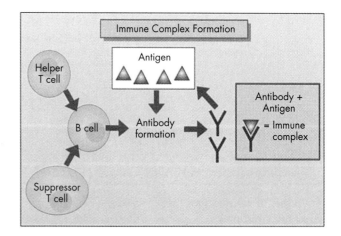

Figure 22-6 The immune system is composed of white blood cells. Four principal classes are involved: phagocytes (including macrophages), natural killer cells, and two kinds of lymphocytes: B cells and T cells. T cells include helper T cells and suppressor T cells. Three different kinds of cells mount attacks against the antigen-studded foreign cell in the center of the diagram. (Modified from Hadi HA, Treadwell EL: Lupus anticoagulant and anticardiolipin antibodies in pregnancy: a review, *Obstet Gynecol Surv* 45:117, 1990.)

These *antinuclear antibodies* are against "self" proteins. The exact trigger for APS is unknown, but it may be viral, hormonal, or stimulated by ultraviolet A and B wavelengths of radiation, with a genetic tendency as an underlying matrix.

Figure 22-7 illustrates how one type of autoimmune antibodies will attack platelets and stimulate formation of thrombi in the vessels, as well as upset the prostacyclin to TXA_2 ratio, which, as discussed earlier, underlies PIH. Thus those who have these antibodies and become pregnant will most likely have PIH as well.

Today a number of syndromes are believed to be associated with thrombosis, including Addison's disease, thromboembolic disorders, certain cerebral infarcts (strokes), and multiple microinfarcts that change mental status. In addition, pathologic conditions that lead to cardiomyopathy, valve obstruction, renal artery occlusion, and LE are antibody-antigen triggered (Asherson and Cervera, 1992). The client will be diagnosed with APS if the anticardiolipin or lupus anticoagulant antibodies are present or if there is repeated fetal loss, thrombotic disease, or thrombocytopenia (Edelman, 1995). About half of the *LE* patients have both of these antibodies. Clinical management is discussed in the section that follows.

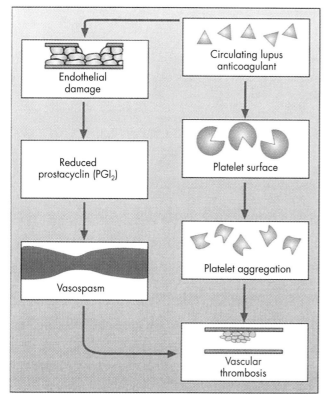

Figure 22-7 Two major pathways whereby lupus anticoagulant produces its thrombotic effect in vivo. (From Hadi HA, Treadwell EL: Lupus anticoagulant and anticardiolipin antibodies in pregnancy: a review, *Obstet Gynecol Surv* 45:117, 1990.)

Lupus Erythematosus

LE is usually diagnosed by a rheumatologist because the most common presenting sign is *migrating arthritis*. Before the autoimmune theory was clarified, a person may have sought many sources for help, each treating only the presenting symptom. Usually damage was well advanced, and kidney failure was a common cause of death. The basic pathology involves production of autoimmune antibodies: antinuclear antibodies (ANA) are present in 100% of lupus clients; APS antibodies are present in about 50% of lupus clients; antiDNA antibodies may be present; and antiRo (Sicca Syndrome [SS A or B]) antibodies are found in 30% of lupus clients. SSA or SSB types will cross the placenta to affect the fetus; SSA is present in fetal heart block and SSB causes neonatal lupus symptoms.

Risk

Pregnancy does not appear to worsen LE (Reece et al, 1992), but if a woman becomes pregnant soon after or just before an episode of LE, of if she already has significant renal damage and hypertension, placental damage can lead to spontaneous abortion. The spontaneous abortion rate is higher after a flare-up during pregnancy. Ideally, a pregnancy should be started only when the woman is clearly in remission for at least 6 months (Lockwood, 1996). There seems to be special risk of a flare-up in the postpartum period, perhaps related to the hormonal changes taking place. Diagnosis is made when 4 out of 11 criteria listed in Table 22-3 are present.

The incidence occurs at a ratio of 10 women to 1 man, which is believed to be related to female hormonal patterns. LE occurs in 1 out of every 700 women between 15 and 65 years of age but is seen in African-American women in a ratio of 1 in 250. In past decades, life expectancy after diagnosis was 5 years. The outcome now depends on early diagnosis and treatment and is much more hopeful. The fetal outcome is less hopeful, however, and loss of the pregnancy occurs in about 30% of first trimester LE cases and in about 20% of second trimester cases (Sala, 1993).

Neonatal risk. The newborn with maternal SSB antibodies will be **photosensitive** and may develop a typical lupus rash in the neonatal period. The infant with SSA antibodies may have congenital heart block. Because these symptoms are caused by maternal antibodies that have crossed the placenta, symptoms gradually diminish in the first few months. The infant *does not* continue to have a lupus syndrome (Sala, 1993).

Signs

Early signs in the client are insidious and may contribute to a diagnosis of APS. These can be malaise, joint aching, low-grade fever, hypertension, and a thrombotic event. In pregnancy, this may easily be confused with PIH. There may be new onset of migraines (see Chapter 23) and *amaurosis fugax*, which is a temporary "white out"

Table **22-3** **Criteria for Lupus Erythematosus***

Sign	Description
Malar rash (butterfly)	Erythema patches on face or hands
Discoid rash	Plaques, spread easily
Photosensitivity	Rash after UV exposure
Oral and nasal ulcers	Painless; on hard or soft palate or nasal septum
Arthritis or arthralgia	Symmetric morning stiffness; swelling in joints
History of pleuritis or pericarditis	Pleurisy, pleural effusion with URI
Proteinuria or renal signs	2-3+ with sediment, RBC, casts, and creatinine >1.6 mg
Psychosis or seizures	Grand mal, organic brain syndrome, CNS problems, microinfarcts
Hematologic disorder	Thrombocytopenia, leukopenia, hemolytic anemia
Immunologic changes	Positive LE factor, Venereal Disease Research Laboratory test; anti-DNA antibodies
Antinuclear antibodies	Abnormal titer

Modified from Hadi HA, Treadwell EL: Lupus anticoagulant and anticardiolipin antibodies in pregnancy: a review, *Obstet Gynecol Surv* 45:117, 1990.
CNS, Central nervous system; *LE*, lupus erythematosus; *RBC*, red blood cell; *URI*, upper respiratory infection; *UV*, ultraviolet.
*Diagnosis of LE made if 4 of 11 signs are present.

with loss of vision in one eye, thought to be caused by platelet clumping in the retinal arteries. Raynaud's disease has also been linked.

When there are flare-ups, antibodies are found in increasing amounts (titers), and antibody titers are followed to show when improvement begins. Because of the migrating character of the symptoms, a client does not know what will occur next. Depending on where thrombi are deposited, renal involvement with signs of damage may be evident. Skin flare-ups include a typical lupus *"butterfly"* rash over the face, chest, and hands, which is triggered by exposure to ultraviolet light from sunlight, fluorescents, or even the light from copy machines (Figure 22-8). All persons with LE can be photosensitive, and they must avoid UV exposure and use a sunscreen with a sun protection factor of 15 to 30 whenever they are exposed to these sources of light.

Clinical management

Antibody levels are followed, along with renal tests and BP checks. Treatment includes a combination of low-dose corticosteroids (15 to 40 mg/day) and low-dose aspirin (75 to 80 mg/day) as an anti-TXA$_2$ agent. If an acute episode with rising antibody titers occurs, hospitalization is required for regulation, with administration of higher doses of IV cortisone and heparin infusion. In very severe cases, human immunoglobulin may be transfused to reduce antibody levels or *plasmapheresis* (plasma exchange transfusion) may be selected to quickly lower levels of antibodies. After birth, immunosuppressive drugs such as azathioprine (Imuran) and cyclophosphamide (Cytoxan) may be used. Blood counts must be monitored closely (Lockwood, 1996).

Pregnancies must be monitored closely. Clients at risk of thromboembolism are treated with subcutaneous heparin throughout the pregnancy, in addition to low-dose aspirin and prednisone as needed (see Drug Profile 22-3).

Nursing responsibilities

The woman with LE who wishes to be pregnant must have preconceptional counseling. She is vulnerable to fetal loss and must understand the grave nature of her disease. Because fatigue and depression are included in her symptoms, the family should be involved in observing the woman's mood and looking for signs of advancing depression or behavioral changes. If she is taking steroids, there may be changes in mood and fluid retention. She will be concerned about the effect of medications on the fetus. The nurse can reassure her that rarely do the prescribed steroid doses (less than 30 mg/day) affect fetal growth and development. Damage to the fetus without these drugs could be significant. Reinforce the client's understanding about the drugs she is using. Because steroids may mask infection, she needs particularly to avoid sources of infection. The nurse should discuss breast-feeding with her, checking dosage with drug tables; steroids doses under 30 mg per day are thought to be acceptable. The infant should be followed-up for growth ratios when the lactating mother is on a daily medication regimen.

Dental care is required. Often there is a lack of saliva and increased caries, bleeding gums, oral ulcers, and candidal infections. The woman should be referred for evaluation and preventive care.

There is an increased potential for exacerbation in the postpartum period. In unusual cases, a woman may have gone through pregnancy with hypertension and given

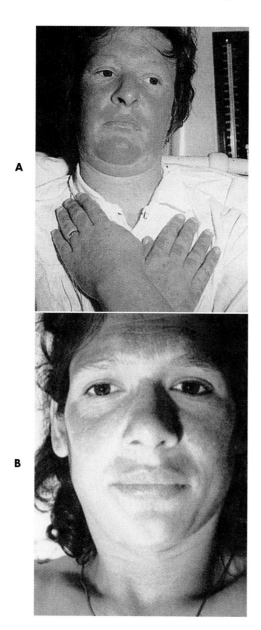

Figure 22-8   Comparison between lupus rash **(A)** and melasma **(B)**. Note that lupus rash is much more reddened than normal melasma and is on the face and chest.
(From Beischer NA, MacKay EV: *Obstetrics and the newborn,* ed 3, Sydney, 1993, WB Saunders. Courtesy Harcourt Brace Jovanovich Group.)

Box **22-3**

DRUG PROFILE

Heparin Sodium

ACTION

Inhibits clotting sequence. Acts at multiple sites. Does not dissolve existing clots. Because large molecule does not cross placenta, it may be used up to 6 hours before birth. Lower molecular weight type has a longer $t_{1/2}$ and can be used as a daily dose. Calcium and weight bearing may limit the osteoporosis effect of heparin.

DOSAGE AND ROUTE

Administered via subcutaneous (SC) route, never intramuscularly. Administer 5000-10,000 U q12hr or as an IV infusion continuously over 24 hours. May be combined with low-dose aspirin and 7500 U heparin. Titrated to partial thromboplastin time levels and clotting time, which are measured regularly.

ANTAGONIST

Protamine sulfate 1 mg/100 U heparin is given over 20-minute interval if bleeding occurs or urgent cesarean.

SIDE EFFECTS AND ADVERSE EFFECTS

Thrombocytopenia, hemorrhage with oozing from mucous membranes, and ecchymosis all possible. Hypersensitivity with fever and urticaria possible. IV site may become locally irritated and SC site may become ecchymotic. Sometimes rash and diarrhea develop. Long-term use (5 to 6 months) may lead to irreversible osteoporosis.

PRECAUTIONS

Rotate SC sites carefully. Do not aspirate or use site with less than one-half inch fatty tissue. Mother may breast-feed. Observe for signs of oozing or hemorrhage. Note laboratory reports.

birth safely, but then she may suddenly become less responsive and have seizures. When seizures occur early in the postpartum period, the first thought is eclampsia, especially if albuminuria accompanies kidney involvement. But LE should be considered as well, since a form of cerebral lupus that results from multiple microinfarcts in the brain occurs in the postpartum period. This cerebral lupus begins with restlessness, confusion, and vague personality changes and may lead to coma and death (Lockwood, 1996).

The woman will benefit by referral to one of the support groups for persons with LE (see Client Resources found before Student Resource Shelf at end of chapter). Certainly, if there is any disability, she will need referrals for rehabilitation and home care follow-up with occupational and physical therapy.

IMMUNE DISORDERS: PLATELET DYSFUNCTION

Thrombocytopenia

The significance of platelet levels has increased because low platelets are found in severe preeclampsia, HELLP syndrome, and systemic lupus erythematosus (SLE).

Thrombocytopenia, low platelet counts, may be the first sign of SLE and HELLP. Levels are followed carefully and are directly related to the severity of these syndromes.

Thrombocytopenia may occur in severe folate deficiencies of because of sepsis, excessive alcohol intake, or idiosyncratic responses to medications. Of special concern is an immunologic disorder that causes *idiopathic (immune) thrombocytopenic purpura* (ITP). Although uncommon, this disorder is found more often in women than in men (3:1). Circulating antiplatelet antibodies, immunoglobin G (IgG), that accelerate the destruction of platelets are formed because of changes in the platelet surface (Giacoia and Azubuike, 1991). The result is a higher risk of hemorrhage and hematoma formation if platelet levels are below 50,000/mm³ (For this reason, anesthesiologists will not use the epidural route if platelet counts are low.)

A second type of immunologic disorder is called *thrombotic thrombocytopenic purpura* (TTP), which is a rare severe form that results in thrombosis in capillaries and in organ damage. The following signs indicate TTP:
- Thrombocytopenia below 50,000/mm³
- Microangiopathic anemia
- Renal abnormalities
- Fever
- Neurologic symptoms

Risk to fetus

The IgG antibody may cross the placenta to affect fetal platelets and cause bleeding. Transient neonatal thrombocytopenia (NAIT) is diagnosed if the neonatal platelet count is below 150,000/mm³ or 150×10^9/L. The major risk is trauma-induced intracranial bleeding during birth. Consequently, in the past it had become the practice in known cases to analyze fetal scalp capillary blood for platelets early in labor. If the count was below 50,000/mm³, a cesarean birth was chosen to avoid trauma to the fetal head. However, the benefit of "rescuing" the fetus by surgical birth is unclear, thus intervention in this way is not usually recommended (Silver, Branch, Scott, 1995). The newborn platelet counts are observed carefully for 72 hours. Very low counts may require therapy with corticosteroids and IV IgG. However, most newborns recover gradually since the cause of the low platelets was maternal antibodies that traversed the placenta, not an intrinsic problem in the infant.

Signs

In addition to low platelets, there may be prolonged bleeding times and petechiae and purpura on the skin and mucous membranes. Any client who has abnormal bleeding from wounds, petechiae, or bruising (signs similar to those for DIC) must be evaluated for ITP.

Clinical management

In chronic ITP, steroids are used to keep platelet levels up. Corticosteroids in the range of 60 to 80 mg per day are given for 1 to 2 weeks, then the dose is tapered to a maintenance level below 30 mg per day. This usual corticosteroid therapy has poor results in managing TTP. A splenectomy may be used to control platelet levels, although this should not be performed during pregnancy. The spleen functions to remove platelets and is believed to contribute to platelet antibody formation (Giacoia and Azubuike, 1991).

High-dose *intravenous immunoglobulin G* (IV IgG) has been useful in managing several immune disorders and is very effective in management of ITP. During the last weeks of pregnancy, infusion of 0.4 g/kg per day for 3 days can raise platelet counts into the normal range, thus protecting the mother against hemorrhage during labor and birth. (IV IgG is also used in Rh-negative women who have been immunized and in SLE cases to reduce antibody levels).

Plasmapheresis is an expensive therapy in which the client's blood is withdrawn and cells (RBCs, white blood cells [WBCs], and platelets) are spun out and resuspended in a new solution. This solution is replaced into the client's circulation. By removing a portion of the client's plasma, adverse substances such as antibodies are removed; thus plasmapheresis is a type of *exchange transfusion*. One or two exchanges often results in rapid improvement (Lockwood, 1996).

THROMBOEMBOLIC DISEASES

Thrombophlebitis (clot formation with inflammation, in the venous system) occurs rarely during early pregnancy; because of hypercoagulability, it is more common in the second half of pregnancy and during recovery. A client with APS may have recurrent early episodes.

Superficial Vein Thrombophlebitis

Superficial vein thrombophlebitis (SVT) is most often seen in saphenous veins. Women who have preexisting varicose veins or prior episodes are at higher risk (see Chapter 9). Other predisposing factors are obesity, high parity, advanced maternal age, and previous heart disease. In addition, bed rest with immobility associated with surgery, anesthesia, or complications can result in thromboembolic disease (TED). Estrogens were once used to suppress lactation but are never used now, because of their association with an increased incidence of emboli.

Signs

SVT is accompanied by moderate to severe inflammation, causing pain and swelling over the site. Sometimes there is a low-grade fever and an elevated pulse.

Deep Vein Thrombosis

The onset of deep vein thrombophlebitis (DVT) varies; a few cases begin during the antepartum period, but most begin within 72 hours of birth, with some occurring as late as 22 days after birth. A related cause is antiphospholipid antibodies (see discussion of LE earlier in this chapter).

Signs

When a large thrombus forms in the deep veins of the leg, the swollen leg becomes cyanotic or may be pale. Reflex arteriolar spasm causes severe pain. The location of the pain depends on the location of the vein involved: in the popliteal and lateral tibial areas, in the low calf and foot, in the inguinal area, or even in the pelvic area. Most often the vein is in the left leg (McPhedran, 1995). Homan's sign tests for the developing presence of DVT (see Figure 17-9).

Risk

Superficial vein thrombophlebitis. SVT occurs in approximately 1.5 out of every 1000 women who have vaginal births and has been reported in slightly higher rates following cesarean birth. It is usually related to prior varicose veins, and often there is a prior history of episodes. Early ambulation has reduced the incidence.

Deep vein thrombophlebitis. Deeper vein embolus has a much lower incidence than SVT, but it is very serious when it occurs because DVT carries a risk of pulmonary embolism. Sometimes the first indication of DVT is when an embolus lodges in the pulmonary circulation. Such embolism is a leading cause of maternal mortality. In addition, Bergquist et al (1990) found that a postphlebotic syndrome could persist in 3.4% of clients. This included intermittent swelling of the extremity, pain, cramping, and, in some cases, later ulceration of the lower leg.

Because *osteoporosis* may occur with prolonged heparin therapy, an oral anticoagulant (warfarin[Coumadin]) is substituted after birth whenever possible (Cosico et al, 1993).

Clinical management

Superficial vein thrombophlebitis. A physical examination can usually pinpoint the trouble. Anticoagulants are rarely used for SVT. The clot is fixed and small, and there is little danger of an embolus to the heart or lungs. Warm soaks are applied to elevated legs, and analgesics may be needed until the clot resolves.

Deep vein thrombophlebitis. Doppler ultrasound, contrast venography, a ventilation/perfusion (V/Q) scan, pulmonary angiography, or a CT scan may be used to diagnose the clot location. Management of DVT includes all the treatment used for SVT, plus anticoagulants, antibiotics, and venous compression with ACE bandages or thromboemolic stockings when the leg improves.

After diagnosis, a heparin loading dose of 100 U/kg is followed by 15 to 20 U/kg per hour until there is a stable *activated partial thromboplastin time* (aPTT) of approximately 1.5 to 2.0 times the control. After 5 to 10 days of IV heparin therapy, subcutaneous therapy every 8 to 12 hours is begun (Drug Profile 22-3). For maintenance, low molecular weight heparin (with a longer half-life of ($t_{1/2}$) may be used as a single daily injection (Hull et al, 1992). Low-dose aspirin with 7500 U heparin twice a day has been suggested as a maintenance regimen (Ginsberg and Hirsch, 1992).

The client should be instructed to administer self-doses at home, or a heparin subcutaneous pump may be used. Anticoagulation must be continued for the entire pregnancy if the episode occurred during pregnancy or if the woman has a history of thrombosis during a prior pregnancy. Anticoagulation is stopped a few hours before birth to allow clearing of the heparin dose (usually within 6 hours). Anticoagulation is begun again in the immediate postpartum period and continued for at least 3 months after an acute episode. Although warfarin is not used orally during pregnancy because of adverse fetal effects, it is the drug of choice in the postpartum period because it does not cross into the breast milk and is much easier to take as an oral dose (Barbour, 1995). Clotting and thromboplastin times are tested at regular intervals, especially during the high-risk period occurring 6 weeks postbirth.

Nursing responsibilities

Supportive interventions of SVT include bed rest until pain and swelling subside. Legs are elevated to reduce edema and to shunt blood into the deep veins. Moist heat is applied to dilate the veins and improve circulation. Analgesics are given for inflammation and pain. Anticoagulants are rarely necessary.

Because varicose veins are so commonly associated with SVT, the client is measured for pressure-gradient elastic stockings and encouraged to ambulate as soon as the swelling decreases. To be effective, these stockings must be applied before the woman sits or stands. Until her custom-fitted stockings arrive, elastic bandaging is used. The woman must learn how to put on the stockings or how to bandage her legs. In addition, she must avoid prolonged standing or sitting with crossed legs.

The client may be anxious about moving because she fears loosening the clot. This usually will not happen with SVT. The nurse helps her to comply with the regimen of bed rest until pain and swelling have disappeared.

The pregnant client with DVT will need to learn self-injection with heparin if she is going home on this therapy regimen. Encourage self-injection, with rotation of sites, during the hospital stay. Teach her not to massage the site and to observe for any signs of bleeding tendency that might develop with prolonged therapy. (See insulin injection techniques in Chapter 24). Women receiving anticoagulants should be observed for evidence of bleeding from mucous membranes, bruising, hematomas, excessive lochia, or hematuria. Finally, the nurse should remain alert to any indications of movement of the clot into vital organs.

Because of prolonged bed rest with DVT, active and passive range of motion exercises are important to enhance venous flow. The extended period of bed rest will be difficult to adjust to and may markedly upset family life (Maloni, 1993). Social service personnel should be involved in arrangements if there are children at home.

> a. List preventive measures to avoid the development of varicose veins during pregnancy.
> b. What would you teach about home care to a woman who is recovering from SVT?
> c. List important teaching points for heparin self-administration.

Obstetric Pulmonary Embolism

In some instances, an embolus breaks off from the deep femoral or pelvic vein thrombosis and migrates to the heart and then to the pulmonary artery. This condition is called **pulmonary embolism** (PE). PE sometimes occurs after the client has returned home; the thrombus either develops late or is undiscovered before she is discharged (see Chapter 25 for septic pelvic thrombophlebitis).

Risk

A client at risk for embolus may have a prior history of thrombophlebitis, varicose veins, or cardiac disease; she may be obese or be an older multipara; or she may have been placed on lengthy bed rest because of complications. Of those women with DVT in the femoral or iliac veins, 10% to 15% will have a pulmonary episode (Beischer and MacKay, 1993). PE was the leading cause of maternal mortality before early ambulation. In many countries, emboli are still a leading cause of maternal death. Today in the United States, PE is the source of two thirds of all embolism deaths and is the third leading cause of maternal mortality (Berg et al, 1996).

Signs

Respiratory signs of PE may be sudden, and the syndrome progresses rapidly. The client may complain of sudden shortness of breath and of a sharp stabbing pain in her chest that mimics a heart attack. She may make statements that she "is going to die." Classic signs are as follows:

- Tachypnea
- Dyspnea
- Rales
- Pleuritic pain
- Cough or hemoptysis
- Apprehension
- Sudden diaphoresis
- Fever

Signs such as sudden shortness of breath, cyanosis, and hemoptysis may be accompanied by a sense of pressure in the bowel or rectum. Collapse may occur within seconds or minutes if a large blood vessel is blocked. If smaller vessels are blocked, lung tissue is deprived of blood and dies (infarct). In this case, signs are tachycardia, tachypnea, and cough with blood-tinged sputum. The clot may break off and reach the vessels in the brain (see discussion on stroke found later in this chapter).

Clinical management

If PE is suspected, clinical therapy should begin immediately. Electrocardiogram, radiograph films, and laboratory tests are not always accurate and take valuable time. Pulmonary arteriography and V/Q scans are diagnostic, but death could occur if treatment is postponed to collect diagnostic data. Strict bed rest in high Fowler's position should be maintained, and nasal oxygen should be administered. As soon as possible, a heparin bolus is given, then heparin infusion is established, and pain medication and sedation are begun. Fibrolytic therapy to lyse a large clot, such as streptokinase, is not usually used until at least 10 days after birth (Barbour, 1995). An embolectomy may be necessary for this critical condition.

Amniotic Fluid Embolism (Anaphylactoid Syndrome)

In very rare instances, amniotic fluid is drawn into the woman's venous circulation (Figure 22-9). The fluid contains debris such as meconium, vernix, and lanugo, which, along with other abnormal substances in the fluid, triggers cardiogenic shock and an *anaphylactoid reaction*. The amniotic fluid triggers the intrinsic clotting system causing rapid defibrination (Resnik, 1996). This syndrome is known as **amniotic fluid embolism** (AFE). There is a striking similarity among signs of septic shock, anaphylaxis, and AFE, often leading to the renaming of this syndrome as *anaphylactoid syndrome*.

AFE may cause anaphylaxis during an apparently normal labor, during artificial rupture of membranes, during placement of an intrauterine catheter (see Chapter 14) or during precipitous birth, or in cases of abruptio placentae. Hypertonic contractions related to oxytocin have been eliminated as a cause (Clark et al, 1995). Other cases have no known associated factors. Two cases have occurred with amnioinfusion when there was thick meconium. A few cases have occurred with dilatation and evacuation of the uterus in the first trimester or with uterine or abdominal trauma. In the postpartum period, most cases occur within a few minutes of birth, though some occur extremely rarely as late as 48 hours after birth (Resnick, 1996). There is a national registry for collating information on cases of AFE (Clark et al, 1995).

AFE and anaphylaxis cannot be predicted or prevented; there are no demographic risk factors to alert the medical staff to the possibility. It constitutes a medical emergency in which every member of the health team must work rapidly to sustain the life of the mother and fetus.

Risk

AFE and anaphylaxis are rare, but currently they have a maternal mortality rate of 60% (Clark et al, 1995). Approximately one third of all deaths from embolism during 1987 to 1990 were from amniotic fluid embolism (Berg et al, 1996). However, diagnosis may not have been

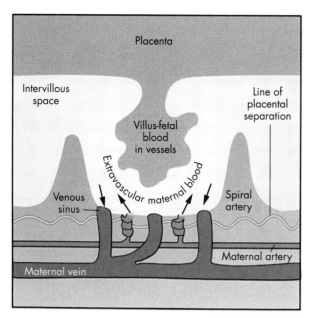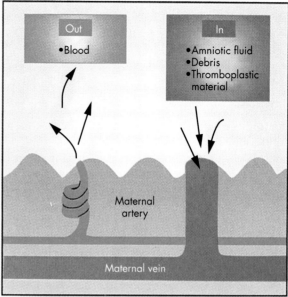

Figure 22-9   Amniotic fluid embolism. The placental circulation may suck amniotic fluid into the venous flow.

made definitively, because DIC, cardiac arrest, and hemorrhage may accompany this syndrome, and deaths may have been listed under other categories. AFE is a leading cause of maternal death in many countries.

Those who survive the acute episode may develop left ventricular failure accompanied by ARDS and DIC and may need intensive care for an extended period of time. Unfortunately, only 15% of those who survive AFE are neurologically intact. The National Registry reports that perinatal mortality is 21%, but 50% of the surviving infants are neurologically impaired from an extended period of hypoxemia. For these reasons, Clark et al (1995) recommend that *perimortem cesarean section* be initiated as soon as possible after maternal cardiac arrest. The relief of pressure may cause improvement in the maternal condition and will certainly give the infant a better chance at survival. See trauma decision making (Figure 23-11) and perimortem delivery in Chapter 23.

Signs

In an otherwise healthy woman, AFE manifests by sudden agitation, dyspnea with a bluish gray pallor, coughing with frothy pink sputum, and hypotension. A seizure may be the first presenting sign. Respiratory collapse and cor pulmonale occur as fluid substances infiltrate the lung circulation. Signs of shock appear, preceded by chills, diaphoresis, and extreme anxiety. Fetal bradycardia and severe variable decelerations are noted. Uterine atony occurs, leading to hemorrhage. Amniotic fluid is thromboplastin rich, which triggers the intrinsic clotting system. There is rapid defibrination, which complicates the treatment of hemorrhage. Cardiac arrest occurred in 87% of cases

reported to the National Registry, and only 8% of these cases survived neurologically intact (Clark et al, 1995).

Clinical management

Cardiopulmonary life support must be started at once, accompanied by endotracheal intubation, high levels of oxygen, and support of blood volume. Hypotension is treated with normal saline, packed cells, and, if DIC is present, platelet infusions. A Swan-Ganz line is placed to monitor pressures and to prevent fluid overload. Because of the possibility of an anaphylactic reaction, hydrocortisone 500 mg every 6 hours may be ordered.

When the woman is stabilized, a cesarean should be performed to save the infant, or if cardiac arrest occurs, a perimortum cesarean may rescue the infant. DIC may develop within 30 minutes of the initial embolus and result in excessive bleeding. Clotting factors must be monitored. Only with skilled, aggressive intervention is there a chance to save the woman's life (Resnick, 1996).

Pulmonary Edema and Adult Respiratory Distress Syndrome

A number of factors predispose the woman to the risk of *pulmonary edema*. First, the physiologic changes of pregnancy include hemodilution caused by physiologic hypervolemia, lowered serum albumin with a lower COP, and renal changes. These normal variations may be exaggerated by hemorrhage and by the too-rapid infusion of crystalloid fluids. Tocolytic therapy with ritodrine or terbutaline has resulted in pulmonary edema. Excessive duration and amount of oxytocin infusion have been implicated in water retention because of an antidiuretic action. When cortico-steroids are used (for asthma or preterm labor), permeability of the lung tissue is affected and the risk increases. Other factors are severe anemia (see Chapter 23), hypokalemia with magnesium sulfate infusion, preeclampsia, chronic cocaine use, and severe cardiac and renal disease. Sepsis may precipitate pulmonary edema from noncardiogenic reasons related to increased permeability of the lung tissue to fluids.

Pulmonary edema may progress to acute lung injury or ARDS, which is characterized by *noncardiogenic* pulmonary edema and is a secondary cause of mortality. ARDS is precipitated by *indirect* injury to the lungs related to preeclampsia, HELLP syndrome, acute fatty liver of pregnancy, AFE, amnionitis, bacterial sepsis, pyelonephritis, and status epilepticus and to injury after aspiration or trauma from motor vehicle accidents (Catanzarite et al, 1991). In these cases, normal blood flow through the lungs is reduced and platelets aggregate, releasing substances (including histamine, serotonin, and bradykinin) that damage alveolar membranes (Shailor, Roach, and Weisnor, 1992).

During pulmonary edema, fluid leaks into the lungs, lung volume decreases, and widespread atelectasis and hypoxia develops. A vicious cycle rapidly develops, as lung damage impairs surfactant supply and gas exchange. Providing oxygen by mask does not correct the worsening hypoxia and respiratory distress. Even with tachypnea, oxygen levels fall, and metabolic acidosis worsens.

Signs

Signs of pulmonary edema are as follows:

- Hypoxemia, cyanosis; oxygen saturation in arterial blood (Pao$_2$) is less than 70 mm Hg on room air
- Tachypnea
- Tachycardia
- Pulmonary infiltration: crackling sounds, wheezing, rales
- Increased BP, depending on precipitating factor
- Cool, moist skin
- Restlessness, confusion
- Nonreassuring fetal heart rhythms

Clinical management of pulmonary edema

Early diagnosis of the susceptible client will prevent iatrogenic causes such as fluid overload. PAC monitoring greatly assists management in most cases (Table 23-1 and Figure 23-1). Oxygen must be delivered by means of intermittent positive pressure, and pulse oximetry must be used. If the cause is fluid imbalance, it must be corrected, either by modifying the IV infusion or by diuretics. Furosemide commonly is used. A Foley catheter with urimeter must be in place for hourly urine output measurements. The causative factors are corrected: vasodilators for vasospasm, antibiotics for infection, and albumin or hetastarch to raise a low COP. Morphine sulfate is given to diminish anxiety

and for its benefit as a vasodilator, thus temporarily reducing preload. If the woman is in labor, epidural anesthesia may help to reduce preload by vasodilation of the circulation in the lower extremities. Rapid reversal of symptoms of pulmonary edema occurs with correct interventions. If the woman's condition deteriorates, ARDS and multiorgan failure must be suspected. (See Surratt and Troiano, 1993; Witry, 1992; and medical texts on pulmonary edema and ARDS for more detailed interventions.)

TEST *Yourself* 22-5 _____

a. Compare presenting signs of pulmonary edema and pulmonary embolism.
b. Twelve hours after birth, if the woman complains of chest pain and is perspiring and anxious, what would your priority nursing interventions be?

Stroke

Although very uncommon, when a stroke occurs during pregnancy, it may progress rapidly to a fatal outcome. The hypercoagulability of blood, especially in the last trimester and the early postbirth period, contributes to the possibility of cerebral arterial infarction or venous thrombosis. In rare instances, the woman has a prior cerebral aneurysm or arteriovenous malformation. The stress of labor and the Valsalva maneuver may place too great a presure on this malformation, causing rupture. An embolus thrown from a DVT site or AFE may lodge in the cerebral circulation. Finally, there may be low-grade DIC and eclamptic seizures plus severe hypertension that may precipitate a cerebral event of infarction or subarachnoid hemorrhage. These events may occur during pregnancy and labor, during early recovery, or after discharge to the home.

Neurosurgical management is the same as for a non-pregnant person. The nurse should be alert to signs of potential cerebral involvement:

- Headache is the most frequent presenting sign—unilateral; limited to forehead, temple, or occiput; may be severe and persistent (see Chapter 23)
- Sensory deficit, usually contralateral
- Increasing motor deficit—facial palsy or weakness in speech, swallowing, or in extremities
- Vomiting, fever, nuchal rigidity
- Seizures—small focal seizures or grand mal seizures—which may be confused with eclampsia
- Varying sites of paralysis develop gradually

Rapid diagnosis by means of magnetic resonance imaging (MRI) and spinal tap are required in order to pinpoint the lesion and decide on interventions. Intensive care is required and prognosis is guarded (Kjas-Wyllie, 1994). Refer to medical-surgical texts for detailed interventions.

Key Points

- Diagnosis of PIH may be difficult because of the prevalence of undiscovered chronic hypertension and APS.
- Prevention of eclampsia is necessary because of the potential of death and cerebral damage associated with vasoconstriction, edema, and seizures. Seizures may occur at any time.
- DIC may be at a low level in preeclampsia or may escalate suddenly in a variety of pregnancy complications.
- Rapid diagnosis of DIC and timely intervention are critical to stop hemorrhage and save the woman's life.
- LE is diagnosed more commonly than in the past, and pregnancy loss, thromboembolism, and hypertension are often related to autoimmune antibody formation.
- Platelet counts have assumed a new importance in PIH, HELLP syndrome, and immune thrombocy-

topenia. Levels below 150,000/mm^3 are considered signals of thrombocytopenia; levels below 50,000/mm^3 carry a serious risk of bleeding.
- Preventive care for SVT and DVT, two types of thromboembolic disease, must be begun before women susceptible to the conditions become pregnant. Pregnancy alters the clotting mechanisms, which increases risk in these cases.
- AFE (anaphylactic syndrome of pregnancy) and PE are critical events for which intense collaborative care is required to prevent maternal or fetal mortality.
- Pulmonary edema may occur with an abnormally low COP or a fluid overload, both of which may occur in crisis situations unless there is very careful monitoring of fluids and hemodynamic status.

Study Questions

22-1. Select the terms that apply to the following statements:
  a. When the hematocrit level is elevated and blood volume lowered there is _____.
  b. A type of edema showing up in the face and hands during pregnancy is _____.
  c. The single sign of hypertension accompanying pregnancy occurs in the condition called _____.
  d. The condition of sudden dyspnea, cyanosis, and hemoptysis after birth could be caused by _____.
  e. A _____ rash forms on the face, chest, or arms when a person with lupus is exposed to ultraviolet rays.
  f. Resulting from PIH, visual changes in one or both eyes is _____.
  g. Change in permeability of tissue barriers is a result of lowered _____.
  h. Lowered platelet counts result in a condition called _____.

22-2. Janice, 33 and para 2010, is admitted to the antepartum unit because of signs of preeclampsia. During the nursing history interview, which of the following information indicates an increased risk of serious hypertension?
  a. She has a previous history of several spontaneous abortions.
  b. Her maternal grandmother died of a cerebrovascular accident.
  c. She has had borderline hypertension for 3 years.
  d. She did not begin prenatal care until 6 weeks before admission.

22-3. In a severe preeclamptic patient, which laboratory findings would indicate vasoconstriction with a lowered blood volume?
  a. Reduced platelet count
  b. Burr cells and elevated hematocrit
  c. Lowered hematocrit and elevated bilirubin
  d. Decreased albumin levels

22-4. Why must the three observations regarding magnesium toxicity be made whenever a woman is being treated for severe preeclampsia?
  a. Magnesium constricts bronchioles and inhibits respirations.
  b. Cumulative effects depress neurologic responses.
  c. Oliguria indicates increasing risk of eclampsia.
  d. Adequate oxygen exchange is always critical.

22-5. Which of the following would indicate that preeclampsia had progressed to eclampsia?
  a. Headaches persisting in spite of analgesia
  b. Oliguria of 800 ml/24 hours
  c. Vasospasm seen in the fundus of the eye
  d. Amnesia leading to coma

22-6. Select the most unusual presenting symptom of DIC.
   a. Bleeding into the urine
   b. Bruising under the BP cuff
   c. Leaking of blood from a venipuncture site
   d. Microemboli causing mental confusion

22-7. Which of the following statements by a postpartum client complaining of pain would be most alarming?
   a. "It's a chest pain that comes and goes."
   b. "It's a sharp chest pain when I burp."
   c. "It's a sharp chest pain, and I can't get my breath."
   d. "It's a catching pain when I breathe deeply."

Answer Key

22-1. *a,* Hemoconcentration; *b,* generalized edema; *c,* gestational hypertension; *d,* obstetric pulmonary embolism; *e,* butterfly rash; *f,* scotoma; *g,* colloid osmotic pressure; *h,* thrombocytopenia. 22-2: c. 22-3: b. 22-4: b. 22-5: d. 22-6: d. 22-7: c.

References

Ament LA: Anticardiolipin antibodies: a review of the literature, *J Nurse Midwifery* 39(1):19, 1994.

American College of Obstetricians and Gynecologists: *Invasive hemodynamic monitoring in obstetrics and gynecology,* Technical Bulletin 175, Dec 1992.

American College of Obstetricians and Gynecologists: *Hypertension in pregnancy,* Technical Bulletin 219, Jan 1996.

Asherson RA, Cervera R: The antiphospholipid syndrome: a syndrome in evolution, *Ann Rheum Dis* 51:147, 1992.

Awada A et al: Stroke and pregnancy, *Int J Gynaecol Obstet* 48:157, 1995.

Barbour LA: Controversies in thromboembolic disease during pregnancy, *Obstet Gynecol* 86(4 pt 1):621, 1995.

Barton JR, Stanziano GJ, Sibai BM: Monitored outpatient management of mild gestational hypertension remote from term, *Am J Obstet Gynecol* 170:765, 1995.

Beischer NA, MacKay EV, eds: *Obstetrics and the newborn,* ed 3, Philadelphia, 1993, WB Saunders.

Berg CJ et al: Pregnancy-related mortality in the United States: 1987-1990, *Obstet Gynecol* 88(2):161, 1996.

Bergquist A et al: Late symptoms after pregnancy-related deep vein thrombosis, *Br J Obstet Gynaecol* 97:338, 1990.

Blackburn ST, Loper DL: *Maternal, fetal, and neonatal physiology,* Philadelphia, 1992, WB Saunders.

Bucher HC et al: Effect of calcium supplementation on pregnancy-induced hypertension and preeclampsia: a meta-analysis of randomized controlled trials, *JAMA* 275:1113, 1996.

Burrows A, Ferris TF, eds: *Medical complications during pregnancy,* ed 4, Philadelphia, 1995, WB Saunders.

Catanzarite V: HELLP syndrome and its complications, *Contemp Ob Gyn* 36(12):13, 1991.

*Chesley L, Cooper D: Genetics of hypertension in pregnancy: possible single gene control of preeclampsia in descendents of eclamptic women, *Br J Obstet Gynaecol* 93:898, 1986.

Childress CH, Katz VL: Nifedipine and its indications in obstetrics and gynecology, *Obstet Gynecol* 83(4):616, 1994.

Clark SL: New concepts of amniotic fluid embolism: a review, *Obstet Gynecol Surv* 45(6):360, 1990.

Clark SL et al: *Handbook of critical care obstetrics,* Cambridge, Mass, 1994, Blackwell Sci Publ.

Clark SL et al: Amniotic fluid embolism: Analysis of the national registry, *Am J Obstet Gynecol* 172:1158, 1995.

Communicable Disease Center: *Morbidity and mortality weekly report* (MMWR) 45(11):235, Atlanta, GA, 1995.

Cosico JN et al: Indications, management and patient education for anticoagulant therapy during pregnancy, *MCN Am J Matern Child Nurs* 17(3):130, 1993.

*Crandon AJ, Isherwood DM: Effect of aspirin on incidence of preeclampsia, *Lancet* 1:1356, 1979.

Dekker GA, Sibai BM: Early detection of preeclampsia, *Am J Obstet Gynecol* 165:160, 1991.

Dekker GA, Sibai BM: Low dose aspirin in the prevention of preeclampsia and fetal growth retardation: rationale, mechanisms and clinical trials, *Am J Obstet Gynecol* 168(1):224, 1993.

Douglas KA, Redman CWG: Eclampsia in the United Kingdom, *Br Med J* 309:1395, 1994.

Easterling TR, Benedetti TJ: Principles of invasive hemodynamic monitoring in pregnancy. In Clark SL et al, eds: *Critical care obstetrics,* Cambridge, Mass, 1991, Blackwell Sci Publ.

Edelman PL: The antiphosphoslipid syndrome, *Curr Opin Obstet Gynecol* 7:427, 1995.

Ferris TF: Hypertension and pre-eclampsia. In Gonik B, Brobrowski RA, eds: *Medical complications of labor and delivery,* Cambridge, Mass, 1996, Blackwell Sci Publ.

Fox D et al: Use of the pulmonary artery catheter in severe preeclampsia: a review, *Obstet Gynecol Surv* 51(11):684, 1996.

Frangieh AY, Sibai BM: Outpatient management of mild gestational hypertension and preeclampsia, *Contemp Ob Gyn* 41(8):67, 1996.

Giacoia GP, Azubuike K: Autoimmune diseases in pregnancy: their effect on the fetus and newborn, *Obstet Gynecol Surv* 46(11):723, 1991.

Gilbert ES, Harmon JS: *High risk pregnancy & delivery,* St Louis, 1993, Mosby.

Ginsberg JS, Hirsch J: Use of antithrombic agents during pregnancy, *Chest* 102(suppl):385, 1992.

Goldberg RL et al: Bedrest in pregnancy, *Obstet Gynecol* 84(1):131, 1994.

Gonik G, Bobrowski RA, eds: *Medical complications of labor and delivery,* Cambridge, Mass, 1996, Blackwell Sci Publ.

Gordon MC, Iams JD: Magnesium sulfate, *Clin Obstet Gynecol,* 38(4):706, 1996.

Grohar J: Nursing protocols for antepartum home care, *J Obstet Gyncecol Neonatal Nurs* 23(8):687, 1994.

Hadi HA, Treadwell EL: Lupus anticoagulant and anticardiolipin antibodies in pregnancy: a review, *Obstet Gynecol Surv* 45:117, 1990.

Helewa J et al: Community based home-care program for the management of preeclampsia: an alternative, *Can Med Assoc J* 149(8):829, 1993.

Hull RD et al: Subcutaneous low-molecular weight heparin compared with continuous intravenous heparin in the treatment of proximal-vein thrombosis, *N Engl J Med* 326:975, 1992.

Ives J: Disseminated intravascular coagulation. In Repke TJ, ed: *Intrapartum obstetrics,* New York, 1996, Churchill Livingstone.

James DK, Steer PJ, Weiner CP: *High risk pregnancy: management options,* Philadelphia, 1994, WB Saunders.

Kajs-Wyllie M: Venous stroke in the pregnant and postpartum patient, *J Neurosci Nurs* 26(4):204, 1994.

Kaplan PS, Repke JT: Eclampsia, *Neurol Clin* 12(3):565, 1994.

Lockwood CJ: Autoimmune disease. In Queenan JT, Hobbins JC, eds: *Protocols for high-risk pregnancy,* Cambridge Mass, 1996, Blackwell Sci Publ.

Maloni JA: Bedrest during pregnancy: implications for nursing, *J Obstet Gynecol Neonatal Nurs* 22(5):422, 1993.

McPhedran P: Venous thromboembolism during pregnancy. In Burrows A, Ferris TF, eds: *Medical complications in pregnancy,* ed 4, Philadelphia, 1995, WB Saunders.

Miles JF et al: Postpartum eclampsia: a recurring perinatal dilemma, *Obstet Gynecol* 76:328, 1990.

Nelson KB, Grether, JK: Can magnesium sulfate reduce the risk of cerebral palsy in very low birthweight infants? *Pediatrics* 95:263, 1995.

*Classic reference.

Perinatal Trial Service: Which anticonvulsant for women with eclampsia? Evidence from the collaborative eclampsia trial, *Lancet* 345:1455, 1995.

Perry KG, Martin JN: Abnormal hemostasis and coagulopathy in preeclampsia and eclampsia, *Clin Obstet Gynecol* 35(2):338, 1992.

Reece EA et al, eds: *Handbook of medicine of the fetus and mother,* Philadelphia, 1995, JB Lippincott.

Repke JT, ed: *Intrapartum obstetrics,* New York, 1996, Churchill Livingstone.

Resnik R: Amniotic fluid embolism. In Queenan JT, Hobbins JC, *Protocols for high-risk pregnancies,* ed 3, Cambridge, Mass, 1996, Blackwell Sci Publ.

Roberts J: Current perspectives on preeclampsia, *J Nurs Midwifery* 39(2):70, 1994.

Ruiz-Irastora G et al: Increased rate of lupus flare during pregnancy and puerperium: a prospective study of 78 pregnancies, *Br J Rheumatol* 35:133, 1996.

Saftlas AF et al: Epidemology of preeclampsia and eclampsia in the United States: 1979-1986, *Am J Obstet Gynecol* 163:460, 1990.

Sala DJ: Effects of lupus erythematosus on pregnancy and the neonate, *J Perinat Neonatal Nurs* 7(3):39, 1993.

Sanches-Ramos S et al: Urinary calcium as an early marker for preeclampsia, *Obstet Gynecol* 77(5):685, 1991.

Seidman DS, Seir DM, Ben-Rafael Z: Renal and ocular manifestations of hypertensive disease of pregnancy, *Obstet Gynecol Surv* 46(2):71, 1991.

Shailor TL, Roach D, Weisnor D: Challenging diagnosis: management of the obstetric patient with adult respiratory distress syndrome, *J Perinat Neonatal Nurs* 6(2):25, 1992.

Sharts-Engle NC: Aspirin for prevention of pregnancy-induced hypertension, *MCN Am J Matern Child Nurs,* 17(3):169, 1993.

Sibai BM et al: Prevention of preeclampsia with low-dose aspirin in healthy, nulliparous pregnant women, *N Engl J Med* 329:1213, 1993.

Silver RM, Branch DW, Scott JR: Maternal thrombocytopenia in pregnancy: time for a reassessment, *Am J Obstet Gynecol* 173:479, 1995.

Simpson K, Creehan P: *AWHONN's perinatal nursing: care of the childbearing woman and the neonate,* Philadelphia, 1995, JB Lippincott.

Suarez VR, Trelles JG, Miyahira JM: Urinary calcium in asymptomatic primigravidas who later developed preeclampsia, *Obstet Gynecol* 87(1):79, 1996.

Surratt N: Severe preeclampsia: implications for critical-care obstetric nursing, *J Obstet Gynecol Neonatal Nurs* 22(6):500, 1993.

Surratt N, Troiano NH: Adult respiratory distress in pregnancy: critical care issues, *J Obstet Gynecol Neonatal Nurs* 23(9):773, 1993.

Tomada S et al: First trimester biological markers for the prediction of pregnancy-induced hypertension, *Am J Perinatol* 13(2):89, 1996.

Ventura SJ et al: Advance report of final natality statistics: 1994, *Monthly Vital Statistics Report* 44(suppl 11):2, 1996.

Visser W, Wallengburg HCS: Temporising management of severe preeclampsia with and without the HELLP syndrome, *Br J Obstet Gynaecol* 102:111, 1995.

Ward K et al: A molecular variant of angiotensinogen associated with preeclampsia, *Nat Genet* 4:59, 1993.

Witry AW: Pulmonary embolus in pregnancy, *J Perinat Neonat Nurs* 6(2):1, 1992.

Witry AW: Pulmonary edema in pregnancy, *J Obstet Gynecol Neonatal Nurs* 21(3):177, 1992.

Working Group: Consensus report: national high blood pressure education program on high blood pressure in pregnancy, *Am J Obstet Gynecol* 163:1689, 1990.

Ziment I et al: Pregnancy and the lungs: cardiopulmonary complications, *J Respir Dis* 15(1):59, 1994.

Client Resources for Lupus

The American Lupus Society
3914 Del Amo Blvd, Suite 922
Torrance, CA 90503
(800)331-1802

Lupus Foundation of America, Inc.
4 Research Place, Suite 180
Rockville, MD 20850-3226
(800)558-0121

 Student Resource Shelf

Harvey M: Critical care for the maternity patient, *MCN Am J Matern Child Nurs* 17(6):296, 1992.
Emphasizes the collaborative role in high-risk care and presents several cases for illustration.

Richardson P: Body experience differences of women with pregnancy induced hypertension, *Matern Child Nursing J* 22(4):121, 1994.
Interesting research on how women with PIH feel about their pregnancies.

Roberts J: Current perspectives on preeclampsia, *J Nurse Midwifery* 39(2):70, 1994.
Complete review of pathophysiology and care for PIH.

Whitmer M: Home care of the patient who has pregnancy induced hypertension, *Home Health Nurse* 12(4):41, 1995.
Management at home involves the client and the nurse.

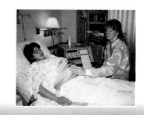

23

Medical Problems *during* Pregnancy

Learning Objectives

- Compare and contrast normal hemodynamic changes of pregnancy with alterations caused by medical problems during pregnancy.
- Apply steps of the nursing process to care of clients with medical problems during pregnancy.
- Describe the usage and risk factors of the various drugs given to a pregnant woman with medical problems.
- Plan care that supports independence in self-care for women with epilepsy, multiple sclerosis, or spinal cord injury.
- Formulate questions that encourage clients to discover their own strengths in self-care and planning for infant care.
- Identify preventive care in cases of maternal-fetal blood incompatibility.
- Identify types of trauma that have special risk for the pregnant woman.
- Describe the necessary adaptations in cardiopulmonary resuscitation for pregnant women.

Key Terms

Alloimmunization
Antiepileptic Drug (AED)
Asthma
Aura
Autonomic Dysreflexia
Erythrocytopoiesis
Generalized Seizure
Hemoglobinopathic Conditions
Isoimmunization
Partial Seizure
Postictal State
Status Asthmaticus
Status Epilepticus

*T*his chapter focuses on the cardiorespiratory, hematologic, and neurologic problems that can complicate pregnancy and delivery. Control of prior chronic illness must be reevaluated as to the effect of medications on the pregnancy and fetus. In some cases women may have improvement of their conditions; in other cases signs may worsen. In every case, self-care may be threatened, and the woman may become anxious about her own health and that of her fetus.

ASTHMA

Bronchial **asthma** is a complex chronic problem that includes airway hyperresponsiveness and obstruction. When airflow through the bronchioles and smaller bronchi is obstructed by bronchospasm, edema and inflammation of the mucous membrane and excessive mucus production result. There also will be wheezing and rhonchi. Major precipitants are inhaled allergens and certain foods. Other precipitants include chemical irritants, emotional stress, exercise, steroid withdrawal, and inhaler abuse.

Risk

Approximately 2% of women of childbearing age have a history of asthma. Approximately 33% to 40% of women have no change in asthma symptoms during pregnancy, 35% to 40% experience worsening of symptoms, and 18% to 30% have improvement (ACOG, 1996b). The risk to the fetus is related to effects of medications and hypoxia that may result from severe attacks. If asthma is poorly controlled during pregnancy, intrauterine growth retardation (IUGR) and low birth weight will occur. A higher risk of pregnancy-induced hypertension (PIH), preterm birth, or perinatal mortality are also present (Mabie et al, 1992).

Effect of asthma on pregnancy

When pregnant women describe an improvement in their breathing during the first trimester it is probably related to the increase in adrenal steroid hormones, cortisol and prednisolone, and to the higher levels of histaminase associated with pregnancy. Other women complain of attacks during the second and third trimesters, perhaps caused by emotional stress, weight gain, the pressure of the uterus against the diaphragm, or in some cases, PIH.

The risk of acute asthmatic attacks is higher during the third trimester. The increase in the severity of asthma symptoms is felt to occur at a time when progesterone, which inhibits glucocorticosteroid receptors, is near its pregnancy peak (Geiger-Bronsky, 1992). Respiratory tract infections should be avoided, and if they occur, they must be aggressively treated.

Although it is not common for a woman to have an asthmatic episode at the time of labor, episodes often will occur after a cesarean delivery and during recovery. An asthmatic woman is likely to repeat the same pattern of exacerbation with each pregnancy. The major risk to the woman is the development of **status asthmaticus**, a sustained period of reduced gas exchange.

Recent data suggest that increased asthma morbidity and mortality may be associated with increased use of bronchodilators in cases of worsening asthma. A woman may reduce regular medications, fearing its effect on the fetus, and thus precipitate asthma symptoms. A severe or even fatal attack can occur if the woman takes aspirin, nonsteroidal antiinflammatory drugs (NSAIDs) or certain prostaglandins.

Signs

During an asthmatic attack, dyspnea with a prolonged expiratory phase is accompanied by a productive cough with thick sputum, wheezing, decreased breath sounds, respiratory distress, and increased anxiety. These symptoms result from bronchospasm, mucosal edema, and increased secretions. Airway obstruction can occur in varying degrees and causes inequality of ventilation and perfusion. The other significant signs and symptoms of asthmatic attack include panic, fear, fatigue, hyperventilation, depression, irritability, anger, hostility, and rapid breathing.

A chest x-ray film is a standard diagnostic tool that reveals hyperinflation of the lungs. Pulmonary function tests are performed to evaluate the degree of obstruction. The usual findings are decreased vital capacity, increased residual volume, and decreased *peak expiratory flow rates* (PEFR). The PEFR is the most useful measurement, which is done by the client at home or in the clinic by exhaling into the portable flow meter. Unless PEFR rates exceed 80% of the best effort, bronchodilators are needed. After an hour of bronchodilator therapy, the PEFR rate should be greater than 40%, and if the rate is not above 70% in 4 hours, the client should be hospitalized (The Working Group, 1993).

To determine the presence of pulmonary infection, a white blood cell count (WBC) and sputum analysis is done. A sustained increase in respiratory distress may result in status asthmaticus. Blood gases become altered and indicate an advanced and dangerous stage of pulmonary obstruction. In these cases fetal oxygenation will be affected. The lives of the mother and fetus are in jeopardy.

Clinical Management

Treatment includes antiinflammatory therapy to decrease airway obstruction and relieve hypoxemia. Without this respite, chronic irreversible hypertrophy and other changes occur, which lead to disability and even death in young persons (Gift, 1991).

Albuterol and metaproterenol are beta$_2$ agonists with bronchodilator activity and are used with a metered-dose inhaler. Medications include other bronchodilators (terbutaline, epinephrine), anticholinergic drugs (aminophylline), cromolyn sodium, and glucocorticoids (beclomethasone, prednisone) (Cahalin and Sandowsky, 1995).

Supportive therapy including oxygen, hydration, and chest physiotherapy are performed. Intermittent monitoring of PEFR is essential to ensure that therapeutic goals are met (Anderson, 1991).

During labor, epidural anesthesia may be chosen. Because of respiratory compromise, narcotics and anesthesia that may depress respirations are used with caution. Fentanyl is safe, while morphine and meperidine should be avoided for epidural analgesia (ACOG, 1996b). Hydrocortisone given intravenously (IV) is used during labor for women who have received corticosteroids during pregnancy. Oxygen levels are monitored by pulse oximeter (SaO$_2$) during labor, and fetal responses are continuously monitored during labor.

Nursing Responsibilities

Nursing assessment and planning for treatment of chronic asthma requires early detection of bronchospasm. The client's self-monitoring of PEFR and comparing its rates with her best efforts will be important. In addition, clients should record events that precipitate attacks so that future attacks may be prevented. Assessment includes taking vital signs and noting the timing and dosage of medications in relation to precipitating events. The woman's compliance, understanding of the stresses of pregnancy, and knowledge of self-care and medication dosage need to be assessed.

Although asthma is a chronic health problem, the nurse should not assume that the client is fully knowledgeable. Some women who have lived with asthma since childhood may have a thorough knowledge of the disease and its required medications. Others may be less aware of self-care requisites or may not follow recommendations. Because an adolescent person with asthma often may be stressed by the chronic nature of the disease, she may not accept the rigorous self-care requirements, as demonstrated by omitting medication, exposing herself to stress or allergens, or overusing bronchodilators. The nurse needs to validate the asthmatic client's understanding of the cause, treatment, and impact of this disease on her present pregnancy.

Self-care should be promoted in every way because the client must manage her condition at home. The nurse can help her with analysis of potential stress areas and engage her in achieving the best prenatal health status for the sake of the developing infant. Because there is a psychosocial component to asthma, it is wise for the plan of care to include only one or two nurses in the woman's primary care (Geiger-Bronsky, 1992).

Box 23-1

CLINICAL DECISION

Randi, 16, tells you that when she gets an asthmatic attack, she puffs on her bronchodilator inhaler like a "house afire." What do you need to know before teaching her its correct use?

CARDIAC DISEASE DURING PREGNANCY

Pregnancy affects the cardiovascular system by normal physiologic changes in blood volume, decreased peripheral resistance, and increased arterial dilation. Blood pressure falls initially, and there is a wider pulse pressure. The increased blood volume may especially be a problem for a woman with cardiac compromise because the peak volume at 28 to 32 weeks of gestation will stress cardiac reserves. In addition, compression of the inferior vena cava by the gravid uterus in the third trimester also may cause significant changes in blood pressure (Roth, Riley, Cohen, 1992). Changes in hemodynamics are shown in Table 23-1.

A woman with a healthy heart can tolerate the stress of pregnancy, but when heart function has been affected by heart disease, pregnancy can be complicated. Major types of heart disease encountered in pregnant women are rheumatic heart disease with mitral stenosis, mitral or

---

Table 23-1 | **Hemodynamics in Pregnant and Postpartum Women**

	Third Trimester	Postpartum
SYSTEMIC CIRCULATION		
Heart rate (beats/min)	83 ± 10	71 ± 10
Central venous pressure (mm Hg)	3.6 ± 2.5	3.7 ± 2.6
Mean arterial pressure (mm Hg)	90.3 ± 5.8	86.4 ± 7.5
Cardiac output (L/min)	6.2 ± 1.0	4.3 ± 0.9
Stroke volume (ml/beat)	74.7	60.6
Systemic vascular resistance (dyne · cm · sec^5)	1210 ± 266	1530 ± 520
PULMONARY CIRCULATION		
Pulmonary capillary wedge pressure (mm Hg)	7.5 ± 1.8	6.3 ± 2.1
Pulmonary vascular resistance (dyne · cm · sec^5)	78 ± 22	119 ± 47

Modified from ACOG (1992), Easterling et al (1990).

aortic regurgitation, congenital heart anomalies, and heart changes resulting from hypertension.

Classification of Disability

An important determinant of whether a pregnant woman with heart disease will experience problems is the degree of disability caused by the heart disease. The following New York Heart Association functional classification of heart disease is accepted as a standard guide:

- *Class I:* No symptoms of cardiac insufficiency on exertion (uncompromised); no limitations on physical activity
- *Class II:* Symptoms felt on ordinary exertion (slightly compromised); slight limitation of physical activity
- *Class III:* Symptoms felt even during limited activity (moderately compromised)
- *Class IV:* Symptoms occurring during any physical activity, even at rest (severely compromised)

Symptoms may be confused with normal effects of pregnancy, and further evaluation is necessary. Signs that a cardiac condition is deteriorating include the following:

- Shortness of breath or fatigue during usual activities of daily living (ADL)
- Frequent coughing, with or without hemoptysis; rales at lung bases
- Feelings of palpitations or recognized arrhythmias
- Development of generalized edema

Overall Risk

It is estimated that some form of heart disease occurs in 1% to 2% of pregnant women. Cardiac disease is a leading cause of indirect maternal mortality (ACOG, 1992). The following four major aspects must be considered for all cardiac clients:

- Increased vascular volume by the third trimester may not be tolerated and may lead to decompensation with heart failure.
- Cardiac output is greatly affected by pregnancy, labor, and the early dramatic changes in blood volume after delivery that result when pressure on the great vessels is suddenly released and blood from the uterus returns to the central circulation.
- Systemic vascular resistance is decreased fostering right-to-left shunts in certain cases.
- Anticoagulants are often prescribed because of the increased risk for thrombus formation, and clients must be observed carefully for hemorrhage.

Rheumatic heart disease

Rheumatic heart disease (RHD) is the most common cause of heart disease encountered in childbearing women. RHD previously accounted for 60% to 80% of all heart disease during pregnancy, but because of improved childhood treatment, its incidence has decreased to less than 50% of these women (Gilbert and Harmon, 1993). RHD must be considered when a pregnant woman complains of chest or joint pains or if she has a history of rheumatic fever or a current unexplained fever, with dyspnea and orthopnea, which are signs of congestive heart failure. RHD sequelae may include mitral valve stenosis, mitral insufficiency or prolapse, or damage to the atrial, triscuspid, or pulmonary valves.

Mitral stenosis. This is a result of recurrent inflammation with group A beta hemolytic streptococcus infection. The resultant scar tissue causes stenosis of the mitral valve, which restricts cardiac output because blood flow from the left atrium to the left ventricle becomes obstructed. Pressures then become elevated in the left atrium, pulmonary veins, and pulmonary capillaries. As the left atrium becomes distended, pulmonary congestion can cause symptoms of dyspnea and orthopnea. Pulmonary artery pressures may increase, causing failure of the right side of the heart. The normal increase in cardiac output, slight tachycardia, and normal fluid retention of pregnancy contribute toward deterioration in the woman's functional status. Because there can be fixed cardiac output, tachycardia results from a stress demand. The greatest risk for these clients occurs immediately postpartum because of the sudden increase in blood volume. In addition, because of the acquired hypercoagulable state of pregnancy, thrombi can form rapidly within the enlarged chamber. Fibrillation can dislodge the thrombi and cause systemic arterial embolism (Kennedy, 1995).

Mitral prolapse or regurgitation. This may be caused by RHD, previous endocarditis, or, rarely, structural factors. The client complains of fatigue related to a decrease in blood flow from the left ventricle. It usually is a much less severe condition than that resulting from mitral stenosis. Some clients with mitral regurgitation remain symptom free for years, even during pregnancy.

Aortic stenosis. This results from RHD. Because cardiac output is limited, the greatest stress is during the highest demand—later pregnancy and birth. Angina, syncope, and even myocardial infarction can occur with severe aortic valve stenosis (ACOG, 1992).

Aortic regurgitation and insufficiency. This occurs as a result of RHD, endocarditis, rheumatic arthritis, systemic lupus erythematosus, or Marfan syndrome. Because of aortic valve incompetence, some of the left ventricle output flows back into the left ventricle during diastole. The left ventricle dilates in an effort to compensate. The increased left ventricle pressure may cause pulmonary congestion. There is a risk of infection related to invasive procedures. With rest, this condition sometimes is tolerated during pregnancy.

Congenital heart disease

The number of women with *congenital heart disease* (CHD) has increased because of better survival as a result of treatment during early childhood. Women with successfully repaired childhood defects will have little or no problem during pregnancy. The degree to which the woman's condition is compromised depends on the defect. Some women have left-to-right shunts because of an atrial septal defect or a patent ductus arteriosus. Some women are unaware of defects until they reach adulthood or become pregnant. These defects often are tolerated by the well-monitored pregnant woman, unless pulmonary hypertension or preeclampsia develops.

Any woman with CHD who shows cyanosis or clubbing of the fingers must be counseled about the risks of pregnancy for herself and her fetus. Management includes symptomatic interventions and curative measures such as repair of the defect, cardiac surgery, and cardiac transplantation. Although the number of cardiac transplants for chronic end-stage disease, CHD, and primary pulmonary hypertension has increased during the past 20 years (Jordan and Pugh, 1996), it is rare for a woman to attempt pregnancy.

Dissecting aortic aneurysm. Aortic aneurysm is a rare but dangerous occurrence in childbearing women. It is associated with Marfan syndrome, an autosomal dominant inherited disorder of the connective tissue. Necrosis and tearing may occur in the aortic wall, possibly resulting from the increased blood volume and a general softening of collagen during pregnancy. Because of the characteristic location, it is thought that these tears are caused by the systolic force. Aortic branches can become occluded, and the aortic valve can become detached. The mortality rate is 25% to 50% (ACOG, 1992).

Heart disease related to hypertension

Women with chronic hypertension may exhibit heart disease. Recently many women have postponed childbearing until their later years. Some of these women have stressful careers, live fast-paced lives, or have poor health habits and are candidates for cardiovascular problems. (See Chapter 22 for discussions on hypertension).

To diagnose hypertension, current studies support the importance of evaluating the client within the context of her clinical symptoms and not by blood pressure changes alone (Green and Froman, 1996). Once the diagnosis is established, maternal and fetal risks of distress will depend upon the severity of the hypertension.

Peripartum cardiomyopathy

In a woman with no prior history of cardiac disease the onset of gradually increasing fatigue, dyspnea, and peripheral or pulmonary edema signals a condition that is puzzling and carries a high risk. This cardiomyopathy may develop in the last month of pregnancy, with a peak at 2 months postpartum and as long as 6 months postpartum. There is evidence in 50% of the women of a pulmonary or systemic embolus. The left atrium and ven-

tricle are dilated, and there is reduced ventricular strength, jugular venous distention, rales, and an S_3 gallop. Pulmonary edema and cardiomegaly are diagnosed by chest x-ray film. Supportive therapy is used because causes are unknown. Digitalis, diuretics, low sodium diet, and bed rest are standard in cardiac care. The condition gradually resolves, but if this condition recurs with another pregnancy, the outcome is grave.

Clinical Management for Cardiac Insufficiency

Clinical management should be directed toward increasing the cardiac output and preventing complications by prompt interventions. An important consideration for clients who have RHD and mitral stenosis is maintenance of left *preload,* or the volume of blood in the left ventricle at end diastole necessary for adequate cardiac output (Kennedy, 1995). If preload is too low, the ventricle cannot contract adequately, and tachycardia follows. If preload is too high, muscle fibers will be overstretched (see Table 23-1). *Afterload* measures the amount of pressure resistance in the aorta as the left ventricle empties and is related to the volume of blood in the system and the degree of vasoconstriction or vasodilation of the vessel walls. Afterload is also called *systemic vascular resistance* and is measured by blood pressure readings. The higher the afterload, the more force is required to open the aortic valve (Gilbert and Harmon, 1993) (Figure 23-1).

Physical examination reveals objective symptoms, such as generalized edema, rales at the lung bases, and cardiac arrhythmias such as murmurs. The clinical diagnosis of heart disease requires a complete physical examination, x-ray films to determine cardiac enlargement, electrocardiogram (ECG), and examination by ultrasound or echocardiogram. Anemia and infection increase cardiac workload; testing is included in prenatal care.

Appointments are scheduled more frequently, especially between 28 and 32 weeks of gestation when blood volume reaches its peak. If cardiac status is deteriorating, hospitalization may be needed for stabilization. Anticoagulants are often prescribed to prevent formation of emboli (see the discussion on heparin in Chapter 22).

There is risk of infection related to invasive procedures. In the presence of cardiac defects or RHD, endocarditis can develop as a result of invasive procedures, including vaginal delivery and cesarean section. Endocarditis might cause further damage to the impaired mitral valve or might injure other vessels or valves (Kennedy, 1995). Therefore prophylaxis against streptococcal endocarditis is indicated whenever there are invasive procedures, even dental work or cleaning tartar off teeth.

General labor precautions

Monitoring during labor of clients with class III or IV disability may include central hemodynamic monitoring

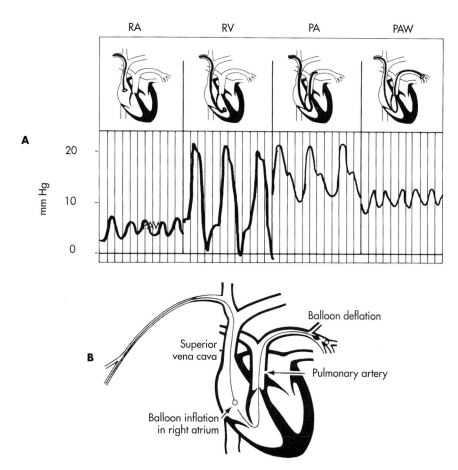

Figure 23-1   A, Flow-directed, balloon-tipped catheter locations with corresponding pressure tracings. **B,** The balloon-tipped catheter enters the right atrium and "floats" through the right ventricle and out to a distal pulmonary artery branch. The balloon is deflated, advanced slightly, and reinflated slightly to obtain a pulmonary artery wedge pressure (PAW). (From Schroeder JS, Daily EK: *Hemodynamic monitoring* (slide series), Tarpon Springs, Fla, 1976, Tampa Tracings.)

(see Figure 23-1) because fluid balance is critical during labor and recovery. Electrocardiographic continuous readings will be noted on the same schedule as fetal monitoring. Positioning to avoid vena caval compression is critical. Semi- or high-Fowler's position may need to be modified with a lateral tilt. Oxygen is delivered by mask, and oxygen saturation is measured by pulse oximeter. Pain must be managed to reduce stress and heart rate. Low-dose morphine and low-dose bupivacaine via epidural catheter have been found useful (see Chapter 16).

Delivery is accomplished as smoothly as possible. Cardiac stress from surgical delivery is *equal to* or *greater than* that from vaginal delivery; therefore operative delivery usually is done only for obstetric reasons (ACOG, 1992). Vaginal birth must be in a semi- or high-Fowler's position. Vaginal birth must be accomplished without intense pushing. Open glottis pushing to prevent Valsalva's maneuver is important. Forceps or vacuum extraction (VE) will be used to reduce maternal efforts at delivery.

Positioning in a semi-Fowler's position, nasal oxygen, and cardiac monitoring will be continued during recovery.

Nursing Responsibilities

Care focuses on assessment, education, and monitoring of compliance, often with restrictive activity levels and medication routines. The woman must be thoroughly involved in care decisions.

NURSING DIAGNOSES

- Activity intolerance related to cardiac limitations, exacerbated by pregnancy
- Altered cardiac output related to infusions during labor or anesthesia and during recovery as a result of fluid shifts.
- Altered comfort related to anxiety, contractions, and central hemodynamic monitoring during labor

- Potential for infection or phlebitis related to method of birth, susceptibility to valvular disease, and thromboembolism
- Altered parenting related to stress, anticipatory grieving, fatigue, and activity restrictions
- Risk for impaired fetal perfusion related to maternal hemodynamics and oxygenation

EXPECTED OUTCOMES

- Maintains health using diet, rest, and medications
- Maintains tissue perfusion and optimum cardiac status at every phase of pregnancy and birth
- Remains free of infection or thromboembolism
- Monitors medications, effects, and cardiac symptoms and reports problems promptly
- Finds ways to cope with stress of pregnancy or anticipatory grief
- Fetal growth and development within normal limits

NURSING INTERVENTION

Nursing interventions are directed primarily at optimizing cardiac output and preventing complications (Kennedy, 1995). The primary nursing problems are alteration in cardiac output and activity intolerance. Activities and interventions include helping the woman to minimize the stress of her pregnancy and to preserve her cardiac function. Assess frequently for vital signs, subjective symptoms, and activity tolerance. An appropriate activity level will be evaluated and established by the physician and supported by the nurse. Counsel the woman about her activity limitation and her needs for sleep and rest periods to improve cardiac reserve. Explore for knowledge deficits about medications and nutritional demands of pregnancy, and reinforce the woman's positive self-care behaviors.

At this time the woman and her family have many concerns about the birth. Anxiety and ineffective coping are common during the third trimester. There may be anticipatory grieving related to the loss of fetal or maternal health (see Chapter 26). The nurse must offer emotional support during such a high-risk pregnancy when the woman may be hospitalized.

Labor and delivery can be stressful for the woman and fetus. The management of the birth depends on the recent functional classification of the woman's disability, the progress of labor, and the response of the woman and fetus to labor stress. The main goals during the intrapartal period are to reduce maternal exertion and promote cardiac reserve. Promote relaxation throughout labor while monitoring maternal vital signs, fetal heart rate, and labor progress. Continuously monitor maternal cardiac status. Position the woman in a lateral position with the head and chest elevated to promote cardiac emptying and placental perfusion. Give oxygen by mask because laboring women usually breathe by mouth. Diuretics, digitalis, and analgesics must be accessible if needed. Monitor IV fluids carefully to prevent fluid overload.

The second stage of labor is especially stressful. The woman who is allowed to push is instructed to prevent the Valsalva maneuver by using shorter open-glottis pushes. She must not become short of oxygen by holding her breath. The woman is encouraged to relax between pushes. She should be allowed to follow her own instinctive desires to push rather than being forced to bear down with each contraction (Cosner and deJong, 1993).

After expulsion of the placenta, even with blood loss during delivery, additional blood volume may strain the woman's cardiac reserves. Extravascular fluid now moves into her bloodstream, and blood flow through the heart is greatly increased for approximately 1 week. Continuous cardiac and postpartum monitoring and laboratory tests are used to assess the maternal condition for at least 48 hours.

Because there is a potential for infection, prophylactic antibiotics are administered during labor and throughout the postpartum period. The woman should be in a private room if possible. She must be protected until clinical evaluation reveals that she is free from bacterial endocarditis. Bed rest is crucial for women with classes II, III, and IV disability until cardiac function is stabilized and increased activity and progressive ambulation are tolerated. This activity limitation poses other problems. Constipation is a particularly serious problem for the woman with cardiac disease because she should not strain during bowel movements. She should receive high-fiber food, adequate fluid intake, and prescribed stool softeners to draw water into the stool. A self-care deficit exists, and total or partial care is necessary, depending on her status.

The nurse will need to work on the alteration in parenting roles related to the separation of the newborn from its mother. If the mother is fatigued, the infant should be kept at the mother's bedside while a nurse or family member provides infant care and feeding. A weak mother should not exert herself or lift the infant. Touching and eye contact are important for establishing an emotional bond between mother and infant. Although women with class I or II disability usually can breast-feed without any problem, antibiotics or other medications must be evaluated for potential effects on the newborn. Usually, because lactation presents increased requirements for rest and nutrition, class III and IV cardiac clients do not breast-feed.

Home care

Discharge requires careful nursing assessment and planning. The mother needs to balance her requirements for rest and her energy potential with her parenting responsibilities. Together, the nurse and woman must evaluate her self-care capability. The available home support for the mother and infant must be evaluated.

Appropriate home referrals must be initiated promptly. In discharge instructions, include the first postpartum visit schedule, newborn care pamphlets, immunization plan, postpartal exercise handout, drug regimen, and dietary allowances. Make sure the written discharge instructions include the telephone numbers of the mother's obstetrician, social worker, liason nurse, and support groups. In addition to normal postpartum blues, the drug regimen may put these clients at greater risk for emotional instability during the immediate postpartum period (Jordan and Pugh, 1996). Encourage the partner to report if there is increased irritability or crying episodes plus marked mood swings (see Chapter 26). The importance of emotional support cannot be overstated (Jordan and Pugh, 1996).

EVALUATION

* Has her cardiac functional status changed and stabilized?
* Did infection or thromboembolism occur?
* Did monitoring detect problems that could be quickly corrected?
* Is the woman knowledgeable regarding self- and infant care?
* Is the infant's growth and development within normal limits?

ANEMIAS DURING PREGNANCY

The major function of red blood cells (RBCs) is to transport oxygen to the tissues. When the number of RBCs is deficient, tissues do not receive enough oxygen because of *anemia*. Inadequate blood production to maintain a normal hemoglobin level may result from a variety of causes including lack of building blocks for blood cells such as iron, folic acid, and vitamin B_{12}. Hormonal stimulation for erythrocyte production also may be inadequate, and the bone marrow structure or the hematopoietic (blood-producing) stem cells in the marrow may be damaged.

Iron Deficiency Anemia

Iron deficiency anemia is 10 times more common than other anemias (Beischer and MacKay, 1993). Iron is essential for oxygen transport and is incorporated into hemoglobin. Iron deficiency is strongly suggested when hemoglobin concentrations are below 11 g/dl and the hematocrit (Hct) value is less than 32%. *Hemoglobin* is the oxygen-carrying pigment of RBCs, and *hematocrit* is a measure of the size, capacity, and number of RBCs, in ratio to plasma. In addition, serum ferritin levels below 12 ng/mL indicate iron depletion (Long, 1995). See Chapter 10 for iron absorption from the diet and the iron stores in an infant at birth. Also see Box 10-3 for a list of teaching points to enhance iron intake during pregnancy.

Risk

Iron deficiency anemia can develop because of inadequate dietary intake, alcohol abuse, increased need for iron as a result of pregnancy, excessive blood loss at birth, and closely spaced pregnancies (Figure 23-2). Populations at greatest risk for iron deficiency anemia are women, minorities, low-income groups, infants younger than the age of 2, and the elderly. Malaria, intestinal parasites, lack of iron-rich foods, poor eating habits, cultural differences, and nonavailability of adequate nutrients increase the risk of iron deficiency in the body. Other factors related to anemia are postpartum hemorrhage, often more than is recorded (see Chapter 21). Insufficient milk in first-time mothers who show signs of dehydration may be a result of anemia (Henly et al, 1995). There is a risk of an increase in preterm labor associated with iron deficiency but not necessarily with low hemoglobin levels (Long, 1995).

Signs

A major symptom of anemia is an activity intolerance. When tissues do not receive enough oxygen, the body attempts to compensate by increasing cardiac output and respirations. The woman may complain of weakness or fatigue when performing normal activities. In addition, she may have sensory-perceptual alterations such as dizziness and light-headedness. She may appear more pale than usual.

There may be a combination of signs such as significant fatigue, fainting, and susceptibility to infection (Henly et al, 1995). The diagnosis is confirmed by looking at the reduced blood values. See Table 23-2 for a list of tests used to determine anemia.

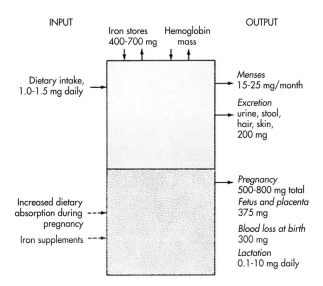

Figure 23-2 Iron balance in nonpregnant women compared with iron demands of pregnancy.

Table 23-2   Tests for Iron Deficiency Anemia

Tests	Normal Results
Hemoglobin	>11 g/dL
Hematocrit (Hct)	>32%
Mean corpuscular volume (MCV)	>82 fl
Mean corpuscular hemoglobin (MCH)	>27pg
Serum iron levels	>30 μg/dL
Serum ferritin	>12 ng/mL
Transferrin levels	>15%
Serum protein/albumin	3.5 g/dL
Red blood cell count	>3.75^6 mm^3
Serum folic acid	>3.5 ng/dL

Clinical management

Usually, an iron supplement of 30 mg/day is recommended during the second and third trimester. Without supplementation or an improvement in dietary iron intake, more severe iron deficiency anemia and decreased fetal iron stores can develop. On rare occasions, parenteral iron is administered IV or intramuscularly (IM) when response to oral intake of iron is poor.

Other authorities do not recommend routine iron supplementation unless the blood studies show a clear indication. In fact, heavy iron intake and a high hematocrit level have been associated with an increase in preterm birth and low birth weight (Enkin et al, 1995). Studies have been conducted regarding daily administration of iron and clients' compliance with the schedule. Recent findings that weekly doses of oral iron were as effective as daily doses may change the methods of administration, cutting down on the side effects and increasing compliance (Stephenson, 1995).

Folic Acid Deficiency

Folic acid is required for the synthesis of deoxyribonucleic acid (DNA) and the maintenance of normal levels of mature RBCs. Folic acid deficiency results in macrocytic or megaloblastic anemia, which is characterized by large immature RBCs. Pregnant women are especially susceptible to this condition because of the increasing demand for this vitamin by the trophoblast, the rapidly developing fetus, and the expanding maternal RBC mass. The normal nonpregnant daily requirement is increased sixfold or sevenfold during pregnancy (see Chapter 10).

Risk

Folate deficiency is common in all parts of the world and is the second most frequent cause of anemia during pregnancy in the United States. It occurs in approximately 15% to 20% of clients who are anemic during pregnancy (Enkin et al, 1995). The studies have shown clear evidence that periconceptional folic acid supplements are associated with a reduction in the risk for first occurrences of neural tube defect and for recurrence of neural tube defects among women with a previously affected pregnancy. The highest rates for neural tube defects occur among certain ethnic groups, such as the Welsh, Irish, and Sikhs (Criezel and Dudas, 1992). The use of periconceptional folic acid can be expected to reduce, but not abolish, the incidence of neural tube defects.

Clinical management

Treatment of folate deficiency consists of oral supplementation of 1 mg/day during pregnancy and lactation. The dosage may be increased up to 4 mg/day in pregnant women with alcohol dependency and in those with chronic infections, hemolytic anemia, or anticonvulsant therapy. Because a woman who has previously had a child with neural tube defects is at higher risk for having an infant with the same problem, she is advised to take 4 mg/day folic acid before becoming pregnant, if she intends to have another pregnancy, then for the first 3 months of pregnancy. Exceptions are women taking the anticonvulsant valproic acid or women with vitamin B$_{12}$ deficiency (Enkin et al, 1995).

Nursing considerations

When a primary health need is information, the nurse and client should collaborate to develop a plan of care. The woman should be instructed to take iron preparations between meals to enhance its absorption (see Box 10-3). She should avoid ingestion of iron with substances such as tea, coffee, and calcium-containing foods, such as milk and milk products, including but not limited to ice cream and cheese. Antacids usually contain calcium and will inhibit iron absorption.

In addition, the nurse identifies foods rich in iron and folic acid and emphasizes the importance of their daily inclusion in the diet. When appropriate, she is given information about the interaction of folic acid with alcohol, antibiotics, chronic infections, and anticonvulsants. Untoward effects such as constipation and gastric irritation should be reviewed, and the client should report these symptoms to her health care provider.

TEST *Yourself* **23-1** _____

a. Which iron-bearing foods would you recommend to a vegetarian?
b. Which substances inhibit iron absorption?
c. Which substances interact negatively with folic acid?

Glucose-6-Phosphate Dehydrogenase

Glucose-6-phosphate dehydrogenase (G6PD) deficiency is an enzyme disorder (enzymopathic condition) that shortens the survival time of RBCs. The deficiency is carried on the female sex chromosome and therefore is expressed more often in male offspring. However, because of its frequent incidence, women also have G6PD.

Risk

G6PD is commonly found in people who have immigrated from the regions shown in Figure 23-3. It is prevalent in southern Europe and northern Africa in much the same pattern as thalassemia. Another variation of G6PD is found in high rates in certain Jewish populations as well.

After insult with a stressor such as a food or chemical, rapid hemolysis of RBCs takes place; the client suddenly becomes anemic. Hemolytic jaundice develops as the bilirubin level rises as a result of the increased rate of RBC destruction.

Diagnosis of G6PD is made by the methemoglobin reduction test. Methemoglobin is an enzyme that helps the hemoglobin of the RBCs to be in the reduced (deoxidized) state to bind with oxygen. The oxidized form of hemoglobin is useless for oxygen transport. Withdrawal of the offending drug, plus folic acid and iron supplementation, nutrition counseling, and drug education, are vital components of care.

Nursing considerations

During the prenatal history of women of African, Mediterranean, Asian, or Middle Eastern descent, the nurse asks about any episodes of jaundice of unknown origin, notes whether the woman has been anemic, and asks if she has ever been tested for G6PD. In addition, the client is assessed for signs of anemia.

The nurse asks the names of prescription and over-the-counter (OTC) medications that the woman is taking or has taken in the past. The nurse should emphasize the following: (1) avoid infections, and get prompt medical attention if infection occurs; (2) review with the client a written list of medications that induce hemolytic anemia, including name, purpose, and potential side effects; (3) identify for the client the problems she will encounter using OTC analgesics such as compounds that contain aspirin or sulfa drugs that may be inadvertently prescribed. Emphasize the importance of follow-up medical care. Finally, all newborn infants are now screened for this enzymopathic condition, and the mother should be informed if her infant has G6PD.

HEMOGLOBINOPATHIES

The impact of hemoglobinopathies during pregnancy generally parallels the severity of the maternal anemia.

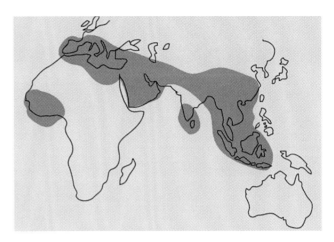

Figure 23-3   Areas where thalassemia is most often found. (Courtesy National Foundation March of Dimes, White Plains, NY)

Pregnancy, with its increase in oxygen consumption, increase in blood viscosity, and increase in red cell mass, may be associated with significant morbidity in women with abnormal hemoglobin (ACOG, 1996a).

Thalassemia (Cooley's Anemia)

Thalassemia has a distinctly different mechanism and effect from iron deficiency anemia. Thalassemia is characterized by anemia caused by decreased or defective production of RBCs. This health deviation is widespread; it is genetically determined and found commonly in 4% to 6% of persons of southern Italian, Greek, or Cypriot origin and in other Mediterranean countries, as well as in persons from Asia (see Figure 23-3). Immigration patterns have made this type of anemia a concern in the United States and Canada (Chui, Wong, Scriver, 1991). Any woman from these areas of the world should be tested for thalassemia if anemia is discovered. The varying severity of anemia is related directly to the degree of defect in either of the alpha or beta chains of the hemoglobin molecule.

Risk

Those with defects in both beta chains of the hemoglobin molecule have *thalassemia major,* a serious chronic disease (Cooley's anemia, Mediterranean anemia), and rarely become pregnant. If only one of the beta chains is affected, the person is heterozygous for beta thalassemia. *Thalassemia minor* is mild, and its signs vary widely. Some persons are completely free of symptoms; others have episodes of severe anemia. This heterozygous form may be combined with sickle cell trait (Figure 23-4) and also may occur in 2% of African-Americans (Mayberry et al, 1990).

Signs

Fewer RBCs are produced, and cells have a shorter life span. As a result hemoglobin values may range from 5 to

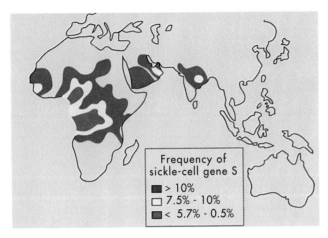

Figure 23-4   Areas where sickle cell S and C disease is seen in greatest numbers. (From Kan YW: *Hemoglobin abnormalities,* New York, 1982, Academic Press.)

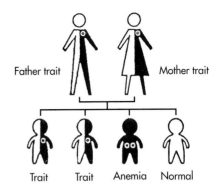

Figure 23-5   Genetic inheritance risk for sickle cell anemia. (Courtesy National Foundation March of Dimes, White Plains, NY)

9 g/dl, and Hct values may range from 15% to 30%. Bilirubin levels may be elevated as well, reflecting RBC destruction. Laboratory tests to establish mean cell volume (MCV) and mean corpuscular hemoglobin (MCH) can detect abnormal erythrocyte populations. Normal MCV range is 82 to 98 fl and the MCH is 27 to 31ng (see Table 23-2). Values below these suggest thalassemia. There may be several anemic episodes during pregnancy plus increased PIH and hemorrhage.

Clinical management

Treatment of thalassemia includes complete blood count (CBC) and skeletal x-ray. Folic acid and vitamin B complex are prescribed because each is necessary to stimulate the production of RBCs, WBCs, and platelets. The woman is checked for many other complications such as enlarged spleen, pain, hepatic failure, cardiac failure, and chronic infection. The couple may be referred to genetic counseling. The client is advised to take pneumococcal and meningococcal vaccines.

Sickle Cell Hemoglobinopathies

More than 1000 possible genetic abnormalities affect the production, structure, and function of hemoglobin, The most common of these are found in clients with sickle cell disease (Hb SS), sickle cell trait (Hb AS), sickle C disease (Hb CC), or a combination of sickle cell with sickle C disease (Hb SC). These **hemoglobinopathic conditions** are inherited equally by men and women.

In the healthy population, approximately 97% of adult hemoglobin is composed of Hb A; the rest is Hb A_2 and Hb F (Table 23-3). In contrast, the person with sickle cell anemia has primarily Hb S. Sickle cells have a half-life ($t_{1/2}$) of 5 to 20 days compared with 120 days for a normal RBC. Thus bilirubin levels are higher, and immature cells are present in larger quantities.

Table 23-3   Hemoglobin Types

Type	Normal (%)	Sickle Cell Anemia (%)	Trait (%)
Hb A (adult)	95	0	60
Hb A_2	2-3	2-3	2-3
Hb F	< 1	< 2	< 1
Hb S	< 1	80-90	35-40

Sickle cell trait

Approximately 8% of African-Americans have only Hb AS and are *carriers* of the affected gene. Hb AS is also found in persons of Mediterranean, Caribbean, Latin American, and Middle Eastern descent. These persons have approximately 35% to 40% Hb S but are symptom-free. Symptoms rarely occur in this relatively benign condition, and pregnancy is not associated with any adverse maternal or fetal effects, unless infection or hypoxia occurs. Pregnant clients with Hb AS, however, have a 13% rate of asymptomatic bacteriuria and should have regular urine cultures during pregnancy (ACOG, 1996a).

Sickle cell disease

Sickle cell disease is genetically inherited and must be carried by both parents (Figure 23-5). It can occur as Hb SS, Hb S–beta-thalassemia, or Hb SC. Hb SS is most commonly seen in African-Americans but is also found in immigrants from the areas shown in Figure 23-4.

If the person has sickle cell anemia there is no Hb A present (see Table 23-3). When oxygen tension is decreased by any cause, RBCs containing Hb S assume a sickle shape and the form of a rigid, semisolid gel (Figure 23-6). Intravascular sickling results in stasis of blood flow, accelerated erythrocyte destruction, and increased blood viscosity, which causes the cells to flow poorly through the vessels. This "sludging" results in tissue hypoxia, ischemia, and microinfarcts in the affected organs, especially the kidney, spleen, bones, lungs, and

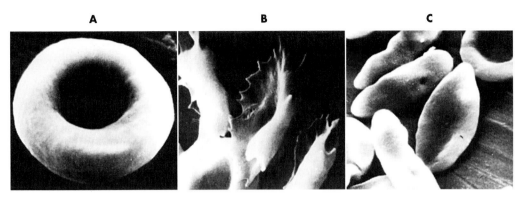

Figure 23-6   Process of sickling and unsickling of red cells. **A,** Stereoscan electron micrograph of normally oxygenated red cell showing classic biconcave disk with central cavity and slight surface irregularity. **B,** Deoxygenated cells take on typical holly-leaf sickle shape. If reoxygenated, cells unsickle. Process may progress to irreversible state. **C,** In oxygenated state, irreversibly sickled cells have characteristic oval or cigar shape with smooth membrane. If deoxygenated and then reoxygenated, cells return to this shape. (From Lessin, Jensen, Klug: Sickling damages red-cell membrane, *Medical World News,* Jan 26, 1973.)

gastrointestinal tract. The diagnosis of vaso-occlusive crises during pregnancy is difficult, because its symptoms may be confused with those of other conditions such as appendicitis, pneumonia, stroke, angina, and infectious arthritis (ACOG, 1996a). Women with vaso-occlusive crisis are also more prone to infections.

Risk. In the United States the incidence of sickle cell anemia is highest among African-Americans. However standard testing of all newborns in the United States shows approximately a 0.3% rate of the trait in the entire group (see Chapter 19).

The impact of the disease on future offspring is a major concern. A child conceived by two parents with Hb AS will have a 50% chance of carrying the trait and a 25% risk of having sickle cell anemia. The same risk accompanies sickle C trait (see Figure 23-5).

Infertility and early abortion are not related to crises and are not increased in clients with Hb SS, but preterm labor and growth restriction are more common than in women with normal hemoglobin. Stillbirths, which are increased in most series of studies, appear to be related to severe maternal vaso-occlusive crises (ACOG, 1996a). The other risk factor can be a reduction in oxygen pressure at high altitude and the risk associated with dehydration. There are dangers of splenic infarcts or dehydration related to the exposure of high altitudes.

Signs. Vaso-occlusive episodes involving multiple organs are the chief problem of sickle cell anemia. The most commonly affected sites are the extremities, joints, and abdomen. However, sickle cell anemia can affect every organ system. Osteomyelitis caused by *Salmonella* organisms can occur. Sickling may occur in the renal medulla, resulting in papillary necrosis. Because of chronic hemolysis and decreased RBC survival, clients often have jaundice. In addition, the increased cardiac work imposed by chronic anemia can cause left ventricular hypertrophy, cardiomegaly, and congestive heart failure.

Clinical management. The care of the pregnant woman with sickle cell anemia requires collaboration among health team members and a thorough understanding of the effect of sickle cell anemia on the woman and the developing fetus. Because of vulnerability to infections, urine cultures should be performed frequently. Any infection should be treated immediately because a hemolytic crisis may be precipitated. The client will be monitored for CBC, hemoglobin, and serum iron studies. Ultrasonography, nonstress testing, and contraction stress testing may evaluate fetal condition. The pregnant woman should be provided with supportive nursing care for pain management, hydration, oxygenation, and bed rest as the need arises during antepartal, intrapartal, and postpartal periods.

As soon as pregnancy is confirmed, a folic acid supplement of 1 mg/day is begun. Although hemoglobin and hematocrit levels are decreased, iron supplements are not routinely given because, according to Enkins et al (1995), heavy iron intake may increase the risk of premature delivery and low birth weight. If, however, serum iron levels (which should be checked monthly) become low, the client may be advised to take daily iron supplementation. The goal is to maintain hemoglobin above 10 mg/dL and hematocrit above 28%.

Additional oral fluids maintain hydration, and fluid intake is a major self-care intervention to prevent the precipitation of a crisis. Hydration is important to decrease viscosity of the blood and to improve circulation. Drinking six to eight glasses of liquids daily is recommended.

Some perinatal centers give *prophylactic* transfusions to pregnant women with sickle cell anemia. Transfusions usually begin after 28 weeks of gestation. Transfusion protocols may administer either simple transfusions or exchange transfusions of RBCs every 4 to 6 weeks, plus erythropoietin to maintain a percentage of HB A of at least 50% and a packed cell volume of at least 25% (ACOG, 1996a).

Erythrocytopoiesis means formation of RBCs, and recombinant erythropoietin is a genetically engineered substance that may be used to stimulate formation of RBCs.

During labor, the client should be in the left lateral recumbent position and receive supplemental oxygen. Adequate hydration should be maintained. Unless complications occur, vaginal delivery is preferable to a cesarean birth.

Hemoglobin C disease

Hemoblobin C disease is a less common hemoglobinopathic condition carried by 1 of 4 persons in some African-American groups and 1 of 50 persons in some Hispanic groups (ACOG, 1996a). Clients with hemoglobin AC have no symptoms. Clients with the combination Hb SC have mild symptoms. Health problems may not be noticed until a hemolytic crisis occurs during pregnancy. Although pregnant women with Hb CC have fewer episodes of illness than do women with Hb SS, an increased incidence of early spontaneous abortion and PIH does occur. Prenatal care should be the same as that provided to clients with Hb SS.

Nursing Responsibilities

ASSESSMENT

Nursing assessment of the client's knowledge of self-care practices and support systems is important. Stress, exertion, and dehydration can increase sickling and precipitate a crisis. Explore with the client which coping mechanisms she has used. Maladaptive behaviors should be evaluated and alternatives suggested. To assess the client's status and to enhance her ability to care for herself, the nurse must know potential risks and complications and interventions that may improve perinatal outcome.

NURSING DIAGNOSES

- Increased risk of infection related to anemia
- Knowledge deficit regarding preventive self-care practices and factors that can precipitate hemolytic crisis
- Potential altered tissue perfusion related to decreased circulation secondary to inflammatory process and occlusion of blood vessels
- Acute pain related to vaso-occlusive episodes
- Altered fetal growth and development related to maternal crises and anemia

EXPECTED OUTCOMES

Depending on the severity of the sickle cell disease the following outcomes may be chosen:

- Exhibits balanced fluid intake and elimination with no infection
- Nutritional intake promotes adequate weight gain and iron intake
- Applies measures that reduce potential for hemolytic crisis
- Complies with treatment regimen
- Fetal growth and development within the normal range

NURSING INTERVENTION

Help the client meet her self-care needs through information, counseling, promotion of self-care, referrals, and collaboration with other health care professionals. Encourage her to take the prescribed medication. She is given information about the interaction of folic acid with alcohol, antibiotics, chronic infections, and anticonvulsants.

Nutritional counseling helps the woman identify foods high in folic acid and iron. Emphasize daily intake of folic acid with vitamin C. If iron supplements are also prescribed, discuss information about self-administration and side effects. Untoward effects such as constipation and gastric irritation can be reviewed, and encourage her to report these problems to her health care provider.

Infection is a major hazard. Explain how to prevent infection by avoiding sick people and crowds. In addition, encourage her to drink adequate fluids; cranberry juice is helpful in changing urinary pH. Clean-catch urines will be collected monthly to monitor for urinary tract infections.

EVALUATION

- Did urinary tract infection occur?
- Has she complied with recommended treatment, and was weight gain adequate?
- Did hemoglobin and hematocrit remain within normal limits for her degree of severity, and were crises avoided?
- Was the infant full term, of average gestational age, and neurologically normal?

MATERNAL AND FETAL BLOOD INCOMPATIBILITY

During pregnancy maternal-fetal blood incompatibility may place the fetus at risk. There are two major types of blood incompatibility between mother and fetus: incompatibility between major blood groups A, B, or O, and the Rh negative factor with the Rh positive (D) factor.

Rh-Factor Incompatibility

The Rh factor is a group made up of the C, D, and E factors of the RBC. Although there are more than 43 blood factors that can cause maternal antibody reactions, the D antigen is

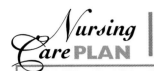 *Nursing Care* PLAN | *Sickle Cell Anemia*

CASE

Naome E. is a 23-year-old African-American woman with sickle cell anemia in her first trimester of pregnancy. Physical examination reveals a short, underweight woman. Vital signs are within normal limits. Laboratory studies reveal a borderline normal erythrocyte count, low hemoglobin and hematocrit values (9.4 g/dl and 28%, respectively). The results of a hemoglobin electrophoresis were Hb F 20%, Hb A$_2$ 3%, Hb S 77%, and Hb A 0%. A peripheral blood smear reveals sickled forms of RBCs, a positive sickle test result, and a blood type of O+.

Assessment

1. Lack of knowledge of precipitating factors or care for hemolytic crisis during pregnancy
2. Verbalizes fear for self and fetus
3. Inadequate dietary and fluid intake; weight gain less than expected
4. Compare urine values, blood values with norms

Nursing Diagnoses

1. Knowledge deficit regarding factors in pregnancy that precipitate hemolytic crises
2. Acute anxiety related to health of developing fetus
3. Alteration in nutrition: less than body requirements
4. Potential for infection related to lowered resistance

Expected Outcomes

1. States factors that precipitate hemolytic crises; identifies measures that prevent episodes, including adequate hydration
2. Gains at least 25 pounds during pregnancy; selects a balanced diet that includes foods rich in folic acid, iron
3. Uses methods to decrease risks of infection; takes in adequate fluids
4. Experiences uneventful pregnancy and successful birth outcome

Nursing Interventions

1. Provide written and verbal information. Discuss effective self-care measures. Provide information about community resources. Review factors that precipitate sickle cell crises.
2. Assist client in identifying ways to decrease anxiety. Help client focus on positive coping behaviors that reduce anxiety.
3. Consult with nutritionist regarding dietary requirements. Perform nutritional assessment at each antepartum visit. Review sources, and reinforce importance of folic acid, dietary iron intake.
4. Identify ways to prevent infection. Review sources of infection and preventive care, including extra fluid intake. Monitor urine during each visit.

Evaluation

1. Can she state causes, signs, and symptoms of sickle cell disease and use of measures to promote health and prevent hemolytic crisis?
2. Has she identified and used community resources?
3. Is her weight gain in the range of at least 25 pounds during pregnancy? Did she report taking folate supplements daily and eating a diet high in iron and folic acid?
4. Were urine specimens free of pathogens?
5. Did hemoglobin levels remain above 10 g/dl and hematocrit above 28%?
6. Was the newborn of average size for gestational age and full term?

the major stimulus. In rare instances, the infant may be affected by C and E factors, Kell antibodies, and other even more rare factors on the blood cell (ACOG, 1990).

Because the Rh-negative cell group is inherited as a *recessive trait,* a child must inherit the same type of genes from both parents to express the Rh-negative trait like the mother. If the father is Rh positive, the child will be heterozygous for the C, D, or E factors (see Chapter 28). There is enough of a difference between positive and negative factors so that if fetal cells enter the maternal blood, an antibody-antigen reaction is set up in the mother in the same way that a reaction to a poorly typed blood transfusion may occur. The fetal cells are recognized as being a "foreign" protein, and specific antibodies are formulated to attach to and destroy these cells. The maternal reticuloendothelial system will now "remember" this reaction, and if similar foreign proteins are again encountered (in the next pregnancy), the system will rush to her defense. Thus if a woman becomes sensitized during one pregnancy, all subsequent pregnancies can be affected if the fetus is a different type from the mother. The mechanism of becoming sensitized or forming antibodies against antigens from the same species is **isoimmunization,** or **alloimmunization.**

Approximately 15% of the European-American population in the United States have the Rh-negative factor. Incidence is lower in the African-American population (5%) and the Asian-American population (1%).

The placenta is usually an effective barrier to the transfer of fetal RBCs. However, fetal RBCs may cross through minute breaks in the placental interface, which may occur in the following:

- Infarction of the placenta
- Trauma during abortion, ectopic pregnancy, and abruptio placentae
- Small tears occurring as the placenta separates from the wall of the uterus during antepartal fetal hemorrhage or at the time of birth
- Amniocentesis

After unusual procedures such as chorionic villus sampling (CVS), percutaneous umbilical cord blood sampling (PUBS), and fetal surgery, most physicians also administer preventive treatment (see Chapter 11).

In addition, a D-negative woman may become sensitized to the D factor if she received a poorly typed blood transfusion containing cells of the wrong type. Finally, if she has received blood products such as platelets or granulocytes, there is a small chance of RBCs being included;

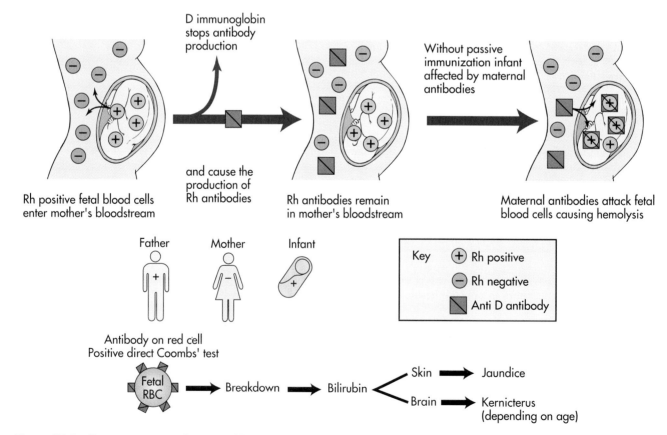

Figure 23-7   D isoimmunization because of Rh incompatibility between a Rh negative mother and a Rh(D) positive fetus.

as little as 0.03 mL of D-positive blood is enough to initiate the reaction (ACOG, 1990) (Figure 23-7).

Risk

There is no risk to the mother. The risk to the fetus varies with the antibody titer; the higher the titer, the more affected the fetus will be. Fetal cells are destroyed by the specific antibodies, and the fetus becomes anemic. (See Chapter 29 for the discussion of care of the newborn). A breakdown product of hemoglobin is bilirubin. The newly born infant will not appear jaundiced because maternal excretion of bilirubin takes place before the birth. Jaundice levels rise sharply in the early hours after birth. The younger the gestational age, the more serious high levels will be because the blood-brain barrier allows easier transfer of bilirubin to deposit in the brain tissue, causing *kernicterus* and brain damage (Figure 23-8).

Clinical management

The best solution to this problem is prevention of the initial reaction. Today few cases of Rh incompatibility are seen in women who receive adequate medical care during their reproductive lives. However women who have immigrated from other countries or have received little or no prenatal care during a prior pregnancy may be vulnerable and already sensitized. All women who receive prenatal care are screened early in pregnancy. ABO and blood type will be tested, and blood will be screened for antibodies against the D factor. At 28 to 29 weeks of pregnancy, D-antibody screening should be done for women who are Rh D negative and whose partners are Rh D positive.

Coombs' test. The Coombs' test detects the presence of antibodies in maternal serum (*indirect* Coombs' test) or detects if antibodies are attached to the infant's RBCs (*direct* Coombs' test). If the woman's indirect Coombs' titer is positive, it is too late to prevent isoimmunization. A positive indirect Coombs' test result means that the mother's body is already producing antibodies against the fetal D factor. If the woman is sensitized already (has formulated anti-D antibodies), her antibody titer is checked as frequently as every 2 to 4 weeks throughout the remainder of the pregnancy. An increase in the titer indicates that the process is worsening, and the fetus will be in jeopardy unless intervention occurs.

Kleihauer-Betke test. The Kleihauer-Betke test is most often used to determine the presence and amount of fetal RBCs transfused into the maternal serum. This test is done when potential fetal-to-maternal-transfusion is possible and serves to determine the dosage of immunoglobulin administered to the mother. Other tests are the Rosette and Fetaldex tests.

Passive immunization. Injection of immunoglobulin prevents isoimmunization of the D-negative woman who bears a D-positive fetus (only if the process has not yet begun). A serum concentrate containing pooled anti-D antibodies (immune globulin) is administered after a potential "insult" or infusion of fetal blood into the maternal system. These *extrinsic* (not the mother's) antibodies will "recognize" the D antigen and begin the destruction of the foreign fetal cells. The maternal system then is protected by this *passive immunization* from receiving an imprint, a code that makes such antibodies again.

The woman must be immunized each time a fetal or maternal transfusion occurs, especially after abortion and other fetal treatment. She must receive the correct dose

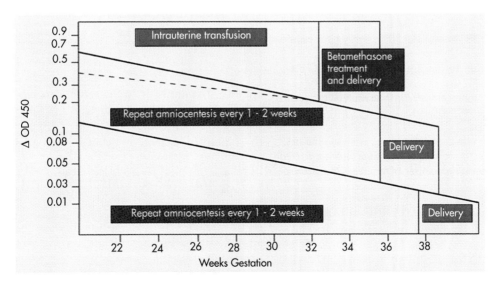

Figure 23-8   Modified Liley curve used for management of the Rh-sensitized fetus. ΔOD 450 of amniotic fluid is plotted against gestational age. Decisions concerning delivery are made on the basis of zone at which coordinates cross. (From Branch DW: Isoimmunization in pregnancy. In Gabbe SG et al: *Obstetrics: normal and problem pregnancies,* New York, 1986, Churchill Livingstone.)

within 48 to 72 hours after birth of a live or stillborn infant of any gestational age. Currently, each D-negative, unsensitized woman receives immunoglobin at 28 to 29 weeks of pregnancy.

Doses of immunoglobulin vary according to the estimate of fetal transfusion (see Drug Profile 23-1). Because 20 µg of immunoglobulin protects against approximately 2 mL D-positive RBC, the larger dose given after delivery protects against 30 mL of fetal blood (ACOG, 1990). The woman's blood is crossmatched with the dose, and the immunoglobulin is given by deep IM injection, using the Z-track method. There should be no side effects. The woman is given complete information about her condition and the injection and takes home a card recording the date of immunization.

Administration of D immunoglobulin is a standard of care; an omission by neglect or error constitutes malpractice (see Chapter 30). Therefore in every case of a D-negative woman's care during pregnancy, birth, and recovery, the following measures must be ensured:

Box 23-1
DRUG PROFILE

Rh$_0$D Immune Globulin (Rh IG)
(Gamulin RH, HypoRho-D, MICRhoGAM, RhoGAM)

ACTION
Suppress immune response of nonsensitized D or D^u negative clients exposed to Rh$_0$, D, or D-positive blood cells.

DOSE AND ROUTE
Deep IM by Z-track method within 48-72 hr of possible exposure.
Prophylaxis: at 28 wk, one vial 300 µg; may be repeated at 34 wk.
After abortion or miscarriage <13 wk: one RhIG dose (50 µg).
After ectopic, amniocentesis, or invasive fetal procedure > 13 wk: one vial (300 µg).
After birth at any age: before 72 hours if negative Coombs' test and D-positive infant, one vial (300 µg).
Dosage adjusted by results of Kleihauer-Betke test (slide smear to determine number of fetal cells in maternal circulation).

SIDE EFFECTS AND ADVERSE EFFECTS
Only local warmth, aching. Rare allergic reaction.

PRECAUTIONS
Must be crossmatched with sample of client's blood. Informed consent; give identification card. Drug repeated as needed during and after each pregnancy with an Rh-positive fetus.

- Check mother's blood type and Rh factor on clinic laboratory reports
- Alert midwife or physician if woman is of D-negative status; flag chart to note Coombs' test results
- Ensure that immunoglobulin is given on schedule if invasive procedure (amniocentesis, CVS) performed during pregnancy
- Ensure correct dose given after abortion at any week
- Alert labor, postpartal, and nursery staff to woman's Rh and Coombs' titer status
- Administer dose within 48 to 72 hours after birth to an Rh-negative, unsensitized (Coombs' negative) woman whose infant is Rh (D) positive. This is important to remember with early discharge of mother and infant.

In cases where sensitization has already occurred, titers are determined biweekly during the third trimester. If titers continue to rise, the woman is scheduled for amniocentesis to obtain amniotic fluid to test for the presence of bilirubin (indicating severe hemolysis of fetal cells). This bilirubin will have been excreted in fetal urine because levels are higher than the maternal excretory processes can handle. Depending on the readings (optical density at 450 nm wavelength) the decision is made regarding an intrauterine fetal blood transfusion to partially correct fetal anemia or early delivery. Hemolytic disease of the newborn (HDN) is rare today, but once the process is activated, the fetus may die from severe anemia or *erythroblastosis fetalis*.

ABO Incompatibility

ABO incompatibility occurs when a woman with type O blood has a child fathered by a man with an A, B, or AB blood type. Genetic inheritance of one factor from each parent leads to these six possible genotypes in the ABO blood groups:

Homozygous	Heterozygous
OO	AO
AA	BO
BB	AB

The antibody in the serum depends on which antigen is in the RBC. For example, if a person has type B antigen, anti-A antibodies are in the serum (Table 23-4). This problem is more frequent in the type O mother because

Table 23-4   ABO Antigen Placement

Type	Antigen in Red Cell	Antibodies in Plasma
O	None	Anti-A, Anti-B
A	A	Anti-B
B	B	Anti-A
AB	A and B	None

she already possesses *a* and *b* agglutinins (i.e., anti-B and anti-B antibodies). These antibodies may cross the placental barrier and interact with the A or B factors in the erythrocytes of the fetus. Interestingly, when D and ABO incompatibility exist at the same time, the anti-A or anti-B antibodies in the maternal serum usually suppress her production of D antibodies (ACOG, 1990).

ABO may account for approximately two thirds of the isoimmunization that leads to neonatal problems, but effects on the infant are much less severe than Rh incompatibility. These combinations are possible:

Mother	Infant
O	A, B, or AB
A	B
B	A

Problems occur most frequently with a type O mother and a type A infant, less commonly with a type O mother and type B infant, and rarely in the other combinations.

Currently no procedure exists for preventing ABO incompatibility. There are no blood or amniotic fluid tests to distinguish between naturally present *a* or *b* agglutinins (antibodies) in a type O mother's serum and an increased titer resulting from introduction of fetal RBC with A or B antigens. Fortunately, ABO incompatibility usually is less severe because these naturally occurring maternal antibodies are weaker in hemolytic effect than are D antibodies. No special testing is done before birth.

Newborns affected by ABO incompatibility will show evidence of problems by a positive direct Coombs' test result and may show jaundice in the first 3 days of life. However, ABO does not lead to pathologic jaundice levels in most instances. See Chapters 18 and 29 for assessment and care of these infants.

NEUROLOGIC PROBLEMS DURING PREGNANCY

Neurologic disorders form a diverse group of health deviations in pregnancy, ranging from annoying conditions (headache) to life-threatening conditions (intracranial hemorrhage).

Epilepsy

Epilepsy is a major neurologic disorder that complicates pregnancy. Epilepsy is characterized by recurrent seizures that are the symptoms of abnormal electrical discharges in the brain. There is a wide variety of seizures that cause problems in motor, sensory, or conscious function. Seizures commonly are classified into two groups: **partial seizures,** which are localized or originate in a specific part of the brain, and **generalized seizures,** which involve the entire brain simultaneously. In pregnant women, generalized tonic-clonic (*grand mal*) or similar convulsive seizures are of greatest concern because of potential harm to the fetus.

Most epilepsy is *idiopathic* (no clearly determined cause), but some cases are due to conditions such as congenital anomalies, head injuries, intracranial tumors, meningitis, hypoxia, toxin exposure, hypoglycemia, hypoparathyroidism, and excessive hydration. In persons with a lowered threshold for seizures, a seizure may be precipitated by bright lights, fatigue, stress, and excessive use of or withdrawal from drugs or alcohol. Finally, psychologic stress, physical fatigue, and anemia may contribute to a lowered seizure threshold.

Risk

Seizures tend to increase during pregnancy in more than one third of epileptic women. Seizure frequency is thought to be related to low levels of **antiepileptic drug** (AED), noncompliance in taking AEDs, and possibly maternal sleep deprivation. The normal physiologic alterations in blood volume during pregnancy can lower the concentration of AEDs in the blood. Nausea and vomiting, decreased gastric motility, and increased extracellular fluid may change the distribution of anticonvulsants and thus lower serum levels.

Not all seizures carry the same threat to the fetus. The potential for hypoxia and acidosis are greatest with generalized convulsive seizures and with **status epilepticus,** a series of seizures with little or no recovery in between.

Antiepiletic drug risks. Noncompliance in taking AEDs may be related to the pregnant woman's concern about teratogenic effects. All AEDs have substantial *teratogenic risks.* Valproic acid has been linked to the higher rate of neural tube defects. Phenytoin has been more frequently associated with fetal malformations than other AEDs, but this may be due to its widespread use. Other drugs used to treat seizures include carbamazepine, phenobarbital, primidone, ethosuximide, and benzodiazepine derivatives such as clonazepam. Women taking anticonvulsants during pregnancy have malformation risk of approximately 5%, which is approximately double the general risk. The defects include neural tube defects, microcephaly, growth deficiency, developmental delays, mental retardation, and dysmorphic craniofacial features (ACOG, 1996c).

AEDs have been associated with depressed folate levels, which can result in anemia and be a possible factor in fetal defects. Long-term use of phenytoin can lower vitamin D levels in the mother. All AEDs depress vitamin K–dependent clotting factors, which can result in fetal and neonatal hemorrhage. The teratogenic risks of these drugs appear to be dose-dependent, so the therapeutic goal is to use the lowest dosage that can adequately control seizures.

Effects on newborn. AEDs may produce neonatal depression, which is characterized by sedation, hypotonia, and poor breathing or sucking. The symptoms appear at birth and disappear within 2 to 8 days. Withdrawal symptoms develop in some newborns, including excessive crying, disturbed sleep, hyperactivity, tremors, myoclonic jerks, hypertonia, hyperreflexia, hyperventilation, hyperphagia, vomiting, sneezing, and yawning.

Breast-feeding is not totally contraindicated for women with epilepsy depending on the specific drug. Many AEDs are excreted in breast milk, which can be a concern. If a mother decides to breast-feed, she should discuss her decision with her physician, observe the suggestions about timing doses in relation to feeding times (see Chapter 17), and observe the infant for any unusual symptoms.

TEST *Yourself* **23-2** _____

> a. Which physiologic changes of pregnancy might lower the AED during pregnancy and thus precipitate a seizure if dosage is not adjusted?
> b. Name two factors that the client herself can control to decrease the likelihood of seizures.
> c. Why is a generalized seizure of greater concern during pregnancy than a partial one?

Clinical management

As indicated, a variety of problems can cause seizures. Consequently, testing is extensive but varies according to individual history and circumstances. Laboratory tests usually include taking electroencephalograms (EEG) with the client awake and asleep, skull x-ray films, and computerized tomography (CT) or magnetic resonance imaging (MRI) scans of the brain to detect skull injury or lesions. Radiation risk from CT scans is minimal when the client is properly shielded. An MRI involves no radiation, and no harmful effects on the fetus have been established. If metabolic problems are the suspected cause of seizures, serum electrolyte, calcium, magnesium, and glucose levels are obtained. Ultrasonic scanning should be done by 16 to 18 weeks' gestation to evaluate the fetus for possible anomalies. Echocardiography, serial ultrasound studies, and amniocentesis also are performed to evaluate the status of the fetus.

If seizure control is not achieved with one drug, others may be added until better control is achieved. However, because teratogenic risks also increase when more than one AED is used, monotherapy is preferred during pregnancy. Treatment of known underlying causes is instituted. Counseling or psychotherapy is recommended when the client has poor coping abilities or low self-esteem related to the disorder.

When possible, the woman should be prepared for conception. Attempts are made to gradually withdraw the anticonvulsant and substitute a less potentially teratogenic drug. During this process of AED adjustment, anticonvulsant drug levels should be monitored weekly until the woman is stable. Once medication doses keep the client within a therapeutic range, she can then be advised to conceive.

In some cases, discontinuation of AED therapy during pregnancy may be possible if the client has been seizure-free for a long period. This is a complex decision that needs to be made after thorough evaluation.

Labor and recovery. Depending on dosage, anticonvulsant drugs continue to be given during labor. In addition, drug levels are monitored frequently during the postpartum period, and the client is carefully observed for warning signs of seizures.

Supplements. Daily vitamin supplements and folic acid should be taken before conception. Women taking AEDs may be given vitamin K supplements in the last month of pregnancy, and neonates may be given additional vitamin K to prevent hemorrhage. Folic acid usually is prescribed. Women who are taking phenytoin should take supplementary vitamin D throughout pregnancy.

Nursing responsibilities

Assessment of status always should include the frequency and type of seizures that have occurred. The characteristics of any warning signs of a seizure, such as eye movement, changes in consciousness and body movement, and the **postical state** (after seizures), are all important observations. The client may be able to provide some of this information. If alteration in consciousness occurs, description must come from observers. The nurse also can explore with the client if there were any precipitating factors before the seizure, such as stress, fatigue, or alcohol ingestion.

Inquire if her family, friends, and co-workers are aware of what to do if a seizure occurs. During pregnancy it is particularly important that the woman with epilepsy has a clear understanding of her prevention and treatment plan, including factors she can control such as stress or fatigue.

Monitoring medications. The nurse must help the client understand the risks and benefits of her AEDs during pregnancy. Plans for testing AED levels, dietary supplements, and follow-up evaluation need to be coordinated with the neurologist and obstetrician so that holistic care is given. Ensure that the client is familiar with warning signs and symptoms of toxicity.

Assessment of AED compliance is crucial. Nonthreatening questions such as, "How are you taking your medications? Is it hard to remember them? Do you have any concerns about your medications?" may elicit more information than accusing a person of failing to take medication. It also is important to assess the client for any signs of drug toxicity and to determine if she knows what those signs are and when to report them to the physician. The following are signs of drug toxicity:

- Ataxia
- Blurred vision or diplopia
- Nausea (may be confused with pregnancy changes)
- Lethargy or other symptoms of the specific AED

Discuss the woman's plans to minimize stress and lack of sleep, and assess how pregnancy is affecting her diet and vitamin intake. Check the early nausea of pregnancy to see if she is tolerating her doses. Encourage her to express fears related to fetal outcome. Additional counseling may be needed if anxiety is overwhelming. Referrals to local epilepsy support groups have been helpful.

After the birth, AED dosage may be continued at the same level, but blood levels must be checked within a few weeks. Be sure the woman is made aware of signs of withdrawal in the infant and when to report the effects to the physician. For the parents whose infant has a congenital defect, special support and information will be needed.

Headache

Almost 30% of women in the United States suffer from headaches that may continue to be a problem during pregnancy. There are a variety of types of headache with varying or unknown causes. Generally, they may be classified as the following:

- Vascular, such as migraine, cluster, or hypertensive headaches
- Muscle contraction tension headaches
- Traction and inflammatory headaches related to brain tumors, cranial hemorrhage, strokes, temporomandibular joint disease, and various other diseases of the ears, eyes, nose, throat, and teeth

Migraine headaches

Because there seems to be a relationship between steroid hormone levels and migraines, pregnancy often affects migraine status. In pregnancy, a complete cessation of migraines or a decrease in frequency often occurs. This usually begins in the third or fourth month and does not seem to be related to emotional status. It is possible, however, for migraines to continue and even become aggravated during pregnancy.

The International Headache Society, aiming at greater precision, renamed migraine categories "migraine with aura" and "migraine without aura" (Silberstein and Niebyl, 1994). Migraine with or without aura may be associated with premonitory sensations that develop hours to days before the headache attack. Examples include hyperactivity and hypoactivity, depression, irritability, difficulty in concentrating, or food cravings, especially chocolate (Silberstein and Niebyl, 1994). Migraines have a wide variety of frequency, duration, and intensity. The headache usually starts on one side of the head and may be accompanied by anorexia and then nausea and vomiting. In classic migraines, a visual, sensory or motor **aura** (sensation) precedes the headache.

Muscle contraction headaches

These are characterized by a sensation of pressure or aching that usually is bilateral and may cover the head like a tight cap. There is a sustained contraction of muscles around the scalp, and no aura precedes the pain, which may last for a few hours or as long as several months. There are many theories about the causes of these headaches, including vascular, muscular, and psychologic factors.

Traction and inflammatory headaches

These are infrequent but can indicate serious problems. They may be caused by inflammation or displacement of cranial structures and are characterized by an ache that becomes continuous and progressively worse. Coughing or straining precipitates or aggravates the pain. Symptoms of neurologic impairment may appear. The cause may be an intracranial tumor, which can grow rapidly during pregnancy because of fluid shifts or hormonal stimulation.

Finally, *intracranial hemorrhage* is characterized by severe explosive headache that requires immediate interventions to avoid death. Headache related to a stroke or cerebrovascular accident is more likely to occur during the puerperium.

Although this last type of headache can have severe, life-threatening causes, it also can be characteristic of more benign disorders of the head and neck. Assessment is needed before any hasty conclusions are drawn. Information to assess origin and significance of the headache is noted in Box 23-1. A headache of acute onset with no previous history and with progressive symptoms is more cause for concern than a characteristic headache in a person who has a history of migraines or muscle contraction headaches that may have been thoroughly evaluated. During pregnancy, increases in frequency or severity of any headaches are signs that need further evaluation.

TEST *Yourself* **23-3** _____

Match the headache type with its typical characteristic.
1. Migraine   a. Coughing makes pain worse
2. Muscle contraction   b. Feels like a tight cap over head
3. Traction-inflammatory   c. Often preceded by an aura

▌ *Box* **23-1** | **Assessment Questions for Headaches**

Is there a history of similar headaches?
If so, have you been seen by a physician?
Describe the onset; was there a prodrome or aura?
Where is the pain located?
How would you describe the character and duration of the pain?

Are there associated symptoms such as photophobia, nausea, vomiting, or neurologic symptoms?
Did you lose vision in part or all of an eye even temporarily?
Can you pinpoint any aggravating factors?
Can you describe any relieving factors you have tried?

Clinical management

When a headache has new onset, a complete health history and physical examination are performed, and laboratory tests such as CBC, sedimentation rate, blood glucose, urinalysis, and ECG may be ordered to rule out systemic causes. Depending on the headache profile, other procedures may be ordered, such as EEG, thermographic examination, x-ray studies of the skull, spine, and paranasal sinuses; CT and MRI scans; and a lumbar puncture.

It is preferable to use nonpharmacologic interventions during pregnancy (Lewith, 1996). Biofeedback and relaxation techniques are effective for both migraine and muscle contraction headaches. During the migraine, comfort measures such as the use of ice packs for at least 12 minutes and rest in a dark quiet room can be helpful. Some migraines have trigger factors that can be minimized; examples are fatigue, heat, and fasting for more than 5 hours during the day or 13 hours at night. Some may find that certain chemicals trigger migraines; these include tyramine, phenylthylamine, nitrites, and monosodium glutamate (MSG). Offending foods include red wine, chocolate, aged cheese, caffeine, alcohol, and hot dogs (Hainline, 1994).

In addition, psychologic interventions such as expressing emotions, adjustment of work patterns, or modification of other stress factors may be useful. Physical interventions such as a cervical collar or dental treatment may help if muscle contraction headaches are caused by a poor alignment.

Drug therapy. When the woman is not pregnant, muscle contraction headaches commonly are treated with acetaminophen, acetylsalicylic acid (ASA), diazepam, and amitriptyline. Except for diazepam and ASA, these are used during the first trimester with minimal risk for the fetus (Khurana, 1992). Of the commonly used migraine drugs, *ergotamine* is avoided because of its oxytocic potential. Meperidine and acetaminophen may be used to treat acute migraine attacks during pregnancy. Propranolol and amitryptyline sometimes are used despite some risk of growth retardation with propranolol. The use of multiple drugs is discouraged, and prophylactic drugs usually are discontinued 2 weeks before delivery. As with any drugs used during pregnancy, a woman should have a clear understanding of the *benefit-to-risk ratio* before taking the drug.

Nursing considerations

A nurse may be the first health care provider contacted regarding a headache. Take a thorough health history to ascertain if further evaluation is needed. Certainly the pregnant client should be referred to her physician for the acute development of a progressively severe headache, especially if there has been no history or work-up in the past. An increase in frequency and severity of any headache should be evaluated.

Even if the headache is benign, the client will need reassurance and education about alternative measures to pharmacotherapy. If drugs have been the only therapy in the past, it may be a daunting prospect to face a headache without such intervention. The client needs to explore ways to reduce stress or identify triggers once she realizes that such factors may contribute to headache. Pregnancy is an opportunity for the women to assume more initiative in preventing and treating her headaches without dependence on drugs. If medication is necessary to achieve adequate relief, describe the risk and appropriate doses. In any case the primary goals are to support the client and assist her in obtaining adequate pain relief while minimizing risk to the fetus.

Box **23-2**

CLINICAL DECISION

Choose the first three questions to ask Debra, 3-months pregnant, who calls to say, "I have a terrible headache! What should I do?"

Peripheral Nervous System Disorders

Two common peripheral nervous system disorders that can occur in pregnancy are carpal tunnel syndrome and Bell's palsy (Table 23-5). These conditions are basically benign but can cause a good deal of discomfort, inconvenience, and even debilitation (Rosenbaum and Donaldson, 1994). Because the initial symptoms may be alarming to the client, prompt diagnosis is helpful. She will need supportive symptomatic care as she waits for her symptoms to resolve (Felsenthal, 1992).

Multiple Sclerosis

The onset of multiple sclerosis (MS) is most common between the ages of 20 and 35, and women are twice as likely to be affected as men. The etiology of MS is unknown, but recent theories suggest that some environmental factor, possibly a viral infection, triggers an autoimmune attack on the central nervous system myelin in a person with a genetic susceptibility. Because treatment is limited and often ineffective and the course of the disease so unpredictable, the psychologic challenge of coping with MS is tremendous. The individual's degree of disability does not necessarily determine the psychosocial problems a person with MS may have. Physical limitations are one factor, but other factors such as social support, how she perceives her condition, and her relationship with care givers and health care providers seem to contribute also. Sometimes a person with minor physical limitations may experience severe psychosocial problems, and a person with pronounced physical limitations may be able to adjust surprisingly well.

Table **23-5**	Bell's Palsy and Carpal Tunnel Syndrome

Characteristic	Effect
BELL'S PALSY	
Unilateral seventh cranial nerve facial weakness	Facial weakness and paralysis of one side of forehead and lower portion of face
Occurs in third trimester or within 2 weeks of third trimester	Client may be concerned she has had a partial stroke; thus prompt diagnosis is helpful
Cause unclear; may be related to edema, hormonal changes in pregnancy, or a virus	Treatment usually is symptomatic, with eye patch, artificial tears, facial massage, and exercises as needed; if lesion is severe, corticosteriods may be used
	Generally resolves in 3-12 weeks after birth.
CARPAL TUNNEL SYNDROME	
Compression of median nerve at the wrist	Burning or numbness in fingers that may arouse client at night and may be relieved by shaking the hands
More often in dominant hand	Weak lifting and grasping ability
Onset is usually between 4-9 months of pregnancy	Splinting the wrist may help; other treatments are nonsteroidal antiinflammatory drugs or local steroid injections
Possible causes: edema, relaxation of transverse carpal ligament	Most cases resolve spontaneously and gradually by 3 months postpartum; surgery may be used in the few cases that do not resolve

Risk

Pregnancy and multiple sclerosis. MS does not affect a woman's fertility and has little impact on the course and outcome of a pregnancy. Pregnancy does not cause MS; in fact the onset of MS is less likely *during* a pregnancy. The condition of most women with MS stabilizes or improves during pregnancy, particularly during the second and third trimesters. This effect is thought to be due to the physiologic *immune suppression* that occurs during pregnancy. At this time, research does not show that pregnancy has any worsening effect on the overall course of MS, but after birth there is a high risk of a relapse or exacerbation in the first 3 to 6 months (Rosenbaum and Donaldson, 1994). This factor is important to consider in planning child care and postpartum work schedules. Although a susceptibility to MS is inherited, the risk of transmitting it to the infant is not present.

Signs

MS is characterized by episodic inflammation and demyelination in the brain, optic nerves, and spinal cord. A wide range of symptoms may result, depending on the specific areas affected. Motor and visual impairment are common. Urinary problems and spasticity can occur, and some clients with MS have impairment of cognitive or emotional functions. The client usually has periods of exacerbation and remission that occur in unpredictable patterns, with a gradual decline in overall neurologic function. In rare cases there is a progressive form that has no remissions and results in death in a few months. The general course of the disease, however, can be long, with an average duration of more than 30 years.

Clinical management

There is no effective treatment in the long-term course of MS. Acute exacerbations may be treated with high-dose corticosteroids or adrenocorticotropic hormone (ACTH) in an attempt to shorten the duration of the event, but these treatments may or may not have any effect. Treatment with immunosuppressive drugs is being tried, but with unclear results. Physical therapy and orthotic devices can help maximize physical abilities. The person with MS also is often advised to obtain adequate rest and avoid excessive exposure to sunlight and heat, factors that may cause exacerbations. Spasticity and bladder dysfunction or infections may be treated with various medications. Psychosocial support and counseling often are important components of adequate care for a person with MS.

The effect on the client's ability to perform self-care and to care for her child is a primary factor to consider in the discussion with the health care provider. Other factors influencing her ability will be the economic situation, social support, and adaptation to the disease. A discussion of MS treatment during pregnancy also is appropriate. Prednisone and ACTH should be avoided if possible, especially in the first trimester. Low doses of prednisone for short periods may be used later. Because the use of immunosuppressive drugs has been associated with some fetal malformations, a careful consideration of the benefit-risk ratio is necessary. Avoidance of anemia is important. Persons with MS tend to have more urinary tract infections and may need prophylaxis with nitrofurantoin or ampicillin.

Labor and delivery are managed routinely. The rate of exhaustion may be higher, resulting in use of VE more often. Because of a possible link with relapse, spinal anesthesia is avoided; epidural is believed to be safer (Goldstein and Stern, 1992). If the woman is being treated with more than 10 to 20 mg prednisone, she must receive steroid coverage during labor and delivery, usually hydrocortisone administered IM or IV.

Breast-feeding is not contraindicated in women with MS. It does not seem to cause or prevent exacerbations. Often, however, the woman is advised to avoid exhaustion, which might mean that night feedings of milk pumped during waking hours be given by someone else. If the mother is being treated with drugs, she should discuss the advisability of breast-feeding because of potential adverse effects on the infant.

TEST *Yourself* 23-4 _____

a. What self-care advice is needed for pregnant women with MS?
b. Which types of infections most frequently affect women with MS?
c. When as a result of pregnancy does risk of MS exacerbation occur?

Spinal Cord Injury

The most common causes of spinal cord injury in women are motor vehicle accidents, followed by falls, acts of violence, and sports-related injuries (Goldstein and Stern, 1992). Some women who have been injured desire to become pregnant, whereas others are injured during the pregnancy. In the latter case the care and needs of the woman are multiplied as she adjusts to her injury and to its impact on her pregnancy.

The challenges faced by a pregnant woman with a spinal cord injury vary, depending on the level of her injury and disability. In addition to the cord level of the lesion, the degree of disability depends on whether the lesion is complete or incomplete, which establishes if some motor or sensory function is left below the level of injury. Paraplegia usually is not a contraindication to vaginal delivery as long as the injury did not include pelvic fractures or occur before puberty, both of which could cause insufficient pelvic diameters. In any case the woman herself is likely to be the most accurate source for information on her abilities and limitations.

Risk

As rescue and treatment modes improve, more victims of trauma are surviving. There are approximately 10,000

spinal cord injuries in the United States every year, and one fifth of those injured are women. Because many are young women, fertility is unaffected and a desire for a family may coexist with varying degrees of motor impairment. Chief problems to be managed during pregnancy are urinary tract infections, autonomic dysreflexia, and decubitus ulcers.

Clinical management

Urinary tract infections are common problems for women with spinal cord injuries, especially because of the use of catheters for bladder management. Because the likelihood of urinary tract infection increases during pregnancy as a result of hormonal changes, frequent urine cultures and sometimes prophylactic antibiotics are used to manage infection. As pregnancy advances, increasing difficulty with self-catheterization and incontinence may occur. Some women may choose to use an indwelling catheter for some time.

Autonomic dysreflexia. A number of stimuli, including labor contractions, may cause muscle spasms related to **autonomic dysreflexia**. This adverse effect occurs most often in persons with lesions located at T6 or higher. Noxious stimuli that cause hyperreflexia include the following:
- Distension, contraction, or manipulation of cervix, rectum, bladder, and uterus
- Excessive deep breathing
- Cold water
- Cold weather

Hyperreflexia is a response of the sympathetic nervous system to noxious sensory stimuli from the skin, a distended bladder, an impacted bowel, a pelvic examination, or labor. Urinary tract infections, pressure ulcers, tight clothing, monitor straps, and even breast-feeding have caused autonomic dysreflexia. Symptoms include a severe pounding headache related to hypertension, profuse sweating; blotching, flushing, and piloerection (erect hairs on skin) above the level of cord lesion; tachycardia; or sometimes bradycardia. The symptoms may be confused with PIH, but the hypertension is transient and episodic; for instance, it may occur during the contraction and subside during the rest period. In severe cases hypertension can result in loss of consciousness, seizures, intracranial bleeding, and death.

Prevention of autonomic dysreflexia is important. Careful attention to bladder and bowel management and maintenance of skin integrity can eliminate the most common prelabor causes. Other preventive measures include the following:
- A semisitting position for a speculum or digital vaginal examination
- Use of an indwelling catheter to avoid bladder distension during labor
- Anesthetic ointments for pelvic examinations or catheter manipulation

If an episode does occur, the woman should be put in a sitting position and any constrictive clothing loosened. Then the primary cause needs to be found and treated; often a distended bladder is the cause. The hypertension is managed pharmacologically during an acute episode or in some cases with epidural analgesia. Epidural anesthesia is favored for the labor and birth.

Labor. Unrecognized labor can be a problem in paraplegia. In women with spinal cord injury, labor usually is painless if the injury is above T10 (Nygaard, Bartscht, Cole, 1991). A gush of amniotic fluid may be confused with incontinence. The first symptoms of labor that some women perceive may be those of autonomic dysreflexia. Others feel back discomfort, nausea, or abdominal spasms. A woman may be taught to feel for a hardening of the uterine muscle. There have been instances of a paraplegic woman delivering an infant at home alone because of little warning of active labor. For this reason some physicians advise admitting paraplegic women at 36 to 37 weeks' gestation or even earlier if there is any indication of early effacement. Others may advocate periodic home uterine monitoring to help detect the onset of contractions.

During the labor process, extra help may be needed for spasms. Frequent positioning will be important, including soft restraints and propping legs with pillows. Note in Figure 23-9 the leg position and padding. A birthing chair may be helpful in adding gravity to the pushing effort and helping to prevent autonomic dysreflexia.

$\mathcal{N}$ursing $\mathcal{R}$esponsibilities

Persons with disabilities often encounter reactions from others who regard them as if they are lacking in intelligence or to be pitied or admired for "courage," as if they are ill or dependent. Conversation may be directed toward a relative or friend rather than to the person herself. A nurse may have common misconceptions—that paraplegic women always need cesarean births, that disabled persons will not be able to parent adequately, or that paraplegic and quadriplegic women will have no pain during labor. A woman with a history of spinal cord injury may be asked to retell "how it happened" to each new nurse that works with her.

Because the woman usually knows best how to handle her disability, collaboratively develop a plan of care that meets the woman's individual needs. Determine how advancing pregnancy changes her activities of daily living. Remember these clients have worked intensely in rehabilitation to become independent in self-care, and this independence must be protected.

ASSESSMENT

Speak frankly and directly to the woman herself, asking her what assistance is needed before assuming she needs help or leaving her alone in a difficult situation. Assessment includes finding out her abilities and how her care can be facilitated by asking questions such as, "What do you find inconvenient in our setup?" or "How can I help?" Nurses have an obligation to become informed about each type of disability when their clients include women with spinal cord injury. Collect data to prepare for a discharge plan.

NURSING DIAGNOSES

A number of diagnoses may apply, depending on the level of injury and the accompanying problems, some of which are listed:

- Alteration in urinary pattern: incontinence secondary to impaired voluntary control
- Risk for urinary tract infection related to changes of pregnancy, weight, difficulty with self-catheterization
- Risk for impaired skin integrity secondary to immobility, edema, incontinence, and impaired vascular tone
- Risk for injury related to altered center of gravity, orthostatic hypotension
- Alteration in self-concept secondary to altered ability for self-care, isolation in managing pregnancy and parenting

EXPECTED OUTCOMES

- Maintains bladder management program
- Maintains nutrition and fluid intake to prevent constipation and urinary tract infection
- Uses methods to prevent edema and skin breakdown
- Exhibits self-confidence in independence of care, seeks support as needed
- Indentifies early signs of labor, knows how to obtain assistance

NURSING INTERVENTION

As weight and size increase with pregnancy, the woman may begin to find her limited mobility further impaired. Transfer may be difficult, for example, even to the point of needing assistance with toileting or driving. An increase in disability, even though temporary, can be traumatic and can feel like regression. Avoiding excessive weight gain and maximizing upper body-strengthening exercises may be helpful. Medical staff members will need to be alert about providing adequate help for transfer to the examination table and toilet during later pregnancy.

Women who spend long hours in a wheelchair may already have orthostatic edema, which can be compounded by pregnancy. Elevating the feet above hip level at regular intervals, wearing elastic support hose, and range-of-motion exercises can help decrease edema. Prevention or treatment of anemia, careful attention to

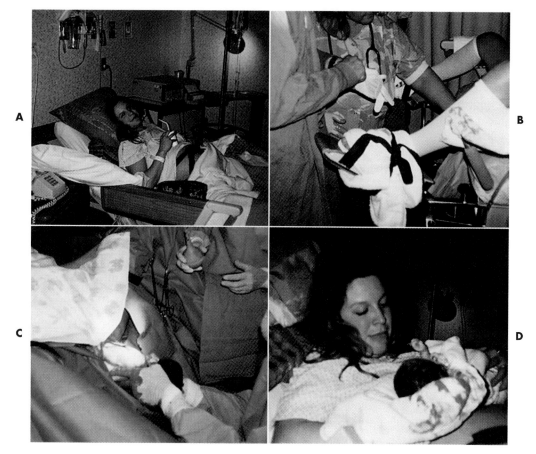

Figure 23-9 Birth sequence of woman with spinal cord injury. **A,** Padding with many pillows makes labor positions more comfortable. **B,** Legs are tied onto the leg holders, and knees are padded against pressure of the birthing bed's side rails. **C,** and **D,** First look at her newborn.

position changes, padding chairs, and daily skin inspection are helpful in preventing skin breakdown. Explain the changes of pregnancy that may affect her established patterns of care, and remind her that constipation can be a major problem for pregnant women, as it may already be for her. Instruct her about the expected urinary changes.

The woman will need a modified version of the warning signs for impending labor. Teach her to look for the signs that can be noticed, such as the mucous plug extrusion, and abdominal contractions that may be palpated and are progressively regular and frequent. Both the woman and her family should be reminded that autonomic dysreflexia, about which she already will be familiar, may be an early sign of labor.

A birth plan should have been devised before labor so that special needs and concerns have been discussed with the woman and solutions found before labor begins (Figure 23-9). Many paraplegic women have felt that no health care providers were prepared for their own special needs. During labor someone should keep careful track of repositioning (every 30 to 60 minutes) to prevent skin pressure. Bladder management usually is han-

dled by an indwelling Foley catheter or by periodic straight catheterization (remember to use anesthetic ointment). Fetal monitoring usually is instituted, but the straps must not be too tight. Internal fetal monitoring or use of a soft stretchable band to hold both tocotransducer and ultrasonic transducer is helpful. Because varying reports indicate that at least half of all paraplegic cases will experience hyperreflexia during labor, the entire staff should be acquainted with the event and planned therapy.

Adequate help for transfers should be arranged, and a physical therapist may be consulted. The use of a birth chair or bed will be helpful in adding gravity to the process, but long periods in one position should be avoided to prevent skin breakdown.

After delivery, mobilization is important to avoid deep vein thrombosis and preserve skin integrity. The assistance of a physical therapist may be appropriate. Bladder management must be carefully followed to avoid new problems with infection. Because lochial flow and sanitary pads may cause skin irritation, commercial disposable diapers and frequent perineal care are advisable.

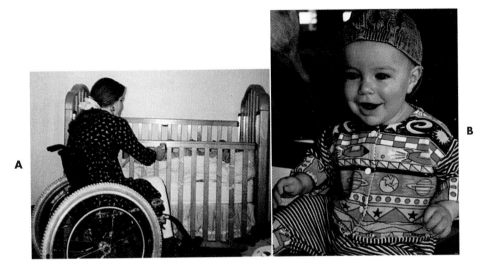

Figure 23-10 **A,** Crib adaptations for a new mother with spinal cord injury. **B,** It is difficult to lift a heavy boy in and out of cribs and car seats, but he is worth it.

In the recovery period the woman will be fatigued, and the nursing care plan should include extra assistance for self-care. The disability should not distract from common needs for adjustment and learning that any new mother has. Rehearsing infant care in the hospital, including baths and hygienic care, is important. Discuss her planning for home care, including how the infant will be placed in a car seat. Referring her to other resources such as other mothers with disabilities, occupational therapy, and appropriate literature may help with practical ideas. (See Figure 23-10 for a crib adaptation.)

EVALUATION

- Is she able to verbalize a positive response to the experience? Did she feel her independence was honored?
- Did planning take place for increased self-care needs and modification of the home for infant care?
- Was hyperreflexia avoided or managed without risk to mother and infant?
- Is she free of bladder infection and pressure sores?

I found out that I was pregnant 7 weeks into the pregnancy. I was extremely excited. My spinal cord injury is at T12 so I have full use and feeling in my arms and torso but no feeling in my legs. I began wondering who I could turn to for advice and realized I would have to blaze my own path, network as best I could, and read what little had been published.

My pregnancy was marked by a series of hard-to-treat urinary tract infections. Life became scientific—tracking intervals between catheterizations, increasing fluid intake to flush the kidneys, and analyzing methods of cleaning catheters for reuse because it is cost-prohibitive to use a new one every time. One way I could tell a urinary tract infection was raging was when involuntary voiding began and was frequent until the infection was under control. I had to have extra supplies (adult superabsorbent diapers) on hand for "accidents."

My greatest fear was that the antibiotic I needed to take would adversely affect the baby. I was assured by my specialist that the risks were small and would be greater if no action were taken. I had to wear clothes and underwear with an access for catheterization when away from home because it became more difficult to remove clothing. I did self-catheterization all during pregnancy with no problems except that I had to watch my balance and recline more fully in the chair to do it.

One piece of advice I would give nurses is not to assume or make decisions for a person with a disability. Sometimes, too, nurses seemed to be intimidated by leg spasms and didn't know what to do. Just ask. If my leg is spasming, it helps if a person holds my leg and bends it at the knee, which usually stops the spasm.

Lower back pain was crippling from time to time, as my weight increased and the center of gravity shifted. The best remedy was a visit out of the chair, lying on a heating pad. If I could not leave the chair, I put my chest on my lap to stretch out the spasm.

Things went smoothly until the seventh month when the excess weight I had gained began to limit my already limited mobility. Transfers from chair to bed and to toilet, and from chair to car, became more strenuous and risky. I was unable to go up even slight uphill slopes like curb cuts. I had to choose carefully for the flattest route anywhere. I gained so much weight, I almost got too big for the wheelchair. Looking back, I would try to limit weight gain because it affected my mobility so greatly.

The worst problem of the last month was edema in my feet. I did elevate my feet at night and wore TED hose. The edema never traveled much past the midcalf, which worried me, because I had previously had deep vein thrombosis in my upper thigh. Exercise such as stretching also might have helped, especially with a partner to assist.

I went to the hospital several times because Braxton-Hicks contractions seemed so strong, but real labor was more painful. We timed the contractions from midnight to 7 AM until the contractions were close and more regular, then went to the hospital. I had a lot of stomach and back pain and asked for pain relief. They gave me intrathecal morphine, which relieved the pain; I was alert, and the labor went well. I did have side effects of itching and a severe headache for 3 days afterward. I wanted my legs secured so if I had spasms they would not get in the way. A birthing chair was available, but it was not offered until late in the labor, and I did not want to transfer then. I was aware of when the contractions began and ended and when the baby's head reached the perineal area, and I was able to push. They did use suction to get the baby's head out. I had a healthy baby boy. The doctor gave me local anesthetic for my episiotomy even though I didn't need it—he couldn't stand doing it without! I felt great all through the labor but was completely exhausted after birth.

Fatigue was one of my biggest problems postpartum. The combination of fatigue, having lots of discharge, and needing to catheterize made perineal care incredibly difficult. Many nurses asked me how my injury happened, when questions about what was happening with me currently would have been more helpful. I didn't get a shower until the second day when someone thought to get a shower chair from another floor. Once I got home, child care seemed overwhelming. Role playing with someone at the hospital might have been helpful. Bathing the baby was difficult because sinks are too high. I couldn't walk or rock the baby to comfort him. So a battery-operated swing really helped. It was difficult to get my baby into his car seat safely while supporting his head. A friend devised a sling to help with this. Disability is often costly, so people don't usually have a lot of extra money for equipment. A crib with a hand-operated gate rather than foot-controlled, as well as a good seamstress, were helpful.

Finally, my advice to nurses is to talk directly to a person with a disability. Feel free to admit, "I don't know—tell me what I can do," as many nurses did with me. Try to think in advance about what special needs may come up and how to address them. An increase in disability, even if temporary, can be frustrating and scary. You can help by being sensitive to needs for assistance and independence.

Nursing Considerations for Women with Disabilities

It may be helpful to explore with the woman her strengths and limitations. She may be facing hostility and emphasis on her disability from other people who disagree with the couple's decision to have a child. An honest exploration of

her physical, emotional, and cognitive status is more likely to occur in an accepting environment. Her need for education or consultation can be assessed through questions such as the following:

1. Have her questions about pregnancy and parenthood been answered adequately?
2. Does she have realistic plans for self-care during pregnancy and for child care?
3. Does she have an active support system, and what is the reaction of significant others to the pregnancy?
4. Is she aware of resources in her community such as support groups and other disabled mothers who can serve as emotional and informational resources?

The time to resolve these questions is before the pregnancy. The nurse's role is to help the client make an informed decision and maximize her potential for self-care and parenting. The way to help a woman consider the decision more thoroughly is by being aware of the questions that a chronic disease raises for the woman contemplating pregnancy (Box 23-2). Although education about medical considerations and drug information and access to articles, books, and community resources are important, the decision to have a child is made by the woman with a disability and her partner.

The client herself may provide an education for the nurse, because she is considering the situation on a personal level. In the hospital setting it is important to accom-

---

Box 23-2   Issues to Consider for Pregnancy with a Disability

DECISION TO BECOME PREGNANT

Will my symptoms get worse with pregnancy?
Will my overall disability be worse as a result of pregnancy?

PREGNANCY

How will my condition affect the medical management of my pregnancy?
Will termination of pregnancy affect my condition?
How will labor and delivery be different?
What drugs are safe during pregnancy and breastfeeding?
Should my current treatments be changed?

POSTPARTUM ISSUES

What assistance will I need to adequately care for my infant?
What adaptations of home and equipment will be needed?
What contingency plans do I have for complications?
How much can I rely on my support systems?
How can I maximize rest?
What community resources and written material are available to provide additional support and information?

modate and assist her when needed but not to take over unnecessarily. The client herself usually is the best person to consult about what is needed because she knows her own abilities. The postpartum nurse will need to carefully assess the woman's comfort level in managing child care and to arrange appropriate referrals if needed (e.g., with a social worker or for occupational therapy). The nurse should remember that some anxiety about caring for the newborn is entirely normal. Encouragement with appropriate humor and a spirit of innovation can go a long way in facing parenthood with a chronic disease.

TRAUMA DURING PREGNANCY

Trauma is a leading cause of nonobstetric maternal and fetal death (ACOG, 1991). The incidence of trauma varies. Minor trauma may be treated in the physician's office. Major trauma is treated in the emergency department. In a study of 441 pregnant trauma clients, Crosby and Costello (1971) defined a list of observations that holds true today:

- Internal injuries often are associated with hidden intraperitoneal bleeding and hypovolemic shock.
- Placental abruption and shock are major causes of fetal death.
- The most common cause of fetal death is maternal death.
- Maternal death is most often from head injuries sustained from automobile accidents.
- Pelvic fractures are extremely hazardous for mother and infant and almost always are associated with placental separation.
- Pelvic fractures carry a high risk of concealed retroperitoneal bleeding. The bladder and urethra may be torn by the fractured bone.

Because two lives are at stake, the following questions take priority:

- Does the injury affect the pregnancy?
- Does being pregnant worsen the effect of the injury?

Remember that the physiologic changes of pregnancy must be considered in trauma treatment. Significant cardiovascular changes that influence care are as follows:

- A higher preload of 40% to 50% greater blood volume is present.
- Before signs of shock will be evident, 30% to 35% of blood volume may have been lost.
- Physiologic alkalemia (higher than normal pH) occurs.
- Physiologic anemia (lower Hct and Hb levels) is present.
- Placental circulation is completely dependent on maternal blood pressure.
- In cases of hypovolemia, shunting of blood to vital organs takes place. The uterus is *not* a vital organ in this process, and blood may be shunted to maintain maternal blood pressure; yet the placental flow is poor.

Thus fetal monitoring often shows signs of distress before any changes in maternal signs. Maternal blood volume must be protected to avoid fetal hypoxia (Table 23-6).

Types of Injury

Falls

Falls tend to result when a pregnant woman loses balance as a result of a shift in weight or orthostatic hypotension. Education for prevention is important (see Chapter 9). Particular attention needs to be paid to whether the woman might be afraid to admit an injury is due to physical abuse (see Chapter 27).

Burns

Burns receive standard burn therapy. Major trauma from fire or electrical burns requires emergency care. If more than one third of the body is affected, the pregnancy will be threatened (Deitch et al, 1989). First-trimester abortion is common. In later pregnancy, preterm labor is frequent. Severe burns require hemodynamic monitoring. Fluid balance is critical especially in the first 24 hours. Output should be more than 50 mL per hour. A high calorie demand may require supplements to reach the 2800 to 3000 kcal per day and 120 g protein requirements. After stabilization, prevention of infection is key in management. Topical preparations with iodine should be avoided (Sherer and Schenker, 1989).

Electric shock

Electric shock usually passes through the hand and then through the fetus on the way to the feet and ground. It has resulted in fetal death, intrauterine growth retardation (IUGR), and oligohydramnios. If electric shock occurs, the woman should be monitored closely for fetal movements. Nonstress test (NST) and amniotic fluid volume measurements may be ordered at regular intervals.

Motor vehicle accidents

Accidents in motor vehicles are the leading cause of accidental injury during pregnancy. How seat belts are used is the primary determinant of the severity of injury (see Chapter 9). Three-point shoulder and lap belts are mandatory, and the lap belt should be located below the abdominal bulge. Correct use of three-point belts has reduced injury to the mother, especially from ejection. The fetus is not so fortunate because the sudden deceleration is powerful enough to throw the fetus against the uterine wall and cause a shearing force to separate the placenta. Normally, amniotic fluid cushions the fetus in the early months, but by the third trimester the infant is larger and there is less fluid. The fetus itself may be injured by blunt trauma; broken bones, skull fracture, and intracranial hemorrhage have been reported.

Table 23-6   Priorities for Trauma Management

Activity	Team A (Mother)	Team B (Fetus)

T = Triage*	Assess ABCs
	  Airway
	  Breathing
	  Circulation
		Assess fetus
		  Cardiac activity
		  Gestational age
		Assess placenta for abruption

R = Resuscitation	Perform CPR Infuse crystalloid fluids Administer oxygen at 8-10 L by mask Administer blood as indicated (in emergency situation, O-negative blood can be used)	Position mother in left lateral tilt
A = Assessment	Assess for maternal injuries (similar to non-pregnant client) Assess vital signs; level of consciousness; respiratory status as to depth, irregularity, and breath sounds	Assess FHR and uterine contractions with EFM Assess for vaginal bleeding and rupture of membranes Kleihauer-Betke test may be done to rule out fetal hemorrhage
U = Ultrasound/uterine evaluation	Evaluate uterine and abdominal cavity for hemorrhage Use peritoneal lavage for penetrating abdominal wounds	Evaluate fundal height Palpate for uterine tenderness, contractions, or irritability Ultrasound may be done to determine placental or fetal injury and placental location Amniocentesis may be done to assess fetal lung maturity or intrauterine bleeding
M = Management/monitor	Decide initial management and needed continual monitoring	Decide to monitor or deliver depending on status of mother and fetus and risk of prematurity
A = Activate transport/transfer	After stabilization, transport/transfer to critical care, operating suite, or level III perinatal unit	Activate neonatal team for consultation, transfer, or transport as necessary

Gilbert ES, Harmon JS: Manual of high risk pregnancy & delivery, St Louis, 1993, Mosby.
*Mother is first priority, then fetus.
CPR, Cardiopulmonary resuscitation; *EFM,* electronic fetal monitor; *FHR,* fetal heart rate.

Gunshot and stab wounds

Gunshot and stab wounds that penetrate the abdomen may injure the fetus more severely than the pregnant woman if the angle is directly into the uterine tissue. Bullets may tumble and cause more extensive damage than is apparent by the wound. If the wound is in the upper or lateral abdomen, the woman's vital organs and intestines may be lacerated. Exploratory surgery is needed.

The puncture stab wound may be less injurious and often must be evaluated by peritoneal lavage before the decision for laparotomy is made. If there is a return of RBCs, leukocytes, or gastrointestinal contents, an exploratory laparotomy is performed.

Physical abuse

Physical abuse may include blows to the pregnant woman's abdomen. The skin surfaces may be bruised, but blunt trauma may have injured underlying tissues and the fetus more severely (see Chapter 27).

Clinical management

Cardiopulmonary resuscitation. In case the pregnant woman has cardiac arrest, the advanced cardiac life support (ACLS) protocol for cardiopulmonary resuscitation (CPR) should be followed. Defibrillation should also be used if appropriate (Mitchell, 1995). The need for CPR always includes initial assessment by evaluating *airway, breathing,* and *circulation* (ABCs), while bleeding is controlled and broken bones are immobilized. The CPR variations for pregnant women recommended by the American Heart Association include steps found in Box 23-3. See Table 23-6 for priorities for perinatal trauma management.

Supporting perfusion. Supporting blood volume and pressure using two large-bore IV lines and a central venous pressure (CVP) line is necessary because pregnancy volumes are critical to support fetal perfusion. Crystalloid fluids (Ringer's lactate or normal saline) are given in a 3:1 ratio to estimated blood loss (ACOG, 1991) plus blood products as needed. Give drugs per ACLS pro-

Box 23-3   Principles of Basic Life Support during Pregnancy

AIRWAY

Determine unresponsiveness.
Call for help.
Position client on firm flat surface.
Displace uterus laterally, either manually or with wedge.
Open the airway with head-tilt and chin-lift or jaw-thrust maneuver.

BREATHING

Look, listen, and feel for air movement.
If breathing is absent, deliver two slow breaths.

CIRCULATION

Feel for presence of carotid pulse.
If pulse is absent, begin external chest compressions at a rate of 80-100/min.
Alternate 15 chest compressions with two slow breaths.
Reassess client after four complete cycles.
If breathing and pulse are absent, continue CPR.

TWO-RESCUER CPR

Same as above, except five compressions are followed by a pause to allow delivery of one slow breath.

INTUBATED CLIENT

Same as for two-rescuer CPR, except compressions and ventilations asynchronous.
Perform compressions at a rate of 80-100/min.
Perform ventilations independently at a rate of 12-15/min.

Modified from American Heart Association: *Textbook of advanced cardiac life support*, Dallas, 1995, The Association.

tocol. To assist with maintaining blood pressure, military antishock trousers (MAST) may be used on the lower extremities but *not* over the abdomen (Sherer and Schenker, 1989). Oxygen at 8 to 10 L/min by mask is started and a pulse oximeter attached. An indwelling Foley catheter is necessary to monitor output and note hematuria. A nasogastric tube decompresses the stomach and prevents aspiration.

The uterus must always be tilted to the side to prevent vena caval and abdominal aortal compression. Placement of a wedge or manual positioning is necessary if the client cannot be in a side-lying position.

Assessing fetal condition. As soon as the woman's condition is initially stabilized, the fetal condition must be monitored. Ultrasonography is used if abdominal wounds prevent placing a belt. Monitoring should continue during any procedure.

Every trauma client should have fetal and contraction monitoring for at least 4 hours in mild cases and continu-

ously until stabilized in more severe cases. Placental separation may be indicated by late decelerations, rising fetal heart baseline, and falling beat-to-beat variability, and in some cases, vaginal bleeding (see Chapter 21).

TEST *Yourself* 23-5

Why does the fetal heart rate show distress signs before the woman's signs of shock become evident?

If CPR is successful and the gestation period is less than 24 weeks the woman is cared for in the intensive care unit (ICU) until stable. On the other hand, if gestation period is more than 24 weeks and CPR is not successful, then thoracotomy with open-chest cardiac massage or bedside perimortem cesarean delivery is recommended (Mitchell, 1995). Perinatal nurses, especially those participating in level III (high risk) perinatal centers should be trained in dysrhythmia recognition and ACLS protocols. Rapid intervention sometimes can save two lives (Mitchell, 1995).

Perimortem cesarean section. In situations in which the woman is brain dead, is dying from fatal head or chest injuries, or has just died, it may be possible to rescue the fetus through a cesarean delivery performed in the emergency department. Choices must be made quickly and, of course, with informed consent of the next of kin if possible. The fetus often does not survive or will be neurologically damaged unless it is "rescued" before 10 to 15 minutes after maternal death.

Sometimes rapid surgery relieves the woman's body of the uterine pressure, and her condition improves. A cesarean should be begun as soon as 5 minutes after onset of cardiac resuscitation to benefit the woman herself (ACOG, 1991). The following criteria are recommended in these cases (Sherer and Schenker, 1989):

- Fetal age more than 28 weeks
- Infant removed less than 15 minutes after maternal clinical death
- Maintaining continuous resuscitation, ventilation, and cardiac massage before and during procedure
- Intensive neonatal care personnel on hand and rapid transport of newborn to the neonatal ICU

A decision tree similar to Figure 23-11 is important to have established in such cases. All health care staff members need to be aware of procedures to be followed in these difficult cases.

Preventing isoimmunization. Often fetomaternal transfusion occurs as placental tissue or the uterus is injured. The fetus may be bleeding. The Kleihauer-Betke test for fetal cells in the maternal circulation may be used to follow the levels. If a woman is Rh-negative, she must receive the correct dose of D immunoglobulin within 48 to 72 hours after the injury. In addition, consideration needs to be given to whether tetanus toxoid is needed.

Decision TREE | *Accidental Injury during Pregnancy*

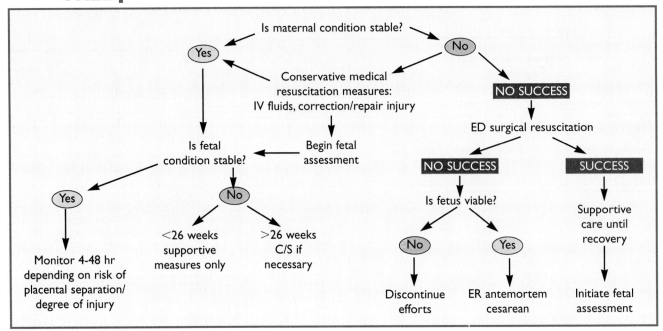

Figure 23-11   Decision tree for accidental injury during pregnancy. If resuscitation of woman is successful, the fetal assessment sequence is followed. (Modified from Sherer DM, Schenker JG: Accidental injury during pregnancy, *Obstet Gynecol Surv* 44(5):330, 1989.)

Nursing considerations

The trauma client will be seen first in the emergency department for evaluation. If any blunt trauma has occurred but is not life threatening, she will be transferred to labor and delivery for fetal and contraction monitoring. Amniocentesis may be used to identify RBCs in the fluid and to determine fetal lung maturity. Monitoring will continue until signs indicate good fetal activity and beat-to-beat variability, without abnormal decelerations. The woman will be instructed in counting fetal movements and asked to return on a regular basis for monitoring. Preventive education concerning preterm labor is included because of the risk of continuing problems.

If major trauma occurs, the maternity nurse works in collaboration with the emergency department team, providing monitoring expertise and assessment of the pregnancy complications. When the client is transferred to the ICU after stabilization, the nurses there may use the maternity nurse's expertise for consultation (Johnson and Oakley, 1991).

Key points

■ Inadequate or noncompliant care for asthma may lead to irreversible hypertrophy, disability, and death.
■ Management of asthma depends primarily on the client's recognition of early changes in her PEFR and use of corrective medication before events escalate.
■ The pregnancy outcome of a client with cardiac disability depends primarily on her functional cardiac status. Special care and monitoring are required during the third trimester, labor, birth, and the recovery periods.

■ Anemia underlies many chronic health problems, and during pregnancy it is intensified by physiologic demands for iron.
■ Anemia related to genetic causes is a widespread problem made worse by poor nutrition in many parts of the world. Because of its prevalence in the United States there is universal newborn testing for the sickle cell trait and G6PD.
■ The importance of maintaining independence in self-care cannot be overemphasized when pregnant women have chronic disease or disabilities.

- Epilepsy is caused by abnormal electrical discharges in the brain and has many trigger events. Generalized convulsive seizures have the greatest potential for harmful impact on the fetus.
- Changes in levels of antiepilepsy drugs during pregnancy may be due to physiologic changes or to noncompliance with medication regimen: all these drugs carry some teratogenic risk.
- The physiologic immune suppression of pregnancy appears to stabilize or improve MS temporarily, but relapses are common in the postpartum period.
- Women with spinal cord injury are fertile, and many retain some sexual feeling; therefore pregnancies can be expected.

- The chief problems when a pregnant woman has a spinal cord injury are preterm labor, autonomic dysreflexia, and need for special assistance with birth.
- After blunt trauma the fetal status should be assessed for at least 4 hours because abruptio placentae is the most common result.
- The Rh status must be assessed after trauma because fetomaternal transfusion is common.
- CPR must be modified for the pregnant woman by ensuring that vena cava syndrome is avoided.
- Perimortem cesarean delivery may improve the condition of a desperately injured woman. A fetus needs to be born less than 15 minutes after CPR has failed in order to survive intact.

Study Questions

23-1. Select the terms that apply to the following statements:
- a. AEDs may depress folic acid levels and can result in _____.
- b. After a seizure a person may be difficult to arouse in the _____ state.
- c. Seizures happen continuously in _____.
- d. When noxious stimuli occur, persons with spinal cord injury may have _____.
- e. Forming antibodies against proteins of the same species is _____.
- f. Sensations that precede certain headaches or seizures are _____.

23-2. Match the description of the management of heart disease in a pregnant woman with the classification of heart disease determined by the New York Heart Association.

- a. Bed rest is necessary for most of the day. Client is hospitalized for final weeks of pregnancy; cardiac symptoms occur during and after labor.
- b. Stress should be limited; additional periods of rest are recommended after meals and at night. Vaginal delivery is planned with use of oxygen and monitoring.
- c. Cardiac signs and symptoms occur at rest.

1. Class I
2. Class II
3. Class III
4. Class IV

23-3. Note if the statements below are true or false:
- a. Pregnancy causes MS to worsen in its overall course.
- b. AEDs should be given during labor even if fluids are being withheld.
- c. Paraplegic women have no pain during labor.
- d. High fluid intake is protective for a client with sickle cell disease.
- e. After trauma the most common cause of fetal death is skull fracture.
- f. D-Immunoglobulin may be administered up to 4 days after the fetal-maternal transfusion.

23-4. Which nursing interventions do not affect autonomic dysreflexia?
- a. Loosen tight clothing.
- b. Move woman to a sitting or high Fowler's position.
- c. Turn woman onto left side, and prop with pillows.
- d. Empty the bladder if full.

23-5. Which intervention is unique for a pregnant woman receiving CPR?
- a. Slightly elevate the legs to increase central circulation.
- b. Use a ratio of chest compression to breaths of 10:1.
- c. Listen for fetal heart rate before using extraordinary methods.
- d. Position so that vena caval compression does not occur.

Answer Key

23-1: *a,* Anemia; *b,* postictal; *c,* status asthmaticus; *d,* autonomic dysreflexia; *e,* isoimmunization; *f,* auras. 23-2: *a,* Class III; *b,* Class II; *c,* Class IV. 23-3: *a,* False; *b,* true; *c,* false; *d,* true; *e,* false. 23-4: *c.* 23-5: *d.*

References

American College of Obstetrics & Gynecology (ACOG): Prevention of D isoimmunization, Technical Bulletin 147, Oct 1990, The College.

ACOG: Trauma during pregnancy, Technical Bulletin 161, Nov 1991, The College.

ACOG: Cardiac disease in pregnancy, Technical Bulletin 168, June 1992, The College.

ACOG Committee Opinion: Obstetric management of patients with spinal cord injury, Committee Opinion, April 1993, The College.

ACOG: Hemoglobinopathies, Technical Bulletin 220, Feb 1996a, The College.

ACOG: Pulmonary disease in pregnancy, Technical Bulletin 224, June 1996b, The College.

ACOG: Seizure disorders in pregnancy, Technical Bulletin 231, December 1996c, The College.

Anderson B: An overview of drug therapy for chronic adult asthma, *Nurse Prac* 16(12):42, 1991.

Beischer NA, MacKay EV: *Obstetrics and the newborn*, ed 2, Philadelphia, 1993, WB Saunders.

Birk K et al: The clinical course of multiple sclerosis during pregnancy and the puerperium, *Arch Neurol* 47:738, 1990.

Cahalin LP, Sadowsky HS: Pulmonary medications, *Phys Ther* 75(5):400, 1995.

Callan N et al: Counseling in congenital heart defects, *Obstet Gynecol Surv* 46(10):651, 1991.

Campbell C: Primary care for women: comprehensive cardiovascular assessment, *J Nurse Midwifery* 40(2):137, 1995.

Carty EM, Conic TA, Hall C: Comprehensive health promotion for the pregnant woman who is disabled: role of the nurse midwife, *J Nurse Midwifery* 35(3):133, 1990.

Chui DHK, Wong SC, Scriver CR: The thalassemias and health care in Canada: a place for genetics in medicine, *Can Med Assoc J* 144(1):21, 1991.

Cosner KR, deJong E: Physiologic second-stage labor, *MCN Am J Matern Child Nurs* 18(1):38, 1993.

Criezel AE, Dudas I: Prevention of the first occurrence of neural tube defects by periconceptional vitamin supplementation, *N Engl J Med* 327:1832, 1992.

*Crosby WM, Costello J: Safety of lap-belt restraint for pregnant victims of automobile collisions, *N Engl J Med* 284:632, 1971.

Davis RK, Maslow AS: Multiple sclerosis in pregnancy: a review, *Obstet Gynecol Surv* 47:190, 1992.

*Deitch EA et al: Management of burns in the pregnant woman, *Am J Obstet Gynecol* 161(1):1, 1989.

Devinsky O, Yerby MS: Women with epilepsy, *Neurol Clin* 12(3):479, 1994.

Easterling TR et al: Maternal hemodynamics in normal and preeclamptic pregnancies: a longitudinal study, *Obstet Gynecol* 76(6):1061, 1990.

Engstrom JL, Sittler CP: Nurse-midwifery management of iron-deficiency anemia during pregnancy, *J Nurse Midwifery* 39(suppl 2):22, 1994.

Enkin M et al: *A guide to effective care in pregnancy*, ed 2, Oxford, 1995, Oxford University Press.

Felsenthal G: Peripheral nervous system disorders and pregnancy. In Goldstein PG, Stein BH, eds: *Neurological disorders of pregnancy*, Mt Kisco, NY, 1992, Future Publishing.

Fleschler RG, Sala DJ: Pregnancy after organ transplantation, *J Obstet Gynecol Neonatal Nurs* 24(5):416, 1995.

Geiger-Bronsky M: Asthma and pregnancy: an opportunity for enhancing outcomes, *J Perinat Neonatal Nurs* 37(9):44, 1992.

Gift AG: Psychologic and physiologic aspects of acute dyspnea in asthmatics, *Nurs Res* 40(4):196, 1991.

Gilbert ES, Harmon JS: *Manual of high risk pregnancy and delivery*, St Louis, 1993, Mosby.

Gilson JG et al: Acute spinal cord injury and neurogenic shock in pregnancy, *Obstet Gynecol Surv* 50(7):556, 1995.

Gobe LI: Pregnancy and movement disorders, *Neurol Clin* 12(3):457, 1994.

*Classic reference.

Goldstein PJ, Stern BJ, eds: Neurological disorders of pregnancy, Mt Kisco, NY, 1992, Future Publishing.

Green LA, Froman RD: Blood pressure measurement, *J Obstet Gynecol Neonatal Nurs* 25(2):155, 1996.

Hainline B: Headache, *Neurol Clin* 12(3):443, 1994.

Harvey M: OB critical care: beyond high-risk pregnancy, *Am J Matern Child Nurs* 17(6):296, 1992.

Hughes SJ et al: Management of the pregnant woman with spinal cord injuries, *Br J Obstet Gynaecol* 948:513, 1991.

Johnson J, Oakley L: Managing minor trauma during pregnancy, *J Obstet Gynecol Neonatal Nurs* 20(5):379, 1991.

Jordan E, Pugh LC: Pregnancy after cardiac transplantation: principles of nursing care, *J Obstet Gynecol Neonatal Nurs* 25(2):132, 1996.

Kennedy BB: Mitral stenosis: implications for critical care obstetric nursing, *J Obstet Gynecol Neonatal Nurs* 24(5):408, 1995.

Khurana R: Headache. In Goldstein PG, Stern BJ, eds: *Neurological disorders of pregnancy*, Mt Kisco, NY, 1992, Future Publishing.

Kirkland CJ: Myocardial infarction during pregnancy, *J Perinat Neonatal Nurs* 5(2):38, 1991.

Konstantinides S et al: Comparison of surgical and medical therapy for arterial septal defect in adults, *N Engl J Med* 333(8):469, 1995.

*Koshy M et al: Prophylactic red-cell transfusions in pregnant patients with sickle cell disease, *N Engl J Med* 319:1447, 1988.

*Lamb M: Myocardial infarction during pregnancy: a team challenge, *Heart Lung,* 16(6):658, 1987.

Lewith GT: Migraine: the complementary approaches considered, *Comp Therapies in Med* 4:26, 1996.

Long PJ: Rethinking iron supplementation during pregnancy, *J Nurse Midwifery* 40(1):36, 1995.

Mabie WC et al: Clinical observations on asthma in pregnancy, *J Maternal-Fetal Med* 1:45, 1992.

Mason JW et al: A clinical trial of immunosuppressive therapy for myocarditis, *N Engl J Med* 333(5):269, 1995.

Mayberry MC et al: Pregnancy complicated by hemoglobin CC and C-thalassemia disease, *Obstet Gynecol* 76(2):324, 1990.

McManus KJ: Effects on the fetus and newborn of medications commonly used during pregnancy, *J Perinat Neonatal Nurs* 3:73, 1990.

Meadow R: Anticonvulsants in pregnancy, *Arch Dis Child* 66:62, 1991.

Nygaard I, Bartscht KD, Cole S: Sexuality and reproduction in spinal cord injured women, *Obstet Gynecol Surv* 46(10):727, 1991.

Pearlman MD et al: Blunt trauma during pregnancy, *N Engl J Med* 323:1069, 1990.

Ritter DC, de Shazo RD: Peripartum complications: hemorrhage, embolism, hypertension, and infection, *Postgrad Med* 95(2):188, 1994.

Rosenbaum RB, Donaldon JO: Peripheral nerve and neuromuscular disorders, *Neurol Clin* 12(3):461, 1994.

Roth CK, Riley B, Cohen SM: Intrapartum care of a woman with aortic aneurysms, *J Obstet Gynecol Neonatal Nurs* 21(4):316, 1992.

*Sherer DM, Schenker JD: Accidental injury during pregnancy, *Obstet Gynecol Surv* 44(5):330, 1989.

Silberstein SD, Niebyl JR: Nature of migraine attacks during pregnancy, *Contemp OB/GYN* 39(5):60, 1994.

Simpson KR: Rupture of a splenic artery aneurysm in pregnancy, *Crit Care Nurse* 25(6):25, 1995.

Stephenson LS: Possible new developments in community control of iron-deficiency anemia, *Nutr Rev* 53(2):23, 1995.

Swain SE: Multiple sclerosis: primary health care implications, *Nurs Practitioner* 21(7):40, 1996.

*Warner MB, Rageth CJ, Zack GA: Pregnancy and autonomic hyper-reflexia in patients with spinal cord injury, *Paraplegia* 25:482, 1987.

Wineman NM: Adaptation to multiple sclerosis: the role of social support, functional disability, and perceived uncertainty, *Nurs Res* 39:294, 1990.

The Working Group Consensus Report: National high blood pressure education program on high blood pressure in pregnancy, *Am J Obstet Gynecol* 163:1689, 1990.

The Working Group Report on Asthma in Pregnancy: *Management of asthma during pregnancy*, NIH publication 93-3279, Bethesda, Md, DHHS 1993.

Student Resource Shelf

Campion JM: *The baby challenge: a handbook on pregnancy for women with a physical disability*, New York, 1990, Tavistock/Routledge.
An exploration of issues from deciding to have a child, to delivery and beyond, including chapters on specific disabilities and one chapter for health professionals.

Henly SJ et al: Anemia and insufficient milk in first-time mothers, *Birth* 22(2):6, 1995.
The study results suggest that anemia is associated with the development of insufficient milk, which in turn, is related to duration of full breast-feeding and to age when weaned.

Mays M, Leiner S: Asthma: a comprehensive review, *J Nurse Midwifery* 40(3):256, 1995.
Review articles bring together all current findings in a succinct manner.

McEwan CE et al: Comprehensive health promotion for the pregnant woman who is disabled, *J Nurse Midwifery* 35:133, 1990.
Considerations for health professionals working with disabled women during pregnancy, labor, and postpartum, with specific discussion of rheumatoid arthritis, spinal cord injury, and hearing and vision impairment.

Mitchell L: Cardiac arrest during pregnancy: maternal-fetal physiology and advanced cardiac life support for the obstetric patient, *Crit Care Nurse* 25(2):56, 1995.
This article reinforces the need for ACLS training for critical care nurses working with pregnant women who have dysrhythmia related to cardiac arrest.

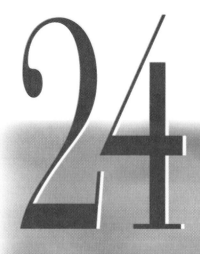

24 Metabolic & Renal Problems Affecting Pregnancy

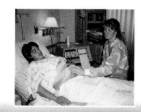

METABOLIC PROBLEMS DURING PREGNANCY

Pregnancy may be considered a laboratory examination of the working order of the female body, testing every organ system and part. Obviously the metabolic system receives its share of work; it is subjected to 40 weeks of stress that often reveals some fascinating reactions and responses. Many of these reactions and responses have appeared so predictably that health care givers are able to act as alert investigators, discovering the first indication that any of these distinctive conditions has appeared, which warrant further scrutiny or treatment.

Obesity

The most common metabolic disorder in the United States is obesity. An estimated 15% of adults are overweight, with women outnumbering men. Simple gain is present when the woman's body weight exceeds the recommended body weight by 10%; obesity is the term used when weight is 20% or more above the ideal weight before pregnancy. The best reproductive outcomes for an obese woman have been associated with a weight gain of 15 to 25 pounds during pregnancy. (See Chapter 10.)

Risk

Invariably, there will be some pregnant women who are obese. Thus their bodies are taxed by two simultaneous stresses: pregnancy and extra weight. Obese women are at higher risk for the following:

- Chronic hypertension
- Latent diabetes with large-for-gestational-age infants
- Uterine dysfunction because of an oversized fetus
- Abnormal presentations and cesarean birth
- Increased anesthetic risk and, in the recovery period, thromboembolism (LeMone and Burke, 1996.)

Additional maternal risks include prolonged operative time (resulting in potential for endometritis and greater blood loss), respiratory complications, and wound infection or dehiscence (separation of suture line) (Zlatnik, 1996).

Women who are obese before pregnancy may have large-for-gestational-age infants. Large birth weight infants tend to be taller and heavier throughout childhood and are at increased risk for obesity in adult life (Binkin, 1988). Women with similar weight gain during pregnancy but who are thinner before pregnancy tend to have smaller babies than do obese women.

Excessive weight gain during pregnancy is associated with increased birth weight of infants and its consequences: risk of fetopelvic disproportion, cesarean delivery, birth trauma, and asphyxia. Excessive weight gain can also place women at a greater risk of continuing to be obese in the future and experiencing its health-related problems, such as hypertension and diabetes.

Nursing responsibilities

Lifestyle issues that are related to excess weight for height should be addressed postpartum, not during pregnancy. However, during prenatal care teach diet-related healthy behaviors such as planning a daily walk. Identify problem areas that affect the client's ability to maintain the desired weight gain as her pregnancy advances. Discuss poor or excessive weight gain on a nonjudgmental basis, and support appropriate changes in the client's diet.

The best indicator for appropriate weight gain during pregnancy is based on the maternal prepregnancy weight (see Chapter 10). Women's weight should be measured at each health care visit, even if the woman is in her second or third trimester at the time of the first encounter. Although prepregnant weights are helpful in assessing gain patterns, women do not always contact a member of the health care team until they are well into their first trimester, or they may report unrealistic prepregnant weights. When abnormal gains in weight are noted, a dis-

cussion with the pregnant woman should be planned to help her establish possible causes to explain the gain in weight, followed by a review of the findings with the health care team.

Severe dietary restrictions should never be attempted during pregnancy. This practice can lead to *catabolism* (breakdown) of fat stores and formation of ketones. Protein restriction, especially during the first trimester, can negatively affect fetal brain cell multiplication and lead to irreversible damage. Dieting and fasting during pregnancy lead to ketone formation and hypoglycemia, conditions that are poorly tolerated by the fetus, and may lead to neurologic impairment.

During pregnancy, women are receptive to nutritional guidance and will attempt dietary behavior changes. Addressing concerns of a pregnant woman's "healthy" balanced diet versus empty calories may have lasting positive effects on health behaviors and dietary practices. Pregnant women may find that an increase in the insoluble fiber content of their diets (wheat bran) will help relieve the common problem of constipation. Nurses should use any situation or "teachable moment" made available to them to promote preventive health patterns to their clients.

Although an obese woman may express interest in changing her diet, you should be aware that it may be difficult for her to change behaviors. Obese women may not be able to follow a diet consistently, even with a support system in place. However, reviews of dietary intake and food preferences are useful tools in establishing expected weight gain during pregnancy.

Maternal Phenylketonuria

Almost all protein sources contain the amino acid phenylalanine, which should be metabolized to tyrosine. The biochemical defect in phenylketonuria (PKU) is a deficiency of the liver enzyme phenylalanine 4-hydroxylase needed to metabolize *phenylalanine.* Excessive accumulation of this amino acid and its abnormal metabolites—phenylpyruvic acid and phenylacetic acid—leads to progressive and irreversible brain damage. This inborn error of metabolism (IEM) is genetically inherited in a recessive pattern; two parents may carry the trait and have a homozygous infant (see Chapter 28). PKU occurs in severe and mild forms. The rate of occurrence is 1 in every 10,000 to 20,000 births, and it occurs equally in male and female infants. It is more commonly found in people of Northern European ancestry. Since 1967 all newborns in the United States and Canada have been screened for PKU. This screening is done 2 to 3 days after birth, after sufficient feeding (a minimum of 120 mL) of breast or bottle milk. Early discharge requires medical follow-up within the specified time period for accurate metabolic screening (see Chapter 19).

An infant diagnosed with PKU is treated with a phenyl-alanine-free diet (see Research Box). Unfortunately, it was thought until the late l970s that one "grew out of" this problem. Today, studies show that a modified diet should be continued throughout life, with a return to a strict diet just before and during pregnancy. Because young women with PKU have been successfully treated with diet modifications and can become pregnant, they believe they are "cured" and begin to loosen diet control. As a result, maternal PKU has arisen as a threat. Some women may not know that as they loosen diet control, rising levels of phenylalanine will have an adverse effect on a fetus.

Risk

The harmful effects of poorly regulated maternal PKU have a teratogenic result: increased incidence of intrauterine growth retardation (IUGR) microcephaly, mental retardation, and a greater risk of heart defects. If the maternal phenylalanine concentration can be kept below 150 μmol/L (<2.0 mg/dl) during pregnancy, there is a better outcome (Acosta and Wright, 1992).

Signs

In the infant with PKU, there is decreased pigmentation, resulting in fair skinned, blond infants often seen with eczema, hypertonicity, irritability, and sometimes with seizures. If the PKU is untreated, severe mental retardation develops.

In the adult, additional signs are a distinct "mousey" or "barnlike" odor, rashes, seizures, or poor coordination (Acosta and Wright, 1992). For instance, it might be possible for a retarded woman to have a diagnosis of epilepsy but actually be an undiagnosed PKU client. Thus screening is important and is performed as it is on the newborn infant.

Clinical management

The data achieved so far by the National Maternal PKU Collaborative Study, which began in l984, have shown that control of maternal blood phenylalanine levels before pregnancy improves pregnancy outcome. More than 3000 women of childbearing age have been successfully treated. Strict dietary treatment of the young infant with PKU has resulted in the child being able to achieve the average intellectual abilities appropriate in his family.

The foundation of treatment is removal from the diet of all protein that contains phenylalanine. A balanced diet is gained by using PHE, a protein-modified supplement. Its use is important especially just before and during pregnancy to keep the blood levels between 60 and 180 μmol/L (Thompson et al, 1991). This medical nutrition is expensive. Supplements for a year cost at least $4500. Women, infants, and children (WIC) assistance programs, insurance company funds, and the Collaborative Study are sources from which to obtain this supplement. The rest of

RESEARCH

PURPOSE OF STUDY

To determine if there is a difference in phenylalanine levels among newborns who are bottle fed with special low phenylalanine (PHE) products and newborns who are breast-fed.

LITERATURE REVIEW

Traditional diets of newborns with PKU include special low PHE products in combination with standard infant formulas to provide sufficient PHE for growth and development. Breast-feeding has been discouraged. The recommended blood level of PHE is under 480 μmol/L.

METHOD

Thirteen infants diagnosed with PKU were included in the study. Nine were breast-fed with supplements of PHE-free formula. Four were fed infant formulas in conjunction with PHE-free formula (standard feeding method).

RESULTS AND IMPLICATIONS FOR NURSING

Overall, no differences were found between the two groups. Initially, the breast-fed newborns had higher levels of PHE. These levels significantly decreased by day 10 as the volume of breast milk increased. The breast-fed newborns drank less PHE-free formula than the bottle-fed newborns. An important finding was that breast milk is lower in PHE than any commercially prepared standard formula. The researchers concluded that breast-feeding can be used to successfully manage the infant with PKU.

Greene L, Wheeler M: Breastfeeding in the management of the newborn with PKU: a practical approach to dietary therapy, *J American Diet Assoc* 94(3):305, 1994.

the diet is made up of low-protein cereals, fruits, fats, and vegetables. Iron and zinc levels are monitored. Blood phenylalanine and tyrosine levels are monitored every 2 to 4 weeks during early pregnancy and may be done every week in later pregnancy.

Nursing responsibilities

Every woman should be asked if she was on special diet in childhood. Any woman who has an infant who is mentally retarded or has microcephaly should be tested. Nutrition counseling and follow-up are critical. The nurse and nutritionist will work as a team in the care of this client.

THYROID PROBLEMS

Circulating iodine from food or iodized salt is synthesized by the thyroid gland into two thyroid hormones: triiodothyronine (T_3) and thyroxine (T_4), controlled by thyroid-releasing factor from the hypothalamus. Thyroid-stimulating hormone (TSH) is produced by the pituitary gland. Balance is maintained by a feedback mechanism, which increases or decreases the amount of T_3 and T_4 for healthy functioning (Figure 24-1).

Normal pregnancy mimics a slightly hyperthyroid state; there is an increase in basal metabolic rate (BMR), cardiac output, heat intolerance, emotional lability, and amenorrhea. The thyroid hormone increases the production of intracellular proteins and energy, which results in increased consumption of carbohydrates, fats, and oxygen and in increased heat production as the BMR is increased.

During pregnancy, maternal thyroid function changes as follows: Serum thyroxine T_4 levels increase during the first trimester because of an increased binding capacity of thyroid-binding globulins (TBG) secondary to the elevated estrogen level. These effects will last 1 to 3 months after birth. Pregnancy, however, may stimulate either remission or exacerbation of certain thyroid disorders.

Fetal thyroid activity usually starts around 2 months' gestation; by the end of the first trimester, the fetal pituitary gland begins secretion of TSH. Apparently, T_4, T_3, and TSH do not cross the placenta in any significant amount.

Hyperthyroid States

Graves' disease, or **hyperthyroidism**, is an autoimmune disorder that occurs in genetically susceptible individuals. Characterized by exacerbations and remissions, the peak incidence occurs during the reproductive years (ACOG, 1993). When a woman with Graves' disease becomes pregnant, there are two patients: the fetus and the woman herself. The woman may be evaluated relatively quickly, but the fetus is at risk because of an abnormal growth environment, and viability is in jeopardy. Fetal loss is common, with some infants stillborn or born prematurely.

Risk

Some newborns are born with Graves' disease, or with a goiter, exophthalamos, and a hypermetabolic state. In most cases, infants have a transient disorder lasting less than 5 months, which is completely treatable.

Signs

Characteristics of hyperthyroidism are listed in Table 24-1. Greatly elevated levels of T_4 and T_3 are found. Diagnostic studies with radioactive iodine (RAI) are not recommended during pregnancy because RAI crosses the placenta and would affect the fetal thyroid gland.

Clinical management

Women with hyperthyroidism may require a diet higher in calories and fluids to compensate for the increased

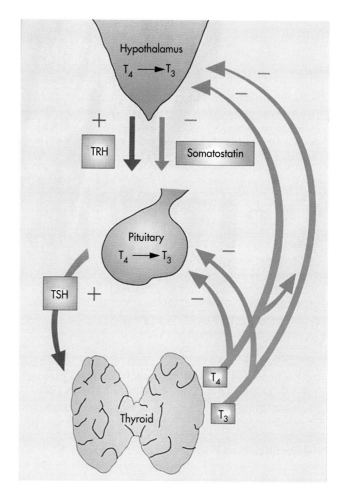

Figure 24-1   Diagram of hypothalamic-pituitary-thyroid axis showing the feedback cycle. (From Martin JB, Reichlin S: *Clinical endocrinology*, ed 2, Philadelphia, 1985, FA Davis.)

metabolic rate. Pregnant women with Graves' disease require medication to control their symptoms. The goal is to achieve acceptable hormone levels for pregnancy to prevent fetal difficulty. Propylthiouracil (PTU) is the drug of choice for women with hyperthyroidism because it crosses the placenta more slowly and blocks synthesis of T_4 and blocks conversion of T_4 to T_3 in peripheral tissues. Breastfeeding has been considered by some practitioners to be contraindicated when the mother is taking antithyroid medications, but drug concentration in breast milk has been found to be low. The American Academy of Pediatrics has stated that neither PTU nor methimazole is a contraindication to breast-feeding (1989).

Women with Graves' disease may improve during pregnancy, experiencing remission or even becoming euthyroid (a return to normal levels) during the third trimester. This improvement occurs because of changes occurring in the immune system that result in lowering of the TSI (thyroid stimulating antigens), thus decreasing thyroid hormone production (Blackburn and Loper, 1992).

Table 24-1	**Signs and Symptoms of Thyroid Imbalances**

Hyperthyroidism	Hypothyroidism
• Nervousness • Hyperactivity • Diaphoresis • Warm, velvety, soft, damp skin texture • Silky hair • Hypersensitivity to heat • Weakness • Fatigue	• Lethargy • Dry skin, thick at knees and elbows • Coarse hair • Cold intolerance • Weakness • Mental impairment (slowed cognitive ability, poor memory, forgetfulness, depressed affect)
• Palpitation • Tachycardia • Dyspnea • Angina • Increased appetite • Weight loss • Absence of forehead wrinkling on upward gaze • Nail loose or detached from bed	• Chest pain • Dyspnea • Anorexia • Weight gain • Facial edema (especially periorbital) • Pale skin (coarse, dry, cold with a yellow tinge [normal sclerae])
• Diarrhea • Eye symptoms (burning, tearing, diplopia, lid lag, prominent eyes [exophthalmia], stare, eyelid tremors when closed) • Hyperreflexia • Goiter • Decreased or absent menses • Susceptibility to infection	• Constipation • Thinned lateral aspect of eyebrows • Sluggish return of reflexes • Diffuse enlargement of thyroid or thyroid is not palpable • Heavy, prolonged menses or infertility • Deafness (occurs in one third of the population)

In most cases thyroid hormone levels are stabilized within 4 weeks. If medical management cannot control hyperthyroidism, surgical management with a subtotal thyroidectomy may be considered only during the second trimester. After birth the infant should be closely observed for signs and symptoms of imbalance.

Nursing Responsibilities

ASSESSMENT

Review the signs of hyperthyroid states, and include observations for these signs in physical assessment and history taking. Determine the type of treatment administered before pregnancy and note its effects, and ascertain nutritional and fluid intake.

NURSING DIAGNOSES

Based on the presenting symptomatology and the woman's history of thyroid problems, the following diagnoses may be chosen.

• Activity intolerance, related to fatigue, weight loss, hyperthermia, and insomnia
• Nutrition: less than body requirements, altered, related to increased metabolic rate resulting in poor weight gain
• Knowledge deficit, related to effect of hyperthyroidism on fetus and new medications
• Self-concept or body image disturbance, related to goiter and exophthalmos

EXPECTED OUTCOMES

• General feelings of health return as noted by temperature stability, normal sleep patterns, and muscle strength.
• Normal weight progression resumes, and appetite returns to normal.
• Ability to discuss feelings about self and body image is present.
• Awareness of treatment plan and medication requirements is present.

NURSING INTERVENTION

During the actual hyperthyroid state, the woman will have increased dietary needs. Guidance as to the appropriate food choices for a well-balanced intake (with suggestions for snacks and extra fluid intake to compensate for increased perspiration, urination, and metabolism) is an important contribution by the nurse counselor. Some women are afflicted with diarrhea. Question the client about particular foods that cause diarrhea for her (highly seasoned and fibrous foods frequently speed peristalsis).

Daily weights should be charted by the client. Instruct her to weigh herself at the same time every morning, after voiding, and before breakfast.

The woman's environment must be made as comfortable as possible. Because there will be initial restlessness, anxiety, insomnia, and diaphoresis, it is important to create a stress-free environment by limiting visitors to those the woman chooses and by reducing noise, dimming lights, and changing linens as needed. Until the treatment plan takes effect, these measures will make the initial period tolerable. Work together with the client to achieve these goals.

Because of the woman's nutritional imbalance, intake and output are important. Vital signs will reflect recovery with a decreased pulse rate and temperature. If an eye condition leads to dryness and discomfort, soothing drops will be ordered and will be administered by either the client or the nurse. The client is included in every step of care, with the nurse giving rational explanations for all questions and providing information to alleviate anxiety or fear. Remember to repeat and reinforce information. When a person is under physiologic stress, ability to retain information is decreased.

Client teaching. When implementing all teaching, including medication information, the following points are helpful:

1. Because the hyperthyroid client may be anxious, go slowly with instruction, repeating information as necessary and have her repeat it for verification of understanding. Personalize instructions, and write out directions.
2. Teach names and dosages of drugs, and specify exact hours for taking each one.
3. Be sure the woman knows she must continue medication as long as the physician considers it necessary. She will soon feel better, but she must not stop medication prematurely. Often, PTU is withdrawn by the physician several weeks before delivery because 30% of gravidas will have returned to a normal thyroid state.
4. Granulocytosis is a rare but serious side effect of PTU. Medication should be stopped promptly with appearance of fever or sore throat and the health care provider contacted immediately.
5. Breast-feeding is not contraindicated if PTU therapy must continue after birth.

EVALUATION

The following questions may be asked:

- Does the woman express satisfaction with environmental comfort?
- Can she state current level of responses to therapy?
- Is weight gain adequate?
- Does she understand the plan of care and precautions about medications at home?
- Has she discussed with the team the implications of thyroid imbalance on the fetus?

TEST *Yourself* 24-1 _____

a. Why should a pregnant woman with hyperthyroidism be carefully monitored during the entire pregnancy?
b. When might surgical correction be indicated?
c. What are the important points to teach about her medications?

Hypothyroidism

Low T_4 levels frequently prevent conception, so **hypothyroidism** is rare in pregnant women. If it occurs, it is usually secondary to a known disorder such as Hashimoto's disease or to prior thyroid gland ablation by RAI or surgery. Any of these disorders may have been diagnosed before pregnancy, with thyroid replacement hormone (TRH) given orally to normalize balance. Because of the demands of pregnancy, however, thyroid replacement may now be inadequate.

Every system of the body is affected by a low thyroxin level (see Table 24-1). Primary hypothyroidism is caused by inability to produce or release thyroid hormones because of irradiation, surgical removal of tissue, or defects in synthesis because of antithyroid drugs or iodine deficiency. This leads to increased secretion of TSH from the pituitary gland without a corresponding release of T_3 and T_4 from the thyroid. Secondary and tertiary hypothyroidism is a result of deficiency in TSH and TRH production and release. Hypothyroid states are more commonly found in whites than in other races.

Risk

A decreased rate of conception is common. Women with untreated hypothyroidism who become pregnant have a greater number of low birth weight and stillborn infants (ACOG, 1993). When the deficient hormone has been adequately replaced, pregnancy outcome appears good. Sensitivity to anesthetic agents is a significant problem in uncorrected hypothyroidism and places the woman at increased risk for complications.

Clinical management

When taken daily, thyroid hormone replacement helps the woman achieve normal thyroid levels. Symptoms of the disorder fade gradually. Pregnant women may need higher doses of hormone replacement than nonpregnant women. Blood levels should be monitored closely by the obstetrician and endocrinologist.

Nursing responsibilities

The woman must understand that a balanced state is achieved slowly. Comfort needs should be given appropriate attention, such as extra clothing if she is cold intolerant, small frequent meals and extra fluids, and fiber in the diet to counteract constipation. Her skin will be dry and itchy, and her hair will be dry, so skin and hair care must be provided. As serum thyroid levels stabilize, symptoms should disappear. The importance of continuing daily medication must be stressed even though signs have resolved. If there are children at home, reinforce safety concerning medications. An intake of thyroid replacement tablets (L-thyroxin, Synthroid) by children can lead to acute hyperthyroidism and all its consequences.

TEST *Yourself* **24-2** _____

When there is a low T$_4$ and high TSH levels, what are the signs?

DIABETES MELLITUS

Diabetes mellitus (DM), from the Greek *diabetes* (siphon) and the Latin *mellitus* (honey-sweet), is the inability to metabolize glucose properly. It is a chronic systemic disease, manifesting metabolic and vascular changes affecting virtually every organ in the body. The basic defect is an absolute or relative lack of insulin, which leads to alterations of carbohydrate, protein, and fat metabolism. The attendant vascular changes include thickening of basement membranes, microaneurysms, peripheral vascular disease, and early and widespread atherosclerosis. Transient and permanent neuropathies commonly develop.

There are several types of DM. Type I **insulin-dependent diabetes mellitus** (IDDM) can occur at any age. This person is dependent on insulin for life; without daily injections, ketoacidosis will develop.

Recently, IDDM has been shown to be linked to the HLA region of chromosome 6, which also has immunologic functions (Reece, Hagay, and Hobbins, 1991).

According to Lipman (1988), DM type I is inherited recessively; 75% of the population is free of diabetes; 20% are not diabetic but are able to transmit the gene; and 5% are diabetic, who, although not necessarily symptomatic, are able to transfer the disease to offspring. Although not specifically race-related, the incidence of diabetes type I is somewhat higher in whites than in African-Americans. DM type I is widely distributed geographically, with the greatest prevalence occurring in northern Europe; its incidence decreases in the Mediterranean region and still further in eastern Asia (Lipman, 1988). (See Table 24-2 for a classification of diabetes existing before pregnancy.)

Type II **non–insulin-dependent diabetes mellitus** (NIDDM) has been called adult or maturity-onset DM and has been further subgrouped into *insulin-requiring* and *non–insulin-requiring*. NIDDM is thought to be a problem of peripheral insulin resistance rather than insulin deficiency. Type II clients are usually middle-aged and overweight at onset. Type II is found more commonly in African-Americans and is also associated with hypertension.

Table **24-2** **Characteristics Associated with Glucose Intolerance**	
Types of Glucose Intolerance	**Characteristics**
DIABETES MELLITUS (DM) *Type I Insulin-Dependent (IDDM)* Insulin deficient	• Prone to produce ketones • Caused by islet cell destruction • Associated with specific HLA types • Common in young, though occurring at any age
Type II Non–insulin-dependent (NIDDM) Insulin resistant	• Is ketosis resistant • Common in adults • Associated with increased basal metabolic rate (overweight) • Seen in families as autosomal dominant recessive trait
DM associated with conditions or syndromes	• Hyperglycemia caused by pancreatic disease • Drug or chemically induced DM • Insulin-receptor disorders • Certain genetic syndromes
IMPAIRED GLUCOSE TOLERANCE (IGT) (Secondary diabetes)	• Abnormal glucose levels but less than those noted in overt DM • Can improve, remain static, or progress to overt DM
GESTATIONAL DIABETES MELLITUS (GDM)	• Glucose intolerance occurring during pregnancy

Modified from Lloyd K et al: Psychosocial factors and complications of IDDM, *J Clin Applied Research and Education in Diabetes Care* 15(2):166, 1992.

Type II diabetes is usually controlled by diet, but women may need insulin when stressed or pregnant (Douglas, 1990). The key difference is that they may require insulin to prevent hyperglycemia but are not insulin dependent to sustain life.

Other types of DM—secondary diabetes—include diseases causing carbohydrate intolerance, such as pancreatic disease, hormonally and chemically induced diabetes, insulin receptor abnormalities, and certain genetic syndromes.

Gestational diabetes mellitus (GDM) is an alteration in carbohydrate intolerance initially noted during pregnancy. It occurs in approximately 3% of pregnant women, and the symptoms and abnormalities in glucose tolerance disappear after delivery. The symptoms of **hyperglycemia** are usually mild, but the risks of this hyperglycemia to the fetus can be serious as with other types of DM. The diagnosis of GDM applies regardless of whether insulin is included in the treatment plan or whether the hyperglycemia persists after delivery. Compare characteristics of these types of DM in Table 24-3.

Impaired glucose tolerance includes a glucose level that is slightly elevated but less than the levels noted in GDM and IDDM. The condition may progress to DM type II, remain static, or disappear (see Table 24-3). Diet and exercise are usually adequate interventions.

Pregnancy Unmasks Diabetes Mellitus

In normal pregnancies, the maternal plasma glucose level fluctuates between 60 and 120 mg/dl. The glucose balance is affected by changes in estrogen and progesterone levels leading to β cell hyperplasia (enlarged insulin-secreting cells in the pancreas). Since peripheral utilization of glucose is increased during pregnancy, this in turn leads to lower glucose levels. Maternal glucose crosses the placenta, but maternal insulin does not. In pregnancies complicated by diabetes, maternal hyperglycemia leads to fetal hyperglycemia. Fetal hyperglycemia in turn stimulates the

fetal pancreas β cells to produce increased insulin. The increased insulin produces β cell hyperplasia and fetal hyperinsulinemia. After the birth and separation from the maternal sources of glucose, the newborn quickly becomes hypoglycemic (see Chapter 29 for treatment of the infant of a diabetic mother.)

Risk

Women with IDDM who have vasculopathy (vascular changes) or unstable diabetes are at the greatest risk for complications and death during pregnancy. Women with progressive vascular disease have a significantly lower rate of conception. Other clients with severe complications of diabetes involving the eyes, kidneys, or heart may be advised not to become pregnant. Most complications, however, are usually not severe enough to preclude pregnancy (Jonaitis, 1995). Benign diabetic retinopathy may worsen during pregnancy but usually will improve following birth. The same cannot be said of women with untreated proliferative retinopathy before pregnancy, since worsening of the condition and vision loss may occur.

Fetal risk from insulin-dependent diabetes mellitus. There is increasing evidence to suggest that the degree of glucose control for an IDDM woman before conception greatly affects the fetal outcome. Studies find that poor maternal glucose control underlies the incidence of congenital malformations in **infants of diabetic mothers** (IDMs) (Box 24-1). Metabolic control during pregnancy reduces the risk of perinatal mortality to the same level of risk experienced by the general population (Fagan, King, Erick, 1995).

The primary problems for an IDM are either **macrosomia** or intrauterine growth retardation (IUGR), intrauterine death, or delayed pulmonary maturation with respiratory distress syndrome. At any age, the IDM is 5 to 6 times more likely to develop respiratory distress syndrome. Why does this happen? Insulin is an important growth factor during fetal development, and hyperinsulinism results in macrosomia (Figure 24-2) but delays pulmonary maturation. The fetus may have adequate

---

Table **24-3**   **Classification of Pregestational Diabetes that Complicate Pregnancy**

Class	Age at Onset	Duration (yr)	Vascular Disease	Therapy A
A	Any	Any	None	A-1, diet only; A-2, add insulin
B	>20	<10	None	Insulin
C	10-19	10-19	None	Insulin
D	<10	>20	Benign retinopathy	Insulin
F	Any	Any	Neuropathy	Insulin
R	Any	Any	Proliferative neuropathy	Insulin
H	Any	Any	Heart disease	Insulin

Landon M: Diabetes in pregnancy, *Clin Perinatol* 20(3):1, 1993.

Box 24-1 Possible Congenital Malformations in Infants of Diabetic Mothers

CARDIOVASCULAR SYSTEM
Transposition of great vessels
Ventral septal defect
Atrial septal defect
Hypoplastic left ventricle

MUSCULOSKELETAL SYSTEM
Cordal regression syndrome
Spina bifida

GASTROINTESTINAL SYSTEM
Tracheoesophageal fistula
Bowel atresia
Imperforate anus

CENTRAL NERVOUS SYSTEM
Meningomyelocele
Anencephaly
Encephalocele
Microcephaly

GENITOURINARY SYSTEM
Absent kidneys
Polycystic kidneys

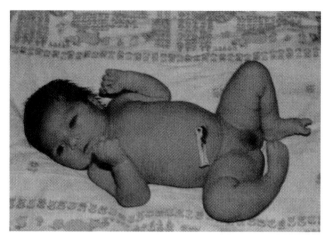

Figure 24-2 Large-for-gestational-age, macrosomic infant of a diabetic mother. (Courtesy Marjorie Pyle, RNC, *Lifecircle*.)

TEST *Yourself* 24-3 _____

a. In IDDM mothers, moderate maternal hyperglycemia may cause what effects in the fetus?
b. For what reasons are IDMs more likely to have respiratory distress?

amounts of lecithin despite limited total surfactant volume because fetal hyperinsulinemia results in inhibition of surfactant synthesis. In pregnancies complicated by diabetes, lecithin to sphingomyelin (L/S) ratios of 3.5 to 4.0:1.0 are more commonly accepted than the standard 2.0:1.0 (Samson, 1992).

Phosphatidylglycerol (PG) appears in amniotic fluid after 35 weeks and is a clear marker of lung maturity. If the woman is a severe diabetic with poor control, the fetus may be IUGR, have mental deficiency, or may die from prolonged exposure to ketonemia. After 36 weeks, the incidence of fetal mortality appears to increase. For this reason, during this period nonstress tests (NSTs) and biophysical profile scores (BPS) are done three to five times a week. Early delivery is not indicated as long as the fetus remains stable (Jovanovic and Peterson, 1992).

Risk for gestational diabetes mellitus infants. Women who have fasting and postprandial glucose elevations are at higher risk for intrauterine or neonatal mortality. Well-controlled glucose levels in maternal GDM leads to less risk. Approximately 25% of infants of GDM mothers have a characteristic triad of problems during recovery: hypoglycemia, hypocalcemia, and hyperbilirubinemia (see Chapter 29). These infants may also have cardiomyopathy, polycythemia, and small left-colon syndrome.

Signs

The symptoms of uncontrolled or new-onset IDDM include excessive thirst, hunger, and weight loss (Box 24-2). There may be blurred vision and possibly recurrent, hard to resolve infections. DM can develop rapidly and lead to hospitalization for acute symptoms. It may also develop slowly, with symptoms appearing gradually so as not to be initially noticed.

On the other hand, GDM women have no overt signs, although hypertension and overweight may be present. An elevated blood glucose (BG) level may be detected only upon testing with a glucose challenge or a glucose tolerance test.

Pregnant women with IDDM are at increased risk for development of diabetic ketoacidosis (DKA). Hyperglycemia related to inadequate insulin production can result in ketoacidosis. Ketone bodies are released into the blood when fatty acids are metabolized. Although (DKA) progresses slowly, it may develop more rapidly in the pregnant client because of the accelerated starvation process that occurs in the nonfed state (Gilbert and Harmon, 1993). DKA may occur with prolonged vomiting or carbohydrate deficiency. The presence of an infection with increased insulin requirements is also a common cause because infection precipitates a rise in plasma glucose levels. If not addressed quickly by increasing the insulin doses, there may be formation of plasma ketones. The pregnant woman will then experience breath with a fruity

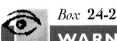

Box 24-2

WARNING SIGNS

Overt Diabetes

Polyuria (excess urination)
Polydipsia (excess thirst and fluid intake)
Polyphagia (excess hunger and food intake)
Neuritis (pain in the fingers and toes)
Skin disturbances (for example, pruritus [itching] and
   slow healing)
Weight loss
Weakness, fatigue, drowsiness

Box 24-3   **General Guidelines for Good Control of Glucose Levels**

	TYPE I	TYPE II
Fasting	<120 mg/dl	<140 mg/dl
Postprandial	<180 mg/dl	<200 mg/dl

Modified from the American Diabetes Association, 1988.

Box 24-4   **Classification of Diabetes Mellitus**

DIABETES MELLITUS
Random plasma glucose level >200 mg/dl with symptoms of diabetes
Fasting plasma glucose level >140 mg/dl on two occasions
Two oral glucose tolerance tests with a 2-hour sample >200 mg/dl and one other value >200 mg/dl repeated in 1 month

GESTATIONAL DIABETES MELLITUS
Two or more plasma glucose levels equal to or greater than those noted below, following a 100 g oral glucose intake:

Fasting	105 mg/dl
1 hour postglucose load	190 mg/dl
2 hour postglucose load	165 mg/dl
3 hour postglucose load	145 mg/dl

Modified from the American Diabetes Association, 1992.

---

odor, dehydration, and blood glucose levels in excess of 300 mg/dL (Gilbert and Harmon, 1993).

When malaise, drowsiness, and hyperventilation are noted, a severe illness requiring hospitalization is present, and an endocrinologist and perinatologist will be needed to treat the mother and fetus. Fluid replacement, stabilization of serum electrolytes, and correction of acidosis are part of the treatment plan for this medical emergency.

Clinical management

The goals of treatment for diabetes are to (1) maintain metabolic control of glucose levels (Box 24-3) and (2) prevent acute and chronic complications.

The American Diabetes Association (ADA) Position Statement on GDM (1990) states that all pregnant women should be screened for glucose intolerance between 24 and 28 weeks of pregnancy. However, a woman with a history of glucose intolerance would be tested in the first trimester. Box 24-4 lists diagnostic criteria, and Figure 24-3 lists decisions based on testing results.

First a *glucose challenge* of 50 g is given, and 1 hour later, blood is drawn for glucose levels. If levels are above 140 mg/dl, the woman is tested with a larger dose in the *glucose tolerance test* (GTT). Three days before a GTT, the client should be put on a diet of 150 g of carbohydrate per day, fasting after midnight on the day of the test and having taken no caffeine or nicotine.

Laboratory tests. A history of elevated glucose may be seen by two laboratory tests. Hemoglobin A_{1c} (HbA_{1c}) is a measure (a "lie detector") used to estimate BG levels during the previous 4 to 6 weeks. HbA_{1c} is an irreversible bond of glucose to a fraction of hemoglobin protein. Because the life cycle of a red blood cell is 120 days, an elevated HbA_{1c} indicates significant *past hyperglycemia*. This test will be used throughout the pregnancy to monitor levels. Levels greater than normal reflect poor control of BG. The following outcomes have been documented by long-term studies (Barss, 1989).

Excellent control <6.9%: outcome has shown no infant malformation

Good control <7 to 8.5%: outcome has shown 5% malformations

Poor control >8.6%: outcome has shown 22% malformations

There may be false low results with anemia and renal failure, and false high results with stress and steroids.

The second measure of elevated glucose levels is the use of fructosamine glycosylated albumin, which indicates the average serum glucose for the last 1 to 3 weeks because the life span of albumin is 28 to 40 days. High fructosamine glycosylated albumin has been seen in women with large infants.

Before conception, the pregnant woman with DM should work together with members of the diabetes health care team, including the obstetrician, a specialist in diabetes, a certified diabetes nurse educator, and a nutritionist. As labor approaches, a perinatologist joins the team. All should agree that the woman is in good control as she plans to conceive. Because she will need extra care, the woman and her partner should understand the cost of the pregnancy in terms of the money and time spent being monitored, both at home and in the hospital.

Decision TREE | *Gestational Diabetes*

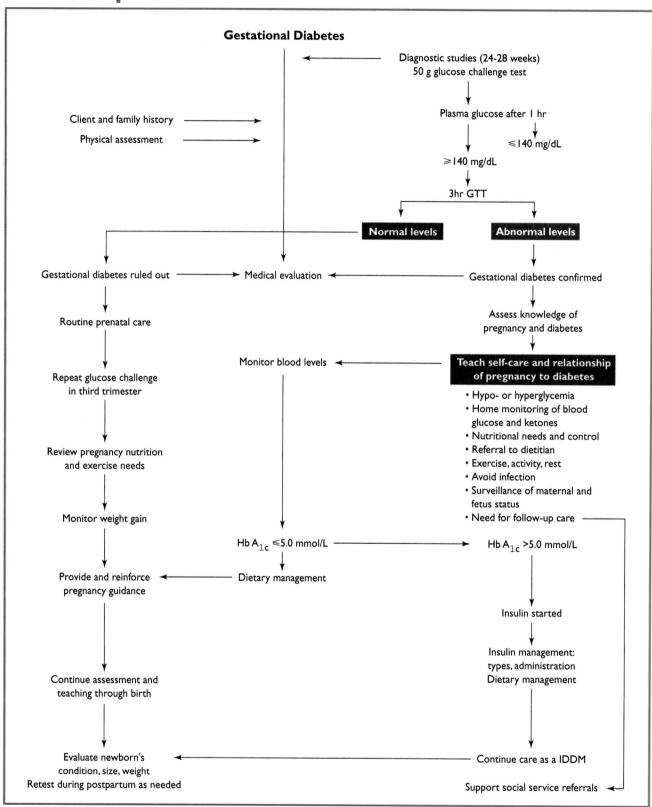

Figure 24-3   Gestational diabetes. *GTT*, Glucose tolerance test; *IDDM*, insulin-dependent diabetes mellitus.

Oral hypoglycemic agents are known to cross the placenta and have adverse effects on fetal development. These drugs should be discontinued before conception. If she is not aware of risks, a woman with type II DM may seek care in the first trimester while still taking oral agents. Risks associated with oral agents will need to be discussed with the client.

The four major areas to be taught in management are BG monitoring, insulin, nutrition, and exercise.

Blood glucose monitoring. Glucose monitoring in the home is essential for pregnant women with DM. Blood glucometers requiring only one drop of blood from a finger-stick sample are easy to use, give rapid results, and are small and portable. Measurements should be taken on a schedule as seen in Box 24-4. Ideally, levels should be checked before meals, two hours postprandial, at bedtime, and around 2 to 3 AM, when there is increased risk of nocturnal hypoglycemia. In reality, it is very difficult for the woman to be so precise. Therefore she needs a number of incentives and much encouragement to inflict needle sticks so many times a day.

The nurse works with the woman to encourage compliance. Keeping a chart is an incentive, especially when the woman brings it to the clinic at each visit. Women soon learn their own patterns and can then omit one or two testing times because they understand the daily fluctuations. Teach the woman that blood is taken only from the side of the finger, using all ten fingers in a rotation so that there is time to heal (see Procedure 24-1). When she is in the hospital, encourage her to continue doing her own checks because she causes herself less pain and can be more consistent. In this way, she keeps a measure of independence in the hospital setting.

Insulin. Most pregnant women have a general lowering of plasma glucose levels during the first trimester for three reasons: levels of human placental lactogen (hPL), an insulin antagonist, are low; energy demands of the embryo are minimal; and the woman is eating less because of nausea and vomiting. Therefore IDDM clients are at greater risk for **hypoglycemia** and insulin shock during the first trimester. The woman will need to know how to adjust insulin levels in response to glucose testing.

PROCEDURE 24-1

Testing for Glucose: Capillary Blood Sugar

1. Wash hands in warm water (warmth promotes circulation).
2. Choose a finger, and, using spring-driven lancet, stick the finger on the side or outer edge (least painful sites).
3. Drop hand to side, below heart. (Perhaps "milk" the finger, using other hand, gently squeezing finger from hand to fingertip.) Be sure there is enough blood to cover both pads on plastic glucose-oxidase impregnated strips.
4. Put drop of blood on strip as instructed by health team, following timing and wiping away excess blood as directed by method.
5. Read visually or on reflectance meter, and record the result.
6. Repeat on recommended schedule.

Urine for glucose and ketones

1. Empty bladder completely (the "long specimen").
2. Using a clean container, void again 30 minutes later, and collect specimen (the "short specimen").
3. Test "short specimen" for glucose and ketones.
4. Repeat in morning each day (or as otherwise instructed).

OPTIONAL ACTIVITY

Write a sample nursing note correctly documenting the performance of this procedure.

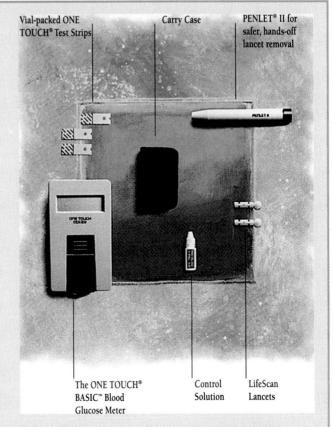

Figure 24-4 One touch glucose testing equipment. (Courtesy Life Scan, Milpitas, Calif.)

During the second half of pregnancy, elevated gestational hormones and increased maternal weight place a demand on the body for greater insulin production. Maternal metabolism usually compensates for this altered state by secreting additional insulin. The client with gestational diabetes demonstrates an elevated blood sugar in the second and third trimesters and progresses to a mild hyperglycemic state.

The woman with IDDM who is under the influence of these metabolic changes in the second and third trimesters will find that her insulin requirement increases as much as two to three times. However, her condition is not becoming worse; insulin needs will return to prepregnancy levels after birth.

However, the IDDM woman's greater need for insulin means administering divided doses, and often three to four injections each day. Thus the woman may begin to feel that she is sick and can become fearful or noncompliant. Nursing intervention is important during these weeks to keep the woman focused on the goal of having a healthy infant.

A number of changes have been made in recommendations for insulin administration, not all of which have been put into practice correctly in hospital units (See annotated reference in Student Resource Shelf from *Diabetes Care*, 1990, for insulin administration recommendations.) In the following list of recommendations, note how the concern to protect tissue integrity overrides certain routine habits of injection.

Human insulin should be used during pregnancy because it has a more rapid onset and a shorter duration of action. Human insulin triggers fewer antibodies and is recommended for women who are beginning insulin treatment, such as for GDM or NIDDM mothers placed on insulin. A pregnant woman already using another type or brand of insulin should remain on that brand, even in the hospital. *Do not change brands without careful supervision because there are different levels of action.*

- Insulin requires refrigeration only for long-term storage. An opened vial should be kept at room temperature for up to 30 days. It has been found that refrigerated, cold insulin irritates the tissue more than that kept at room temperature.
- Neutral protamine Hagedorn (NPH) and regular insulin may be premixed into the same syringe without any change in stability. At home, these may be mixed in the morning and given at the specified intervals throughout the day.
- At home, insulin needles and syringes may be reused until the needle is dull. This is true as long as the needle is recapped *immediately* after use. Do not wipe needle with alcohol because alcohol removes the silicone covering that prevents trauma during injection.
- Insulin should be given at a 90-degree angle without aspiration or massage of the site. It is not necessary to cleanse the skin with alcohol because alcohol tracked

down with the needle irritates the tissue. If alcohol is used, *be sure the skin is dry before injection.*

- The site of insulin administration and exercise following administration will affect the rate of absorption. In a crisis, if insulin is not given intravenously, the intramuscular (IM) route has the fastest absorption rate.
- Sites should be used for a week, with *rotation within the site*. This allows an area to completely heal in 3 to 4 weeks before being used again.
- Whenever possible, insulin should be self-injected by the client, even in hospital or during labor. Always ask her to inject herself, and only do it for her at her request.

Insulin pump. In certain cases, a woman may not be able to achieve a balanced glucose level—**euglycemia**—with the standard administration regimen. The continuous subcutaneous insulin infusion (CSII) pump is often a lifesaver for these women. The CSII pump has a small syringe that holds a 2-day supply of insulin. A thin catheter attaches to the insulin syringe in the pump. The end of the catheter has a small subcutaneous needle that is placed in recommended sites. The pump is programmed to deliver a basal rate of insulin in units an hour. The pump user programs the desired bolus of insulin before meals and snacks. Multiple BG measurements are needed to ensure that the basal rates and the dose of insulin are appropriate. Because CSII pumps require precise control, their use can only be an option for a select group of compliant pregnant women with DM. Cost is also a factor in availability for use.

Nutrition. The nutritional recommendations for pregnant women with DM are similar to those of the American Heart Association, though the proportions change slightly. Total calories are calculated to achieve desired body weight and the weight gain needed during pregnancy. The distribution of calories recommended by the ADA (1990) is as follows:

Carbohydrates 55% to 60% of caloric intake, with most in the form of complex carbohydrates

Fats < 30% of caloric intake

Protein 0.8 g/kg of body weight, unless renal disease is present

The average daily intake should be between 2000 and 2500 kcal. A gravida should be encouraged to increase the amount of fiber to at least 30 g per day to assist in glycemic control, relieve constipation, and satisfy the appetite.

Fiber. Addition of certain forms of dietary fiber to the diet of diabetics significantly *decreases* postprandial hyperglycemia. The ADA suggests a fiber intake as high as 20 to 30 g per 1000 calories. This amount would be derived from complex, unrefined carbohydrates, and from a generous amount of vegetables, salads, and fresh fruits.

The absorption rate of glucose into the blood has led to the labeling of carbohydrates as "slowly absorbed" and "rapidly absorbed." The slowly absorbed carbohydrates (complex, high in fiber) are preferred above the rapidly absorbed carbohydrates (simple sugars and disaccharides).

Because pregnancy is a dynamic state, frequent adjustments to the diet are made as gestation advances. Attention is focused on food preferences and lifestyle to increase the woman's ability to maintain appropriate intake. A daily planned pattern of three meals and three to four snacks is essential whether or not nausea is present (Table 24-4). Because nocturnal hypoglycemia is common in IDDM women, emphasis is placed on the importance of the bedtime snack. If the woman is in the hospital, she should participate in meal and snack planning because the snacks usually provided are often inadequate for her.

Obese pregnant women with NIDDM present a problem regarding diet and glucose levels. Because NIDDM is usually symptom-free, they may not be as motivated to make lifestyle changes early in pregnancy. Since this type of DM is related to insulin resistance, glucose regulation is difficult. The woman may be placed on insulin; she then must learn all the self-care factors. Under no condition should any weight loss be considered during pregnancy.

Women with GDM should follow the same general nutrition guidelines as seen in Table 24-4. Dietary modification is the first step in controlling hyperglycemia. In general, attempts are made to maintain BG between 60 mg/dl and 120 mg/dl. Although the woman may not need insulin, she should divide food intake into three meals and three snacks and maintain the ratio of fats, protein, and complex carbohydrates.

Exercise. Pregnant women with DM should begin exercise programs only after discussing the frequency, intensity, and duration of the exercise with the diabetes care team. Hopefully, a woman with IDDM has already been using a personal exercise program. Exercise lowers BG levels and decreases cardiovascular risk factors such as high blood pressure and hyperlipidemia. It also affects fuel use and insulin sensitivity in Type II diabetes, thus low-

---

▮ *Table* **24-4**	**Sample Menu and Distribution of Food with Insulin**[*]

Time	Menu
MORNING MEAL[†]	
Split between 7:30 AM and 10 AM	2 slices low-fat cheese or ¹/₂ cup cottage cheese
7 AM glucose test and insulin—regular and long-acting	2 slices wheat or rye bread or 1 cup oatmeal
	2 tsp margarine or butter
	1 cup skim milk
	1 serving fresh fruit
NOON MEAL	
Split between 12:30 PM and 3 PM	3 oz of fish, poultry, or meat (trim fat)
Noon glucose test	1 serving mixed salad
	2 slices wheat or rye bread or 1 cup rice
	2 tsp of margarine or mayonnaise
	1 cup skim milk or plain low-fat yogurt
	1 serving fresh fruit
EVENING MEAL	
Split between 5:30 PM and 8 PM	4 oz fish, poultry, or meat (trim fat)
5 PM glucose test and regular insulin	¹/₂ to 1 cup cooked vegetables
	1 serving mixed salad
	1 cup corn or lima beans
	2 tsp margarine or oil
	1 cup skim milk or buttermilk
BEDTIME SNACK	
10:30 PM	¹/₂ cup cottage cheese, 2 slices low-fat cheese,
Some clients need to be tested at night.	or 2 tsp of peanut butter
	1 slice wheat or rye bread
	1 serving fresh fruit

Available from the American Dietetic Association (216 West Jackson Boulevard, Chicago, Illinois 60606), the "diabetic exchange list" can be used as a guide to high-fiber foods.
[*]2000 Calories.
[†] Reduce carbohydrates in morning meal. Distribute food from each list between the meal and the snack after the meal.

ering insulin requirements. Regular exercise sessions rather than sporadic exercise are more effective in regulating BG levels. The benefits of exercise can be obtained through scheduled sessions lasting 20 to 45 minutes, 3 days a week.

Intrapartum management. Infants of well-controlled DM women are usually delivered just before or at term. Acceptable results of weekly and then biweekly NSTs and of an L/S ratio greater than 3.5 to 4.0:1 or a positive PG level are indicators of fetal well-being and pulmonary maturity.

Regardless of what a fetal maturity test may show, early delivery is required when pregnancy-induced hypertension (PIH), repeated ketoacidosis, increasing polyhydramnios, advancing maternal retinopathy or preexisting renal disease with hypertension or albuminuria occurs. Sonography should aid the obstetrician in identifying the infant who may require a cesarean birth because of macrosomia.

Intrapartum management of an IDDM woman requires attention to glucose levels, glucose infusion rates, and insulin dosage. Bedside BG testing during labor is mandatory on a schedule of every 2 hours in early labor and every hour in late labor and immediate recovery. Labor is equivalent to moderate exercise; thus less insulin is needed for control. An IDDM patient will usually have an intravenous (IV) infusion of 1000 ml D$_5$LR with 10 U regular insulin, to run at 100 ml per hour. This rate provides 1 U per hour. An additional bolus may be given as needed.

If the plan is for cesarean birth, it should be done early in the morning, with no glucose or insulin administered until after delivery if blood sugar is 80 to 120 mg/dl. The woman's glucose level should be checked before and immediately following delivery. If necessary, IV glucose will be administered. A neonatologist must be present at the delivery.

Postpartum management. BG management following birth can be difficult because of endocrine and metabolic changes. When the placenta separates, insulin antagonists (hPL, estrogen, and progesterone), are removed and there is a reduction in plasma cortisol; thus there is a reduced need for insulin. After the second day, hPL is gone, and insulin shock is possible if usual doses of insulin are continued. Therefore, during the first 24 hours, long-acting insulin is not given. Monitoring BG levels every 4 hours will determine the need for additional cover regular insulin. The prepregnancy amount of long-acting insulin is usually ordered by the second morning after birth.

Breast-feeding is encouraged as beneficial for both mother and infant. Breast milk is not altered by diabetes. The breast-feeding diabetic mother may have a lower BG level because glucose is transferred from blood to the breast to be converted into lactose. Production of milk also expends energy. During lactation, calorie needs increase 500 to 800 kcal above prepregnant requirements (see Chapter 10). Insulin dosage will be recalculated

according to the individual's needs. Home BG monitoring should continue for the breast-feeding IDDM mother. Hypoglycemia decreases milk supply and inhibits the letdown reflex. If ketonuria is present and persists, breast-feeding must be discontinued.

Barrier methods are preferable for contraception. Oral contraception may change insulin requirements as a result of altered carbohydrate metabolism. Many diabetic women eventually choose tubal ligation.

Gestational diabetes mellitus management. The majority of women with GDM revert to a condition of euglycemia after delivery. Nonetheless, it is important after delivery to reassess women with an abnormal glucose tolerance to determine whether it returns to normal. The test is best repeated 6 weeks after birth. The woman should be warned that there is a strong possibility that diabetes will recur in each subsequent pregnancy. If she remains overweight, there is a greater chance of developing diabetes later in life (Coustan, 1993). All these factors make pregnancy an ideal time for teaching nutrition and self-care.

Nursing Responsibilities

ASSESSMENT

Never assume that a pregnant woman with known diabetes is fully knowledgeable about her survival needs. Glucose monitoring, insulin administration and adjustment, meal planning and timing, nutritional balance, health habits, and management of acute imbalance of glucose should be reviewed. In the same way, a client with a prior experience with GDM should be carefully assessed. She may be much more aware of her own needs than the nurse is, but she may also be ignorant in some surprising areas. Nursing assessments and intervention assume significant proportions because women who are diagnosed for the first time as type II DM or as GDM will need the complete range of teaching. The nurse may use the Diabetes Knowledge Screen in the initial assessment (Box 24-5).

NURSING DIAGNOSES

Depending on data collection, you may choose nursing diagnoses similar to the following for a pregnant woman identified as a diabetic.

- Anxiety over implications of diagnosis, related to risks for self and fetus, testing, and cost of pregnancy.
- Health-seeking behaviors, related to need to manage diabetic self-care.
- Injury, risk for maternal or fetal, related to glucose imbalance.

Box 24-5   Diabetes in Pregnancy Knowledge Screen

Below are questions about diabetes during pregnancy. Answering these questions will help us determine your current knowledge about diabetes during pregnancy and enable us to provide the best care possible during your pregnancy. Many questions have more than one answer; therefore circle "I don't know" rather than guessing. By answering to the best of your knowledge, we will be better able to counsel you effectively about diabetes during your pregnancy.

1. **Which of the following feelings may result from a reaction? (Circle all that might happen, not just those that have happened to you)**
   a. Difficulty thinking
   b. Blurred vision
   c. Nervousness or shaky
   d. Numbness
   e. Sweating
   f. I don't know.

2. **What should you do if you have a reaction? (Circle all that apply)**
   a. Walk it off.
   b. Sit down and rest.
   c. Eat crackers or cheese.
   d. Drink milk.
   e. I don't know.

3. **Glycosylated hemoglobin levels are drawn about once a month during pregnancy. Why are these levels taken?**
   a. They measure previous blood sugar control.
   b. They measure the amount of iron in your blood.
   c. They measure how helpful your diet is in controlling your blood sugar.
   d. I don't know.

4. **When planning vigorous exercise (e.g., swimming, playing tennis), what changes should you make in your daily routine? (Circle all that apply)**
   a. Decrease insulin.
   b. Carefully time when to do your exercising.
   c. Increase the amount of carbohydrates (e.g., bread, fruits) you eat.
   d. Increase the amount of protein (e.g., meat, cheese) you eat.
   e. I don't know.

5. **On days when you are sick, what steps should you take to control your diabetes?**
   a. Increase the amount of water or other fluids.
   b. Stop your insulin.
   c. Call your doctor.
   d. I don't know.

6. **The normal range for blood sugar during pregnancy is:**
   a. 40-150 mg/dl
   b. 60-120 mg/dl
   c. 100-200 mg/dl
   d. I don't know.

7. **A specific meal plan has been devised for you by the dietitian. Which of the following statements about your meal plan are correct? (Circle all that apply)**
   a. You should eat everything on your meal plan.
   b. You can reduce the amount of food you eat if you're not hungry.
   c. You should control the amount of food you eat all the time.
   d. You can eat your meals any time during the day as long as you eat everything on your plan.
   e. I don't know.

8. **Bedtime snacks are an important part of your meal plan because they help you avoid having reactions overnight. True or False?**

9. **Margarine is mainly: (Circle one)**
   a. Protein
   b. Carbohydrate
   c. Fat
   d. Mineral and vitamin
   e. I don't know.

10. **Rice is mainly: (Circle one)**
    a. Protein
    b. Carbohydrate
    c. Fat
    d. Mineral and vitamin
    e. I don't know.

11. **If you don't feel like having the egg on your diet for breakfast, you can: (Circle two)**
    a. Have extra toast.
    b. Substitute one small chop.
    c. Have one ounce of cheese instead.
    d. Skip the egg, and don't eat anything else.
    e. I don't know.

12. **If you have problems controlling your blood sugar during pregnancy, what are some of the possible effects on your infant after birth? (Circle all that apply)**
    a. Could be born with low blood sugar (hypoglycemia)
    b. Could be a large infant, making delivery more difficult
    c. Could have breathing problems after birth
    d. I don't know.

13. **What does glucagon do?**
    a. Helps the liver release more sugar into the blood
    b. Makes the liver stop releasing sugar into the blood
    c. Helps the pancreas release more insulin
    d. Stops the pancreas from releasing insulin
    e. I don't know.

14. **After using glucagon, it is most important to:**
    a. Drink plenty of fluids.
    b. Get plenty of rest.

Spirito A et al: Screening measure to assess knowledge of diabetes in pregnancy, *Diabetes Care* 13(7):712, 1990.

Box 24-1

CLINICAL DECISION

Debra, an IDDM woman, is scheduled for induction at 8 AM. She is anxious about the preparation for labor. Explain why each of these plans would be either helpful or harmful.
  a. Give her nothing by mouth after midnight, and draw fasting blood sugar before transfer to the labor area.
  b. Give both insulin and glucose by IV pump during labor.
  c. Provide a special high protein early breakfast.
  d. Begin IV therapy with D₅W, 1000 mL before the onset of labor.

- Noncompliance, risk for, related to restrictions in diet, frequent glucose measurements, lifestyle changes.
- Infection, risk for, caused by hyperglycemic state.

EXPECTED OUTCOMES

All of the outcomes center on the woman learning self-monitoring and self-care well enough that she can manage "day-to-day operations."
- Discusses the plan of care to determine fetal status and outcome.
- Verbalizes her understanding of how the pregnancy changes DM control.
- Demonstrates dietary control, insulin self-medication and glucose regulation.
- Maintains BG within advised range as seen by HbA$_{1c}$ tests.
- Persists with skin care, infection prevention, and exercise requirements.

NURSING INTERVENTION

The nurse plays an important role in the care and counseling of a pregnant DM woman. The woman may be eager to learn, or she may be angry and resistant because of the diagnosis. Whatever the case, it is essential that she soon learn how to manage her situation. She may need hospitalization during this learning interval, for regulation is difficult in the first trimester. She will need frequent prenatal visits and supervision by a diabetologist and nutritionist. Reinforce the idea that the health care team also desires a stable pregnancy and a healthy infant. Help her understand the ways hyperglycemia or hypoglycemia may injure her or her fetus. Without raising severe anxiety, help her understand the daily need for euglycemia. With good control, fetal defects and intrauterine deaths are practically at the same levels as for nondiabetic pregnancies.

The woman should be made aware of the potential signs of complications from infection, hypertension, and vascular disease. She should keep a record of insulin intake, glucose monitoring, and dietary schedules and amounts, noting her own ups and downs. She brings this record with her at each visit. Weight gain should follow the normal pattern, based on the BMI (see Chapter 10). With counseling from the nutritionist, the woman's cultural and ethnic patterns will be considered. The nurse can reinforce her nutritional choices.

Urinary ketones should be monitored daily by dipstick, since ketonuria may occur in the third trimester. A pregnant woman is more likely to spill ketones because calories from glucose and amino acids are diverted to the fetus, leading to increased breakdown of maternal fats. Significant ketonuria can alert the woman to the possibility of DKA, which carries an increased risk of fetal death.

Education is the key to a successful pregnancy. The woman must learn all signs of hyperglycemia and ketosis and how to use emergency treatment for hypoglycemia. At home or in the hospital, the *first line of defense* for hypoglycemia is a *glass of milk* because protein sustains a glucose level for a longer period than do simple sugars. If the BG level has dropped below 50 mg/dl and the woman is becoming confused, a rapid simple sugar such as orange juice can be offered. This should be followed by a protein, such as peanut butter with crackers, to prevent the BG level from rapidly dropping again. For a labile diabetic, **glucagon** may be administered IM by a nurse or a family member who has been instructed. Finally, IV glucose may be administered, usually by the physician. Venous and capillary blood sugars should be tested 30 minutes to 1 hour after such administrations; capillary levels are slightly below venous blood levels.

Client teaching. The following areas must be part of the teaching plan for the newly pregnant diabetic:
- Importance of early prenatal care and keeping all appointments
- Role of the diet for good nutrition and diabetic control
- Meals and snacks must be eaten on time and never skipped. Keeping a diet diary is a useful tool for learning or reviewing meal planning, calorie counting, and food values.
- Importance of consistent testing of capillary blood sugar and urine for ketones
- Ability to recognize the signs and symptoms of hypoglycemia and hyperglycemia, and understand why she may be more labile
- Friends and colleagues should be told of her diabetes, and she should wear identification as a diabetic.
- Need to carry fast-acting carbohydrate for emergency use and to use milk as the first choice when hypoglycemic
- Importance of care of teeth, skin, feet, and personal hygiene and of avoiding vaginal infections

- Importance of exercise and rest
- The woman should exercise after a meal, not when her blood sugar may be low. Do not administer insulin into an extremity that will immediately be used in exercise, and monitor BG to determine its variations with exercise.
- Method of administration of insulin (if applicable)
- The woman must have knowledge of type or types of insulin to be used. She must also be aware of protocol for sites of injection, rotation of sites, and skin inspection. She must demonstrate the technique for preparing materials and injection skills.
- In last trimester, ability to monitor and record level of fetal movements 3 times a day for 1 hour and report any changes.
- Reasons for referral to other health professionals (such as visiting nurse, ADA, homemaker, dietitian or nutritionist, social worker, other physicians, childbirth educator)

EVALUATION

- Did the woman demonstrate understanding of and compliance with plan of care in maintaining diabetic diet and following insulin requirements?
- Did the woman avoid injury to self and infant by maintaining adequate glucose balance?
- Were abnormal symptoms reported promptly and appropriately?
- Did family coping mechanisms appear positive?

RENAL ALTERATIONS DURING PREGNANCY

Renal plasma flow and glomerular filtration rates increase greatly during pregnancy. This increase begins in the first trimester and increases until just after delivery and is related to the increased cardiac output and decreased vascular resistance (Figure 24-5).

Infection

Women seem to be at a greater risk than men for developing urinary tract infections (UTIs), probably because of anatomic factors, as well as personal hygiene and sexual practices. The progression of enteric bacteria into the bladder is thought to occur by bowel flora (bacteria) colonizing in the perineum, vaginal vestibule, urethra, and bladder. The proximity of the anus, vagina, and urethra aids this process. Therefore routine hygiene factors after toileting and sexual intercourse are important to reinforce during pregnancy (Box 24-6).

Asymptomatic bacteriuria

Asymptomatic bacteriuria (ASB) is defined by the presence of more than 100,000 organisms/mm^3 in urine,

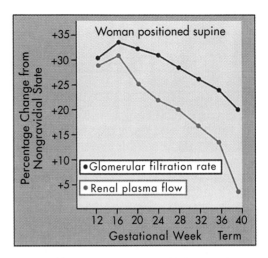

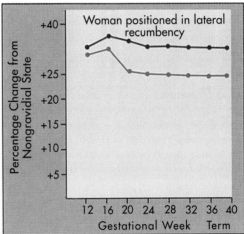

Figure 24-5   Renal hemodynamics in pregnancy. Differences in glomerular filtration rate and renal plasma flow in supine and lateral positions. Increases occur early in pregnancy and are sustained to term if women maintain lateral recumbency position. (From Lindheimer M, Katz A: Renal hemodynamics in pregnancy, *Contemp Obstet Gynecol* 3[1]:49, 1974.)

Box 24-6	**Perineal Hygiene**

Wipe front to back with a fresh tissue after each bowel movement.
Cleanse the urethral area with a fresh tissue.
Maintain adequate fluid intake.
Do not douche.
Flush perineum with warm water.
Void after intercourse.

without symptoms of fever, dysuria, urinary frequency, or flank pain. A great deal of research has been directed toward UTI because of a link with preterm labor, but ASB does not in itself appear to be causative. However, ASB may develop into **acute cystitis** (AC), and then a positive link with preterm labor becomes present (see Chapter 21).

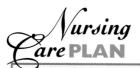

Nursing Care PLAN | *Diabetes during Pregnancy*

CASE

Denise, Para 2002, was a type II DM who managed on diet alone until this pregnancy. She is 130% of baseline weight. She earns a small weekly income and is a single parent living with her two active sons at her mother's home. At her eighth week visit, she was placed on insulin because of a high HbA$_{1c}$. She was counseled regarding risk of defects, and she needs extensive support and teaching about using insulin. She is to begin medication for bacteriuria.

Assessment

1. Has prior knowledge of diabetes and self-care with nutrition and exercise
2. Makes inaccurate choices in diet plan
3. Is new to insulin; has used only urine dipstick for checking glucose
4. Is now being treated for bacteriuria
5. Life situation indicates need for extensive support during this pregnancy

Nursing Diagnoses

1. Knowledge deficit, related to meaning of diagnosis, testing, and management throughout pregnancy
2. Noncompliance, risk for, related to lack of adequate support systems, anxiety, and need to work full time
3. Injury, risk for fetal or maternal, related to hyperglycemia
4. Infection, risk for, related to glycosuria and inadequate knowledge of preventive measures
5. Individual coping, ineffective, related to increased risk of diagnosis, stress of pregnancy and lack of resources.

Expected Outcomes

1. Maintains euglycemia at 60-120 mg/dl as seen by periodic HbA$_{1c}$ testing.
2. Keeps accurate records of glucose tests and dietary intake.
3. Masters insulin requirements and methods.
4. Identifies self-care requirements during pregnancy, and demonstrates prevention of infection, increased exercise, and good skin care.
5. Participates in planning care, keeps clinic appointments, and follows through on referrals for additional assistance.

Nursing Interventions

1. Engage Denise in reviewing what she knows and in identifying areas that need improved monitoring. Review learning needs for this pregnancy as well.
2. Determine her understanding of warning signs of hypoglycemia or hyperglycemia and which interventions to use. Ascertain if she knows when to call physician or nurses for questions.
3. Review customary diet, and help plan modifications.
4. Ensure her understanding of relationships between calories, fiber, exercise, and insulin balance.
5. Instruct her in record keeping and the Dextrostix procedure.
6. Demonstrate and then determine ability to select, measure, draw, and administer insulin injection.
7. Refer her for assistance in obtaining supplies, glucometer, test strips, lancets, syringes, and insulin. Refer her to social services and WIC program.
8. Review self-care needs for skin, infection prevention, adequate sleep and rest, and social support. Discuss ways she handles single parenting and full-time work. Set up a home care liaison if possible.
9. Refer her for identified coping problems and reinforce positive behaviors. Assign her to a contact person in the office or clinic setting, and exchange telephone numbers.

Evaluation

1. Is there appropriate weight gain for gestational age?
2. Has Denise maintained euglycemia? Did she accurately manage diet modifications, glucose testing, and insulin?
3. Did infection or other signs of complications occur?
4. Has she managed her social environment satisfactorily with referrals and support?

Acute cystitis

In approximately 1% of pregnant women, signs of bladder infection become evident. Symptoms include the classic signs of urgency, frequency, dysuria, and pyuria. Suprapubic tenderness is present, but fever and flank pain are absent. There may be a strong unpleasant odor to the urine and blood on the toilet tissues. Urine cultures test positive for the same organisms as those found in ASB.

Approximately 30% of women with acute symptoms may have sterile urine cultures. In this case, they are considered to have **acute urethral syndrome**, a condition most commonly associated with *Chlamydia trachomatis* infection (see Chapter 25), and they require treatment for that condition.

Acute pyelonephritis

Women with AC may progress to develop acute **pyelonephritis**. Acute pyelonephritis is the most common, nonobstetric cause for hospitalization during pregnancy.

Risk. The risk of maternal and fetal morbidity from acute pyelonephritis is significant. Up to 10% of pregnant women with acute pyelonephritis have bacteremia (positive blood cultures). Recurrent pyelonephritis, chronic renal disease, septicemia, septic shock, and adult respiratory distress syndrome are potential complications. In addition, the fetus is at risk from preterm labor and birth and potential teratogenic effects of maternal fever and antibiotic therapy (Gilbert and Harmon, 1993).

The presence of asymptomatic bacteriuria is the most common risk factor during pregnancy. Other risk factors are the same as for ASB (lower socioeconomic status, increasing age, parity, sickle cell trait, and chronic medical illness).

Signs. The clinical diagnosis of acute pyelonephritis is based on subjective complaints of chills, fever, back pain, dysuria, urgency, frequency, nausea and vomiting; physical findings of temperature greater than 101° F and costovertebral angle tenderness; and laboratory findings of pyuria and bacteriuria. During the early clinical course, the client may be afebrile but may still complain of these symptoms.

Clinical management. Because almost one half of the pregnant women with ASB will develop an acute infection if left untreated, most obstetricians believe that treatment is warranted (Davison et al, 1994). Women should have urine recultured within 3 to 4 days after the antibiotic course is completed and regularly throughout the rest of the pregnancy. Pregnant women must have a midstream, clean voided specimen or a straight catheterized specimen to avoid mixing urine with vaginal mucus. The woman should be taught to complete the course of antibiotics, which sometimes causes nausea. For ASB and AC, treatment is recommended for 10 to 14 days with nitrofurantoins, Gantrisin, or ampicillin. Sulfonamide antibiotics such as Gantrisin are avoided in the third trimester of pregnancy because of the association between their use and newborn hyperbilirubinemia.

Some authorities recommend that women with recurrent ASB during pregnancy should be given antimicrobial suppression by low doses of antimicrobials daily for the remainder of the pregnancy (Enkin et al, 1995).

Pregnant women with pyelonephritis require hospitalization and close monitoring of maternal status, IV hydration, and antibiotic therapy. Choice of antibiotics includes broad spectrum antibiotics or those that provide coverage for the microorganisms most often found. Combinations of ampicillin or a cephalosporin with an aminoglycoside are usually initiated. This combination therapy is recommended because microorganisms resistant to ampicillin and cephalosporins are often recovered from women with pyelonephritis. The high incidence of bacteremia and the potential for endotoxin sepsis warrants the use of broad spectrum antimicrobial agents. Ampicillin is indicated because a small portion of pyelonephritis is associated with group B streptococci and Enterococcus. IV antibiotics are generally continued until the client is afebrile for at least 24 hours and able to tolerate oral medication. The majority of clients are usually afebrile within 48 hours of treatment onset. If the client continues to be febrile, a repeat urine culture for antimicrobial sensitivities is performed to evaluate for the presence of microorganism resistance. Frequently, a change or addition of antibiotics is then made. After discontinuation of IV antibiotics, the client continues oral antibiotics for 10 to 14 days on an outpatient basis.

Chronic Renal Problems

Among the background renal conditions that may be complicated by pregnancy are chronic glomerulonephritis, nephrotic syndrome, polycystic kidney, class F diabetes, solitary kidney, and kidney transplant. Significant proteinuria will invariably accompany these conditions, leading the physician to investigate. Normally the BP falls during early pregnancy. An elevated BP and serum urea may be the earliest signs of a developing renal problem. Accompanying acute renal failure may be abruptio placentae and severe preeclampsia.

Chronic glomerulonephritis

Ranging in severity from tolerable impairment of kidney function to severe disability, *chronic glomerulonephritis* was once incompatible with pregnancy. Now it is considered manageable in a cooperative client. Usually a sequel to a severe systemic disease (most notably streptococcal glomerulonephritis) chronic glomerulonephritis results in proteinuria or persistent urinary sediment. Because streptococcal infections are now treated aggressively, this condition is becoming less prevalent. In pregnancy, it produces palpitation, visual disturbances, headaches, fatigue, dizziness, nausea, vomiting, edema, hypertension, and eventually some degree of cardiovascular disease and renal insufficiency. Anemia is usually severe enough to require transfusion. After pregnancy, the mother's condition returns to the state present at conception.

Nephrotic syndrome

If nephrotic syndrome appears during pregnancy, the findings may seem to indicate preeclampsia—edema, massive protein in the urine, low blood protein, and lipidemia, with or without hypertension. Renal biopsy is required for definitive diagnosis. Usually the kidney functions enough to allow the pregnancy to continue; interruption is indicated by severe malfunction, hypertension, or uremia. Thromboembolism (caused by an elevated fibrinogen or depressed antithrombin level) and infection as a consequence of low gamma globulin level must also be anticipated. Depending on the cause, recovery may occur, or the disease may progress to renal failure and death. Pregnancy seems to have no serious effect on the course of the disease.

Solitary kidney or kidney transplant

Traditionally, a woman with one functioning kidney would be discouraged from conceiving because of the strain pregnancy places on the remaining kidney.

When only one kidney is present, it will enlarge to compensate for the extra demands of pregnancy. Pregnancy does not seem to cause any other special problems. The duration of the solitary kidney condition, the present ability of that kidney to function, and the cause of the condition must be taken into account.

Following renal transplantation, renal and endocrine functions return to normal quickly. Most centers advise that the woman be 2 years posttransplant before she considers becoming pregnant.

Currently, the following criteria may be applied to a woman with a kidney transplant to assess eligibility for becoming pregnant (Pritchard, 1993):
1. Good general health
2. No elevation in BP for 2 years after treatment
3. No evidence of graft reaction
4. No persisting proteinuria

If for any reason a cesarean birth is needed, a midline incision is preferable because it minimizes danger to the transplanted kidney if it is pelvically located.

Risk. Davison and Lindheimer (1996) state that the ability of women with renal disease to sustain an uncomplicated pregnancy is related to the absence or presence of hypertension and to the degree of organ system impairment. Women who have mildly impaired renal function and no hypertension generally have successful pregnancy outcomes. Pregnancy does not seem to adversely affect their underlying disease. Perinatal mortality is less than 3% (Davison and Lindheimer, 1996). The risk is much greater for a woman with moderate or severe dysfunction. The risk to the mother is considerable, but the fetal risk is even higher. About one third of those with moderate renal problems experience escalating hypertension, and one fourth suffer an irreversible decrease in renal function (Davison and Lindheimer, 1996). Along with the hypertension, superimposed preeclampsia develops in 80% of women (see Chapter 22). Women with severe dysfunction rarely become pregnant.

Fertility is decreased as renal function decreases. If a woman with renal disease becomes pregnant before speaking with her physicians, the question of whether the pregnancy should continue must be answered.

Clinical management. A woman with chronic renal disease should have a counseling session with her obstetrician and nephrologist before considering a pregnancy. Complete renal function studies, including creatinine clearance with protein excretion, should be obtained before conception so that studies taken during pregnancy can be compared to the prepregnant state. There is an increased incidence of renal infections in these women, and frequent urine cultures are followed for infection. Ultrasound studies assist in the evaluation of fetal growth during the pregnancy. Diastolic BP should be below 90 mm Hg before a pregnancy is considered (Davison and Lindheimer, 1996). The development of superimposed preeclampsia may lead to the need for an emergency preterm delivery.

Women with chronic renal disease should be followed more closely than other pregnant women. Their needs include evaluation of the following:
1. *Renal function.* To monitor the status of renal function frequently (monthly), 24-hour urine collections should be followed, assessing both creatinine clearance and protein excretion. If deterioration is noted, further studies must be planned. Serum urea nitrogen, albumin, and cholesterol concentrations are followed.
2. *Blood pressure.* Most of the risks of hypertension are secondary to superimposed preeclampsia. High BP is treated aggressively during pregnancy to preserve renal function.
3. *Fetal growth and development.* Measurements of fetal well-being are important, since there is an association between renal disease and IUGR. Fetal surveillance is started by 28 weeks.

Provided that no infection or hypertension intervenes, pregnancy will progress to term. If renal function deteriorates at any stage of gestation, reversible causes, such as UTI, subtle dehydration, and electrolyte imbalance, should be sought. Failure to find such a reversible cause may be grounds for recommending termination of the pregnancy. In general, for glomerulonephritis, therapy includes administration of antihypertensive agents and, with cardiac insufficiency, digitalis and perhaps diuretics.

When modification of the customary prenatal diet is indicated, it should be undertaken, guided by the principles of good nutrition. Diet prescription for a pregnant woman with kidney disease is for adequate protein, allowing for fetal growth and maternal needs. Sodium may be restricted. Consideration should be given to avoid dehydration, electrolyte imbalance, and anemia.

Preeclampsia necessitates hospitalization. Azotemia (nitrogen in the blood), hyperkalemia (high potassium content in the blood), and a continuing rise in BP indicate the need to interrupt the pregnancy. Nephrotic syndrome is treated according to symptoms and the other conditions accompanying it. Bed rest in the lateral recumbent position is necessary. Steroids are contraindicated during the first 2 months of gestation. Infections must be vigorously treated.

Barbara, para 0040, had severe chronic hypertension related to renal disease. When she became pregnant, a home health aide was assigned to her because she had to be on modified bed rest for the last 15 weeks of pregnancy. She delivered a 33-week-old IUGR 1800 g boy who did well. She decided that she wanted a second child and became pregnant within 6 weeks, without discussing this decision with her physician. However, she did decide on a bilateral tubal ligation after this birth. She again needed home nursing visits and a homemaker. At 30 weeks' gestation, she called the nurse to report swollen, painful legs. Hospitalization showed severe superimposed preeclampsia and a soaring hypertension. The baby was born by cesarean and survived only 20 days in NICU. Although she had a great deal of support from her family and from church members, she grieved a long time because she had already gone ahead with the tubal ligation.

Nursing responsibilities. All pregnant women should be screened for asymptomatic bacteriuria at specific times during prenatal visits. Waiting for acute symptoms to develop may have serious consequences for the mother and fetus. Women with high risk for UTIs should provide clean-catch urine samples for culture. Women at high risk include those with history of UTIs, sickle cell trait, or renal stones.

Pregnant women with acute cystitis are usually uncomfortable, and they need to be reassured that the symptoms will lessen within 48 hours. As in the treatment of any infection, the woman must understand the importance of following the dosing schedule and completing the entire course of treatment in order to prevent relapse, recurrence, or worsening of this infection. Increased fluid intake is usually recommended to ensure hydration and to help flush the urinary system.

The nurse's role in working with pregnant women with chronic renal disease is to help identify gaps in the client's knowledge base that may affect completion of a successful pregnancy. Nutrition knowledge and dietary changes, such as appropriate protein intake and sodium requirements, must be addressed throughout pregnancy. Proper technique and timing of urine collections should be reviewed. Home care referrals should be made as appropriate for women whose activities have been restricted. Emotional and social support systems should be developed to aid in the woman's adherence to the treatment plan.

The woman may require interpretation and teaching about all the drugs she may be given (such as digitalis, diuretics, antihypertensives, steroids, and antibiotics), whether she is going to take them at home or receive them as an inpatient. If bed rest has been prescribed, she will need to explore her emotional response to this order and to discover activities that can keep her from boredom. The side-lying position is critical for her (see Figure 24-5). If the infant has a problem, the nurse can provide support and information and help during the grief process.

key points

- Metabolic changes accompanying pregnancy may complicate a preexisting disease or unmask potential problems in glucose or thyroid balance.
- Assessment during prenatal care always includes measurements for glucose levels, weight gain, and the presence of infection.
- Self-monitoring is the key to effective control of diabetes and overweight.
- After diagnosis of glucose imbalance, an intensive educational program is required so that the woman can manage her daily care.

- Nutrition is the key to control in PKU and diabetes.
- Clients must have sufficient knowledge of prescribed medications because of the potential for adverse effects.
- Because pregnancy alters insulin effects, the woman requires increased doses as gestation progresses.
- After birth, insulin needs drop swiftly and overdose is a risk. Careful intrapartal monitoring is required.
- The team approach is extremely important in caring for metabolic and renal problems during pregnancy.

Study Questions

24-1. Select the terms that apply to the following statements:
   a. A test that gives evidence of hyperglycemia within the previous 6 weeks is _____.
   b. When hyperglycemia is unmasked by the metabolic changes of the second and third trimesters, it is called _____.
   c. A hormone of pregnancy that acts as a direct insulin antagonist is _____.
   d. The definition for _____ is, "A body weight that is more than 20% over the normal weight for height."
   e. A balanced, normal amount of glucose in the blood is _____.
   f. When signs of frequency, dysuria, and urgency occur, infection is causing _____.
24-2. Which of the following are true regarding the effect of pregnancy on insulin and carbohydrate metabolism?
   a. The fasting blood sugar is higher in pregnancy.
   b. Estrogen and progesterone reduce insulin production.
   c. As pregnancy progresses, maternal insulin requirements are lower.
   d. hPL and estrogen are insulin antagonists.
24-3. If a diabetic woman shows signs of insulin overdose because she did not adjust her insulin dosage, which change in her normal pattern has probably occurred?
   a. She added extra simple sugars to her diet.
   b. She has had nausea, vomiting, and loss of appetite for a week.
   c. It rained all week so she omitted exercise.
   d. She had an additional intake of high sodium at dinner.
24-4. Birth several weeks before the due date may be induced for a diabetic woman to:
   a. Prevent hypoglycemia in the fetus.
   b. Reduce the chances of neonatal respiratory difficulty.
   c. Provide an easier labor and birth because infants tend to be larger.
   d. Avoid the chance of unexpected intrauterine fetal death.
24-5. When a woman has a urine laboratory report of 100,000 organisms/mm^3 with no other symptoms, the understood diagnosis would be:
   a. Urethritis.
   b. Asymptomatic bacteriuria.
   c. Cystitis.
   d. Pyelonephritis.
24-6. When a woman in her second trimester begins to experience urinary frequency and dysuria, she should:
   a. Drink more fluids.
   b. Call her health care provider for advice.
   c. Try resting and call her health care provider if the symptoms do not pass.
   d. Realize that these are expected sensations during advanced pregnancy.

Answer Key

24-1: *a*, HbA$_{1c}$; *b*, gestational (GDM); *c*, hPL; *d*, obesity; *e*, euglycemia; *f*, cystitis. 24-2: d. 24-3: b. 24-4: d. 24-5: b. 24-6: a and b.

References

Acosta PB, Wright L: Nurses' role in preventing birth defects in offspring of women with phenylketonuria, *J Obstet Gynecol Neonatal Nurs* 21(14):270, 1992.

ADA Position Statement: Office guide to diagnosis and classification of diabetes mellitus and other categories of glucose intolerance, *Diabetes Care* 13 (suppl 1):3, 1990.

ADA Position Statement: Gestational diabetes mellitus, *Diabetes Care* 13(suppl 1):5, 1990.

American College of Obstetricians and Gynecologists (ACOG): *Fetal macrosomia*, Technical Bulletin 159, Washington, DC, 1991, The College.

ACOG: *Thyroid disease in pregnancy*, Technical Bulletin 181, Washington, DC, 1993, The College.

ACOG: *Diabetes and pregnancy*, Technical Bulletin 200, Washington, DC, 1994, The College.

Avery M, Rossi M: Gestational diabetes, *J Nurse Midwifery* 39(2 suppl):9, 1994.

*Barss V: Diabetes and pregnancy, *Med Clin North Am* 73:685, 1989.

*Binkin NJ et al: Birth weight and childhood growth, *Pediatrics* 82:828, 1988.

Blackburn ST, Loper DL: *Maternal, fetal, and neonatal physiology*, Philadelphia, 1992, WB Saunders.

Coustan DR: Gestational diabetes. In Queenan JT, Hobbins JC, eds: *Protocols for high-risk pregnancies*, Cambridge, Mass, 1996, Blackwell Science.

Criezal AE, Dudas I: Prevention of the first occurrence of neural tube defects by periconceptional vitamin supplementation, *N Engl J Med* 327(26):1832, 1992.

*Davis LE, Leven KJ, Cunningham FG: Hypothyroidism complicating pregnancy, *Obstet Gynecol* 72(1):108, 1988.

Davison JM, Lindheimer MD: Renal disorders. In Creasy R, Resnick R, eds: *Maternal-fetal medicine: principles and practice*, ed 2, Philadelphia, 1994, WB Saunders.

Davison JM, Lindheimer MD: Renal disease. In Queenan JT, Hobbins JC, eds: *Protocols for high-risk pregnancies*, Cambridge, Mass, 1996, Blackwell Science.

Douglas JG: Hypertension and diabetes in blacks, *Diabetes Care* 13(1suppl 4): 1191, 1990.

Enkin M et al: *A guide to effective care during pregnancy*, ed 2, Oxford, 1995, Oxford University Press.

Fagan C, King J, Erick M: Nutrition management in women with gestational diabetes mellitus: a review by ADA's diabetes care and education dietetic practice group, *J Am Diet Assoc* 95(4):461, 1995.

Gabbe SG: Diabetes mellitus. In Queenan JT, Hobbins JC, eds: *Protocols for high-risk pregnancies*, Cambridge, Mass, 1996, Blackwell Science.

Gilbert ES, Harmon J: *Manual of high risk pregnancy and delivery*, St Louis, 1993, Mosby.

*Guthrie R: Maternal PKU—a continuing problem, *Am J Public Health* 78(7):771, 1988.

Herbert V: Folate and neural tube defects, *Nutrition Today* 27(66):30, 1992.

Insulin administration, *Diabetes Care* 13(suppl 1):28, 1990.

Jonaitis MA: Diabetes 2000: complications during pregnancy, *RN* 58(10):40, 1995.

*Classic reference.

Jovanovic L, Peterson C: Pregnancy in the diabetic woman, *Endocrinol Metab Clin North Am* 21(2):433, 1992.

Landon M, ed: Diabetes in pregnancy, *Clin Perinatol* 20(3):515, 1993.

LeMone R, Burke K: *Medical-surgical nursing: critical thinking in client care*, New York, 1996, Addison-Wesley.

*Lipman T: What causes diabetes? *MCN Am J Matern Child Nurs* 18(1):40, 1988.

Macheca MK: Diabetic hypoglycemia: how to keep the threat at bay, *Am J Nurs* 93(4)26, 1993.

National Academy of Sciences, Committee on Nutritional Status During Pregnancy and Lactation: *Nutrition during pregnancy, part 1: weight gain*, Washington, DC, 1990, National Academy Press.

Perlow JH: Obstetric managment of the obese patient, *Contemp OB/GYN* 40(11):15, 1995.

Pritchard JA et al: Metabolic conditions in pregnancy. In Cunningham et al, eds: *Williams obstetrics*, ed 17, East Norwalk, Conn, 1993, Appleton-Century-Crofts.

Reece EA et al: Assessment of carbohydrate tolerance in pregnancy, *Obstet Gynecol Surv* 46(1):1, 1991.

Reece EA, ed: Diabetes in pregnancy, *Obstet Gynecol Clin North Am* 23(1):273, 1996.

Reece EA, Hagay Z, Hobbins JC: Insulin-dependent diabetes mellitus and immunogenetics: maternal and fetal considerations, *Obstet Gynecol Surv* 46(5):255, 1991.

Samson L: Infants of diabetic mothers: current perspectives, *J Perinat Neonat Nurs* 6(1):61, 1992.

Smith JE: Pregnancy complicated by thyroid disease, *J Nurse Midwifery* 35(3):143, 1990.

Spirito A et al: Screening measure to assess knowledge of diabetes in pregnancy, *Diabetes Care* 11(7):712, 1990.

Thompson GN et al: Pregnancy in phenylketonuria: dietary treatment aimed at normalizing maternal plasma phenylalanine, *Arch Dis Child* 66:1346, 1991.

*White P: Classification of obstetrical diabetes, *Am J Obstet Gynecol* 130:228, 1978.

Zlatnik FJ: Obesity. In Queenan JT, Hobbins JC, eds: *Protocols for high-risk pregnancies*, Cambridge, Mass, 1996, Blackwell Science.

Student Resource Shelf

Acosta PB, Wright L: Nurses' role in preventing birth defects in offspring of women with phenylketonuria, *J Obstet Gynecol Neonatal Nurs* 21(4):270, 1992.
Describes diagnosis and treatment of varying degrees of PKU. Precautions given for the pregnant woman will often ensure a healthy outcome.

ADA: Insulin administration, *Diabetes Care* 13(suppl 1):28, 1990.
These recommendations were made in 1990. Each student should read this article and then compare what is said here with practices in the hospital setting.

ADA Position Statement: Nutritional recommendations and principles for individuals with diabetes mellitus, *Diabetes Care* 13(suppl 1):18, 1990.
A clear description of the recommendations for each type of diabetes.

Caldwell J: Hyperthyroidism during pregnancy: nursing care issues, *J Obstet Gynecol Neonatal Nurs* 26(6):395, 1996.
Review of effects of hyperthyroidism during pregnancy with nursing interventions.

25 Infectious Diseases & Pregnancy

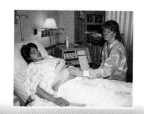

*P*regnant women may acquire any infectious disease. Infectious diseases during pregnancy are of special concern because they may occur more frequently or more severely in pregnant women. This is because pregnant women have less efficient and less protective immunologic defense systems. Infections may also threaten the well-being of the fetus or newborn with little or no physiologic effect on the mother, or the fetus and mother may both be seriously affected. Most importantly, the presence of any active infections may complicate the usually normal events related to sexuality, pregnancy, and the birth experience.

Infectious diseases are caused by a wide variety of microorganisms, including bacteria, viruses, fungi, rickettsiae, protozoa, and parasites. Depending upon the competency of the host's immune system, microorganisms may cause disease under appropriate circumstances. For infection to develop, the following must be present:

- Sufficient numbers of the invading virulent microorganism
- Conditions favoring transmission of the microorganism
- Entry of the microorganism into the body

The immune status of the woman ultimately governs whether the **pathogen** is to survive, reproduce, and cause damage. Initiatives to combat infection are directed toward each of these steps in the pathogenic process.

HOST DEFENSE MECHANISMS

All organisms have evolved a variety of mechanisms by which they protect themselves from hostile agents in their environment. Alterations in the maternal host defense mechanisms are crucial for continuation of the pregnancy. These mechanisms may be inborn or acquired, nonspecific or specific. *Nonspecific protective mechanisms* are numerous and frequently taken for granted. Examples include the intact skin and mucous membranes, ciliated epithelial cells of the respiratory tract, secretions that bathe mucous membrane surfaces, and "normal flora," microorganisms that colonize body surfaces but do not cause disease. The nonspecific host defense mechanisms generally are not altered during pregnancy (Blackburn and Loper, 1992).

Specific **host defense mechanisms** remain responsive to invading microorganisms during pregnancy, while at the same time allowing the fetus to develop and thrive. Complex alterations within the cell-mediated immune system appear to occur primarily locally in the uterus and are regulated in part by placental and sex steroid hormones. The specific host defense mechanisms—**humoral** and **cell-mediated immune responses**—are depressed during pregnancy. This depression and other changes allow the fetus to survive, while continuing to allow the woman's immune system to respond to microorganisms. However, these immunologic changes may in fact *impair* the pregnant woman's response to some infections. Table 25-1 lists examples of mechanisms by which human beings resist microbial infections.

Vaginal microbiology is complex. During pregnancy, the normal flora of the vagina undergoes a shift in the type of microorganisms that predominate. A wide variety of microorganisms colonize the vagina, including mainly nonpathogenic *Lactobacillus* species and some potentially pathogenic aerobic and anaerobic bacteria. As gestation progresses, vaginal *Lactobacillus* species increase in number, and anaerobic bacteria decrease in number. This shift in vaginal flora prepares a benign microbial environment for birth. As an additional protection, amniotic fluid contains substances that inhibit the growth of many pathogenic bacteria, and the maternal serum leukocyte count increases. Finally, increased numbers of neutrophils are found in the cervix and uterine decidua during labor (Figure 25-1).

Extra Risk during Labor

The processes of labor challenge the host defense systems. Loss of the cervical mucous plug, cervical dilation, and rupture of the fetal membranes allow microorganisms of the vagina to ascend to the uterus and fetus. The pH of amniotic fluid is considerably more basic than that of the normal vagina; this high pH favors the growth of anaerobic bacteria higher in pathogens.

Obstetric practices during pregnancy may disrupt natural defenses. Interventions such as amniocentesis, cervical examinations, artificial rupture of membranes (AROM), intrauterine monitoring, fetal blood sampling, and fetal operative procedures may introduce bacteria into the amniotic fluid. General anesthesia and cesarean birth are also associated with increased risk of postpartum infection.

Immunization during Pregnancy

When a foreign substance enters the body, there is a series of complex interactions—the immune response (see Table 25-1). The immune system response is modulated not only by pregnancy but also by the individual's age, sex, nutritional status, and genetic background (McCance and Huether, 1994). This response occurs when microorganisms invade the body from the environment or are purposefully induced through immunization.

Active immunity

Vaccination is the most effective means of disease prevention. **Active immunity** occurs when an individual produces antibodies in response to a specific infectious agent. Active immunity may be induced by administration of the following:

- Toxoids: bacterial extracellular toxin (exotoxin) that has been altered to retain antigenicity without toxicity (for example, tetanus-diphtheria toxoid)
- Whole organisms or portions of killed bacteria or virus administered to induce immunity (for example, typhoid)
- Attenuated live virus vaccines created by repeated inoculation of the virus through animals or tissue culture until it loses its virulence (for example, rubella, measles, and mumps)

Vaccinations should be given *before conception*. Only after evaluation of the woman's risk of exposure, susceptibility to the disease, gestational age, and type of vaccine will any vaccine be given during pregnancy because *live attenuated vaccines* generally cause a *subclinical* or mild illness, as well as transplacental passage and possible fetal infection. Women who are inadvertently immunized with *live virus vaccines* within 3 months before or after conception should be reported to the Centers for Disease Control (CDC) in Atlanta, Georgia, so that their infants may be followed up closely for potential adverse effects. If deemed necessary, *killed virus or bacteria* preparations are probably safe for use during pregnancy.

Table 25-1	Host Defense Mechanisms
Nonspecific and Specific Host Defense Mechanisms	**Mechanisms of Protection**

NONSPECIFIC RESPONSES

Physical Barriers

Epithelial surfaces	Cell turnover and sloughing remove adherent microorganisms.
Unidirectional flow of fluid within organs or on mucosal surfaces	Unidirectional flow washes microorganisms away.
Mucociliary system	Cilia on mucous membranes trap microorganisms and carry them out of the body.
Cervical mucus	Mucus blocks cervical opening and helps to prevent ascent of microorganisms into uterine cavity.
Amniochorion	This structure aids in prevention of ascent of microorganisms into uterine cavity.

Biochemical Mechanisms

Secretory products in mucosal surface fluids	Lysozyme is a bactericidal substance. Lactoferrin, an iron-binding protein, competes with bacteria for iron, which bacteria require for growth.
Variation in pH	This inhibits microorganisms.
Unsaturated fatty acids	This inhibits many microorganisms.
Amniotic fluid—antibacterial system	This inhibits growth of microorganisms.

MICROORGANISM COLONIZATION

Colonization response	Colonization of epithelial and mucosal surfaces with nonpathogenic bacteria helps to inhibit growth of pathogenic bacteria. This likely occurs by production of antibacterial substances, competition for host receptors, and alteration of microenvironment.
Inflammatory response	Microorganism invasion of tissue leads to dilation of blood vessels (redness). It also causes capillary permeability (edema) and migration of neutrophils and macrophages to area.
Neutrophils, monocytes, and macrophages	These phagocytize (ingest) and destroy microorganisms.
Complement	This responds to certain microorganisms' surface structures or antigen-antibody complexes. It promotes chemotaxis, opsonization, and microorganism lysis.

SPECIFIC RESPONSES

Secretory immunoglobulin A (IgA) and other immunoglobulins in mucosal surface fluids	These inhibit attachment of bacteria and viruses to cell surfaces.
Immune response	
Humoral immune response	This causes production of specific antibodies to microorganisms by B cell lymphocytes. Antibodies and complement coat microorganisms to enhance phagocytosis (ingestion of leukocytes).
Cell-mediated immune response	Sensitized lymphocytes release factors that stimulate macrophages to migrate to area and enhance phagocytosis; sensitized lymphocytes stimulate multiplication of other T cell and B cell lymphocytes, which destroy and produce antibody to the microorganisms, respectively. As infection is contained, biologically active substances released in this response stimulate T cell lymphocytes to halt response. Memory T cells and B cell lymphocytes remain in circulation.

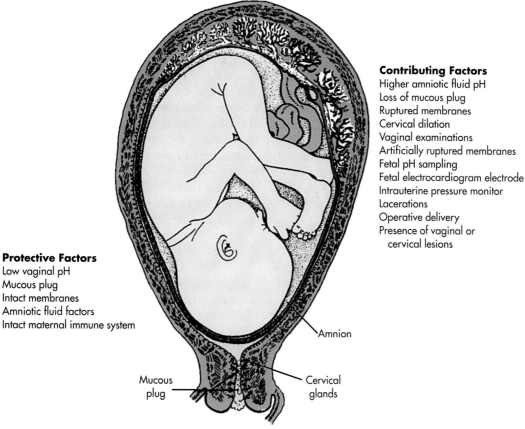

Contributing Factors
Higher amniotic fluid pH
Loss of mucous plug
Ruptured membranes
Cervical dilation
Vaginal examinations
Artificially ruptured membranes
Fetal pH sampling
Fetal electrocardiogram electrode
Intrauterine pressure monitor
Lacerations
Operative delivery
Presence of vaginal or
   cervical lesions

Protective Factors
Low vaginal pH
Mucous plug
Intact membranes
Amniotic fluid factors
Intact maternal immune system

Amnion

Mucous
plug

Cervical
glands

Figure 25-1 Ascending infection during labor. (Modified from Corliss CE: *Patten's human embryology,* ed 4, New York, 1976, McGraw-Hill.)

Passive immunity

To prevent illness, **passive immunity** is achieved by administration of antibody that is derived from human or animal sources. Immunity is immediate *but transient.* Immune serum globulin may be given to provide nonspecific immunity, or a specific **hyperimmune globulin** may be given to provide postexposure immunity against specific infections such as varicella-zoster and hepatitis. Appendix 3B lists immunization recommendations for the most commonly encountered infectious agents for which vaccinations are available.

TEST *Yourself* **25-1**

a. List one difference among the following immunizing agents:
  • Toxoids
  • Attenuated live virus
  • Killed bacteria
b. Which type of immunizing agent is not recommended during pregnancy and why?

Antimicrobial Use during Pregnancy

More than one third of all pregnant women will receive some form of antimicrobial treatment during pregnancy. Antibiotics should be used with discretion because toxic side effects and development of resistant bacterial strains may result (Sulis, 1995).

Antibiotics may be given either in full therapeutic doses for infection or prophylactically for a shorter duration to reduce the risk of infection. No antibiotic is approved by the Food and Drug Administration (FDA) for use during pregnancy, largely because of the lack of research that exists on safety for pregnant women and fetuses. Such research is unlikely to occur because of ethical reasons. In practice, however, antimicrobial agents are among the most commonly used drugs by pregnant women. Accordingly, this long-time use of selected antibiotics during pregnancy provides enough information to suggest that they may be used with confidence.

Antibiotic *pharmacokinetics* are altered by the physiologic changes of pregnancy. Antibiotics must be distributed over a larger area within the body; thus the overall concentration of circulating antibiotic will be *reduced* if usual adult dosages are given. Because of increased glomerular filtration and expanded blood volume in pregnancy, the effective serum levels of many antibiotics are lower than those in nonpregnant women. These physiologic changes facilitate an increased renal clearance of the drugs. The increased rate of hepatic breakdown may further interfere with obtaining effective serum antibiotic levels. Overall, circulating antibiotic levels are *lower* among pregnant women than among nonpregnant women (ACOG, 1988). In addition, placental transport of antimicrobial agents generally increases as gestation progresses because of progressive thinning of the placental membrane.

Isolation Procedures

Isolation procedures are implemented to prevent transmission of the microorganism or disease. Basic medical-surgical isolation procedures also apply to obstetric clients with infectious diseases. Guidelines for whether mother and infant are isolated are listed in boxes that accompany description of each infection. These guidelines are based on recommendations by the most current protocols of the American College of Obstetricians and Gynecologists (ACOG), the American Academy of Pediatrics, and the Communicable Disease Center. The purpose of isolation procedures and precautions is to prevent the transmission of disease. The rationales for these procedures are explained in Box 25-1.

Universal precautions required for the human immunodeficiency virus (HIV) and hepatitis B virus (HBV), discussed in Chapter 13, include blood and body fluid precautions. Universal precautions are intended to *supplement, not eliminate,* other types of isolation precautions. Each infection listed in this chapter identifies those fluids that contain infectious material. For instance, the rate of transmission of HIV through tears and saliva seems very low. The nursing responsibility for precautions is primary: first, to arrange for acquisition of correct protective clothing and devices and for disposal of these, and second, to follow the precautions and insist that others do so as well. Finally, every health care worker should monitor her or his own hand washing practice and the practices of coworkers.

Risks to Health Care Workers

Compliance with universal precautions has often been inconsistent in labor and delivery units, perhaps because of an attitude of denial or because of being rushed. In addition, in areas of the country in which prevalence of HIV, HBV, and herpes simplex virus (HSV) are lower, an intensive level of infection control may not be considered necessary. Noncompliance is found among both nursing and medical personnel, especially in starting intravenous (IV) infusions, in hand washing, in eye or hair protection, and in *double gloving* (Morrison et al, 1991). Although double gloving does not completely protect against needlestick injuries, it is thought to decrease latex glove fatigue, especially during long procedures. See Box 25-2 for risk of seroconversion.

COMMUNITY-ACQUIRED INFECTIONS

Community-acquired infections are acquired by an individual from the environment. These infections may be

---

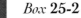

Box 25-1　Isolation Procedures and Precautions

RESPIRATORY ISOLATION
Reduces risk of transmission of organisms by droplets dispersed into the environment from the upper respiratory tract or lungs

ENTERIC PRECAUTIONS
Avoids contact with feces or objects contaminated with feces

WOUND PRECAUTIONS
Avoids contact with contaminated wounds or secretions from contaminated wounds

BLOOD PRECAUTIONS
Avoids contact with blood or objects contaminated with blood

BODY FLUIDS
Usually added to blood precautions, ensuring prevention against contact with additional body fluids—urine, sweat, saliva, and tears

---

Box 25-2　Health Care Workers Acquiring HIV through the Work Setting*

The following factors confer an increased risk of HIV infection above the usual 0.3% risk for an exposure event (a 0.3% risk means that 3 out of every 1000 nurses exposed to bloodborne exposures will become infected with HIV):
• Deep injury
• Visible blood on device
• Procedure involving needle placed directly in a vein or artery
• Terminal illness in source patient

*From Morbidity and Mortality Weekly Report, *MMWR* 44(50):929, Dec 22, 1995.

spread or acquired by a wide variety of mechanisms, including direct person-to-person contact, hand-to-mouth contact, or sexual contact; by carriage through air (coughing, talking), water, soil, foods, or contaminated fomites; or by infected animals and insect bites. Knowledge of the incidence of infections in the community, mode of transmission, potential risks, signs and symptoms, preventive strategies, treatments, and follow-up care will aid the nurse in asking directed questions, making observations, reviewing records, and obtaining physical findings and laboratory data so that actual and potential problems or needs may be identified. Nursing care plans may then be developed to address these problems (Figure 25-2).

Sexually Transmitted Diseases

Sexually transmitted diseases (STDs) are specific infections or syndromes transmitted primarily during sexual contact. STDs may be caused by bacteria, viruses, protozoa, fungal agents, or ectoparasites. More than 20 different diseases are recognized as being sexually trans-

mitted. Although STDs were traditionally considered to most commonly afflict men, it is young women and their unborn or newly born infants who especially suffer the most severe symptoms and complications. A wide variety of STDs have been associated with serious complications during pregnancy, including spontaneous abortion, preterm birth, intrauterine growth retardation (IUGR), stillbirth, neonatal death, congenital infection, and postpartum endometritis. As a group, STDs constitute a major, largely *preventable health threat* to women and infants. Public health initiatives for STD prevention have been directed at the primary areas of health education, disease detection, optimal treatment, partner tracing, and research. Health care providers and the public at large should apply this information more effectively.

Transcultural note

Nurses have the necessary task of delivering the educational information related to STDs in a culturally competent manner in order for it to be effective and humane. Surrounding the mysteries of life attached to fertility, sex, and giving birth are cultural beliefs and behaviors for

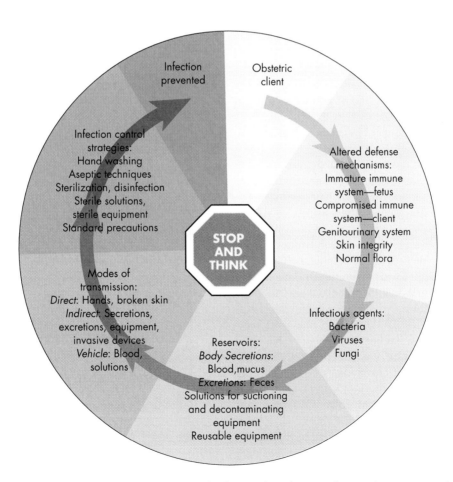

Figure 25-2   Factors affecting the obstetric client leading to the selection of strategies to prevent infectious complications. (From Schaffer S: *Infection prevention and safe practice,* St Louis, 1996, Mosby.)

women in a nurse's care. Becoming aware of the existence and importance of these beliefs and behaviors is essential in achieving cultural literacy, a necessity for planning patient care (Giger and Davidhizar, 1995). STDs, for example, are viewed in many cultures as an unnatural illness and may be perceived as a punishment from God or the work of the devil, placing these women in great need of psychosocial support and health education throughout their pregnancies. Much of what is labeled as "noncompliant" client behavior can be attributed to the disparity between traditionally held client beliefs and medical regimens. Culturally sensitive health education delivered by a nurse can address this disparity.

Chlamydia

Today, infection with the bacteria *Chlamydia trachomatis* is a widespread STD in the United States; an estimated 4 million persons are affected annually. The infection has not been a reportable disease; therefore the actual incidence is difficult to determine, though it has been found to be as low as 3% in asymptomatic women and as high as 20% in clients attending an STD clinic. Chlamydial and gonorrheal infections are the two most prevalent sexually transmitted bacterial infections in the United States today. Women at high risk during pregnancy include those who are young (less than 25 years old), poor, have a past history of the disease or have other STDs, have had a new sexual partner within the preceding 3 months, have multiple sexual partners, or are using an oral contraceptive method or nonbarrier contraceptive method (Fogel, 1995).

There are three major groups of infection associated with chlamydia: (1) lymphogranuloma venereum, (2) trachoma (an eye disease), and (3) the oculogenital disease discussed in this chapter. The chlamydia organisms invade and reproduce inside the cells that line the cervix, endometrium, fallopian tubes, and urethra, among other tissues.

Risk. Chlamydia causes a variety of clinical conditions, including cervicitis, endometritis, pelvic inflammatory disease (PID), irregular menses, acute salpingitis, urethritis, bartholinitis, Fitz-Hugh–Curtis syndrome (perihepatitis), and possibly infertility. Women with chlamydia infections have two to three times the risk of ectopic pregnancy (Pearlman and McNeeley, 1992). During pregnancy, cervical chlamydial infection has been associated with premature labor, premature rupture of membranes (PROM), and preterm birth. Treatment of chlamydial infections during pregnancy has been found to result in better obstetric outcomes and can prevent neonatal chlamydial infections (Peter, 1994).

Neonatal risk. If chlamydiae are present at the time of vaginal birth, 50% to 60% of infants become infected. Chlamydial conjunctivitis develops within the first week of life among 25% to 50% of exposed infants, and pneumonia will develop in 5% to 20% of exposed infants with-

in the first 3 months of life. Even infants delivered via cesarean section have acquired the infection (Peter, 1994).

Signs. Women with cervical chlamydial infection frequently are symptom-free or may have nonspecific symptoms such as increased discharge. The presence of a mucopurulent cervical discharge and *friable cervix* (bleeding when cervix is touched) upon pelvic examination indicates chlamydial infection. Signs of endometritis are evident about 2 days after vaginal delivery.

In the neonate, conjunctivitis consists of edema of eyelids, conjunctival redness, and mucopurulent discharge. Untreated, the cornea may become scarred (Figure 25-3). Chlamydial pneumonia occurs within 2 to 3 months of birth. Signs are afebrile cough, tachypnea, malaise, cyanosis, and poor weight gain. Diffuse bacterial infiltrates appear on the chest radiograph film.

Clinical management. Because evidence of chlamydial infection often is not apparent by clinical examination, laboratory methods such as cell culture, antigen detection, or the enzyme-linked immunosorbent assay (ELISA) are required to identify infection. The partner will usually be infected and should also be treated. Condoms must be used during treatment to prevent **reinfection**, although sexual intercourse should be avoided during treatment. Recommendations for treatment during pregnancy are

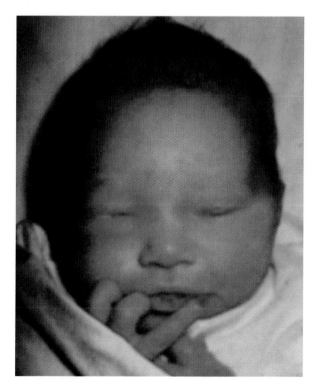

Figure 25-3 *Chlamydia trachomatis* eye infection. Note puffy, bruised-looking eyelid. (From Beischer NA, MacKay EV: *Obstetrics and the newborn,* ed 3, Sydney, 1993, WB Saunders. Courtesy Harcourt, Brace, Jovanovich Group.)

shown in Box 25-3. In addition to primary prevention strategies, screening all pregnant women for chlamydial cervical infection at their first prenatal visit has been recommended. Additional screening at 36 weeks for high-risk women is also recommended.

The best prevention for neonates is maternal treatment in the last trimester. Topical chlamydia prophylaxis with the mandated erythromycin opthalmic ointment does not treat other sites of infection. Once *conjunctivitis* is diagnosed, the treatment in Box 25-3 is recommended.

Nursing responsibilities

Client teaching. The woman being treated for chlamydia should be instructed to be persistent in insisting that a condom be used and in encouraging her partner to go for treatment. If he does not, condom prophylaxis (including perhaps the use of the female condom) should be continued during pregnancy. The woman should be informed about signs of recurrence: increased vaginal mucus, abdominal aching, and preterm labor. She must be taught that chlamydial infection leads to PID, ectopic pregnancy, and spontaneous abortion. After the birth, she should be instructed to look for signs of infection in herself and in her infant.

Collaborative referral. When the infant is diagnosed with chlamydial infection, the parents should also be referred for examination, treatment, and counseling.

Isolation precautions. See Box 25-4 for a list of isolation precautions.

Gonorrhea

Gonorrhea is one of the most commonly reported communicable diseases in the United States (along with chlamydia). Up to 3 million cases of gonorrhea are thought to occur annually in the United States in males and females, and up to 7% of pregnant women are infected with gonorrhea. The bacteria *Neisseria gonorrhoeae* lives preferentially in the types of cells that line the cervix, endometrium, fallopian tubes, and urethra.

Gonorrhea may cause uncomplicated genitourinary tract infection (urethritis and cervicitis) and upper genital tract infections such as endometritis and PID. Urethritis, epididymitis, and prostatitis occur in men. Gonorrhea may also cause Fitz-Hugh–Curtis syndrome, disseminated gonorrhea with associated arthritis, and rarely, endocarditis or meningitis. Disseminated gonorrhea appears to be more frequent among pregnant women than among nonpregnant women, but the reason for this is unknown.

Risk. Untreated gonorrhea during pregnancy has also been associated with increased risk of PROM, preterm birth, chorioamnionitis, neonatal sepsis, and puerperal sepsis. Neonatal gonococcal ophthalmia, **ophthalmia neonatorum**, is a serious complication of gonorrhea infection during pregnancy. Newborns acquire the infection during passage through the infected cervix.

Signs. Nonpregnant women with gonorrhea may be symptom-free, or they may have dysuria, urinary frequency, increased vaginal discharge, or abnormal uterine bleeding, whereas pregnant women most commonly have no symptoms.

In the newborn, purulent conjunctivitis usually occurs within 4 days of birth and without treatment may progress rapidly to cause corneal ulcerations and, ultimately, blindness. In a review of neonates with gonococcal infection, Desenclos (1992) found that 81% had ophthalmia neonatorum, 6% had genital infection, 3% showed infection in gastric or respiratory aspirates, and 1% had skin infection, scalp abscesses, or ear infection.

Clinical management. Most gonococcal strains are sensitive to penicillins and are eradicated by a single-dose therapy of ampicillin 3.5 g or amoxicillin 3.0 g orally followed by probenecid 1.0 g by mouth. Probenecid inhibits renal excretion of penicillins and usually increases plasma levels of these antibiotics, enhancing their action. Because of penicillin resistance, the current CDC recommendations for treatment of gonorrhea are shown in Box 25-5 (Sulis,

---

Box 25-3   **Pharmacologic Treatment of Chlamydial Infection during Pregnancy**

One of the following is used:
Erythromycin base 500 mg PO q6h for 7 days
Sulfisoxazole 500 mg PO q6h for 7 days
Amoxicillin 500 mg PO q8h for 7 days
Clindamycin 300 mg PO q8h for 7 days
Note: Quinolines are contraindicated in those < 17 years and in pregnancy.

NEONATAL TREATMENT
Erythromycin 50 mg/kg per day PO in 4 doses for 7 to 14 days

PNEUMONIA TREATMENT
Erythromycin 50 mg/kg per day PO in 4 doses for 14 to 21 days or 15 to 20 mg/kg per day IV in 4 to 6 divided doses

---

Box 25-4   **Isolation Precautions: Chlamydia**

INFECTED MOTHER AND INFANT
No isolation
Careful hand washing
Prevent contact with vaginal fluids

BREAST-FEEDING
Permitted if antibiotic regimen safe for breast-feeding

Box 25-5   Pharmacologic Treatment of Gonorrhea

Penicillin-resistant gonorrhea
Ceftriaxone 250 mg IM as a single dose
For women who cannot take ceftriaxone:
Spectinomycin 2 g IM as a single dose
When type of gonorrhea is not resistant to penicillin:
Amoxicillin 3 g PO, with 1 g probenecid

Box 25-6   Isolation Precautions: Gonorrhea

MATERNAL AND INFANT ISOLATION
Careful hand washing
Avoid genital contact until initiation of therapy

BREAST-FEEDING
Permitted if antibiotic regimen safe for breast-feeding

1995). Compliance with treatment is usually achieved because only one dose is needed. Nonetheless, a follow-up culture is needed to test the cure. The *reinfection* rate is estimated to be 5% to 8% (Cavenee et al, 1993).

Nursing considerations

Client teaching. Strategies to prevent gonorrhea infection involve methods of personal prevention (see Box 25-13). Secondary prevention includes education and screening all pregnant women for gonococcal infection early in pregnancy and screening those women of high-risk populations again during the third trimester.

Collaborative referral. Women with positive cultures are reported to the state health department to ensure treatment and counseling of sexual contacts.

Isolation precautions. Isolation precautions are listed in Box 25-6.

Herpes simplex virus

HSV is a member of the herpesvirus group, which includes varicella-zoster virus, cytomegalovirus, and Epstein-Barr virus.

Transmission of HSV infection occurs by direct contact of the virus onto susceptible mucosal tissues (oropharynx, labia, cervix, vagina, or conjunctiva) or onto broken skin. (Spread by fomites or aerosol is unlikely *because HSV does not survive drying and room temperature.*) Historically, herpes lesions "above the waist" were attributed to HSV type 1 (HSV-1), and genital herpes "below the waist" was attributed to HSV type 2 (HSV-2). For reasons that are not completely understood but likely involve changes in sexual practices, the number of persons with genital HSV-1 infection or oral HSV-2 infection has increased. The distinction between HSV-1 and HSV-2 genital infections is of

little value, since both virus types may cause significant neonatal illness.

Risk. It is estimated that 20 million people in the United States have genital HSV (ACOG, 1988). Transmission to the infant occurs during passage through the infected birth canal or by ascending infection after rupture of membranes. Rarely has transplacental infection been noted. Transmission through close contact with an infected mother, relative, or health care provider may occur if simple precautions are not followed (Table 25-2).

Primary HSV infection poses the greatest risk to the pregnancy. Primary HSV infection has been associated with increased risk of spontaneous abortion, low birth weight, and preterm delivery. The rate of transmission is approximately 50% if the infection is a primary one (Sulis, 1995). Recurrent HSV disease has not been associated with adverse outcome other than neonatal infection and has a transmission rate of 5%.

Neonatal risk. Although the clinical course of the infection in pregnant women does not appear to be different from that of nonpregnant women, without treatment approximately 50% of HSV-infected newborns die. An additional 50% of the survivors experience significant neurologic or ocular damage.

It has been determined that 60% of infants with neonatal HSV infection are born to women with no history of HSV and no lesions at the time of delivery. Because of the close relationship between HSV and varicella zoster, the Immunization Practice Advisory Committee recommends administration of varicella zoster immunoglobulin (VZIG) to the newborn if the mother develops chickenpox within 5 days before or 2 days after delivery.

Signs. After inoculation with HSV, the infected person may have symptoms or be asymptomatic. In either case, during primary (initial) HSV infection, the virus ascends along peripheral sensory nerves, enters sensory or autonomic nerve root ganglia, and establishes latent infection (Figure 25-4). Symptomatic *primary genital HSV infection* is often accompanied by prolonged systemic and local symptoms. Fever, headache, malaise, and myalgias are common and may persist for the 3 to 4 days after lesions develop. Local symptoms include severe pain, itching, dysuria, vaginal or urethral discharge, and tender inguinal lymph nodes. Typical lesions appear as papules and progress to vesicles, which rupture and ulcerate. Lesions may spread over the genital area. Ulcerated lesions of primary herpes may persist for 4 to 15 days before healing. HSV cervicitis occurs among 70% to 90% of women with primary HSV infection. In some cases there is increased and abnormal vaginal discharge and mucopurulent cervicitis.

Nonspecific stimuli, including fever, sunlight, and stress, have been associated with triggering recurrences of oral HSV-1. Stress may be a trigger mechanism for HSV-2 infection. Signs and symptoms of *recurrent genital HSV* are

Table 25-2	Guidelines for Prevention of Perinatal Transmission of Herpes Simplex Virus

Recommendation	Rationale
PRENATAL	

Carefully question all pregnant women about:
  History of HSV infection
  Sores or lesions that recur in the same places
  Sexual contact (past or present) with a partner with history of HSV infection or sores that recur in same location
  Prior affected infant
	Identifies women with history of HSV infection, history that suggests HSV infection, or risk for acquiring infection. Allows for education about signs and symptoms of infection and guidelines for prevention of transmission (interpersonal and perinatal).

INTRAPARTUM	
If no lesions are visible or no prodrome is occurring during labor, vaginal delivery is allowed.	Risk of perinatal transmission is small.
To ensure absence of virus at time of vaginal delivery, women with active lesions close to term and before labor or rupture of membranes may have cultures obtained every 3 to 5 days until one is negative.	
Culture of mother's cervix and vulva or the newborns mouth, umbilicus, and rectum may be obtained at time of delivery.	May aid the pediatrician in determining need for newborn therapy. This protocol, however, may not prove beneficial because 70% of neonatal infections occur in women with no history of HSV.
Women in labor at term or with ruptured membranes at term who have visible lesions should have cesarean delivery (regardless of the duration of ruptured membranes).	Cesarean delivery will reduce the risk of neonatal herpes infection.
Women with premature rupture of membranes and active lesions should be managed individually, with the risk of prematurity weighed against the risks of HSV.	Little information is available to provide universal recommendations.
POSTPARTUM	

Infant does not need to be isolated from mother.
  Avoid direct contact with lesions. Mother should avoid kissing infant if oral-labial lesion present.
  Wash hands carefully before handling infant. Do not place child in parent's bed.
	Risk of transmission is low with careful hygiene precautions.

Breast-feeding is not contraindicated unless visible lesions are present on the breast.	Risk transmission is low with avoidance of direct contact with lesions and careful hand washing.
Infected health care providers should not be prohibited from caring for these clients as long as direct contact with lesions is avoided and scrupulous hand washing is followed.	Risk of transmission from health care workers is low.
Private room is not required.	HSV infection is transmitted by direct contact with secretions from open lesions, not by fomites or casual contact.

Data from ACOG: *Perinatal herpes simplex virus infection,* ACOG Technical Bulletin 122, Nov 1988; Gibbs RS et al: Management of genital herpes infection in pregnancy, *Obstet Gynecol* 71(5):779, 1988.
HSV, Herpes simplex virus.

localized to the genital region and generally are less severe than those of primary HSV. Lesions may last 4 to 10 days. Up to 50% of persons with **recurrent** HSV **infection** may note warning symptoms, including local tingling, itching, or shooting pains in buttocks, legs, or hips. Frequency of recurrences differs, and in some persons, severity of individual recurrent episodes varies. HSV infection may involve the cervix only, without external genital or extragenital lesions being noted. Viral shedding from the cervix may occur, without symptoms, at any time during the course of HSV infection. Cervical viral shedding is detected among 70% to 90% of women during primary infection and among 15% to 30% of women with recurrent vulvar lesions. Up to 5% of women excrete the virus

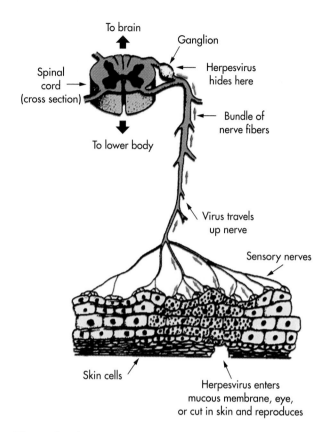

To brain

Ganglion

Spinal cord (cross section)

Herpesvirus hides here

Bundle of nerve fibers

To lower body

Virus travels up nerve

Sensory nerves

Skin cells

Herpesvirus enters mucous membrane, eye, or cut in skin and reproduces

Figure 25-4   Path of the herpesvirus. The virus ascends to hide in the nerve ganglion. (Courtesy National Foundation March of Dimes, White Plains, NY)

between recurrent episodes. Latex condoms may provide some protection.

Neonatal HSV is secondary to infection from either ascending infection with ruptured membranes or from exposure to infectious material during the birth process. Neonatal HSV is a serious disease, with a 60% mortality rate. If an infant survives, serious sequelae follow, such as microcephaly, retinal dysplasia, and encephalitis. Although one third of infected newborns will not demonstrate either cutaneous, ocular, or oral symptoms of HSV infection, they may develop more severe systemic infection later in the neonatal period. All infants born to mothers with genital HSV infection must be monitored carefully during the first few months of life for signs of either local or systemic infection (Peter, 1994).

Clinical management. Diagnosis of HSV infection is made based on a history of tingling, itching, or painful lesions on the genital area, thigh, or buttocks, which appear as blisters that burst and ulcerate, then crust over and heal. These lesions tend to recur periodically in the same location. Confirmation of HSV infection is best made by recovery of HSV from a viral culture of vesicle fluid. The ELISA test is also used.

HSV infection is currently *incurable.* Acyclovir antiviral therapy shows promise in lessening the severity of pri-

mary illness and in preventing recurrences among nonpregnant women. No teratogenic effects have been demonstrated in work with laboratory animals, but its use in human beings has been limited. Currently it is not recommended for use during pregnancy except in life-threatening, disseminated infection (see information on management of varicella-zoster virus found in this chapter). Administration of VZIG within 96 hours of exposure to HSV may prevent or lessen the severity of maternal disease (Sulis, 1995).

Current recommendations for prenatal screening, method of delivery, and postpartum care are outlined in Table 25-2.

Nursing responsibilities

Client teaching. Pregnant women should be carefully questioned regarding a history of (1) genital or oral HSV (sores that seem to come and go in the same general place), (2) sexual contact with a current or past partner with a history of HSV infection or recurrent sores in the genital region, thigh, or buttocks, and (3) a previous infant with HSV infection. Women who have no history of HSV or no history of possible contact with HSV should be counseled in ways to reduce their risk of acquiring HSV during pregnancy, as appropriate. Women who experience true primary infection during pregnancy will require considerable emotional support and information about HSV infection (see Table 25-2). Women should be counseled about their somewhat increased risk for pregnancy complications, including spontaneous abortion, preterm birth, and IUGR. Strategies for preventing perinatal HSV transmission should be carefully discussed.

Palliative nursing interventions. HSV is a very painful infection, with pain disproportionate to the size of the lesions. Palliative measures such as the application of cool tea or milk compresses or the use of warm-to-cool sitz baths may relieve lesion discomfort. Goldenseal sitz baths (1 tablespoon of Goldenseal powder in warm bath) are very soothing to irritated perineal lesions (Denenberg, 1994). Urination into bath water may allow women who have severe dysuria to avoid catheterization. Analgesic medications may also be required.

Isolation precautions. See Box 25-7 for isolation precautions.

Human papillomavirus

Human papillomavirus (HPV) is the most common *viral STD,* with approximately 20 million Americans infected and with an estimated 1 million new cases occurring annually. The CDC reports an increase in a particular type of HPV, *condyloma acuminatum,* to be nearly 460% over the last 25 years. More than 70 types of HPV have been identified by laboratory techniques. Infections are categorized into latent (asymptomatic), subclinical, or clinical. Latent infections may not be visible to the naked eye, detectable only by DNA tests (ACOG, 1994). Different skin manifestations are asso-

| **Box 25-7** | **Isolation Precautions: Herpes Simplex** |

ACTIVE GENITAL LESIONS AT BIRTH
See Table 25-2

HISTORY OF GENITAL LESIONS BUT NONE ACTIVE AT BIRTH
Careful hand washing
Gloves for perineal care or lochia contact

ORAL HERPES LESIONS
No general isolation
Mother wears mask and prevents infant's contact with
   oral secretions until lesions heal

ciated with different viral types, although mixed infections are common (HPV types 6, 11, 42, 43, and 44 are most commonly associated with condylomata acuminata, whereas severe lesions are more often associated with HPV types 16, 18, 31, 33, and 35). Genital warts are the most common sign. In addition to causing complications during birth (cervical lesions can block the birth canal, transmit infection to the newborn, and retard healing after the birth), there seems to be a direct role for HPV in lower genital tract cancer. It has also been determined that heavy cigarette smoking among women with HPV infection increases their risk for cervical cancer (Hellberg et al, 1988). Coinfection with chlamydia and herpesvirus may have a synergistic effect. Considerable research is ongoing, directed toward understanding HPV infection, diagnosis, and treatment.

Risk. The virus can be transmitted through sexual intercourse (vaginal, oral, or anal) but also through other acts of intimacy involving *any contact* with the infected person's genital or perianal region. It has even been transmitted through contact with fomites, such as an infected person's underwear. The overall infection rate is thought to be as high as 20% in pregnant women. During pregnancy, papillary lesions of HPV infection may increase in size and number. Lesions may become more vascular and friable during pregnancy, and, in a few cases, extreme growth on vulva and vagina may be noted. HPV is so highly contagious that barrier contraceptives such as male condoms offer only limited protection from the virus, protecting only the covered mucosal area. Female condoms may offer more effective barrier protection since they cover the vaginal vault mucosa, but their effectiveness remains to be tested against HPV (see Figure 5-9 for a graphic of a female condom).

HPV and cervical cancer. Epidemiologic research has shown that a diagnosis of HPV is associated with a tenfold or greater increase in the risk for cervical cancer (Schiffman, 1992). Not all cases, however, necessarily lead to cervical cancer. Millions of women harbor the virus in

their bodies, and yet only 13,000 cases of cervical cancer are diagnosed annually in the United States.

Neonatal risk. HPV is highly contagious, and transmission occurs primarily during passage through the contaminated birth canal, although viral ascent from the cervix and vagina into the uterus, transplacental passage, and postnatal transmission are also possible (Wood, 1991). Children born to mothers with HPV infection may have the virus in their respiratory tract, and it may progress to serious illness if the lesions develop in the lungs. Infants born via cesarean section rarely get the infection, leading experts to believe that the neonate is infected through a contaminated birth canal (Gerchufsky, 1996).

Signs. HPV cannot be cultured in the laboratory. DNA testing is possible but expensive (Gerchufsky, 1996). When lesions are visible, diagnosis of clinical HPV infection is made by identification of the characteristic appearance of lesions. The lesions are most common on moist areas and may occur in the vagina or on the cervix. They may appear as soft, pink, white, or tan cauliflower-like (papillary) masses and may be single or multiple or the size of a small pinhead, or they may cover several centimeters in area. The papules may also look like skin warts or be flat.

The neonate is usually asymptomatic at birth; symptoms do not often appear until later in life, sometimes years later. It is thought that childhood laryngeal papillomas are the result of aspiration of infected secretions in the birth canal. It should be carefully documented on the newborn's chart that the mother was infected with HPV so that subsequent monitoring of the infant can include this potential diagnosis. Often misdiagnosed, recurrent respiratory papillomatosis (RRP) can involve any or all of the child's entire respiratory tract, from the mouth to the alveoli, causing respiratory distress. RRP can also develop later on in life (see Student Resource Shelf for the address of the RRP Foundation).

Clinical management. Recommendations for follow-up care and treatment of HPV infection are likely to change in the next few years as more is learned about HPV pathogenesis. Pap smears taken on a regular basis are commonly used, easy, inexpensive, and highly accurate if sent to a quality laboratory. Because these tests are not definitive, patients with an abnormal test result should also have a colposcopic biopsy. Treatment of HPV infection during pregnancy is controversial and problematic, with cases of recurrence even after treatment. In many cases, the warts associated with HPV resolve spontaneously. If they do not, the type of treatment depends upon the location of the lesions. Since specific antiviral therapy is not available, treatment includes destroying visible lesions, followed by controlling the virus in the host. A mixture of chemical, mechanical, and surgical interventions are used to treat genital warts. Topical concentrated trichloroacetic or bichloroacetic acids are nontoxic, can be used during pregnancy, and work best on moist mucosal warts. Topical podophyllin or podofilox has been a frequent treatment among nonpregnant women but is contraindicated during pregnancy and lactation because of increased potential for maternal and fetal neurotoxicity. Topical 5-fluorouracil is not used in pregnancy because of its reported teratogenicity. Excision of lesions with cryosurgery (freezing), laser, electrocautery, sharp excision, or Cavitron ultrasonic suction aspiration is used. Interferon has been used for persistent disease but is controversial for use during pregnancy because its safety for mother and fetus are unknown.

Recently, podofilex 0.5% solution has been found effective and practical. It is not yet approved for use during pregnancy, however, because of its potential for bone marrow and central nervous system (CNS) toxicity (ACOG, 1994). Treatment in nonpregnant women consists of topical application by the woman herself, twice a day for 3 days (Figure 25-5). After a 4-day rest the cycle is repeated for 2 or 3 more weeks. No systemic effects have been reported (Patsner, 1991). Local effects—pain, burning, stinging, itching, edema, and some sloughing of skin, with odor—diminish over the 3 weeks but are uncomfortable (Baker et al, 1990).

Human immunodeficiency virus

HIV is an RNA retrovirus that establishes a chronic infection with a long latency period before causing progressive immunodeficiency. HIV attaches to and invades selected host cells. This RNA retrovirus may remain latent, it may reproduce, or it may cause cell destruction. However, it appears to replicate only in certain white blood cell types, including cells of the CNS, intestinal tract, and possibly bone marrow. HIV is unique among human viruses in that it infects and destroys helper T lymphocytes and macrophages, cells that are integral to the body's defense system. Viral replication appears to occur more slowly among other cell types and interferes with function rather than causing cell death.

Risk. Women represent the most rapidly growing category of persons with HIV infection in the United States. By the year 2000, it is estimated that *more women than men will have become infected* in the United States, thereby more closely resembling the worldwide pattern (Cotton,

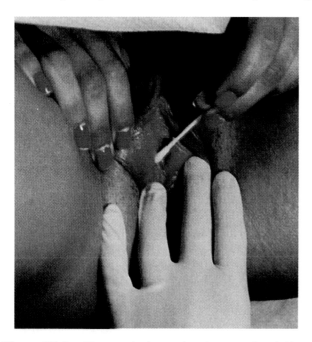

Figure 25-5 Client-applied topical application of podofilex for human papillomavirus (HPV) warts. (Courtesy Patsner B: A patient-applied topical solution for genital warts, *Contemp Ob Gyn* 36:12, 27, 1991.)

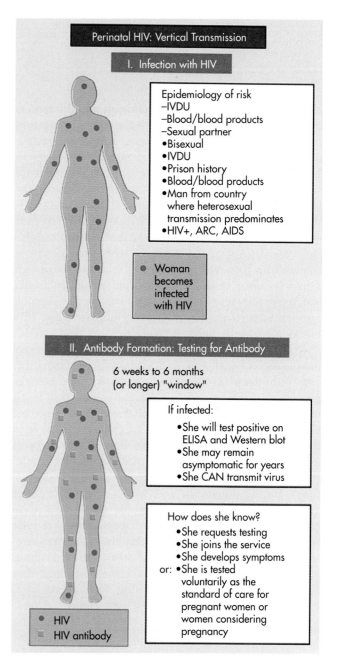

Figure 25-6 Vertical transmission of perinatal human immunodeficiency virus. (*AIDS*, Acquired immunodeficiency syndrome; *ARC*, AIDS-related complex; *HIV*, human immunodeficiency virus; *IVDU*, intravenous drug user.)

1995). Demographically, the features of women infected with HIV are different than those of men infected with the virus. The majority of women are women of color (52% African-American, 21% Hispanic, 27% white) and are less likely than men to be IV drug users (51% for women vs. 70% for men), but they are more likely to be the sex partner of IV drug users (21% vs 3%). Thus, drug abuse directly or indirectly contributes to a total of 70% of the HIV infection risk for women (Kazanjian and Eisenstat, 1995). However, heterosexual transmission is a rapidly growing means of infection for women. In addition, pregnant women have the potential to transmit the virus to their children, placing these children in a unique position in the epidemic.

HIV may be transmitted by sexual penetration between women and men, between men, and between women. Nonsexual transmission may occur by inoculation with contaminated blood, blood products, and possibly other selected bodily fluids. Inoculation with large numbers of virus during transfusion of contaminated blood or blood products almost always causes HIV infection in the recipient. HIV has been detected in other body fluids, including saliva, tears, amniotic fluid, cerebrospinal fluid (CSF), synovial fluid, and peritoneal fluid; however, evidence of transmission by contamination with these fluids is considered inefficient. Intact skin appears to be an effective barrier to HIV infection. As the second decade of coping with HIV progresses, studies continue to probe the nature of the transfer of the organism from one person to another and the state of infection that causes disease states.

Pregnancy is associated with a modest suppression of cell-mediated immunity or a decrease in helper T cells. Most women with HIV infection are of reproductive age and therefore also risk transmitting HIV perinatally. **Vertical transmission** from mother to infant may occur *transplacentally*, during the *intrapartum* period from contamination with vaginal secretions and blood or during *breast-feeding* (Figure 25-6).

Fetal and neonatal risk. Exact modes of vertical transmission are unclear. All infants of HIV-positive women show maternal antibodies at birth (Box 25-8), but 70% will show seroconversion to negative before 2 years of age because there is no viral infection in their systems. Zidovudine (ZDV) therapy is being offered to pregnant women with HIV infection beginning at 13 weeks and also during labor and delivery. ZDV therapy for infants begins the day of birth (at 12 hours) and continues for the first 6 weeks of life. Infants who do have HIV infection appear to develop end-stage disease or acquired immunodeficiency syndrome (AIDS) after a much shorter incubation period (less than 1 year) than do adults (Figure 25-7).

Box 25-8   **Perinatal Transmissions— Possible Outcomes (HIV-Positive Mother)**

INFANT 1 (approximately 70%)

Has positive HIV antibody test (will have negative polymerase chain reaction [PCR] test by 3 months)

Has only maternal HIV antibody

Does not have HIV virus

Will show seroconversion to antibody-negative before 2 years of age or by 3 months with PCR test

INFANT 2 (approximately 30% or approximately 8% if mother is taking zidovudine [ZDV])

Has positive HIV antibody test result (will continue to test positive by PCR test)

Has HIV antibody and virus infection from mother

Has virus, is infected, and will develop symptoms

Will continue to show positive HIV antibody test result after 2 years of age and will continue to test positive for PCR beyond 3 months of age

---

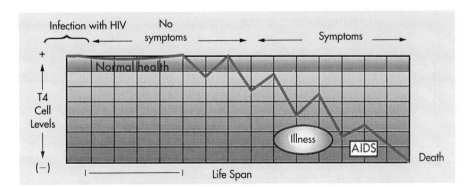

Figure 25-7   Life span comparison between those with neonatal human immunodeficiency virus infection and those with adult onset infection. Newborn early onset results in illness within 2 to 3 months. Late onset results in illness after 15 months. In an adult, illness begins 8 to 10 years after the onset of infection. T4 cell levels below 200 usually signal the beginning of acquired immunodeficiency syndrome.

Currently it is believed that HIV is transmitted to the fetus if the maternal viral load is high, such as that which occurs at the beginning of the infection, and when the T4 helper cell count is low, such as toward the period when AIDS symptoms appear. Maternal viral load is now measurable and may become an important diagnostic tool for determining pregnancy outcomes and treatment (Volberding, 1996). In addition, it is now clear that *at the time of birth the infant may be inoculated with a virus load by contact with maternal blood and vaginal fluids.*

Since 1989 recommendations have been made to guard skin integrity in infants at risk of HIV contamination (Connor et al, 1989) (Box 25-9). Recent recommendations continue to advocate for discouragement of invasive monitoring techniques (Ross and Dickason, 1992; Schaffer et al, 1996). Puncture of the fetal scalp to attach the internal electrocardiogram electrode or to monitor scalp pH is a means of contamination from mother to fetus. In addition, immediately after birth, nurses must advocate for procedures to accomplish the following for the newborn. These added precautions may be termed "newborn universal precautions."

1. No skin puncture before skin cleansing
2. Early bath with soap or dilute chlorhexidine (Hibiclens) before eye prophylaxis or intramuscular (IM) injection

Signs. Initial HIV infection may be accompanied by a mononucleosis-like illness, with symptoms that include fatigue, fever, and swollen glands. A rash may develop. The initial viral-like symptoms resolve completely within 3 to 14 days. HIV infection may remain silent, yet transmissible, for 2 to 10 years in a **latent period** before progressive symptoms of immunodeficiency develop. As this period ends, the person develops weight loss, malaise, lethargy, CNS dysfunction, unexplained fever, and generalized lymphadenopathy. Opportunistic infections—infections that *take advantage of the opportunity* to invade or reactivate while the immune system is weakened—will develop.

> ▌ *Box* **25-9**   **Isolation Precautions: HIV**

MOTHER
Universal precautions
Careful hand washing
Avoid newborn contact with blood, blood products, or lochia

INFANT
Universal precautions
Bathe child promptly with soap and water before skin puncture or eye prophylaxis

BREAST-FEEDING
Contraindicated

AIDS is the end stage of HIV. Persons with AIDS show evidence of a severely compromised immune system and have life-threatening illnesses from microorganisms or malignancies that seldom cause problems among healthy persons. Evidence of immunodeficiency in the absence of other known causes and the presence of **opportunistic infection(s)**, severe neurologic disease, HIV antibody, or a positive polymerase chain reaction (PCR) test constitute the definition of AIDS.

Neonatal signs. Most infected infants are clinically and immunologically intact at birth. Although still not completely understood, the mechanisms for transmission of the virus seem to correlate with onset of symptoms. For example, those infants who contract HIV infection in utero appear to be symptomatic at 4 to 12 weeks after birth (Oxtoby, 1994). Those who are infected intrapartally or early in life by breast-feeding have a median symptom onset at 3 years. Recent data suggest that the majority of vertical transmission of HIV infection is intrapartal. Now that ZDV is being administered to mothers and infants, it is expected that there will be lower vertical transmission rates and a reduction in the incidence of pediatric HIV infection. The CDC (1995) recommends that infants born to HIV-infected mothers also receive prophylaxis for *pneumocystis carinii* pneumonia (PCP) with Bactrim, beginning when the 6 weeks of newborn administration of ZDV ends, to avoid possible hematologic toxicity. Bactrim doses continue until it is determined that the infant is not infected.

Clinical management. Currently, there are several tests that are used to identify persons with HIV infection. *Antibodies* to the virus develop and are detectable within the first 6 months of infection, again demonstrating a window in which infection is present but antibody formation is inadequate to trigger a positive test response. As the infection progresses, the amount of virus in the body increases and is measured as the **viral load** by an HIV RNA assay, possibly predicting which HIV-infected pregnant women are most likely to transmit the infection to their infants and which infants are most likely to develop progressive disease states (Volberding, 1996).

Two antibody methods, used together, detect and confirm the presence of HIV-1. The ELISA is relatively easy to perform and is inexpensive. It is highly sensitive in detecting the HIV antibody for many people. A single, positive ELISA test result is not absolute evidence of HIV infection. If the ELISA shows a positive reaction, the test is repeated on the same serum sample. Confirmation of a twice-positive ELISA test result is achieved with a second antibody test (Western blot), which is specific for antibody to the HIV protein coat. The Western blot test is difficult to perform and therefore is less suited for wide screening. Persons whose test reaction is negative with the ELISA method and who have not been exposed or potentially exposed to the virus within the previous 6 months are considered free of HIV-1 infection. However, some clinicians recommend a second confirmatory negative ELISA test at least 3 months following the first negative test.

Other HIV-related tests are the PCR assay, which is a method for amplifying proviral DNA 1 million times or more to increase the probability of detection. Recently, PCR has replaced ELISA/Western blot as the "gold standard" of pediatric HIV testing. The advantage of this test in infants (older than 3 months) is that the PCR allows detection of the infant's *own HIV status* by age 3 to 4 months, rather than the 18 to 24 month period for the infant to shed maternal HIV antibodies. PCR sensitivity is close to 100% at age 2 to 3 months. Although also used, HIV cultures and P24 antigen are less useful than the PCR assay because they are problematic as a result of lengthy waiting periods (Rogers et al, 1994).

Maternal signs in antepartum and intrapartum periods are confirmed by blood work, with the **T4 lymphocyte** (T helper lymphocyte) counts being followed at regular intervals. Regular fetal assessment will be increased because of the potential for IUGR. Intrapartal management differs from standard care only in that efforts to minimize ascending infection and vaginal examinations, avoid premature rupture of membranes, and maintain frequent perineal hygiene are all *emphasized* in the HIV-infected woman in labor. Laboratory reports for potential thrombocytopenia and anemia will be followed, especially if the woman is on a medication regimen.

HIV infection currently is incurable. Pregnant women are treated when the T4 counts fall below 200 cells per microliter (Sperling, Stratton, and Working Group of AIDS Clinical Trials Group, 1992). Some controversy surrounds the use of the combination drug sulfamethoxazole-trimethoprim (Bactrim or Septra) that is given during pregnancy to women whose need for prophylaxis against PCP requires treatment. The dilemma is that PCP is a life-threatening disease which is extremely treatable with Bactrim, a drug with theoretical potential for side effects in the fetus. Bactrim is a folate antagonist, and because marginal folate levels in pregnancy may cause neural tube defects, it should be avoided when possible. However, its use is justified in high-risk situations in which the mother's life may be threatened by PCP (Toltzis, 1993). The rationale is that appropriate prophylaxis should be used in the mother, because severe disease is also being prevented in the infant (Baker, 1994).

Nursing responsibilities. Preconceptional screening is the ideal for women who are at increased risk for HIV infection (Box 25-10). It would, of course, be best to delay pregnancy until effective treatments for HIV infection are developed. However, reality is different. Serologic screening is advised for women who are already pregnant and belong to a high-risk group. Nonjudgmental counseling before and after HIV antibody testing is of extreme importance.

Screening involves obtaining a history for risk-taking behaviors, signs and symptoms of illness, physical exami-

nations, and serologic testing. To identify those at risk for HIV infection, careful history taking includes specific questions in the *language and terms familiar to the individual* (see Box 25-10). Nurses who are culturally "competent" will use appropriately phrased questions.

Client teaching. Women are advised about their risks for HIV infection, the benefits of antibody testing, the procedure for testing, the meaning of possible test results, the confidentiality of results, and the psychologic and social impact of a positive result. The client's consent to perform the test is almost universally required. Post-test counseling includes discussion of the meaning of the results, limits of the test, psychologic and social implications of the results, and a pointed discussion on behaviors to reduce future risk of infection for the client and others. In addition, if the woman is infected with HIV, the importance of continuing medical care is stressed and resources for psychologic support are given. Persons at risk for HIV infection should be counseled about their high-risk behaviors and the specific means they may use to decrease this risk.

Individualized antepartum management after screening is important. The psychosocial impact of discovering a positive test result may be intense. The woman may have been infected by a partner whose own status was unknown. In other cases, it may be found that the HIV-positive man refuses to tell his partner or to use a condom for fear that when she learns of his status, she will leave

---

▌ *Box* **25-10**   **Suggested Questions for Screening Persons at Risk for HIV Infection**

Do you inject drugs in your veins or under your skin?
Do you share needles?
Have you ever had sex with someone who used needles to inject drugs?
Have you ever had sex with someone who has AIDS or had a positive test reaction for the AIDS virus?
Were you born in or have you had sex with someone from an area where infection with the AIDS virus is common?
Have you ever had sex with a man who has also had sex with other men or prostitutes?
Do you have or have you ever had sex with someone who is a bleeder (or who has hemophilia)?
Have you ever had sex for money or ever traded sex to get drugs?
Have you had sex with someone who has sex for money or to get drugs?
Have you or your sex partner received blood or blood products between 1977 and 1985?
Have you had sex with more than 5 different people in the last 12 months?
Have you had sex without a condom?

him. This tragic situation is not uncommon, especially among immigrant women who come from patriarchal societies in which discussion of sexual habits is avoided and unquestioning obedience to the husband is the norm. In a number of instances, the first sign of parental HIV infection is the admission of the infant for AIDS-related symptoms. The woman in this situation needs careful counseling. Because confidentiality is a major ethical and legal issue, the nurse may not disclose a client's HIV status to *any* members of her family without the client's permission, not even to a spouse. Disclosure of HIV status to others is a justifiable fear: women have been known to suffer abuse, discrimination, stigma, and loss of children, jobs, and homes as a result of being HIV-positive.

Self-Discovery

Your client in labor is Mrs. R, whose HIV seroconversion occurred because her husband "went with prostitutes" before she arrived in this country. She is resigned to her situation but worried about the infant. As a nurse, how do you feel about this situation? If you were in her situation, how might you feel? What would you like the nurse to help you with? ~

Breast-feeding by the HIV-positive mother is not advised by the CDC, as it has been shown to be a *source of postnatal infection.* Formula feeding should be used in the United States. However, in countries where there are no safe alternatives available, breast milk may be the *only* life-sustaining choice, and breast-feeding is permitted on a risk-benefit ratio for the infant (Mofenson and Wolinsky, 1994).

Collaborative referral. Post-test counseling may go for three sessions. After that, the woman may need to be referred to a mental health professional to assist in adjusting to the diagnosis and to plan for her family's future. Advanced placement (foster care choices made by the mother for her children before she dies) is a very arduous task and must be undertaken only after intensive counseling.

A multidisciplinary approach to follow-up care is appropriate because of the complex needs of the woman with HIV infection. The advent of the HIV epidemic has allowed comprehensive planning for care in ways that longer-standing and less life-threatening problems have not evoked. Pediatric follow-up for the infant and home care by providers familiar with the stigma of HIV should be standard practices today.

Isolation precautions. See Box 25-9 for guidelines.

Syphilis

Syphilis is a chronic infection, recognized since antiquity as "the great pox." The spirochete *Treponema pallidum*

TEST *Yourself* 25-2 _____

a. Identify how obstetric procedures may cause the fetus or newborn to receive a higher viral load for its HIV-positive mother than it would receive if the care were different.
b. What purpose is served by cleansing newborn skin before eye prophylaxis or infection? Have you observed this precaution carried out in your clinical setting?

is capable of penetrating intact skin or mucous membranes and is transmitted by direct contact with skin lesions or blood, primarily during sexual intimacy, including kissing. The incidence of primary and secondary syphilis infection has been increasing rapidly since the 1980s, especially in areas with high prevalence for HIV infection (Masci, 1996). Consequently, additional numbers of infants have been born with congenital and acquired syphilis. Women aged 15 to 24 have experienced the greatest increase in the incidence of syphilis. In the United States, syphilis is most frequently reported among young, urban, poor, and unmarried persons. Syphilis is more prevalent in developing nations than in industrialized nations, because treatment is not as widely available.

Risk. The rate of primary and secondary syphilis has increased 75% since 1985, with most of the increase in lower socioeconomic groups; 44% of these cases occurred in women (Tillman, 1991). The rise in rates for women has been linked to the convergence of substance abuse, HIV infection, and limited access to care in medically under-served areas. Delays in treatment occur for several reasons, especially because the woman may perceive a loss of her emotional relationship related to the diagnosis. A sense of shame and guilt may allow her to deny the mild symptomatology, causing her to avoid seeking medical care in a timely fashion. Reinfection is common (Fogel, 1995). Pregnancy itself does not affect the disease course, but the fetus may be severely infected during pregnancy, including stillborn births and multiple manifestations in the survivors.

Treponema pallidum can cross the placenta and invade the fetus *at any gestational age.* Fetal infection may result directly in spontaneous abortion, intrauterine fetal death (IUFD), premature labor and birth, neonatal death, and clinically evident congenital syphilis. Newborns can also become infected by coming into direct contact with the organism during the birth process. Infants of women with untreated or inadequately treated primary or secondary syphilis are at greatest risk for congenital infection, preterm birth, or perinatal death.

Congenital syphilis is a preventable disease, avoided by early identification and treatment of maternal syphilis during pregnancy. The population most at risk for developing syphilis is also the population at risk for HIV infection, with the resultant burden that congenital syphilis falls upon infants of women who are also HIV infected. Therefore mothers and infants who are infected with either syphilis or HIV should be thoroughly evaluated for both infections (Gutman, 1994). The fetus may be severely infected before treatment, however, and may show the signs described in the text that follows even after treatment. Congenital syphilis may also occur because of inadequate treatment, maternal relapses, or reinfection from an untreated partner. Treatment before 15 weeks' gestation may prevent congenital syphilis (Tillman, 1991).

Signs. If not adequately treated, syphilis is a progressive, chronic infectious process. After the initial infection, syphilis is described as *primary, secondary, latent,* and *tertiary,* depending on the duration of the infection, the symptoms, and the organ systems involved.

After the usual incubation period of several weeks to up to 90 days, *primary* syphilis develops with a painless **chancre**—an ulcerated, firm lesion with a raised border. It may not be observable if it occurs on the cervix or vagina rather than on external genitalia and produces no irritating symptoms. Lasting 1 to 2 months or longer, this chancre is highly infectious, but it resolves spontaneously without treatment.

Secondary symptoms of syphilis develop 6 to 8 weeks later and include bacteremia and involvement of all organ systems. Short-lived malaise, fever, sore throat, headache, anorexia, and arthralgia, as well as a maculopapular rash involving palms and soles, are identifying signs, but these mimic many other dermatologic lesions. Later, elevated, white, moist papules (condyloma latum) occur on labia, groin, and anal regions.

Latent syphilis has an early stage (usually asymptomatic) lasting up to a year, during which time syphilis is transmitted to the fetus through blood and placenta. Late-stage latent syphilis is not seen in pregnancy, since the woman in this stage is usually not able to get pregnant or carry a pregnancy.

Infants with congenital syphilis are most often symptom-free at birth. Symptoms often appear by 10 days to 2 weeks and nearly always within the first 2 to 3 months of life. Clinical symptoms initially may be nonspecific:
- Profuse serous rhinorrhea
- Enlarged liver or spleen
- Mucocutaneous rash or patches

Clinical management

Diagnostic testing. Syphilis is diagnosed by serologic tests or by direct microscopic examination of lesion exudate for spirochetes. Serologic tests—Venereal Disease Research Laboratory (VDRL), rapid plasma reagin (RPR), automated reagin test (ART), fluorescent treponemal antibody-absorption test (FTA-ABS)—detect the presence of antibodies to the spirochete. Unfortunately, antibody test reactions will be negative for 4 to 6 weeks after exposure to the infection; false-negative test results occur at this time.

Evaluation includes two types of serologic tests. Nonspecific screening tests or *nontreponemal tests* include the VDRL, RPR, and ART. Because these tests are *nonspecific,* other diseases (e.g., acute febrile illness, immunization, Epstein-Barr virus infections, malaria, leprosy, autoimmune diseases such as lupus erythematosus, and pregnancy itself) may cause false-positive results in these nontreponemal tests. Any positive nontreponemal test reaction must be confirmed by a *treponemal serologic test.* The FTA-ABS is the most commonly used *specific* test. Results of the FTA-ABS remain positive for the person's lifetime despite adequate treatment.

In other areas of the world, where other *Treponema* species cause infections such as pinta, yaws, and bejel, persons who have had these infections will show positive reactions on both treponema-specific and nonspecific serologic tests. These women are often given antibiotic treatment as if they have syphilis.

In all cases where a neonate is being screened serologically for possible congenital syphilis, the blood of choice is maternal blood, not cord blood. A maternal VDRL is drawn in the clinic or on admission to labor. If the result is positive, the infant is treated (Box 25-11). The CDC recommends that newborns not be discharged until the maternal VDRL results are known. Early discharge is a threat to full evaluation of newborns at risk, necessitating discharge protocols that *must* include a mechanism for serologic screening and prompt treatment of all newborns. There is potential for a gap in the care of newborns between care in the hospital unit and pediatric follow-up care.

Because of the *window* in antibody formation, newborns have manifested congenital syphilis when the maternal VDRL response was negative. In these cases, the women became infected within 4 to 6 weeks of birth, before antibody levels were significant (see HIV testing for the same problem).

Treatment. The drug of choice to treat syphilis at any stage is penicillin (see Box 25-11). Recommended treatment for primary, secondary, and early latent syphilis is a one-time, IM dose of benzathine penicillin G. HIV-infected women or those with latent syphilis or syphilis infections of unknown duration are often treated for 3 consecutive weeks. Because of the pharmacokinetic alterations that occur during pregnancy, it is recommended that all pregnant women be treated with parenteral penicillin G. Pregnant women who are allergic to penicillin should be *desensitized* and treated with penicillin in the hospital, since there is no proven alternative. Tetracycline cannot be used because of potential deleterious effects upon the fetus. Erythromycin therapy in a pregnant woman with syphilis cannot be considered a reliable cure for the fetus (Peter, 1994). All pregnant HIV-positive women should be retested after the course of treatment, since even the increased doses of penicillin given to them may not be adequate.

Box 25-11 | Treatment of Syphilis during Pregnancy

PRIMARY, SECONDARY, AND EARLY LATENT (LESS THAN 1 YEAR)

2.4 million units benzathine penicillin G IM
Rescreen at 3 and 6 months

LATE LATENT AND GUMMA-AFFECTED CARDIOVASCULAR SYSTEM

7.2 million units benzathine penicillin G IM in three
   divided weekly doses
Rescreen at 6 and 12 months

TREATMENT OF CONGENITAL SYPHILIS

100,000 to 150,000 U/kg aqueous crystalline penicillin G
   IV daily for 10 to 14 days
(Procaine penicillin IM every day for 10 to 14 days has
   been used, but there is risk of damage to small
   muscle sites)
Rescreen at 1, 2, 3, 6, and 12 months

Box 25-12 | Isolation Precautions: Syphilis

MOTHER
Avoid contact with body fluids or chancre mucous
   patches
Blood precautions
Careful hand washing

INFANT
Infant is isolated with mother

BREAST-FEEDING
Breast-feeding permitted after treatment

TEST *Yourself* 25-3 _____

a. Test-of-cure after treatment for syphilis is performed
   with which type of screening test?
b. Why is this test especially important for newborns and
   HIV-positive women?

Spirochete reactions. At times, after initiating penicillin treatment against spirochetes such as those causing syphilis and Lyme disease, an adverse event called *Jarisch-Herxheimer* reaction occurs (Peter, 1994). The sudden release of spirochete cell wall lipids into the maternal and fetal bloodstream as the microorganisms are killed is the most likely explanation. Within hours of treatment, high fever, chills, malaise, myalgia, tachycardia, and occasionally shock may occur. This reaction is usually self-limited, and treatment is symptomatic with antipyretics, bed rest, emotional support, and fetal monitoring.

After antibiotic treatment, pregnant clients should receive follow-up with monthly quantitative nontreponemal antibody tests such as VDRL and RPR titers for the remainder of the pregnancy and should be retreated if a four-fold rise in antibody titer occurs. Long-term follow-up care includes quantitative VDRL and RPR titers at 3, 6, 9, and 12 months after therapy. With successful therapy, the nontreponemal tests will become nonreactive after 1 year for primary syphilis and within 2 years for secondary syphilis (Peter, 1994).

Isolation precautions. While in the hospital unit, use isolation precautions listed in Box 25-12.

Nursing Responsibilities

In the antenatal clinic setting, nursing care often includes obtaining information about current problems and a detailed health history. Assessment of a woman's risk of acquiring or having an STD is essential, but since it is a form of compulsory intimacy between nurse and client, trust and confidentiality are the cornerstones of a good assessment. It is accomplished by *tactfully* asking very specific, nonjudgmental questions about the person's (1) sexual practices—whether she participates in vaginal, oral-genital, anal, or oral-anal sex, her use of sexual devices, or other types of sexual expression, (2) the gender of her sexual partner, (3) whether she has had a new partner in the past 3 months, (4) the number of partners in the past month, year, and in her lifetime, and (5) history of any STDs. When eliciting information on STDs, questions about each type of infection should be asked separately, using language and body clues that are appropriate to the educational level and cultural background of the woman. If using a translator to elicit sexual data for an assessment, do not use a family member, including a husband. In addition to being culturally incorrect, the woman's *sexual confidentiality* may be compromised with those upon whom she most depends. Nurses should advocate for trained objective translators who are not known by the client.

A few examples of the questions to ask during the assessment include: Have you noticed any increased vaginal discharge? Does your discharge burn, itch, or have an odor? Do you notice the vaginal odor at any particular time (e.g., after intercourse)? What color is your discharge? Are there any sores or bumps that you notice today or that come and go? Do you have any pain, burning, or discomfort with intercourse?

NURSING DIAGNOSES

Using the nursing process, the information gathered from an interview and a review of the records is used by the nurse to consider several nursing diagnoses, depending on whether a potential or actual problem is identified. For example, if a woman is found to be at high risk for STDs, the following nursing diagnoses may apply:

- Altered health maintenance related to the effects of the STD
- Knowledge deficit regarding the risk of acquiring STDs
- Risk for infection related to exposure to a sexual partner without using an effective barrier method

When a sexually transmitted infection has been identified after assessment, nursing diagnoses may be directed toward increasing the woman's knowledge and understanding of the infection, treatment, and follow-up care; actual and potential physical symptoms; psychologic and social responses to having the infection; or prevention of potential complications from the infection. The following examples of nursing diagnoses may apply:

- Knowledge deficit, regarding risks of STD during pregnancy, spread of disease, and reinfection
- Body image disturbance or self-esteem disturbance, related to acquiring a sexually transmitted infection
- Injury, risk for, fetal, related to congenital infection
- Ineffective individual coping mechanisms, related to effects of disease state on mother or infant
- Social isolation, related to significant other's response to diagnosis

EXPECTED OUTCOMES

Depending upon the type and stage of the STD, outcomes will vary. Some respond quickly to treatment, whereas others may continue to be long-term problems, presenting treatment challenges and relapses. Some of the following examples may apply:

- Gains cooperation of partner in safe sex and preventive measures (may need professional assistance).
- Uses methods to relieve discomforts during treatment.
- Follows precautions to prevent reinfection.
- Can identify signs and symptoms of relapse or reinfection and seeks appropriate treatment.
- Infant exhibits negative laboratory test results.

NURSING INTERVENTION

Client teaching

Nurses adopt an assertive role in STD care. Syphilis is a reportable communicable disease with a potential impact upon the health of the fetus. This fact, and the importance

of eradicating the infection, should be explained to the client. Education to reduce personal risk is especially important because it can prevent the disease and potentially fatal maternal-child events (Box 25-13). Knowledge of the resources in the community is essential for anyone engaged in counseling. The nurse is often the advocate for the client in finding other support. The nurse practices as part of a team because social problems, drug use, and distress often accompany an STD and require complex approaches to the problem. Clients may also be referred to the free CDC National Hotline (1-800-227-8922) for information and confidential referral services for STDs. The following are elements of client education for the treatment and prevention of STD spread.

- Client is educated about the importance of completing the full course of antibiotic therapy. Report any side effects, recurrence, or increase in symptoms.
- The woman with primary or secondary syphilis is reassured that symptoms such as skin lesions and other manifestations of infection will decrease and that serology will ultimately demonstrate a cure for her and protection for the fetus. Individualizing each client's education plan will help ensure understanding and compliance.
- The client is advised to abstain (if possible) from sexual contact with partner(s) until each has been treated. Offer to instruct the woman's partner about STDs, the importance of treatment, reinfection, and potential danger to the fetus.
- The woman with an STD needs to negotiate for condom use if her partner will not abstain from sex. *Nurses who instruct women to use condoms must be aware that this request may put the woman's safety at risk in some cases* (Cotton, 1995). Her partner may react to her request by feeling his authority is being questioned, may force her to have sex without a condom anyway, or may physically abuse her in other ways. Asking the client to describe in advance her partner's probable reaction to using a condom will cue the nurse's response, including a possible client teaching session with the partner.

A successful pregnancy is a developmental task for women of childbearing age that may be jeopardized by having an STD. As a result of the STD diagnosis, the pregnant woman may have additional anxiety about the infant, and, in vulnerable women, feelings of self-blame, humiliation, and lowered self-esteem may be present. Nurses need to know how the STD affects fetus and newborn health, as well as be aware of the effect of the medications the woman must take. Finally, appropriate universal and isolation precautions must be taught and followed.

Collaborative referrals

Each client encounter is an opportunity to assess the pregnant woman's physical and mental status. Additional

Box 25-13

TEACHING PLAN *for* HOME CARE

Risk Reduction for Acquiring Sexually Transmitted Diseases

CAREFUL CONSIDERATION OF SEXUAL ACTIVITY

Abstinence and restriction to a single (uninfected) partner or partners reduce the risk of all sexually transmitted diseases (STDs) to a minimum. Increased numbers of partners, especially unfamiliar ones, increase risks.

PRACTICE OF SEXUAL ACTIVITIES THAT DO NOT EXCHANGE BODILY FLUIDS WITH UNFAMILIAR PARTNERS (E.G., MASSAGE, MASTURBATION)

STD pathogens are transmitted by direct contact of microorganisms with mucosal surfaces or open skin.

USE OF BARRIER FORMS OF CONTRACEPTION WITH SPERMICIDAL AGENTS

Properly used, condoms (and possibly diaphragms) combined with spermicides reduce the risks of many STDs. They will not work if infectious lesions or secretions are not covered or contained. Women may think they are protected from STDs because they are taking oral contraceptive pills or have had a tubal ligation. These measures do avoid conception but *they do not protect mucosal surfaces* from infective microorganisms.

AVOIDANCE OF "UNSAFE SEX" PRACTICES

Avoid practices that cause local skin or mucosal membrane trauma and increase direct inoculation of pathogens. Avoid oroanal contact and anal intercourse altogether. Avoid sexual activities that cause bleeding.

PERIODIC SCREENING FOR STDS

Persons at increased risk should be screened at intervals corresponding to their risk. (Young persons, persons with a prior STD, and persons with more than three partners in the last 6 months should be screened frequently.)

ENSURING PARTNER'S TREATMENT OR COMPLIANCE WITH SAFE SEX

Partners of persons with gonorrhea or *Chlamydia* infection have a 50% to 56% risk of becoming infected. Many are symptom-free.

WHEN AT RISK FOR AIDS

Practice sexual activities that do not include exchange of body fluids. Do not share IV needles. Do not donate blood or other body fluids or organs. If female, discuss pregnancy risk with counselor.

Data from Fogel C: Sexually transmitted diseases. In McElmurry B, Parker R, eds: *Annual review of women's health,* NY, 1995, National League for Nursing Press; Cotton D: AIDS in women. In Sachs B, ed: *Reproductive health care for women and babies,* NY, 1995, Oxford University Press.

treatment referrals to the appropriate physician will be necessary should any of the tests for STD monitoring indicate recurring infection. In addition, women who demonstrate signs and symptoms of psychosocial distress or of being physically abused need immediate referral to social work colleagues. Spiritual distress could generate a referral by the nurse to a pastor of the woman's choice. Cultural distress could be alleviated by referral to a community-based organization operated by the same culture.

Cultural aspects

A woman's culture forms the framework within which her pregnancy experience takes place. In some cultures, women are not supposed to speak of sexual matters, birth control, condoms, or even the names of body parts. Many women exist in traditional relationships in which their male partners make the decisions, including reproductive decisions. Within this framework, the diagnosis of an STD may present a *crisis* for the woman. The crisis may take many forms. The woman may even be blamed for contracting the illness and threatening the life of the fetus, even though it was probably the male partner who infected her. In order for the nurse to plan interventions

for the client, *he or she must become familiar with the cultural framework within which the client lives and operates.* Only when cultural literacy and nursing interventions are appropriately congruent will effective nurse-client communication, care, and advocacy take place.

EVALUATION

- Were precautions followed and was transmission prevented? If not, were barriers identified?
- Does the woman know infection outcome, signs of recurrence, and preventive actions?
- Is there any evidence of perinatal transmission?

TEST *Yourself* 25-4

Make a chart for these major STDs and compare and contrast:
a. Fetal risk and newborn outcome
b. Effect of treatments in prevention of newborn disease
c. Isolation precautions
d. Risk of acquiring STD because of breast-feeding

- If no cure is possible (HIV, HSV), has she followed through on supportive treatment?

PERINATAL INFECTIONS

Perinatal infections are acquired by transmission before, during, or shortly after birth. They may be caused by bacteria, viruses, protozoa, or fungi. Intrauterine transmission of these infections may occur across the placenta via the maternal bloodstream, by ascent of microorganisms from the vagina, or possibly by descent from infected fallopian tubes. The infant may become infected during passage through the infected birth canal or from maternal blood during birth or by maternal-infant contact after birth. It is important to remember that infections such as HBV and cytomegalovirus may be sexually transmitted.

Enterovirus

Enteroviruses are RNA viruses that occur worldwide and are spread from person to person by fecal-oral or possibly oral-oral routes. Each of the three major enteroviruses— poliovirus, coxsackievirus, and echovirus—has been associated with serious neonatal disease. Enterovirus may be transmitted transplacentally or by contamination during birth.

Poliovirus

In the United States where poliomyelitis is rare, routine immunization of pregnant women is not recommended (ACOG, 1991). However, in persons at risk for exposure, such as pregnant women traveling in areas where the disease is endemic, it can be given. Two doses of enhanced inactivated poliomyelitis vaccine (e-IPV) should be injected SC at 4- to 8-week intervals, followed by a third dose 6 to 12 months after the second dose. There is an oral polio vaccine (OPV), which is a live attenuated virus that affords immediate protection, but it has associated risks. The HIV-positive woman and the members of her household should *not* receive OPV; instead the injectable inactivated vaccine must be used. Her children who receive OPV may shed virus for 1 to 2 weeks, placing her at great risk of becoming ill with poliovirus.

Coxsackievirus and echovirus

Coxsackievirus is implicated in nonspecific neonatal febrile illnesses, sudden infant death syndrome (SIDS), gastrointestinal malformations, and serious neonatal morbidity and mortality. Shortly after birth, neonatal echovirus infection may cause fever, cyanosis, hypothermia, bradycardia, hepatic necrosis, disseminated intravascular coagulopathy (DIC), and death. There are no specific treatments or vaccines for echovirus or coxsackievirus infections.

TORCH Infections

TORCH is a classic acronym for several infections that cause severe developmental congenital anomalies when the embryo or fetus is exposed to them via the pregnant woman anytime during her first 12 weeks of gestation: **TO:** toxoplasmosis; **R:** rubella; **C:** cytomegalovirus; **H:** herpes simplex (covered earlier in this chapter with the information on STDs).

Toxoplasmosis

Toxoplasmosis is a systemic, usually asymptomatic, illness caused by the protozoan parasite *Toxoplasma gondii*, which infects most mammalian species. Approximately one third of adult women in the United States have antibodies for toxoplasma, which means they have had a previous infection. The *Toxoplasma* tachyzoite invades muscle and CNS tissues and forms cysts in tissue after the development of the host immune response. These cysts remain viable for the person's lifetime. Acquired toxoplasmosis is usually asymptomatic. If symptoms do occur, they are nonspecific and self-limited. Complications can occur in chronically infected immunocompromised patients, such as those with AIDS, who can experience a reactivation of CNS disease or systemic disease. Infrequently, infants born to immunocompromised mothers, including those with HIV infection who also have chronic *Toxoplasma* infection, have been known to develop congenital toxoplasmosis because of their mother's reactivated disease state (Peter, 1994). During pregnancy, *Toxoplasma* may be transmitted across the placenta and cause severe infection in the developing embryo or fetus. Early treatment of the pregnant woman often prevents infection of the fetus. Those fetuses affected early may spontaneously abort.

Human beings acquire toxoplamosis in the following ways: (1) ingesting the tissue cyst stage from inadequately cooked meat or other animal products, including eggs and milk, (2) ingesting or inhaling the oocyst stage excreted in feline feces from contaminated soil or food (e.g., pica or poorly washed root vegetables), or (3) transplacental or blood-product transmission or tachyzoites. Serologic evidence suggests that 30% to 60% of domestic cats have had *Toxoplasma* infection. *Toxoplasma* tissue cysts can be isolated from the muscle of 25% to 30% of swine and sheep and from 1% of cattle (Freij and Sever, 1991). With the exception of the rare occurrence of infected organ donors, blood transfusion donors, and transplacental infection from mother to fetus, toxoplasmosis is not a disease that is communicated from person to person (Peter, 1994).

Risk. Toxoplasmosis is transmitted to the fetus across the placenta when the organism is spread through the bloodstream during *primary* or *reactivated* maternal infection (as in the case of HIV-infected mothers or mothers who are immunosuppressed for other reasons). In most cases, prior **toxoplasma** infection appears to offer nearly complete protection against intrauterine infection.

Newborn risk. Manifestations of congenital toxoplasmosis can include hepatosplenomegaly, generalized lymphadenopathy, a maculopapular rash, jaundice, or thrombocytopenia. The occurrence of intrauterine transmission of toxoplasmosis is related to the stage of pregnancy at the time of maternal infection. The incidence of congenital infection is less in mothers infected early in the pregnancy, but their infants have a greater risk of developing early symptomatic disease. These infants develop cerebritis with intracranial calcifications, hydrocephalus, chorioretinitis, hepatosplenomegaly, and thrombocytopenia. Most infected infants are born without symptoms (70% to 90%), but many will go on to develop symptoms after a period of months or even years later. The consequences of congenital infection in these infants range from mild to serious and can include seizure, mental retardation, deafness, and blindness (Mitchell, 1994).

Nursing considerations

Client teaching. Diagnosis of toxoplasmosis is often problematic. Clinical signs and symptoms are not specific and are often attributed to influenza or mononucleosis. Instruction for all HIV-1 positive pregnant women should include information about the potential for toxoplasmosis, as well as advocating for testing for *Toxoplasma*-specific immunoglobin G (IgG). By educating pregnant women about prevention methods for toxoplasmosis, the nurse plays a vital role in preventing infection in both the mother and her infant. Methods of prevention are listed in Box 25-14.

Rubella

Rubella is caused by the rubivirus and is spread by oral droplets and transplacentally. Currently, most cases are seen in the teenage and young adult group who were not immunized as children, before the availability of the vaccine. In a pregnant woman, rubella can produce devastating congenital abnormalities. The incubation period is 2 to 3 weeks.

Risk. Young women 15 years of age or older who were not targeted for vaccination during their childhood are at extreme risk for rubella. The risk of congenital defects in the developing fetus is greatest when maternal infection occurs in the first trimester, then the risk gradually grows less until it is considered rare after 16 to 20 weeks (Sulis, 1995). The most commonly occurring anomalies are congenital cataracts, patent ductus arteriosus, sensorineural deafness, and meningoencephalitis. Other frequently reported defects are growth retardation, radiolucent bone disease, hepatosplenomegaly, thrombocytopenia, jaundice, and purpuric skin manifestations that are described as resembling "blueberry muffins" (Aronoff, 1994).

Signs. Usually a mild disease, rubella is characterized by a low-grade fever and tender, swollen lymph nodes, followed by a rash lasting 3 days that appears over the face and spreads to the trunk in a lacy pattern. Polyarthritis, especially in teenage girls and young women, has been reported, and it lasts for several days to several weeks (Aronoff, 1994). Supportive care includes rest, fluids, and maintenance of isolation precautions (Box 25-15).

Maternal infection resulting in congenital rubella after 16 to 20 weeks is rare (ACOG, 1992). Infants with congenital rubella infection are deemed *to be contagious* until they are 12 months old, except those who have negative

Box 25-14

TEACHING PLAN *for* HOME CARE

Prevention of Congenital Toxoplasmosis

PREVENTION OF INFECTION IN PREGNANT WOMEN

The woman should take these precautions:

Cook meat at a temperature higher than 66° C, smoke it, or cure it in brine.

Use frozen meats kept at −20° C for at least 24 hours. Home refrigerators may not achieve −20° C.

Avoid touching mucous membranes of mouth and eyes while handling raw meat.

Wash hands thoroughly after handling raw meat.

Avoid eating uncooked eggs and unpasteurized milk.

Wash fruits and vegetables before consumption.

Prevent access of flies and cockroaches to fruit and vegetables.

Avoid contact with materials that are potentially contaminated with cat feces (e.g., cat litter boxes, sand boxes, or garden)

Wear gloves and wash hands for tasks if exposure to cat feces cannot be avoided.

SECONDARY PREVENTION

Serologic screening for toxoplasma antibodies in women during pregnancy is not currently recommended but may be selectively performed.

If acute toxoplasma infection is a real possibility in pregnancy, expert advice should be sought to help to determine which, if any, tests should be ordered and what, if any, treatment should be considered.

Box 25-15   Isolation Precautions: Rubella

MOTHER AND INFANT

Respiratory isolation

Infant isolated with mother

Mask for 3 to 4 days after rash appears

Careful hand washing

BREAST-FEEDING

Breast-feed with mask

nasopharyngeal and urine cultures after 3 months of age (Peter, 1994). All efforts to diagnose congenital rubella should be made, and infections should be reported to local, state, and CDC authorities. Infants diagnosed with, or suspected of having, congenital rubella should be isolated with contact isolation. Congenital rubella is pictured in Figure 25-8.

Nursing considerations. Prevention of rubella infection in women of childbearing age is crucial for preventing potentially damaging effects to the fetus. To accomplish this, all susceptible young persons should be immunized before considering sexual activity. Pregnant women should not receive the rubella vaccine because of the theoretical risk to the fetus, estimated at 1.6%. However, should a pregnant woman inadvertently receive rubella vaccine, it is not an indication to terminate the pregnancy (Peter, 1994). Ideally, all pregnant women are tested for rubella antibodies as early as possible in prenatal care. A negative titer signals that the woman is susceptible and must receive instructions to do the following:

1. Avoid exposure during pregnancy.
2. Be immunized just after the birth. (Vaccination is done only after birth to avoid the chance of viral infection of the fetus.)
3. Delay any future pregnancy for 3 months after immunization.

Side effects of the vaccine may include transient muscle and joint pain and paresthesias. Small amounts of virus may be excreted into breast milk, but this does not contraindicate breast-feeding. Immunization with Rho(D) immune globulin does not appear to interfere with rubella immunization, but some delay giving the dose of rubella.

Client teaching. All children (12 to 15 months of age or older) of pregnant women should receive their immunizations according to schedule, since there is no definitive evidence that the vaccine virus is transmitted from person to

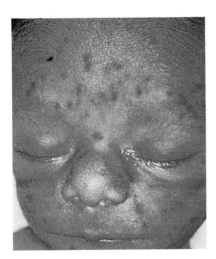

Figure 25-8 Congenital rubella. (Courtesy Donald C Anderson, MD, Baylor College of Medicine, Houston, Texas)

person (ACOG, 1992). For many women, going for prenatal and obstetric care is their first entrance into the health care system as adults, and this visit affords the nurse an opportunity to offer rubella education and timely vaccination.

Cytomegalovirus infection

Cytomegalovirus (CMV) is a member of the *herpesvirus* family. Like other viruses of this type, CMV initially establishes a *primary* infection, then a *latent* infection with persistent shedding of the virus. CMV is commonly asymptomatic or has mononucleosis-like symptoms. CMV has been isolated from urine, saliva, blood, cervical mucus, semen, breast milk, and stool. Transmission may occur from contamination of any of these bodily fluids, close interpersonal contact, and sexual contact. Infection with CMV appears to increase with age and varies with socioeconomic group. Approximately 40% of women of childbearing age in the United States have antibodies for CMV (ACOG, 1993). Approximately 1% of pregnant women have detectable cervical CMV during the first trimester; increased viral shedding occurs as pregnancy progresses. CMV may be transmitted across the placenta even if the woman has no overt signs. Vertical transmission at birth also occurs from contaminated cervical and vaginal fluids, blood, and later, through breast milk.

Risk. Approximately 6% of all pregnant women become infected with CMV. Approximately 40% of women with *primary* CMV infection will have an infected fetus. Newborns infected with CMV in utero excrete CMV at birth. Only 10% to 15% of these infected infants demonstrate characteristics associated with congenital CMV. Congenital CMV is characterized by an enlarged spleen and liver, microcephaly, hyperbilirubinemia, motor impairment, hematologic dysfunction, cerebral calcifications, and eye defects.

About 5% of those infected but *symptom-free* at birth develop varying degrees of neurologic deficits by 48 months, including hearing loss and learning and visual difficulties. Symptom-free children may excrete the virus in urine and saliva for a long time and may infect others, especially in day-care centers (Peter, 1994). Preventive care includes good hygiene: careful washing of hands after changing and disposing of diapers and adequate washing of any dishes, utensils, or toys in contact with saliva, especially for pregnant caregivers. Health care workers are exposed to CMV, and most demonstrate antibodies against it. The development of a vaccination is under way (Peter, 1994).

The following are ways in which CMV may be transmitted to an infant:

- In utero through transplacental passage of maternal blood-borne virus
- During the birth process by passing through an infected maternal genital tract
- After birth by ingesting CMV-infected milk

Clinical management. Treatment is reserved for severe infections because of the potential toxicity of the medications used. Currently, the drug ganciclovir is used to treat CMV retinitis in AIDS patients and is combined with CMV immune globulin (IV) for the treatment of severe CMV infections.

Other Infections in the Perinatal Period

Influenza

Influenza is an epidemic disease caused by viruses, especially types A and B. It is spread by direct contact, airborne droplets, or articles contaminated by infected secretions. These viruses are capable of altering their antigen structure frequently to protect themselves from the human host defense system. Influenza epidemics in the past have been associated with significantly increased maternal mortality. Whether pregnant women are more susceptible to influenza or to influenzal pneumonia is unclear. If, however, influenzal pneumonia develops in pregnant women, they are more severely affected.

During pregnancy, potential increases in morbidity and mortality exist during the epidemic of a newly evolved antigenic strain. Increased abortion rates have been reported during these times. Yearly immunization with inactivated virus vaccine to women with serious underlying disease states is recommended to reduce risks (ACOG, 1991).

Lyme disease

A tick-borne disease spread worldwide, Lyme disease may be the cause of increased fetal loss and widely diverse malformations, as well as neonatal illness (Peter, 1994). Several types of ticks carry the spirochete, which acts somewhat like the syphilis spirochete. Mice and deer are carriers, as are other wild and domesticated animals that roam wooded areas. Protective clothing (with snug fitting sleeves and pantlegs), showers after outdoor activity, and examination of skin for tick sites are recommended.

The tick must stay attached for 12 to 24 hours for transmission to occur. Lyme disease is most prevalent in late spring or early summer (Peter, 1994). It is a complex syndrome with many varied expressions, making diagnosis difficult, especially in the early stage.

Stage I signs are *erythema migrans*, the characteristic "bulls-eye" skin lesions consisting of small papular or macular patterns that occur in 60% to 80% of patients. Lesions most commonly occur on the thighs, groin, and axilla. In stage I, there may be flulike symptoms with headache and arthralgia.

Stage II occurs when the disease continues undiagnosed and untreated. The lesions show neurologic signs of cranial nerve palsy (Bell's palsy is most common), but third and sixth cranial nerves may involve eye function. Meningitis may occur. Cardiac manifestations may begin 4 to 6 weeks after exposure. Chronic fatigue and cognitive problems may develop. Peripheral nerve involvement leads to weakness, reduced reflexes, and pain.

Stage III involves joint arthritis, ranging from arthralgia to chronic destructive joint disease.

Prevention is crucial for those in areas of tick infestation. Since early serologic tests are negative (until enough antibody has formed to turn the test positive), the question is whether to treat pregnant women who are suspected of having been exposed but are seronegative. Prophylactic antibiotic during pregnancy and treatment of suspected early disease consist of a three week course of either amoxicillin or erythromycin. Information for clients is available from Lyme Disease Education Project, PO Box 55412, Madison, Wisc, 53705.

Termination of pregnancy because of Lyme disease is not recommended. The infant's health care provider should be told that maternal disease is suspected. A vaccine is being prepared but is not yet available.

Measles

The incidence of measles (rubeola) has been increasing in recent years. Fortunately it is not common for measles to occur during pregnancy, but when it does, it can be extremely serious, especially if pneumonia develops. Though it has the potential to increase premature labor, there are no definitive reports of other adverse effects.

Immunization. The measles vaccine should be given postpartum to those clients born after 1957 who did not receive the live vaccine version (live vaccine became available only in 1967) and to those who do not have a history of measles infection (conferring natural immunity) (ACOG, 1991). The client should receive 2 injections at least 1 month apart. Clients without any previous immunizations who may be entering college or who are employed in areas such as child care or health care need the vaccine. Many outbreaks occur among unimmunized preschool children, children of newly arrived immigrants, or among infants too young for current immunization (less than 15 months). Since childbearing families are likely to come in contact with small children and be exposed to childhood illnesses such as measles, the nurse should be aware of the signs and symptoms of infection, the mode of transmission, the incubation period, and the potential complications of measles during pregnancy.

The measles virus can be transmitted to the fetus across the placenta at any gestational age. Intrauterine infection is associated with spontaneous abortion, IUFD, premature birth, perinatal death, and congenital measles. Infants may have the characteristic rash at birth, or it may develop within the first days of life. Mortality rates may be as high as 20%. Associations between intrauterine measles and fetal anomalies are inconclusive. (See Box 25-16 for isolation precautions.)

> **Box 25-16** | **Isolation Precautions: Measles**

MOTHER

No history of measles:
  No isolation for first 7 days; respiratory isolation for next 7 days
Mask until 4 days after onset of rash
Careful hand washing
Cover gown
Avoid contact with lesions and fomites

INFANT

None for first 5 days after exposure; respiratory isolation for next 7 days
Give measles hyperimmune globulin

BREAST-FEEDING

Not recommended by some authorities, though little information available

> **Box 25-17** | **Isolation Precautions: Mumps**

MOTHER AND INFANT

No isolation for first 7 days after exposure
Respiratory isolation for 2 weeks or until 9 days after swelling starts
Mother wears mask with infant for 1 week after swelling starts
Careful hand washing

BREAST-FEEDING

Breast-feeding permitted

Mumps

As the result of childhood immunization with live attenuated mumps vaccine in the United States, mumps is not a common infection during pregnancy. Among susceptible adults, person-to-person infection rates are low. Intrauterine infection in the first trimester has resulted in loss of the fetus, and isolated cases of fetal abnormalities have been reported (ACOG, 1991). However, there are no conclusive associations between specific fetal abnormalities and mumps. The infection is caused by a paramyxovirus, a virus that is transmitted by respiratory droplets. Exposure of susceptible persons to the mumps virus results in unilateral or bilateral parotitis after an 18-day incubation period. In adult infections, the disease course is self-limited, and management focuses on relief of symptoms.

Adults suffer more mumps-related complications than do children, including meningoencephalitis, oophoritis, orchitis, (inflammation of ovaries or testes), and neurosensory deafness. Women of childbearing age should not be vaccinated if known to be pregnant; the live virus vaccine has been known to infect the placenta. Theoretically, women who have been recently vaccinated should avoid becoming pregnant for 3 months to avoid risk (Peter, 1994). Isolation recommendations are noted in Box 25-17.

Tuberculosis

The agent of infection is *Mycobacterium tuberculosis*, an acid-fast bacillus (AFB). *Tuberculous (TB) disease* must be differentiated from having the *infection*. In the disease process, there are clinical symptoms present such as lymphadenopathy, a chest radiograph demonstrating pulmonary involvement of TB, a cough, night sweats, fever, loss of weight, and fatigue. There may also be clin-

ical signs of extrapulmonary TB disease involvement. In patients with a low-grade infection, the tuberculin skin test is positive but the chest radiograph is normal, and there are no clinical signs or symptoms of tuberculosis.

The most effective mode of transmission is airborne through the inhalation of infectious droplets, which are aerosolized by sneezing, coughing, or talking. When a susceptible person inhales infectious particulates, the organisms gravitate toward the distal air tubules where they proliferate. The bacilli reproduce in the lung alveoli and cause an acute inflammatory response that surrounds the bacilli, forming a *tubercle*. During this initial infection—primary tuberculosis—microorganisms may spread to other organs of the body. Fortunately, most bacilli are killed or encapsulated into *granulomas* without causing disease; others may progress or become quiescent. In the event of lowered resistance or a high bacilli count, the infection may become widespread and cause symptoms of the *disease*. It is estimated that the infection progresses to disease in 5% to 10% of initially infected persons. Social conditions such as poverty, malnutrition, and crowded living conditions contribute to disease spread. Recent trends in immigration and international travel, with movement of infected persons to the United States from areas where tuberculosis is endemic, have increased the incidence of the infection in several cities and have made it more common in all segments of society. AIDS patients often have tuberculosis as a presenting sign of disease.

Risk. Increased risk for tuberculosis occurs in late pregnancy and postpartum, in the newborn, and during postpubertal adolescence (Summers, 1992). Tuberculosis during pregnancy places mother and fetus at significant risk because of diminished resistance. Pregnant women are susceptible to the development of two forms of tuberculosis: (1) primary infection with pulmonary involvement or (2) reactivation of previously controlled primary infection. Newborns are capable of acquiring tuberculosis by inhalation of infectious respiratory droplets from their mother, a household member, or hospital attendant after birth. Newborns and infants appear *especially susceptible* to tuberculosis for reasons not yet fully understood. Rarely, tuberculosis can be transmitted to the fetus transplacentally or by infected amniotic fluid. If an infectious mother remains untreated, *there is a 50% chance that her newborn will be infected within the neonatal period.* Newborns and infants are at high risk for progressive dissemination, which is frequently fatal if inadequately treated (Peter, 1994).

Neither tuberculosis nor antituberculosis treatment is an indication for pregnancy termination. If necessary, pregnant women may be treated with isoniazid (INH), rifampin, and ethambutol without teratogenic effects, and breast-feeding is permissible with these drugs (American Thoracic Society, 1986; Peter, 1994).

Signs. The incubation period for tuberculosis is 2 to 10 weeks. Every positive tuberculosis skin test reaction is verified by a chest film. In endemic areas, the patient is isolated until the chest film is read. Sputum is sent for acid-fast stain. A sputum smear report is available within few days, and if positive, it indicates that mycobacteria is present, although it may not necessarily be *Mycobacterium tuberculosis.* (If the chest film is consistent with pulmonary TB, the patient is kept in isolation until three negative smears are obtained.) Final identification of the organism is confirmed by culture, and final reports may take up to 6 weeks. Overt change may be minimal, except for the presence of a chronic cough with sputum. Pleuritic chest pain is sometimes present. Weight loss, anorexia, fatigue, and night sweating may occur. Because of the known coexistence of tuberculosis and HIV, all women with tuberculous disease should be offered HIV testing, with pretest and posttest counseling.

Because tuberculosis is often an asymptomatic infection, all women obtaining prenatal care or appearing for a delivery without prenatal care should be screened for *Mycobacterium tuberculosis* infection with the intradermal Mantoux test. Pregnancy itself does not alter test reactivity. Women with a positive skin test reaction should receive a standard chest radiograph examination, with abdominal shielding.

Mantoux test. A 0.1 ml dose of freshly mixed and stabilized purified protein derivative (PPD) (Tween 80) containing 5 tuberculin units (TU) should be placed intradermally on the lower aspect of the forearm, and the skin test should be examined 48 to 72 hours later. *The diameter of test-site induration,* not the reddened skin (erythema), is measured, and is considered positive if the induration is greater than or equal to 10 mm. Induration of less than 5 mm indicates negative test result. Induration between 5 and 9 mm may be caused by infection with atypical mycobacteria, prior bacillus Calmette-Guérin (BCG) vaccination, or recent tuberculosis exposure and infection.

Newborn implications. Infants of mothers with untreated pulmonary tuberculosis are at very high risk for

---

▌ *Box* **25-18** ▏ **Pharmacologic Treatment of Tuberculosis**

> INH, rifampin, and ethambutol for 2 months
> INH and rifampin for 4 to 7 months (9 months total)
> If PPD reaction is positive but no disease is evident, INH alone may be used for 6 months
> For resistance to INH, ethambutol or newer drugs are used

(Peters, 1994; Summers, 1992)
INH, Isoniazid; *PPD,* purified protein derivative.

contracting the disease, given their close contact to the infected mother's droplet secretions and their innate susceptibility. If an infant is suspected of having congenital tuberculosis, a Mantoux intradermal test with 5 TU/PPD should be performed. In addition, a chest radiograph, lumbar puncture, and appropriate cultures should be executed promptly. Regardless of the skin test results (infants begin reactivity to PPDs at 3 to 6 weeks), INH should be started immediately with rifampin, pyrazinamide, and streptomycin (Peter, 1994).

Clinical management. During pregnancy, screening, diagnosis, and treatment are ideally accomplished as a component of antenatal outpatient care. In the case of active disease, a 9-month course of INH and rifampin is supplemented by an initial (first 2 months) course of ethambutol if drug resistance is suspected. Because treatment must be extended over 6 months to 1 year, compliance may be a problem. Medications, often used in combination, are shown in Box 25-18. (For the wide spectrum of additional drugs used in resistant tuberculosis types, see the CDC reference [1990] on screening for tuberculosis and tuberculosis infection at the end of this chapter.) Tuberculosis has become a major problem in HIV immunosuppression. With multidrug resistant types of TB, there may be severe and rapidly progressive fatal cases. Health care personnel who have been exposed to these TB types are susceptible to infection. Currently, preventive therapy with INH or a similar drug is recommended for persons in high-risk groups. The drug must be taken consistently; noncompliance can promote increased drug resistance in the organism.

Nursing responsibilities

Client teaching. Teaching pregnant or postpartal clients about the transmission factors and the dangers of tuberculosis to both themselves and their families will advance compliance with interventions. Identification of barriers to treatment is the first step in the teaching process. Nurses should clarify misconceptions held by clients about tuberculosis, since a stigma is still attached to the disease and myths related to tuberculosis still abound.

Collaborative referral. Nurses caring for antepartal and postpartal women identified as having tuberculosis

Table 25-3	**Isolation Precautions: Tuberculosis**		

Tuberculosis Stage	Maternal or Infant Isolation	Infant Interaction	Breast-feeding
Positive reaction to PPD; no evidence of current disease	None	Routine	Permitted
Mother with disease on treatment regimen for more than 2 weeks at delivery	None	Routine	Permitted if medication safe for breast-feeding
Mother with current pulmonary disease suspected to be contagious	Respiratory isolation	None until mother completes 2 weeks' treatment with appropriate medications or has two negative sputum tests Careful hand washing; neonatal and maternal treatment with appropriate medications	Pump and discard milk, reestablish in 2 weeks if medications do not contraindicate Permitted if medications do not contraindicate

PPD, Purified protein derivative.

must recommend that all the client's household members be screened and treated if necessary. Interdisciplinary referral to departments of health for family screening and to social services for help with overcrowded housing conditions and malnutrition issues may be indicated.

Isolation precautions. Because of the risk to self and others, each nurse is responsible for following respiratory isolation procedures when caring for clients at high risk for tuberculosis and those with known tuberculosis cases (Table 25-3).

TEST *Yourself* 25-5 ⎯⎯⎯⎯⎯

a. What are the fetal risks for Jane, who was exposed to rubella at 14 weeks?
b. What are the risks of toxoplasmosis for Ann, who has always had a cat in the house?
c. What are the risks of maternal active pulmonary tuberculosis for the fetus? What are the risks for the newborn?

Varicella-zoster virus: chickenpox

Varicella-zoster virus (VZV) is a member of the herpesvirus family, a group that includes CMV, Epstein-Barr virus, and HSV-1 and HSV-2. VZV is responsible for two infections: varicella (chickenpox) and herpes zoster (shingles).

Varicella-zoster and herpes zoster are two clinical variations of the same virus. Varicella is the form of primary infection known as chickenpox. Herpes zoster is a reactivation of a previous infection. The virus is extremely contagious and is transmitted through direct contact, droplet, or airborne means. Although uncommon in pregnancy, maternal chickenpox may lead to serious maternal illness, preterm labor, and transplacental viral transmission. Pneumonia is the most common complication of varicella among adults, with a significant rate of mortality.

Risk. Pregnant women who are varicella-susceptible may be at higher risk for serious complications than adults in general. Respiratory collapse and death have been noted. A major concern is the transmission of congenital varicella syndrome to the newborn, especially when the mother contracts varicella in the first half of the pregnancy (Peter, 1994). Second- or third-trimester maternal varicella appears to be less often associated with birth defects. Onset of maternal infection in the days just before or 2 days after delivery places the newborn at increased risk of transplacentally acquired neonatal varicella (Aronoff, 1994). A person is infectious 2 days before vesicles appear until the time all vesicles have dried and are crusted over (Figure 25-9). Chickenpox is transmitted by airborne droplet and from discharge from vesicles and mucous membranes (Box 25-19).

Signs. The incubation period is 10 to 21 days, with mild symptoms, such as fever, malaise, and anorexia, preceding the rash. Vesicles begin on the trunk and spread to head and limbs. Lesions, the characteristic teardrop vesicle upon an erythematous base, are always present at various stages of healing. A dangerous complication is pneumonia, which occurs in about 15% of adult cases. Pleuritic chest pains signal a worsening state. A live attenuated varicella vaccine has been

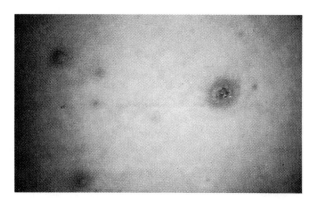

Figure 25-9   Chickenpox lesions usually occur in successive outbreaks, with several stages of maturity present at one time. The lesions start on the scalp and trunk and spread centrifugally to the extremities. (Courtesy Walter Tunnessen, MD, The Johns Hopkins University School of Medicine, Baltimore, Md; From Seidel HM et al: *Mosby's guide to physical examination*, St Louis, 1991, Mosby.)

Box 25-19	**Isolation Precautions: Chickenpox**

MOTHER

Strict isolation (gown, mask, gloves)

Private room with special ventilation, preferably in area remote from immunocompromised clients or susceptible staff members until 7 days after onset of rash or all lesions crusted

No contact until newborn receives VZIG or mother out of isolation

INFANT

None for the first 7 days after exposure

Strict isolation (gown, mask, gloves) for subsequent 2 weeks

If mother contracted varicella less than 5 days before delivery or within 48 hours after delivery, VZIG is promptly administered to newborn

BREAST-FEEDING

Facilitate as soon as all lesions have crusted

Early milk is pumped and possibly discarded (information unavailable to evaluate safety of giving milk to infant)

VZIG, Varicella-zoster immunoglobin.

---

developed, but its use in pregnancy is new and results are unknown.

Congenital varicella-zoster syndrome is characterized by skin scarring, hypoplastic limbs, eye abnormalities, microcephaly, neurologic damage, and motor and growth retardation. Neonatal varicella is frequently associated with complications, including pneumonia, that may be fatal in up to 30% of cases. Because of the protective effect of maternal antibodies that cross the placenta, neonatal varicella is less common when maternal infection occurs more than 5 days before delivery. If the mother has natural immunity to varicella (having had chickenpox) or has had the VZIG, she will have antibodies. When maternal antibodies are present, not all infants develop the infection. Because signs of neonatal infection may be delayed for 1 week or 10 days after birth, careful monitoring of the newborn is required. When it is unclear whether the infant has acquired passive antibody protection to varicella or when the infection occurs at the time of labor, the newborn can receive VZIG to afford passive immunity.

Clinical management. Exposure should be reported, and the susceptible pregnant woman without antibodies to varicella should receive VZIG within 96 hours of exposure. This expensive injection is available from the American Red Cross and can prevent or modify the course of the disease. Used only after the woman has been exposed, it is not effective once the disease is established. Pregnant women with known immunity to varicella are considered protected against reinfection (Sulis, 1995).

Management of chickenpox depends partially on the time in pregnancy it occurs. Although acyclovir is the drug of choice for treatment of varicella, the oral form of acyclovir is *not* recommended in the pregnant adolescent or adult without disease complications, since the risks for both mother and fetus are unknown. However, if severe symptoms occur, intravenously administered acyclovir is used. Prevention of preterm labor is important to allow time for maternal antibodies to be transferred to the fetus.

Nursing considerations. Health care workers should be aware of their immune status for varicella. If susceptible, they should avoid contact with infected persons and receive VZIG if exposure occurs. Nonimmune nurses must report exposure and should not work in maternity areas after exposure until it is clear they will not be affected. (See the isolation precautions for chickenpox in Box 25-19.)

Client teaching. Antepartal disease prevention teaching includes checking immunity before pregnancy or at an early visit. Instruct women that those exposed to preschool or school-age children are at most risk, as well as health care workers. Postpartal women with newborns should be taught the precautions in Box 25-19 and their rationales to lessen any potential feelings of emotional isolation. Vaccines currently being introduced will reduce these risks in the future.

Varicella-zoster virus: *shingles*

Shingles, also called *herpes zoster* or *zoster*, is a reactivation of latent VZV, which establishes a lifelong infection of dorsal root ganglia (Aronoff, 1994). The virus reactivates and causes pain along the dermatome served by the ganglion (see Figure 25-4). Within days of the pain, vesicular lesions appear in the dermatome, lasting for 5 to 10 days and accompanied by localized lymphadenopathy. The pathophysiologic mechanisms that allow development of latent infection and that trigger reactivation are largely unknown.

Risk. Herpes zoster infection is generally considered to pose little risk to the unborn fetus. Because it is a recurrent infection, it is presumed that maternal antibodies provide protection for the fetus and greatly reduce the risk for congenital varicella-zoster syndrome. Though there are a few reports of infant varicella-zoster after the mother has shingles during the pregnancy, it is rare.

Signs. A prodrome of fever, malaise, and headache may occur 1 to 4 days before eruption of typical skin lesions. Vesicular lesions on an erythematous base appear in groups and follow dermatome lines. Lesions may last 2 to 3 weeks, but pain may persist for 2 to 3 weeks after the vesicles resolve. Shingles is especially serious in HIV-immunosuppressed clients; for these women, it may be severe and persist for long periods. Because the fluid from the vesicles contains infectious material, precautions should be followed.

Viral hepatitis: A and C

Hepatitis, or infection of the liver, can have several causes. *Hepatitis A virus* (HAV) has also been called *infectious hepatitis*. Associated with poor hygiene, HAV transmission occurs mainly by fecal-oral contamination, but it is also passed through contaminated food, shellfish, and water. Its incubation period is approximately 15 to 50 days. A person does not have to contain a reservoir of virus to continue to be a *carrier* after symptoms are resolved. Infection may often be asymptomatic. When present, symptoms are mild and nonspecific. HAV infection is not a usual complication of pregnancy, and transmission to the fetus has not been reported. An inactivated vaccine for HAV has recently been developed. It has been found to be free of side effects in field trials and is presumed to be safe for use in pregnancy (ACOG, 1992).

Hepatitis C virus (HCV), formerly called non-A, non-B hepatitis, is a blood-borne infection (like HBV), often transferred through needle sharing and sexual contact. Unfortunately, HCV is associated with perinatal transmission, and there is no immunoprophylaxis currently available. *Hepatitis D* is uncommon in this country, and fortunately, immunization against HBV also provides protection against vertical transmission of HDV.

Hepatitis B virus

Highly pathogenic as well as infectious, HBV is the most common cause of hepatitis worldwide. HBV is highly contagious when transmitted by direct contact with the blood or bodily fluids of infected persons. The rationale for preventing transmission, screening pregnant women, and vaccinating susceptible newborns is to avoid the chronic infection state of HBV, which causes increased morbidity and mortality from chronic liver disease (hepatitis and cirrhosis), as well as primary hepatocellular carcinoma. The earlier in life one is infected, the higher the risk of death from liver disease later on in life.

The blood of an infected person or a carrier contains up to 1 million viral particles per ml, a much higher viral density than HIV-infected blood. Despite the availability of the vaccine for more than 6 years, there are 300,000 new cases of HBV annually, and it is estimated that there are more than 1 million chronic carriers. In pregnancies, acute infection of HBV occurs in 1 to 2 out of every 1000 cases, whereas chronic infection occurs in 5 to 15 out of every 1000 cases (ACOG, 1992). HBV must also be thought of as an STD (transmitted by blood and body fluids) because of its increased associated risk with IV drug abuse (20%) and multiple heterosexual or homosexual partners (Peter, 1994). In addition, immigrants from endemic parts of the world have higher infection rates (70% to 90%) and higher carrier rates. Indochina (14%), the Pacific Islands and Alaska (10%), Haiti, certain Caribbean areas, South America, and certain areas of Africa have high rates (CDC, 1990).

Risk. In the United States, pregnancy in previously healthy, well-nourished women does not appear to be adversely affected by hepatitis, nor is the course of the disease altered by pregnancy. However, in certain developing nations, pregnant women appear to be more susceptible to hepatitis and may have significant maternal complications, including severe disease or death, as well as perinatal morbidity or mortality. Women can be exposed to HBV by substance abuse involving needle exchange, sexual contact with an infected partner, tattooing, working in a setting caring for chronically infected patients, or household contact with an HBV carrier.

Hepatitis is so infectious that the rate of health care worker infection after needle stick or contamination has been 7% to 30%, in contrast with the HIV infection rate of 0.3%. Mandatory vaccination is now required and is available, free of charge, in three injections: initial injection, injection 30 days later, and injection 6 months later. When there is universal vaccination of health care workers and all children, transmission rates should drop dramatically.

Vertical transmission. Perinatal infection continues to occur with regularity despite the availability of the HBV vaccine for women of childbearing age. The onset of acute HBV infection during pregnancy may be associated with increases in spontaneous abortion during the first trimester and premature labor in later months. The primary concern during pregnancy in the presence of HBV infection or in the carrier state is of vertical transmission to the newborn at the time of birth. Even if the pathogen has not passed through the placenta during fetal life (this occurs at a rate of 5% to 10%), the infant has a 70% to 90% chance of becoming infected at the time of birth because of the high viral load in maternal blood and secretions. Neonates may also become infected through breast milk or maternal contact after birth. Newborns infected with HBV at birth are less able to clear the virus, and they more frequently become chronic carriers of HBV. Being a chronic carrier is now linked with a much higher risk of *future liver cancer* and *cirrhosis;* therefore immunization of all children is now being implemented in the United States (ACOG, 1992).

Signs. Hepatitis may range in severity from a mild flu-like episode to a fulminating, lethal infection. Low-grade signs are malaise, fever, headache, enlarged liver, dark urine, and light stools, and jaundice of varying degrees. In addition, severe hepatitis manifests markedly altered liver enzyme levels, anorexia, and epigastric pain, and it can progress to liver coma and death. Carriers show no signs.

Infants and young children commonly have asymptomatic infection without jaundice. Infants with symptoms show fever, poor feeding, malaise, emesis, and abdominal discomfort. Symptoms may be severe enough to include involvement of skin joints. Elevation of liver enzymes, particularly ALT, is often the first clinical evidence of HBV, occurring just before the onset of clinical symptoms. Skin lesions may include urticaria, purpura, macular or maculopapular rashes, and jaundice (Snyder and Pickering, 1996).

Clinical management: Hepatitis A virus. Once active HAV disease has begun, supportive care with nutrition, analgesics tolerated by the liver, and fluids is important. Infection may be rendered less acute by immune globulin.

Clinical infection with HAV may be prevented by administration of the newly developed safe formalin-killed vaccine for HAV. Vaccination of the general population is not necessary because of the mildness of the disease and the fact that it confers lifelong immunity. Pooled immune globulin given within 2 weeks of exposure can be used for passive immunity as an alternative to the vaccine and is effective in modifying clinical manifestations of the disease (Snyder and Pickering, 1996). Pregnant women who are exposed to HAV in the following settings should receive either passive immunization or the vaccine:

1. Household contact with infected person
2. Children in diapers who attend day care settings with HAV outbreaks
3. Employee with close contact to infected person (e.g., health care or day care worker)
4. Travel to or residence in developing countries with poor sanitation

Clinical management: hepatitis B virus. At present, no specific treatment exists for HBV. The clinical management is similar to that for HAV. Hepatitis B immunoglobulin (HBIG) is used to promote immunoprophylaxis in both preexposure and postexposure situations, and it provides short-term immunity. Use of HBIG during pregnancy has shown no untoward effects upon the devel-

oping fetus, and since severe HBV infection in the mother and chronic infection in the infant may be avoided, it is recommended. Lactation is not a contraindication. In the United States, all pregnant women receiving prenatal care are screened early and treated with HBIG if positive. Women who enter the labor area without prenatal care should be tested and should receive immunoglobulin before the test results are returned. The same problem that exists with other types of screening exists with hepatitis antibody screening—testing that occurs within the period when antibodies are not present. Only 2 to 4 weeks after an acute infection may antihepatitis antibodies be found.

In addition, as was mentioned in the information on HIV care, the newborn must be guarded against inoculation with large amounts of virus by implementing "newborn universal precautions," which include cleansing infant skin of maternal blood and secretions as soon as is possible by gloved attendant's hands and avoiding puncture of newborn skin until the skin surface is clean. (Ross and Dickason, 1992). The blood of these infants should always be handled with universal precautions, since approximately 3% are congenitally infected.

Infants born to mothers who are positive for hepatitis B surface antigen (HB$_s$Ag) are at highest risk for HBV infection and must receive HBIG immediately. Vaccination of infants born to HB$_s$Ag *positive* mothers is also recommended, and infants need the initial dose of HBV vaccine followed by administration of HBIG within 12 hours of birth, concurrently, each at a different site. *Active vaccination with HBV vaccine,* given at birth and at 1 and 6 months, provides additional protection against **horizontal transmission** from mother to infant during the postpartum period and childhood. Universal vaccination of all infants born to HB$_s$Ag negative mothers is recommended to provide long-term immunity.

Breast-feeding by HB$_s$Ag positive women does not significantly increase the danger of transmission to the infant (Peter, 1994). However, temporary discontinuation of breast-feeding is recommended, even for immunized newborns, if nipple cracking or bleeding develops.

Nursing responsibilities

Client teaching. Educating childbearing women concerning primary prevention of hepatitis of all forms is essential. Perinatal transmission of HBV may be largely prevented by maternal prenatal screening, the importance of which is explained by the nurse. Outlining the rationale for immunization of the infant in the hospital and the importance of follow-up care to complete infant immunization will help the mother produce a favorable health outcome for her infant. Follow-through with previously unregistered clients is important so that immunoglobulin and vaccination are not forgotten.

Teaching the mother body fluid precautions is an effective way to reduce horizontal transmission. Hand washing effectively reduces the transfer of organisms. The nurse

Box 25-20 Isolation Precautions: Hepatitis

MOTHER

Universal precautions

Blood and enteric precautions for hepatitis B and hepatitis C; enteric for hepatitis A

Careful hand washing

Avoid newborn contact with blood, blood products, or lochia

Gown and gloves when handling infant

INFANT

Universal precautions

Blood and enteric precautions

Isolation with mother

Passive and active immunization for hepatitis B required

BREAST-FEEDING

Hepatitis A

Permitted

Emphasize good hand washing

Hepatitis B

Passive and active immunization for the neonate is required before initiating breast-feeding

Hepatitis C

Permitted (no information available on risk of transmission to newborn)

must be a model for the client and her family by scrupulously adhering to hand washing protocol (Box 25-20).

Collaborative referral. Refer susceptible family members, household contacts, or health care workers to their health care providers for vaccination as is appropriate. In addition, each nurse is responsible for being vaccinated against HBV, with self-referral to the Employee Health Service, as well as encouraging other health care providers to become vaccinated.

Isolation precautions. Because maternity care is a high-risk area, the nurse must follow universal precautions for *each person* to whom she gives care, not just the women who have already been diagnosed with a blood-borne infection (see Box 25-20).

TEST Yourself 25-6

a. Why is hepatitis B so much more infectious than other viral diseases?

b. What are the risks for the nurse using only universal precautions with those women or infants who have definite diagnoses of blood-borne infections?

Intrapartum Infections

The woman in labor is at risk for infections that may be linked to events associated with labor and delivery or ones that are the result of stresses on the maternal defense mechanisms caused by pregnancy. Urinary tract infections are discussed in detail in Chapter 24. Clinically evident antepartum or intrapartum intrauterine infection may be called *amnionitis, chorioamnionitis, intramniotic infection,* or *amniotic fluid infection.* The uterine cavity is usually sterile before labor and rupture of membranes, and the cervical mucous plug and chorioamniotic membrane usually serve as efficient barriers to infection. In a healthy woman, even after rupture of membranes, intrauterine infection is infrequent because of the combined efforts of polymorphonuclear leukocytes, nonspecific biochemical host defense mechanisms, immunoglobulins, and other, as yet unknown, antibacterial properties of the amniotic fluid. In HIV-infected women whose membranes ruptured more than four hours before delivery, risk for vertical transmission of HIV is almost doubled, suggesting that an intact chorioamniotic membrane acts as an additional barrier to infection (Landesman et al, 1996).

Chorioamnionitis is a polymicrobial infection and can occur as a result of infective activity of the bacterial organisms, both aerobic and anaerobic, normally found in the vagina and cervix. Other microorganisms, including especially *group B streptococcus* (see information on streptococcal infections on following pages), *Listeria monocytogenes, Neisseria gonorrhoeae,* and *Escherichia coli* may also be involved. Although bacteria may gain entrance to the uterus by ascent from the vagina and cervix before labor and rupture of membranes, the risk of bacterial ascent greatly increases after rupture of membranes and labor. Infection may also occur from maternal infection spread across the placenta or by means of amniocentesis. Of special interest to the nurse is the fact that *obstetric practices may induce chorioamnionitis by ascending infection* (see Figure 25-1). These practices include AROM to hasten delivery, cervical circlage, frequent cervical examinations, and intrauterine fetal and contraction monitoring.

Risk. Uterine infection risk increases 10 to 20 times when there are ruptured membranes (especially related to AROM). As the infection process progresses, the uterine musculature is unable to contract normally, and women may experience a long labor and a subsequent increase in cesarean delivery. Preterm labor (at less than 37 weeks) is associated with increased risk of chorioamnionitis (see Chapter 21).

Signs. Chorioamnionitis often begins with fetal tachycardia, occurring *before* maternal tachycardia and fever, accompanied by irritability of the uterus. Labor nurses will look for signs of increasingly dysfunctional labor as the infection causes the uterus to lose its ability to contract efficiently. Late signs of uterine tenderness or foul odor of amniotic fluid may not be apparent until the infectious process is well established.

Newborn implications. Preterm infants of mothers who had chorioamnionitis suffer increased incidence of pneumonia, meningitis, septicemia, respiratory distress syndrome (RDS), and perinatal death as compared to infants of similar gestational ages without exposure to chorioamnionitis.

Clinical management. Maternal and fetal complications from chorioamnionitis may be minimized if it is identified in those women at risk and early antibiotic treatment is initiated. If the membranes are intact, samples of amniotic fluid may be obtained by amniocentesis to be cultured and examined microscopically for bacteria and leukocytes. Bacteria may gain entrance to the uterus during labor, *even with intact membranes*, and the recovery of bacteria is not always associated with clinical evidence of infection. Though it is normal for the peripheral white blood cell count to increase during labor, counts greater than 18,000/mm³ are frequently viewed as suggestive of chorioamnionitis.

Administration of combined broad-spectrum antibiotics to cover most of the pathogenic bacteria has been shown to reduce the incidence of neonatal sepsis. Delivery is usually expedited, by cesarean delivery if necessary, to avoid prolonged intrauterine exposure to infection and significant neonatal morbidity or mortality. However, some authors believe when a cesarean delivery is performed, maternal postpartum infectious complications (including septic shock), prolonged antibiotic requirements with possible resistant organisms, and prolonged hospitalizations are more likely (ACOG, 1992). In addition, cesarean sections performed on women with HIV infection may be associated with an increased risk of infectious complications because of their severely compromised immune system (Semprini et al, 1995).

Nursing responsibilities. The nurse is frequently the one who identifies the first evidence of chorioamnionitis. When signs occur, the nurse should eliminate other sources for the altered vital signs. For example, the nurse should ensure adequate hydration, relieve maternal anxiety, and provide pain relief and proper positioning to ensure adequate fetal oxygenation. When evidence of chorioamnionitis is detected, the care provider managing the woman's labor should be notified of the altered maternal and fetal response, the nursing actions that were taken, and the response. After the diagnosis of chorioamnionitis has been made, promptly initiate any antimicrobial therapy ordered, maintain close monitoring of maternal and fetal status for the remainder of labor, and ensure that the mother and family have received full explanations about the nature of the infection, likely causes, risks for herself and her infant, and treatments and expected outcomes. The labor nurses must be alert for the

signs of infection: fetal tachycardia, changed beat-to-beat variability, and increasing maternal fever (see Clinical Decision 25-1). It is important that the infant's pediatrician be notified that maternal chorioamnionitis was present during labor and birth.

Box **25-1**

CLINICAL DECISION

The mother has been in labor for 16 hours with ruptured membranes. She has reached 8 cm dilation and a +1 station. Her temperature began to rise 1 hour ago and is now 100.2° F. You see the reading in (A) on the accompanying strip chart. Describe it as you would on a nursing note. Now look at (B), the reading taken 30 minutes later when her temperature was 101° F. What interventions should now be taking place?

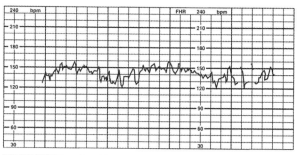

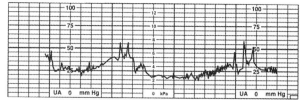

A

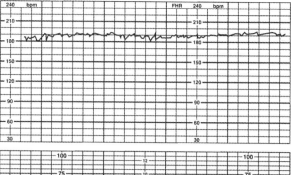

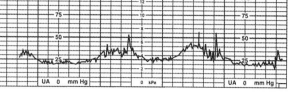

B

Streptococcal Infections

Streptococcal infection is the leading cause of life-threatening infections. It is associated with a spectrum of increased morbidity and mortality related to maternal endometritis, postcesarean endometritis, bacteremia, chorioamnionitis, neonatal sepsis, pneumonia, meningitis, PROM, preterm birth, and neonatal death.

Streptococcal microorganisms are gram-positive cocci or spherical bacteria that appear as chains on microscopic examination. Streptococci are categorized by their ability to break down or hemolyze red blood cells. Of the different streptococci, only groups A, B, and D are associated with significant human illness. Groups A and B are nearly always β-hemolytic, and group D streptococcus varies in its ability to hemolyze blood cells.

Group A β-hemolytic streptococcus most commonly causes streptococcal sore throat, scarlet fever, skin infection, impetigo, erysipelas, and puerperal sepsis. Its sequelae are rheumatic fever and glomerulonephritis. Although it is an infrequent cause of postpartum infection today, the classic works of Holmes and Semmelweis, which describe the epidemic of childbed fever, demonstrate the seriousness of group A streptococcal infection among pregnant women. *Group D streptococcus* causes maternal urinary tract infections and may be associated with neonatal sepsis and maternal postpartum endometritis.

Group B Streptococcal Infection

Over the past 30 years *group B streptococcus* (GBS) has emerged as the leading cause of newborn sepsis and meningitis and also is associated with significant maternal and fetal infection. GBS can be the cause of chorioamnionitis, endomyometritis, urinary tract infection, pyelonephritis, asymptomatic bacteriuria, postpartum and postcesarean endometritis, bacteremia, and puerperal sepsis.

GBS may be isolated from the lower genital tract of 15% to 40% of pregnant women. Most of these women are symptom-free. The bacteria are thought to spread from the intestinal tract reservoir to the perineum, vagina, and cervix.

Risk. There is a direct association between prolonged rupture of membranes (more than 12 hours) and transmission of infection. Prolonged labor, intrapartum maternal infection, postpartum infection, and preterm delivery are associated with increased likelihood of *early onset* of the disease. GBS initiates local inflammation of the intact fetal membranes, resulting in weakness and rupture of these amniotic membranes, causing premature labor (Gotoff, 1996). If the maternal genitourinary tract is heavily colonized there is greater risk for ascending infection through ruptured membranes. Among newborns, GBS is one of two common causes of septicemia and meningitis, often leading to severe neurologic impairment and death. From 40% to 72% of newborns exposed to GBS-infected mothers will become colonized (Greenspoon, Wilcox, and

Kirschbaum, 1991). Most of these infants remain symptom-free, with clinical infection developing in somewhat less than 1 in 200 exposed infants.

With GBS, *early-onset* newborn infection occurs rapidly, within the first 5 days of life. Early-onset disease occurs more frequently among preterm or low birth weight infants. Early-onset GBS disease is associated with rapid deterioration of the newborn, often taking the form of pneumonia with bacteremia, complicated by pulmonary hypertension. Early-onset GBS disease is associated with immature host defense immune systems among low birthweight infants, and it can lead to death or severe neurologic damage in up to 55% of infants, even when appropriate antibiotics are given.

Late-onset GBS infection occurs after the first week of life, and it is thought to be related not to obstetric factors but rather with horizontal transmission of the organism. Community acquisition from mother, siblings, or other contacts may be sources of late-onset infection, which can occur as late as 7 months after birth. Signs are irritability, poor appetite, fever, conjunctivitis, and ear infections progressing to potentially severe neurologic involvement.

Clinical management. It is currently recommended that every pregnant woman be screened at 26 to 32 weeks for group B β-hemolytic streptococcus infection. Antepartum cultures that identify her as a carrier can partially predict colonization at birth. Diagnosis is made difficult by the fact the infection is unpredictable and may be present at one visit but not at the next (Greenspoon, Wilcox, and Kirschbaum, 1991).

Whenever there is a risk of preterm labor, PROM of more than 12 hours, or intrapartum fever, GBS must be considered. Because of the devastating effects on the newborn, most units now do a "rapid" test (which takes 4 to 5 hours, but may sometimes take only 1 hour) to determine if infection is present in high-risk clients at the start of labor. This test must also be performed whenever fever develops, and antibiotics must be started before results are returned.

Ampicillin or *penicillin G* is used for both maternal and infant treatment, with the addition of an aminoglycoside if needed. *Erythromycin* or *clindamycin* may be used for mothers who have penicillin or ampicillin allergies. Higher-than-usual doses must be used because of the virulence of the organism. If chorioamnionitis is present, broader-spectrum antibiotics will be needed to cover both GBS and any other penicillin-resistant bacteria that may be present in the host. Newborns do not develop penicillin or ampicillin allergies, so it is safe to treat them with these parenteral antibiotics. With postpartal infections, such as endomyometritis, the antibiotic treatment should be continued until the client is free of fever and symptoms for at least 24 hours (ACOG, 1992).

Nursing responsibilities

Client teaching. Clients must be adequately counseled about their risk of infection and must be taught to recognize signs and symptoms and to seek prompt medical attention if they occur. Health care providers must be taught to thoroughly evaluate symptoms and to provide adequate therapy and follow-up care. Reassuring the pregnant woman and her family about effective treatment for GBS, should she be diagnosed, will reduce anxiety and increase nurse-patient dialogue.

Collaborative referral. All women seen in admission screening, especially those women experiencing preterm labor or PROM who have no prenatal GBS tests, should be referred to the physician for testing, either for rapid antigen testing, ELISA (which can sometimes be obtained in less than 1 hour), or by culture (ACOG, 1992). Collaboration with the Infection Control Nurse in a hospital setting is useful in planning care.

Isolation precautions. These are necessary only in rare instances of hospital nursery outbreaks; otherwise, no special precautions are necessary for newborn or mother (Peter, 1994). Routine hand washing by all personnel caring for women and their newborns is always necessary to prevent nosocomial disease spread.

Postpartum Infections

Infection during the postpartum period may occur in the genital tract (endometritis or vaginitis), urinary tract, breast, or episiotomy or wound, or it may occur as complication of anesthesia (pneumonia). The rate of infection following vaginal deliveries is 3%, whereas rates following cesarean section are 12% to 25%.

Endometritis

The mucous membrane lining the uterus—the endometrium—becomes inflamed as the result of an acute infection immediately after delivery. Intrauterine infection is the most common infection in the postpartum period. Uterine infection frequently involves the endometrium first and may spread to the myometrium, parametrium, fallopian tubes, ovaries, pelvic peritoneum, and the blood. Thus intrauterine infection may lead to pelvic abscess, septic pelvic thrombophlebitis, or septicemia (sepsis). Theoretically, immunocompromised persons, such as those with HIV infection or those who have undergone invasive monitoring, are at increased risk for developing endometritis.

Postpartum endometritis is most commonly associated with a mixture of bacterial species (polymicrobial) that may arise from the gatrointestinal tract (group D streptococcus, *E. coli*, or *Klebsiella*) or from the lower genital tract (aerobic and anaerobic bacteria, GBS, chlamydia, and gonorrhea).

Maternal sepsis—septic shock. This is defined as a systemic response to infection causing peripheral circulatory collapse and resultant poor tissue perfusion. Although maternal death because of pregnancy is infrequent in the United States, sepsis remains a leading cause of maternal mortality (Thomason, 1993). Maternal sepsis may occur as a disease progresses to an overwhelming infection, such as that caused by gram-negative or anaerobic infection or may occur after abortions, vaginal births, or cesarean births. Endometritis after cesarean section delivery is the most common cause of septic shock. Early signs of shock are tachypnea and hypotension, and if supportive measures are not successful, the syndrome progresses to respiratory distress, renal insufficiency, DIC, and death. The nurse monitors early signs of life-threatening septic chock and intervenes by obtaining immediate medical attention for the client (see signs of endometritis).

Risk. Predicting precisely which patients will develop endometritis is difficult. Four major factors are repeatedly associated with endometritis:

- *Length of labor*—Those clients who have a long labor generally have a higher risk than those clients with a normal span of labor.
- *Rupture of membranes*—The longer the time since rupture of membranes, the greater is the risk for finding microorganisms in the amniotic cavity. Ordinarily, the amniotic fluid is sterile, but once the integrity of the membrane is broken, invading organisms may enter the amniotic cavity.
- *Multiple vaginal examinations*—The frequency of vaginal examinations increases the risk of infection. Most protocols list three vaginal examinations as the critical number before the incidence rate for infections rises sharply. There is no difference in infection rates between vaginal and rectal examinations. Although it is important that the nurse advocate for a minimum amount of manual examinations, it is the length of labor that has a higher correlation with infection than does the number of examinations.
- *Cesarean section—Cesarean section is the primary risk factor for uterine infection* (Buckley, 1993). The highest infection rate is described after emergency or nonelective cesarean sections. Elective cesarean sections (whether primary or repeat) with no labor and intact membranes have lower infection rates than do emergency cesarean sections. Determining the length of labor before cesarean section is the single most important factor for predicting the development of infection after cesarean section.

Other factors associated with endometritis include the following:
- Low economic status
- Lack of prenatal care
- Adolescence

These factors do not cause postpartum infection. Rather, these factors are markers for those women at risk. Susceptibility to infection among these women may involve overall nutritional status, hygienic factors, differences in host defense mechanisms and cervical and vaginal microorganisms, iatrogenic factors, and other unknown factors. Immunosuppression, clients on steroids, and serious maternal disease (e.g., diabetes) are also factors which facilitate infection rates.

Signs. Symptoms heralding endometritis include delayed uterine involution, abdominal pain, tachycardia, temperature elevations (often spiking) between 101.4° F and 104° F, and chills. Early fevers are associated with early onset of ruptured membranes and infection before labor. Fever begins by 24 to 48 hours if infection began at the time of birth. The white blood cell count may be increased beyond the usual physiologic elevation. Lochia may be scant, purulent, and foul-smelling.

Clinical management. All other sources of infection, including urinary tract infection, wound infection, episiotomy infection, mastitis, and IV site phlebitis, should be evaluated in postpartum women as sources of infection. Antibiotic therapy with broad-spectrum agents is initiated, and the identification of the microorganism is accomplished by sending specimens of urine, wound secretions, or lochia for culture. Prompt intervention usually results in effective treatment of the infection. Lack of clinical improvement within 48 hours requires reevaluation for other sources of infection and addition of antibiotics to cover presumed *anaerobic* infection. Failure to respond clinically to aggressive intravenously administered antibiotics may be caused by pelvic abscess, septic pelvic thrombophlebitis, another site of infection, or a noninfectious source of fever, including drug reaction (drug fever) (Buckley, 1993).

Nursing responsibilities. Nursing care for women with postpartum endometritis includes bed rest in Fowler's position to facilitate drainage and lessen congestion, maintaining adequate hydration (3000 to 4000 ml/day), and providing analgesia; administration of the appropriate antibiotic regimen is effective for 95% of women. Monitoring physical response to therapy and psychologic adaptation to complications are ongoing functions of the nurse in the postpartum period. As previously mentioned, the alert nurse will take note of any signs of impending septic shock and take immediate action. *Breast-feeding* is usually continued; maternal medications will be transmitted through breast milk to the nursing infant. Observation of the infant for evidence of medication intolerance is required. If breast-feeding is interrupted during therapy, breasts should be emptied by other means to maintain the milk supply (see Chapter 17).

Client teaching. Full explanations of the cause of infection and the expected outcomes should be given. Maternal contact with and care for the infant are encouraged as the woman's condition allows. Normal postpartum and newborn teaching should be included in the client's care as her condition improves.

Septic pelvic thrombophlebitis

Women with postcesarean endometritis are at increased risk for septic pelvic thrombophlebitis. Septic pelvic thrombophlebitis is the formation of clots within the pelvic veins because of infection. Although rare, pelvic vein thrombophlebitis occurs more frequently after obstetric procedures than after other types of pelvic surgery or with pelvic inflammatory disease. Bacterial species implicated in this disease are common vaginal pathogens, including aerobic and anaerobic streptococci, staphylococci, *Bacteroides* species, and yeast.

Risk. Pregnancy causes an increase in certain clotting factors, and when it is accompanied by decreased venous return from the legs and pelvis from the pressure of the enlarging uterus, these together predispose the development of thrombophlebitis (see Chapter 22). Contributing risk factors include the relaxation of the blood vessel smooth muscle because of progesterone, the presenting part of the infant causing trauma to the pelvic blood vessels during the birth, and intraoperative trauma. Most maternal deaths caused by thromboembolism occur postpartum. Postcesarean section clients who manifest signs of infection should especially be considered to be at risk for septic pelvic vein thrombophlebitis. The overall incidence is low in postpartum women—less than 1%—but there is an increase of up to 2% after cesarean section (Buckley, 1993). Women with septic pelvic thrombophlebitis are at risk for further complications, which include septic embolus, lung abscess, empyema, and acute endocarditis.

Signs. Pelvic vein thrombophlebitis should be suspected in any client who is receiving appropriate broad-spectrum antibiotic treatment for postpartum intrauterine infection and whose symptoms *are not resolving.* Septic pelvic thrombophlebitis most often occurs within 1 day to 6 weeks after delivery. The medical diagnosis is based largely on the client's clinical history and physical examination. The woman continues to have temperature elevations and worsening, constant, localized abdominal pain even on an appropriate antibiotic regimen. She may appear acutely ill with fever, shaking chills, tachycardia, nausea, vomiting, and tachypnea, or she may have improved clinical signs of infection with the exception of temperature elevations, which continue to climb as high as 103° to 104° F (Humphrey, 1995).

Clinical management. Medical treatment includes use of broad-spectrum antibiotics and anticoagulation therapy with intravenously administered heparin and bed rest. Temperature is usually normal within 24 to 48 hours of therapeutic heparin. Heparin may be continued for 2 to 6 weeks afterward (see Chapter 22 and Drug Profile 22-3). Surgery may be required if the client remains critically ill despite adequate antimicrobial and anticoagulation therapies (Humphrey, 1995).

Nursing responsibilities. Nursing care for women with septic pelvic thrombophlebitis includes the following interventions:

- Provide antibiotic and anticoagulation therapy as ordered. Observe for any signs and symptoms of medication side effects, including heparin overdose such as uterine bleeding or bleeding from IV site.
- Assess breath sounds every 4 hours to monitor for signs of pulmonary embolism or infection.
- Monitor for chest pain that may also be related to pulmonary emboli.
- Facilitate the patient with turning, coughing, and deep breathing every 4 hours.
- Check vital signs every 4 hours to monitor response to therapy. Do not take rectal temperatures as this might prompt rectal or hemorrhoidal bleeding.
- Provide analgesic medications as needed.
- Provide contexts for maternal-infant bonding.

Client teaching. Determine the patient's level of understanding of the medications she is taking, including dose, time of administration, therapeutic purpose, and side effects. Instruct the patient regarding anticoagulant precautions. Clarify the fact that she must avoid over-the-counter medications that might augment the anticoagulent effects of her prescribed drugs, such as aspirin or nonsteroidal anti-inflammatory drugs. Teach the client the signs of anticoagulant side effects, and instruct her to call the doctor immediately should any of the following signs occur: bleeding gums, hematuria, heavy menstrual flow, easy bruising, epistaxis, abdominal pain, vomiting, fever, chest pain, or shortness of breath.

Collaborative referral. Refer patient to home care to assess the mother's compliance with medications and to evaluate both the mother's ability to carry out newborn care and her psychosocial adjustment to the maternal role after being ill.

Breast-feeding is not contraindicated in either heparin or warfarin anticoagulation therapy. Because warfarin is tightly bound to plasma proteins, it does not cross the lipid barrier into milk, and heparin is a large molecule that also does not cross the lipid barrier to enter breast milk.

Key points

- Defense systems are altered by pregnancy, making both mother and newborn more vulnerable to infection.
- Certain infections during pregnancy pose a special risk of fetal malformation, congenital infection, IUGR, or death.
- Risk of transmission of HIV from mother to infant increases when the fetal membranes rupture more than 4 hours before delivery.
- Vertical transmission during fetal life depends on the size of the microorganism, the actual number (count), and the placental integrity.
- Vertical transmission during the birth process has been documented, especially for human HIV, HBV, HSV, and chlamydial and gonorrheal infection.
- Universal precautions are key to reducing the risk of horizontal transmission during care.

- Nurses are responsible for consistent use of universal precautions and for insisting that other health care workers also do so.
- Culturally sensitive education is essential to reduce the risk of STDs.
- Handwashing is the best line of defense in protecting mother, infant, and the nurse from nosocomial infection.
- Perinatal infections may be prevented in some instances by immunization before pregnancy.
- In the United States, all health care workers and all children should be vaccinated against HBV infection.
- Endometritis poses a risk to mother and infant because of the rapid rate of ascending infection in the birth canal. Especially dangerous are CMV and β-streptococcal infections.

Study Questions

25-1. Select the terms that apply to the following statements:
   a. The humoral response includes production of specific _____ to microorganisms.
   b. The cell-mediated immune response stimulates multiplication of _____ and lymphocytes.
   c. A toxin may be a _____ antigen or an _____ antigen called a toxoid.
   d. _____ is perinatal infection that establishes a lifelong infection of the sensory nerve ganglia.
   e. HBV infection can be prevented in the newborn by _____.
   f. Infection of the newborn at the time of birth by a staff member is an example of _____.

25-2. An infant was born with congenital rubella after the mother acquired the infection at week 30 of pregnancy. This route of infection describes:
   a. Nosocomial infection.
   b. Autoinfection.
   c. Vertical transmission.
   d. Placental insufficiency.

25-3. Untreated, gonorrhea may be linked to neonatal gonococcal ophthalmia and maternal:
   a. Bladder infections.
   b. Pruritic rashes.
   c. Painless chancres.
   d. Postpartum endometritis.

25-4. If chlamydial infection is diagnosed at 28 weeks, the most important reason that Rhonda should be treated now is to prevent:
   a. PROM.
   b. Sexual transmission to her boyfriend.
   c. Infant blindness.
   d. Maternal sepsis.

25-5. Rose, 23, has had multiple sexual partners, and at 14 weeks' gestation, she has a positive FTA-ABS test result. She will be treated with penicillin. Therefore you must include instructions to report which of the following signs of Jarisch-Herxheimer reaction:
   a. Hypotension and cyanosis.
   b. Increase in fetal movements.
   c. Onset of uterine contractions and high fever.
   d. Maternal bradycardia and anxiety.

25-6. You will teach Rose that her condition will be followed with the VDRL titer instead of the FTS-ABS test at 3, 6, 9, and 12 months because the FTA-ABS test:
   a. Results are altered by penicillin.
   b. Reaction remains positive even after treatment.
   c. Is expensive.
   d. May alter the results of other diseases.

25-7. Why is isolation of the infant from the mother not practiced for most perinatally acquired infections?
   a. The infant's immunologic response is immature.
   b. Maternal antibodies protect the infant.
   c. The infant already has received pathogens in most cases.
   d. Breast-feeding conveys immunities.

25-8. Which sign or symptom would not occur if a woman in labor has chorioamnionitis?
   a. Fetal tachycardia
   b. Prolonged, more difficult labor
   c. Decrease in blood pressure
   d. Increase in white blood cell count

Answer Key

25-1: *a,* Antibodies; *b,* macrophages; *c,* pathogenic; altered; *d,* herpesvirus; *e,* vaccination; *f,* horizontal transmission. 25-2: c. 25-3: d. 25-4: a. 25-5: c. 25-6: b. 25-7: c. 25-8: c.

References

*American College of Obstetricians and Gynecologists: *Antimicrobial therapy for obstetric patients,* ACOG Technical Bulletin 117, June 1988.

*American College of Obstetricians and Gynecologists: *Perinatal herpes simplex virus infections,* ACOG Technical Bulletin 122, November 1988.

American College of Obstetricians and Gynecologists: *Antimicrobial therapy for gynecologic infections,* ACOG Technical Bulletin 153, March 1991.

American College of Obstetricians and Gynecologists: *Immunization during pregnancy,* ACOG Technical Bulletin 160, October 1991.

American College of Obstetricians and Gynecologists: *Group B streptococcal infections in pregnancy,* ACOG Technical Bulletin 170, July 1992.

American College of Obstetricians and Gynecologists: *Rubella and pregnancy,* ACOG Technical Bulletin 171, August 1992.

American College of Obstetricians and Gynecologists: *Hepatitis in pregnancy,* ACOG Technical Bulletin 174, November 1992.

American College of Obstetricians and Gynecologists: *Perinatal viral and parasitic infections,* ACOG Technical Bulletin 177, February 1993.

American College of Obstetricians and Gynecologists: *Gonorrhea and chlamydial infections,* ACOG Technical Bulletin 190, March 1994.

American College of Obstetricians and Gynecologists: *Genital human papilloma virus infections,* ACOG Technical Bulletin 193, June 1994.

American College of Obstetricians and Gynecologists: *Septic shock,* ACOG Technical Bulletin 204, April 1995.

*American Thoracic Society: Treatment of tuberculosis and tuberculosis infection in adults and children, *Am Rev Respir Dis* 143:355, 1986.

Aronoff S et al: Infectious diseases. In Rudolph A, Kamei R, eds: *Fundamentals of pediatrics,* Stanford, Conn, 1994, Appleton & Lange.

Baker DA: Management of the female HIV-infected patient, *AIDS Res Hum Retroviruses* 10:935, 1994.

Baker DA et al: Topical podofilox for the treatment of condylomata acuminata in women, *Obstet Gynecol* 76:656, 1990.

Blackburn ST, Loper DL, eds: *Maternal, fetal, and neonatal physiology: a clinical perspective,* Philadelphia, 1992, WB Saunders.

Buckley K: Deviations of postpartum period. In Buckley K, Kulb N, eds: *High risk maternity manual,* ed 2, Baltimore, 1993, Williams & Wilkins.

Cavenee MR et al: Treatment of gonorrhea in pregnancy, *Obstet Gynecol* 81:33, 1993.

Centers for Disease Control: Screening for tuberculosis and tuberculous infection in high-risk populations, and the use of preventive therapy for tuberculous infection in the United States: recommendations of the Advisory Committee for the Elimination of Tuberculosis, *MMWR* 39(RR-8):1, 1990.

Centers for Disease Control: Immunization Practices Committee: Hepatitis B virus: a comprehensive strategy for eliminating transmission in the US through universal childhood vaccination, *MMWR* 40:1, 1991.

Centers for Disease Control: Update on adult immunization: recommendations of the immunization practices advisory committee, *MMWR* 40:1, 1991.

Centers for Disease Control: 1993 sexually transmitted diseases treatment guidelines, *MMWR* 42:1, 1993.

Centers for Disease Control: Revised guidelines for prophylaxis against *Pneumocystic carinii* pneumonia for children infected with or perinatally exposed to human immunodeficiency virus, *MMWR* 44:1, 1995.

*Connor E et al: The intrapartum management of the HIV-infected mother and her infant, *Clin Perinatol* 16:899, 1989.

Cotton D: AIDS in women. In Sachs B, ed: *Reproductive health care for women and babies,* New York, 1995, Oxford University Press.

Crane MJ: The diagnosis and management of maternal and congenital syphilis, *J Nurse Midwifery* 37(1):4, 1992.

Dempster JS: STDs: a contemporary epidemic, *Am Acad Nurse Pract* 7(3):133, 1995.

Denenberg R: *Gynecological care manual for HIV positive women,* Durant, Okla, 1994, Essential Medical Informations, Inc.

Desenclos JC: Gonococcal infection of the newborn in Florida: 1984-1989, *Sex Transm Dis* 19:105, 1992.

Faro S, Pastorek J: Perinatal infections. In Knuppel R, Drukker J, eds: *High-risk pregnancy: a team approach,* Philadelphia, 1993, WB Saunders.

Fogel C: Sexually transmitted diseases. In McElmurry B, Parker R, eds: *Annual review of women's health,* vol VII, New York, 1995, Pub 19-2669, National League for Nursing Press.

Freij BJ, Sever JL: Toxoplasmosis, *Pediatr Rev* 12(8):227, 1991.

*Gerberding JL: Risks to health care workers from occupational exposure to hepatitis B virus, human immunodeficiency virus, and cytomegalovirus, *Infect Dis Clin North Am* 3:735, 1989.

Gerchufsky M: Human papilloma virus, *Advance for Nurse Practitioners* 4:21, 1996.

Ginsberg HM: Occupational exposure to bloodborne pathogens: the new OSHA regulations, *Pediatr AIDS HIV Infect: Fetus Adolesc* 2(1):31, 1991.

Gotoff S: Neonatal sepsis and meningitis. In Nelson W, ed: *Textbook of pediatrics,* ed, 2, Philadelphia, 1996, WB Saunders.

Greenspoon JS, Wilcox JG, Kirschbaum TH: Group B streptococcus: the effectiveness of screening and chemoprophylaxis, *Obstet Gynecol Surv* 46:499, 1991.

Gutman LT: Sexually transmitted diseases in children and adolescents with HIV infection. In Pizzo P, Wilfert C, eds: *Pediatric AIDS,* ed 2, Baltimore, 1994, Williams & Wilkins.

*Hellberg D et al: Smoking and cervical neoplasia, *Am J Obstet Gynecol* 158:910, 1988.

Humphrey MD: Postpartum abnormalities. In Humphrey MD, ed: *The obstetrics manual,* New York, 1995, McGraw-Hill.

International Registry of HIV-exposed twins, and others: high risk of HIV-1 infection for first-born twins, *Lancet* 338:1471, 1991.

Kazanjian PH, Eisenstat SA: Human immunodeficiency virus. In Carlson K, Eisenstat S, eds: *Primary care of women,* St Louis, 1995, Mosby.

Kelley KF, Galbraith MA, Vermund SH: Genital human papillomavirus infection in women, *J Obstet Gynecol Neonatal Nurs* 21(6):503, 1992.

Krivine A et al: HIV replication during the first weeks of life, *Lancet* 339:1187, 1992.

Landesman SH et al: Obstetrical factors and the transmission of human immunodeficiency virus type 1 from mother to child, *N Engl J Med* 334:1617, 1996.

Linscott DA: Pregnancy and immunosuppressive drug therapy, *Journal of Perinat Neonat Nurs* Frederick, Maryland, Aspen Publishers, 1996.

Masci J: *Outpatient management of HIV infection,* St Louis, 1996, Mosby.

McCance S, Huether S: *Pathophysiology: the biological basis for disease in adults and children,* St Louis, 1994, Mosby.

Mitchell CD: Toxoplasmosis. In Pizzo P, Wilfert C, eds: *Pediatric AIDS,* ed 2, Baltimore, 1994, Williams & Wilkins.

Mofenson LM, Wolinsky SM: Current insights regarding vertical transmission. In Pizzo P, Wilfert C, eds: *Pediatric AIDS,* ed 2, Baltimore, 1994, Williams & Wilkins.

Morrison JC et al: Universal precautions in an obstetric population to prevent health care provider infection with human immunodeficiency virus, *Pediatr AIDS HIV Infect: Fetus Adolesc* 2(4):161, 1991.

Oxtoby M: Vertically acquired HIV infection in the United States. In Pizzo P, Wilfert C, eds: *Pediatric AIDS,* ed 2 Baltimore, 1994, Williams & Wilkins.

Patsner B: A patient-applied topical solution for genital warts, *Contemp Ob Gyn* 12:27, 1991.

Pearlman MD, McNeeley SG: A review of the microbiology, immunology and clinical implications of *Chlamydia trachomatis* infections, *Obstet Gynecol Surv* 47(7):448, 1992.

Peter G, ed: *Red book report of the committee on infectious diseases,* Elk Grove Village, Ill, 1994.

Rogers MF et al: Advances in diagnosis of HIV infection in infants. In Pizzo P, Wilfert C, eds: *Pediatric AIDS,* ed 2, Baltimore, 1994, Williams & Wilkins.

Ross T, Dickason EJ: Nursing alert: vertical transmission of HIV and HBV, *MCN Am J Matern Child Nurs* 17(4):192, 1992.

Schaffer S et al: *Obstetrical procedures: infection prevention and safe practice,* St Louis, 1996, Mosby.

Schiffman MH: Recent progress in defining the epidemiology of human papillomavirus infection and cervical neoplasia, *J Natl Cancer Inst* 84:394, 1992.

Semprini AE et al: The incidence of complications after cesarean section in 156 HIV-positive women, *AIDS* 9:913, 1995.

*Classic reference.

Serrano C et al: Surgical glove perforation in obstetrics, *Obstet Gynecol* 77(4):525, 1990.

Snyder JD, Pickering LK: Hepatitis A through E. In Nelson W, ed: *Textbook of pediatrics,* Philadelphia, 1996, WB Saunders.

Sperling RS, Stratton P, and Working Group of AIDS Clinical Trials Group, National Institute of Allergy and Infectious Diseases: Treatment options for human immunodeficiency virus-infected women, *Obstet Gynecol* 79(3):443, 1992.

Sulis C: Infectious disease in pregnancy. In Carr P, Freund K, Somani S, eds: *The medical care of women,* Philadelphia, 1995, WB Saunders.

Summers L: Understanding tuberculosis: implications for pregnancy, *J Perinat Neonat Nurs* 6(2):12, 1992.

Thaler MM et al: Vertical transmission of hepatitis C virus, *Lancet* 338:17, 1991.

Thomason JL: Peripartum infections. In Shaver D et al, eds: *Clinical manual of obstetrics,* ed 2, New York, 1993, McGraw-Hill.

Tillman J: Syphilis: an old disease, a contemporary perinatal problem, *J Obstet Gynecol Neonatal Nurs* 21(3):209, 1991.

Toltzis P: Rationales for treating the human immunodeficiency virus-infected woman during pregnancy, *Clin Perinatol* 20:47, 1993.

Volberding PA: The HIV RNA assay: a valuable new diagnostic tool, *HIV Newsline* 2:27, 1996.

Wong D, Nye K, Hollis P: Microbial flora in doctors' white coats, *BMJ* 303:1602, 1991.

Wood CL: Laryngeal papillomas in infants and children, *J Nurse Midwifery* 36(5):430, 1991.

World Wide Web (Internet) Resources

(1) Video catalog—parenting/family planning/pediatrics.
Includes understanding maternal grief, loss of an infant, death of a dream, infertility and adaptation, miscarriage and stillbirth, and many more choices.
http://www.cmil.unex.berkley.edu/video_catalog/8_health_med_sci/I_parent_fam_plan_ped.html

(2) http://www.slackinc.com/intromed.html
This internet address provides a link to vast internet resources of interest to students and practitioners alike, with more than 20 million users and 20 thousand networks.

 Student Resource Shelf

Gallagher M, Klima C: Patient focus: the challenge of maternal-infant transmission of HIV, *JANAC* 7(1):47, 1996.
A nursing update on new guidelines of vertical transmission including nurse's responsibilities for patient information, medications, ethical considerations, partnership, and empowerment.

Giger JN, Davidhizar RE, eds: *Transcultural nursing: assessment and intervention,* St Louis, 1995, Mosby
The authors provide students and practitioners with a template for systematically exploring how caregivers' responses, recipients of care, contexts of care, and goals of care may vary, given the cultural diversity in the United States.

Jones DA: HIV-seropositive childbearing women: nursing management, *J Obstet Gynecol Neonatal Nurs* 20(6):446, 1991.
Details the nursing process for assessment and care planning for the HIV-positive pregnant women.

Recurrent Respiratory Papillomatosis Foundation, Telephone (609) 890-0502 or write
Marlene Stern, President
RRP Foundation
50 Wesleyan Drive
Hamilton Square, NJ
08690.
Parent and founder of the foundation, Ms. Stern will send information about current diagnosis and treatment to interested students and practitioners.

Russell LK: Management of varicella-zoster virus infection during pregnancy and the peripartum, *J Nurse Midwifery* 37(1):17, 1992.
Discussion of the difficulties in care for the client with VZV, including isolation precautions.

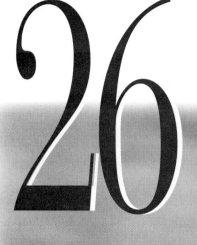

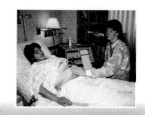

26

The Childbearing Family *at* Psychologic Risk

Learning Objectives

- Identify elements in the crisis of high-risk pregnancy.
- Describe use of therapeutic communication with women and their partners who are experiencing loss.
- Identify defining characteristics of spiritual distress.
- Describe the phases of perinatal grief.
- Investigate the work of a perinatal grief team in your setting.
- Discuss how grief stresses the family system.
- Describe the role of the nurse in facilitating healthy grieving.
- Summarize the differences between postpartum blues and depression.
- Describe nursing interventions for the woman at risk for postpartum depression.

Key Terms

Anxiety
Fetal Demise
Grief Resolution
Incongruent Grieving
Loss
Neonatal Death
Pathologic Mourning
Perinatal Grief
Postpartum Depression
Postpartum Psychosis
Spiritual Distress
Stillbirth

*T*oday parents expect more from a pregnancy than ever before. Many carefully choose their care provider and plan the birthing experience. When expectations are not met because of complications of pregnancy or labor, the birth of an imperfect child, a cesarean birth when a natural birth was planned, the death of the infant, or postpartum depression, parents experience feelings of loss and crisis.

This chapter explores the nursing role with parents experiencing loss as a result of high-risk pregnancy, perinatal death, or postpartum depression. Nurses play a critical role in providing support, counseling, and teaching for these families. Nurses must be knowledgeable to provide optimal care.

ANXIETY

When a situational crisis such as preterm labor or maternal illness occurs during pregnancy, anxiety will result. Excessive preoccupation with the problem, extreme overinvestment in certain aspects of care, continual questioning, and a need for constant reminders and immediate reassurance are common signs of parental anxiety. Some fears are expected, but irrational fears often surface. Mild to moderate **anxiety** levels may be beneficial because these motivate a person to action and increase the ability to perceive details. Moderate to severe anxiety levels, however, can narrow perceptions and render a client and family unable to focus on other aspects of care, to understand the problem, to make decisions, or to carry out instructions. In 1961 Hays described anxiety levels, their effect on the client, and the type of nursing care required. Nearly four decades later, anxiety is a major nursing diagnostic category.

Table 26-1 serves as a useful guide to planning nursing care for clients with anxiety. Note the differences in operations (client behavior), variations (signs), and learning tasks (interventions) required in each anxiety state. Mild to moderate levels of anxiety facilitate learning. Severe anxiety and panic impede learning.

CRISIS INTERVENTION

Crisis applies to a state or to an individual's reaction to a perceived threatening situation (Infante, 1982). A crisis may be maturational *(developmental)*, such as new parenthood, or accidental *(situational)*, such as in the birth and care of an infant with a defect. A life situation may not pose a negative threat when preparation and adequate support are available. Instead it may become a positive growth-producing experience if the person is enabled to cope effectively. Crisis contains both *opportunity* and *danger* (Baird, 1986). It is useful to consider crisis inter-

Table 26-1	**Level of Anxiety and Its Implications for Nursing Care**	
Operations (Client Behavior)	**Variations (Signs)**	**Learning Tasks (Interventions)**
MILD ANXIETY		
Alertness	Noises seeming louder Restlessness Irritability	Recognition of anxiety as a warning sign that something is not going as expected. This can be done by: 1. Observing what goes on 2. Describing what was observed 3. Analyzing what was expected 4. Analyzing how expectations and what went on in the event differed 5. Formulating what can be done about the situation in terms of changing the situation or expectations 6. Validating with others
MODERATE ANXIETY		
Reduced ability to perceive and communicate Increased tension	Concentration on a problem Possible inability to hear someone talking Possible inability to notice part of the room Muscular tension, pounding heart, perspiration, gastric discomfort	Recognition that in moderate and severe anxiety the focus is reduced and connections may not be seen between details; anxiety provides energy that can be reduced to mild anxiety and then used to find out what went wrong
SEVERE ANXIETY		
Perception of details only Physical discomfort Emotional discomfort	Connections between details not seen Headaches, nausea, trembling, dizziness Awe, dread, loathing, horror	Moderate to severe anxiety may be reduced by: 1. Working at a simple, concrete task 2. Talking to someone who can listen 3. Playing a simple game 4. Walking 5. Crying
PANIC		
Elaboration and blowing up of perceived detail	Inability to communicate or function	The person experiencing panic needs help in getting more comfortable. (In this stage learning cannot be expected to take place.)

From Hays D: Teaching a concept of anxiety, *Nurs Res* 10(2):109, 1961.

vention in terms of the self-care conceptual framework described by Aguilera (1994):

> A crisis is a danger because it threatens to overwhelm the individual or his family. . . . It is also an opportunity because during times of crisis individuals are more receptive to therapeutic influence. Prompt and skillful intervention may not only prevent the development of a serious long-term disability, but may also allow new coping patterns to emerge that can help the individual function at a higher level of equilibrium than before the crisis.

A pregnant woman in crisis is at a turning point. She faces a problem that cannot readily be solved by using the coping mechanisms that have worked for her in the past. Tension and anxiety increase as she becomes caught in a state of great emotional upset and is unable to take action to solve the problem (Aguilera, 1994).

Nursing Responsibilities

ASSESSMENT

To assess how best to help clients in these situations, the nurse collects the usual background data and ascertains the client's expectations of the pregnancy. Crisis is related to the degree to which those expectations differ from what is actually happening or going to happen. Learning how she has helped herself during other upsetting events may be useful. Past maladaptive coping behaviors such as avoidance or denial are not desirable and should not be supported. Questions concerning those to whom the client and family turn for support are helpful (e.g., friends, other family members, clergy or church groups, and other professionals such as social workers).

The nurse strives to understand what the diagnosis and consequences of a high-risk pregnancy mean from both the client's and family's perspective. What concerns or frightens them? Fears should be elicited by the use of open-ended questions, reflection, and careful listening, for example, "Many women have a lot of questions or concerns during a time like this. What are yours?" or, "You say that you feel frightened," or "I can understand that you feel angry and upset." This therapeutic interaction encourages the client to express her fears and concerns and prevents the nurse from imposing personal fears and concerns. The woman then may provide clues to her self-care needs, priorities, support system or lack thereof, and barriers to obtaining needed tangible and psychologic care. It may take several interactions to develop enough trust to allow the client to talk freely. Acknowledge her fears. Dispel irrational concerns by giving correct information or referring her to someone who can.

Never give false hope or reassurance. It is far better to tell the client that you do not know than to give inaccu-

rate information. A client may cling to false reassurance to facilitate denial or avoidance behavior, and you should not encourage this behavior in any way.

Anger and mistrust will develop if concerns, even minor ones, are brushed aside or if the client feels she cannot believe what she is being told.

NURSING DIAGNOSES

Depending on assessment findings, the following diagnoses are possible:
- Decisional conflict related to several unacceptable alternatives
- Individual or family coping: potential for growth
- Anxiety related to threat to self, the ideal pregnancy, or to the fetus
- Knowledge deficit because of pregnancy crisis and unknown outcomes
- Powerlessness over outcome despite following care regimen

EXPECTED OUTCOMES

Outcomes can be stated in numerous ways and often are difficult to evaluate because resolution may take time.
- Client will be enabled to make decisions.
- Family support and coping will be strengthened.
- Knowledge will reduce anxiety.
- Alternative ways of coping with powerlessness and fear will be discovered.

NURSING INTERVENTION

Aguilera (1994) provides a four-step outline for intervention. First, the person needs to gain an intellectual understanding of the situation. All family members and friends who need to know should be told what is happening and, if possible, why. The nurse should give as detailed an explanation of the problem, probable causes, treatment risks, benefits, and consequences as can be understood. When this information cannot be provided the nurse is responsible for seeing that another professional talks with the family. The interdisciplinary team consists of many providers, including nurses, nurse-midwives, physicians, physician's assistants, social workers, and dietitians. There are appropriate times for each team member to be the primary provider of care or information. The nurse who spends the most time with the client may be the best person to coordinate the provision of care.

Second, the client should be encouraged to express her feelings. The nurse, by providing an open, nonjudgmental climate, may afford an opportunity for the client to express her feelings of anger, guilt, shame, and fear. These feelings should be affirmed as normal and expected.

Third, the nurse helps the client to examine alternative ways of coping because past coping mechanisms are failing to work. The client is encouraged to avoid maladaptive coping behaviors such as denial and to develop new, more healthy coping behaviors (Aguilera, 1994). Comments that may help when a client is having trouble accepting a diagnosis include a statement such as, "Most people want to ignore unpleasant topics and focus on happy ones." In this way the woman may begin to recognize if she is using avoidance behavior.

Fourth is the "reopening of the social world." This might include helping a family plan to bring their congenitally malformed infant to see relatives or giving a picture or a lock of hair of an ill or stillborn infant to the family so they can show it to relatives and friends.

Whenever possible, the nurse can help the woman regain a sense of control and mastery. For example, allowing a diabetic client to make meal choices may seem simplistic, but the independence and freedom she regains from this is important for her. Praising small accomplishments helps the client. Often, undesirable behavior disappears more rapidly if it is ignored because it may be a mechanism the client is using to gain attention.

The nurse may feel anxious and unable to do anything to ease the client's pain or anxiety. In reality, little can be done for some clients in some situations. For example, when an infant dies of a congenital abnormality, the pain cannot be erased. Clients have shown that the availabilty of the nurse, along with listening, information giving, support, and encouragement to express feelings have been of great assistance. Clients have found assistance with

problem solving and reassurance to be the most supportive and helpful aids, according to Wheeler and Gardner (1987).

The nurse encourages clients to use family and community supports. Clients may feel embarrassed and reluctant to ask for help but should understand that seeking support and assistance from friends, family members, and health care providers usually draws people together.

EVALUATION

Interventions in crises that involve loss and grief cannot be evaluated in a short period. With that in mind, the following questions can be asked:

- Was the client able to articulate her needs and seek assistance?
- Did she understand the normality of the mourning process and allow herself to journey through it?
- Was there support from her network of family and friends?

LOSS AND GRIEF

Feelings of **loss** come when a person recognizes that a desired, valuable goal has been missed, spoiled, or taken away. *Grief* describes the person's emotional response to loss. *Mourning* is the process by which a person goes through the phases of **grief resolution** and accepts the loss. Types of grief are described in Table 26-2.

It should be kept in mind that the loss of *any* desired experience, such as a vaginal delivery or the birth of a child

Table **26-2**   **Types of Grief**

Type of Grief	Description	Responses	Examples
Acute grief	Occurs after a sudden death or major insult to body or psyche	Symptoms of somatic distress occur each time loss acknowledged	Late miscarriage, stillbirth
Anticipatory grief	Response to event that has not yet occurred	Person preoccupied with loss event; a mental rehearsal Premature detachment and altered parent-infant attachment may occur	Preterm labor, prenatal diagnosis of neonatal anomaly
Pathologic or chronic grief	Grief blocked or delayed; person usually not aware of need for professional help	Exaggerated symptoms of anxiety, depression, anger; obsessive thinking	Woman with depression and anger 6 years after perinatal loss at 34 weeks gestation. Family does not acknowledge her feelings of loss

with even a minor congenital problem, can trigger a grief response. According to Peretz (1970), any loss is both a reality and a perceptual or symbolic event. The nurse must remember that each couple's perception will differ based on their unique life experiences. For example, the reality for two women who have each had a cesarean birth is the same. However, each woman's experience of the birth will differ based on her perception of the event. The first woman may respond by grieving over the lost experience she had hoped for—a "natural" birth. The second woman may have a history of infertility or perinatal death. She is satisfied to have a healthy infant and expresses no feelings of loss related to the cesarean (Kowalski, 1996).

Denial

When there is real or perceived loss, one of the first manifestations is *denial,* the "not me" response. For example, a client with recently diagnosed diabetes or preeclampsia may refuse to follow instructions because she feels well and cannot believe that something could be wrong. She may even seek another caregiver to tell her that everything is all right. A mother who is told that her unborn fetus has died may refuse to believe it and continue to state that she feels fetal movement. During this phase, parents feel helpless and anxious.

Anger

The next phase is *anger,* or the "why me" stage. When the obvious no longer can be ignored or occasionally while the client drifts in and out of the denial stage, she may show anger toward caregivers, her partner, or her family. Outbursts of accusations and threats may occur. If she becomes angry at herself, anger turns inward and results in depression. Anger heralds the onset of *guilt.*

The client may think of many reasons to blame herself. Most of the reasons are unfounded and may seem irrational. They are, nonetheless, real to her and should be acknowledged and discussed. If fears are unfounded, the client should be reassured. At the same time she should be reassured that her guilt feelings are normal and expected and that she is not "crazy."

Bargaining

The next step is *bargaining:* "If only I had chosen another doctor!" "If only I had asked before I took that drug!" "God, if you can make this go away, I will never be a bad person again!" "What did I do to deserve this?" These are some of the common responses to which the nurse can offer little response but should listen and show concern in whatever way is appropriate. Irrational feelings can be dispelled partially by providing information. Social service and psychiatric referral may be indicated.

Acceptance

After the client passes through all these stages, she arrives at a relatively peaceful *acceptance.* That does not mean that her sadness disappears; it will always be there, awakened by an anniversary, thought, or similar experience. Acceptance does not mean that the client comes to see the loss as a good event; rather she will see it as a tragedy that occurred, that she lived through, and that made her stronger. The true resolution of a crisis is to turn a bad situation into a growth experience.

Risk Related to Maternal or Fetal Complications

Maternal or fetal complications represent the realization of the worst fears of the pregnant woman and her family. Although ambivalence and concern are typical in the normal pregnancy, when a problem occurs the woman, her partner, and her family may feel guilty. They assume that the problem may have been caused by a thought they had (or did not have), an action they took (or did not take), or a decision they made (or did not make). Providers can unwittingly reinforce these feelings by asking questions or making statements that imply blame such as "Why didn't you come in sooner?" or "Why did you do that?" To learn to avoid the process of blame, the nurse can record several interviews and listen to other nurses' responses to the client.

Body-image disturbance

Women experience both physical and psychologic changes during normal pregnancy. Sometimes these changes in body image cause feelings of loss. Early-pregnancy morning sickness, in the absence of other perceptible signs of pregnancy, can make a woman feel ill, not pregnant. Normal hormonal shifts may cause tremendous mood swings, which intensify anxiety and lead to fears that something is wrong. During these times, women and their partners normally may wonder if the pregnancy is worth all the trouble, even if it has been eagerly anticipated and planned. These feelings may be more intense in cases of unintended pregnancy (Richardson, 1996).

Changes in the urinary, cardiopulmonary, musculoskeletal, and integumentary systems in normal pregnancy often cause *body-image disturbances.* Women with medical problems existing before pregnancy have additional concerns about how the pregnancy will affect them: "Will my diabetes go out of control?" "Will my heart disease become fatal?" This anxiety may lead to excessive focus on symptoms (i.e., hypochondriasis) because the basic safety needs are threatened. Severe levels of anxiety may result.

When a medical problem first appears during pregnancy, a dual crisis has to be faced. The client must deal with the problem (e.g., her newly diagnosed gestational diabetes or hypertensive disease). Her body is failing her:

"Will I need surgery or die?" "Will this be a lifelong problem?" "Will I ever be normal again?" "Will I ever be able to eat what I want, exercise at the gym, have sexual relations?" "How can I cope with labor, delivery, and a new baby when I also have to cope with an illness?" The severity of her reaction often is not in proportion to the problem. Her support systems, her cultural and ethnic background, her expectations of herself, and her hopes for the pregnancy all affect her response.

Box 26-1

CLINICAL DECISION

A woman's status is designated as high risk because of gestational diabetes. The client and her husband question staff members constantly and refuse to continue with the diet and blood glucose monitoring that has been recommended. They are upset that they have been transferred from the alternative birth center to the hospital center. Explain their responses. Suggest nursing interventions.

Fears for fetal safety

When fetal complications occur (e.g., genetic disorders or the threat of preterm labor) normal fears about fetal well-being and guilt are intensified. The anxiety over even routine diagnostic tests is considerable, and when tests confirm a problem, the worst fears of the parents are realized. "Will our baby be OK?" "I knew I shouldn't have taken that exercise class!" "There is something wrong with me. I can't even take care of my baby before it's born!"

Clients and their partners rarely express their concerns directly. Their need for information, counseling, and assistance may be expressed in many often covert ways. They may not discuss fears or problems with family or friends. Even in normal pregnancy, expression of fears may not be well accepted by the family.

Interrupted parent-infant attachment

Stress that leaves the parents feeling unsupported or that causes real or imagined concerns for their infant's health or survival interferes with attachment. Anxiety over health or psychosocial problems during pregnancy may also interfere with attachment. A threatened miscarriage or a history of previous miscarriage threatens a woman's self-image. Fearing for the survival of her infant and protecting herself from feelings of loss if she miscarries, she unconsciously delays forming an image of herself as a mother. Illness or traumatic delivery may leave her with little energy for interaction with her infant. Similarly, pain (e.g., after a cesarean birth) can distract from her interaction.

When the unexpected outcome is a problem with the infant, the difficulty of attachment will be compounded.

The mother needs to mourn the loss of the anticipated "perfect" infant; in addition, attachment may be delayed if the infant must be immediately transported to the special care nursery or to another facility because of medical problems. This separation means that her sense of herself as important to the infant is immediately cast aside. Without contact, she fears that her need to be close to the infant is in jeopardy, and thus she may begin to detach from her pregnancy relationship. Early contact with her infant is essential because she is eager to identify, claim, and attach to her child (Figure 26-1).

If the mother cannot be brought to the special care nursery within a few hours of the birth (e.g., if she is ill or the infant is transferred to another hospital), she should be given a picture of her infant and unlimited access to the nursery by telephone to help her maintain a sense of being important to the infant.

PERINATAL GRIEF

The death of an infant is not the natural order of life. Children are not supposed to die before their parents. When an infant dies, parents are faced with a devastating crisis for which they are totally unprepared.

The grief response following a perinatal death is often as severe, and sometimes more severe, than that following the death of an adult. Yet many parents do not receive adequate support. After a few weeks, well-meaning family and friends may avoid discussing the infant, believing that they are sparing the parents from further pain. Some persons who are uncomfortable talking about death will avoid the parents. Parents feel isolated. They want and need to talk about their infant. They know that others care, but few, if any, truly understand. They often are left to deal with their grief alone.

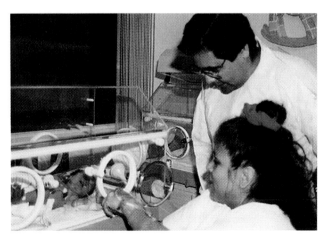

Figure 26-1   Parents should be encouraged to visit their infant in the neonatal intensive care unit as early as possible. (Courtesy Marjorie Pyle, RNC, *Lifecircle*.)

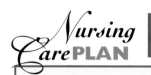
Nursing Care PLAN | *Loss and Grief*

CASE

Jane, 34, para 0010, has recently been separated from her spouse. Her own family lives in the next state. She had hoped for a normal child to fill an emotional vacuum in her life. Diagnosis at 32 weeks shows that the male infant has a defect but will survive. At 34 weeks she gives birth prematurely to a healthy boy with a cleft lip and palate.

Assessment

1. Level of expressed anxiety about infant; hopes for the infant's place in family
   Past and present coping mechanisms
   Actual family support, friends
2. Phase of grief response: diagnosis known since 32 weeks
   Expressions of hopes and fears about future
   Understanding of normality of grieving in situation
3. Knowledge about future treatment, length of stay in neonatal intensive care unit (NICU)
   Ability to understand explanations given by physician and nurses
   Ability to participate in decision making about future
   Knowledge of resources for self and infant care; support

Nursing Diagnoses

1. Anxiety related to perceived threats to self and infant
2. Risk for dysfunctional grieving and depression over infant's condition, loss of partner
3. Altered body image related to perceived inability to have normal infant
4. Spiritual distress related to questioning outcome of pregnancy

Expected Outcomes

1. Anxiety will be managed with effective coping mechanisms.
2. Client moves through grief process at an acceptable pace and finds ongoing support.
3. She asks for clarification of causes and treatment for infant.
4. She expresses concerns about body image, self-esteem, and spiritual distress.
5. She participates in planning for future and seeks additional counseling and resources

Nursing Interventions

1. Maintain calm, safe environment. Encourage nurse-client relationship by assigning primary nurse.
2. Assess anxiety level, and support her in seeking personal resources for coping. Identify phase of grief, and assure her of normality of feelings.
3. Give understandable information at a pace she can accept. Provide written information for going home. Work toward well-informed decisions. Provide telephone numbers for professional assistance as required.
4. Engage in therapeutic listening. Encourage attachment by frequent visits to NICU. Use open-ended statements to elicit spiritual or self-esteem concerns. Refer to additional counseling or clergy as appropriate.
5. Praise constructive problem solving. Be sure sequence of infant recovery, surgery, and home care is explained and understood by the mother. Identify financial resources by referral to appropriate persons. Refer for home care when infant is ready. Follow through with her own recovery with the home care nurse.

Evaluation

1. Did she increase coping skills? Have symptoms of anxiety been recognized and reduced?
2. Has she expressed feelings about crisis and loss? Does she realize the phases of grief through which she will be going? Can she identify support persons in her situation?
3. Is attachment to the infant established? Does this attachment appear to overcome any feelings of lowered self-esteem? Does there appear to be adequate emotional support for her in her home setting?
4. Is she clear about the planning for care of the defect, recovery times, and home care of the infant? Does she know about resources?

This "conspiracy of silence" described by so many parents after the loss of an infant is due in large part to the unique nature of **perinatal grief.** Nurses need to understand the unique characteristics of this type of loss if they are to be effective caregivers.

It is the memory of a person that produces our emotional response to their death. The intensity of grief is related to the relationship each one had with the deceased. When an infant dies, either before or shortly after birth, there are few people other than the infant's parents who have any memory of that child. Sadness, emptiness, and feelings of intense loss are emotions felt primarily by the child's parents. Friends and relatives feel sadness for the grief of the parents and helplessness because they cannot erase their pain.

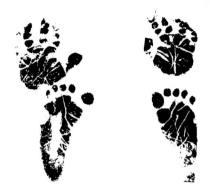

Figure 26-2   Tiny hand and footprints are some of the precious memories grieving parents appreciate.

Types of Perinatal Loss

It is important that the health professional be knowledgeable about the types of perinatal loss. While each type of death is different, the grief response is essentially the same. The nurse plays a critical role in facilitating healthy parental grieving.

Early loss

Spontaneous abortion, or miscarriage, is the termination of pregnancy by natural causes before 20 weeks of pregnancy and before the infant can survive outside the uterus. It is the most commonly experienced form of perinatal loss. Statistics show that 15% of all pregnancies end in miscarriage (see Chapter 21). The grief response felt by parents seems to be the same, regardless of gestational age. A history of previous miscarriage, stillbirth, or neonatal death is the one factor that may alter the intensity of the reaction. It is insignificant to parents who have this kind of experience to point out that their child was very young or may not have been completely formed because they grieve the infant they had envisioned. Therefore, whenever possible, visualization and gender identification will help to confirm the loss and facilitate the grieving process. The inability to visually bond with a young fetus may alter healthy grieving because there are no memories to rely on for comfort. Providing a set of footprints may be helpful (Figure 26-2).

Elective abortion or termination, either with or without genetic anomalies as a factor in decision making, also causes a grief response. Although these families have made a choice, there are often feelings of guilt, regret, and psychologic disturbance that can complicate healthy grieving. Frequently, these parents experience an intense, prolonged grief. After elective termination, teenagers are more likely to suffer distress than adults (Ney et al, 1994).

Ectopic pregnancy, commonly termed *tubal pregnancy,* is a less common form of fetal loss. Ectopic, or extrauterine, pregnancy occurs when a fertilized egg is implanted outside the uterus. Fewer than one third of women who have an ectopic pregnancy have a successful subsequent pregnancy. Many are unable to conceive at all. One in four of those who do will have another ectopic pregnancy (Caron and Buster, 1993).

Grief after an early loss.   Following an early loss, it is important to assess its meaning for the woman and her partner. Listen carefully to her. Does she use the words "pregnancy" or "baby" when referring to her loss? Avoid terms such as "products of conception," which tend to devalue the loss.

Pregnancy loss, however early, can cause later physical and psychologic health problems if grieving does not occur. In one study, approximately 25% of the women felt the need for professional help after a loss (Ney et al, 1994). Single women, including teenagers, may be alone as they experience the loss of their pregnancy. It is important that the nurse assess the woman's support system because women with an inadequate support system are more likely to experience pathologic grief (Ney et al, 1994) (see Table 26-2).

Death after age of viability: later loss

The discussion below will focus on the loss of a fetus before birth, a **stillbirth,** or immediate loss of the neonate, either at the time of birth or shortly afterwards. See Yoder (1994) and others for infant death after a period of time in a pediatric setting.

Stillbirth.   An infant is stillborn if it died between the twentieth week of pregnancy and the time of birth and is termed an intrauterine fetal death (IUFD). The parents must go through the difficult period of labor, knowing the fetus is not viable, or if the death occurs during labor, they experience the panic of discovery and the rescue attempts. if resuscitation was attempted, the parents should not be excluded. Watching the intense involvement of staff makes the parents feel involved and that "they did everything possible for my baby" (Yoder, 1994).

For the parents the pain and anguish of grief are intensified by the absence of being able to visually bond while the infant was alive. Parents of a stillborn infant or **fetal demise** are denied the memories of hearing the infant cry or looking at and holding a warm body.

Neonatal death. Neonatal death encompasses death of an infant between birth and 1 month of life. The most common cause of neonatal death is prematurity with its complications. However, congenital anomalies, infections, birth trauma, and complications of pregnancy are also factors. When death after a live birth occurs, the parents have the opportunity to see and touch their child. This beginning interaction aids memory formation and brings comfort to those families once the infant dies. Although much of the time spent together may be painful, parents manage to cling to the positive aspects of this time together. They view it as an opportunity to acquaint themselves and others with the infant who was with them only briefly.

Physical and Emotional Responses to Grief

This is the darkest moment, so parents think. Upon hearing the news that the infant has died, parents believe that the pain of the moment could not possibly get any worse. Unfortunately, the agony of living through the days and months ahead and the effort to rejoin the "world of the living" will provide tougher challenges than with which parents are prepared to deal. There is no greater task in life than facing death, dealing with death, and learning to happily live again despite the death of someone so special.

Physical responses

Physical symptoms of grief may include a feeling of severe physical exhaustion, perhaps further aggravated by a difficult delivery, heaviness in the chest, need to take deep sighing breaths, palpitations, aching arms, anorexia, sleep disturbances, nightmares, and dreams of the deceased. All of these symptoms reflect a normal initial response to the process of grieving. Although symptoms affect the parents' physical sense of well being, these reactions play an important role in allowing the body to experience the pain. It is only in feeling and dealing with the pain that parents will eventually be able to let this pain go in grief resolution. The physical symptoms are only temporary and will diminish with time.

Although light sleep sedation may be necessary to guard against chronic fatigue, other forms of antidepressants and antianxiety drugs are not recommended during this early stage of grieving. Being tranquilized only postpones and prolongs the real pain. It is better for parents to face reality while family and friends are close by to help.

Emotional responses

Parental emotional responses to the loss of an infant are numerous and may occur in varying order on many different levels of intensity. Some of these responses may not be experienced at all. Many of these feelings may cause parents to think they are "going crazy," and they may appreciate professional reassurance. Especially now, parents need reassurance that they are behaving in a healthy way. A clue to healthy recovery through this time is the length of good time experienced each day. As time goes by, and it goes by slowly, parents will recognize that they have smiled, hummed a tune, or even had a pleasant thought. The event may have been brief, but it may mark the beginning of healing that will progress through grief resolution.

Intense feelings of loss and emptiness are the primary emotions initially. The loneliness is magnified by the constant reminder of a recent birth, as evidenced by the mother's engorged breasts. An overwhelming sense of anxiety, alarm, and restlessness soon surfaces. Couples find it difficult to reestablish normal routines, have problems with concentration and decision making, and may lose interest in projects that once held their attention. Forgetfulness is another disturbing element of grief and the most common complaint of the parents who return to work too soon. Anger and hostility may develop as thoughts of "Why?" begin to overwhelm them. Eventually, depression unveils itself and usually remains in varying degrees of intensity for a prolonged period. Every couple, especially mothers, experience some form of guilt in the primary stages of crisis. The common question, "What if I had . . . ?" haunts parents. An answer is never found.

Phases of Bereavement

To more fully understand the process related to perinatal grief, four phases of bereavement have been identified by John Bowlby and C. Murray Parkes (Kellner and Lake, 1993).

Shock and *numbness* predominate during the first 2 weeks after a loss. During this phase, denial serves a useful, self-protective function by allowing the parents time to mobilize their resources to cope with their loss. Parents often feel unaware of their environment, are unable to make decisions, and need much assistance in performing even the simplest tasks. Crying may or may not be present, and emotional outbursts may occur.

The next phase, *searching* and *yearning,* surfaces approximately 3 to 7 days following the infant's death and peaks from 2 weeks to 4 months later. During this phase parents yearn for their infant, and search for answers. Consequently, they have many questions and often experience anger that may be directed at professionals. Feelings of restlessness and guilt are common. Physical symptoms may surface at this time. A mother's arms may "ache" to hold her infant. This appears to be the longest phase of bereavement, gradually declining as resolution approaches.

Disorientation occurs during the first week following the death, magnifies and subsides at varying intervals for months to years afterward, and intensifies briefly during the infant's first anniversary. Depression is the primary symptom. Parents begin to feel guilty about their inability to recover from their loss and may take on a role of sickness to mask their depression and avoid criticism. The mourner may lose her or his appetite and fail to maintain personal care. Introduction into a support group at this time can be crucial to avoid parental suspicions of going crazy.

Reorganization, the final phase of bereavement, indicates that the grief response is approaching completion and that the parents are close to total healing and recovery. Parents are taking care of themselves physically and are able to participate in activities of daily living without the oppressive feelings of the earlier phases. While memories of their infant continue, they are able to feel sadness that doesn't immobilize them (Kellner and Lake, 1993).

It is important to consider that, although the phases of grief are presented here in an orderly time frame, characteristics of each phase overlap one another. In addition, clients pass through the stages of the grief process at different rates, and each individual's response will be unique. Advances and regressions typically occur. The degree of support that the client and family receive influences the rate at which they progress. Full resolution may take 18 months to 2 years.

Pathologic grief reactions

When events occur that inhibit or block the grieving process described earlier, **pathologic mourning** may occur. The risk of this occurring increases when well-meaning friends and relatives avoid discussing the pregnancy, the delivery, and the infant with the parents. Two groups of women are at particularly high risk: those who become pregnant within 6 months following a stillbirth and those who give birth to twins with only one surviving twin (Kellner and Lake, 1993). These women are at higher risk because it is difficult to mourn a death and attach to a new pregnancy or infant at the same time. Women with an inadequate or absent support system are also at greater risk.

Differences between maternal and paternal grief

Studies tell us that mothers and fathers grieve differently. To understand this difference it is important to first appreciate the differences between maternal and paternal bonding. During pregnancy, because the infant is growing within her, the mother's attachment to her fetus is generally greater than the father's. Certain events, such as hearing the infant's heartbeat and quickening (feeling fetal movement) strengthen this bond. A father's attachment "catches up" to hers at birth when both partners see and hold their infant. Peppers and Knapp (1980) termed this "incongruent bonding." When a loss occurs, mothers and fathers tend to grieve differently. Men are more likely to

suppress their grief. They may use work to cope with feelings and "get on with things." Women tend to cry more and often want to talk more about the loss. This **incongruent grieving** can cause communication difficulties at a time when couples need each other most (May, 1996).

Another aspect of perinatal grief is that fathers are often the comforter while also the bereaved. Fathers interviewed following the stillbirth of their infant have described feeling helpless and overwhelmed while also feeling a responsibility to support their wives (Page-Lieberman and Hughes, 1990). This conflict can complicate their own ability to grieve.

Nursing Considerations

Confirming the loss

Helping parents to confirm their loss is the first step in the grieving process. There is an abundance of literature supporting the importance of the bereaved parents' need to see and hold the dead infant. Seeing and holding their infant makes the child real and enhances bonding. If the parents wish, the nurse can unwrap blankets so that parents see all of the infant. Pointing out the positive features of the child is comforting to parents. The nurse may also suggest that the mother or father bathe, diaper, and dress the infant, thus easing the need to nurture their child (Yoder, 1994).

To say goodbye, parents should have as much private time alone with the infant as they need. This time together provides an opportunity for parents to incorporate this child into their lives. One nurse should be the liaison between parents and the rest of the staff. The person can see to their physical needs such as a telephone, tissues, and coffee or juice, if helpful.

The nurse should prepare parents for the infant's appearance if the infant is macerated, cold, or malformed. Bereaved parents need to see and hold their child regardless of any physical deformity or malformation in order to have a sense of reality. A parent's fantasy of the imagined deformity will usually be much worse than what is seen. By verbally preparing the parents for what the infant will look like, the nurse can allay unnecessary fears. Of course, some parents will not want to see or hold the infant. In such cases the nurse should take pictures of the infant to keep on file. Most families will later request the pictures.

Naming the infant

Although parents may be reluctant to use a chosen name for an infant who has died, they should be encouraged to do so. The name will identify the infant as an integral part of the family who can be remembered and loved.

Providing keepsakes

Following an infant's death, tangible memories provide the greatest source of comfort for parents as time passes.

Having something to touch, smell, and look at will keep the infant close to the parents and alleviate some of the loneliness and emptiness. Helpful keepsakes may include the birth certificate, footprints, cribcard, name bracelet, lock of hair, articles of clothing, infant hat, blankets and fleece, ultrasound pictures, fetal heart rate strip, infant photos, or videos. A memory book is a way to organize these keepsakes (Figure 26-3).

Photos and videos. Pictures and videos can be comforting to parents, especially as time passes and the vivid memory of the infant begins to fade. Pictures also provide parents with a means of having friends and family become acquainted with the deceased child if they haven't already done so. The display of the photos is a personal and private choice made by the family. Many choose to frame and display the pictures along with other family photos; others will tuck the pictures privately into a drawer or wallet.

Encourage parents to take many different pictures of the infant, both wrapped and unwrapped. Parents may appreciate help with picture taking. Pictures of the infant with the family, including siblings, are of enormous benefit in preserving the memory of the family unit. Anyone present and significant to the parents may participate in the picture taking. The use of stuffed animals can soften the photo and make the pictures more appealing.

Baptism and prayers for the infant

When appropriate, the rite of baptism, the Sacrament of the Sick, or a blessing by a chosen clergy member should be offered as an option to parents to facilitate spiritual healing. Allow them the choice of clergy, and encourage participation of siblings, grandparents, godparents, and significant others. If the rite of baptism is performed, provide the family with a baptismal certificate stating the date, time, and child's name. In emergencies, and if so desired by the parents, any lay person can bap-

tize the infant. Use water and touch the infant's head while saying, "I baptize you in the Name of the Father, Son, and Holy Spirit," adding any prayer you wish. Most Christian groups recognize this emergency baptism and will honor the rite as if it had been performed by clergy. Muslim parents may appreciate a prayer commending the infant to Allah, the All-Merciful.

Family needs

When crisis occurs, some families will turn inward in an attempt to isolate themselves so that others will not have to experience pain. The nursing goal for these families is to maximize their support systems.

Siblings. Children grieve for their lost siblings, even if they never knew them. Parents should be encouraged to tell their children about the death of the infant and to allow for expressions of sadness. When the parents are sad, the children should be told that it is because of the death of the infant. Parents need especially to clarify that the sibling in no way affected the death. Children often imagine that they caused the death by an angry thought or response. Young children may be afraid that the same thing will happen to them. Reassurance that their parents will take care of them is essential. For this reason, explanations such as, "An angel took the baby," are not helpful and should be rephrased.

Sisters and brothers should always be included in the birth and death of an infant, including the funeral. Although the events are difficult, research has shown that exclusion of siblings creates feelings of isolation and confusion in these children. Shared tears are far more therapeutic for both parents and siblings and allow each the opportunity to help the other through the grieving process. There are a number of books for children to assist them in voicing concerns.

Grandparents. When the opportunity exists, grandparents also need to be included in discussions of grieving and have their own loss acknowledged. The nurse can facilitate family coping by talking openly with grandparents and providing guidance. Grandparents should know that their support and willingness to discuss their grandchild can be extremely therapeutic to the grieving couple.

Autopsy and funeral

Parents will be faced with decisions regarding an autopsy. The nurse's role is to make sure that this decision is not rushed by other health professionals and that parents are aware of the autopsy options available. The consent form is signed by the parents and the requesting physician. When the cause of death is unclear, parents may be anxious to hear the findings. They should be informed in person by the physician. They need to be informed when the infant's body will be ready for the funeral.

Both parents are encouraged to plan for their infant's funeral. They should be advised to disassemble the infant's

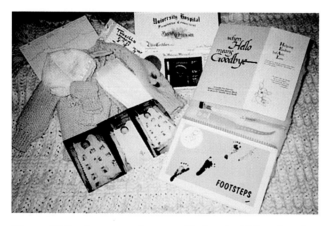

Figure 26-3 A memory kit assembled at the University of Connecticut Health Center, Farmington, Conn. It includes pictures of the infant, clothing, death certificate, footprints, ID bands, fetal monitor printout, and ultrasound picture.

room together. Although both processes are painful, they are therapeutic. Saying goodbye provides the parents with the opportunity to make choices in what has been, to this point, a helpless situation.

Parental education. Preparing bereaved parents for the emotional experience of the days following the funeral should include information about normal grief responses. Information about grief responses is important; it reassures them that their behavior is normal and expected and prevents the confusion and fear that arises when parents are faced with unfamiliar feelings.

The nurse can also facilitate coping by preparing parents for reactions of family and friends, differences in grieving between men and women, care of surviving siblings, living through the holidays, and thoughts about a future pregnancy. When appropriate, significant others should be part of this education to facilitate their efforts in supporting the grieving family. Nurses should stress that there is no time limit on grieving and that, although the pain does not always remain as intense, the experience will be one that will change the parents' lives forever. With reassurance, families will understand that getting through the due date (in the case of the premature birth) and the first year will be the most intense emotional time. They

will ultimately learn how to incorporate their infant's death into their lives, and they will, subsequently, reacquire happiness.

Finally, parents should be given adequate information about appropriate support systems within their community. Support groups and counseling can be a tremendous source of stability when experiencing grief. Referrals should be made as soon as possible. These nursing interventions are summarized in Box 26-1.

Remembering the infant. Most hospitals today have a perinatal bereavement committee that advocates for the needs of families who have experienced a loss. Some hospitals follow up with the family by phone several days after discharge and send monthly letters that contain information to assist the family in their journey (Stewart, 1995). Others send a card at the infant's 1-month or 1-year anniversary. Parents appreciate it anytime their infant is acknowledged and remembered by others (Figure 26-4). Many parents state that "everyone forgets and goes on with life, except us." Yoder (1994) encourages health providers to do the following whenever possible:
- Do not use platitudes, which minimize individuality of the parent's loss
- Do not identify with the parents' loss; don't share similar situations
- Attend the wake, or funeral if possible, especially if a nurse has been a primary care person in the NICU
- Reach out to the family without waiting for them to ask for help (see Figure 26-4)

Pregnancy after perinatal loss

When a couple achieves pregnancy again after a previous loss they may still be grieving the infant who died while also attaching to the new pregnancy. The nursing assessment should include a complete obstetric history, a description of each partner's response to the previous loss, and the meaning of the loss to each of them. Such an assessment gets their fears and concerns out in the open and allows the nurse to address each one (Brost and Kenney, 1992).

To establish the meaning of the loss the nurse acknowledges the loss and then uses an open-ended statement to encourage communication. For example, "I'm sorry to hear you've had a miscarriage (or your baby was stillborn). How are you doing now?"

Brost and Kenney further suggest referring to an early miscarriage as a "loss" rather than a "baby" until the meaning of the loss to the parents is clarified. Parents who have experienced a later loss should be asked about the experience. Did they see and hold their infant? Were pictures taken? Which other family members saw and held the child? The nurse can also ask parents to share pictures of their child.

Fear of another pregnancy loss and heightened anxiety are common. An atmosphere of trust where the woman

---

Box 26-1 — Perinatal Bereavement: Nursing Interventions during Shock and Numbness Phase

- Assess impact of loss on the client and her significant other.
- Acknowledge their loss.
- Communicate a willingness to listen; allow repetitious review of death events.
- Allow silence; use touch and eye contact to convey continued interest and caring without interrupting thought processes.
- Be prepared to repeat information several times (remember thought processes are slowed).
- Provide opportunity for parents to see, hold, and touch their infant. Include other family members (siblings, grandparents) as parents desire.
- Prepare them for appearance of the infant (cold, malformed).
- Use the infant's name and comment on any positive characteristics.
- Provide privacy and time alone with their infant when they are ready.
- Provide as many mementos as are available.
- Help parents to observe cultural and spiritual practices.
- Prepare parents for the grieving process and for possible differences in their grieving.
- Make referrals to community support groups such as SHARE.

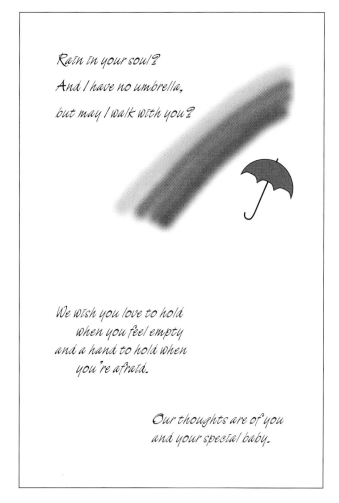

Rain in your soul?

And I have no umbrella,

but may I walk with you?

We wish you love to hold
when you feel empty
and a hand to hold when
you're afraid.

Our thoughts are of you
and your special baby.

Figure 26-4   Bereavement card sent at 1 month after infant death by hospital bereavement team. (Courtesy Margaret Bovard.)

feels safe to share her fears is important. The nurse can then clear up any misconceptions and provide appropriate reassurance.

Because perinatal loss often leaves parents feeling a loss of control, gaining a sense of control in the new pregnancy is therapeutic. Providing information, allowing them to participate in decisions, and more frequent prenatal visits are all helpful interventions.

Finally, it is important to assess maternal attachment to the new pregnancy. Who has she told about the pregnancy? Has she made any plans for the infant? If there seems to be delayed attachment, the nurse may open a discussion about her fears and concerns.

SPIRITUAL DISTRESS

Each person has spiritual needs, which if unmet may cause restlessness, unhappiness, and a sense of lack of purpose in life, or **spiritual distress**. A state of crisis often

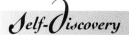

intensifies such feelings. Spiritual distress can be thought of as the state in which an individual experiences, or is at risk for experiencing, a disturbance in the belief or value system that provides strength, hope, and meaning to life (Carpenito, 1993). Spiritual needs may be expressed in a variety of ways. Depending upon exposure to and acceptance of a set of religious beliefs, an individual may turn to those who seem to have faith or may seek help with basic questions of, "Why me?," "What purpose?," and "Who can help me?"

One's spirituality may seek expression through practice of a specific religion. It is, however, a much wider concept, expressed in one writer's words as "in Whom we live and move and have our being" or by another as "Our hearts are restless until they find their rest in Thee." Through faith a person finds meaning in life and life's difficulties, understands personal growth, and achieves healing and hope.

Holistic nursing involves the client's whole being. It is important that nurses in maternal-child health care become knowledgeable about spiritual distress as a nursing diagnosis and learn to use it appropriately; see its defining characteristics (Box 26-2).

In an inner-city setting in which a group of nurses (Corrine et al, 1992) encountered expressions of deep spiritual distress, spiritual interventions were found to be important in maternal-child health care. The concept of a *life journey* was a useful way to indicate the dynamic character of faith development and influence on life decisions. Using questions, such as the following, the nurse may help the person tap into these spiritual needs.

- "How did you cope with the loss?," when discussing a miscarriage or death
- "Where did you find the strength to do what you did?," when leaving an abusive relationship or dealing with a difficult life situation
- "How are your spirits today?," when the client has been depressed
- "Whom do you turn to when problems seem too much?," helps identify resources
- "To whom do you pray?," when better acquainted with the client, opens the doors to discuss faith resources
- "Where do you seem to be on your journey?," to a mother grieving over a stillbirth

Cultural variations in the area in which a nurse works need to be studied and understood before wrong conclusions are drawn. For instance, in some Hispanic subgroups, *mal oho,* or the evil eye, is feared, and precautions are taken. A family will have a specific saint as a protector, and colored beads, a *sabache,* may be attached to a bracelet or necklace as a protection. Others may protect the infant by saying, "Que Dios lo bendiga" (God bless him) when they see the infant (Corrine et al, 1992).

Interventions go beyond a simple referral to a clergy person. The nurse may offer suggestions of activities that others have found helpful. Clergy can provide reading material to help the person become centered and think about spiritual needs. Writing down feelings in a journal often is a powerful tool, especially during mourning. To assist the woman in mobilizing her own resources, the nurse can suggest walking, meaningful activities with friends, and conversation to identify her helpful supports. Mainly, it is the nurse's caring attitude that indicates to the client that her spiritual distress is taken seriously and deserves attention.

POSTPARTUM AFFECTIVE DISORDERS

After giving birth, many women experience alterations in affect or mood. For some women, this may be as mild as one isolated crying episode. For others, episodes continue for weeks, becoming more severe and disruptive. Postpartum affective disorders can have a significant impact on family adaptation. At a time when many families are already stressed, depression in the new mother burdens the entire family with additional stress and increases the risk of dysfunction.

Types of Affective Disorders

Postpartum affective disorders are commonly organized into three categories: transitory postpartum depression, or "baby blues," postpartum depression, and postpartum psychosis.

The baby blues affect 50% to 75% of new mothers (Casiano, 1990). Women with the baby blues experience crying spells, labile moods, irritability, and changes in appetite and ability to sleep. The blues typically occur 3 to 5 days postpartum and last only a few days. The leading causes are the sudden drop in estrogen and progesterone levels plus the discomforts, fatigue, interrupted sleep, and change in role that new motherhood brings.

While the blues are temporary, **postpartum depression** is not. It may last as long as a year or more. It can start anytime during the year after the birth, and its symptoms are much more severe and disruptive (Box 26-3). Approximately 10% to 15% of new mothers will develop varying degrees of postpartum depression.

Some researchers see the baby blues and postpartum depression as existing on a continuum. Women who experience the blues and have extra stressors, such as marital or financial concerns, may be at greater risk for more severe postpartum depression.

Postpartum psychosis occurs in only 1 or 2 out of every 1000 postpartum women. Symptoms can vary greatly. Some women exhibit maniclike symptoms such as racing thoughts, hyperactivity, and extreme mood swings. In others the psychosis resembles a delirious state (with waxing and waning confusion and dissociative episodes). Still others display symptoms resembling psychotic depression, such as psychomotor retardation and delusions (Casiano, 1990).

There is controversy about whether postpartum psychosis is distinct from nonpostpartum psychosis. Much of the research to date does not suggest a distinction other than the fact that postpartum psychosis occurs after childbirth. The International Classification of Diseases (ICD) and the Diagnostic and Statistical Manual (DSM-IV) no longer list postpartum psychosis as a separate diagnostic category. Currently, diagnosis and treatment are the same as for nonpostpartum psychosis. Hospitalization and antipsychotic medications are generally required (Kendall-Tackett and Kantor, 1993).

Clinical significance of postpartum depression

Maternal depression often has a negative impact on the family, especially the children. Studies show that depressed

| *Box* 26-3 | **Symptoms of Postpartum Depression** |

Restlessness
Irritability
Crying spells
Loss of control over emotions, thought, and actions
Obsessive thinking
Anxiety attacks
Impaired concentration
Anger directed at family members including infant
Inability to cope with care of infant
Isolation of self
Contemplation of or attempting self-destruction

mothers tend to interact with their children differently than nondepressed mothers. They tend to be less spontaneous, less happy, less vocal, and less close with their infants. Infants of depressed mothers have been found to express more negative emotions than infants of nondepressed mothers. Most disturbing of all, Zuravan (1989) found that moderately depressed mothers are at increased risk for physical aggression, and severely depressed mothers are more likely to be verbally aggressive with their children. Beck (1995) explored postpartum depressed mothers' experiences interacting with their children.

Jane had a difficult birth with her first child. She was angry and depressed although she tried to be the perfect mother, going through breast-feeding and infant care punctiliously. She did not like the infant and showed no warm feelings toward him nor talked with him. At 3 months this infant was listless, never smiled, and had no verbalization. Her friends "ordered" her to play a series of games with the infant for stimulation (counting toes and fingers, peek-a-boo). Gradually, with continued family support, she became acquainted with and enjoyed interacting with her son.

Maternal depression also interferes with the couple's relationship. The father is likely to feel confused by his partner's behavior. Confusion over what is happening, as well as lack of knowledge about how he can help, often leaves the man feeling frightened and helpless.

"Lived experience" of postpartum depression. What is it like to have postpartum depression? To answer this question, Beck (1992) interviewed mothers with postpartum depression who described having feelings of anxiety, obsessive thoughts of being a bad mother, loss of control, and thoughts of hurting the infant. Overwhelmed by the responsibility of motherhood, some said they lacked feelings of love for their infant. Many said that when they tried to tell those around them of their need for help, they were ignored. Feeling that no one understood what they were experiencing led to severe loneliness and isolation. Several women said they contemplated death as

a way out of their "living nightmare." As recovery came, women grieved over the early time lost with the infant, which never could be recovered (Beck, 1993).

Nursing Responsibilities

ASSESSMENT

Certain risk factors or predictors of postpartum depression have been identified. While further study is needed, women who experience especially severe "blues" seem to be a greater risk (Beck, Reynolds, and Rutowski, 1992). Additional risk factors include: (1) history of major depression or bipolar disorder; (2) premenstrual syndrome; (3) antepartum depression; (4) history of early childhood loss, such as death of a parent; (5) history of physical or sexual abuse; (6) socioeconomic disadvantage; (7) traumatic birth experience; and (8) lack of social support, especially from the father of the infant.

Assessment for risk factors should begin during pregnancy and continue during labor, delivery, and the postpartum period. Women at risk may benefit from additional emotional support.

Identifying postpartum depression

Nurses in obstetric and pediatric offices and who practice home care need to be alert when talking with women to recognize symptoms of postpartum depression. Symptoms can begin anytime during the first year. Symptoms that deserve attention include women's feelings of being overwhelmed, hopeless, or out of control. Descriptions of anxiety, nervousness, or insomnia should also be investigated (Kendall-Tackett and Kantor, 1993).

Nonspecific questions such as, "How are you doing?" often elicit vague responses such as "OK" or "Fine." Asking direct questions such as, "Have you been feeling sad?," "Have you been crying lately?," "How much?," and "Are you enjoying the baby?" are more effective because they validate the woman's experience and give her permission to share how she feels (Kendall-Tackett and Kantor, 1993). The nurse may also choose to use a questionnaire such as the Edinburgh Postnatal Depression Scale (Box 26-4).

NURSING DIAGNOSES

The following nursing diagnoses may be appropriate for women with postpartum depression:
- Risk for ineffective individual coping related to depressed symptoms
- Knowledge deficit about the difference between blues and depression and when to seek professional help
- Risk for altered parenting related to postpartum affective disorder

■ *Box* 26-4   **Edinburgh Postnatal Depression Scale (Department of Psychiatry, University of Edinburgh)**

Name:
Address:
Infant's age:
Because you have recently had an infant, we would like to know how you are feeling. Please *underline* the answer that comes closest to how you have felt *in the past 7 days,* not just how you feel today.

Here is an example, already completed:

I have felt happy:

    All the time
    <u>Most of the time</u>
    Not very often
    Not at all

This choice means: "I have felt happy most of the time during the past week." Please complete the other questions in the same way.

In the past 7 days:

1. I have been able to laugh and see the funny side of things:
    As much as I always could
    Not quite so much now
    Definitely not so much now
    Not at all

2. I have looked forward with enjoyment to things:
    As much as I ever did
    Rather less than before
    Definitely less than before
    Hardly at all

*3. I have blamed myself unnecessarily when things went wrong:
    Most of the time
    Some of the time
    Not very often
    Never

4. I have been anxious or worried for no good reason:
    Not at all
    Hardly ever
    Sometimes
    Very often

*5. I have felt scared or panicky for no very good reason:
    Quite a lot
    Sometimes
    Not much
    Not at all

*6. Things have been getting on top of me:
    Most of the time I haven't been able to cope at all.
    Sometimes I haven't been coping as well as usual.
    Most of the time I have coped quite well.
    I have been coping as well as ever.

*7. I have been so unhappy that I have had difficulty sleeping:
    Most of the time
    Sometimes
    Not very often
    Not at all

*8. I have felt sad or miserable:
    Most of the time
    Quite often
    Not very often
    Not at all

*9. I have been so unhappy that I have been crying:
    Most of the time
    Quite often
    Only occasionally
    Never

*10. The thought of harming myself has occurred to me:
    Quite often
    Sometimes
    Hardly ever
    Never

Instructions for use:

1. The mother is asked to underline the response that comes closest to how she has been feeling in the previous 7 days.
2. All 10 items must be completed.
3. Care should be taken to avoid the possibility of the mother discussing her answers with others.
4. The mother should complete the scale herself, unless she has limited English or has difficulty with reading.
5. The EPDS may be used at 6 to 8 weeks to screen postnatal women. The child health clinic, postnatal check-up, or a home visit may provide suitable opportunities for its completion.

From Cox JL, Holden JM, Sagovsky R: Edinburgh postnatal depression scale, *Br J Psych* 150:782, 1989.
The EPDS was developed to assist primary care health professionals to detect mothers suffering from postnatal depression: a distressing disorder more prolonged than the 'blues' (which occur in the first week after delivery) but less severe than puerperal psychosis. The validation study showed that mothers who scored above a threshold 12/13 were likely to be suffering from a depressive illness of varying severity. Nevertheless, the EPDS score should *not* override clinical judgment. A careful clinical assessment should be performed to confirm the diagnosis. The scale indicates how the mother has felt *during the previous week,* and in doubtful cases it may be usefully repeated after 2 weeks. The scale will not detect mothers with anxiety neuroses, phobias, or personality disorders.
*Response categories are scored 0, 1, 2, and 3 according to increased severity of the symptoms. Items marked with an asterisk are reverse scored (i.e., 3, 2, 1, 0). The total score is calculated by adding together the scores for each of the 10 items.

EXPECTED OUTCOMES

- The client can describe self-care measures that may help coping and postpartum adjustment.
- The client can describe the difference between the "blues" and depression and knows when to seek help.
- Postpartum depression is recognized, and treatment is initiated.
- The mother receives adequate support in caring for her newborn.

NURSING INTERVENTION

Because nurses cannot predict with certainty which mothers will develop postpartum depression, it is important that all postpartum women and their families be educated. Ideally, this education begins in childbirth preparation classes and is reinforced during the postpartum period. The nurse's role includes teaching parents what the blues encompass and the difference between blues and depression. We know that more than half of all new mothers will experience the "blues." If the family is prepared, they can support the mother through this difficult time. Knowing that the "blues" are mild and temporary will enhance their seeking professional help early should the mother's depression become more severe or last longer than expected.

Health care providers need to focus special attention on the family and strengthen social supports so that the new mother gets adequate sleep, nutrition, and emotional support. After delivery of a new infant, the entire family's adaptation is best facilitated when the mother receives "mothering." While nurses often begin this nurturing process in the hospital, early discharge necessitates that the woman's supporters understand how to continue her care at home. Hansen (1990) advocates the following strategies:

- Get plenty of rest.
- Let friends and family help.
- Eat a well balanced diet that is low in salt and sugar and high in protein, complex carbohydrates, and green, leafy vegetables.
- Limit caffeine.
- Continue taking prenatal vitamins (extra B-complex may also help).
- Exercise briefly daily (one or two short walks a day to start).
- Take time for yourself.
- Make time for adult relationships.

Educating the family

Educating the client and family about signs and symptoms of postpartum blues and depression is critical. In general, clients should be told to seek help from their care-provider for symptoms that last longer than 2 weeks or seem to be getting worse. In addition, thoughts of harming oneself or the infant always warrant medical evaluation. Women and their partners need to know that they will not be labeled as "crazy," that depressive illness is fairly common, and that there is help available.

Support groups

Groups such as Depression After Delivery (DAD) and Postpartum Support International offer support to women experiencing postpartum depression. Many women find participation in a group helpful to their recovery. Being able to openly discuss fears and concerns with other mothers who have had similar experiences decreases the sense of isolation. Women experience increased hope that change and recovery are possible. Also, the partner may receive support and information about how he can help his partner (Berchtold and Burrough, 1990). Nurses who have contact with postpartum women should be prepared to make appropriate referrals to support groups.

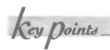

Key Points

- There are developmental crises and situational crises. Pregnancy is a developmental crisis in that it demands growth and coping in new ways. It may become a situational crisis if high-risk conditions are present.
- Spiritual distress arises from the deepest core of one's being and can be recognized by defining characteristics.
- Anxiety reduces the ability to perceive and communicate. Interventions are aimed at reducing anxiety to a level at which the client may cope with the threatening situation.

- Crisis presents an opportunity for growth or a danger of reduced functioning. Nursing interventions support coping.
- After any significant loss, some degree of grief and grief work is normal.
- Mothers and fathers grieve differently, and one parent may progress through the phases of grief more rapidly than the other, placing strain on the relationship.
- Nurses play an important role in facilitating healthy grieving by helping to create memories of the infant.

- Parents and their families need education about the grief process, autopsy, and funeral arrangements. A perinatal grieving team will prepare materials and provide support in a hospital setting.
- Postpartum depression often has a profoundly negative effect on the family, especially children.

- Nurses can facilitate the woman's physical and emotional recovery during the postpartum by teaching families how to support and care for the new mother at home.
- Postpartum families need to know the difference between the "baby blues" and postpartum depression so that they recognize when to seek professional help.

Study Questions

26-1. Select the terms that apply to the following statements:
   a. A state in which an individual experiences a disturbance in the belief or value system that supplies strength, hope, and meaning to life is called _____.
   b. An example of _____ occurs when a client promises to improve behavior in the future if the current distress will go away.
   c. The unexpected birth of an infant with a defect is a _____ crisis.
   d. Seeing and holding the dead infant helps parents to _____.
   e. Death of a fetus after the age of viability and before birth is a _____.
   f. Death of a live-born fetus, even though only a few breaths were taken, is termed a _____.
   g. When phases of grief differ in each parent problems may arise because of _____.

26-2. Choose a characteristic of the client who is experiencing moderate anxiety levels:
   a. Learns easily because this level increases activation and awareness
   b. Will forget instructions because of poor perception
   c. Requires a calming agent
   d. Needs a quiet, undemanding environment until levels diminish

26-3. It is important to teach women and their families about "baby blues" and postpartum depression because:
   a. Postpartum depression always requires hospitalization.
   b. Without early intervention, the "baby blues" will progress to postpartum psychosis.
   c. Postpartum depression occurs in the majority of postpartum women.
   d. The development of symptoms may confuse the family and lead to feelings of helplessness.

26-4. Choose whether the following statements are true or false.
   a. The "baby blues" generally last no longer than 5 days.
   b. Postpartum depression occurs in 25% of postpartum women.
   c. Children under the age of 5 should be protected from the facts of an infant's death.
   d. Excessive focus on symptoms indicates unresolved anxiety.

Answer Key

26-1: *a*, Spiritual distress; *b*, bargaining; *c*, situational crisis; *d*, confirm the loss; *e*, stillbirth or fetal demise; *f*, neonatal death; *g*, incongruent grieving. 26-2: *b*. 26-3: *d*. 26-4: *a*, True; *b*, False; *c*, False; *d*, true.

References

Aguilera DC: *Crisis intervention: theory and methodology,* ed 7, St Louis, 1994, Mosby.

*Baird SF: Crisis intervention strategies. In Johnson SH, ed: *Nursing assessment and strategies for the family at risk: high risk parenting,* ed 2, Philadelphia, 1986, Lippincott.

Beck C: Teetering on the edge: a substantive theory of postpartum depression, *Nurs Res* 42(1):42, 1992.

Beck C: The lived experience of postpartum depression: a phenomenological study, *Nurs Res* 41(3):166, 1993.

*Classic reference.

Beck C: Perceptions of nurses' caring by mothers experiencing postpartum depression, *J Obstet Gynecol Neonatal Nurse* 24(5):819, 1995.

Beck C, Reynolds M, Rutowski P: Maternity blues and postpartum depression, *J Obstet Gynecol Neonatal Nurs* 21(4):287, 1992.

Berchtold N, Burrough M: Reaching out: depression after delivery support group network, *NAACOG's Clinical Issues in Perinatal and Women's Health Nursing* 1(3):385, 1990.

Birenbaum L, Stewart B, Phillips D: Health status of bereaved parents, *Nurs Res* 45(2):105, 1996.

Boyer D: Prediction of postpartum depression, *NAACOG's clinical issues in perinatal and women's health nursing* 1(3):359, 1990.

Brost L, Kenney J: Pregnancy after perinatal loss: parental reactions and nursing interventions, *J Obstet Gynecol Neonatal Nurs* 21(6):457, 1992.

Caron S, Buster JE: Ectopic pregnancy, *N Engl J Med* 329:1174, 1993.

Carpenito L: *Nursing diagnosis: application to clinical practice,* ed 5, Philadelphia, 1993, Lippincott.

Casiano M: Outpatient medical management of postpartum psychiatric disorders, *NAACOG's clinical issues in perinatal and women's health nursing* 1(3):395, 1990.

Clement S: Listening visits in pregnancy: a strategy for preventing postnatal depression, *Midwifery* 11:75, 1995.

Corrine L et al: The unheard voices of women: spiritual interventions in maternal-child health, *MCN Am J Matern Child Nurs* 17(3):141, 1992.

Enkin M et al: *A guide to effective care in pregnancy and childbirth,* ed 2, Oxford, 1995, Oxford Univ Press.

Hansen C: Baby blues: identification and intervention, *NAACOG's clinical issues in perinatal and women's health nursing* 1(3):369, 1990.

*Hays D: Teaching a concept of anxiety, *Nurs Res* 10(2):108, 1961.

Ilse S: Reproductive losses: June 1990, Proceedings of the Hartford Hospital's Conference. Empty arms: the caregiver's role after miscarriage—stillbirth and infant death, Hartford, Conn,

*Infante MS: *Crisis theory: a framework for nursing practice,* Reston, Va, 1982, Reston.

Kellner R, Lake M: Grief counseling. In Knuppel RA, Drukker, JE, eds: *High-risk pregnancy: a team approach,* St Louis, 1993, Mosby.

Kendall-Tackett K, Kantor G: *Postpartum depression: a comprehensive approach for nurses,* Newbury Park, 1993, Sage Publications.

Kim MJ, McFarland GK, McLane AM: *Pocket guide to nursing diagnoses,* ed 5, St Louis, 1993, Mosby.

*Klaus MH, Kennell JH: Caring for the parents of a stillborn or an infant who dies. In Klaus MH, Kennell JH, eds: *Parent-infant bonding,* St Louis, 1982, Mosby.

Kowalski K: Loss and bereavement: psychological, sociological, spiritual, and ontological perspectives. In Simpson KR, Creehan PA, eds: *AWHONN's perinatal nursing,* AWHONN, 1996.

Lepper H, DiMatteo R, Tinsley B: Postpartum depression: How much do obstetric nurses and obstetricians know? *Birth* 21:149, 1994.

May A: Group work 2: using exercise to tackle postnatal depression, *Health Visitor* 69:146, 1995.

May J: Fathers: the forgotten parent, *Pediatr Nurs* 22(3):243, 1996.

*Nagai-Jacobson MG, Buckhardt MA: Spirituality cornerstone of holistic nursing practice, *Holist Nurs Pract* 3:18, 1989.

Ney P et al: The effects of pregnancy loss on women's health, *Soc Sci Med* 9:1193, 1994.

Page-Lieberman J, Hughes C: How fathers perceive perinatal death, *MCN Am J Maternal Child Nurs* 15:320, 1990.

*Peppers L, Knapp R: *Motherhood and mourning,* New York, 1980, Praeger.

*Peretz D: Development object relationships and loss. In Schoenberg B et al: *Loss and grief: psychological management in medical practice,* New York, 1970, Columbia Univ Press.

*Classic reference.

Price J, Stevens H, LaBarre M: Spiritual caregiving in nursing practice, *J Psychosoc Nurs* 33(1):5, 1995.

Richardson P: Women's experiences of body change during normal pregnancy, *Matern Child Nurs J* 19:93, 1990.

Richardson P: Body experience differences of women with pregnancy induced hypertension, *Matern Child Nurs J* 22:121, 1994.

Richardson P: Body experience differences of women with preterm labor, *Matern Child Nurs J* 24:5, 1996.

Ross L: The spiritual dimension: its importance to patients' well-being and quality of life, *Int J Nurs Stud* 32:457, 1995.

Stewart ES: Family centered care for the bereaved, *Pediatr Nurs* 21(2):181, 1995.

Stiles MK: The shining stranger: nurse-family spiritual relationship, *Cancer Nurs* 13(4):235, 1990.

Tunis SL, Golbus MS: Assessing mood states in pregnancy: survey of the literature, *Obstet Gynecol Surv* 46(6):340, 1991.

Ugarriza D: A descriptive study of postpartum depression, *Perspect Psychiatr Care* 31(1):25, 1995.

Van der Zalm J: The perinatal death of a twin: Karla's story of attaching and detaching, *J Nurse Midwife* 40:335. 1995.

Wheeler E, Gardner K: Nurses' and patients' perceptions of supportive nursing, *J NY State Nurses Assoc* 18(2):33, 1987.

Widerquist J, Davidhizar R: The ministry of nursing, *J Adv Nurs* 19:647, 1994.

*Zuravan S: Severity of maternal depression and three types of mother to child aggression, *Am J Orthopsychiatry* 59:377, 1989.

 Student Resource Shelf

Kendall-Tackett K: *Postpartum depression: a comprehensive approach for nurses,* Newbury Park, 1993, Sage Publications.
Written for nurses who work directly with or have contact with new mothers. A comprehensive discussion of the multifactoral causes of postpartum depression and specific nursing interventions that may help.

Lawson LV: Culturally sensitive support for grieving parents, *MCN Am J Matern Child Nurs* 15(2):76, 1990.
Identifies the cultural beliefs of Native American, Mexican-American, and Southeast Asian-American people and how these beliefs affect the grieving of parents following the death of an infant.

Yoder L: Comfort and consolation: a nursing perspective on parental bereavement, *Pediatric Nursing* 20(5):473, 1994.
Summarizes many aspects of nursing interventions for loss of a child, including questions about organ donation.

Resources for Parents

Depression After Delivery (DAD)
P.O. Box 1282
Morrisville, PA 19067

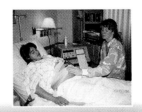

27

The Socially High-Risk Client

Learning Objectives

- Apply Maslow's theory of needs to the psychosocial care of women at high risk and to their families.
- Identify factors that place a woman at social high risk.
- Discuss differences between the adolescent woman and the adult woman who is abused or homeless.
- Identify the common licit and illicit drugs that are abused by the pregnant woman.
- Use findings from the woman's health history, physical examination, laboratory data, and screening instruments to identify pregnant women who abuse alcohol, tobacco, or other drugs.
- Structure a plan of care, including referral to other members of the health care team, for the abused woman.
- Discuss appropriate nursing interventions for the client who is pregnant and continuing to use alcohol, tobacco, and illicit drugs.
- Practice elements of the therapeutic nurse-client relationship with the socially high-risk client.

Key Terms

Developmental Crisis
Enabling and Empowering Model
Help-giver
Help-seeker
Hierarchy of Needs Theory
Illicit Drugs
Licit Drugs
Polydrug User
Self-Blame
Situational Crisis
Socially High-Risk Client
Substance Abuse

THE SOCIALLY HIGH-RISK PREGNANT CLIENT

One of the accepted roles of the nurse is that of help-giver. This role takes on additional significance when the nurse is caring for the **socially high-risk client.** For the purposes of this chapter, the socially high-risk client includes adolescents who are pregnant, those who have been victims of violence, homeless pregnant women, and those individuals who abuse substances. In addition, many of these adolescents and women may also have major concerns about their economic status and may have experienced educational or intellectual deprivation.

Basic Concepts

Abraham Maslow first described his **hierarchy of needs theory** in 1954. He stated that human beings have dynamic and fluid needs that motivate them to action and help create their personalities. The categories of need in Maslow's hierarchical list are (1) physiologic, (2) safety, (3) belongingness and love, (4) esteem, and (5) self-actualization. These needs are met in ascending order of importance. Until lower level needs are met, more advanced needs cannot be addressed.

The most basic needs are physiologic; if these are not met, disability or death can result. Safety needs constitute the next category. People who feel physically or psychologically threatened are unable to consider anything else unless they feel safe. The need for belongingness and love makes up the next level. People need to feel that they are cared for by others and crave the security of warm, close relationships. Esteem needs, which make up the next category, reflect human desire for self-respect. These needs also include the desire for strength, adequacy, mastery, competence, and independence and freedom (Maslow, 1970). As Maslow points out: "Satisfaction of these needs leads to feelings of self-confidence, worth, strength, capability and adequacy, of being useful and necessary in the world. Thwarting of these needs produces feelings of inferiority, of weakness, and of helplessness."

According to Maslow, the highest level need, which he identifies as interpersonal, is for self-actualization: the desire for self-fulfillment and the full use of one's talents, capacities, and potentialities. The expression of this need varies with the individual's situation. Figure 27-1 illustrates a conceptualization of the Maslow schema in which Mitchell (1973) arranged the needs in the shape of a pyramid to illustrate how they build on each other. An individual moves from one level to another and is influenced by positive and negative life events. Any crisis, whether it is a **developmental crisis** (graduating from college, entering adolescence) or **situational crisis** (loss of a job, marital discord leading to violence), can precipitate movement.

The **enabling and empowering model** was developed by Dunst, Trivette, and Deal (1988) as a model for use by health care providers working in the field of early intervention. This model has application to the care of the client (or family) who is characterized as "socially high-risk." Developed from a social systems perspective, this model takes a proactive approach to the helping relationship that values individual differences and builds on the strengths of each individual (family). It also focuses on the needs of the individuals (families) and not on those of the professional. Recognizing that all individuals (families) have strengths, efforts are made to build on these strengths to help the individuals (families) meet their identified needs.

The major emphases of the model are strengthening families and their natural support networks and enhancing families' abilities to acquire a wide variety of competencies to meet their needs by mobilizing their social support systems. Nurses caring for the pregnant woman are in a position to enable and empower this family or "family to be." Within this model, the client would be identified as the **help-seeker** and the nurse would be the **help-giver**. Help-givers should demonstrate behaviors that are likely to evoke positive, nondefensive attitudes in the help-seeker. These behaviors include providing positive help-giver attributions toward the help-seeker, limiting threats to the autonomy and self-esteem of the help-seeker, and giving help in a cooperative manner.

Application of Concepts to Nursing Role

It is recognized that many women identified as socially high-risk clients share a number of characteristics, such as low self-esteem, a history of substance abuse or violence, and poverty or homelessness. By blending the concepts of Maslow and Dunst, Trivette, and Deal, the nurse can provide a supportive, client-centered model of care. The nurse must establish a nurse-client relationship built on trust. Initially, this is accomplished by assessing whether the clients' basic needs for food, safety, positive relationships, and self-esteem are met. After this assessment, the nurse, as help-giver, can then utilize the enabling and empowering model to assist the help-seeker with appropriate interventions. Areas that the help-giver may focus on include identifying the clients' needs and aspirations, building on the individual's strengths in order to promote the client's mobilization of resources, assisting the client to strengthen personal and social networks, and, when appropriate, promoting the client's acquisition and use of competencies and necessary skills to become more self-confident and self-sustaining. It is recognized that the

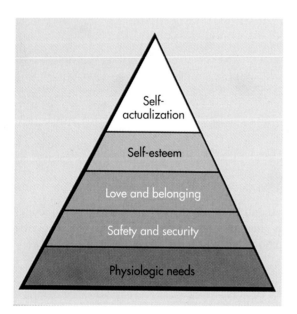

Figure 27-1 The Maslow model is pyramid-shaped, with the most basic needs forming the foundation. Needs are met in ascending order of importance.

person-in-environment must be seen as a whole. Thus it becomes apparent that poverty, racial barriers, drug abuse, and abuse within a family grouping have complex interacting factors. As a result, both the help-seeker and the help-giver must realize that care requires an on-going commitment from both the client and the nurse and that accomplishments are often small, occurring over an extended period of time.

Case example

Tanya comes into the prenatal clinic with her three-year-old child. She tells you she is 5 months pregnant. Her significant other was arrested yesterday and is in jail. Today when she went out to run an errand, her landlord locked her out. History reveals that she has not had any prenatal care and that she had a previous preterm infant who required 6 weeks' care in the neonatal intensive care unit (NICU). She indicates she is frantic because she has no place to go nor any funds. It is obvious that Tanya's basic needs are not being met. The initial need identified by Tanya and the nurse is for the provision of food and shelter. Tanya is referred to the local women's shelter, and arrangements are made for transportation. She is also seen by the nurse practitioner, and after an initial prenatal examination is conducted, it is determined she does not have a medical emergency. Appointments are made for follow-up for Tanya and her daughter.

The nature of the nurse-client relationship is best fostered by an objective, caring professional who helps the client identify self-care needs and the deficits in meeting those needs. The nurse plans *with*, not *for*, the client and family, thus helping the client move toward self-fulfillment. When these interventions reflect the client's resources and sociocultural network, the best result is obtained. The goal is to work with client, family, and community resources to formulate realistic plans, foster growth and independence, and prevent further disability, disease, or dysfunction, which is often accompanied by feelings of helplessness and hopelessness. Much of this theory is taught in social work programs. Nurses must recognize the client in a more holistic way, seeing each one as a person-in-environment (Figure 27-2).

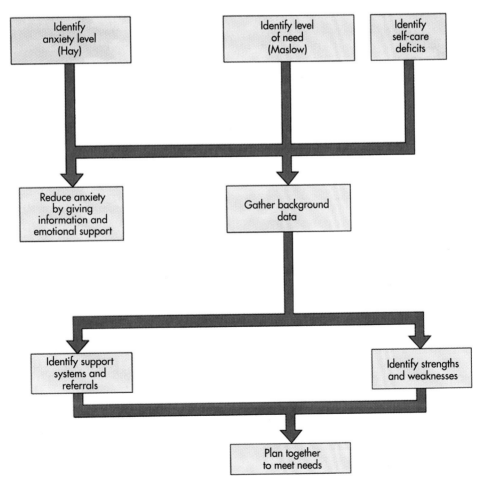

Figure 27-2   Model for provision of psychosocial care. (Courtesy JD Virzi and CA Moleti.)

Case example

Tanya continues to come to the prenatal clinic and is now in her eighth month of pregnancy. She continues to use the services provided by the shelter and is now living in a safe environment. Her daughter is well and "thriving." Tanya has developed a trusting relationship with the nurse practitioner and today reveals that she was abused during her last pregnancy and early in this pregnancy. She tells the nurse practitioner that her significant other is a drug dealer and has been sentenced to the state prison. Tanya has terminated this relationship. She is concerned how she will care for her daughter and the new infant. With the nurse practitioner's encouragement, Tanya develops a list of concerns. The practitioner helps Tanya develop a list of community resources, and the contact persons are provided. Tanya is encouraged to prioritize her concerns. She admits that she is unsure which concern is most important but says she will make one call before her visit next week.

Gutiérrez (1990) defines an escape from helplessness and hopelessness as a process of increasing personal, interpersonal, or political power so that individual persons can take action to improve their life situations. She identifies four associated psychologic interventions for moving the individual from apathy to action, which have application to the nurse's role in empowering clients:

1. *Increasing self-efficacy or the belief in one's own ability to act and regulate life events* (Bandura, 1982). Self-efficacy (a term also applied to early parenting behaviors) includes developing an increased ability to act because there is some success gained by action. For a person to have success, information is often a key: How to access the health care system? How to get food stamps? Who can help with a referral? Nurses are often involved with providing information that results in increased self-efficacy. Group discussions, interaction, and problem-solving strategies can empower members by allowing them to share problems and solutions, sympathy, and determination to improve a situation.

2. *Developing group consciousness.* The woman sees that she is not alone or stranded in an unintelligible, uncaring society. She begins to focus on causes of problems, not simply on results and her own feelings. She begins to seek ways of altering life situations.

3. *Reducing self-blame.* By raising consciousness, a person learns that outside forces may also be causing the current distress. Abused women may blame themselves for their abuse. **Self-blame** is often at the root of depression. A glimpse of an alternative way may start a person on health-seeking behaviors and may help separate false guilt from actual guilt.

4. *Recognizing personal accountability to change a situation.* A healthy response to a life problem is to begin looking for causes and solutions. Changing one's view of *self-as-victim* creates powerful energy for positive action.

It is also important to acknowledge that the nurse's needs cannot be neglected in this framework. Nurses who are unable to understand their own functioning when attempting to meet a client's needs may be unable to provide adequate care by assuming the role of help-giver. For example, a nurse's problems at home can be a stress factor as the nurse struggles to meet her own personal self-esteem and belongingness needs. Fear of physical harm may bring safety needs to the forefront and thus limit the nurse's ability to care for substance abusers who are at high risk for violent behavior and communicable diseases. Nurses must know their needs in order to choose the setting in which they can best work. As part of their professional education, they must learn how their own needs will affect their work. Judgmental behavior can result from fear for safety or a fear that similar problems can happen to oneself. The desire to *rescue* all clients (and the subsequent disappointment of failure) may result from intense self-esteem needs. Though this behavior is understandable and normal, it does get in the way of providing care. Maslow (1970) points out that most *need-motivated behavior is unconscious.* Thus nurses should become aware of their needs and the forces that drive them; then they can take action to satisfy them or prevent them from interfering with nursing care. For example, Selleck and Redding (1995) documented that many nurses who work with perinatal clients who abuse substances have negative attitudes that influence the quality of care they provide to their clients.

A nurse carries personal, racial, ethnic, and cultural biases into nursing practice. When a person is raised in a particular environment, it is often difficult to understand other lifestyles, belief systems, and customs. Again, nurses must learn to identify conflicts between their beliefs and clients' beliefs and deal with them rather than try to force personal beliefs, suggestions, or solutions on a client and family. Acquiring cultural competence is a lifelong process. The nurse must be willing to continue to improve his or her cultural awareness and to learn about clients. As society changes, populations within a community change, and there is a need to continue to learn both formally and informally. Box 2-3 identifies the characteristics of the culturally competent practitioner that are an essential component of the nursing role. The Maslow framework and the enabling and empowering model of Dunst, Trivette, and Deal provide a guide to understanding the care requirements for a client and family, their responses, and a workable approach to planning and interventions.

Overview of the Socially High-Risk Client

A variety of situations and social problems identify pregnant clients as socially high risk. For some clients, this designation is one that they have had for their entire life; for others, this designation will be temporary. Some clients do not see themselves in this high-risk category even though they have all the characteristics that identify them as socially high risk. These individuals may have accepted this situation as their fate in life, whereas others have learned to use the "system" effectively and are moving toward "self-actualization" as described by Maslow.

Many high-risk clients have had multiple social problems over a long time. The compounding factors may exacerbate each other. For example, the pregnant homeless mother may experience chronic deprivation in many areas of life, such as sexual abuse as a child, single parenthood, inadequate nutrition, and unemployment. Familial support systems are often nonexistent, overtaxed, or quite vulnerable to collapse under the burden of additional problems.

Being socially high risk may also be a complicating factor in women at risk for medical, surgical, or age-related complications. Being socially high risk can contribute directly or indirectly to the development of physical high-risk problems. For example, intravenous (IV) drug users are at physical risk for human immunodeficiency virus (HIV) infection and at psychosocial risk for child abuse and neglect.

Most socially high-risk clients are poor and members of minority groups. They may be recent immigrants who have entered the country illegally and are often afraid of being discovered. They may be unable to speak English. Their ethnic and cultural beliefs about health care and therefore their priorities are often not harmonious with those of their care providers. These clients are vulnerable to communicable diseases, substance abuse, inadequate housing, and inadequate nutrition. They are often reluctant to seek care because they do not perceive the need for it, are fearful, or cannot negotiate through the complex health care system because of language, literacy, or financial barriers.

Many clients and their families are in a continuous crisis. One problem may lead directly or indirectly to another. There is disorganization, anxiety, and irrational behavior, some of it violent. These clients present a great challenge to the help-givers, who are frequently overwhelmed by their clients' needs, the severity of their problems, and the lack of resources. Clients may be able to do little to help themselves or to seek help from others. They may be viewed as hostile, irresponsible, and seemingly disinterested, missing appointments and not following through with aspects of care. Help-givers must understand that this is not irresponsibility but rather a *manifestation of underlying hopelessness, helplessness, and depression*. Working with these clients who have such overwhelming needs and who may not trust the health care system becomes a real challenge for the help-giver. It is important to remember that it is not always possible to intervene with each client. What *is* important is to make the effort. Many times, repeated contacts are necessary before the client is able to trust in and accept assistance from a help-giver.

Adolescents

Adolescence is a period in which individuals experience many physical and emotional changes. Adolescents are especially influenced by their peers, and they experience great peer pressure to experiment with the "privileges" associated with impending adulthood. These "privileges" include using cigarettes, alcohol, and drugs; having sex; driving a car; becoming pregnant; getting married; and experiencing violence in many forms. In the world of the adolescent, these are identified as "risk-taking behaviors," which are considered a hallmark of their adolescence. Adolescents may rebel against the rules and regulations set by their parents, or if there is little structure in their lives, they may try to do things differently from the way they experienced things at home. As a result, they may seek alternatives that they believe will provide more stability, such as early marriage or pregnancy.

Early pregnancy, delinquency, poverty, and substance abuse are major health and social concerns for adolescents. *Healthy People 2000* (1991) has addressed all of these concerns related to the adolescent population. As a result, there is increased effort at the national level to improve the quality of the health of adolescents in these specific areas. As adolescents strive toward becoming self-actualized, they are faced with a variety of developmental crises. Families and communities must assist them by serving as role models and by providing the resources needed to support their self-esteem and movement toward maturity.

Factors that may result in adolescent pregnancy include risk taking, impulsiveness, lack of knowledge about contraception, substance abuse, and lack of communication between partners. Adolescent pregnancy occurs in all ethnic groups, and the rate continues to increase. As reported in *Healthy People 2000: Midcourse Review and 1995 Revisions*, the birth rate for girls aged 15 to 17 in 1985 was 70.9 per 1000, whereas in 1990 it was 74.3 per 1000. Pregnancy rates are higher among Hispanic and African-American girls, indicating that poverty has an influence on the pregnancy rates.

Koniak-Griffin and Brecht (1995) report that "being pregnant was highly predictive of the adolescent's engaging in unprotected sex *and* not having multiple sexual partners." The lack of condom use continues to be a major concern because of the risk of HIV transmission, as well as the risk of contracting sexually transmitted diseases (STDs).

The use of alcohol and other drugs plays a part in the incidence of adolescent pregnancy. Many individuals, including adolescents, view alcohol as enhancing their sexual performance and pleasure. Thus alcohol use might be considered a risk-taking behavior and may lead to pregnancy. Among adolescents, substance abuse is higher in white girls than in African-American girls, although sexual activity is higher in African-American girls. Alcohol, tobacco, and marijuana are the drugs used most frequently by pregnant adolescents. In general, there is a decrease in the use of alcohol and drugs during pregnancy (Cornelius et al, 1993; Koniak-Griffin and Brecht, 1995).

Adolescents are especially vulnerable to abuse and violence. It has been estimated that more than 50% of adolescents had children by men 20 years old or older. In some instances, the age span between the girl and boy is 3 to 4 years, but in others, the age span is greater. The sexual abuser may be a stepfather, a mother's partner, or a man who offers shelter to the homeless adolescent. Adolescent girls may also be the victim of incest involving fathers or brothers. The rate of incest is estimated to be 4% to 12%, although it is probably higher because of underreporting. Date rape is another cause of violence, which begins in middle school and continues into the college years, with few of these ever reported to authorities. The risk factors for date rape include the fact that it is a first date, a male-initiated date, the boy is the car driver, or the date is paid for by the boy. Alcohol and other drugs are frequently used by the perpetrator in these episodes of abuse or violence.

Abused women

Healthy People 2000 (1991) lists prevention of violence as one of the top 21 priorities for the nation. It is estimated that between 2 and 4 million women are physically abused each year by men, including husbands, former husbands, and significant others. Mental abuse and intimidation are components of many abuse incidents. Although the majority of studies have focused on a single ethnic group or women in poverty, it is estimated that approximately 11% to 23% of women have been assaulted. Abuse does not cease in pregnancy, and in those situations where abuse occurred before pregnancy, the abuse may actually escalate during pregnancy.

Poverty and homelessness

It is estimated that 1 of every 8 American individuals lives below the poverty line as a result of economic or immigration status. In addition, there is a large group of individuals and families who may fall below the poverty line as a result of the current trend during downsizing and elimination of some job categories. Poverty makes individuals and families vulnerable to injuries, disease, violence, poor nutrition, and poor pregnancy outcomes. In a study describing empowerment for women of color (e.g., Asian-Americans, Latinos, Native Americans, and African-Americans), Gutiérrez (1990) notes that among African-American women and Latinos, the poverty rate is 32% and 26%, respectively.

As a result of their poverty status, an increasing number of individuals and families are finding themselves homeless. The homeless are individuals who do not have a stable residence or a place where they can sleep and receive mail. The homeless population is estimated to be from 350,000 to 2 million, with families and children among the fastest growing group (25% of the total). The overwhelming majority of this fast-growing group is single women with children, many who are dependent on welfare.

Homeless women represent a vulnerable group who engage in high-risk behaviors, resulting in an increased risk for health-related disorders. Homeless mothers with children are less likely to have problems with alcohol abuse and psychiatric hospitalization. However, these same women appear to have less family or nonfamily ties and, as a result, less access to relatives who might serve as a safety net.

The adolescent homeless population may occur because of voluntary homelessness (runaways) (possibly the result of adolescents that leave abusive families or families that force them out), failures in the foster care system, and those living with homeless families (Institute of Medicine, 1988). Adolescents may have difficulty acquiring services because of their age and the possible need for parents' permission. In addition, if adolescents have a substance abuse problem, they are frequently excluded from treatment programs because of their age. Because most of these homeless adolescents have few marketable skills, they are frequently victimized, which places them at risk for participating in illicit activities. As a result, they are at high risk for physical and sexual abuse, STDs, and breaking the law.

Many of these socially high-risk women express feelings of hopelessness, helplessness, and depression. Maslow (1970) points out that *depression* can occur when the defensive efforts of a person fail because of overwhelming outside pressure or weak defense mechanisms. Deep hopelessness and discouragement have been described in people who have been exposed to extended disappointment, deprivation, or trauma. They often just give up trying because they see no benefit from their efforts. As previously stated, these clients pose a challenge to the help-giver, and the need for referral must be considered.

A person living in inadequate housing without sufficient food is meeting only basic physiologic and safety needs. To expect this person to be concerned about needs above this level (e.g., prenatal care) is not realistic. Unless she becomes so ill that it affects her daily functioning, the client will deal with the most pressing needs first. She cannot deal with well-child care and immunizations. Her primary concern is feeding her family and finding a safe place to live. The help-giver may find this client overwhelmed, anxious, and unable to focus on problem solving. She often is withdrawn. She denies her problems and deals only with what cannot be ignored. She often is angry at others, and this anger can lead to hostility or suicidal behavior, which may manifest in ways such as refusing treatment for life-threatening conditions or continuing to abuse alcohol and drugs. On the other hand, some socially high-risk clients are skilled manipulators who have survived by outsmarting others, including the legal system. Although illegal activities cannot be overlooked, the help-giver should acknowledge that manipulation may be the only coping strategy that some clients have.

Abuse during Pregnancy

When discussing abuse, a variety of terms are used, including spousal abuse, physical and emotional abuse, incest, rape, battering, violence, and assault. In each of these instances, it is most frequently the woman who is abused. Abuse occurs across every socioeconomic level; however, it is more prevalent where poverty, drug abuse, and racial barriers frustrate normal family life. In situations where abuse occurs, there is frequently a history of drug and alcohol abuse, often by both partners. When pregnancy occurs, it is a crisis that increases stress in an already stressed situation.

A deeply rooted feeling still exists that men are justified in abusing women because of an implicit right to control what is "theirs." Women who make and carry out choices may find themselves victims of violence as their partners feel threatened by their move toward independence. Only recently have abusive men begun to be punished, and this is done unevenly at best. Restraining orders are available for spouse abuse, but the deep-rooted causes of abuse will often reassert themselves despite these restraints. Indeed, it is often after a woman leaves the abusive spouse that he attempts to severely injure or kill her.

The problem of abused women, children, and elders did not suddenly escalate in this society. It has always been present, but it was largely ignored until recently. Mandatory reporting of child abuse is now the law. Because the urban setting reduces neighborliness, spousal violence is less often reported. There is now increased recognition of elder abuse, which occurs in the family setting and in institutional settings.

Physical abuse during pregnancy has been identified as a form of child abuse. Another form of prenatal child abuse is Munchausen syndrome, in which the mother induces preterm delivery. If the infant does survive the effects of prematurity, the mother may then fabricate illnesses in the child, which continue until the intervention or death of the child. This type of abuse is known as Munchausen syndrome by proxy, in which the mother is seen as the child's advocate and suggests a variety of treatments. When this syndrome is recognized and the child is protected from the mother, the child usually recovers.

Women who have been abused before pregnancy may continue to be abused throughout the pregnancy. In some instances, there may be an increase in violence, occurring in any or all trimesters of pregnancy. Common sites for abuse include the head, abdomen, breasts, and extremities.

Risk factors

Although abuse occurs at every socioeconomic level of society, it is recognized that there is a variety of factors other than pregnancy that places the woman at risk for abuse. Parker, McFarlane, and Soeken (1994) differenti-

ated between factors for adolescents and factors for adult women (Box 27-1). Additional factors include prior abuse, alcohol or drug dependence in the male partner, violence in the family of origin of either partner, low socioeconomic status, unemployment, violence directed toward the fetus, sexual frustration, stress of family transition, biochemical changes, defenselessness of the pregnant women, or the woman being divorced or separated.

Differences between adolescents and adult women. There are some differences between the adolescent woman and the adult woman who is abused. As noted in Box 27-1, there are different risk factors. Parker et al (1993) found an abuse rate during pregnancy of 21.7% for adolescents and 15.9% for adult women. Adolescents were abused by a nonintimate partner more frequently than were adult women.

Adult women are often the victims of more severe physical violence and more mental abuse than adolescents. They are also more prone to injury as they attempt to protect themselves, suffering additional injuries as a result. These injuries often occur to extremities as they try to protect themselves from blows.

Nursing interventions

Pregnancy may be the only time in her life that a healthy woman seeks health supervision. For the abused woman, this is an opportune time to assess and intervene in a private, confidential manner. The woman can be counseled about personal safety and be given information about options for dealing with the abuse. Assessment for abuse must be a standard of care for all pregnant women. It is important for the nurse to ask the woman about abuse at each prenatal visit, at delivery, and during the postpartum period, because it may occur at any point during the childbearing cycle.

During the taking of admission history and the physical examination, the nurse uses a screening tool such as the *Abuse Assessment Screen* in Figure 27-3. This screening tool allows the nurse to bring up the subject with the client, remembering the concept of the person-in-environment, to discover what feelings the woman may be able to

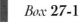

Box 27-1	Differences in Risk Factors for Abuse During Pregnancy

ADOLESCENTS	ADULT WOMEN
Poor weight gain	Poor obstetric history
First or second trimester bleeding	Infections
	Short interpregnancy interval (less than 24 months)
Smoking	Anemia
Alcohol or drug use	Smoking
	Alcohol or drug use

Modified from Parker, McFarlane, Soeken (1994).

share. It is important to remember that these questions should be asked at each visit. As a help-giver, the nurse is in a position to assist the help-seeker build on personal strengths, however limited they may be.

The nurse uses strategies such as the following to assess the woman's situation:

1. *Help the client identify the most serious problem from her point of view.*

2. *With the client, identify support systems in her family and the community.* Does she have family, friends, or a church group to which she belongs? Is she connected to the social service system for public assistance, Medicaid, or food stamps?

3. *Help her differentiate between chronic and acute problems.* The problems that have existed for an extended time, although serious, generally will not be the client's priority. Often asking, "What brought you in today?" will help elicit this information.

4. *Ask her to identify how she has coped with similar problems.* Her resourcefulness is often amazing, and any positive coping strategies should be identified and encouraged. Past maladaptive coping behaviors such as avoidance or denial are not desirable and should not be supported.

5. *Strive to understand what the diagnosis and consequences of a high-risk pregnancy mean from the client's and the family's perspective.* Ask the woman to describe what the physician has told her. Clarify information. Find out how her partner feels about the situation.

6. *Encourage clients to use their extended family and community supports.*

By using these strategies during assessment, the nurse can enable and empower her client. In addition, the concept of Maslow's hierarchy of needs should be kept in mind so that assessment as to where the woman is on the continuum of needs can begin. Next, the level of anxiety must be assessed. In cases of severe anxiety or panic, before any other thing can be accomplished, this level must be reduced by giving support and information that address concerns. General background data must be gathered to identify needs or potential problems that may interrupt a healthy outcome of the pregnancy. It is always helpful to write a list of the problems and issues and make a note of which of these demonstrate strengths, which are weaknesses, and which are merely neutral. The strengths should be built upon. The weaknesses must be addressed and modified to lessen their impact. Neutral factors have the potential to become strengths or weaknesses.

ABUSE ASSESSMENT SCREEN

1. Have you ever been emotionally or physically abused by your partner or someone important to you?

YES ☐

NO ☐

2. Within the last year, have you been hit, slapped, kicked, or otherwise physically hurt by someone?

YES ☐

NO ☐

If YES, by whom _____

Number of times _____

Mark the area of injury on body map.

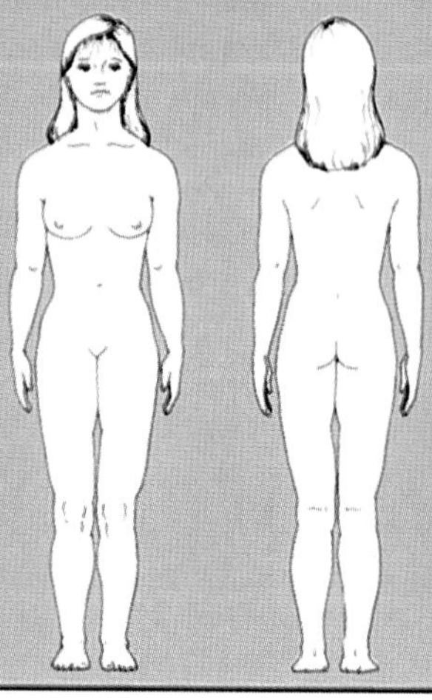

3. Within the last year, has anyone forced you to have sexual activities?

If YES, whom _____

Number of times _____

4. Are you afraid of your partner or anyone you listed above?

YES ☐

NO ☐

Figure 27-3 Abuse Assessment Screen. Developed by the Nursing Research Consortium on Violence and Abuse 1989. Readers are encouraged to reproduce and use this assessment tool.

After assessment, the help-giver plans care with the client. It is important to assist the client in identifying realistic short-term goals. It is not appropriate to expect quick solutions for chronic problems. The nurse cannot rescue the client or remove the pain and anxiety she and her family may feel. She *can*, however, facilitate the family's development of coping skills by using the techniques of crisis intervention. The client should be encouraged to take charge of her life and begin solving the less-pressing problems. When the client meets her own goals, these small victories will increase her self-esteem and create a positive outlook. The process is continuous. The input of other care providers is vital. In many constructive care situations, the nurse will simply be the coordinator or case manager. Figure 27-2 illustrates this model for psychosocial care.

Not all clients will accept help, and some refuse it or will not comply. Many more will respond to what is often one of the first instances of understanding they have experienced and may be motivated to make real and lasting changes in their lives. Although care of high-risk clients is difficult, the rewards are great.

Specific nursing interventions for the woman who is in an abusive situation include the following: care for any acute injuries, discussion of an exit plan, information on how to seek assistance if injured, and availability of community resources including shelters and the legal system. Many of these women do not want to leave their home or seek legal intervention. However, the help-giver must provide information so that the woman is enabled to seek assistance when needed. If the woman has access to all of this information, it will be readily available to her when she is in a crisis situation. It is also recommended that the abused pregnant woman be seen more frequently by health care providers so that the woman has consistent access to a support system.

Poverty and Homelessness

Receiving adequate nutrition and prenatal monitoring and controlling gynecologic disease and hypertension are important factors of a healthy pregnancy. Many women in poverty and those who are homeless have limited or no access to any health care. As noted by Gutiérrez (1990), the poverty rate is above 25% among African-American women and Latinos. Poverty and powerlessness are often linked.

Pregnancy in a homeless individual is indeed a high-risk situation. It is estimated that the pregnancy rate among homeless women is twice as high as the rate for the general population. Possible reasons include uncertain fertility, limited access to contraception, rape, and the use of sex to gain necessities. Some of the women also feel empowered by pregnancy and a sense of control and ownership engendered by being pregnant and giving birth (Killion, 1995).

Adverse pregnancy outcomes occur with homeless women because they have less access to health care, are poorly nourished, and have limited access to substance treatment programs. In addition, the physiologic changes of pregnancy are often burdensome. Discomforts are more pronounced; for instance, feelings of needing to void frequently are a problem when the woman must use a communal bathroom or public facilities, which are often at a distance and not clean. As a result, there is increased incidence of urinary tract infections, which may precipitate preterm delivery (Killion, 1995). (See Research Box.)

Risk factors

There is a variety of risk factors that places adolescents and women at risk for homelessness. These factors include poorly paid jobs, unemployment, substandard housing, low educational levels, substance abuse, mental illness, and single parent families. Minority populations and recent immigrants are also at risk. For example, 32% of African-Americans live below the poverty line, and the Laotians also have a high poverty rate (*Healthy People 2000*, 1991).

RESEARCH

PURPOSE OF STUDY
To examine the relationship between abuse during pregnancy and acknowledged risk factors for low birth weight.

LITERATURE REVIEW
Many risk factors have been associated with low birth weight, including demographic factors such as age, race, education, and marital status; prepregnancy medical risks such as poor weight gain, anemia, and infections; medical risks in pregnancy; behavioral risks such as smoking and alcohol; and health risks such as abuse or limited prenatal care.

METHOD
A sample of 1203 pregnant women with a mean age of 20 to 29 years was included in this study. The Abuse Assessment Screen determined the frequency and severity of abuse and injuries. The Conflict Tactics Scale measured the self-reported frequency of conflict resolution tactics.

FINDINGS AND IMPLICATIONS FOR PRACTICE
Abused women are more likely to begin prenatal care during the third trimester of pregnancy. Abuse during pregnancy is a significant risk factor for maternal complications in pregnancy and low infant birth weight. Strategies for effective interventions include education for women, advocacy for safe living, and community referrals.

McFarlane J, Parker B, Soeken K: Abuse during pregnancy: associations with maternal health and infant birth weight, *Nurs Res* 45(1):37, 1996.

Differences between adolescents and adult women.
There is little literature available about homeless women who are pregnant. Adolescents and adult women who are homeless have the same basic needs. Adult women may have more life experiences and, if they have had other children, more knowledge of pregnancy itself. In addition, they may have had more experience with the health care system and are better able to access care. Because of her lack of role models and lack of health care and pregnancy experiences, the adolescent who is pregnant and homeless is more vulnerable to obstetric complications and preterm delivery.

Pregnant homeless adolescents report higher rates of abuse, suicide attempts, depression, family conflict, and drug use than do those who are not homeless. Because of substance abuse, they often fail to access prenatal care. One reason for this is that the homeless adolescent is less likely to stop using alcohol or drugs than the adolescent who is not homeless. STDs are common among homeless adolescents. As a result, they are at a high risk for infection with and transmission of HIV. Providing free services to street youth on a voluntary basis, which allows care to be immediately accessible and on site, is one method of care that continues to be effective with adolescents.

Nursing interventions

Homeless people will use services if they are readily available and offered in a nonjudgmental manner. Because of the overwhelming problems of safety, transportation, lack of finances to purchase needed medications and equipment, frequent change of sleeping arrangements, and distrust of the health care system, services may go unused or underused. The concept of "one-stop shopping" for services, such as the placement of services in a shelter or next to a soup kitchen or the availability of a mobile clinic, seems to increase use (Figure 27-4). Help-givers must show respect for the homeless person as an individual who has dignity and self-worth.

Making services available on site recognizes that each person can be enabled and empowered. Assessing at what level of Maslow's hierarchy the individual is will help the nurse meet the woman's needs at the appropriate level. In addition, on-site services recognize that there is a need to establish trust with the homeless individual in her own "place." In addition, some of the help-giver barriers are lowered as the help-seeker is met on her own "turf."

Initial assessment and physical examination provides an opportunity to establish a connection with the health care system. Standard history formats that include infor-

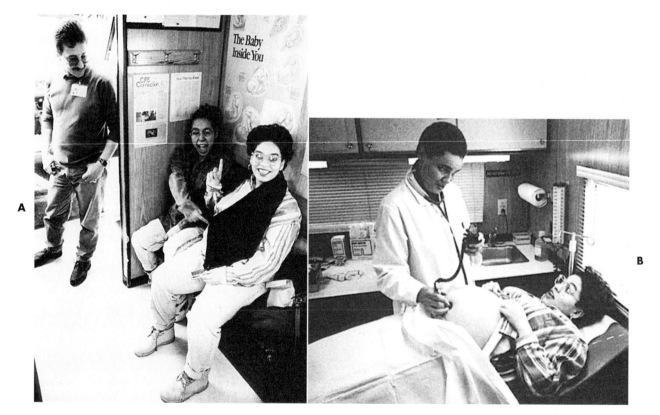

Figure 27-4 All prenatal services are located in the mobile clinic so that homeless women on the street and in shelters do not have to wait long hours for care. (Courtesy Ross Whitaker, Community Family Planning Council, New York, NY.)

mation on high-risk behaviors should be used. The help-giver should be comfortable with asking questions regarding all high-risk behaviors, including those specific to substance abuse and sexual practices. By asking questions, the help-giver is actually helping the client identify high-risk behaviors, often resulting in opportunities to initiate discussions regarding "safe" practices.

Instructions given regarding medications and treatments should be realistic within the limitations of the client's situation. For instance, clients may not have a watch to take medications every 8 hours. Giving direc-

tions to take them upon arising, before going to bed, and sometime in between will be more realistic.

For the pregnant client who is homeless, critical information and strategies for self-care as a person-in-environment should be provided. Providing information on available community resources is important. The nurse should find ways to assist the client in reconnecting to previous support systems. More frequent contact with the health care system may be one method of providing a link to a caring environment (see the Nursing Care Plan).

Nursing Care PLAN | *Pregnancy of the Abused Woman*

CASE
Molly A, 28, arrives for her first prenatal visit, accompanied by her 3-year-old daughter. She is in her third trimester. Physical examination reveals large bruises on her abdomen, breasts, and arms. When questioned, Molly initially indicates she fell down the stairs. As the nurse practitioner continues with the examination, Molly admits that her husband, who has a history of alcohol abuse, beat her.

Assessment
1. Health history, including use of Abuse Assessment Screening instrument
2. Physical examination
3. Does Molly have access to a safe place?
4. Does Molly use alcohol, tobacco, or drugs?

Nursing Diagnoses
1. Anxiety, related to physical abuse by husband
2. Denial, ineffective, related to delay in seeking prenatal care
3. Family process, altered, related to unmet need for security
4. Injury, risk for, related to actual abuse by husband

Expected Outcomes
1. Anxiety will be managed with continuing contact with her nurse practitioner.
2. Client acknowledges that she is in danger.
3. Client develops a plan for personal safety for self and child.
4. Client accepts referral information for social worker, police, and shelter.

Nursing Interventions
1. Assess potential for violence using screening instruments (Abuse Assessment Screen)
2. Provide supportive environment through use of nurse-client relationship
3. Assess if client has a plan for personal safety of self and child
4. Provide information on resources specific to personal safety
5. Help client develop a plan for personal safety
6. Refer client to local Al-Anon meeting for information and support
7. Provide client with phone numbers in the event of imminent threat to her survival
8. Provide referral to community resources: legal aid, domestic violence program, shelter, police

Evaluation
1. Did client acknowledge that she is in an unsafe environment?
2. Did client realize that she alone is not the cause of the abuse?
3. Did client receive adequate information on community resources to make a contact?
4. Has client prepared a plan for personal safety?
5. Has client identified a support person (neighbor) who will serve as her personal contact?
6. Did client need to implement her exit plan?
7. Does client have phone numbers of contacts: police, legal aid, shelter?

Substance Abuse

Substance abuse occurs in all socioeconomic and all cultural groups for a variety of reasons. When substance abuse occurs in a woman who is pregnant, there is concern for her and her unborn child. It is suggested that the woman who is planning a pregnancy should abstain from alcohol, tobacco, and other drugs for several months before pregnancy. All of these substances are teratogenic and may cause problems in the pregnancy itself and in the fetus during the "critical periods" of development (see Chapter 28 for a discussion of teratogens).

Licit drugs are those that, though legal, are often abused and lead to a high-risk situation for the pregnant woman, such as alcohol abuse and nicotine use. **Illicit drugs** are those that are not legal and include cocaine, marijuana, and opiates. It is also important to recognize that many individuals who abuse drugs are **polydrug users,** that is, using more than one drug at the same time. In fact, most have a drug of choice but will use another when their drug is unavailable, often combining licit and illicit drugs.

The following facts provided by the 1992 National Household Survey on Drug Abuse are specific to women of childbearing age:

- Although there has been a decrease in the use of alcohol and drugs by American women in the past 16 years, the rate of alcohol and marijuana use by adolescents has increased.
- An estimated 2.2 million women 12 years of age and older have engaged in heavy alcohol use during the previous 30 days (5 or more drinks per occasion on 5 or more days).
- Women in their prime childbearing years (18 to 25 years) are most likely to have engaged in heavy drinking (6.5% versus 2.1% for women overall).
- It is estimated that 10.7 million American women over age 12 may abuse alcohol.
- Caucasian women are slightly more likely to use alcohol once a week or more than are African-American women (12.3% compared to 10.4%) and much more likely than are Hispanic women (8%).
- Of the survey respondents, 14.1% reported using an illicit drug during the preceding month, 2.9% had used marijuana, and an estimated 0.4% had used cocaine (US Department of Health and Human Services, 1993). Finally, it is estimated that 375,000 newborns are born each year who have been prenatally exposed to at least one illegal drug.

Risk factors

There are a variety of risk factors identified with substance abuse by women of childbearing age. Many of these risk factors can be identified and include the following:

- Family history of substance abuse
- History of physical, sexual, or emotional abuse
- History of partner or significant other using alcohol or drugs
- History of chaotic, unstable lifestyle (homelessness)
- History of conflict, lack of cohesion, and poor parenting role models
- History of problems in school or with the law
- History of suffering from poor self-esteem, hopelessness, helplessness, and depression

Common licit drugs of abuse

For many women, it may be the use of alcohol and nicotine that affects the outcome of a pregnancy. Both of these drugs are an integral part of our society and are used without legal consequences. The use of these drugs in the first 8 weeks places the fetus at risk for a variety of problems, which may include obvious birth defects and subtle behavioral and developmental abnormalities. Some of these defects may be obvious at birth, but many may not be recognized until the child enters the school system.

Alcohol. Alcohol is considered a central nervous system depressant. In small amounts it induces feelings of relaxation and a sense of well-being. In large amounts, it may lead to intoxication, respiratory depression, and even death. Women who are chronic users of alcohol experience many medical complications that place a fetus at risk for fetal alcohol syndrome or alcohol-related effects. Alcohol readily crosses the placenta. Alcohol and its primary metabolite, acetaldehyde, are directly toxic to the fetus. (See Table 27-1 for further effects on the pregnancy, fetus, and the infant.) In 1994 53% of mothers reported taking one drink or less per week. There is no "safe" time to consume alcohol or "safe" amount to consume. Alcohol use is underreported, and there is risk of low birth weight infants when mothers drink several times per week (Ventura et al, 1996).

Nicotine. In 1995, cigarettes were added to the list of substances tracked as part of the *Healthy People 2000* study. The rationale for this addition is that tobacco use has been identified as a "gateway" to the use of alcohol and other drugs (*Healthy People 2000: Midcourse Review and 1995 Revisions*). It is estimated that 20% to 30% of all low birth weight infants are the result of maternal cigarette smoking. In 1990, the U.S. Department of Health and Human Services attributed 10% of all fetal deaths to cigarette smoking. It is estimated that 14% of pregnant women smoke (Ventura et al, 1996).

 Box 27-1

CLINICAL DECISION

Betty R. is in her fifth month of pregnancy. During your initial assessment, she tells you that she enjoys having a glass of wine on the weekend. What strategies would you include in her plan of care and why?

Table 27-1   Effects of Selected Drugs on Pregnancy, the Fetus, and the Newborn or Infant

Pregnancy	The Fetus	Newborn or Infant
ALCOHOL		
Abruptio placentae	Fetal demise	Hypertonia
IUGR		Low birth weight
Spontaneous abortion		Poor habituation
Vaginal bleeding		Poor sucking
		Sleeping disorders
		Tremors
		Withdrawal

CHARACTERISTICS OF FETAL ALCOHOL SYNDROME
- Prenatal or postnatal growth retardation: weight, length, or head circumference below tenth percentile
- Central nervous system involvement: neurologic abnormality, developmental delay, or intellectual impairment
- Characteristic facial dysmorphology: small palpebral fissure, fat maxillary area, microcephaly, poorly developed philtrum, thin upper lip

Pregnancy	The Fetus	Newborn or Infant
COCAINE		
Abruptio placentae	Fetal growth retardation	Increased congenital anomalies
Premature rupture of membranes	Fetal hyperactivity	Increased muscle tone
Preterm labor	Fetal hypoxia	Increased risk of SIDS
Poor weight gain	Fetal tachycardia	Inconsolability
		Irritability
		Low birth weight
		Reduced head circumference
		Tremors
MARIJUANA		
Spontaneous abortion	None identified	Altered visual response pattern
Stillbirth with high doses		Exaggerated startle response
		Increased tremulousness
		Low birth weight
		Marked epicanthal folds
		Poor habituation
		Withdrawal-like crying
NICOTINE		
Abruptio placentae	Blood vessel constriction leading to hypoxia	Birth weight less than 7 lbs
Increased frequency of spontaneous abortion	Fetal demise	Decreased head circumference
Placenta previa		Decreased length
Premature rupture of membranes		Developmental lag
Preterm labor		Increased incidence of SIDS
Vaginal bleeding		Increased respiratory difficulties
OPIATES		
Increased risk of abruptio placentae	Fetal demise	Brain hemorrhage
Breech presentation	IUGR	Cardiac and genitourinary infection
Placental insufficiency	Meconium aspiration	Increased risk of HIV infection
Preterm labor		Small head circumference
Risk of STD or HIV infection		Respiratory distress syndrome

CNS, Central nervous system; *GI*, gastrointestinal; *HIV*, human immunodeficiency virus; *IUGR*, intrauterine growth retardation; *NS*, nervous system; *SIDS*, sudden infant death syndrome; *STD*, sexually transmitted disease.

Continued.

| Table **27-1** | Effects of Selected Drugs on Pregnancy, the Fetus, and the Newborn or Infant—cont'd |

Pregnancy	The Fetus	Newborn or Infant
OPIATES—CONT'D		Neonatal abstinence syndrome CNS: Abnormal suck, hyperirritability, hypertonia, irritability, poor feeding, seizures Skin: Abrasions GI: Diarrhea or vomiting Respiratory: Hyperapnea, respiratory alkalosis tachycardia Autonomic NS: Hyperpyrexia, lacrimation, sneezing, sweating, yawning,
METHADONE	IUGR	Neonatal abstinence syndrome Hyperthyroid state Seizures SIDS Thrombocytosis

Nicotine is the psychoactive substance found in cigarettes. As a drug, it produces both stimulation and relaxation. Nicotine crosses the placenta and is able to produce harmful effects to the blood vessels, resulting in fetal hypoxia. (See Table 27-1.)

Researchers are finding that combining nicotine and alcohol may result in additional risks for the fetus. For example, both of these drugs result in low birth weight, and the infant born to the woman who uses both drugs may be lower in weight than the infant born when only one of the drugs is used. The pregnant woman who smokes and consumes alcohol should be informed of the risks and should be encouraged to decrease or stop alcohol and nicotine intake (Box 27-2).

Common illicit drug use

The use of illicit drugs varies somewhat by geographic area. For the purpose of this chapter, cocaine, marijuana, and the opiates, including narcotics, heroin, and methadone, are discussed.

Cocaine. Cocaine, a stimulant drug, affects the central nervous system by blocking the reuptake of neurotransmitters. Cocaine can be used intranasally, subcutaneously, intravascularly, or intramuscularly. Crack is a form of cocaine that is smoked. The cocaine user experiences a

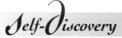

Self-Discovery

How do you respond to this photograph? How does the media glamorize smoking among young women? ~

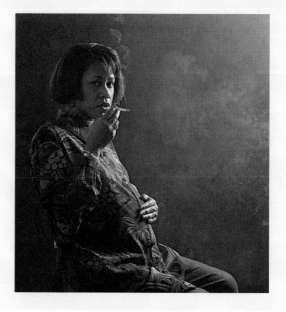

(Courtesy American Cancer Society, Inc.)

Box **27-2**

TEACHING PLAN *for* HOME CARE

Guide for Smoking Cessation for Pregnant Adolescents

INCIDENCE
- 25% to 30% of women of reproductive age smoke
- Number of female adolescents who smoke continues to increase
- Percentage of women who quit smoking during pregnancy continues to decrease: 39% in 1985 versus 31% in 1991

POSITIVE OUTCOME FOR SMOKING CESSATION
- If a pregnant woman stops smoking by 16 weeks of gestation, she has no greater risk of having a low birth weight infant than does the woman who does not smoke

DANGERS OF NICOTINE USE
- Cigarette smoking is the single most preventable cause of death in the United States
- Smoking is strongly associated with other substance use
- Increased risk of spontaneous abortion, abruptio placentae, premature rupture of membranes, preterm delivery
- Increase in number of obstetric complications
- Lower birth weight (mean difference 200 g), shorter body length, smaller head circumference
- 40% increase in perinatal mortality rate
- Increased risk of sudden infant death syndrome (SIDS) in infant
- Increased risk of vascular-related diseases later in child's life
- Increased rate of hospitalization of infants for pneumonia and bronchitis during first year
- Increased incidence of upper respiratory and middle ear infections in children exposed to cigarette smoke

WITHDRAWAL SYMPTOMS FROM NICOTINE
- Usually occur within 24 hours of smoking cessation
- Usually appear if the client attempts to decrease the number of cigarettes to 10 or fewer per day
- Actually indicate that the body is recovering from the effects of nicotine

- The smoker who stops or cuts down will have the following symptoms of withdrawal:
  Dizziness
  Headache
  Tiredness
  Coughing
  Tightness in the chest
  Sleeping difficulties
  Constipation
  Hunger
  Lack of concentration
  Craving for cigarettes
  Possible depression

INTERVENTIONS THAT MAY HELP TO DECREASE THE SYMPTOMS:
- Relaxing, exercising, sipping or drinking lots of water, eating low-calorie snacks, avoiding caffeine drinks in the evening

IF THE CLIENT HAS *STOPPED* SMOKING
- Nicotine gum may help reduce the symptoms of withdrawal
- Refer client to physician or nurse practitioner for treatment of symptoms if they persist or if the client does not find relief from supportive interventions

INTERVENTIONS THAT MAY SUPPORT THE CLIENT IN BREAKING THE SMOKING HABIT:
- Help client identify cues associated with smoking and modify cues
- Avoid individuals who continue to smoke
- Avoid places where smoking occurred
- Establish rewards for nonsmoking
- Ask friends and family not to offer cigarettes
- Engage in activities that keep hands busy
- Change routines during high-risk situations
- Declare certain places nonsmoking
- Encourage partner to provide support for the client who is attempting to cut down on or stop smoking

---

rush of pleasurable sensations and mood elevation. These pleasurable sensations soon give way to depression, fatigue, and the desire for more cocaine. Physical effects of cocaine use include vasoconstriction, hypertension, and tachycardia, which may lead to arrhythmias, cerebrovascular accidents, myocardial infarction, pulmonary edema, and death (Figure 27-5).

Readily crossing the placenta, cocaine and its metabolites act as a vasoconstrictor and may cause atresias, infarcts, and terminal limb defects in the fetus. Neurobehaviorally, these infants may have cerebral irritability with abnormal elec-

troencephalograms (EEGs), although most EEGs are normal by 3 to 12 months. Infants may be stressed at birth with irritability, abnormal cries, and abnormal state behaviors (Cook, Peterson, Moore, 1990). (See Table 27-1 for further effects on the pregnancy, fetus, and the infant.)

Marijuana. Marijuana is the most frequently used illicit drug in the United States. The use of marijuana usually decreases with the diagnosis of pregnancy, and this decrease continues throughout pregnancy. Marijuana may be ingested or smoked. Heavy users are at risk for respiratory problems similar to those experienced by cigarette smokers.

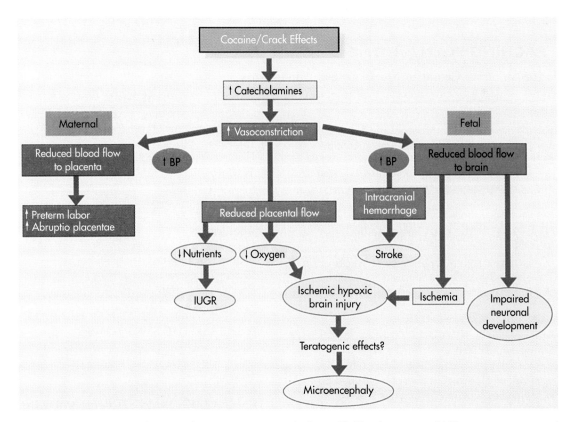

Figure 27-5   Pathway of injuries from cocaine or crack abuse. *BP,* Blood pressure; *IUGR,* intrauterine growth retardation.

The major psychoactive ingredient is delta-9 tetrahydro-cannabinol (THC). Marijuana readily crosses the placenta, although the drug level is much lower for the fetus. (See Table 27-1.)

Opiates. Opiates, also known as narcotics, act primarily on the central nervous system. These illicit drugs include therapeutic medications such as codeine, morphine, and methadone (used to treat opiate dependency) and heroin. Effects of opiate drugs include drowsiness, mental changes, and pain reduction. They cross the placenta, but their level is lower in the fetus than in the mother. As a result, opiates produce an unstable uterine environment that puts the fetus at risk.

Heroin can be inhaled, smoked, or injected under the skin. It is a potent analgesic, producing respiratory depression and euphoria. As the drug is metabolized, the user has a strong desire to repeat these sensations, followed by a feeling of physical discomfort. The drive to use heroin soon supersedes all other drives, leading to social isolation from anything not associated with drug use. Physical dependence follows, and because heroin easily crosses to the fetus, fetal dependence is also created. Heroin is also an appetite suppressant, and as a result, the fetus may receive inadequate nourishment. In addition, there is increased risk of HIV transmission because the woman may be sharing needles for drug use.

Methadone. Methadone is used to treat heroin addiction. Because it is similar to morphine and heroin but has a much longer half-life, it may be given once a day. Methadone maintenance (MM) programs are functioning in most larger cities in the United States. Methadone has been used successfully with pregnant women. However, close supervision is indicated. Methadone obtained from a maintenance program increases the woman's contact with health care providers, which should improve the woman's participation in prenatal care. With methadone, fetal weight is less severely affected and fetal demise is lessened. However, both heroin and methadone result in withdrawal in the newborn. (See Table 27-1.)

Nursing interventions

Working with pregnant women who abuse drugs is often frustrating. Many of these women have difficult life circumstances and appear uncooperative, hostile, and suspicious of the help-giver. The ability to recognize the client's basic needs on her first contact with the health care system is essential. The establishment of a positive nurse-client relationship may be a slow and sometimes unrewarding process for both parties. The use of a nonjudgmental, nonpunitive attitude by the help-giver will allay some of the anxieties anticipated by the help-seeker. However, the ultimate goal for both the help-seeker and the help-giver is a positive environment for the infant.

Prenatal care. When caring for a pregnant woman who abuses drugs, both the prenatal period and the postnatal period are important times. Because the client has come in for prenatal care, it can be assumed that she has made the choice to come of her own accord for the sake of her infant. This initial visit provides a window of opportunity for encouraging the woman to decrease or stop her substance abuse. It is during this time that the woman is more motivated to change her behavior. During the postnatal period, emphasis is placed on supporting the woman as she continues treatment and on her interactions with her infant.

Some women who abuse substances may seek prenatal care late in pregnancy or not at all. Others may seek care early in their pregnancy because they are concerned about the effect of their substance use on their unborn child. The initial step in the assessment process includes screening and identification. When taking the family and psychosocial history, the nurse should explore the risk factors previously identified. The nurse should also explore additional psychosocial factors, which may include past and current marital or family problems, work performance, involvement with the legal system, and financial difficulties. The nurse should explore a history of the woman's previous infections including cellulitis, hepatitis, STDs, and HIV. The past obstetric history should be reviewed with specific questions regarding lack of prenatal care, poor weight gain, obstetric complications (including spontaneous abortion), abruptio placentae, preterm labor, meconium staining, low birth weight infants, and fetal death. Information about the use of alcohol, tobacco, and other drugs should be obtained. The nurse should determine the client's willingness to cooperate before gathering this information. Initially, some general questions should be asked, and the more sensitive areas can be explored on succeeding visits. Questions about the use of caffeine and nicotine should be asked, leading up to questions about the use of alcohol and illicit drugs. The amount of each drug used should be assessed, keeping in mind that the amount used is often greater than the client recalls. There are several screening instruments that can be used. These screening instruments are brief, simple to administer, and easy to score. The CAGE, T-ACE (Box 27-3), and TWEAK screening instruments, among others, have been used successfully to identify substance abuse problems in the prenatal client. It is important to be familiar with the specific use of each instrument and to ask the questions as designed. The T-ACE is specifically designed for risk-drinking among prenatal clients (Russell, 1994).

Health history taking and screening should be followed by a physical examination. The nurse should observe for evidence of poor hygiene, confusion, inappropriate behavior, dilated or pinpoint pupils, needle marks, scars,

---

Box 27-3   **T-ACE Questionnaire**

T How many drinks does it take to make you feel high (TOLERANCE)?
A Have people ANNOYED you by criticizing your drinking?
C Have you felt that you ought to CUT DOWN on your drinking?
E Have you ever had a drink first thing in the morning to steady your nerves or get rid of a hangover (EYE OPENER)?

From Sokol RJ, Martier SA, Ager JW: The T-ACE questions: practical prenatal detection of risk-drinking, *Am J Obstet Gynecol* 160:863, 1989.

Box 27-4   **Positive Urine Test Result after Last Adult Use**

Alcohol 8-16 hr
Amphetamines 24-72 hr
Benzodiazepines 2-3 wk
Cocaine 24-72 hr
LSD 2-3 days
Marijuana 1-2 wk
Meperidine 2-4 days (5-7 in infant)
Methadone 1 wk or longer
Phencyclidine 3-7 days

Data from Evans and Gilloghey, 1991.

---

abscesses, slurred speech, hypertension, tachycardia or bradycardia, weight loss, anxiety, panic, or depression. It should be noted that none of these findings may be present in the early stages of substance abuse.

Laboratory tests may also be useful. Some women do not admit to drug use or to the amount of drugs used, and laboratory tests provide data independent of self-report. At each prenatal visit and on admission to labor and during the early recovery period, a urine specimen is obtained for toxicologic examination. Urine drug screens can also be performed on the newborn infant. Results of these urine screens are dependent on the half-life of the drug (Box 27-4). Protocols for drug screening vary from state to state and from hospital to hospital. Some protocols allow for the mother and infant to be screened if overt signs are identified, such as a lack of prenatal care, an altered mental state, or the inability of the infant to be consoled. The nurse must be familiar with the laws of the state in which he or she is practicing. In some states, mandatory reporting of drug-exposed infants to child protective services is required; in others, involuntary testing of pregnant women is permitted, while in others, substance-abusing pregnant women can be criminally prosecuted. All of these actions and more are practiced throughout state and local authorities. These situations present the nurse with both an ethical and legal dilemma. The primary concern should be the health of the woman and her unborn child. Equal access to health care and treatment for recovery should be the basis for nursing interventions.

New techniques of hair and meconium analysis are used to determine the woman's cocaine use. These techniques are much more accurate, rapid, and easier to do. Using radioimmunoassay, hair closest to the scalp is analyzed for a history of drug use, though it is recognized that radioimmunoassay's use may be limited because of the variability in hair texture and hair problems associated with cutting, perming, and other chemical treatments. Meconium tests are not invasive and allow for rapid and accurate (87% to 95%) screening. Sampling of the first stool is preferred because the presence of the metabolite for cocaine is diluted as new stool is formed.

Another important factor during the prenatal period includes the care of the pregnant woman. Any medical complication resulting from substance abuse should be addressed. This involves care for any infection, treatment of hypertension or cardiac involvement, and any obstetric complication.

General counseling regarding personal care, rest, and care of self is provided. If the woman is without adequate resources, referrals are initiated to deal with housing needs and with maintaining access to the health care system. Adequate nutritional intake is critical. The mother should be encouraged to increase her protein intake in every possible way. Dietary substitutions that are realistic should be in keeping with her food preferences. Vitamins, folic acid, and iron are prescribed, and it should be stressed that these supplements are necessary for the infant's health.

In addition, every effort should be made to encourage the mother to cut down or discontinue her abuse of alcohol, tobacco, or other drugs. However, the priority is to have the mother continue with her prenatal care. Frequently, as the mother continues into her second trimester, she may become increasingly concerned for her unborn child and consider treatment. The help-giver should be supportive of any effort the mother makes, stressing that treatment is available but her access to care is not dependent on it.

Other aspects of prenatal care, such as attendance at childbirth classes and parenting classes, should be encouraged. As previously discussed, many of these women have had little support and are at high-risk for poor parenting. Attendance at these classes provides not only much needed knowledge but also a social support system that boosts the women's self-esteem. It may be necessary to provide transportation and child care for these women and the opportunity for them to address their individual needs.

Toward the latter part of pregnancy, the delivery process should be discussed with the client. The mother who continues to use illicit drugs should be informed that regional rather than general anesthesia is usually used because of the inability to determine how much drug is in her system. In response to the client's concern about the infant's response to drugs, information about the drug's effect on the infant should be given in a straightforward manner. If the mother has continued to use drugs during her pregnancy, she should know that the infant will be passively addicted and that the infant's degree of difficulty will depend on the extent of her habit. The nurse should reassure the woman that because of the absence of psychologic dependency in the infant, medical treatment usually alleviates withdrawal symptoms.

Postnatal care. The postnatal care of the client will depend upon whether she is drug free, in treatment, or continuing to use. If the client is drug free or in treatment, her postnatal care is the same as for any mother who has had an uncomplicated delivery. The management of post-delivery pain should have been discussed with the physician before delivery. For the woman in treatment, the care of her infant following discharge may be a concern if she cannot take her infant into the treatment facility. This may be the situation in many geographic areas because treatment facilities for women and their children are limited.

The mother needs a great deal of support during the period following delivery. The time with her infant should be "quality" time in which bonding between them is supported. Frequently, the mother is ambivalent about continuing treatment if she cannot take her infant with her, and she will consider returning to her home environment where a return to drug use is inevitable.

For the client who is continuing to use, her first concern after delivery is usually to satisfy her need for drugs. A heroin user, if she is not on a methadone regimen or receiving tranquilizers, will make attempts to acquire drugs through outside visitors to avoid withdrawal symptoms (e.g., nausea, tremors, sweating, abdominal pain, cramps, yawning). These symptoms may appear 2 or 3 hours after delivery, depending on the time of her last use. When indicated, the nurse must be alert to the possibility of the client stealing from other clients and must not leave medication rooms or carts unlocked. There should be unobtrusive surveillance of visitors to a drug-addicted client when she is not separated from other clients. When early discharge of the mother is possible, she may choose to leave the hospital to secure her drugs.

Fears of separation from the infant may be intensified after delivery because, in most instances, the infant is placed in an intensive care unit for observation and treatment (see Chapter 28). In instances in which the mother has had several children placed in foster care, she may attempt to remove this child from the nursery setting.

A social worker will be involved in the placement of the infant following delivery. There is great variability in state laws regarding placement of the infant. The infant may be placed in foster care, with the woman's relatives, or in the woman's home if someone can assume the major portion of the care. When treatment facilities are available that allow the mother to care for her infant, the infant will be discharged to the mother. In all cases in which the mother has been known to abuse drugs, child protection agencies should be involved as soon as the infant is born. Although confidentiality is an issue, it is the responsibility of the professional, and in some states a legal responsibility, to report the suspicion of child abuse or neglect to the proper authorities for further investigation. In cases in which the nurse is unsure of how to proceed, the agency administration, legal or risk management department, and ethics committee should be consulted (see Chapter 30).

An essential component of care in the immediate postpartum period is the promotion of bonding, which is even more critical when there is a potential for mother-infant attachment disorders. The way in which this is accomplished depends on the individual institution, such as the presence of mother-baby units, rooming-in, or visits in the special care nursery. Every effort should be made to facilitate the mother's efforts to bond with the infant and to modify the social situation to provide opportunities for mother-infant interaction. The client needs to know that staff members care about her and are willing to help her in any way that supports mother-infant interaction. When limits are set for her, such as the state's refusal to discharge an infant for social reasons, the client often feels punished, which reinforces her feelings of hopelessness and loss of control. She needs to be reminded that the infant is hers and that, by taking the steps prescribed, she will be able to take the infant home as soon as the social situation is stable. *This client cannot tolerate surprise.* She should be warned long in advance about delays in infant discharge, which can help restore some sense of control and offer her the guidance and support she needs to begin learning to meet her self-care needs.

Newborn care. The care of the newborn of a substance-abusing mother is dependent upon the condition of the newborn because there is great variability in the outcome of each pregnancy. As noted in Table 27-1, the effects of the drug abuse may be similar for different drugs, and the manifestations are dependent on factors within the pregnancy. Timing of drug use, dosage, and individual susceptibilities all affect the outcome in the newborn. The ingestion of alcohol may result in fetal alcohol effects (FAE) and other alcohol-related effects. The use of many other drugs may express itself in a drug-exposed infant, and when the mother uses any drug, especially heroin, or is in a methadone treatment program, the infant may experience neonatal abstinence syndrome. Breast-feeding is contraindicated in all mothers who are using drugs except for the mother who is on a methadone maintenance program, unless this mother is a polydrug user or is HIV positive.

Fetal alcohol syndrome and alcohol-related effects

First described in 1973 in the United States, fetal alcohol syndrome (FAS) occurs in infants of women who are chronic alcoholics and in women who drink five or more drinks per day throughout pregnancy. This completely preventable condition is the most common cause of mental retardation. It occurs in 1 to 3 newborns per 1000 live births, and its rate continues to increase (*Healthy People 2000*, 1996).

Alcohol is the most common human teratogen and produces a variety of effects in the infant. The syndrome is identified by the presence of three characteristics: growth retardation, central nervous system manifestations, and distinct facial dysmorphology (Figure 27-6) (see Table 27-1). The Institute of Medicine (1996) has recommended a revision to the diagnostic criteria for FAS: FAS confirmed with maternal exposure, FAS without confirmed alcohol exposure, and partial FAS with confirmed alcohol exposure. The Institute of Medicine also recommends that the terminology of FAE be revised. In this revision, there are two groups identified, and there must be a confirmed history of maternal alcohol exposure. In those infants who have physical anomalies, the term "alcohol-related birth defect" (ARBD) is recommended, and in those infants with neurodevelopmental problems, the term "alcohol-related neurodevelopmental disorder" (ARND) is recommended.

The diagnosis of FAS is difficult unless there is a positive history of alcohol abuse during pregnancy. Initially, many children fail to thrive despite adequate food intake. FAS is difficult to diagnose before the age of 2 because infants do not have all of the facial features that make diagnosis easier. Children suspected of having FAS, ARBD, or ARND should be evaluated by a developmental pediatrician or a dysmorphologist.

Newborns show difficulties in regulating states, have tremors and poor sucking ability, and are unable to shut out sounds in the environment. Infants and toddlers show neurobehavioral manifestations that include abnormal EEGs, decreased motor skills, hyperactivity, or speech delays. Neurobehavioral problems continue into the school-age and adolescent years. More than half of adolescents with FAS and alcohol-related effects have significant levels of maladaptive behavior.

Infants with FAS, ARBD, or ARND benefit from early intervention and infant stimulation programs. In addition, any physical problems should be addressed. These children have additional major and minor congenital anomalies, including cardiac defects, dental malalignments, microcephaly, and minor genital anomalies. In those instances where the mother is unable to provide care, alternative placement is sought. Many of these children experience multiple placements, resulting in inconsistency in their lives.

The drug-exposed infant. The drug-exposed infant (DEI) is a vulnerable infant. Nationally there are approx-

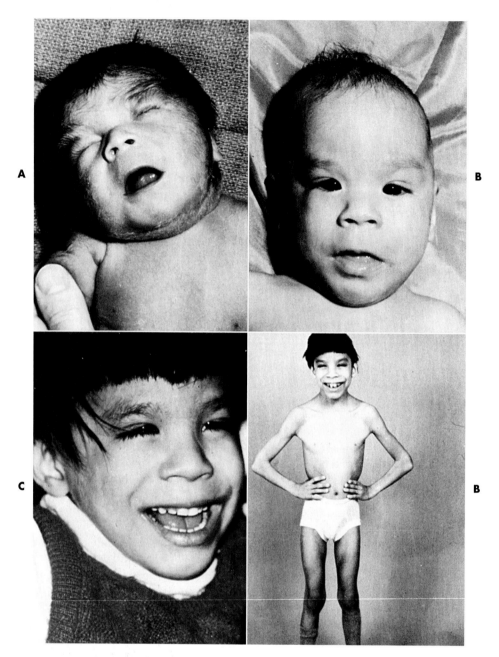

Figure 27-6   Fetal alcohol syndrome (FAS). **A** to **D,** Child of chronically alcoholic mother, diagnosed at birth with FAS. Although he was raised his entire life in one excellent foster home and participated in various remediation programs, he continues to have an IQ around 45 (more severe retardation than most FAS children), with accompanying hyperactivity and distractibility. (From Streissguth AP: *Ciba Foundation Symposium No 105: mechanisms of alcohol damage in utero.* Courtesy AP Streissguth and the Ciba Foundation, Pitman, London.)

imately 350,000 DEIs born each year. Many of these infants are preterm and have a variety of health problems. As noted in Table 27-1, each drug produces certain manifestations, and a child may have all or none of the manifestations noted. A mother who is a polydrug user exposes her child to a wide variety of manifestations, often compounded by the combinations of drugs.

DEIs often have respiratory problems, diarrhea, and other medical problems, and they are at risk for HIV infection and hepatitis B. Some of these children will have developmental delays, which may become more severe as they enter school.

Health assessment, developmental assessment, and physical examination are all indicated in planning a program for intervention. These children benefit from an early intervention program that is structured. Referral to appropriate community services is indicated.

Neonatal abstinence syndrome. Neonatal abstinence syndrome can occur within the first month of life in any infant who has been exposed to drugs in utero. The longer the exposure and the greater the amount of the drug used by the mother, the greater the possibility the infant will experience withdrawal. With today's early discharge of mothers and infants, it is possible that these infants may go home before showing signs of withdrawal. The time when the infant experiences withdrawal varies for individual drugs. For example, withdrawal from alcohol has been reported in infants within 6 to 12 hours after delivery.

Heroin and methadone both produce withdrawal in the newborn; heroin withdrawal occurs in 42% to 68% of newborns, and methadone withdrawal occurs in 63% to 85% of newborns whose mothers are being treated with methadone. If the infant is experiencing severe signs of distress, admission to the NICU is indicated (see Table 27-1: opiates). Priorities of care include thermoregulation, respiratory and cardiac stabilization, and interventions for any congenital anomalies. Nursing interventions include modulation of the infant's environment, swaddling, and the use of a pacifier. If nursing measures are not effective, pharmacologic intervention may be indicated; phenobarbital or Paregoric may be used.

Mothers whose infants are experiencing withdrawal require a great deal of support. Their infants are frequently irritable and inconsolable, and the mother experiences a great deal of guilt. Mother-infant interactions are often strained, and both mother and infant need the support of a caring nurse. Mothers should be taught comforting techniques, such as quieting the environment, swaddling, using a pacifier, and using a front infant carrier. In addition, mothers should be taught how to recognize their infants' cues. Positive reinforcement by the nurse will increase these mothers' self-esteem.

Prevention of Substance Abuse

Prevention of substance abuse by the pregnant client is an important focus of obstetric care. There are actually three levels of prevention, and nurses can be involved at each level. Primary prevention involves getting information to those individuals who have not yet begun to experiment or use or those who have problems with alcohol, tobacco, or other drugs. For example, nurses can speak to adolescents about the dangers of substance abuse. Secondary prevention involves case finding and treatment for problematic users. Nurses can screen their clients using the CAGE, T-ACE (see Box 27-3), or TWEAK instruments. Nurses can recommend treatment options or refer clients to those places where treatment is indicated, such as 12-step programs or inpatient facilities. Tertiary treatment involves preventing substance abuse and treating complications of this abuse. One example of treatment would be the nurse who counsels the pregnant woman about the dangers of alcohol use. If all nurses who have contact with a pregnant woman would assume an

active role in prevention, perhaps the goals established in *Healthy People 2000* (1991) could be met.

Model of care

Much has been written about home care and follow-up care, and the practical application of care has taken several creative directions. What follows is a model of care that illustrates that nurses and the health care team have not yet found an ideal approach but that they are trying to reach the perinatal client in a holistic, person-in-environment way.

Incorporating spirituality into the program: Boston*

Boston Department of Health and Hospitals' Healthy Baby and Healthy Child Programs are designed to reduce the unacceptably high infant mortality in Boston's poor neighborhoods. The black infant mortality rate in these neighborhoods was 20.9 per 1000 in 1988, as opposed to 8.11 in the white, more affluent areas of Boston. Public health nurses, neighborhood health advocates, and neighborhood health centers have collaborated closely to follow high-risk pregnant women and their children for up to 3 years.

Since many of the risk factors are psychosocial and economic, traditional prenatal care hasn't sufficed for this population. In 1989, only 50.1% of black pregnant women got prenatal care, as compared with 80.1% of white pregnant women in Boston (The Task Force, 1991). We widened the focus of care to recognize culture and spirituality of those we serve. We also included advocacy to help clients meet basic needs like food and housing. We have found that if we pay attention to these aspects of their lives, many more women develop trust in their providers and seek and remain in care. Home visiting, teaching, support, and advocacy are the program's major interventions.

An important step in designing a program like this was to recruit and retain a multicultural staff that reflects the composition of the community. Nurses and neighborhood health advocates thus provide the client with a more familiar, comfortable link to the often-intimidating health care system.

The program provided training that explored and promoted respect for everyone's cultural background. When white European-American nurses met with staff from Haitian, Hispanic, and African-American cultures, they often became more aware of their own ethnic background.

Public health nurses in urban areas increasingly confront problems of drugs, alcohol, disorganization, and violence that touch a growing number of families. Not only do they see the effects on their clients but may fear for their own safety. Nurses in a recent study said they continued this work, often at the expense of their souls.

Staff and administration need to be honest about the spiritual drain of the work and take steps to maintain and promote staff well-being. Simple measures that recognize each staff member as an individual help counteract the spiritual drain and strengthen the nurse's ability to extend oneself to the client. A structure that promotes sharing,

*Reprinted from Corrine L et al: The unheard voices of women: spiritual interventions in maternal-child health, *MCN Am J Matern Child Nurs* 17(3):145, 1992.

mutual support, and recognition of spirituality can be developed. For example, at the beginning of selected meetings, a "check-in time" is held so all staff persons can relate whatever they wish about job or personal events. Team meetings begin with staff volunteering to lead a moment of meditation or prayer or read a passage from booklets with affirmations like the ones put out by 12-step programs.

Relating case stories informally or at case conferences validates the spiritual aspect of nursing practice and illustrates that the expression of spiritual needs is not an isolated or infrequent part of the client's care. Inservice education programs can contribute to increased awareness and comfort with the topic. A staff that can appreciate cultural diversity and maintain its own well-being can address the spiritual needs of its clients.

Key Points

- Each person functions to meet basic needs according to a hierarchy of needs that requires that physiologic and safety needs be met first.
- Without the basic needs of belongingness and love, both children and adults become angry and depressed, feeling that no one cares about them. Esteem and self-actualization needs, however, cannot be addressed while the more basic needs are unmet.
- For the woman who is considered socially high risk, pregnancy is a situational crisis.
- Pregnancy in socially high-risk clients is complicated by social problems that have chronic roots and thus are difficult to solve. The help-giver must have patience in these interactions.
- Underlying hopelessness, depression, and despair may prevent a client from taking actions that could empower her to change a situation.
- Empowerment as a way out of despair includes increasing personal, interpersonal, or political power to improve a situation.

- Four changes appear to be necessary to improve a situation: increase self-efficacy, develop group consciousness, reduce self-blame, and assume personal accountability to change a situation.
- The use of alcohol and other drugs plays a part in the occurrence of adolescent pregnancy.
- Poverty makes individuals and families vulnerable to homelessness, violence, and poor pregnancy outcomes.
- Women who are abused by their partners are at greater risk for abuse during pregnancy.
- Substance abuse in clients illustrates the need for crisis intervention and long-term involvement in change.
- Nurse advocacy for change is an important part of planning nursing support of clients who are socially at high risk.
- Nurse involvement in prevention of substance abuse can occur at three levels of prevention.

Study Questions

27-1. Select the terms that apply to the following statements:
   a. Inability to deal with a situation or follow advice because more pressing needs are present is an example of _____.
   b. A child feels _____ especially when incest or sexual abuse occurs.
   c. Being enabled to take action to improve one's life situation is to experience _____.
   d. The unexpected birth of an infant with a defect is a _____ crisis.
   e. Alcohol is an example of a _____ drug.
   f. A person who uses alcohol and cocaine is labeled a _____.
27-2. Select true or false for the following statements.
   a. Instructions for the woman who is pregnant and homeless should focus on the common discomforts of pregnancy.
   b. Hair analysis as a method of detecting cocaine use is more reliable than collection of a urine sample.
   c. Alcohol use by the pregnant woman can be detected in a urine sample for 2 to 4 days.
   d. The priority in care of the pregnant woman who is using alcohol, tobacco, and other drugs is prenatal care.
   e. Fetal alcohol syndrome is a completely preventable cause of mental retardation.

27-3. When a client is abusing illegal drugs, you should:
　a. Inform her that she will have to be reported to the police.
　b. Counsel her on possible effects of the drugs on her body and fetus and offer assistance in finding a treatment program.
　c. Maintain confidentiality even if she is observed using or selling illegal substances.
　d. Ignore the situation because paying attention to the problem reinforces negative behavior.

27-4. Cocaine may cause:
　a. Hypotension and syncope.
　b. EEG changes and dilated pupils.
　c. Tachycardia and hypertension.
　d. Hypoglycemia.

27-5. The fetus is affected most seriously by maternal crack use because of
　a. Cerebral anoxia.
　b. Vasoconstriction.
　c. Reduction in amniotic fluid volumes.
　d. Delayed or postmature birth.

27-6. When working with the pregnant woman who has been abused, the priority of care is to
　a. Review with her ways to manage her partner.
　b. Counsel her to leave her husband.
　c. Assist her with an exit plan.
　d. Encourage her to get a restraining order.

Answer Key

27-1: a, Hierarchy of needs; b, self-blame; c, empowerment; d, situational; e, licit; f, polydrug user. 27-2: a, F; b, T; c, F; d, T; e, F. 27-3: b, 27-4: c, 27-5: b, 27-6: c.

References

Aase JM: Clinical recognition of FAS: difficulties of detection and diagnosis, *Alcohol Health & Research World* 18:5, 1994.
Amaro H et al: Violence during pregnancy and substance abuse, *Am J Public Health* 80:575, 1990.
Andrews AD, Patterson EG: Searching solutions to alcohol and other drug abuse during pregnancy: ethics values, and constitutional principles, *Soc Work* 40(1):56, 1995.
*Bandura A: Self-efficacy mechanisms in human agency, *Am Psychol* 31:122, 1982.
Bell GL, Lau K: Perinatal and neonatal issues of substance abuse, *Pediatr Clin North Amer* 42:261, 1995.
Butler MJ: Domestic violence: a nursing imperative, *J Holistic Nurs* 13:54, 1995.
Cook P, Petersen RC, Moore DT: Alcohol, tobacco and other drugs may harm the unborn, Rockville, Md, 1990, US Department of Health and Human Services, Office for Substance Abuse.
Cornelius M et al: Drinking patterns and correlates of drinking among pregnant teenagers, *Alcohol Clin Exp Res* 17(2):290, 1993.
Day NL, Cottreau CM, Richardson GA: The epidemiology of alcohol, marijuana, and cocaine use among women of childbearing age and pregnant women, *Clin Obstet Gynecol* 36:232, 1993.
*Dunst C, Trivette C, Deal A: *Enabling & empowering families,* Cambridge, Mass, 1988, Brookline Books.
Evans AT, Gilloghey KM: Drug use in pregnancy: obstetrical perspectives, *Clin Perinatol* 18(1):25, 1991.
*Ewing JA: Detecting alcoholism: the CAGE questionnaire, *JAMA* 252:1905, 1984.
Forrest DC: The cocaine-exposed infant, part I: identification and assessment, *J Pediatr Health Care* 8:3, 1994.
Forrest DC: The cocaine-exposed infant, part II: intervention and teaching, *J Pediatr Health Care* 8:7, 1994.

Grant T et al: Cocaine exposure during pregnancy: improving assessment with radioimmunoassay of maternal hair, *Obstet Gynecol* 83:525, 1994.
Gutiérrez LM: Working with women of color: an empowerment perspective, *Soc Work* 35:149, 1990.
Healthy People 2000: national health promotion and disease prevention objectives, Washington, DC, 1991, Public Health Service, US Department of Health and Human Services.
Healthy People 2000: midcourse review and 1995 revisions, Washington, DC, 1996, Public Health Service, US Department of Health and Human Services.
Hofkosh D et al: Early interactions between drug-involved mother and infants, *Arch Pediatr Adolesc Med* 149:665, 1995.
*Institute of Medicine: *Homelessness, health, and human needs,* Washington, DC, 1988, National Academic Press.
Jezierski M: Abuse of women by male partners: basic knowledge for emergency nurses, *J Emerg Nurs* 20(5):361, 1994.
Johnson MO, Lobo ML: Case study of the home health management of a child with congenital anomalies associated with perinatal cocaine abuse, *J Pediatr Nurs* 10:375, 1995.
Killion CM: Special health care needs of homeless pregnant women, *ANS Adv Nurs Sci* 18(2):44, 1995.
Kleinfeld J, Wescott S, eds: *Fantastic Antone succeeds: experiences in educating children with fetal alcohol syndrome,* Fairbanks, 1993, University of Alaska Press.
Koniak-Griffin D, Brecht ML: Linkages between sexual risk taking, substance use, and AIDS knowledge among pregnant adolescents and young mothers, *Nurs Res* 44: 340, 1995.
Lewis KD: *Infants and children with prenatal alcohol and drug exposure: a guide to identification and intervention,* North Branch, Minn, 1995, Sunrise River Press.

*Classic reference.

Lex BW: Alcohol and other drug abuse among women, *Alcohol Health & Research World* 18(3):212, 1994.

*Maslow A: *Motivation and personality,* ed 2, New York, 1970, Harper & Row.

Maternal substance use assessment methods reference manual, Rockville, Md, 1993, Center for Substance Abuse Prevention, US Department of Health and Human Services.

McFarlane J, Parker B, Soeken K: Abuse during pregnancy: frequency, severity, perpetrator, and risk factors of homicide, *Public Health Nurs* 12(5):284, 1995.

Mitchell JL: *Pregnant, substance-using women,* Rockville, Md, 1993, US Department of Health and Human Services.

*Mitchell PH: *Concepts basic to nursing,* New York, 1973, McGraw-Hill.

National household survey on drug abuse: population estimates 1992, Rockville, Md, 1993, Substance Abuse and Mental Health Services Administration.

Oyemade UJ et al: Prenatal substance abuse and pregnancy outcomes among African American women, *J Nutr* 124:994S, 1994.

Parker B, McFarlane J, Soeken K: Abuse during pregnancy: effects on maternal complications and birth weight in adult and teenage women, *Obstet Gynecol* 84(3):323, 1994.

Parker B et al: Physical and emotional abuse in pregnancy: a comparison of adult and teenage women, *Nurs Res* 42:173, 1993.

Peipert JF, Domagalski LR: Epidemiology of adolescent sexual assault, *Obstet Gynecol* 84(5):867, 1994.

Practical approaches to the treatment of women who abuse alcohol and other drugs, Rockville, Md, 1994, Center for Substance Abuse Treatment, US Department of Health and Human Services.

Redding BA, Selleck CS: Perinatal substance abuse: assessment and management of the pregnant woman and her children, *Nurse Pract Forum* 4:216, 1993.

Rosengren SS, Longobucco DB, Bernstein BA: Meconium testing for cocaine metabolite: prevalence, perceptions, and pitfalls, *Am J Obstet Gynecol* 168:1449, 1993.

Russell M: New assessment tools for drinking during pregnancy: T-ACE, TWEAK, and others, *Alcohol Health & Research World,* 18:55, 1994.

Selleck CS, Redding BA: *Knowledge and attitudes of registered nurses toward perinatal substance abuse,* Tampa, Fla, 1995, University of South Florida.

Smitherman CH: The lasting impact of fetal alcohol syndrome and fetal alcohol effect on children and adolescents, *J Pediatr Health Care* 8:121, 1994.

Stratton K, Howe C, Battaglia F, eds: *Fetal alcohol syndrome: diagnosis, epidemiology, prevention, and treatment,* Washington, DC, 1996, Institute of Medicine, National Academic Press.

Streissguth AP: A long-term perspective of FAS, *Alcohol Health & Research World* 18:74, 1994.

Ventura SJ et al: Advance report of final natality statistics: 1994, *Monthly Vital Statistics Report (MVSR)* 44(lls):1, 1996.

Student Resource Shelf

Burian J: Helping survivors of sexual abuse through labor, *MCN Am J Matern Child Nurs* 20(5):252, 1995.
Discussion of the common characteristics that serve as guides for identifying in labor sexual abuse survivors and the strategies for providing sensitive care during labor.

Campbell JC et al: Battered women's experiences in the emergency department, *J Emerg Nurs* 20(4):280, 1994.
Presentation of a research-based model policy and procedure for care of battered women in the emergency department.

Cole JG: Intervention strategies for infants with prenatal drug exposure, *Infants Young Child* 8(3):35, 1996.
Discussion of intervention strategies for hospital and home care of infants exposed prenatally to drugs.

Dorris M: *The broken cord,* New York, 1989, Harper & Row.
This nonfiction, autobiographic book is written by the father of Adam, a child with fetal alcohol syndrome.

Newborn *at* Risk

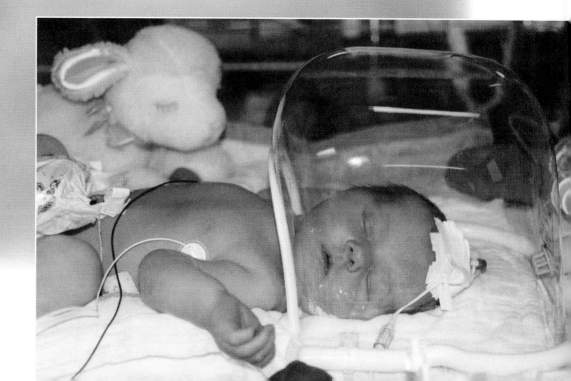

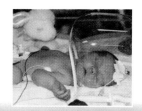

28 Birth Defects

When an infant is born with a **birth defect**, the parents are shocked and upset and ask for reasons. The medical staff investigates possible causes, and nurses care for the parents and infant. Thus it is important to have an overview of the events that can change the normal pattern of fetal growth and development. These adverse changes may occur through genetic inheritance or result from teratogenic factors during pregnancy. When an infant is born with a defect, the parents need support, information, and counseling. This role may be difficult, but its function is essential with these parents.

From the time of Mendel in 1865 until the early 1900s, few people understood the significance of genetic inheritance. It was not even described until 1941 when Beadle and Tatum hypothesized that "one **gene** controlled one enzyme." This new concept became an essential principle in current genetic research. In addition, it was not understood until 1956 that chromosomal makeup consisted of 22 matched pairs of **autosomes** and 1 pair of sex **chromosomes** in each body cell (Figure 28-1).

The major groups of chromosomes were first recognized in 1960 at a meeting of cytogeneticists in Denver. The length of each chromosome and the placement of the centromere (a small constriction separating the chromosome's short and long arms) are used to arrange them in the order of descending size. Pairs of autosomes are numbered serially from 1 to 22; the two sex chromosomes become pair 23. A high-powered microscope is used to photograph the darkly stained chromosomes. The classification devised in Denver arranges them into a **karyotype**.

Chromosome banding took the research a step further. The technique of banding allows researchers to identify regions of each chromosome. Large deletions and duplications are seen as abnormal bands. Regions of particular chromosomes can be correlated with known defects (e.g., retinoblastoma). In this manner many diseases can be classified as genetic in origin and can be assigned to a particular chromosome. Currently a large-scale effort is under way using deoxyribonucleic acid (DNA) technology to map the location of every gene in the human **genome** (complete set of genes in each cell) to provide detailed knowledge of the genetic basis for many diseases, some of which may not now be considered to have a genetic cause.

IMPORTANCE OF GENETIC STUDIES

Because of advances in technology, the basic principles of genetics can be applied to human beings; as a result gene mapping leads to a series of positive applications and to many ethical questions. Research in molecular genetics has already resulted in gene therapy, or the introduction of normal genes where nonoperative genes exist (Rosenfeld et al, 1992). Such techniques also lead to important questions of normalcy because, currently, normal genes can be inserted only into cells of an affected organ, not into sex cells (oocytes or spermatozoa).

In the last few years research has identified gene groups that indicate susceptibility to heart attack, emphysema, multiple sclerosis, insulin-dependent diabetes, schizophrenia, and some types of cancer. It is known that chromosomal defects exist in many neoplastic conditions. For example, there is a missing piece of chromosome 22 in the bone marrow cells of persons with chronic myelogenous leukemia; this piece has been found attached to chromosome 9. Mental retardation, which affects 3% of the population in the United States, is thought to be related in 80% of cases to a genetic cause. A high rate of spontaneous first-trimester abortion (50%) is related to chromosome abnormality. In addition, some cases of infertility and many disorders of polygenic origin have genetic bases. Thus it is apparent that genetic disorders cause a significant portion of health deficits.

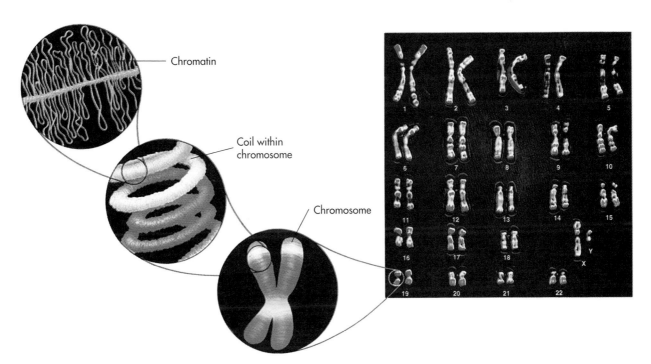

Figure 28-1   Human chromosomes. Each of the 46 human chromosomes, arranged here in numbered pairs—called a karyotype—is a coiled mass of chromatin (DNA). (From Rolin Graphics and CNRI/Science Photo Library.)

In this age of rapid change, health professionals must advocate positive support of persons with genetic disorders while working to reduce the potential occurrence of defects. Because of pollutants and radioactivity in the environment, new mutations may occur. The task of prevention has a number of aspects; certainly preventive care is important to reduce the incidence of mental retardation.

Genetics must be a major focus in maternal and infant care. Concerned parents are seeking preconception, prenatal, and postnatal counseling. An understanding of genetic inheritance is required to know about basic defects, their frequency, and the referral process for counseling when parents ask for help during pregnancy or after birth.

Genetic Code

DNA carries the genetic information that will be passed to each generation of cells. It is a blueprint for the production of proteins, both structural and functional (enzymes). If the DNA in one human cell could be unraveled and stretched, it would be more than 2 yards long. The structure, however, is actually two molecules built like two spiral staircases circling one another. The backbone of each spiral is made of a sugar called *deoxyribose*. One of four nucleic acids is attached to each sugar; the acids form pairs across the staircase to the complementing strand to make a double helix. The acids always pair in the same way: *adenine* (A) with *thymine* (T) and *cytosine* (C) with *guanine* (G) (Figure 28-2). When a cell divides, the DNA must be replicated. The double helix is pulled apart while a new strand from each of the old strands is synthesized (Figure 28-3).

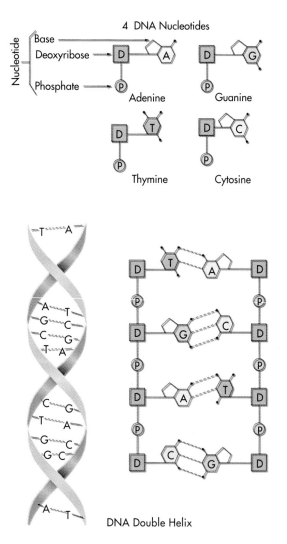

Figure 28-2   Base pairings between two nucleotides from double helix of DNA. *A,* Adenine; *C,* cytosine; *D,* deoxyribose; *G,* guanine; *P,* phosphate; *T,* thymine. (From Vander AJ, Sherman JH, Luciano DS: *Human physiology,* ed 4, New York, 1986, McGraw-Hill.)

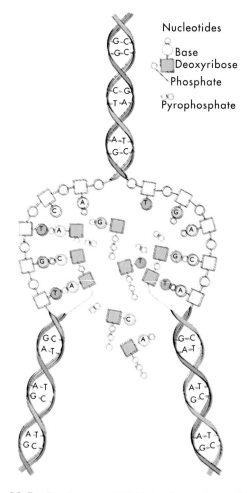

Figure 28-3   Replication of DNA involves pairing of free nucleotides with bases of each DNA strand. Result is two new DNA molecules, each containing one old and one new strand. *A,* Adenine; *C,* cytosine; *D,* deoxyribose; *G,* guanine; *T,* thymine. (From Vander AJ, Sherman JH, Luciano DS: *Human physiology,* ed 4, New York, 1986, McGraw-Hill.)

The easiest way to think about the function of DNA is by analogy. DNA can be thought of as a language. A gene is a sentence, whereas a chromosome is a letter packaged in an envelope. For replication, the information carried in DNA must be transcribed into another language to be read; this language is ribonucleic acid (RNA). Each gene is transcribed individually into RNA by a complex array of highly specific enzymes. RNA is a molecule closely related to DNA but is much less stable. DNA and RNA are "read" in groups of three nucleic acids called **codons.** Each codon designates an amino acid. Because there are 4 nucleic acids and they are read in groups of 3, 64 combinations are possible. Different enzymes in the cell then translate the RNA into protein (Figure 28-4), which provides structure and function for the cell. An absent or dysfunctional protein may cause the cell to be unable to carry out its task or to die prematurely. This molecular defect may cause a physical defect; for example, muscular dystrophy is a single-gene defect that causes muscle cells to malfunction.

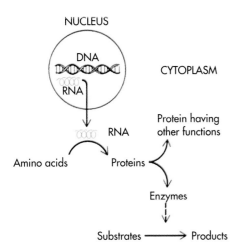

Figure 28-4   Expression of genetic information occurs throughout transcription from DNA to RNA in nucleus followed by translation of this RNA information to proteins in cytoplasm. (From Vander AJ, Sherman JH, Luciano DS: *Human physiology,* ed 4, New York, 1986, McGraw-Hill.)

This analogy also helps to explain the reasons that **inversions, deletions,** and **translocations** result in abnormalities; these are rearrangements of pieces of chromosomes that cannot be read in a meaningful way. It is comparable to splicing together two sentences that do not make sense when read.

More than 100,000 genes in the human chromosomes provide codes for RNA to produce protein and enzymes, and it is within these structural genes that the recognized genetic defects seem to occur and where new mutations have their effect. The position of a specific gene on a chromosome is called a **locus** (pl., loci). The rest of DNA seems to be involved in a regulatory role or in reproducing and recombining chromosomes (Thompson and Thompson, 1986).

Mutations

Sometimes mistakes are made in duplication or external factors change certain codons. The result is a faulty message transmitted by messenger RNA (mRNA) to all subsequent replications. Mutations arise when a change occurs in the sequence of base pairs by one of the following means:

- *Substitution* of one base pair by another
- *Insertion* of an extra base pair
- *Deletion* of a required base pair

The result is an altered reading. Thus another amino acid is encoded, possibly changing the protein's function, or the amount of a protein with the correct amino acid sequence is reduced or suppressed. For example, this sequence of bases

CATTCACCTGTA

would be read as

CAT/TCA/CCT/GTA.

If the second T is deleted, the sequence becomes

CATCACCTGTA,

which is read as

CAT/CAC/CTG/TA.

Note that the code has changed and that the new code may cause defects in protein synthesis. The result may be

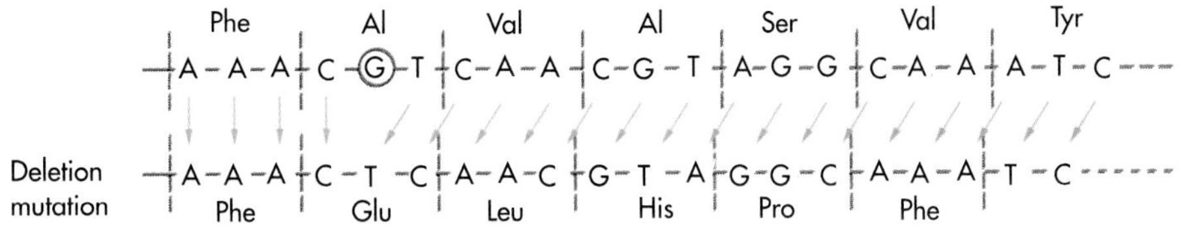

Phe   Al   Val   Al   Ser   Val   Tyr
—A-A-A—C-(G)-T—C-A-A—C-G-T—A-G-G—C-A-A—A-T-C———

Deletion   —A-A-A—C-T—C—A-A-C—G-T-A—G-G-C—A-A-A—T-C——
mutation   Phe   Glu   Leu   His   Pro   Phe

Figure 28-5   Mutation caused by deletion of single base G in DNA sequence, resulting in other code words also being misread. *A,* Adenine; *C,* cytosine; *G,* guanine; *T,* thymine. (From Vander AJ, Sherman JH, Luciano DS: *Human physiology,* ed 4, New York, 1986, McGraw-Hill.)

partial or complete absence of the gene product. Thus a mutation is a change in genetic material that possibly, but not always, leads to a change in gene function. For example, Figure 28-5 shows deletion of a single base (*G*); instead of CGT, the new product is CTC.

Mutations can arise spontaneously, or they can be induced by *mutagens,* substances in the environment that cause genetic changes in certain (target) cells. Genetic diseases that occur in families for the first time often are the result of new mutations. Under certain circumstances, however, the presence of an undesirable trait provides some survival advantage. This may cause the trait to be preserved or promoted within a population. For example, a mutation in the beta-hemoglobin gene (which causes sickle cell trait) also provides some protection against death from malaria in persons with *one* copy of the gene. However, sickle cell anemia develops in those persons with *two* copies of the mutant gene. Mutations like these also tend to occur in higher concentrations in ethnic groups that have been isolated geographically and as a result have intermarried with more frequency. Examples of other deleterious mutations that become concentrated in ethnic groups are cystic fibrosis in the Irish and northern Europeans, Tay-Sachs disease in Ashkenazic Jews and French Canadians, and phenylketonuria (PKU) in the Amish.

TEST *Yourself* 28-1 _____

    a. The normal male karyotype consists of _____
       autosomes and _____ sex chromosomes,
       _____ and _____ .
    b. A group of three nucleic acids is called a _____ .
    c. Describe how a mutation can alter protein synthesis.

SINGLE-GENE INHERITANCE PATTERNS

A human being is a diploid organism; that is, he or she carries a set of chromosomes from the mother and a set from the father. Therefore each person carries two copies of each gene, although only one of the copies may be expressed. These two copies are **alleles** of the same gene, each at the same locus (location) on the chromosome pair (Table 28-1). If a person carries one *recessive* allele, the trait for that allele is not observable because of the presence of the *dominant* allele. If, however, a person carries two copies of a recessive allele, the trait *will* be expressed. The **phenotype** of an organism is an *observable trait* that depends on the expression of these alleles. For example, the color of a person's eyes or the hair texture is the phenotype of that person. A **genotype** on the other hand, is the combination of alleles. For example, brown eyes are dominant (B), whereas blue eyes are recessive (b) (Table 28-2). If a person has alleles for brown and blue eyes, this **heterozygous** genotype (Bb) shows a phenotype of brown

eyes because the gene for brown eyes is dominant. If both parents have brown eyes, the child might inherit both dominant alleles; in this case the phenotype is brown eyes, but the genotype is **homozygous** dominant (BB). The person whose genotype is blue eyes is homozygous recessive (bb). Recessive alleles may not become apparent for generations and then only if the partner carries similar genes. Of course, there are several genes for eye color and hair characteristics; as a result, many phenotypical and genotypical gradations are observed.

During meiosis there is a 50% chance that the X or the Y chromosome will be placed in the sperm or egg. This **segregation** is true for each of the 23 pairs of chromosomes, thus allowing a wide variation in the genetic makeup of each sperm or egg. The degree of variation is further increased because of the normal crossing over between members of a chromosome pair (see Figure 7-2). The segregation and **independent assortment** reduce chances of inheriting gene defects and contribute to the variety in individual appearances and abilities.

Charting Genotypes

When a family genetic history is taken, a specific protocol is used. The result should be an indication of the proba-

Table **28-1**   **Mendel's Laws of Dominance**

| Gene | Genotype | | Phenotype |
	Allele		Expression
Dominant (D)	Dominant (D)		Dominant (DD)
Recessive (r)	Recessive (r)		Recessive (rr)
Dominant (D)	Recessive (r)		Dominant (Dr)

Table **28-2**   **Inheritance of Eye Color**[*]

Parent	Parent	Children
Brown (B, B)	Brown (B, B)	Brown (B, B)
Blue (b, b)	Blue (b, b)	Blue (b, b)
Brown (B, B)	Blue (b, b)	Brown (B, b)
		Brown (B, b)
Brown (B, b)	Blue (b, b)	Brown (B, b)
		Blue (b, b)
Brown (B, b)	Brown (B, b)	Brown (B, B)
		Brown (B, b)
		Brown (B, b)
		Blue (b, b)

[*]According to Mendel's laws, brown (B) is dominant and blue (b) is recessive.

bility of passing a particular problem to the unborn child. Of course, it is only a *probability* because of the randomness of gene distribution and the presence of other factors that influence the child's phenotype. The protocol is as follows:

1. Use a **Punnett square**, or mating diagram, to indicate the risk of passing a problem to offspring.
2. Use a lowercase letter when a gene is not expressed alone in the phenotype (i.e., when it is a recessive gene).
3. Use a capital letter when the single gene is expressed in the phenotype (i.e., a dominant gene), whether it is disease producing or normal.
4. Use a slash mark between alleles.
5. Use the standard symbols as in Figure 28-6 to draw a family history, or **pedigree** chart.

Genetic Results of Consanguinity

Matings of first- and second-degree relatives such as half-siblings, double first cousins, parent and child, brother and sister, and uncle and niece unfortunately do occur. When a man and woman of **consanguine** (related by blood) pairings have a child, one fourth to one half of all the genes are homozygous; therefore the chance for abnormal genes to be expressed in the phenotype is greater. In descriptive studies a higher incidence of

defects, mental retardation, prematurity, and intrauterine growth retardation (IUGR) have occurred.

Dominant Patterns of Inheritance

When a single allele is expressed in the phenotype, it is **dominant**. Both normal and abnormal genes may be dominant. In dominant disorders the signs of abnormality appear when the person is a heterozygote; however, many dominant disorders do not become apparent until later in life, often after childbearing years. Dominant disorders occur mainly in nonenzyme structural proteins such as hemoglobins, collagens, or regulator proteins.

T E S T *Yourself* 28-2 _____

  a. Differentiate between a dominant and recessive gene.
  b. What is consanguinity? How does it increase the chances of genetic disease in the offspring?

Characteristics of autosomal dominant patterns

1. There is a 50% risk of disorder in the infant *with each pregnancy*. This occurs when the affected parent passes the gene to the child. The child who does not receive the affected gene from the parent will neither have the disorder nor pass it on to offspring.

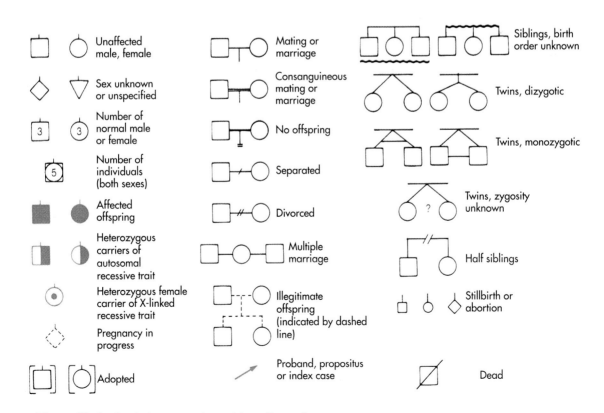

Figure 28-6   Symbols commonly used in pedigree charts.

2. An apparently unaffected parent (normal phenotype) who has the affected gene (abnormal genotype) can pass the disorder to the child. This possibility results from lack of gene **penetrance** in the parent where the gene is present but is not yet expressed.
3. The severity of the disorder may vary among persons with the gene. This is called **expressivity**.
4. Both sexes are equally affected.

Examples of autosomal dominant disorders

More than 1800 recognized problems are caused by autosomal dominant inheritance. Although most are not

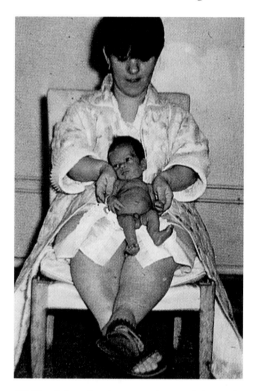

Figure 28-7 Achondroplastic mother with her achondroplastic child, the result of a dominant pattern of inheritance. (From O'Doherty N: *Atlas of the newborn,* ed 2, The Hague, 1985, Kluwer Academic Publishers Group.)

lethal, some reduce the affected person's ability to reproduce, decreasing chances of passing the gene to children. Achondroplasia is an example of a defect that causes dwarfism but usually does not affect intelligence or primary human functions. The arms and legs are short, but the head is normal size. These children may lead normal lives (Figure 28-7).

Other disorders become evident in adulthood during or after the reproductive period; thus they may be passed to offspring by the affected parent. Hyperlipoproteinemia in the dominant form is common. The narrowing of blood vessels with fatty deposits may precipitate early heart attacks. Gastrointestinal polyposis predisposes the host to gastrointestinal cancer. Multiple neurofibromatosis type I (von Recklinghausen's disease) may show up later in life with multiple neurofibromas of the skin that are benign but disfiguring; the accompanying severe hypertension may be dangerous. Figure 28-8 shows the inheritance pattern.

Huntington's chorea. An example of a late-onset dominant disorder is Huntington's chorea. Huntington's chorea is found in many parts of the world, possibly traced to a mutation originating in northern Europe. Currently 25,000 adults have overt signs. In this country the incidence of carriers is thought to be between 1 in 5000 and 1 in 15,000. The problem for carriers is the knowledge that the expression of the trait may begin any time after age 30. By 40, half the persons heterozygous for Huntington's chorea will show overt signs, including slow, progressive degeneration of the nervous system, and will require complete care for long periods before eventual death. Preconception testing is now possible for couples who have a family history of Huntington's chorea. This produces a dilemma for the family: Would you want to know that you will develop Huntington's chorea in 20 years?

Homozygous dominant disorders

When both parents pass a dominant trait for a disease, the expression of the disease will be more severe in its effect than if the child inherited a dominant trait from only one parent.

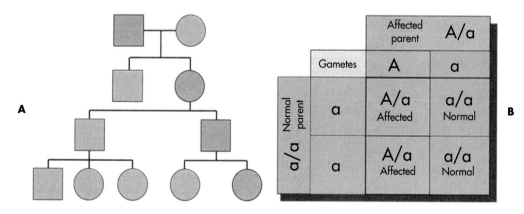

Figure 28-8 Dominant pattern. **A,** Pedigree chart, **B,** Punnett square.

Codominance

In some cases both alleles are present in the genotype and both are expressed in the phenotype. One of the main blood groups is an example of **codominance**; a person inheriting the gene for blood type A from the mother and the gene for B from the father will demonstrate a phenotype of AB. Type O, however, is recessive if combined with A or B. Thus a person with blood type O must be homozygous for O to have that type expressed (Table 28-3).

TEST *Yourself* 28-3 _____

a. In autosomal dominant disease there is a ___% chance that an affected parent will pass the gene to the child.
b. Why is the inheritance of blood types said to be codominant?
c. Why does a person with blood type O have to be homozygous for O alleles?

Recessive Patterns

An allele that is expressed in the phenotype only when it is homozygous is called a **recessive** trait (Figure 28-9). Thus two recessive genes must be present for a disorder to be expressed. In recessive disorders, if one of the alleles is normal, the normal enzyme will be produced. If there is only one abnormal gene, the person is a *carrier* of the trait. In recessive disorders the gene products usually are enzymes. Therefore many recessive disorders affect the metabolic cycle.

Characteristics of autosomal recessive inheritance

1. The condition appears to skip generations.
2. The condition appears only in the child's phenotype when both parents carry the same recessive gene.
3. There is a 25% risk of disorder in the infant *with each pregnancy*. This occurs when both parents who carry the recessive gene pass it to the child.
4. Both sexes are affected equally.
5. The risk is greatly increased if there is consanguinity.

Examples of autosomal recessive disorders

Because the gene product is an enzyme in most of these disorders, these conditions are called inborn errors of metabolism (IEM). The main groups are deficiencies in amino acid, carbohydrate, or lipid metabolism. When an enzyme needed for a metabolic pathway is absent or suppressed, the pathway may change or partially metabolized products may accumulate in the system, causing damage or affecting other functions.

Inborn errors of metabolism

Amino acid metabolism. PKU is probably the best known of these disorders because it was one of the first to be reversed with strict dietary treatment. The carrier incidence is only 1 in 16,000 in the United States but increases to 1 in 50 for persons of northern European ancestry. The child with PKU often has decreased pigmentation with light skin and hair and blue eyes. Classic PKU results from absence of the hepatic enzyme phenylalanine 4-hydroxylase, which is necessary to convert the essential amino acid, phenylalanine, into tyrosine. When this does not happen, the normal metabolic route is changed and partial phenylalanine metabolites build up and injure the infant; phenylpyruvic acid and phenylacetic acid blood levels increase, cross the blood-brain

Table **28-3**	**ABO Blood Groups**			
	O	A	B	AB
Genotype	OO	AA AO	BB BO	AB
Antigens on red cells	Neither	A	B	A and B
Antibodies in serum	Anti-A, Anti-B	Anti-B	Anti-A	Neither

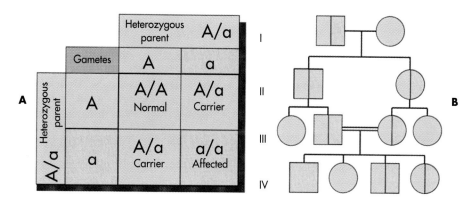

Figure 28-9   Autosomal recessive inheritance pattern. **A,** Punnett square. **B,** Pedigree chart.

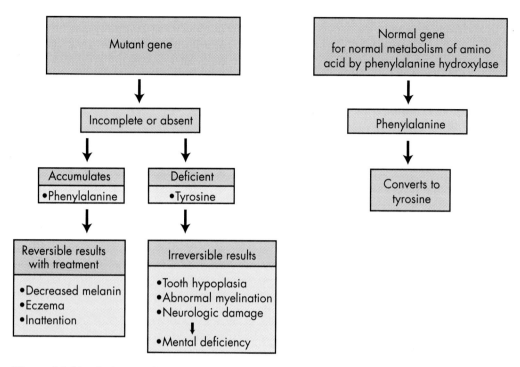

Figure 28-10 Pathways of PKU damage.

barrier to stop myelinization in the central nervous system, and thus damage the brain (Figure 28-10). Without strict dietary control, the child will become severely retarded. However, with treatment a fairly normal life is possible. Early diagnosis is important, and although the overall rate is low, all newborns are tested (see Chapter 19). It is important to test after the infant has sufficient amounts of proteins to begin the build-up of phenylketones. Thus if an infant is discharged within 72 hours or is breast-feeding, follow-up assessment should be done. Dietary control is normally continued until neurologic development is completed in early adulthood. This mandated screening program has therefore allowed many women with PKU to develop normally and subsequently have children. However, during pregnancy, PKU levels will quickly become elevated unless they resume strict dietary control. The developing fetus will then be exposed to high levels of phenylalanine metabolites and suffer neurologic damage *even if the fetal genotype is normal.* Nutritional counseling with the goals of adequate protein intake and strict phenylalanine control are vital for the pregnant PKU woman (see Chapter 24 for maternal PKU treatment).

Maple syrup urine disease, so called because the infant's urine has a maple syrup smell, results in failure to thrive, metabolic imbalance, and seizures. There is a defect in the metabolism of the amino acids leucine, isoleucine, and valine. Untreated, the infant becomes severely retarded and dies. Dietary treatment that omits these amino acids is required.

Histidinemia and *homocystinuria* result from defects in the metabolism of histidine and methionine. Unless treated by a diet free of these amino acids, the infant may be retarded and, with homocystinuria, may develop eye defects.

Carbohydrate metabolism. *Galactosemia* results from a missing enzyme necessary to metabolize galactose, one step of lactose metabolism. High levels of galactose produce severe vomiting and refusal to eat with resulting failure to thrive, weight loss, dehydration, seizures, hepatosplenomegaly, and cataracts. Symptoms may begin after the first feeding of almost any milk formula but especially after breast milk because of its higher lactose content.

If symptoms are recognized early and treatment is initiated, brain damage, metal retardation, and blindness can be prevented. Treatment consists of a low-galactose formula at first. As the infant matures, puddings, cake mixes, cream soups, meat from milk-fed animals (veal), or any commercial foods containing galactose (or lactose) must be avoided. The mother must be taught to read labels carefully.

Lactose intolerance. Problems with digestion of lactose follow geographic lines. A persistence into adulthood of the lactase enzyme, important in digestion of milk, is found in many parts of northern Europe, northern Africa, and Arabia among milk-dependent populations.

Much of the rest of the world's population has a lactase restriction by early adulthood because of poor ability to digest milk. In this country many persons refuse milk saying that it upsets their digestion. If tested these persons would probably show some inability to digest lactose.

Generally those of the following racial origins have adult lactase deficiency to some degree (Flatz, 1986):

- Vietnamese, Thai, Chinese, Taiwanese, Indonesian, and Japanese
- Alaskan, Central American, Native American, and Mexican Indian
- South Americans of Indian origin
- South Sea Islanders
- Afghan and persons from Middle East countries such as the Jordan, Syria, Lebanon, Israel, and Egypt
- Ashkenazic Jews
- Asian Indian (varied)
- Middle and Southern Africans, except for milk-dependent tribes

Lipid metabolism. Tay-Sachs disease is a recessive disorder carried in 1 in 25 Ashkenazic Jews and at a much lower rate in other populations. Before pregnancy, couples may seek blood tests to determine whether they are carriers of this deleterious gene.

The homozygous child appears normal at birth, but as poorly metabolized lipid substances accumulate, fatty deposits in the brain cause degeneration of neural tissue. There is failure to thrive by 6 months, and by 1 year, progressive degeneration leads to blindness, muscle weakness, excessive production of mucus, and seizures, with death before 5 years of age. Families trying to care for the infant at home will need a great deal of support, in-home equipment, and nursing care.

One of the most common lipid disorders is *hyperlipoproteinemia*, which leads to high levels of cholesterol and triglycerides. There are many recessive single-gene forms, and some forms are dominant in expression. One heterozygous form occurs as frequently as 1 in 500 in the general population. Because elevated cholesterol and triglyceride levels underlie many types of coronary artery disease, evaluation for elevated levels is a routine part of most complete physical examinations.

Summary of inborn errors of metabolism. In all cases of enzyme deficiency the infant will not thrive, will be irritable, may have changes in stool, and will suffer from colic or vomiting with weight loss. Any infant not doing well on usual formulas or breast milk should be evaluated for some type of IEM. All infants in the nursery are tested for the metabolic problems listed in Chapter 19. The nursery or home care nurse may notice an irritable infant, or shortly after discharge to the home, signs of difficulty may appear.

Other recessive disorders

Sickle cell disease. Sickle cell disease is a recessively inherited disorder that involves a structural change in the hemoglobin molecule. Substitution of one of the 146 amino acids in the beta-chain with another amino acid is the only difference between normal hemoglobin A and hemoglobin S, the sickle cell hemoglobin. The heterozygous person is a carrier (i.e., he or she can pass the trait to a child who will show signs of difficulty early if homozygous). Those who inherit a homozygous pattern for hemoglobin S will experience the crisis of sickling; the cell changes into a sickle shape when low oxygen tension is present (see Chapter 23).

The incidence of the trait is widespread throughout Africa and Asia. The mutation appears to offer protection from death from malaria. More than 150 variations of beta-chain defect are recognized. Because many persons in this country carry the trait, it is estimated that 1 in 500 newborns (from the groups that migrated to this country from Africa and Asia) will be homozygous for the sickle gene. Therefore all newborns are tested before discharge from the nursery.

Thalassemias. Thalassemic defects in the hemoglobin molecule are the most common gene disorder and originate from the Mediterranean basin, Africa, and parts of India and Asia. There are two types; the defect is in the alpha- or beta-chain hemoglobin molecule. Four genes are involved in alpha-thalassemia; two pairs may be variously affected. A person may have one, two, or three faulty genes with increasingly severe degrees of anemia. If, however, a fetus is homozygous for this thalassemia (i.e., all four genes are dysfunctional), it will not survive gestation (see Chapter 23).

TEST *Yourself* 28-4

a. Describe how an inborn error of metabolism may affect a newborn infant.
b. Those affected with sickle cell disease carry one or more copies of the affected genes. How does the hemoglobin in sickle cell anemia differ from normal hemoglobin?

Cystic fibrosis. Cystic fibrosis (CF) has a carrier rate among Irish people of 1 in 30 and a general occurrence rate of 1 in 2000 in other northern Europeans.

CF is another example of **genetic drift**; as people intermarry and move geographically, defects once found only in isolated ethnic groups are now scattered into the general population. Because these recessive disorders need inheritance from father and mother, the incidence should gradually diminish as the gene pool is diluted.

In CF the passage of chloride ions into cells is altered. This affects the exocrine, gastrointestinal, and respiratory systems. Abnormal secretions occur from exocrine glands, including sweat glands; viscid (sticky) secretions are produced in the pancreas, liver, duodenum, and small intestine. A classic sign is a *meconium plug* passed into the diaper before the first stool. Meconium ileus is often present at birth. However, the respiratory effects are the most lethal. Thick, viscid secretions from the lungs complicate respiration and are intensified by respiratory infection.

Until recently prenatal diagnosis was limited to evaluation of amniotic fluid for levels of certain intestinal enzymes with a high prediction rate. In 1986 the gene that codes for the defective protein in CF was located on the seventh chromosome. This led to the use of *gene markers* (series of

codons that are found near the CF gene), which allow the CF gene to be tracked in families with a known history of the disease. DNA analysis with gene markers may be performed early in pregnancy by means of chorionic villus biopsy. When this is done during the second trimester by amniocentesis, the amniotic fluid also is analyzed for intestinal enzymes, further confirming the diagnosis. Currently many states mandate screening of newborns for CF at the time blood is drawn for other metabolic testing. There is an enormous research effort for CF treatment, including both gene therapy and "tricking" respiratory viruses to deliver normal genes to lung cells (Alton, 1995).

X-Linked Inheritance

A gene on the X chromosome may carry a defect. Figure 28-11 is a map of the X chromosome, showing several X-linked disorders. Because the male has only one X chromosome, any disorder carried on that X is expressed in his phenotype and thus follows a dominant pattern. In this case the male is **hemizygous**. On the other hand, a female has two X chromosomes, but in this case an interesting change occurs; one of the two Xs becomes inactivated, or "silent," early in the development of the embryo. This inactivation is random within the cells and is seen as the Barr chromatin body, a dark staining spot on the cell. After one X is inactivated, its cell retains the activity of the other X in all future replications. Therefore in some cells the maternal X is active, whereas the paternal X is active in other cells. These females have a mixed chromosome pattern; that is, they are **mosaic** for the active X. Thus if a gene mutation occurs on one of the X chromosomes, it is muted by the presence of a normal gene in half of her other cells. *Therefore the female usually must be homozygous for a disorder to be fully expressed in her phenotype.* As a result, females are spoken of as carriers of X-linked traits. Homozygosity is rather unusual in females (Figure 28-12) but is seen with color blindness, a common, non-lethal **X-linked defect.**

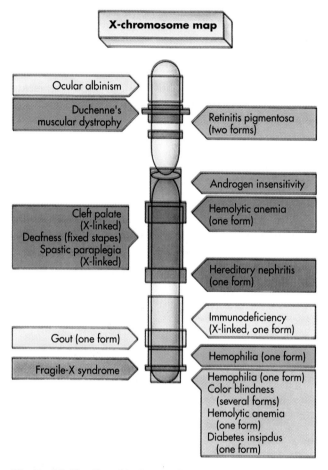

Figure 28-11   Simplified map of the X chromosome. This diagram shows only a few of the many regions of the X chromosome that have been identified to contain specific bits of genetic information. (Courtesy Rolin Graphics.)

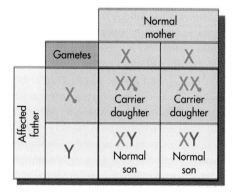

Figure 28-12   X-linked recessive inheritance pattern. Sex differences in offspring ratios in X-linked recessive inheritance. •, Recessive allele on X chromosome.

X-linked dominant patterns

There are few X-linked dominant disorders. In these cases an affected father may have an affected daughter but no affected son. Mothers may pass to daughters or sons.

X-linked recessive patterns

Characteristics of X-linked recessive patterns:

1. A male is hemizygous, inheriting one X. If the defective gene is on that X, the male will have the disorder. Many X-linked recessive traits are severe enough to prevent reproduction by affected males.
2. A female may be heterozygous or homozygous for the gene and usually follows the autosomal recessive pattern.
3. There is only one active X in each female cell; the other X is inactivated.
4. Because maternal or paternal X may be activated in a mosaic pattern, any disorder may be muted or silent in the female.
5. *With each pregnancy* the risk for infants of carrier females is 50% for a male to be affected and 50% for a female to be a carrier.
6. Affected males do not pass the disorder to their sons.

Fragile X syndrome. Breakage may occur at fragile sites on chromosomes. The classic example is the **fragile X** (fra X), a cause of mental retardation second only to Down syndrome. As more has been recognized about fragile chromosomes, diagnosis of fra X syndrome has been made in many puzzling cases of mental retardation. Currently the estimate is that 100,000 males and a smaller number of females are affected. The occurrence rate is 1 in 1000 male births (Laxova, 1994).

The defect is passed by X-linked inheritance or may be a mutation in the sperm. Approximately one third of carrier mothers may have mild retardation. Males with normal genotypes and phenotypes also may cause a fra X chromosome to be passed to their daughters when an as yet unknown factor creates the fragile site after formation of the female zygote.

Fra X is a leading cause of mental retardation (Nelson, 1995), and most fra X males have moderate to severe retardation. They also may have organic brain disease, seizures, and self-mutilating and hyperactive behavior. Signs are delayed speech and mild enlargement of the chin, ears, and testes. For carrier females the range of intelligence is broad. Learning difficulties may occur; only one third have mild mental retardation.

Pattern. The pattern for fra X syndrome follows:

1. The fra X is not completely recessive because one third of heterozygous females are affected.
2. An apparently normal male may transmit fra X to his daughter.
3. The mutation rate is high for the sperm and low for the ovum.

The breakage of the affected chromosome is shown in a culture medium that lacks folate. Therefore some cen-

ters have tried folic acid supplement in early treatment, and some children have shown improvement in behavior. Others believe that folic acid supplements have no benefit.

Genetic counseling is important and may take time. The child may have been misdiagnosed with autism, cerebral palsy, or a birth injury. It is recommended that all family members at risk be tested, including the siblings of the parents and the child.

Other fragile sites. Fragile sites on autosomes are being linked with cancer. Researchers have identified 30 **oncogenes**, genetic mutations that change cellular behavior by changing the structure or amount of protein produced by the cell. Although normal cells have tumor-suppressing abilities, affected cells lose the ability to regulate their rate of growth. This unrestrained growth is the beginning of cancer. An example of this is the **retinoblastoma** gene (Rb), the first oncogene to be identified. Retinoblastoma occurs when a *single* mutant gene on chromosome 13 is passed on from a carrier parent, followed by a *second* mutation within a fetal or infant retinal cell. This mutation also predisposes children with Rb to other tumors such as osteosarcoma. Although in the past these young persons did not live to reproduce, advances in treatment now allow more survivors to pass the gene on to their children. Other tumors, such as lung and colon carcinomas and Wilms' tumor, are associated with the absence of normal alleles at specific loci. Researchers expect to find many more sites that are correlated with cancer.

Hemophilia. Used as the classic illustration of X-linked recessive disease, hemophilia is a deficiency of antihemophilic globulin, a problem in the clotting cycle (factor VIII). The gene was often found among royal families in Europe. It appears to be more prevalent in northern Europeans. Recently, because a replacement for the missing clotting factor has become more available, males with hemophilia survived long enough to become fathers. A female could thus be a hemophiliac if she inherited the defect from both parents.

Glucose-6-phosphate dehydrogenase. The most common X-linked problems are color blindness and glucose-6-phosphate dehydrogenase (G6PD) deficiency. G6PD is an enzyme involved in glucose metabolism. It is more common in males but also can be found in females. When a person with G6PD deficiency ingests certain drugs or foods, red blood cells are destroyed, resulting in severe anemia. Drugs and foods that precipitate breakdown of red blood cells are listed in Chapter 23. It is important to check drug interactions for any person with G6PD deficiency, and all newborns are now tested for it.

Color blindness. One in ten males from Mediterranean countries and Ashkenazic Jewish groups is color blind, and many other groups in the world also have frequent color blindness disorders. The locus of the genes is near that of G6PD on the X chromosome. Because color blindness is not fatal and occurs frequently, females may be homozygous and thus also color blind. Other X-linked recessive problems are Duchenne's muscular dystrophy and the rare Lesch-Nyhan syndrome.

TEST *Yourself* 28-5

a. A color blind man and a woman who sees normally have a daughter who is color blind. What is the child's genotype?
b. Why are only males affected by X-linked recessive traits?
c. Give two examples of a fragile site on a chromosome causing disease or disability.

Polygenic Inheritance

When more than one pair of genes plays a role in disease, the cause is **polygenic inheritance**. More often, multiple genes and environmental influences precipitate disorders. In this case the cause is **multifactorial inheritance**. Certain disorders seem to run in families and yet do not occur as often as those inherited according to Mendel's patterns. Although polygenic and multifactorial problems do not follow Mendel's dominant and recessive patterns, the overall risk for the problem to develop is increased if there is a history in close relatives. Therefore clients are asked about their medical history to ascertain whether close relatives have problems that follow this pattern of inheritance.

Certain disorders show up during fetal development; for instance, the cleft lip and palate fail to fuse by about 35 days of development. Congenital dislocation of the hip and certain heart defects also follow the multifactorial distribution. Several disorders may become apparent at birth or during infancy, whereas others are not expressed unless environmental factors precipitate symptoms. Hypertension is an example of a late-developing disorder.

Because many factors contribute to multifactorial defects, precise prevention is difficult. Avoidance of environmental exposure that may precipitate problems and ensuring adequate diet and vitamin intake are important during pregnancy.

Diabetes mellitus

Poorly controlled diabetes mellitus increases the risk of anomalies two or three times that of the general population. Organs most affected are the spine, lower limbs, heart, kidneys, and external genitalia. Before the use of folic acid, neural tube defects were seen 20 times more frequently in fetuses of mothers with insulin-dependent diabetes mellitus (IDDM). Good glucose control and folic acid are important for this reason.

Structural Birth Defects

The overall incidence of birth defects is approximately 3%, and defects remain a leading cause of infant mortality.

Birth defects are reported to several data banks, such as the Centers for Disease Control and Prevention (CDC), Metropolitan Atlanta Congenital Defects Program, and the California Birth Defects Monitoring Program. Major hospitals report occurrences; health care providers submit case reports to journals. From these data, projections are made, and any increase in a specific malformation is noted. In this way a newly emerging problem may be brought to the attention of practitioners, and epidemiologic studies can be undertaken.

Although in the past more attention has been given to maternal risk factors for birth defects, it is now recognized that paternal risk factors such as age and occupational exposures must also be considered (Schnitzer et al, 1995; McIntosh et al, 1995). Teen mothers as well as those more than 35 years of age are at increased risk for having offspring with congenital malformations (Croen and Shaw, 1995).

Defects in structure occur when some factor alters the progress of normal fetal development. The part may stop developing and remain in an immature form, accessory structures may be produced, or cells may be organized in an abnormal way. The cause of these changes may be genetic, environmental, or multifactorial. An essentially normal fetus may be deformed or misshapen because of intrauterine crowding as a result of multiple gestation or an abnormally small amount of amniotic fluid. In most cases, however, the cause remains unknown.

Defects may be found alone (isolates) or as part of a syndrome—a group of signs. In general the more severe defects arise earlier in gestation (Table 28-4). It is important that an infant with a defect be assessed for the presence of other system defects because multiple organs may be affected. In this chapter, only those defects that can be detected at birth or soon after are discussed.

| *Table* **28-4** | **Timing of Selected Malformations** |

Malformation	Time of Development
Anencephaly	Day 26
Spina bifida	Day 28
Tracheoesophageal fistula	Day 30
Renal agenesis (Potter's syndrome)	Day 34
Transposition of great vessels	Day 36
Cleft lip and palate	Day 36
Ventriculoseptal defect	Week 6
Duodenal atresia	Week 7-8
Urethral obstruction	Week 9

Data from Brent RL: Evaluating alleged teratogenicity of environmental agents, *Clin Perinatol* 13:609, 1986; Moore KL: *The developing human: clinically oriented embryology*, ed 4, Philadelphia, 1988, WB Saunders.

Cardiovascular defects

The cardiovascular system is the first to function in the embryo with defects arising early in gestation. Although even major defects are compatible with fetal life, such defects are life threatening to the newborn. Some are isolated defects; others are part of known syndromes caused by genetic or environmental hazards. Recent research indicates that the risk for cardiac and other birth defects is decreased in women who use multivitamin supplements, especially those including folic acid (Shaw et al, 1995). Cardiovascular defects are discussed in detail in Chapter 29 because they are a large part of care of the newborn at high risk.

Cleft lip and palate

Failure of fusion of the lip or palate may be unilateral or bilateral. Lack of fusion may be limited to the lip or soft palate, or a combined lip and hard and soft palate cleft may occur (Figure 28-13). Cleft lip with palate is often found as an isolated defect or as part of trisomy 13. Rates of occurrence seem to be higher in agricultural areas where there are high levels of toxic materials (Das et al, 1995). Treatment is directed toward supporting the

infant's status until the surgical decision is made. Repair is usually successful, and cosmetic surgery may be performed later to improve facial contours, which may reassure parents. Until surgical repair is completed (a series of operations may be required), the infant is fed in an upright position with use of a special nipple. Even breastfeeding may be possible, depending on the degree of cleft. The student should consult a pediatrics nursing text for further details of nursing care.

Gastrointestinal atresias

Gastrointestinal defects of the esophagus or intestine may be life threatening. In *tracheoesophageal fistula,* a communication between the trachea and esophagus, the esophagus may be patent or end in a blind sac. Swallowing any liquid results in regurgitation and danger of aspiration (Figure 28-14). Tracheoesophageal fistula may be complicated by rectal atresia or imperforate anus (Figure 28-15). In any case surgical repair is extensive.

Intestinal obstruction may be caused by *atresia,* which is narrowing anywhere below the stomach. Before birth gastrointestinal atresias produce polyhydramnios because

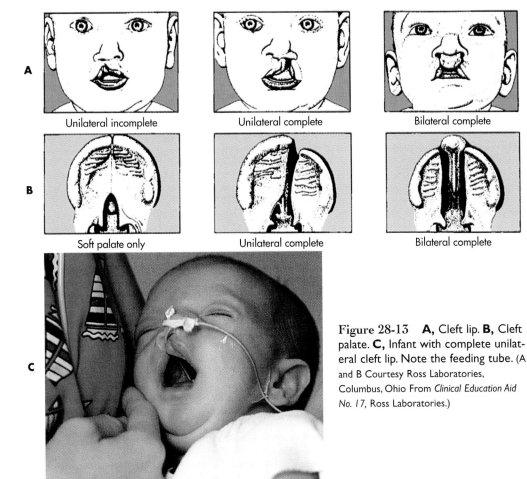

Unilateral incomplete	Unilateral complete	Bilateral complete
Soft palate only	Unilateral complete	Bilateral complete

Figure 28-13   A, Cleft lip. **B,** Cleft palate. **C,** Infant with complete unilateral cleft lip. Note the feeding tube. (A and B Courtesy Ross Laboratories, Columbus, Ohio From *Clinical Education Aid No. 17,* Ross Laboratories.)

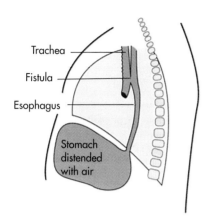

Figure 28-14   One type of tracheoesophageal fistula. (From Corliss CE: *Patten's human embryology*, ed 4, New York, 1976, McGraw-Hill.)

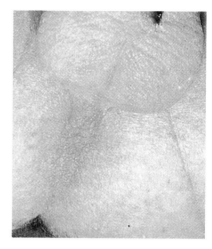

Figure 28-15   Imperforate anus. (From Chessell GSJ et al: *Diagnostic picture tests in clinical medicine*, vol 2, 1984, Mosby-Wolfe.)

the fetus is unable to swallow amniotic fluid. Duodenal atresia causes symptoms of vomiting and distension soon after birth. It is commonly seen with other conditions such as Down syndrome and cardiovascular abnormalities. Atresias of the large intestine, rectum, and anus will cause distension and failure to pass meconium. Repair of the most common types of anal and rectal defects may be simple or may require colostomy for a period.

Renal defects

When an obstructive malformation limits the flow of urine into the amniotic fluid, the infant's distended kidneys, ureters, and bladder may be seen on ultrasound, depending on the location of the obstruction. Some degree of oligohydramnios will occur if urine is not passing freely. In rare instances the kidneys will completely fail to develop. Severe oligohydramnios results, and the excessive pressure on the fetal body prevents normal lung and skeletal development. The resulting Potter's syndrome is fatal (Figure 28-16).

Neural tube defects

Anencephaly. Defects of the central nervous system can be of varying severity. The most severe is **anencephaly**, absence of all brain but the medulla. Anencephaly is caused by failure of fusion of the cranial end of the neural tube before day 26 of gestation. There is no cranium or cerebrum, although the rest of the body usually is well formed. The condition is found more frequently in certain families, and two of three cases are female infants. Many are stillborn or survive for only hours or days. *Hydranencephaly* is the absence of cerebral hemispheres but a normal skull (Figure 28-17).

Meningomyelocele. Spina bifida, a failure of fusion of the lower neural tube, may occur in many degrees of severity (Figure 28-18). The condition is now linked with inadequate folic acid intake before and during early preg-

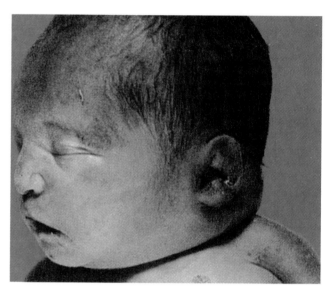

Figure 28-16   Potter facies. This infant with bilateral multicystic dysplasia died of pulmonary insufficiency 12 hours after birth. The altered facies produced by the fetal compression syndrome of oligohydramnios includes small, posteriorly rotated ears, micrognathia, a beaked nose, and wide-set eyes. (Courtesy Dr. MacPherson, Magee-Women's Hospital, Pittsburgh, Penn.)

nancy (MMWR, 1992). Other research has linked maternal hyperthermia and neural tube defects (Hoyme, 1990). A maternal core temperature over 38.9° C may be teratogenic. Other central nervous system (CNS) and facial defects also possibly are linked to hyperthermia. The highest risk seems to be for pregnant women who use hot tubs or who have sustained fevers.

Neonates with meningomyelocele are at risk for infection (meningitis and urinary tract infection), neurologic deficit, and hydrocephalus. The risk of meningitis is decreased if the sac has not been ruptured during delivery (cesarean birth is preferred). Repair of this form of neural

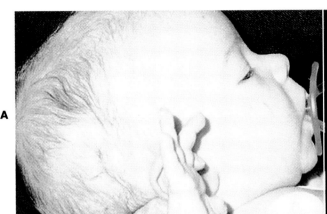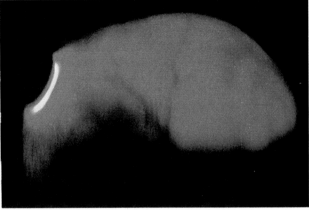

Figure 28-17 **A,** Hydranencephaly. Infant 3 weeks after birth has a deceptively normal appearance with little to suggest a severe brain abnormality. **B,** Transillumination of the skull lights up the calvarium, suggesting the diagnosis. (From Zitelli BJ, Davis HW: *Atlas of pediatric physical diagnosis,* ed 3, St Louis, 1997, Mosby-Wolfe.)

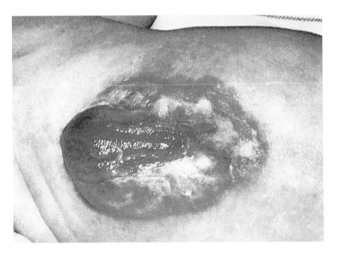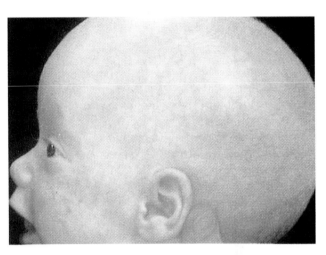

Figure 28-18 Meningomyelocele (spina bifida). (From Zitelli BJ, Davis HW: *Atlas of pediatric physical diagnosis,* ed 3, St Louis, 1997, Mosby-Wolfe.)

Figure 28-19 Infantile hydrocephalus. The characteristic appearance is an enlarged head, thinning of the scalp, distended scalp veins, and a full fontanelle. (From Booth IW, Wozniak ER: *Pediatrics,* Baltimore, 1984, Williams & Wilkins.)

tube defect is accomplished as soon as the infant's condition is stable.

A high defect (high lumbar to low thoracic), hydrocephalus, and other bony abnormalities of the spine increase the probability that the infant will have significant motor and mental neurologic deficits. Many ethical problems affect the extent to which these infants should be treated. These decisions are made with input from the parents and the agency's infant care review board.

Other central nervous system defects

Hydrocephaly. Hydrocephaly is an abnormal accumulation of cerebrospinal fluid (CSF) within ventricles of the brain (Figure 28-19). The cause is varied; it can result from a congenital malformation (it often is associated with meningomyelocele) or an infectious or hemorrhagic process that blocks the flow or alters the absorption of CSF. Increased pressure of the fluid prevents normal growth and development of the brain.

The fetus with hydrocephaly may be identified prenatally by means of ultrasound. Cesarean birth may be necessary when the head size is greatly increased. The hydrocephalic neonate may have a head circumference far larger than the percentile for birth weight and height, although this varies depending on the onset. In extreme forms the head circumference can exceed 42 cm (normal maximum for a full-term infant is 37 cm). The sun-setting sign may be present, (look at the infant's eyes—a rim of sclera will be visable *above* the iris) and the skull feels soft and thin, similar to a ping-pong ball.

Newborn infants with hydrocephaly initially may behave fairly normally or be severely affected. Without treatment, however, progressive damage to the brain is a certain outcome. Computerized tomography (CT) scans and ultrasound are used to assess the extent to which brain growth has been disrupted. Therapy consists of measures to drain the excessive CSF and lessen intracranial pressure. Fetal therapy attempts to relieve intracranial pressure earlier in development, allowing brain growth to proceed normally.

Microcephaly. Microcephaly may occur because of a reduced number of brain cells or because of space restrictions imposed on a normal number of cells. Cells may be reduced in number by congenital syndromes such as trisomy 21 or because of intrauterine infections, especially viral. Premature closure of the cranial sutures (*craniosynostosis*) restricts the space available for brain growth. The prognosis depends on the cause because there can be no increase in cellular number after birth.

Autosomal Disorders

Often chromosome defects result from a 45 or 47 chromosome pattern in which each cell contains one less or one more than the normal 46. On other occasions defects result from loss of part of a chromosome (**deletion**) or by exchange of one piece of a chromosome to another chromosome (**translocation**); translocation is a rare cause of Down syndrome in which chromosomes 21 and 14 exchange a block of material. There also may be an extra portion of some chromosome material (**duplication**); duplications result in additional material and seem to be less harmful than deletions.

Finally, when division of chromosomes takes place and separation, which should occur longitudinally at the centromere, instead occurs laterally between the short arms (p) and the long arms (q), the result is an **isochromosome**. The child may have trisomy for the material on the long arms and be missing the material on the short arms. The X chromosome most often is involved because monosomy in the autosomes (resulting from lack of the short arm material) is not compatible with survival. Women with Turner's syndrome (45, X syndrome) may have this variation.

Nondisjunction

Nondisjunction is the most common cause of chromosomal abnormalities. During the first and second steps of meiosis and even during mitosis, a chromosome pair can refuse to separate to the poles (at anaphase). The resulting daughter cells will have an extra chromosome (**trisomy**) or be missing a chromosome (**monosomy**). The karyotype of an individual is labeled by the affected pair (e.g., 47, XX+21 or 47, XY+21). This set of numbers and letters means that in either a male (XY) or female (XX), there are 47 chromosomes instead of 46 with the extra at pair 21 (Figure 28-20).

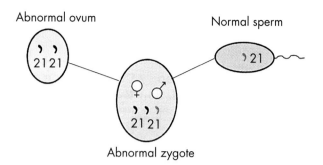

Figure 28-20   After fertilization with normal sperm, oocyte with double chromosome at 21 becomes zygote with three chromosomes (trisomy 21). (From March of Dimes Birth Defects Foundation, White Plains, NY)

Table **28-5**	**Risk of Trisomy 21 Resulting from Nondisjunction in Relation to Mother's Age**
Mother's Age	**Risk**
Less than 29	1 in 1500
30 to 34	1 in 700
35 to 39	1 in 250
40 to 44	1 in 100
Greater than 45	1 in 25-40

Mosaicism

Mosaicism is the presence of different patterns of gene expression in tissue within the same organism. For example, a person may have one brown eye and one blue eye pattern with some cells containing Bb and others BB. Such variation indicates a mosaic gene.

If nondisjunction occurs during early mitosis, a mosaic for an entire chromosome may occur. Because the mosaic individual contains two cell lines in the body, the proportion is variable, and the phenotypical signs are usually milder because the normal cells modify expression of the problem cells. Sometimes the abnormal cells are "ignored," and normal cells seem to duplicate more readily with resultant later improvement in signs of the defect.

Causes. As with mutation of genetic material in single-gene defects, certain risk factors accompany chromosomal abnormality. The aging parent seems to be linked most often with chromosome defects. Sufficient evidence exists that the older a woman is, the higher the risk of a trisomy (Table 28-5). For example, for Down syndrome, which has been studied most thoroughly, the risk is approximately 1 in 1500 for women younger than 30 and 1 in 100 for women older than 40. Radiation also increases the incidence of nondisjunction in experimental animals. In humans it is difficult to know whether it is just "wear and tear" or the accumulation of environmental exposures like radiation that causes the risk to increase so dramatically with age.

Nondisjunction composes the greater part of trisomy cases, and in Down syndrome, nondisjunction is thought to occur during the first stage of meiosis. Because the oocyte began this stage in the last third of the mother's own fetal life and completes it 30 or 40 years later, there may be a slower separation of chromosome material in the aging ovum. Trisomy incidence is not solely connected to the older woman; it is now known that 20% of the cases of nondisjunction are in the spermatocyte. This nondisjunction is illustrated with some of the sex chromosome trisomies.

Trisomies

Trisomy 21 (Down syndrome). Down syndrome (47, XX+21 or 47, XY+21) is the most frequently occurring trisomy (perhaps because the 21 chromosome is so small). Described in 1866 by John L. H. Down, the syndrome stems from nondisjunction (95%), translocation (4%), or mosaicism (1%). Most pregnant women younger than 35 and all older than 35 are encouraged to have prenatal screening for alpha-fetoprotein levels, which show much lower levels than normal if the syndrome is present. Testing is confirmed with amniocentesis with karyotype preparation and by triple analyte screen.

Signs of Down syndrome are usually observable at birth in facial features, fingerprints and footprints, and body tone.
- Body tone is markedly hypotonic.
- The iris of the eye has speckles (Brushfield's spots).
- The lids have epicanthal folds beginning at the inner canthus of the eye as a thickened lid.
- The upper insertion of the ear should be parallel to the inner canthus of the eye, but in a child with Down syndrome it is set low.
- The bridge of the nose is flat and easy to miss because all babies have a somewhat low bridge (Figure 28-21, *A*).
- The tongue is thickened and may protrude; macroglossia interferes with feeding in severe cases.
- Characteristic hand structures and dermal patterns are similar in every affected baby. The simian line across the palm can be observed in the initial physical assessment (Figure 28-21, *B*).
- Similarly, footprints are different.
- Developmental delays vary widely, with an intelligence quotient (IQ) from 25 to 100.
- Children with Down syndrome may have heart defects and many require surgery.

The capability of each affected infant must be discovered because of the wide range of ability seen with this syn-

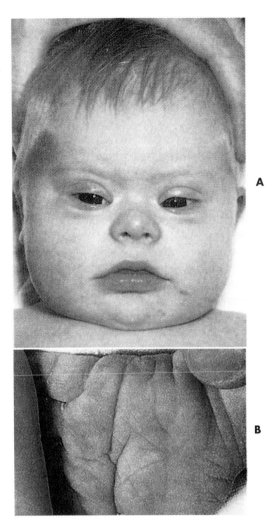

Figure 28-21   Two minor anomalies associated with Down syndrome. **A,** Typical facies (note epicanthal folds). **B,** Simian crease in palm. (From Zitelli BJ, David HW: *Atlas of pediatric physical diagnosis,* ed 3, St Louis, 1997, Mosby-Wolfe.)

drome. The best outcome is obtained when early training and intensive stimulation are provided. When a parent is unable to cope with this regimen, special institutions are available to work with the child. Life expectancy is variable and depends on defects accompanying Down syndrome; usually these children do not have a normal life span.

Trisomy 18 syndrome. Trisomy 18 (Edwards' syndrome) (47, XX+18 or 47, XY+18) occurs as rarely as 1 in 8000 births because only 5% of these conceptions survive. Most cases are due to nondisjunction in older mothers. A few have mosaicism and live slightly longer with less severe abnormalities. The survival period may be 2 to 6 months.

Characteristics can be seen at birth; hypertonia, low-set and malformed ears, a small chin, and a large occiput are the obvious facial characteristics. Hands show simian lines and unusual fingerprints, and the infant makes fists with

TEST *Yourself* **28-6**

Describe the clinical findings characteristic of a newborn with Down syndrome.

the second and fifth fingers overlapping the third and fourth. Feet show "rocker bottoms" with the arch appearing to be rounded below the heel. Severe cardiac defects also may be present. The infant is severely mentally retarded, has trouble feeding, and therefore fails to thrive.

Trisomy 13 syndrome. The incidence of trisomy 13 (Patau syndrome) (47, XX+13 or 47, XY+13) is rare, and survival is short. Ethical questions arise about the amount of intervention to provide for a child with such a poor prognosis.

Many of the defects of trisomy 18 syndrome show in the child with trisomy 13 syndrome and include mental retardation, hand and foot abnormalities, simian line abnormalities, and cardiac defects. Other malformations also are present, the most obvious of which are severe cleft lip and palate and eye deformities (Figure 28-22).

Deletion: cri du chat syndrome

The cat-cry syndrome is caused by a deletion; chromosome 5 is missing a short arm (p) so that the karyotype is

written 46,XX,5p- or 46,XY,5p-. Signs at birth are the "cat cry," like the mewing of a cat, wide-spaced eyes with a slant and epicanthal fold, low-set ears, small head, and mental retardation. In addition, these children have unusual fingerprints and footprints, and simian lines may be present on the palms.

TEST *Yourself* **28-7**

a. Name three causes of structural birth defects.
b. Nondisjunction occurs when a pair of chromosomes fail to _____ during meiosis.
c. The most common trisomy, _____, also is called _____ syndrome.

Sex Chromosome Disorders

Monosomy

Turner syndrome. Monosomy is always lethal in autosomes. However, sex chromosome monosomy (Turner syndrome, or 45, XO) is possible; remember that in all normal female cells one X is active and the other is inactive. Thus cell lines can survive a single active X. Even so, 99% of monosomy 45,X fetuses are spontaneously

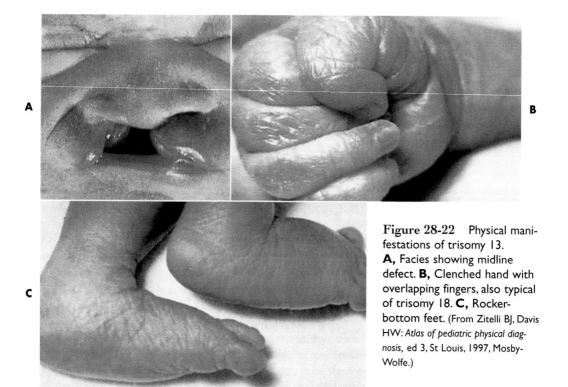

Figure 28-22 Physical manifestations of trisomy 13. **A,** Facies showing midline defect. **B,** Clenched hand with overlapping fingers, also typical of trisomy 18. **C,** Rocker-bottom feet. (From Zitelli BJ, Davis HW: *Atlas of pediatric physical diagnosis,* ed 3, St Louis, 1997, Mosby-Wolfe.)

aborted; the incidence of live births is only about 1 in 10,000. Some of these have isochromosomes or mosaicism. Mosaic fetuses will have X/XX; that is, some cells in the body have only one X, and others have two normal Xs.

Signs present at birth are webbing of the skin at the sides of the neck, a low hairline at the back of the neck (hard to distinguish in many infants), puffy hands and feet (lymphedema), and a broad chest with widely spaced nipples (Figure 28-23). In some children there may be coarctation of the aorta. At puberty secondary sex characteristics are not developed, and the girl is sterile (unless a mosaic pattern). Because intelligence is usually in the normal range, counseling and hormonal therapy are used to help with psychosocial adjustment and body growth.

Sex trisomies

The incidence of sex chromosome trisomy syndrome is rather frequent for males and females (1 in 1000). The infant usually does not show phenotypical changes at birth, but the changes appear by puberty when gonads should be directing the development of secondary sex characteristics. Mosaicism is common in these sex chromosome trisomies and will lessen the phenotypic effect.

Klinefelter syndrome. Nondisjunction in the older mother appears to be the cause of approximately 60% of males with Klinefelter syndrome. The rest are due to paternal nondisjunction. Although the karyotype is written as 47,XXY, approximately 15% of these males have a mosaic pattern, XY/XXY.

Because a trisomy may be from either parent, the sex chromosomes letters are labeled with "m" or "p" to indicate origin of the problem. Thus an infant with an extra X from the mother would be identified as XX_mY, and when the X comes from the father it is XX_pY.

There are few clinical signs at birth, but at puberty the secondary sex characteristics show poor development. Skeletal height is not reduced, and many boys are tall and lanky. There may be some breast development and neuromuscular difficulty. Head size is smaller than normal in many boys, and there are some learning difficulties related to language skills. There may be accompanying psychosocial difficulties from peer criticism, and the boy may have a poor sense of body image. At the time of puberty the boy may be given androgens to assist in development of secondary sex characteristics. Because the testes remain small and no sperm are produced, the man is sterile but not impotent. Therefore in a few cases the first recognition of the problem may occur when a man comes in for infertility testing.

XYY syndrome. Parental nondisjunction during the second stage of meiosis can cause production of a sperm bearing two Y chromosomes. The result in the fertilized

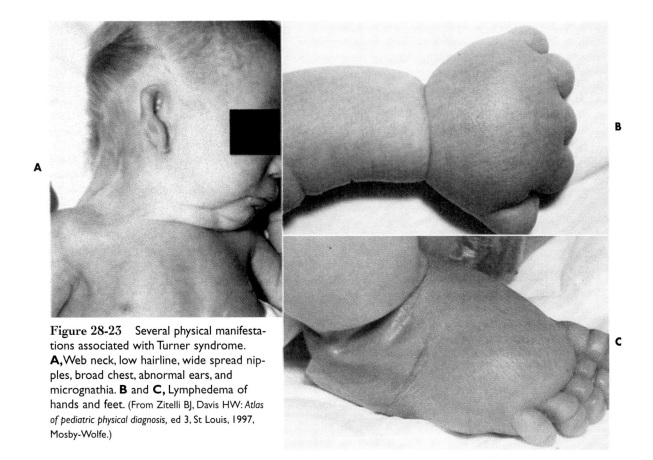

Figure 28-23 Several physical manifestations associated with Turner syndrome. **A,** Web neck, low hairline, wide spread nipples, broad chest, abnormal ears, and micrognathia. **B** and **C,** Lymphedema of hands and feet. (From Zitelli BJ, Davis HW: *Atlas of pediatric physical diagnosis,* ed 3, St Louis, 1997, Mosby-Wolfe.)

ovum is XYY. Because initial studies of XYY involved a prison population, early studies linked XYY with criminal behavior (Hook, 1973). The boy with XYY syndrome tends to be tall and weigh more than the XXY boy. He is fertile. Intelligence is usually in a normal range, but about half have learning problems related to language, motor, and reading skills.

XXX syndrome. Girls with XXX syndrome are usually fertile and taller than average. Head size may be somewhat smaller than usual. Some XXX girls have a lower IQ, and many have trouble with verbal skills and interpersonal relationships. There is a wide range of learning, verbal ability, and neuromotor coordination problems. Like trisomies in boys, signs are usually not evident at birth. Thus many XXX girls go on to marry, have children, and lead fairly normal lives. If, however, there is more than one extra X—for example, XXXX or XXXXX—mental retardation occurs on a fairly severe level.

Early parental intervention may improve the potential of these children. Early diagnosis is important, and referral to speech therapists, child psychologists, and others may help in development. Research shows that although children may have trouble learning or mastering a psychomotor skill, a supportive, loving environment may be the crucial factor in their optimal development.

Ambiguous Genitalia

On rare occasions genital indication of sex is unclear in an infant (Figure 28-24). The presence of ambiguous genitalia has an immediate impact on the parents because their first question after birth is, "Is it a boy or a girl?" When the answer is not known, the parents are stunned. The most important intervention after support of the parents and care of the infant is interpretation of the possible causes and the methods of evaluation. Because people are gender conscious, the parents will be distressed until the

issue is settled. Knowledge of the possible causes of poor differentiation of genitalia and potential interventions will help the nurse to be supportive during the investigation. For a few infants reconstructive surgery is the choice; for others, gonadal tissue may be removed to allow the remaining gonads to develop.

Hermaphroditism

On rare occasions a child has ovarian and testicular tissue; this is *hermaphroditism.* The external genitalia are usually ambiguous. Most of these children have an XX pattern, and the gonads have been inhibited in the phase of differentiation. Others show mosaicism with XX/XY cell lines. The gonads usually are not functional; therefore the sex of rearing must be determined in other ways. The gender of the child must be decided early because it is very traumatic to change gender during rearing. The genetic sex may not be the deciding factor because it is difficult to "reconstruct" a male who will function normally. Usually the child is raised as a female with estrogen treatment at puberty.

Pseudohermaphroditism

Children with pseudohermaphroditism have testicular or ovarian tissue and corresponding chromosomes, but the genitalia are ambiguous at birth. There are several causes of *pseudohermaphroditism,* including mosaicism, gene defects changing androgen production or sensitivity, or teratogens interrupting crucial growth sequences.

The most common of these uncommon disorders is androgen insensitivity, an X-linked inherited problem in a boy with normal chromosome makeup. He has testes, but the external genitalia may show hypospadias, small penis and scrotal sac, or even female genitalia. At puberty, depending on a number of factors, secondary sex characteristics may or may not develop.

Female pseudohermaphroditism often occurs as a result of adrenal hyperplasia, which is inherited as an

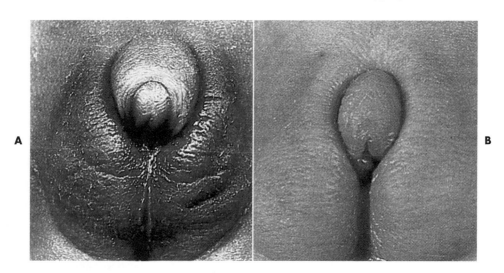

Figure 28-24   Ambiguous genitalia. **A** and **B,** Congenital virilizing adrenal hyperplasia. (Courtesy Dr. Becker. From Zitelli BJ, Davis HW: *Atlas of pediatric physical diagnosis,* ed 3, St Louis, 1997, Mosby-Wolfe.)

autosomal recessive gene defect. The girl has excess levels of adrenocorticotropic hormone (ACTH), which, by a series of effects, produces an enlarged clitoris and fusion of the labia. This syndrome needs immediate medical attention because ACTH has many other adverse effects when present in elevated amounts. Finally, it is possible that a teratogen such as a drug may have affected the development of the infant's genitalia.

THE ENVIRONMENT AND BIRTH DEFECTS

The developing embryo is sensitive to environmental influences, but susceptibility varies because of genetic differences. **Teratogens** cause birth defects in those fetuses who are susceptible to the effect of the exposure. The specific effects vary with the timing of exposure during the pregnancy. To fully appreciate this influence, one's concept of the environment must be expanded to include anything that can alter fetal development—substances in the atmosphere, the mother's metabolic state, the food she eats.

Wilson (1977) defines teratogens as "any factor or mechanism that causes cells to die, change their rate of proliferation or biosynthesis, or otherwise fail to follow the prescribed course in development." A wide range of injury may result when a teratogen impinges on fetal development. This variation is the result of one or more of the following as defined by Brent (1986):

1. There are different periods of cell susceptibility to injury. During the preimplantation period the free floating fertilized zygote in body fluids in the tube or uterus is too small to be only partly affected. An "all or nothing" effect occurs.
   a. After implantation, with a few exceptions, whatever is in the maternal environment or circulation will pass through the placenta to the fetus: "the placenta is a sieve."
   b. During organogenesis in the 60 days after implantation, differentiation may be distorted, slowed, or stopped, resulting in structural changes.
   c. During the second and third trimesters, teratogens may continue to inhibit differentiation and may cause cell death, retard growth, or distort biochemical development.
   d. Certain changes may be carcinogenic but show up in later childhood.
2. A genetic variability exists in which one fetus will be affected if subjected to the same teratogen; the other fetus will not be affected.
3. There is usually a dose-response effect with a correlation of dose to severity of effect. Fetal alcohol syndrome (FAS) illustrates dose-response effects.
4. The environment has so many factors that may interact or potentiate the effects of teratogens that tracing the cause is often difficult if not impossible.

It is difficult to trace a cause and effect because animal research does not often apply to human embryos. The dosages used in animal studies are extremely high, much higher than might be found in the environment. Because it is impossible to experiment on the human fetus, information often comes from retrospective studies after the injury has occurred.

The thalidomide tragedy illustrates these points all too well. Only the timely action of Frances O. Kelsey, the science officer of the Food and Drug Administration (FDA) in 1960, prevented the approval of this potent teratogen for use in the United States. Kelsey's suspicions were aroused by case reports from Germany and Australia of an epidemic of limb defects associated with maternal use of the sedative (Figure 28-25) (Lappe, 1991). It is interesting to note that this drug is a teratogen only in some mammals. Currently all drugs are classified as to teratogenicity by means of data from animal and epidemiologic studies (see Table 16-1).

It is estimated that only 2% to 3% of defects result from known teratogens such as drugs, chemicals, and infections and that 50% to 60% of human malformations cannot be traced to direct causes such as genetic disease or teratogens.

Because the causes of these defects are largely unknown, most probably they should be regarded as resulting from multifactorial reasons, including environmental factors and gene abnormalities; preventive measures should be used when possible. These measures, summarized by Brent in 1986, remain relevant:
1. Balanced nutrition before and during pregnancy
   a. Avoidance of overnutrition or undernutrition and weight gain of at least 25 to 30 lb
2. Avoidance of known teratogens during pregnancy

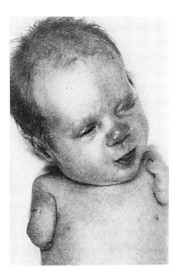

Figure 28-25   Thalidomide embryopathy. Neonate with bilateral phocomelia, each hand with three three-segmented fingers and nevus flammeus of the medial region of the face. (From Wiedemann HR et al: *Atlas of clinical syndromes: a visual aid to diagnosis*, St Louis, 1992, Mosby.)

a. Elevated body temperature from sauna, hot tub, or work environment
b. Nonprescription, over-the-counter, or self-medication with formerly prescribed drugs
c. Potentially infecting agents of any kind
d. Contact with heavy metals, polychlorinated biphenyl (PCB) agents, and dioxin
e. Exposure to sources of high doses of ionizing radiation
f. Use of cigarettes, alcohol, and drugs of abuse
3. Prevention of chronic, prolonged hypoxia in utero and acute distress during labor and birth
4. Prevention of trauma during pregnancy or birth

Susceptibility to Teratogens

The nurse who cares for the pregnant couple must be aware of current research to help the parents arrive at some important decisions. Parents motivated to receive information about medications or other factors affecting the growth of their infant tend to ingest fewer drugs and follow more health-promoting practices during pregnancy.

The stage of development determines the susceptibility of the growing infant to teratogens (Figure 28-26). The period of development from fertilization until the formation of the three germ layers has been thought to be relatively resistant to teratogenic influences because either the teratogen is powerful enough to destroy the entire conceptus or most of the cells compensate for injury to a few cells. However, in several animal studies, early exposure (before formation of the three germ layers) has resulted in

birth defects. Whether this also occurs in humans is yet to be determined. The embryonic period is one of the most highly susceptible to the influence of teratogens because the cells are undergoing rapid and intensive differentiation. The type of injury that may occur, however, depends on the organ undergoing the most rapid differentiation at the time the teratogen is introduced. During the fetal period of development, the susceptibility to teratogens diminishes, but the cerebellum, cerebral cortex, eyes, and parts of the urinary tract continue to develop rapidly. Therefore these organs are susceptible to teratogens even in late pregnancy. A growing concern is the effect of teratogens on function, even when structure appears normal. This has created a new field—behavioral teratology.

The effect of certain teratogens depends on the susceptibility of the genes. That is, some families have genes that are unable to withstand influences that other families are able to resist. In addition the teratogen acts in a specific way on specific aspects of cell metabolism. It is difficult to predict how a teratogen will affect an organ because sometimes it is not known whether the teratogen will alter the cell membrane, change the nucleic acid, or change the entire cellular structure. The result of exposure to a teratogen (even with only one or two doses) may delay, distort, or divert the development of one group of cells. For example, the use of alcohol in differing amounts at the time of conception or throughout the embryonic period may result in FAS. Many medications, including aspirin or drugs such as cocaine, when used close to labor may affect the fetus's ability to adapt to the environment after birth.

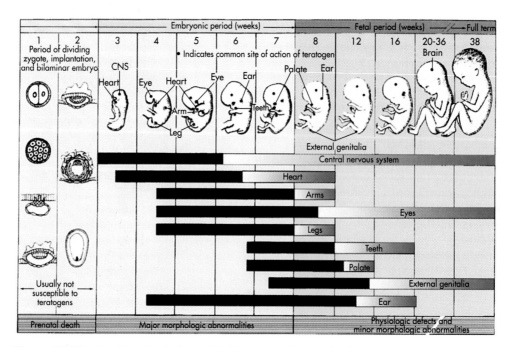

Figure 28-26   Sensitive *(shaded)* or critical periods in human development. (From Moore KL: *The developing human: clinically oriented embryology,* ed 4, Philadelphia, 1988, WB Saunders.)

Environmental pollutants

Society becomes aware of the toxic effects of environmental pollutants when people are exposed to high levels and become dramatically ill or die. Exposure may occur when in the workplace, when participating in hobbies, or from the general environment (air, water, food). Warnings about potentially harmful exposures come from animal (toxicology) and human (epidemiology) research. The lay public as well as health professionals are often confused by the results, which are obtained in different ways. Toxicologists use animals to evaluate exposures by giving them high, short-term doses because of the animal's shorter life span. Epidemiologists study humans, whose life style cannot be controlled and are not "pure bred" laboratory animals. There are therefore more uncertainties in human (epidemiologic) research. These include our inability to know the exact dose of exposure.

It is a challenge for scientists to balance out the pros and cons of both types of research when addressing the public. Health care professionals often get caught in between them and concerned people. Being alert and knowledgeable about the strengths and weaknesses of research is as important as being knowledgeable about specific exposures.

Workplace exposures. Workplace exposure (e.g., asbestos, coal dust, or lead) or contamination of the water supply by a chemical such as dioxin or a metal such as methyl mercury provides evidence too clear to ignore, and public health measures must be taken. Both men *and* women should be concerned about workplace exposures for several reasons. First, exposure to the family results when contaminants are brought home on clothing. Second, from 1977 to 1980 it was established that workplace exposure to three pesticides (dibromochloropropane, ethylene dibromide, and chlordecone) caused male infertility (Paul, 1993). Last, agents can enter the semen and alter fetal development. Nurses also must be alert to sources of information concerning possible workplace teratogens. One source is the Material Safety Data Sheets (MSDS) prepared by chemical manufacturers. Employers are required by law to keep these and make them available to employees on request. These are highly informative but complex, therefore interpretation should be left to a trained professional. Although the Occupational Safety and Health Administration (OSHA) determines exposure standards for the workplace, these are appropriate for the general population, and may not be stringent enough to protect the growing fetus (Risklines, 1994).

Health workers and reproductive hazards. There are certain health risks in caring for the sick. It is well known that workers need to protect themselves from infection. The risk of working with anesthetic and chemotherapeutic agents is less understood. Early in the 1970s an awareness developed that anesthetic gases led to a higher miscarriage rate among nurses and physicians working in operating rooms.

Anesthesiologists carried gas effects home, and before implementation of safety precautions, some excreted gas up to 30 hours after leaving the operating room. After these studies standards of ventilation were reconsidered, and most hospitals today follow these standards. Those working in small agencies (e.g., dental practices) should ask whether these standards are being followed.

Cytotoxic drugs are given to as many as 400,000 clients each year. There have been reports of increased abortions among health personnel handling these drugs. Guidelines for drug handling and administration have been formulated by OSHA (OSHA, 1986). Health workers need to follow these guidelines and question the workplace policies if evidence of noncompliance becomes apparent.

Recreational exposures. Exposures while engaging in hobbies, although more "voluntary" than those sustained while employed, can be equally as harmful. Exposure to paint thinners and removers, lead (from stained glass assembly), or restoration of older homes can be significant for the "do-it-your-selfer" (Paul, 1993). Nursing assessment for exposure to pollutants should therefore include questions about hobbies as well as employment.

Specific environmental exposures. Although most of the research has been done regarding exposures to high doses of environmental teratogens, there are numerous low levels of pollutants to which mother and fetus are exposed from the general environment. The United States has banned many developmental toxins, such as DDT, from use in this country. However, these are still used in other countries and enter residents of the Untied States via the food chain and through the air and water. Control of these exposures requires international effort and cooperation. However, it is obvious that there is much that can be done right here at home. More research into the effects of low-level chronic exposure is needed because these are the exposures that affect most of our population. Nurses should be alert to government action and participate in political action for tighter controls on pollution and standards that protect maternal-fetal health.

A listing of several major teratogens is shown in Box 28-1. It is important to note that several environmental exposures are currently being investigated as *possible* reproductive hazards. These include video display terminals, electromagnetic waves (from heating blankets, water beds, and cellular telephones) and by-products of water disinfection.

Lead. Lead inhibits synthesis of the heme fraction of hemoglobin and affects neural, gastrointestinal, and kidney function. It causes changes in the electroencephalogram (EEG), as well as fatigue and depression on a dose-related level; it accumulates in the body over a lifetime.

Lead enters the environment in many ways, primarily into the air through gas emissions. Lead then precipitates into soil and water and enters the food chain to be taken up by plants, which in turn are eaten by animals. Human

Box 28-1   Human Teratogenic Agents

KNOWN TERATOGENS

Radiation

High doses of ionizing radiation

Drugs and Chemical Agents

Ingestion of heavy metals, mercury, lead, cadmium, polychlorinated biphenyls, and pesticides
Medications such as steroid hormones
Androgens
Diethylstilbestrol
Oral progestogens
Thalidomide
Antineoplastic medications
Tetracyclines
Antithyroid agents
Anticoagulants such as warfarin
Folic acid antagonists
Isotretinoin (Accutane)

Biologic Agents

Viral diseases such as rubella, cytomegalovirus disease, and herpes simplex
Toxoplasmosis
Syphilis, varicella
Hyperthermia as a result of infection or use of hot tub

PROBABLE OR SUSPECTED TERATOGENIC AGENTS

Drugs or Chemical Agents

Anticonvulsants
Streptomycin
Appetite suppressants
Antianxiety medications such as chlordiazepoxide (Librium), diazepam (Valium), or meprobamate
Sulfonylurea hypoglycemics

Maternal Illness or Deficiency

Diabetes of long duration or severity
Epilepsy
Severe anemia
Thyroid disease of long duration or severity
Severe vitamin or mineral deficiencies
Alcohol use
Maternal hypertension
Drug abuse, especially cocaine
Uncontrolled phenylketonuria

AGENTS REQUIRING CAUTION

Excessive caffeine
Decongestants
Barbiturates
Most diuretics
Antituberculosis medications
Imipramine
Sulfonamides
Amphetamines
Antiemetics
Tranquilizers
Salicylates
Narcotics
Quinine
Cimetidine
Laxatives such as mineral oil or castor oil
Aminopterin
Nicotine
Cortisone

Data from Pregnancy labeling, *FDA Drug Bull* 9:23, 1979; Brent RL: Evaluating the alleged teratogenicity of environmental agents, *Clin Perinatol* 13:609, 1986.

beings ingest plants and milk from animals grazing in polluted fields, drink water, and inhale lead in polluted air. Lead also has been used in paint, pottery, and tin. Workers in industries that use lead have had high rates of illness, stillbirth, and children with neurologic deficits. In this country, some industrial controls protect workers, and leaded gasoline is being phased out. In other areas of the world, people may be required to work without protection.

Another source of lead is glaze on ceramic ware. Improperly fired glazes may leak lead into food, especially when acidic foods like vinegar or citrus juices are used. The FDA regulates the amount of lead that is permissible but cannot test all items made for sale in the United States. Imported ceramic products may have poorly glazed fin-

ishes. Therefore such items should not be used for cooking or serving salads or juices.

A lead level of 10 µg/dl is considered toxic to children less than 5 years of age. Previous research indicates a relationship between social class and lead toxicity, with 2-year-olds of lower socioeconomic status showing deficits at lead levels of 6 to 7 µg/dl (Lappe, 1991). However, more recently, researchers have been measuring levels of lead in the dentin of deciduous (baby) teeth, which indicates exposure after birth. Bellinger and colleagues (1994) found more behavioral problems in children with elevated dentin levels than with elevated cord blood levels. Because neurologic development is a process beginning at conception and lasting into early adulthood, it may be impossible to separate out the effects of prenatal and postnatal exposure. It is also important to remember that many lead exposed children come from social environments that also have an effect on development.

Mercury. Mercury compounds were shown to have devastating effects on growth and development before and after birth after people in Minimata, Japan were poisoned by fish that contained a high level of methyl mercury. The effects on fetal development included microcephaly and mental and motor impairments. Unfortunately, low levels of mercury compounds are not an unusual finding in fish. This environmental pollutant needs additional study. Pregnant women especially should not ingest potentially contaminated fish.

Polychlorinated biphenyls. Polychlorinated biphenyls (PCBs), common components of transformer fluids, dyes, and inks, are potent teratogens in large doses. This was demonstrated in Japan in 1968 and again in Taiwan in 1979 after pregnant women used PCB-contaminated rice oil in cooking. Their children, affected by a disorder called Yusho, had abnormal pigmentation ("cocoa-colored"), low birth weight, prematurely erupted teeth, malformed gums, abnormal skull calcification, and rocker-bottom feet. Aside from these two dramatic events, PCBs are found throughout the food chain because of their persistence in the fat cells of animals. Research indicates that persons with higher than normal PCB levels suffer ill effects such as pregnancy failure, infertility, and preeclampsia (Lappe, 1991). Although in 1976 the Toxic Substance Control Act attempted to stop production of PCBs, there are still almost 750 million pounds left in the environment. Current research indicates that male fetuses of women who eat sport fish contaminated with PCBs during pregnancy may have an increased risk for birth defects (Mendola et al, 1996).

Ionizing radiation. The first studies on the effects of radiation on fetal development arose from the dramatic exposure of thousands of women in Hiroshima and Nagasaki at the end of World War II. Exposure was associated with microcephaly and delayed development. More recently the explosion of the nuclear reactors in Chernobyl in 1986 has provided a tragic natural experiment. An increased incidence of birth defects has not been observed; however, this may be due to poor reporting of pregnancy outcomes in the affected areas (Little, 1993).

Fortunately, the more common scenario for radiation exposure is for diagnosis or therapy. When diagnostic tests or therapeutic radiation is indicated, the mother and her family should be fully informed before the procedure. Although there is no lower level of exposure that can be considered safe, it is thought that radiation doses of less than 5 to 10 rad do not increase risk for developmental defects (Scialli, 1992).

In this case, as with other therapeutic or diagnostic exposures, the risk to the mother from not being treated or diagnosed must be balanced with the risk of exposure for the fetus. Before studies or therapies are initiated, all factors should be discussed openly with the couple with documentation in the chart to indicate discussion and response. (Lawsuits often are precipitated by anger ["If you had only told me"] and failure to communicate the benefit-to-risk of a procedure.)

TEST *Yourself* **28-8**

a. What is a teratogen?
b. What is the most important determination of the degree to which a fetus may be harmed by a teratogen?
c. Name three environmental pollutants that are teratogenic.

Infectious agents

Intrauterine damage from infection is hard to prevent. Many infections are spread venereally; others such as rubella, cytomegalovirus (CMV), and varicella are acquired through close contact. Currently immunization exists only for rubella. Careful avoidance of infection during pregnancy seems best. (See Chapter 25 for full discussion of effects of infection on pregnancy and the fetus.)

Human immunodeficiency virus. A possible syndrome of congenital malformations in infants born to mothers with human immunodeficiency virus (HIV) has been reported. Characteristics of the syndrome include IUGR, microcephaly, a flat nasal bridge, wide-spaced and up-slanting eyes, prominent forehead, and fullness of the upper lip. More research is necessary, however, to determine if these are racial variations or due to the virus (Hoyme, 1990).

Syphilis. The rate of syphilis is rising; lack of prenatal care is an important factor in the rise in congenital syphilis. In contrast to what had been formerly thought, *Treponema* organisms can cross the placenta at any age. Although not as common as later transmission, early syphilis infection in the fetus leads to abortion, stillbirth, and premature labor. Approximately one half of the fetuses infected early in gestation and 10% infected later will have signs such as maculopapular rash; hepatosplenomegaly; nail, skeletal, and tooth deformities; and neurologic and ocular involvement.

Toxoplasmosis, rubella, cytomegalovirus, herpes simplex (TORCH)

Toxoplasmosis. Primary infection with the *Toxoplasma* parasite during pregnancy causes congenital infection in 60% of the infants. The most severe disease occurs in those infected earliest in gestation. Effects include chorioretinitis, intracranial calcification, hydrocephaly, and microcephaly. Affected infants suffer psychomotor delay, severe visual impairment, and hearing loss.

Rubella. Although vaccination for rubella is available, many women are not immunized. Approximately 85% of the fetuses infected with the virus during the first 8 weeks of gestation will have anomalies such as cataracts, deafness, glaucoma, and congenital heart disease (Hoyme, 1990). The later in the pregnancy the infection occurs, the fewer the malformations. (See Chapter 25 for more details about neonatal rubella.)

Cytomegalovirus. CMV infection is a strong teratogen. Approximately 65% of infants infected with CMV at *any time* during gestation will have some form of visual, hearing, or learning disability. The signs of congenital CMV infection are similar to other congenital infections; therefore laboratory confirmation often is needed for diagnosis.

Herpes. Early fetal herpes infections are rare, but teratogenic effects are similar to toxoplasmosis. The risk for spontaneous abortion and preterm labor is connected to severe infection. The newborn can acquire ascending infection at birth with a localized infection about the mouth and eyes and on skin. A generalized sepsis with CNS involvement results in high mortality, and survivors may show eye or neurologic defect.

Varicella. Only a few of the infants born after maternal chickenpox demonstrate congenital defects. Of these, growth retardation, eye, limb, and gastrointestinal and genitourinary anomalies have been reported (Hoyme, 1990).

Therapeutic and diagnostic agents. Use of therapeutic agents in pregnancy always presents a dilemma inasmuch as the benefits must be weighed against the possible risk. Unfortunately, when a pregnant woman abuses drugs and has poor nutrition, infection, and lack of prenatal care, the multiple factors increase risk of fetal injury. Through careful observation, however, it is possible to identify specific patterns of malformations that are associated with individual drugs.

Anticonvulsants. In general, women with epilepsy have two to three times the general risk for congenital malformations. Many diseases, some of which have a genetic component, are grouped under the label "epilepsy." Although use of anticonvulsant agents increases the teratogenic risk of neural tube defects, discontinuing therapy may lead to seizures (see Chapter 23).

Diethylstilbestrol. Diethylstilbestrol (DES) was prescribed for thousands of women in the 1950s and 1960s in an effort to save pregnancies threatened by spontaneous abortion. The efficacy of this treatment is questionable but not its effects on fetal development. Early observations were of ambiguous genitalia in newborn girls. Later, cases of a previously rare cancer—*clear cell adenocarcinoma* of the vagina—were seen in young teen-age girls. Both groups had been exposed to DES before week 18 of development. Further studies have demonstrated that actual risk of cancer is small. As the girls approached childbearing age, however, structural defects of the reproductive system were identified. There is controversy concerning the effects of DES on the reproductive system of male offspring. At this time DES-related anomalies are known to contribute to perinatal mortality by increasing the risk of spontaneous abortion, ectopic pregnancy, and premature delivery.

Folic acid antagonists and antineoplastic agents. Folic acid antagonists and antineoplastic agents cause cell death and therefore have teratogenic potential. Women at risk include those receiving therapy as well as those administering therapy. For the clients treatment regimens may be varied to decrease fetal risk. Accurate assessment of the risk to personnel is difficult because of the variety of drugs that are administered. Malformations of the CNS and face and IUGR have been observed after aminopterin exposure. Methotrexate use has been associated with absent digits.

Isotretinoin (Accutane). Isotretinoin is an effective treatment for severe acne. It also is a potent teratogen. Fetal exposure to this and other vitamin A analogs produces a pattern of anomalies now termed *retinoic acid embryopathy.* Infants with this syndrome have craniofacial defects, malformed or absent ears, cardiac defects, and altered CNS development. The risk of spontaneous abortion also is increased. Women who are planning a pregnancy and those who are pregnant should avoid use of vitamin A analogs because of their unusually long half-life (Hoyme, 1990).

Lithium. The fetus exposed to lithium is at risk for cardiac defects. Lithium does not appear to harm other developing organs and therefore may be taken after the period of cardiogenesis (after 45 days of gestation).

Tetracycline. Infants exposed to tetracycline after the fourth month of gestation have brown staining of the primary teeth and may have some staining of permanent teeth. There may be hypoplastic enamel and an increased risk for dental caries.

Warfarin (Coumadin). Warfarin is an anticoagulant that causes a pattern of anomalies with fetal exposure. The fetal warfarin syndrome includes IUGR, developmental delays, seizures, a malformed nose, and abnormal bone development. Heparin, a molecule too large to pass the placental barrier, is the anticoagulant best used during pregnancy.

Drugs of abuse. Although drug abuse is voluntary, the resulting addiction makes avoidance of alcohol, cocaine, and other substances most difficult for a small but significant number of pregnant women. Because drug abuse is a psychosocial as well as physical problem, it is discussed in Chapter 27.

TEST *Yourself* 28-9 _____

a. The decision to use a medication during pregnancy must be made by weighing the _____ vs the _____.

b. How would you advise a pregnant woman with severe acne about exposure to Accutane?

GENETIC THERAPY

Genetic therapy consists of several classes of care, ranging from the familiar to the "cutting edge." Those in Class I are familiar:

1. Organ transplantation such as kidney transplant is used for clients with inherited kidney disease.
2. Drug therapy is used to induce the production of certain enzymes.
3. General surgery can alter malformed tissues.
4. Fetal surgery is an exciting advance that has been used to correct diaphragmatic hernia and hydrocephalus before further damage can occur.
5. Dietary changes also can be used to treat many inherited inborn errors of metabolism.

Class II interventions involve administration of enzymes and protein factors to those with inherited deficiencies. Injections of insulin and blood factor VII are examples. Class III genetic therapy attempts to insert a normal gene into cells with a genetic defect. The proposed new treatment for CF will attempt to do this (Rosenfeld et al, 1992). Nurses may be caring for families whose infants are in therapy and should have basic knowledge about various interventions.

GENETIC COUNSELING

Couples who seek genetic counseling begin with some information, enough to form questions about their reproductive future. One of the many reasons they seek guidance is a history of genetic problems in the family.

After an affected infant is born, couples may seek guidance about the risks of the defect in a future pregnancy. For some, the defect (e.g., an IEM) did not become evident until after the second child was conceived.

Parental attitudes toward abortion influence their readiness to seek a diagnosis through chorionic villus sampling (CVS) or amniocentesis. In a number of studies of parents' attitudes in counseling, the groups were almost evenly divided among those strongly opposed, partially opposed, and in favor of abortion in cases of diagnosed defects. Thus the nurse should not *assume* any attitude about outcome when working with parents who are in counseling.

It is important to differentiate among the decisions made during the planning phase, before pregnancy has begun, and after pregnancy has been confirmed. The options before pregnancy are as follows:

1. Not to risk pregnancy
   a. For the first time (to remain childless)
   b. After having an affected child
2. To try to conceive and make the decision to retain or abort the fetus depending on test results (risk rates and personal values will influence this decision)
3. To conceive and carry the pregnancy to term, regardless of genetic findings (in this case, after counseling,

many parents decide not to have prenatal testing because they will not abort)

After the pregnancy has begun, decisions that initially confront the couple are more difficult. In most cases the couple did not suspect that there would be any problem or had not supposed that they were even at risk; they are stunned to receive the results of ultrasound evaluation or amniocentesis. Couples may be confronted with other test results such as a low or high alpha-fetoprotein level and, depending on interpretation of information, may be confused and panicked.

These couples must face the loss of the fantasized "perfect" child. Their sense of coherence as a couple is threatened. Grief may absorb their emotional energy. The genetic counselor must work with them to think through the decision, within a certain time limit, to end the pregnancy or to retain it. If they choose to end the pregnancy, it must be done promptly after the amniocentesis.

The couples who seek counseling before pregnancy work on a more theoretic level and have time to reach a considered decision. The couples who have had one affected child and seek counseling and amniocentesis are intensely concerned. They know what it means to live and work with a handicapped child. They may feel they must not bring another child into the world who has the same problems. If they have decided to risk another pregnancy, they may experience great tension until the test results come back.

Work of Counseling

It is important to understand what genetic counselors offer and to realize that geographic location may prevent a couple from seeking their resources. Physicians may not be aware of genetic counseling centers or do not refer their clients.

Counselors should know about the risks of genetic disease and the status of environmental teratogens. When given the test results or family genetic history, they should be able to guide the couple in decision making without influencing them for or against pregnancy termination. This is difficult because people in crisis often seek advice from an expert and may expect to be told what to do. An experienced counselor will prevent client dependency in this way. It is vitally important for the couple to make their own decision and to have gone through the process of making it. If they do not, they may blame each other, the counselor, the physician, or others who gave advice. They may come to feel that someone "talked them into" their decision. To recover from the grief of having an infant with a defect, the couple must feel that they made the best decision about the future of their family.

Nursing Responsibilities

Nurses meet pregnant couples who are waiting for or after they have received the results of amniocentesis. They may also meet new parents who have been given very distressing news about their newborn. They must be supportive and aware of the process that counseling has initiated. There are several levels of decision making, and the partners may be together or struggling at different places in the process. Many do not receive appropriate support but instead receive information that they find hard to integrate. In working with these couples, the nurse should be knowledgeable and use therapeutic support, which follows the same principles as support for the grieving person (see Chapter 26).

However, we should not overlook the tremendous influence the nurse can have in prevention and detection of birth defects. The following are strategies that nurses can employ:

Increase your knowledge base about birth defects so that you are able to discuss these with parents. Be alert to factors that increase the risk of birth defects and be able to discriminate between those that can be changed (maternal illness or substance abuse) and those that cannot (advanced maternal or paternal age). Teach women of childbearing age the risk of exposures to teratogens, especially in the peri-conceptual period. The time for this action is well before the pregnancy is conceived if possible.

Be aware of signs that a fetus or newborn may have a birth defect, especially prior history of a child with a birth defect, poor intrauterine growth, oligohydramnios, decreased fetal movement, abnormal presentation during labor, or a newborn who has an unusual appearance or is not adjusting normally to extrauterine life. It is commonly thought that prior knowledge exists only to allow parents the opportunity to continue or terminate the pregnancy. On the contrary, this allows parents to prepare for the birth of a child with a health problem. In addition, health care professionals can make plans for early specialized care (such as an abdominal delivery for a child with meningomyelocele).

TEST *Yourself* **28-10**

a. List three examples of genetic therapy in use today.
b. Describe nursing responsibilities for the family receiving genetic counseling.

Key points

- Congenital and genetic anomalies are the fifth leading cause of years of potential life lost (YPLL). As such, these defects are a major cause of death and disability.
- Varying degrees of developmental disabilities are present in more than 3% of the population.
- One gene, one function describes the inborn errors of metabolism that are carried by recessive inheritance. These may cause disability or death, but many can be treated today.
- Dominantly inherited gene defects may be fatal or may not appear until later in life, allowing reproduction and passing on of the gene.
- These gene defects tend to be concentrated in racial groups, although genetic drift is "diluting" the gene pool.
- Autosomal defects generally are devastating, and many result in loss of the embryo before maturation. Others result in trisomy with multiorgan effects.
- The most common of the trisomies, Down syndrome, may be severe or modified, and early intervention provides the best possible chance of development.
- Sex chromosome trisomies often do not show signs at birth but usually affect intelligence and reproductive function.

- Only one monosomy is possible; children with Turner syndrome survive with fairly normal intelligence but without development of secondary sex characteristics, unless mosaic.
- Prenatal genetic screening is available to couples with a potential for single gene and chromosomal defects. Amniocentesis and maternal serum alpha-fetoprotein are standards of care for pregnant women.
- For a couple who find elective abortion morally unacceptable, these screening tests will be useful only in cases for which fetal therapy is possible or if the family wishes to prepare for the birth of a child with special needs.
- Environmental pollutants have been recognized for years, but escalating levels in the air and water are major health problems to be addressed.
- Nurses, as health educators, must participate in appropriate community and political action to improve the environment.
- Genetic counseling is available in larger urban settings and should be offered to any couple with a history of defects in family or in offspring.

Study Questions

28-1. Select the terms that apply to the following statements:
  a. Exchange of genetic material between chromosomes is _____.
  b. Loss of part of a chromosome is called _____.
  c. An extra chromosome in the ovum results in a _____.
  d. Nonsex chromosomes are called _____.
  e. Change in genetic material as a result of radiation or other factor is a _____.
  f. An environmental toxin is called a _____.

28-2. Note the following statements as either *true* or *false*.
  a. Major structural birth defects arise in the third trimester.
  b. Only substances that a pregnant woman breathes, ingests, or injects can be teratogenic.
  c. If a man fathers one child with a heterozygous autosomal dominant gene disorder, he himself must have this disorder.

28-3. There is evidence that maternal hyperthermia in the first trimester increases the risk for which of the following problems?
  a. Anencephaly
  b. Cleft lip and palate
  c. Gastroschisis
  d. Potter syndrome

28-4. Baby Ann is diagnosed with Turner's syndrome. Which statement most completely describes this variation?
  a. Severe mental and physical retardation will be evident.
  b. The female infant will show an extra chromosome and neural tube defects.
  c. Wide-spaced nipples, web neck, and future sterility occur.
  d. Ambiguous genitalia are present as a result of altered sex chromosome pattern.

28-5. Choose two of the following terms to correctly complete this sentence: genotype, phenotype, homozygous, heterozygous.
  Blue eye color is the _____ that is observed in those who are _____ for the gene for blue eyes.

28-6. Joe carries one dominant gene for brown eyes and a blue recessive gene. Jane's eyes are blue. What is their chance to have a blue-eyed baby? Draw a Punnett square to discover the answer.

28-7. Mary has blood type AA and Jim's type is BO. Do they have any chance of having an infant with a homozygous blood type? Use a Punnett square.

28-8. Mr. Ahmed is color blind and his wife has a completely normal genotype. The couple asks if their newborn son will be color blind. Which response by the nurse is most accurate?
  a. The child will be completely normal.
  b. The child has a one in four chance of being color blind.
  c. Only if the child were a girl would she be color blind.
  d. Mrs. Ahmed would have to be color blind for the son to have the defect.

28-9. Characteristics of fetal alcohol syndrome include all of the following except:
  a. Microcephaly
  b. Symmetric prenatal growth retardation
  c. Hemangioma
  d. Low bridge of nose, smooth upper lip line

Answer Key

28-1: *a,* Independent assortment; *b,* deletion; *c,* trisomy; *d,* autosomes; *e,* mutation; *f,* teratogen. **28-2:** *a,* False; *b,* false; *c,* false. **28-3:** *a.* **28-4:** *c.* **28-5:** Phenotype, homozygous. **28-6:** 2 in 4 chances. **28-7:** No chance. **28-8:** *a.* **28-9:** *c.*

References

Alton EW: Gene therapy for cystic fibrosis, *J Inherit Metab Dis,* 18(4):501, 1995.

Bellinger D et al: Pre- and postnatal lead exposure and behavior problems in school-aged children, *Environ Res* 66(1):12, 1994.

*Brent RL: Evaluating the alleged teratogenicity of environmental agents, *Clin Perinatol* 13(3):609, 1986.

Croen LA, Shaw GM: Young maternal age and congenital malformations: a population-based study, *Am J Public Health* 85(5):710, 1995.

Das SK et al: Epidemiology of cleft lip and palate in Mississippi, *South Med J* 88(4):437, 1995.

*Hook EB: Behavioral implications of the human XYY genotype, *Science* 179:139, 1973.

Hoyme HG: Teratogenetically induced fetal anomalies, I: fetal dysmorphology, *Clin Perinatol* 17(3):547, 1990.

Lappe M: *Chemical deception: the toxic threat to health and the environment,* San Francisco, 1991, Sierra Club Books.

Laxova R: Fragile X syndrome, *Adv Pediatr* 41:305, 1994.

Little J: The Chernobyl accident, congenital anomalies and other reproductive outcomes, *Paediatr Perinat Epidemiol* 7(2):121, 1993.

McIntosh GC et al: Paternal age and the risk of birth defects in offspring, *Epidemiology* 6(3):282, 1995.

Mendola P et al: Maternal consumption of contaminated sport fish during pregnancy and risk of major congenital malformations in male children- work in progress. Poster presented at Society for Pediatric Epidemiology Research, June 11-12, 1996.

*Moore KL: *The developing human: clinically oriented embryology,* ed 4, Philadelphia, 1988, WB Saunders.

Nelson DL: The fragile X syndromes, *Semin Cell Bio* 6(1):5, 1995.

*OSHA work-practice guidelines for personnel dealing with cytotoxic drugs, *Am J Hosp Pharm* 43:1193, 1986.

Paul M, ed: *Occupational and environmental reproductive hazards: a guide for clinicians,* Baltimore, 1993, Williams & Wilkins.

Recommendations for the use of folic acid to reduce the number of cases of spina bifida and other neural tube defects, *MMWR Morb and Mortal W Rep* 41(RR-14):1, 1992.

Risklines: *Screening patients for occupational exposures,* University of Connecticut Health Center, Pregnancy Exposure Information Service, 3(2), June 1994.

Rosenfeld MA et al: In vivo transfer of the human CF transmembrane regulation gene to the airway epithelium, *Cell* 68:143, 1992.

Schnitzer PG et al: Paternal occupation and risk of birth defects in offspring, *Epidemiology* 6(6):577, 1995.

Scialli A: *A clinical guide to reproductive and developmental toxicology,* Boca Raton, 1992, CRC Press.

Shaw GM et al: Maternal periconceptual use of multivitamins and reduced risk for conotruncal heart defects and limb deficiencies among offspring. *Am J Med Genet* 59(4):536, 1995.

*Thompson JS, Thompson M: *Genetics in medicine,* Philadelphia, 1986, WB Saunders.

*Wilson JG: *Environment and birth defects,* New York, 1977, Academic Press.

*Classic reference.

Resources for Parents

National Center for Education in Maternal and Child Health (NCEMCH)
38th and R Streets, NW
Washington, DC 20013-1133
(202)625-8400
> *Funded by the Division of Maternal and Child Health, Department of Health and Human Services, to be a channel of communication and to build networks and coordinate public- and private-sector efforts in maternal and child health.*

Sample publications
> *Reaching out: a directory of voluntary organizations in maternal and child health*
> *A reader's guide for parents of children with mental, physical or emotional disabilities*
> *Comprehensive clinical genetic services centers: a national directory*

National Center for Orphan Drugs and Rare Diseases (NCODARD)
P.O. Box 1133
Washington, DC 20013-1133
> *Funded by the Food and Drug Administration, Division of Health and Human Services*

National Institutes of Health
Public Inquiries Office
Bethesda, MD 20205

March of Dimes Birth Defects Foundation
1275 Mamaroneck Ave.
White Plains, NY 10605

 Student Resource Shelf

Graham JM, ed: Fetal dysmorphology, Pt I, *Clin Perinatol* 14:3, 1990.
Graham JM, ed: Fetal clinical genetics, Pt II, *Clin Perinatol* 14:4, 1990.
> *These symposia include major research reports on abnormal fetal development. Both genetic and environmental influences are considered with many illustrations of mechanisms and effects.*

Lappe M: *Chemical deception: the toxic threat to health and the environment,* San Francisco, 1991, Sierra Club Books.
> *Reviews 10 myths about the human response to environmental toxins; not limited to the effects on the fetus.*

Moore KL: *The developing human: clinically oriented embryology,* ed 4, Philadelphia, 1988, WB Saunders.
> *A standard work in the area of genetics and embryology.*

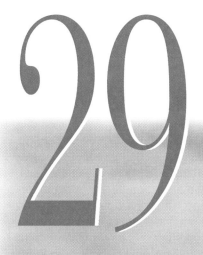

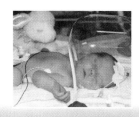

Nursing Care *of the* High-Risk Newborn

*H*igh-risk infants are newborns who are compromised because of prematurity, congenital anomalies, postmaturity, or many other factors, all of which prevent normal transition to extrauterine life. Because multiple risk factors cause problems in normal adaptation, this neonate needs special care.

Since the early 1900s, significant improvements have been made in the care of the newborn at risk. From the development of the first incubator and respirator to the introduction of surfactant replacement therapy and specially designed premature formulas, there has been a dramatic increase in infant survival.

The high-level technology that is commonplace in neonatal intensive care units (NICUs) places tremendous demands on neonatal nurses. The nurse must have an understanding of physiology and pathophysiology. The lines between medicine and nursing are often blurred in the NICU. Care is primarily collaborative, with overlapping, shared responsibilities. The entry level nurse observes and intervenes with much guidance from more experienced staff members. The NICU is often a noisy, bright, chaotic environment that is stressful for both the staff and their tiny clients. Learning to deal with the environmental stress and the emotional stress of caring for critically ill newborns is essential for the neonatal nurse.

CLASSIFICATIONS OF HIGH-RISK INFANTS

Size

The term **low birth weight** (LBW) is defined as a birth weight less than 2500 g. Initially, LBW was considered a manifestation of prematurity, but in 1963, Lubchencho introduced growth curves that illustrated the relationship between gestational age and birth weight. From these curves, LBW includes both premature infants and growth-retarded term infants (Figure 29-1).

Small-for-gestational age

Small-for-gestational age (SGA) infants have birth weights less than the 10th percentile for their gestational age on the intrauterine growth curve. The factors that influence fetal growth are outlined in Box 29-1. SGA infants are characterized as *symmetric,* where birth weight, length, and head circumference are proportionately small, or *asymmetric,* where the head circumference is proportionately larger than expected for birth weight or length. Fetal factors are more often a cause of symmetric SGA infants, whereas maternal factors are associated with asymmetric SGA infants. SGA infants are at risk for asphyxia, hypoglycemia, polycythemia, and hypothermia in the immediate postnatal period.

Large-for-gestational age

An infant whose birth weight is greater than the 90th percentile for gestational age on the intrauterine growth curve is considered **large-for-gestational age** (LGA). LGA infants are at risk for difficult deliveries and birth trauma,

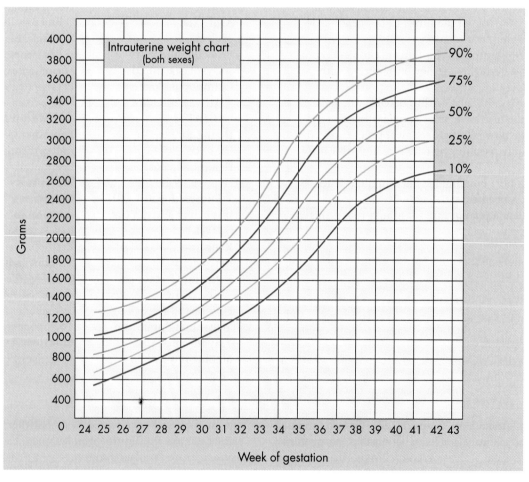

Figure 29-1 Intrauterine growth curve. The weights of liveborn Caucasian infants at gestational ages from 24 to 42 weeks are graphed as percentiles. Based on this intrauterine growth curve, the Ballard tool is commonly used to determine appropriateness of weight with gestational age. There are several modified forms. (From Lubchenko L et al: Intrauterine growth as estimated from birth weight data, *Pediatrics* 32:795, 1963).

which may result in asphyxia or birth injuries (i.e., fracture of the clavicle, brachial plexus palsy). LGA infants are at high risk for developing hypoglycemia shortly after birth. Figure 29-2 shows three infants of the same gestational age but of markedly different sizes.

Gestational Age or Maturity

Postmaturity

Postmaturity is gestation lasting beyond 42 weeks. The incidence of postmaturity varies with its causes. Prolonged pregnancy may be a normal variant because some women routinely deliver as much as 2 to 3 weeks after the estimated date of delivery (EDD). A postmature infant has normal length and head circumference but may have lost weight in utero as a result of poor placental function after 42 weeks. This placental insufficiency may result in fetal distress during labor. Signs of postmaturity are listed and contrasted with prematurity signs in Table 29-1. Postmature infants are at risk for birth asphyxia and hypoxic-ischemic encephalopathy (HIE), meconium aspiration, hypoglycemia, hypothermia, hypocalcemia, and polycythemia.

Prematurity

Premature birth is defined as any delivery that occurs after the twentieth week and before 37 completed weeks of gestation, regardless of birth weight. **Prematurity** is the primary cause of admission to NICUs in the United States. Despite advances in medical management, premature infants continue to be at increased risk for illness and death as a direct result of their incomplete development.

Characteristics of prematurity are compared with postmaturity in Table 29-1. Premature infants are at risk for problems with respiratory, metabolic, hematologic, immunologic, neurologic, and gastrointestinal functions.

Box 29-1 Factors that Influence Fetal Growth

FETAL FACTORS
Genetic anomalies
Congenital infections
Multiple gestation

MATERNAL FACTORS
Age
Smoking
Substance abuse
Hypertension
Diabetes mellitus
Poor nutrition
Uteroplacental insufficiency

DELIVERY OF THE HIGH-RISK INFANT

During fetal life, the placenta is the organ for gas exchange (i.e., oxygen and carbon dioxide). At birth, the lungs and circulation go through a series of changes until, ultimately, the lungs provide the neonate with oxygen and remove the by-products of respiration. A more complete description of the cardiorespiratory transition can be found in Chapter 18. If there is a problem with the normal transition, an infant can be depressed, which could lead to asphyxia.

Asphyxia

Asphyxia is a direct result of respiratory dysfunction, whether from alterations in uteroplacental function or from alterations in the neonate's ability to breathe independently. Asphyxia is the triad of *hypoxia, hypercapnia,* and *acidosis* (metabolic and respiratory) that may occur in the uterus or after birth. Typically, something prevents the delivery of oxygen to the tissues, causing the body to convert from aerobic to anaerobic metabolism. Lactic acid builds up, causing metabolic acidosis because whatever prevented the delivery of oxygen also prevents the removal of carbon dioxide. Respiratory acidosis is also present.

Asphyxia stimulates the primitive **diving reflex** during which blood is shunted from the periphery to more "valuable" organs. For a short time, the brain, heart, and adrenal glands are preferentially perfused at the expense of the intestine, kidneys, liver, and other organs. If, however, asphyxia is not corrected promptly, even vital organs suffer from hypoxia and ischemia. Hypoxia, hypercapnia, and resulting acidosis affect the function of several body systems (Box 29-2).

Fetal asphyxia can occur any time during gestation but is more common during labor and delivery (see Chapter 14). Many factors during pregnancy, labor, and delivery that can contribute to intrapartum asphyxia are listed in

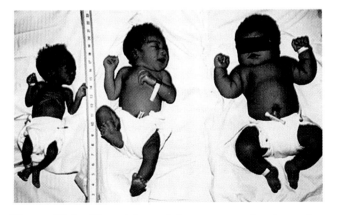

Figure 29-2 Three infants of the same gestational age who are large-for-gestational age *(right),* appropriate-for-gestational age *(middle),* and small-for-gestational age *(left).* (From *Perinatal assessment of maturation,* National Audiovisual Center, Washington, DC.)

Table 29-1   Physical and Neurologic Findings of Postmaturity Contrasted with Findings of Prematurity

Postmature	Premature
HEAD	**HEAD**
No lanugo on face; edges of skull bones firm with small fontanelles	Head seems small; fine, "wooly," bunchy hair
Hair smooth but may be receding from forehead	Lanugo on face, edges of fontanelles soft
Pinna incurved to lobe, firm with cartilage	Ear pinna flat to slightly curved, soft, less spring
Appears alert; eyes wide open, gazing at objects	Lids may be fused in immature infant (Figure 7-22)
Face appears thin, "little old man" look	
CHEST	**CHEST**
May have respiratory distress if meconium was aspirated	Respiratory distress as evidenced by retractions, nasal flaring, grunting; higher resting heart rate
Bony prominences evident—caused by loss of weight	
Low resting heart rate	
ABDOMEN	**ABDOMEN**
May be flattened if meconium passed; appears sunken in, not protuberant	May be distended if bag-mask ventilation required at birth; otherwise, flat
Cord may be thin with little Wharton's jelly and may be meconium stained	Cord has thick Wharton's jelly
GENITALIA	**GENITALIA**
Pendulous scrotum with descended testes	Scrotum empty or testes in upper inguinal canal; no rugae
Labia cover clitoris but may show signs of subcutaneous loss of fatty tissue	Prominent clitoris; labia flat or small labia minora
SKIN	**SKIN**
Degrees of dry, peeling skin evident	Gelatinous, translucent
No lanugo or vernix	Smooth, pink
Poor skin turgor	Sparse to abundant lanugo
EXTREMITIES	**EXTREMITIES**
Loss of subcutaneous tissue makes legs and arms look wasted	Thin; lack of subcutaneous tissue
Nails long and may be meconium stained	Nails do not reach end of finger or toe
Deep sole creases	Smooth or faint red marks on plantar creases
Ankle flexion at zero angle	
CENTRAL NERVOUS SYSTEM	**CENTRAL NERVOUS SYSTEM**
Hypertonic	Flaccid tone
All reflexes readily elicited	Weak Moro and grasp, poor suck
Vigorous suck; often appears hungry	Reflexes not elicted or weak
Tremors of hypoglycemia or hypocalcemia are frequent	

From Ballard JL et al: New Ballard Score, expanded to include extremely premature infants, *J Pediatr* 119(3):417, 1991.

Box 29-3. Because of the risk of asphyxia, the high-risk infant should be identified before birth and closely monitored during labor and delivery.

Prenatal birth asphyxia is caused by factors that disrupt uteroplacental circulation. When a neonate is asphyxiated, the acidosis reverses the normally high affinity of fetal hemoglobin for oxygen, resulting in reduction of tissue oxygenation. Asphyxia may also prevent normal dilation of pulmonary blood vessels. This perpet-uates the normal fetal *right-to-left shunt* in the heart and further prevents blood from reaching the lungs.

Risk

Most infants cry vigorously at birth, which establishes adequate respiratory effort and heart rate. However, some infants may be depressed at birth with a poor respiratory effort and decreased muscle tone. Factors associated with an increased risk for asphyxia in an infant at birth include

▌ *Box* **29-2**	**Multisystem Effects of Perinatal Asphyxia**

RESPIRATORY SYSTEM
Meconium aspiration
Increased severity of respiratory distress syndrome
Respiratory acidosis

CARDIOVASCULAR SYSTEM
Persistent pulmonary hypertension
Myocardial dysfunction

METABOLIC SYSTEM
Ineffective thermoregulation
Hypoglycemia
Hypocalcemia
Metabolic acidosis

CENTRAL NERVOUS SYSTEM
Hypoxic-ischemic encephalopathy
Intraventricular hemorrhage
Stroke or infarction

RENAL SYSTEM
Acute tubular necrosis

GASTROINTESTINAL SYSTEM
Necrotizing enterocolitis

HEMATOLOGIC SYSTEM
Disseminated intravascular coagulation

▌ *Box* **29-3**	**Factors Placing Infant at Risk for Birth Asphyxia**

MATERNAL FACTORS
Diabetes mellitus
Isoimmunization
Infection
Third-trimester bleeding
Pregnancy-induced or chronic hypertension
Drug abuse
Abruptio placentae
Placenta previa
Oligohydramnios
Polyhydramnios
Preterm labor

FETAL FACTORS
Multiple gestation
Congenital anomalies
Intrauterine growth retardation
Cord prolapse
Prematurity or postmaturity
Prolonged rupture of membranes
Operative delivery
Poor biophysical profile score
Nonreassuring heart rate for extended time
Meconium-stained amniotic fluid
Macrosomia

uteroplacental insufficiency, prematurity and postmaturity, in utero passage of meconium, maternal drugs administered during labor, and congenital anomaly.

Signs

Asphyxial episodes before or after birth trigger central nervous system (CNS) dysfunction because of disturbances in cerebral blood flow, which may result in infarction (i.e., stroke) or intraventricular hemorrhage. Myocardial ischemia, necrotizing enterocolitis, acute tubular necrosis, and persistent fetal circulation may also develop because of asphyxial insult to specific organs.

Perinatal asphyxia causes syndromes of cardiovascular and respiratory alterations called *primary* and *secondary* apnea (Figure 29-3). Primary apnea begins with an acute episode of asphyxia. Initially the fetus makes several gasping motions, and the heart rate and blood pressure (BP) rise in an attempt to maintain oxygenation and perfusion. Respiratory effort, heart rate, and BP then fall as the infant becomes more acidotic. Primary apnea ends (approximately 7 minutes after it began) with the last gasp when the infant progresses to secondary apnea. Frequently it is impossible to know which stage of apnea affects a depressed infant at birth; thus resuscitative efforts should *never* be delayed.

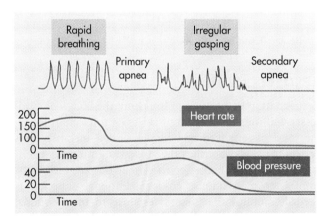

Figure 29-3   Physiologic changes that occur during primary and secondary apnea. (Modified from Bloom RS, Cropley C: *Textbook of neonatal resuscitation,* Dallas, 1994, American Heart Association.)

Clinical management

Management of the infant with asphyxia follows the ABCs (airway, breathing, and circulation) of cardiac resuscitation, with modifications in technique because of differences in neonatal physiology. The delivery of a high-risk infant may be an unexpected event. Therefore procedures for resuscitation must be reviewed regularly, and personnel trained to perform neonatal resuscitation should be present at *every* delivery. All emergency equipment should be inspected regularly for contents, expired medications, sterile

Decision TREE | *Resuscitation*

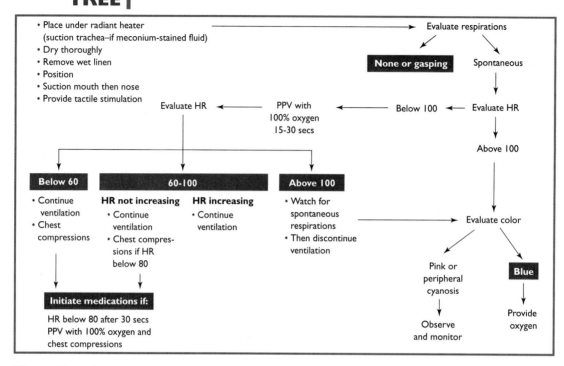

* Place under radiant heater
  (suction trachea–if meconium-stained fluid) ————————————→ Evaluate respirations
* Dry thoroughly
* Remove wet linen   **None or gasping**   Spontaneous
* Position
* Suction mouth then nose
* Provide tactile stimulation

Evaluate HR ←——— PPV with ←——— Below 100 ←——— Evaluate HR
                  100% oxygen
                  15-30 secs   Above 100

Below 60   **60-100**   **Above 100**

* Continue   **HR not increasing**   **HR increasing**   * Watch for
  ventilation   spontaneous
* Chest   * Continue   * Continue   respirations   ——————→ Evaluate color
  compressions   ventilation   ventilation   * Then discontinue
              * Chest compres-   ventilation   Pink or   **Blue**
                sions if HR   peripheral
                below 80   cyanosis   ↓
                                                                                                     Provide
Initiate medications if: ↓   oxygen
                                                                                    Observe
HR below 80 after 30 secs   and monitor
PPV with 100% oxygen and
chest compressions

Figure 29-4   Decision tree for resuscitation. (Modified from Bloom RS, Cropley C: *Textbook of neonatal resuscitation*, Dallas, 1994, American Heart Association.)

supplies, and working order. Documentation is essential for medicolegal and accreditative reasons.

RESUSCITATION

Resuscitation is the attempt to restore the body's life processes and thus reverse asphyxia. It is a team effort led by the most experienced and highly skilled member. This person usually establishes the airway and provides respiratory support. Others support cardiac output, prepare or administer medications, go for additional supplies as needed, monitor the infant's response to interventions, and document the events as they occur. Resuscitation is a stressful procedure for the infant, family, and staff. Ethical and medicolegal issues are woven into a highly complex physiologic situation. In the midst of the high-technology atmosphere, it is easy to forget touch; thus make a conscious effort to humanize nursing care.

Basic Steps

The American Heart Association (AHA) and the American Academy of Pediatrics (AAP) have designed a standardized program for neonatal resuscitation, which is available as an instructional textbook (Bloom and Cropley, 1995). Hospital-based programs certify staff members to perform

neonatal resuscitation; an overview of the basic steps of resuscitation is presented here.

Preparation for high-risk delivery includes the following steps.

1. Turn on the warmer. Have warmed blankets or towels ready.
2. Have bulb suction and meconium suction device available. Connect suction catheter (size 8 French for preterm and 10 French for term infant) to wall suction, turn suction on, and set at less than or equal to 100 mm Hg.
3. Connect oxygen source to ventilation bag; add pressure manometer. Attach appropriate size face mask to ventilation bag.
4. Place stylet in appropriately sized endotracheal tube (size 2.5 to 3.0 French for preterm and 3.0 to 3.5 French for term infants).
5. Attach appropriate laryngoscope blade (Miller 0 for preterm and Miller 1 for term infants) to handle. Check for bright light; replace bulb or battery if needed.
6. Drugs, intravenous (IV) fluids, or volume expanders, such as 5.0% albumin or 0.9% sodium chloride, may be readied for use in certain situations.
7. Umbilical catheterization tray and catheters sizes 3.5, 5.0, and 8.0 French.

Although the Apgar score provides guidelines for management of asphyxia, never wait until 1 minute has

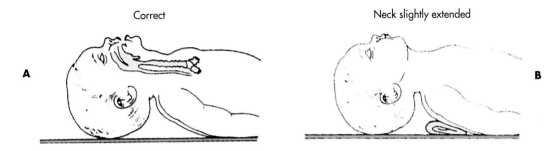

Correct   Neck slightly extended

Figure 29-5   Positions for resuscitation. **A,** The neonate should be placed on his or her back or side, with the neck slightly extended. **B,** To help maintain the correct position, a rolled blanket or towel may be placed under the shoulders, elevating them slightly off the mattress. (From Bloom RS, Cropley C: *Textbook of neonatal resuscitation*, Dallas, 1994, American Heart Association.)

passed to intervene. Resuscitation efforts should begin as soon as the infant is born (see the Decision Tree for resuscitation, Figure 29-4). The *first steps of resuscitation* include the following:

1. To prevent cold stress from heat loss, place the infant under a prewarmed radiant heat source.
2. Thoroughly dry the infant and discard the wet linen to reduce heat loss.
3. Position the infant flat, either supine or side-lying, with the neck slightly extended. A shoulder roll may be helpful in maintaining the correct position to open the airway (Figure 29-5).
4. Use the bulb syringe to suction secretions from the mouth and nose.
5. Evaluate the infant for respiratory effort, heart rate, and color.
6. Provide a brief period of tactile stimulation (gently slap or flick foot or rub back), and provide free-flow oxygen if the infant is apneic or gasping.
7. If there is no response to stimulation or if the heart rate is below 100 beats per minute, positive pressure ventilation (PPV) should be initiated. PPV can be provided with a resuscitation bag and mask or with a resuscitation bag and endotracheal tube (see Figure 29-6 for correct placement of mask).
8. If the infant is breathing spontaneously but there is cyanosis of the lips and mucous membranes, provide supplemental oxygen at a flow of 5 L per minute.

Ventilation and oxygenation

As Bloom and Cropley (1995) point out in *Textbook of Neonatal Resuscitation*, the single most important procedure used in neonatal resuscitation is PPV. In the majority of cases, proper oxygenation can be restored with the bag and mask if it is used promptly and properly.

Once it has been determined that the infant requires PPV, position the infant in the supine position with the neck slightly hyperextended to maintain patency of the airway. Position the mask on the infant's face, forming a seal; ventilate two to three times and observe for a rise in the chest to check the seal (Figure 29-6). Once there is

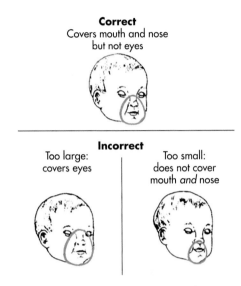

Correct
Covers mouth and nose
but not eyes

Incorrect

Too large: Too small:
covers eyes   does not cover
                    mouth *and* nose

Figure 29-6   Correct placement of mask during resuscitation. (From Bloom RS, Cropley C: *Textbook of neonatal resuscitation*, Dallas, 1994, American Heart Association.)

adequate chest movement, ventilate the infant for 15 to 30 seconds at a rate of 40 to 60 breaths per minute. The amount of pressure required to provide adequate ventilation will vary, depending on whether you are providing the initial breath after delivery (which requires higher pressure) or the subsequent breaths.

Another member of the team listens for breath sounds, which should be heard equally at each axilla, and monitors the heart rate when auscultating the chest or by palpating the cord. This should be done every 30 seconds. Tapping the index finger in synchrony with the heart rate easily communicates the rate to the other members of the team. If the heart rate remains above 100 beats per minute, continue to support respirations while watching for the return of spontaneous respirations. It may be necessary to insert an orogastric tube so that air introduced into the stomach by the positive pressure can be removed. This should be done if an infant receives bag-and-mask ventilation for longer than 2 minutes. If bag-and-mask ventilation is inadequate or if the infant requires ventilation for longer than several minutes, endotracheal intubation will be necessary.

Chest compressions

Infants with severe asphyxia need vigorous resuscitation. At least three persons are needed at this time: one manages the airway, another starts cardiac compressions, and a third monitors the heart rate and listens for breath sounds. The infant will require prompt intubation by a skilled person. The endotracheal tube will deliver oxygen into the lungs. Chest compressions are indicated if, after 15 to 30 seconds of bag-and-mask ventilation with 100% oxygen, the heart rate is below 60 or between 60 and 80 beats per minute but not increasing. Once the heart rate is above 80 beats per minute, chest compressions should be discontinued (Bloom and Cropley, 1995). Chest compressions must always be accompanied by PPV with 100% oxygen. Two techniques may be used (Figure 29-7). Holding the infant's chest between two hands is preferred to control the depth of compression. Once your fingers and hands are positioned, compress the sternum ¹/₂ to ³/₄ of an inch, then release to allow the heart chambers to refill. Ventilations are interposed between compressions. A ventilation follows every third compression. The ratio of compressions to ventilations is 3 to 1, with 90 compressions and 30 ventilations occurring in 1 minute. The heart rate should be checked after an initial 30 seconds of chest compressions and then periodically. Chest compressions should be stopped when the heart rate is 80 beats per minute or above.

Medications

For most infants, effective ventilation and oxygenation are all that are necessary during resuscitation. The routes for administration of resuscitation medications include the umbilical vein, a peripheral vein, or the endotracheal tube. Some infants may require epinephrine for cardiac stimulation. However, the infant whose heart rate remains less than 100 beats per minute after effective ventilation has been established will need sodium bicarbonate to |correct acidosis. Acidosis depresses the myocardial response to epinephrine and also depresses efforts by the infant's own sympathetic nervous system to increase the heart rate.

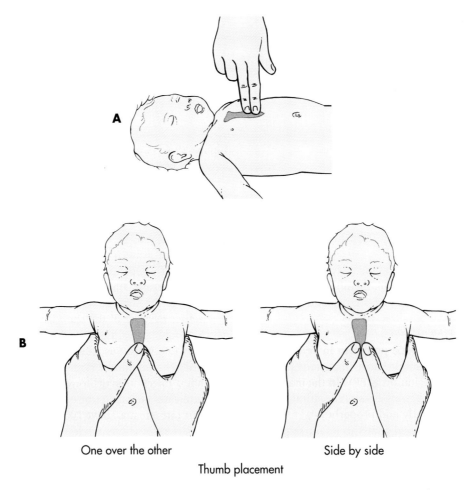

A

B

One over the other   Side by side

Thumb placement

Figure 29-7   Position for cardiac compressions. **A,** Two finger method; **B,** Thumbs used for compression of the chest. (From Bloom RS, Cropley C: *Textbook of neonatal resuscitation,* Dallas, 1994, American Heart Association.)

Resuscitation will be ineffective if the infant's perfusion is decreased; thus the intravascular volume must be expanded. Fluids are administered to restore the blood's osmotic pressure (the force that keeps the fluid component within the intravascular space). Medications used for neonatal resuscitation are summarized in Drug Profile 29-1.

Discontinuing Resuscitation

A difficult decision with obvious ethical and legal ramifications results when resuscitation efforts are unsuccessful.

One guideline is to end resuscitation if no vital signs can be detected after 20 minutes of vigorous physical and chemical resuscitation. The gestational age of the infant and the presence of major malformations may influence the course of action. The decision to discontinue resuscitation is made by the attending neonatologist or pediatrician.

Special Situations: Meconium Aspiration

Special situations require alterations in the usual process of resuscitation. Meconium aspiration causes a mechan-

Box **29-1**

DRUG PROFILE

Medications for Neonatal Resuscitation

Medication	Indications	Concentration to Administer	Dosage/Route/ Rate	Precautions/ Effects
EPINEPHRINE				
	Heart rate < 80 despite 30 seconds of adequate ventilation with 100% oxygen and chest compressions	1:10,000	0.1-0.3 ml/kg IV or ET Give rapidly	Increases strength and rate of cardiac concentration. Causes peripheral vasoconstriction.
VOLUME EXPANDERS				
	Hypovolemia	Whole blood, 5% albumin, normal saline, Ringer's lactate solution	10 ml/kg IV Give for 5-10 minutes	Increases vascular volume. Decreases metabolic acidosis by increasing tissue perfusion.
SODIUM BICARBONATE				
	Falling pH, low blood volume	0.5 mEq/ml (4.2% solution)	2 mEq/kg IV Give *slowly,* for at least 2 minutes	Give only if infant is being effectively ventilated. Corrects metabolic acidosis by raising the pH in the presence of adequate ventilation.
NALOXONE HYDROCHLORIDE				
	Maternal narcotic intake, depression	0.4 mg/ml	0.1 mg/kg (0.25 ml/kg) IV, ET, IM, SQ Give rapidly	IV, ET preferred; IM, SQ acceptable, may be repeated.
		1.0 mg/ml	0.1 mg/kg (0.1 ml/kg) IV, ET, IM, SQ	

From Bloom RS, Cropley C: *Textbook of neonatal resuscitation,* Dallas, 1994, American Heart Association.
ET, Endotracheal; *IM,* intramuscular; *IV,* intravenous; *SQ,* subcutaneous.

ical obstruction that allows air to reach the alveoli during inspiration but then traps it in the air sacs behind the sticky meconium. These alveoli may then rupture, causing a pneumothorax and further compromising resuscitation. If the amniotic fluid is thickly meconium stained, every effort must be made to minimize aspiration. The birth attendant must thoroughly suction the infant's mouth and nose immediately after the head is delivered but before the first breath is taken. The infant is quickly placed under the radiant warmer and intubated, and the trachea is visualized and suctioned with the use of an endotracheal tube. The infant is not stimulated to cry until the trachea has been thoroughly suctioned. If the infant's heart rate drops below 100 beats per minute, ventilation is begun. Infants who are delivered through thin meconium staining or infants who cry vigorously at birth may not receive suctioning in this manner, depending on agency policy.

Box 29-1

CLINICAL DECISION

A 16-year-old arrives in the labor and delivery area at 30 weeks' gestation in preterm labor. Her pregnancy has been uncomplicated until the onset of labor today. She is dilated to 8 cm. What preparations should you make for the delivery of the infant?

RESPIRATORY DYSFUNCTION

Respiratory Distress Syndrome

Respiratory distress syndrome (RDS) is a disease of prematurity caused by a lack of pulmonary **surfactant.** Production of surfactant, a surface tension-reducing substance, by type II pneumocytes increases with gestational age. A lack of surfactant causes alveoli to collapse with each expiration; therefore unlike the normal lung, no residual capacity is established. For the infant with RDS, each breath is like the first, requiring high pressures to reopen the collapsed alveoli. Scattered **atelectasis** (collapsed alveoli) and areas of overinflation occur because some alveoli have more surfactant than others. Damage to the alveoli and pulmonary capillary epithelium resulting from surfactant deficiency causes the formation of a **hyaline membrane**, which consists of fibrin and sloughed cells. This further compromises gas exchange.

Risk

Prematurity is the single most common factor associated with the occurrence of RDS. The incidence is 10% to 15% in infants with a birth weight less than 2500 g. The incidence is more than 80% for infants who are less than 28 weeks' gestation, but it is only approximately 2%

for those at 37 weeks or more. RDS occurs more frequently in males (2:1) and more often in infants born to women with gestational or insulin-dependent diabetes (Hicks, 1995).

Signs

Clinical signs of RDS may occur immediately after birth or not until several hours have passed. Grunting, cyanosis in room air, tachypnea, pallor, retractions, and nasal flaring may be evident. There will be decreased breath sounds and scattered rales. Vital signs will be altered; tachycardia or bradycardia, hypotension, and hypothermia may be observed. The Silverman score (Figure 29-8) may be used to assess the severity of the distress. The infant will become progressively hypotonic. A chest radiograph will show a typical reticulogranular or ground glass pattern caused by air in the bronchi and bronchioles contrasted against areas of atelectasis. As the disease progresses, the hallmark manifestations of hypoxia, hypercapnia, and acidosis become more pronounced.

Infants with RDS will get progressively worse for the first 48 hours, then they will begin to improve as the type II cells produce surfactant. Dramatic improvement often occurs in infants with better prognoses. Other infants, usually those of smaller birth weight and lesser gestational age, require longer periods of respiratory assistance and may fail to improve as expected.

Clinical management

Ventilatory support and supplemental oxygen are the principle therapies for RDS that improve oxygenation and maintain lung volume. Minimizing oxygen consumption by maintaining body temperature, BP, and blood sugar within a normal range will assist with the management of RDS.

Surfactant replacement therapy provides hope for treatment of RDS. The Food and Drug Administration (FDA) has approved the use of two commercially prepared surfactant products: Survanta, a modified natural product, and Exosurf, a synthetic product (Prevost, 1991). The dosage and methods of administration vary for the different products, but both are administered through the endotracheal tube of an intubated infant (Drug Profile 29-2).

Transient Tachypnea of the Newborn

Transient tachypnea of the newborn (TTN) results from delayed reabsorption of pulmonary lung fluid. TTN typically occurs in infants delivered by cesarean section or precipitous delivery, where there is absence of the compression (or "squeeze") of the chest wall during delivery.

Tachypnea, retractions, grunting, nasal flaring, and cyanosis may be present. In general, the infant with TTN will require supplemental oxygen; on occasion, ventilatory support will be necessary.

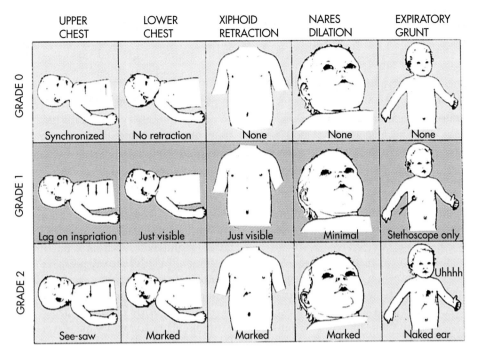

	UPPER CHEST	LOWER CHEST	XIPHOID RETRACTION	NARES DILATION	EXPIRATORY GRUNT
GRADE 0	Synchronized	No retraction	None	None	None
GRADE 1	Lag on inspriation	Just visible	Just visible	Minimal	Stethoscope only
GRADE 2	See-saw	Marked	Marked	Marked	Naked ear

Figure 29-8   Silverman score. Observations indicating presence and severity of respiratory distress. (From *Pediatrics* 24:194, 1959.)

Box **29-2**

DRUG PROFILE

Surfactant Replacement

Bovine lung extract: Beractant (Survanta)
Artificial surfactant: Colfosceril (Exosurf)

INDICATIONS
Prevention and treatment of respiratory distress syndrome in premature infants
- For *prevention,* drug is administered within 15 minutes of birth to infants with clinical manifestations of surfactant deficiency or with birth weight less than 1250 g.
- For *treatment,* drug is administered to infant with confirmed diagnosis of respiratory distress syndrome, preferably within 8 hours of birth.

DOSAGE AND ROUTE
Depends upon drug used. Administer via endotracheal tube.

SIDE EFFECTS AND ADVERSE EFFECTS
Bradycardia and oxygen desaturation after administration
Respiratory distress immediately after administration

Pneumonia

Pneumonia may result from prenatal aspiration of infected amniotic or cervical fluids or blood-borne infection. The common causative organisms are group B *b*-hemolytic streptococci, *Escherichia coli,* and viral agents. After delivery, pathogens such as coagulase-positive staphylococci or group A streptococci are most often carried to newborns by the caregiver's hands. This type of pneumonia starts as a local infection that is not contained. Other organisms (*Klebsiella* and *Pseudomonas aeruginosa*) grow in water used in respiratory therapy equipment and gain entry to the respiratory tract.

Risk

There is a strong association between premature birth and neonatal pneumonia. Infection of amniotic fluid may precipitate preterm delivery. Other risk factors for pneumonia include chorioamnionitis, prolonged rupture of the membranes, cervical colonization (group B *b*-hemolytic streptococcus), and maternal fever.

Signs

Signs of pneumonia may be seen soon after birth or may be delayed as the organisms incubate. The infant will appear lethargic and demonstrate hypothermia, hypotonia, or jaundice. Grunting, nasal flaring, costal retractions, and tachypnea may be present. Alterations in vital signs, arterial blood gas levels, and respiratory function are similar to those that accompany RDS—so similar that any infant with RDS is assumed to have a prenatally acquired pneumonia and is treated with antibiotics until infection is ruled out.

Clinical management

Support of respiratory function and correction of asphyxia are important. The normal arterial blood gas values for newborns are different from adult values (Table 29-2). Blood cultures, cerebrospinal fluid examination and cultures, and other diagnostic tests will direct the therapy. Treatment usually begins with broad-spectrum antibiotics until the culture report returns. The cultures demonstrate which organism is present, and the most effective antibiotic can then be prescribed.

Apnea

Apnea is the cessation of respiration for 15 or more seconds, or the cessation of respiration for any amount of time when cyanosis, bradycardia, hypotonia, or metabolic acidosis occur. This differs from **periodic breathing**, during which respiration ceases for 5 to 10 seconds without pathophysiologic changes. The risk factors associated with apnea are outlined in Box 29-4. Periodic breathing is a normal respiratory pattern in the preterm infant but should approach normal full-term characteristics by 40 weeks.

Risk

Apnea occurs more frequently in premature infants. It is an important sign that may be caused by a disease process or may occur because of immaturity of the respiratory and neurologic systems. Any infant who becomes apneic should be examined for the underlying cause. Apnea is significant when there is a lack of gas exchange for more than 15 seconds, accompanied by bradycardia or oxygen desaturation. Apnea may be induced by hypothermia and hyperthermia, sepsis, hypoglycemia, and intracranial hemorrhage.

Table **29-2**	**Normal Arterial Blood Gas Values for Neonates**

Value	Range
pH	7.33-7.42
Arterial oxygen pressure (PaO$_2$)	50-80 mm Hg
Carbon dioxide pressure (PaCO$_2$)	38-48 mm Hg
Bicarbonate (HCO$_3$.)	20-24 mEq/L
Oxygen saturation	> 90%

Clinical management

Infants less than 1750 g or 34 weeks' gestation are at high risk for apneic episodes. They should have cardiac and respiratory rates and oxygen saturation monitored continuously for the first 2 weeks of life or until 5 to 10 days have passed without any apnea. The apneic infant should be quickly evaluated for bradycardia and cyanosis. Immediate gentle tactile stimulation, such as rubbing the back or flicking the soles of the feet, stimulates respiration in most infants. A bag and mask connected to an oxygen source and equipment for suctioning should be at the bedside and ready for use as indicated. The underlying cause of apnea must be determined and treated promptly.

Apnea of prematurity may be treated with other forms of tactile stimulation, such as a pulsating water mattress or **continuous positive airway pressure** (CPAP); an increase in environmental oxygen may be needed. Research into biobehavioral methods of treating apnea of prematurity involves placing a "regularly breathing" teddy bear in the incubator with the infant. It appears that the stimulation provided by the breathing bear encourages cerebral development and regulation of respiration. Methylxanthines, a group of drugs including aminophylline, theophylline, and caffeine, are used to treat apnea of prematurity. Theophylline is a potent CNS stimulant and bronchodilator. For infants who do not respond to theophylline therapy or who have side effects to the drug, caffeine can be used instead (Drug Profile 29-3).

Meconium Aspiration Syndrome

Prenatal passage of meconium usually occurs in postmature pregnancies or when there is intrauterine growth retardation (IUGR). Infants aspirate meconium either in utero or during delivery and develop respiratory complications from **meconium aspiration syndrome** (MAS).

Risk

Infants with MAS are usually either postterm or growth retarded. MAS is often associated with fetal distress and in utero hypoxia. The meconium that has been passed into the amniotic fluid can be swallowed and aspirated. Meconium may obstruct the airway at any level.

Signs

Amniotic fluid stained with meconium is usually noticed before delivery. (Appropriate delivery room management has been discussed previously in this chapter.) Typically, infants with MAS manifest signs of respiratory distress, including tachypnea, grunting, nasal flaring, retractions, and cyanosis. Rales may be audible upon chest auscultation. Progressive overinflation of the chest may be evident. MAS may be complicated by the development of persistent pulmonary hypertension of the newborn (discussed later in this section).

Clinical management

The major problem present with MAS is hypoxemia; therefore the goal of treatment is to improve oxygenation. Ventilatory support is frequently needed. Maintenance of acid-base balance may prevent the development of pulmonary hypertension.

Box 29-3

DRUG PROFILE

Methylxanthines

ACTION
Cardiac, respiratory, and central nervous system stimulation and smooth muscle relaxation

DOSAGE AND ROUTE
Aminophylline
   Loading: 6 mg/kg IV or PO
   Maintenance: 3-5 mg/kg/day IV or PO in divided doses
   Therapeutic range: 6-12 µg/ml
Theophylline
   Loading: 5 mg/kg IV or PO
   Maintenance: 2-5 mg/kg/day IV or PO in divided doses
   Therapeutic range: 6-12 µg/ml
Caffeine
   Loading: 10 mg/kg (or 20 mg/kg of caffeine citrate) PO
   Maintenance: 2.5 mg/kg PO daily
   Therapeutic range: 5-25 µg/ml

SIDE EFFECTS AND ADVERSE EFFECTS
Tachycardia, dysrhythmias, hypotension, vomiting, diarrhea, hemorrhagic gastritis, irritability, jitteriness, restlessness

---

Box 29-4   Risks for Apnea

Bacterial or viral infection
Hypoxia
Neurologic alterations: asphyxia, intraventricular hemorrhage, subarachnoid hemorrhage, seizures, congenital malformations
Altered metabolic function: temperature instability, hypoglycemia
Fluid and electrolyte imbalance
Maternal, fetal, or neonatal medications
Prematurity: respiratory and neurologic immaturity
Airway obstruction: choanal atresia or stenosis, nasopharyngeal mass
Anemia

Persistent Pulmonary Hypertension of the Newborn

The normally low fetal oxygen tension keeps the pulmonary vascular bed constricted in utero so that less than 10% of the circulating blood goes to the lungs. Factors such as intrauterine hypoxia, RDS, polycythemia, and meconium aspiration can cause pulmonary vasoconstriction to persist after birth. Circulation to the alveoli is decreased because of vasoconstriction. The pressure within the pulmonary arteries remains high. The ductus arteriosus fails to constrict. Blood, therefore, is shunted from the right to the left side of the heart through the ductus arteriosus and foramen ovale. This occurs because there is a higher pressure on the right side of the heart. The alterations worsen the hypoxia and result in **persistent pulmonary hypertension of the newborn** (PPHN). Both prenatal and postnatal factors are associated with the incidence of PPHN.

Signs

Neonates with PPHN are usually full term or postterm, with persistent cyanosis, tachypnea, altered cardiac sounds, and congestive heart failure present. Arterial blood gases will demonstrate acidosis.

Clinical management

Treatment focuses on the underlying condition. Mechanical ventilation is necessary in most cases of PPHN. A vasodilator medication (e.g., tolazoline) may be given IV to reduce pulmonary vascular resistance. Newer methods of ventilation maintain partial pressure of carbon dioxide (P_{CO_2}) levels within a normal range, and drugs such as sodium bicarbonate are given to create a metabolic alkalosis that can dilate the pulmonary blood vessels. The use of sodium bicarbonate to achieve alkalosis has been shown to improve pulmonary blood flow.

Systemic BP is supported with volume expanders. Vasopressors such as dopamine may also be needed to maintain systemic perfusion. Extracorporeal membrane oxygenation (ECMO), a technique that allows blood to bypass the lungs, has been used with success for infants with PPHN.

TEST Yourself 29-1 _____

   a. Name three underlying factors for RDS.
   b. What does surfactant replacement allow to happen in the newborn lung?

Ventilatory Interventions

Oxygen therapy

Infants who have cyanosis, hypoxemia, apnea, and respiratory difficulty will require supplemental oxygen therapy. An *oxygen hood (oxyhood)* delivers warm, humidified oxygen to the infant at measured concentrations. A *nasal cannula* delivers humidified oxygen to the nares of the infant; it provides low concentrations of oxygen (Figure 29-9, *A* and *B*).

Continuous positive airway pressure

CPAP delivers a constant pressure into the infant's lungs throughout the respiratory cycle, thereby preventing alveoli from collapsing during expiration. An infant receiving this form of respiratory therapy is breathing spontaneously and receiving only additional pressure and increased inspired oxygen. CPAP decreases the effort required to breathe and may be delivered through an endotracheal or pharyngeal tube or nasal prongs. Nasal prongs, the most commonly used system in the NICU, resemble the standard nasal cannula used to deliver oxygen except that they fit tightly against the nares. Pharyngeal tubes are threaded nasally or orally into the pharynx (Figure 29-10).

Intermittent mandatory ventilation

Neonates require endotracheal intubation and mechanical ventilation when there are problems with oxygenation, ventilation, or respiratory effort. *Intermittent mandatory ventilation* (IMV) provides a continuous flow of warm, humidified oxygen and periodic breaths to lessen the infant's work of breathing. It provides both continuous distending pressure and intermittent inflating pressure to the alveoli (Figure 29-11).

New technologies

High-frequency ventilation. High-frequency ventilation (HFV) was designed to ventilate infants with respiratory dysfunction while avoiding the complications of conventional mechanical ventilation, such as those encountered with IMV. HFV delivers breaths at a high rate while using low inflating pressures.

Extracorporeal membrane oxygenation. ECMO is a form of prolonged cardiopulmonary bypass used for infants

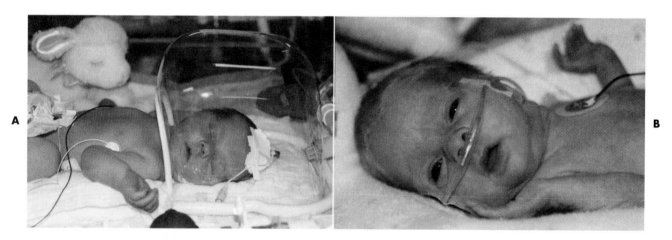

Figure 29-9 **A,** Infant under oxyhood. **B,** Infant with nasal cannula. (Courtesy Victoria Langer, RNC, MSN, NNP.)

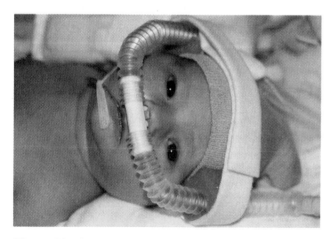

Figure 29-10 Infant receiving ventilatory assistance with nasal continuous positive airway pressure. (Courtesy Victoria Langer, RNC, MSN, NNP.)

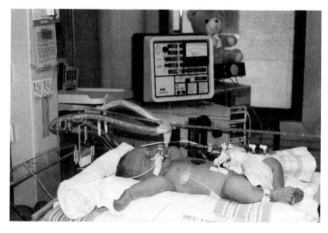

Figure 29-11 Infant intubated and on ventilator. (Courtesy Victoria Langer, RNC, MSN, NNP.)

with severe hypoxemia that does not improve with aggressive ventilatory management. Neonates with MAS, pneumonia or sepsis, RDS, and congenital diaphragmatic hernia may meet the criteria for treatment with ECMO. Unfortunately, morbidity and mortality rates associated with the use of ECMO are high.

Nitric oxide. Nitric oxide (NO) is the newest technology introduced to neonatal medicine. It is a gas that may be a useful therapy in infants with PPHN because it is a pulmonary vasodilator. It is still being used in clinical trials to determine its efficacy (Miller, 1995).

T E S T *Yourself* 29-2 _____

Match the terms with the statements that best apply.
a. CPAP   ____ Provides warm, humidified oxygen only
b. Oxyhood   ____ Requires endotracheal intubation
c. Mechanical   ____ Delivers only distending pressure to the airways

Complications of Interventions

Respiratory support for newborns has become possible only in the last two to three decades. With the advancements in neonatal pulmonary medicine, many complications have arisen (Box 29-5). Although hypoxia still damages many high-risk infants, medical and nursing personnel are now faced with complications resulting from *hyperoxia,* which mainly affects the developing eyes and lungs. Although hyperoxia is a sustained PO_2 level over 100 mm Hg, small infants may be adversely affected by lower levels in the "normal" range.

Retinopathy of prematurity

Although **retinopathy of prematurity** (ROP) may occur in premature infants of varying gestational ages and weights, it is more common in infants of lower birth weight. ROP describes the pathologic fibrous process that may affect the blood vessels of the retina in neonates. It was formerly referred to as *retrolental fibroplasia* (RLF). It has been found to occur as a result of vasoconstriction of retinal blood vessels in response to high oxygen levels. Researchers believe that prematurity is the primary risk factor because ROP has also developed in some preterm infants who have not received supplemental oxygen. Retinal vasoconstriction is followed by obliteration and then proliferation of the affected vessels. These vessels are abnormal and leak blood and serum into the retina. Retinal detachment and myopia follow. Early in the disease, these changes are seen only in the periphery of the retina. As the process worsens, the entire retina may be involved. In some affected infants, laser photocoagulation or cryotherapy may be used during the active phase of ROP (Gracey, 1991).

Prevention still focuses on strict control of arterial oxygen tension below the level that stimulates vasoconstriction. However, there is no agreement on safe levels of PO_2; in fact, variables such as duration of oxygen therapy also influence the development of ROP. Continuous monitoring of oxygen saturation may reduce the incidence of hyperoxemia, thereby reducing the incidence of ROP. LBW infants are always evaluated by a pediatric ophthalmologist before discharge.

Bronchopulmonary dysplasia

Bronchopulmonary dysplasia (BPD) is a chronic disease of the infant lung caused by the effects of oxygen delivered over time at high pressures. The epithelium lining of the bronchi and alveoli become necrotic. A process of regeneration follows but is complicated by interstitial fibrosis and metaplasia of the bronchial lining. Infants who recover do so because alveoli continue to multiply into the eighth postnatal year. However, respiratory deficits are common.

Infants with BPD have chronic oxygen hunger, hypercapnia, psychosocial and physical delay, feeding intolerance, and oral aversion. Respiratory infections are frequent complications. Many medications, including antibiotics, diuretics, steroids, and vitamin supplements, are used to treat the infant with chronic lung disease. It is difficult to provide adequate nutrition; fluid restrictions are necessary to control pulmonary edema, and much energy is spent on

 Box 29-5   **Complications Associated with Assisted Ventilation**

OXYHOOD
Hyperoxia

NASAL CANNULA
Hyperoxia
Pressure-related tissue damage (nares, nasal septum)

CONTINUOUS POSITIVE AIRWAY PRESSURE
Hyperoxia
Hyperexpansion of the lungs
Air leaks (e.g., pneumothorax)
Pressure-related tissue damage

ENDOTRACHEAL INTUBATION
Trauma
Infection
Pulmonary air leaks
Mucous plugs
Subglottic stenosis
Laryngomalacia
Tracheomalacia
Bronchopulmonary dysplasia and retinopathy of prematurity related to hyperoxia

the increased work of breathing. Gastrointestinal reflux is common. The resulting growth failure compounds the respiratory difficulty. It is possible and usually preferable to care for these infants at home. A healthy home environment stimulates normal growth and development and avoids contact with nosocomial pathogens.

Box 29-2

CLINICAL DECISION

You are caring for a full-term infant with pneumonia. He is in an oxyhood, receiving 60% O_2. Arterial blood gas levels are pH, 7.28; Po_2, 52 mm Hg; Pco_2 60 mm Hg. You should:

1. Recognize that these values are not normal and that the infant needs more respiratory assistance.
2. Determine that these values must not be correct because the infant is breathing spontaneously.
3. Continue to observe the infant, monitoring vital signs until the next blood gases are drawn.

CARDIOVASCULAR DYSFUNCTION

Most common alterations in neonatal cardiovascular function are caused by congenital defects in structure or function or by failure of transition from fetal to adult circulation (see Figure 18-5). It often is difficult to identify the infant with congenital heart disease (CHD) because the signs (tachypnea, cardiac murmur, and cyanosis) are also seen with respiratory dysfunction or sepsis. Neonatal health care providers now evaluate infants for cardiac disease earlier because survival is more likely with earlier diagnosis and treatment.

Congenital Cardiac Defects

CHD occurs in 7.5 to 8.0 infants out of every 1000 live births. It is a major cause of death in full-term infants. (Because a full discussion is beyond the scope of this text, the reader should consult textbooks of pediatric nursing.) The occurrence of congenital heart defects is multifactorial. Though genetic and environmental factors influence the occurrence of CHD, the cause is usually unknown. Certain defects occur more in males, whereas others occur more in females.

Signs

Infants with CHD may have all or some of the following signs: cyanosis, respiratory distress, congestive heart failure (CHF), and abnormal cardiac rhythm and sounds (murmurs). One important clue is cyanosis that is *out of proportion* to the degree of respiratory distress. Another sign is CHF, which can appear slowly in early stages. A heart defect

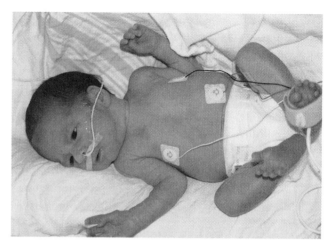

Figure 29-12   Infant on cardiac monitor. Note placement of monitor leads. (Courtesy Victoria Langer, RNC, MSN, NNP.)

should be suspected in any infant with tachypnea, tachycardia, oliguria, edema, hepatomegaly, abnormal cardiac rhythm, diminished peripheral perfusion, and difficulty in feeding (Figure 29-12). Cyanosis is a predominant feature in some cardiac defects. When cyanosis is present, it is because desaturated venous blood is shunted from the right to the left side of the heart without passing through the lungs to become oxygenated. CHD defects are classified as cyanotic or acyanotic (Flyer and Lang, 1993).

Cyanotic Congenital Heart Defects

Transposition of the great vessels

The cardiac defect most commonly diagnosed during the first week of life is *transposition of the great arteries* (TGA). The aorta arises from the right ventricle and the pulmonary artery from the left. As a result, desaturated venous blood returning to the right atrium and ventricle is recirculated to the body without having been oxygenated. Highly saturated arterial blood returning to the left atrium and ventricle is then recirculated through the lungs instead of supplying the body's oxygen needs. Mixing of these two circulations must take place if the infant is to survive after birth (Figure 29-13, *A*).

TGA causes cyanosis soon after delivery. It is diagnosed by echocardiogram and chest radiograph. Treatment attempts to establish mixing of the saturated and desaturated bloodstreams by maintaining *patency* of the ductus arteriosus through the use of prostaglandin E_1. Palliative surgery increases the mixing through an artificially created atrial septal defect (ASD). Corrective surgery is usually delayed until the infant is more stable. A newer procedure may be performed within the first few days of life. The great arteries are "switched" so that the pulmonary artery will arise from the right ventricle and the aorta will arise from the left.

Cyanotic Defects

A

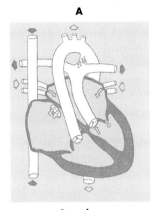

B

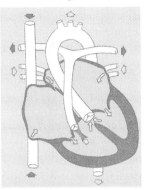

Complete Transposition of Great Arteries (TGA)

The aorta originates from the right ventricle, and the pulmonary artery originates from the left ventricle. An abnormal communication between the two circulations must be present to sustain life.

Tetralogy of Fallot (TOF)

Tetralogy of Fallot is characterized by the combination of four defects: (1) pulmonary stenosis, (2) ventricular septal defect, (3) overriding aorta, (4) hypertrophy of the right ventricle.

C

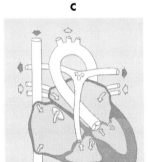

Tricuspid Atresia

Tricuspid valvular atresia is characterized by a small right ventricle, large left ventricle, and usually a diminished pulmonary circulation. The lungs may receive blood through one of three routes: (1) a small ventricular septal defect, (2) patent ductus arteriosus, (3) bronchial vessels.

Acyanotic Defects

D

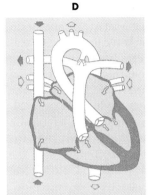

E

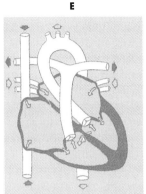

Patent Ductus Arteriosus

Functional closure of the ductus normally occurs soon after birth. If the ductus remains patent after birth, the direction of blood flow in the ductus is reversed by the higher pressure in the aorta.

Ventricular Septal Defect

A ventricular septal defect is an abnormal opening between the right and left ventricles. Ventricular septal defects vary in size and may occur in either the membranous or muscular portion of the ventricular septum. Because of higher pressure in the left ventricle, a shunting of blood from the left to right ventricle occurs during systole.

F

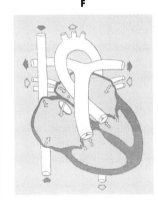

Atrial Septal Defect

An atrial septal defect is an abnormal opening between the right and left atria. Basically, three types of abnormalities result from incorrect development of the atrial septum. An incompetent foramen ovale is the most common defect. In general, left to right shunting of blood occurs in all atrial septal defects.

Figure 29-13   A-F, Congenital heart defects.

Tetralogy of Fallot

Tetralogy of Fallot (TOF) is a syndrome of four associated cardiac lesions, including ventricular septal defect, an aorta that overrides the interventricular septum, pulmonary stenosis, and right ventricular hypertrophy (Figure 29-13, *B*). Infants with TOF exhibit cyanosis that depends on the degree of the pulmonary stenosis. Hypercyanotic or "tet" spells can occur when pulmonary flow is obstructed even further by the muscular area at the root of the pulmonary artery. These episodes are unusual in the first month of life. Surgical repair is usually delayed beyond the neonatal period.

Tricuspid atresia

Tricuspid atresia is a failure of the development of the tricuspid valve. The normal flow of blood from the right atrium to the right ventricle is therefore prevented. Blood entering the right atrium is shunted through the foramen ovale to the left atrium and left ventricle and then out through the aorta to the systemic circulation. A ventricular septal defect (VSD) is commonly present (Figure 29-13, *C*). Cyanosis will be present shortly after birth and will worsen when the ductus arteriosus closes. CHF may occur if there is a large VSD. Initial management includes oxygen and prostaglandin to maintain patency of the ductus arteriosus. Surgical repair is required.

Acyanotic Congenital Heart Defects

Patent ductus arteriosus

Patent ductus arteriosus (PDA) may be an isolated finding in infants of varying gestational age or may occur with RDS in an ill premature infant. It can also be seen as part of a syndrome of complex heart disease. In the infant with a PDA, blood will shunt from the aorta (left side of the heart) to the pulmonary artery (right side of the heart) and cause overcirculation to the lungs (Figure 29-13, *D*). An increase in blood returning to the left atrium and ventricle occurs, increasing the workload on the heart and leading to CHF. The systolic BP increases, the pulse pressure widens, and the peripheral pulses feel "bounding" as a result. A characteristic "machine" murmur is heard.

Management of a PDA depends upon the hemodynamic significance of the shunt. Conservative measures include fluid restriction, diuretics, and digoxin. A prostaglandin inhibitor (indomethacin) may cause spontaneous closure. Surgical intervention involves ligation of the ductus arteriosus.

Ventricular septal defect

VSD is the most common congenital heart defect. It may occur as an isolated cardiac defect or as part of a complex of defects. A characteristic murmur is heard. Larger defects cause more severe symptoms. After birth, blood will shunt from the left to the right ventricle through the VSD, overloading the right side (Figure 29-13, *E*). There is increased blood flow to the lungs, followed by increased blood returning to the left atrium and ventricle. Symptoms such as pneumonia and CHF result. Infants whose CHF does not improve with medical treatment or who have repeated bouts of pulmonary infections are candidates for surgery. Small VSDs may close spontaneously and require no treatment.

Atrial septal defect

Incomplete formation of the septum during fetal cardiac development results in an opening between the two atria (Figure 29-13, *F*). A characteristic heart murmur is heard. Although an ASD is usually asymptomatic, CHF may result from shunting of blood from the left to the right atrium. If CHF does not respond to medical management, the ASD might be closed by a special procedure performed during cardiac catheterization. Surgical repair takes place if the catheterization procedure is not possible.

Coarctation of the aorta

Coarctation (constriction) *of the aorta* may occur with varying degrees of severity. The coarctation may occur alone or as part of a complex cardiac defect. Simple coarctation causes CHF because the heart attempts to maintain output against the obstruction. The defect may be located near the ductus arteriosus. As the ductus closes, the obstruction worsens. Pulses and BP in the upper extremities far exceed values in the lower extremities, and signs of CHF soon develop. Treatment includes stabilization with prostaglandin E$_1$ to keep the ductus arteriosus open until surgical repair can be accomplished.

If the coarctation does not require surgery in the neonatal period, treatment includes stabilization with digitalis and diuretics to prevent CHF. Repair is electively scheduled between the ages of 1 and 3 years.

Hypoplastic left-heart syndrome

Hypoplastic left-heart syndrome (HLHS) includes a small (hypoplastic) ascending aorta and left ventricle and atresia of the aortic and mitral valves. Symptoms begin when the ductus arteriosus constricts, leading to a decrease in systemic circulation. The infant will become ashen in color with poor capillary filling and weak pulses. Metabolic acidosis and progressively worsening CHF accompany the shock. If HLHS is recognized promptly, the infant's condition may be temporarily stabilized by maintaining patency of the ductus arteriosus.

Although HLHS affects 7% to 9% of infants with CHD, it accounts for as many as 22% of infant deaths as a result of cardiac disease in the neonatal period (Long, 1990). Surgical intervention involves cardiac transplantation or a two-stage palliative and then corrective repair. Mortality rates are high.

Clinical management

Management is dependent upon the specific defect that is present and the manifestations. Administration of oxygen, diuretics, and digoxin may adequately treat CHF. Prostaglandin E$_1$ will dilate the ductus arteriosus to maintain patency, necessary for cardiac lesions where there is minimal or no pulmonary blood flow (Paul, 1995). Surgical procedures are specific to the defect.

TEST *Yourself* 29-3

a. List three manifestations of cyanotic CHD and the cyanotic defects.
b. List two characteristics of acyanotic CHD and the acyanotic defects.

Nursing Responsibilities

CARDIOPULMONARY DYSFUNCTION

ASSESSMENT

A complete physical examination should include observation of color, respiratory effort, and posture; auscultation of lung and heart sounds; and palpation of skin and peripheral pulses. The cardiorespiratory monitor will demonstrate the cardiac rhythm and respiratory pattern, whereas the pulse oximeter will determine oxygen saturation.

NURSING DIAGNOSES

- Impaired gas exchange
- Ineffective breathing pattern; related to apnea or tachypnea; related to CHF
- Ineffective airway clearance
- Risk for injury related to hypoxemia or hyperoxemia
- Decreased cardiac output, related to CHD
- Parental anxiety and fear, related to infant compromise
- Knowledge deficit (parental)

EXPECTED OUTCOMES

- Vital signs and blood gases are within normal limits.
- Exhibits satisfactory oxygenation as evidenced by color, oxygen saturation, blood gas levels.
- Exhibits spontaneous respiratory effort within expected normal parameters.
- Perfusion is adequate to meet baseline requirements.
- Parents verbalize understanding of infant's status.
- Parents demonstrate ability to administer medications and treatments.

NURSING INTERVENTION

Infants are usually intubated by the orotracheal route. On rare occasions (i.e., when an obstructive oral mass is present), the nasotracheal route is used for intubation. Pulmonary hygiene maintains the patency of the endotracheal tube and the airways. The ill neonate is less able to maintain patency because of the small airway diameter, inadequate cough reflex, poor respiratory effort, and inability to change position. Chest physiotherapy and suctioning provide the infant with mechanisms for maintenance of airway patency, prevention of infection, and adequate ventilation. Infants with respiratory or cardiovascular compromise will frequently have an umbilical artery catheter inserted to monitor blood gases and BP (Figure 29-14).

Assessment of heart sounds, breath sounds, oxygen saturation, and capillary perfusion is performed frequently. Observe the infant for signs of worsening respiratory distress, increasing frequency of apnea, and signs of CHF. It is important to provide the infant with the minimal level of oxygen needed to maintain oxygenation without causing complications.

An effort should be made to organize care in such a manner as to decrease the workload on the cardiopulmonary system. Ill neonates are extremely sensitive to the stresses of handling and manipulation; they require min-

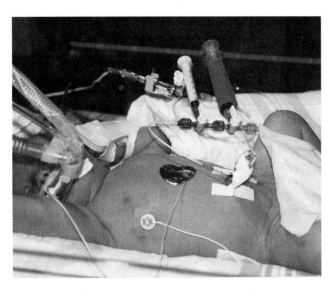

Figure 29-14 Infant with umbilical artery catheter. (Courtesy Victoria Langer, RNC, MSN, NNP.)

imal stimulation. Some infants will benefit from sedation with a narcotic analgesic.

EVALUATION

- Has the infant demonstrated improvement in oxygenation or ventilation?
- Does the infant who is diagnosed with RDS show improvement in respiratory function by the fifth day of life?
- Will the infant require oxygen therapy or respiratory treatments at home?
- Has the occurrence of apnea in the infant improved by 35 to 37 weeks' postconceptional age?
- Were the signs of hypoxia identified before the infant suffered injury?
- Did the infant have adverse sequelae from the treatment?
- Are the parents able to safely provide the necessary therapies before discharge to home?

FLUID, ELECTROLYTE, AND NUTRITIONAL IMBALANCE

Problems in fluid, electrolyte, and nutritional balance are common for the preterm infant. Immature structures, hormones, and behaviors make regulation difficult. It is important to observe for imbalances because they can compromise the functions of other systems. Overhydration can cause pulmonary or cerebral edema and maintain a PDA; underhydration can lead to renal failure. Nutritional deficiencies can affect the infant's ability to fight infection and decrease the rate of growth and development.

Fluid Balance

Fluid balance in the preterm infant is tenuous at best. At 24 weeks' gestation, 85% of the infant's total body weight is water. Most of this is contained in the extracellular space; the remainder is intracellular fluid. Total body water decreases with increasing gestational age. By the second postnatal month, there are equal amounts of intracellular and extracellular water until, in the months to follow, most body water is found in the intracellular space.

Regulation of body water is primarily the responsibility of the kidneys. Renal function, however, is immature, even at term. Antidiuretic hormone (ADH) controls the amount of water excreted or retained by the kidneys. When ADH levels are elevated, the kidneys excrete less water. When ADH levels are diminished, the kidneys excrete more water. At term, ADH levels are only one fifth of adult levels. Preterm infants do not respond well to overhydration or underhydration because of the inadequate levels of ADH. They cannot concentrate urine as well as term infants do. They also cannot produce dilute urine quickly; therefore they will retain excessive water loads. Term and preterm infants who have been asphyxiated can have symptoms of inappropriate ADH secretion.

The glomerular filtration rate (GFR) determines the amount of blood filtered by the kidneys and, therefore, the amount of urine produced. This rate is limited in the neonate but increases after birth. Preterm infants have fewer nephrons and much lower filtration rates than do term infants, affecting their ability to excrete water.

Risk

Neonates lose water easily by a variety of mechanisms. The kidneys, sweat glands, and gastrointestinal tract are obvious routes for water loss. Water is also lost through the lungs and skin by a process called **insensible water loss** (IWL). The amount of water lost via this route varies with gestational age and body weight. The preterm infant's thin skin and larger ratio of body surface area to body weight allows for greater water loss. The factors that influence water loss are listed in Box 29-6.

Clinical management

Fluid requirements vary for the newborn. These may be met by enteral or parenteral fluids. On the first day of life, the healthy full-term newborn needs 65 to 80 ml/kg per day; this gradually increases to 100 to 150 ml/kg per day by the end of the first week. Because preterm infants have higher fluid requirements, factors that increase IWL are figured into the total fluid requirement. Preterm infants weighing between 1000 and 1500 g may need up to 120 ml/kg per day in the first 2 days, with an increase to 150 ml/kg per day by the end of the first week. Infants who weigh less than 1000 g will require more fluid because of increased IWL. Fluid, electrolyte, and nutritional requirements are calculated at least once daily.

Box 29-6	**Factors Affecting Water Loss**

INCREASED LOSS
Low gestational age
Radiant warmer
Hyperthermia
Phototherapy
Activity
Tachypnea
Inadequate humidification

DECREASED LOSS
High humidity in incubator via assisted ventilation
Double-walled incubator
Plastic heat shield
Plastic blanket
Clothes

Requirements for ill infants are recalculated more often (Darby and Loughead, 1996).

Electrolyte Balance

Electrolyte requirements vary with age. No supplementation is needed unless symptoms of deficiency occur. Preterm infants lose sodium easily, which causes hyponatremia, even when they receive an average sodium intake. Hyponatremia is usually due to excessive retention of water. In some cases, unusually large amounts of sodium may be retained (hypernatremia), especially if insensible fluid loss is high. Sodium and potassium are absorbed by the gastrointestinal tract and excreted by the kidneys. Both sodium and potassium can be lost by the kidneys because of the administration of certain diuretics, such as furosemide. Potassium is needed for normal neuromuscular functioning. *Hypokalemia* (low potassium level) may result from excessive losses through the gastrointestinal or renal route, whereas infants with acidosis may have *hyperkalemia*.

Nutritional Balance

Weight gain should approximate that which occurs during normal intrauterine growth. Intrauterine growth curves are widely accepted for use in measuring the adequacy of the postnatal growth of premature infants (see Figure 29-1). Weight is plotted on a graph that correlates with gestational age. Many factors make it difficult for the preterm infant to gain adequate weight. For example, nutritional deficits may exist because of increased metabolic demands placed on the preterm infant by thermoregulation, work of respiration and feeding, and decreased ability to absorb nutrients. The preterm infant's ability to adequately digest lactose and fats is also compromised by inadequate production of lactase, bile acids, and pancreatic lipase.

The ability to coordinate the suck-swallow-breathing complex matures at approximately 34 weeks of gestation. Many preterm infants have respiratory disease, which further hampers the ability to feed.

Clinical management

Calories. Caloric requirements are calculated from the sum of needs for the basal metabolic rate, plus needs for activity, cold stress, loss via feces, digestive and metabolic processes, and growth (Table 29-3). Just after birth, 90 to 100 kcal/kg per day are needed; this increases to 120 kcal/kg per day in a few days. Certain infants will require 150 kcal/kg per day or more for growth. Formulas with caloric densities of 20, 24, and 27 calories per ounce are available.

Most often a 24 kcal per ounce formula is provided to preterm infants, compared with a 20 kcal per ounce formula for the term infant. Human milk does not have a constant caloric density because the fat content varies both from the beginning to the end of any one feeding and diurnally. However, the calories are easier to digest. Women are encouraged to lactate with a breast pump until the preterm infant can nurse (Figure 29-15). Human Milk Fortifier (Mead Johnson, Evansville, Indiana) and Natural Care (Ross Laboratories, Columbus, Ohio) may be added to breast milk to increase the protein and carbohydrate content and to provide supplemental vitamins, minerals, and electrolytes. This provides the preterm infant with a controlled level of necessary nutrients, in addition to the benefits of human milk.

Protein. Optimal growth should occur with a protein intake of 2.5 to 4.0 g/kg/per day (8% to 12% of total daily caloric intake). Casein is the predominant protein in most cow milk formulas, whereas human milk protein is mostly whey. The balance of amino acids in whey protein is suited for human infants. Milk from mothers who have given birth to premature infants also contains more protein than milk at term. The additional benefits of immunologic factors makes human milk the preferred food for preterm infants (and for term infants as well).

Fat. Fat is the major source of energy for the premature infant. The preterm infant has not had the benefit of the caloric intake of the third trimester of gestation. Therefore for weight gain, fat should make up 35% to 55% of intake; 3% of this should be linoleic acid. The fat in human milk is more easily digested by low birth weight infants.

Carbohydrates. Carbohydrates are stored as glycogen during gestation to provide reserves of energy; however, preterm, SGA, or asphyxiated infants have inadequate stores. Lactose and other glucose polymers provide carbohydrates. Breast milk and some prepared formulas are lactose based; other formulas use lactose and glucose polymers as carbohydrate sources. Most infants tolerate lactose well,

Table **29-3**	**Daily Caloric Requirements for Preterm Infants**
Caloric Requirement	**Kcal/kg/day**
Basic metabolic rate	35-50
Day 1	35
Day 2	45
Day 28	50
Intermittent activity (highly variable)	15
Occasional cold stress	10
Fecal loss	8
Specific dynamic action (energy cost of digestion and metabolism)	12
Growth	25
Total calories	105-120
Nutritional Requirements for Growth	**Amount**
Fluid	150-180 ml/kg/day
Protein	2.5-4.0 g/kg/day (7%-12% of kcal)
Fat	3-4 g/kg/day (35%-55% of kcal)
Carbohydrate	35%-55% of kcal

From Merenstein GB, Gardner SL: *Handbook of neonatal intensive care,* ed 32, St Louis, 1993, Mosby.

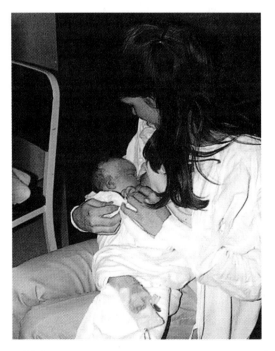

Figure 29-15   Graduating to breast-feeding in the NICU. (Courtesy Marjorie Pyle, RNC, *Lifecircle*.)

even though lactase levels are subnormal. Carbohydrates should account for 35% to 55% of total calories per day.

Minerals and vitamins. The exact requirements of vitamins and minerals for premature neonates have not been determined. Fat-soluble vitamin absorption is unknown. Calcium, phosphorus, and magnesium are needed for bone mineralization. Iron is important for the synthesis of hemoglobin, but anemia of prematurity will not improve with iron replacement therapy.

Minerals are supplied in adequate amounts by prepared formulas and human milk. Formulas have varying amounts of additional iron. The calcium/phosphorus ratio (2.2:1.0) found in human milk has been approximated in most premature infant formulas. Vitamins are found in adequate amounts in premature infant formulas and in human milk when it is fortified. Special formulas for preterm infants provide the additional minerals, vitamins, and trace elements required. (See Chapter 17 for a comparison between cow milk and human milk.)

TEST *Yourself* **29-4** _____

A 1-week-old infant born at 31 weeks' gestation weighs 1200 g. What are the fluid and caloric requirements?

Enteral Nutrition

Infants who are too immature to feed orally may be fed by gavage with orogastric or nasogastric tubes passed into the stomach, duodenum, or jejunum. Intermittent (bolus) feedings are preferred because they stimulate normal postprandial enzyme release and gastrointestinal motility. The amount of the feeding and the intervals are slowly increased, which follows the normal progression of feeding behavior. Parenteral nutrition may be needed to supplement enteral feedings initially. Parents may learn to assist with these feedings (Figure 29-16, *A*).

Certain infants demonstrate a vagal stimulation response from bolus feedings that results in bradycardia. Others may have esophageal reflux and an increased risk of aspiration. Continuous feedings are offered in these cases. In some NICUs, continuous gavage feeding tubes are gradually advanced through the pyloric valve; in others, they are placed in the stomach, as they are for bolus feedings (see Procedure 29-1, which includes Figure 29-16, *B*). Equipment other than the actual feeding tube is changed often to reduce the danger of infection.

Nonnutritive sucking (NNS)—sucking on a pacifier during gavage feeding—has many benefits. NNS promotes the release of gastric hormones and enzymes, thus improving motility. It has been shown to improve transi-

tion to oral feedings and to increase the infant's level of alertness before oral feedings.

Feeding by nipple or breast should be encouraged because it encourages growth and maturity of the gastrointestinal tract. It also provides comfort for hunger and oral gratification. Oral feeding is slowly introduced when the infant is mature enough to use a nipple. Cardiorespiratory status does not need to be completely normal; however, the respiratory rate should be less than 60 breaths per minute with only minimal amounts of supplemental oxygen. Cardiorespriatory and pulse oximetry monitors are used to determine an infant's stability while feeding.

Complications of enteral feedings

Assessment of feeding tolerance is essential. Before every feeding, the nurse should assess the infant for the presence of bowel sounds, observe the abdomen for gastric distention, check the placement of the feeding tube, measure the abdominal girth, and determine the amount of gastric residual that is present. A large gastric residual (more than 20% of a feeding volume) and vomiting are indications of feeding intolerance, which may require a decrease in feeding volume. Gastric residuals should be refed to the infant to avoid fluid and electrolyte imbalances.

Parenteral Nutrition

The infant who cannot be fed enterally is fed by the IV route. The usual basic solution is 10% dextrose in increasing amounts (see section on fluid requirements) with appropriate additives. During the first 24 hours of life, the newborn's serum electrolyte balance reflects that of the mother. On the second day, infants receiving IV therapy are given supplemental electrolytes, sodium chloride, and potassium chloride. The amounts are determined after serum electrolyte levels have been measured. Solutions are infused via sites found in veins of the hands, arms, feet, or scalp. Extremely small (as small as 27-gauge) needles or IV catheters are used. Control of infusion rates is *always* maintained by an electric infusion pump, never by gravity. Careful attention for signs of infiltration is vital because extravasated solutions cause tissue necrosis.

Infants who are unable to take enteral feedings after the first 1 to 2 days of life will require hyperalimentation or total parenteral nutrition (TPN) to meet basic nutritional needs. Dextrose (10% to 30%) supplies carbohydrates, an amino acid solution provides precursors for protein synthesis, and fats are added through an emulsified solution. Electrolytes, minerals, and vitamins are added to the solution as needed. The TPN solution is prepared in the pharmacy, with strict attention to sterility.

PROCEDURE 29-1

Feeding Tube Placement for Intermittent or Continuous Gavage Feedings

1. Prepare feeding, and place adjacent to work area.
   Rationale: Minimize stress on infant when you are prepared.
2. Select No. 5, No. 6, or No. 8 French feeding tube according to infant size.
   Rationale: Choose size that is appropriate to prevent trauma to the nares.
3. Determine appropriate distance of insertion by measuring length from tip of nose (for nasogastric) or from mouth (orogastric) to the earlobe and then to the end of the xiphoid process. (Alternate method: measure length from the bridge of the nose to the umbilicus.)
   Rationale: Tip of catheter must be in stomach for feedings.
4. Place a short length of tape at the measured point.
   Rationale: Tape will mark the distance for insertion and can also be used to stabilize tube once it is in place.
5. Insert tube: nasal route may occlude air passage; oral route is more difficult to insert and may interfere with oral feeding. Choose route according to infant's condition and responses.
6. Tape tube securely to face (use skin protective dressing first).

   Rationale: Catheter must be stable to avoid aspiration during feeding.
7. Confirm placement of tube in stomach by injecting small amount of air while listening to characteristic sound with stethoscope placed just under left costal margin.
8. For intermittent feeding: aspirate residual stomach contents, and note amount and color of aspirate. If green (bile) or if brown or red (blood), report at once and delay feeding (necrotizing enterocolitis [NEC] may be occurring). Unusually large aspirate may be caused by overfeeding or intestinal obstruction, NEC, or infection.
9. Measure and refeed normal gastric aspirate. Record aspirate and feeding totals.
   Rationale: The volume of the gastric residual will determine how well the infant is tolerating the feedings.
10. Proceed with new feeding by gravity administration; avoid "pushing" feeding. Place infant on right side to enhance gastric emptying and avoid aspiration with regurgitation. The feeding should infuse at a rate of 1 mL per 30 to 60 seconds.

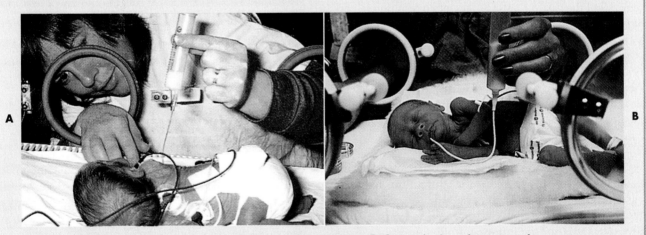

Figure 29-16   A, Mother has learned to feed her infant by gavage. **B,** Gavage feeding of preterm infant. (**A,** From Beischer NA, MacKay EV: *Obstetrics and the newborn,* ed 3, Sydney, 1993, WB Saunders. Courtesy Harcourt, Brace Jovanovich Group, Australia. **B,** Courtesy Ross Laboratories, Columbus, Ohio.)

OPTIONAL ACTIVITY

Write a sample nursing note correctly documenting the performance of this procedure.

It may be administered through a peripheral infusion if the dextrose concentration is not over 12.5%. A central venous catheter is needed to infuse higher dextrose concentrations.

Percutaneous central venous catheters are often placed in premature infants within the first week of life to provide the much needed parenteral nutrition. Complications of TPN include hypoglycemia or hyperglycemia, hyperammonemia, cholestatic jaundice, hyperlipidemia, and increased risk of kernicterus.

GASTROINTESTINAL DYSFUNCTION

Nutritional intake is necessary for survival. Many complex metabolic processes are involved, but ultimately, the gastrointestinal tract must be structurally intact in order to maintain adequate nutrition. The majority of disorders of the gastrointestinal tract result from congenital anomalies, including abdominal wall defects, esophageal atresia and tracheoesophageal fistula, cleft lip and palate (see Chapter 28), congenital diaphragmatic hernia, and Hirschsprung's disease. **Necrotizing enterocolitis** (NEC) is a gastrointestinal disorder that occurs predominantly in preterm infants.

Necrotizing Enterocolitis

NEC is an acquired disorder characterized by ischemia and necrosis of the gastrointestinal tract, often resulting in perforation of the intestine. It occurs predominantly in the sick premature infant. The etiology of NEC is unclear; there are many theories, none of which is definitive (Parker, 1995). The underlying risk factor is prematurity. Any condition that causes ischemia and growth of bacteria in the presence of formula feedings is an additional risk factor (Box 29-7).

Signs

The infant with NEC has signs that are indistinguishable from sepsis. Abdominal distention, lethargy, gastric residual effects, vomiting, and gastrointestinal bleeding are common. Gas produced by intestinal organisms dissects the intestinal wall, producing a characteristic radiograph pattern. Varying areas of the gastrointestinal tract may be affected; however, the ileum and proximal colon are the usual sites. Rupture of the diseased intestine may result in free air in the peritoneum (pneumoperitoneum).

Clinical management

The infant with NEC will have a gastric tube inserted to decompress the stomach. Antibiotics, usually ampicillin, gentamicin, and clindamycin, are started. The infant should have nothing by mouth but will have a greater than usual fluid requirement. Blood transfusions

Box 29-7	Risk Factors of Necrotizing Enterocolitis

Placental abruption
Infection
Asphyxia or hypoxia
Hypovolemia
Hypotension
Umbilical line
Hypertonic feeding
Apnea
Exchange transfusion

may be necessary to control anemia and aid coagulation. Surgery—a resection of necrotic bowel—is performed on infants with intestinal gangrene or perforation; a temporary colostomy may be necessary. Hyperalimentation is used to support nutrition. The complications of NEC (short bowel syndrome resulting from surgery and intestinal strictures) affect many survivors.

The infant may have nothing by mouth for an extended period while the repaired bowel regains normal function. The reintroduction of feedings is a slow process.

 Box **29-3**

CLINICAL DECISION

The 1100 g infant you are caring for has been on a schedule to advance feedings. Currently, she is receiving 24 cal/oz formula, 10 ml every 2 hours. How would you determine that she is ready to have the feeding volume advanced again?

METABOLIC DYSFUNCTION

Preterm, SGA, LGA, and postterm infants and any infant who has had intrauterine stress is at risk for altered metabolic function. Infants may show signs of hypothermia, hypoglycemia, and hypocalcemia from decreased glycogen and fat stores, poor CNS control, and endocrine imbalance.

Hypothermia

Hypothermia, a body temperature that is below normal, is a problem often seen in LBW infants. Premature and SGA infants are not able to control body temperature but instead reflect the environmental temperature. LBW neonates have a large surface area in relation to mass, a limited ability to produce heat, and minimal subcutaneous fat, all of which contribute to the occurrence of hypothermia. Premature infants also have thin skin, resulting in increased evaporative heat loss. Hypothermia can be an early indication of sepsis (see Chapters 18 and 19).

Signs

Initially, the infant may develop pallor and cyanosis in an attempt to conserve heat by peripheral vasoconstriction. Respiratory distress, lethargy, hypotonia, or difficulty feeding can occur.

Clinical management

Treatment consists of gradual rewarming; warming too rapidly may cause apnea. The cause of the heat loss must be searched. Monitor the infant's axillary temperature and the environmental temperature every 15 to 30 minutes until the axillary temperature is within normal range. The goal is to achieve a **neutral thermal environment** (NTE) for the infant, the temperature where heat balance is maintained. The NTE will differ according to gestational age and weight. High-risk infants are cared for under radiant warmers or in incubators. Radiant warmers allow convenient access to the infant but do contribute to IWL (refer to the section on maintaining fluid balance) and hypothermia. Single- or double-walled incubators allow control for both. It is important to note the amount of heat needed to maintain an infant's temperature in the normal range. Comparison to established normal ranges will reveal the infant who is hypothermic but is artificially warmed by an over-heated environment.

Hypoglycemia

Hypoglycemia is a blood glucose level of less than 40 mg/dl. Hypoglycemia is often associated with an *infant of a diabetic mother* (IDM) and is frequently seen with LGA, SGA, preterm, postterm, and polycythemic infants. SGA and preterm infants are at risk for hypoglycemia because of reduced glycogen stores. An infant who has an elevated hematocrit level (polycythemia) may also have hypoglycemia because of increased glucose consumption by red blood cells.

These infants have been exposed to elevated maternal glucose levels in utero. In most pregnancies, glucose readily diffuses across the placenta into the fetal circulation, causing increased insulin production. Prenatally, the excess glucose and insulin cause increased fetal growth. At delivery the maternal supply of glucose ends, but neonatal insulin production continues at the previous rate, causing hypoglycemia. This may last 1 to 5 days.

Finally, if an infant has nothing by mouth for hours after birth (a common practice in past years), hypoglycemia may develop. Prevention is vital because unchecked hypoglycemia causes seizures and brain damage.

Signs

Although a blood glucose value below 40 mg/dl is considered hypoglycemia, some infants may have symptoms

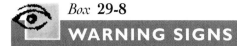

Box 29-8

WARNING SIGNS

Hypoglycemia

> Tremors
> Jitteriness
> Apnea
> Cyanosis
> Respiratory distress
> Diaphoresis

at lower or higher levels. Because signs of hypoglycemia (Box 29-8) may mimic other conditions, it should always be considered.

Frequent assessment of serum glucose levels for infants at risk can identify the hypoglycemic infant before signs are seen. Capillary blood from a heel stick (Procedure 29-2) is tested in the nursery by any of the available test strip kits (see Chapter 19). If levels are below normal, the reading is usually confirmed by laboratory analysis of blood, but you should not wait for laboratory results to intervene.

Clinical management

Treatment consists of oral or parenteral glucose. If the infant has only mild symptoms (without respiratory distress or seizures), 10% oral dextrose is given. These infants are usually hungry and will feed well. Retest the serum glucose within 30 minutes and again 1 hour after offering the feeding. Early feedings of breast milk or formula should be offered every 2 to 3 hours to supply needed calories and glucose.

Infants with major symptoms such as respiratory distress or seizure will need glucose infusions. A peripheral IV infusion is started with 10% dextrose. A slow push of 200 mg/kg (2 ml/kg) of 10% dextrose may be given over 2 to 3 minutes. The bolus should be followed by a maintenance infusion of 7 to 8 mg/kg per minute of dextrose. The serum glucose levels are then closely followed.

TEST *Yourself* **29-5** _____

a. To give a 200 mg/kg bolus to a 2.5 kg infant, how much 10% glucose should be administered?
  1. 2.5 ml   3. 10 ml
  2. 5.0 ml   4. 20 ml
b. What is the *maximum* concentration of dextrose that can be infused through a peripheral IV line?

PROCEDURE 29-2

Capillary Blood Sampling

1. Warm heel with prepackaged heel warmer or warmed diaper soak.
2. Cleanse with alcohol preparation depending on protocol. Allow to air dry.
   Rationale: Alcohol must dry for at least 1 min to be effective.
3. Puncture site perpendicular to skin with sterile lancet (Figure 29-17). Do not puncture bottom or back of heel.
   Rationale: To avoid damage to nerves, arteries, and heel fat pad that could affect walking in later years.
4. Wipe away first drop of blood.
5. Gently squeeze ankle and foot above puncture site to increase flow.
6. Place one bead of blood on test strip.
7. Follow timing directions.

Capillary Blood Gas Sampling

Technique is similar to routine sampling except as follows:
1. Hold heel horizontal with body to avoid venous stasis.
2. Fill anticoagulant tube and hold tube horizontal. Check for bubbles.
   Rationale: Bubbles affect reading. Discard tube if air or bubbles get into tube.
3. Cap end after filling. Mix blood to ensure anticoagulation (may use magnet and metal chip to mix blood).
4. Place in cup with crushed ice. Take to lab as soon as possible.

Omit step 4 if analyzed within 5 minutes.

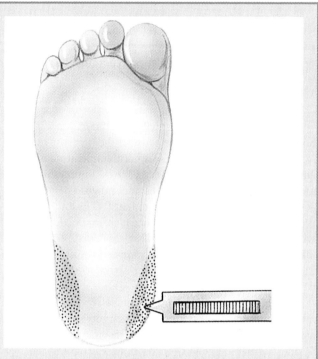

Figure 29-17 Capillary sampling from the heel. Stippled areas indicate correct sites.

OPTIONAL ACTIVITY

Write a nursing note that accurately describes this procedure.

Hypocalcemia

Calcium is important for many metabolic functions. Hypocalcemia is present when the serum calcium level is less than 7 mg/dl. Premature infants and infants of diabetic mothers have a higher incidence of hypocalcemia. Infants who are hypoglycemic are also at risk for hypocalcemia. Placental insufficiency, birth asphyxia and stress, and inadequate dietary calcium are other risk factors for hypocalcemia. Hypocalcemic infants are jittery and tremulous. Symptoms may be seen during the first days or the first week.

Clinical management

Mild hypocalcemia may resolve without treatment. Treatment consists of adding calcium gluconate to parenteral IV fluids or supplementing enteral feedings with additional calcium. Parenteral calcium should be infused through a central catheter; subcutaneous infiltration of calcium causes necrosis and sloughing of tissue.

Nursing Responsibilities

FLUID, ELECTROLYTE, NUTRITIONAL, AND METABOLIC DYSFUNCTION

ASSESSMENT

Adequacy of nutrition by either route is assessed by measuring the progress of growth and development. In addition, a careful record of assessments of nutrition and fluid balance is kept. The infant should be growing in length and weight; weight gain alone may indicate edema. Fluid and caloric intake is reordered every day depending on approximate visible and insensible fluid loss. The following parameters are measured:

- Daily weights: ideal gain is 15 to 20 g per day
- Weekly length: plotted on chart for intrauterine growth curve

- Weekly head circumference: up to 1 cm per week; plotted on chart for intrauterine growth curve
- Urine output: 1 to 3 ml/kg per hour
- Urine specific gravity: 1.002 to 1.010
- Adequate skin turgor and capillary refill: within 3 seconds
- Serum electrolytes: sodium (Na) (135 to 145 mEq/L), potassium (K) (3.5 to 7.0 mEq/L), colloidal iron (CI) (100 to 117 mEq/L), glucose (70 to 100 mg/dl), calcium (7 to 11 mg/dl)
- Blood urea nitrogen (BUN): 3.1 to 25.5 mg/dl
- Normal vital signs, including BP

Once an infant is receiving enteral feedings, the nurse must assess feeding tolerance. Neutral thermal environment must be maintained for the body to function normally.

NURSING DIAGNOSES

- Risk for fluid volume excess or deficit related to fluid demand and immature renal function
- Altered nutrition: less than body requirements; related to intolerance or need for parenteral nutrition, resulting in hypoglycemia
- Risk for trauma to gastrointestinal tract, related to hypoxemia and underperfusion of bowel, especially in premature infant
- Altered growth and development
- Ineffective thermoregulation related to immaturity, size, disease, and environment
- Parental knowledge deficit regarding nutritional needs, modes of parenteral and enteral nutrition, and special needs of premature, SGA, and IDM infants

EXPECTED OUTCOMES

- Fluid balance is achieved and maintained.
- Maintains serum glucose and calcium levels within normal parameters.
- Exhibits feeding tolerance by lack of emesis and gastric residuals.
- Exhibits progress consistent with expected growth parameters (i.e., fetal growth rate).
- Maintains stable body temperature in a neutral thermal environment.
- Parents verbalize understanding of infant's fluid and nutritional requirements and understand maintenance of normal body temperature of infant.

NURSING INTERVENTION

The nurse is responsible for monitoring fluid intake every hour. Urine output must be carefully measured, usually by weighing diapers. Urine dipstick and specific gravity tests should be performed every shift. Infants are usually weighed daily; extremely LBW infants may be weighed twice a day.

Assess the infant receiving enteral feedings for the presence of bowel sounds, measure the abdominal girth and compare it with the previous measurement, and check for gastric residuals before every feeding. Stools should be tested for the presence of occult blood.

If the temperature is unstable, make appropriate adjustments in the environmental temperature to correct the problem. Observe the infant for further signs of the cause of temperature instability. Monitor the infant's temperature frequently, and observe for signs of complications from hypothermia, such as apnea and hypoglycemia.

The nurse is often responsible for obtaining laboratory specimens to determine glucose and calcium levels. Frequent blood glucose levels are necessary after treatment for hypoglycemia. Maintain the patency of the IV access for dextrose infusion. When the infant is clinically stable, provide feedings on time to prevent further hypoglycemia.

EVALUATION

- Has the infant's growth paralleled the intrauterine growth chart?
- Did the infant experience complications from inadequate nutrition?
- Are the parents knowledgeable about the necessary aspects of maintenance of growth and development before the infant's discharge?

HEMATOLOGIC DYSFUNCTION

Hyperbilirubinemia

Of the many hematology problems faced by neonates, *hyperbilirubinemia* is certainly the most common. All infants experience changes in the metabolism of bilirubin after birth. In the neonate, most bilirubin is produced from the destruction of red blood cells. There are two types of bilirubin. *Direct bilirubin,* also called *conjugated* bilirubin, is water soluble; therefore it is more easily handled by the neonatal metabolism. It is excreted in bile via the small intestine or by the kidneys. Indirect, or *unconjugated* bilirubin is lipid soluble and therefore cannot be excreted. When indirect bilirubin builds up, it can be deposited in the skin (causing jaundice) or in the brain (causing kernicterus). Indirect bilirubin must be metabolized by the liver into direct bilirubin before it can be excreted.

The terms *physiologic jaundice* and *nonphysiologic* (or pathologic) *jaundice* refer to the underlying cause of the jaundice. Physiologic jaundice is a normal process that occurs within the first week of life. Pathologic jaundice results from factors, such as blood group incompatibility, sepsis, or bruising, that alter the mechanism for bilirubin metabolism. An explanation of bilirubin metabolism is found in Chapter 18.

Physiologic hyperbilirubinemia

The infant with physiologic hyperbilirubinemia has elevated bilirubin levels because the *normally* elevated red blood cell mass of the fetus is being *normally* reduced after birth. Physiologic jaundice is also caused by the deficiency of an enzyme needed for the metabolism of bilirubin by the liver. The risk factors associated with the incidence of physiologic jaundice are compared with the causes of nonphysiologic jaundice in Table 29-4.

Nonphysiologic (pathologic) hyperbilirubinemia

Bilirubin levels that are elevated within the first 24 hours of life or levels that exceed 12.9 mg/dl are abnormal for a term infant. The pathologic level in small or sick preterm infants is lower and can cause **kernicterus**, deposits of bilirubin in the brain. The most frequent reasons for abnormally elevated bilirubin levels are as follows (Blackburn, 1995):

- The normally elevated red blood cell mass is being abnormally reduced after birth because of some pathologic process, as in isoimmunization and sepsis.
- An abnormally elevated red blood cell mass (see section on polycythemia) may be present for a variety of reasons.
- Abnormalities of red blood cell structure or enzyme systems (glucose-6-phosphate dehydrogenase [G6PD] deficiency) make the cells more prone to hemolysis and increase bilirubin production.
- Abnormal enzyme activity can result from inborn errors of metabolism (IEM).

Breast milk jaundice

Breast milk jaundice may become evident after as little as 3 to 5 days of life or it may not be evident until the second or third week of life. Bilirubin levels exceed 12 mg/dl and may be as high as 20 mg/dl. The levels remain elevated for a prolonged time, up to 2 months of age. The jaundice is thought to be caused by substances in breast milk that either interfere with bilirubin conjugation or cause increased reabsorption of bilirubin from the intestines. Fortunately, despite elevated levels of bilirubin, most infants with breast milk jaundice do not develop kernicterus.

Isoimmunization

Severe fetal hemolysis may result from maternal-fetal Rh incompatibilities. ABO or minor blood groups contribute, but they usually do not cause such severe problems (see Chapter 23). The fetus of an isoimmunized mother is at risk for intrauterine hemolysis, anemia, and hyperbilirubinemia. The consequences for the affected fetus may range from mild to fatal if untreated.

An increasing anemia stimulates the production of immature erythrocytes, thus the name *erythroblastosis fetalis*. A varying amount of bilirubin is excreted into the amniotic fluid through fetal urine production. Serial measurements of amniotic fluid bilirubin from amniocentesis are used to evaluate the severity of fetal involvement (see Chapter 23). The results will determine the need for intrauterine intervention with packed red blood cell transfusion via the umbilical cord (PUBS) (see Chapter 11). Premature delivery may be necessary for the life of the fetus.

In severely affected fetuses, a syndrome of massive edema, pleural effusions, and ascites called *hydrops fetalis* may develop, which frequently leads to intrauterine fetal death (IUFD). At birth, less severely affected infants may appear pale but not jaundiced because most of the by-products of fetal red blood cell breakdown (bilirubin) have been excreted by the mother. Once separated from the mother's efficient metabolic system, however, the newborn will quickly become jaundiced.

Clinical management

Prevention of hyperbilirubinemia may be achieved for Rh-positive infants of Rh-negative mothers with administration of Rh(D) immune globulin to eligible mothers after every potential "insult" (see Chapter 23). Early initiation

---

Table **29-4**   **Factors Associated with Physiologic Jaundice and Pathologic Jaundice**

Physiologic Jaundice	Nonphysiologic Jaundice
Increased red blood cell volume	Blood group incompatibilities or isoimmunization
Shortened lifespan of fetal red blood cells	Hereditary disorders: galactosemia
Delayed passage of meconium	Infection: intrauterine viral infection (TORCH), neonatal bacterial or viral infection
Prematurity	Maternal drugs: sulfonamides, aspirin
Inadequate enteral nutrition	Acidosis and hypoxia
Breast-feeding	Prematurity

of enteral feedings in neonates helps to eliminate bilirubin that is in stool; meconium is passed quickly and gastrointestinal function is established. The preterm or ill infant may not have enteral feedings at first, thus retaining some of this bilirubin as well.

Exchange transfusion. An exchange transfusion may be needed for an infant with severe hemolytic disease. During exchange transfusion, the antibody-coated red blood cells and excess bilirubin are removed, and the volume is replaced with noncoated red cells. Today the procedure is done less often because of better intrauterine diagnosis and postnatal treatment. If the procedure is needed, the parents should understand that it is done by means of an umbilical venous catheter connected to a four-way stopcock, which allows a few milliliters of blood to be withdrawn, discarded, and replaced by correctly typed blood. The process is repeated for some time until the infant's total blood volume has been "diluted" with the fresh blood.

Phototherapy. Phototherapy is the most common method of treatment for hyperbilirubinemia. Phototherapy facilitates biliary excretion of unconjugated bilirubin. Phototherapy can prevent bilirubin toxicity, but it does not treat the cause of hyperbilirubinemia (Figure 29-18, *A* and *B*).

Phototherapy reduces bilirubin levels by effects created at the skin level; therefore exposure of skin to the light is necessary. In most cases, infants receiving phototherapy will be in an incubator, naked except for eye shields and a covering over the genitalia. Phototherapy increases IWL and causes increased bowel motility resulting in watery stools. Frequent oral/enteral feedings or IV fluids are needed to prevent dehydration. Other problems associated with phototherapy include temperature instability, rashes, and irritability.

Serum bilirubin will be measured every 8 to 24 hours and more frequently for infants whose levels rise rapidly. When phototherapy is discontinued, bilirubin levels will be monitored for at least 24 hours because these may again revert to a level needing treatment.

Nursing responsibilities

It is frequently the nurse caring for the infant who is first to recognize jaundice, pallor, or signs of bleeding. In the case of jaundice, it is important to closely monitor vital signs, especially temperature, while an infant is under phototherapy lights. The eyes must be covered because an infant will gaze into the light and eyes may be damaged. The patches can be removed occasionally to check the eyes for exudate and to provide the infant with visual stimulation. Creams should not be used on the skin while the infant is under phototherapy lights. Fluid balance is important since IWL is increased, and stools may be loose and more frequent.

TEST *Yourself* 29-6 _____

  a. Which type of bilirubin is water soluble and easily excreted by the neonate?
  b. In which ways does phototherapy assist the excretion of bilirubin?
  c. List nursing interventions to prevent complications of phototherapy.

Anemia

Anemia may begin in utero as a result of isoimmunization, fetomaternal transfusion, twin-to-twin transfusion, or puncture of the placenta or umbilical cord during an amniocentesis. After birth, infants may become anemic

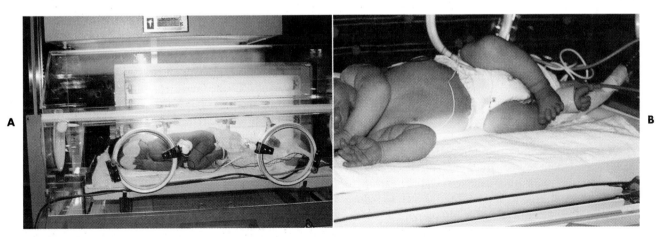

Figure 29-18   Phototherapy. Note eye coverings. **A,** Traditional overhead phototherapy unit. **B,** Phototherapy blanket enables infant to be treated in a crib; infant can be wrapped in phototherapy blanket for feedings and to be held. (Courtesy Victoria Langer, RNC, MSN, NNP.)

because of continued hemolysis from isoimmunization, intracranial or gastrointestinal bleeding, sepsis, or iatrogenic blood loss as a result of repeated laboratory work. Preterm infants are at risk for anemia of prematurity, which is an exaggeration of physiologic anemia. Finally, infants of any gestational age can suffer from hereditary defects in hemoglobin synthesis or hemoglobinopathies.

Healthy full-term infants have sufficient iron stores for synthesis of red blood cells until the third to fourth month after birth. Although supplemental iron is not needed in these first few months, most formulas now contain it. Therefore full-term formula-fed infants generally do not have problems with anemia. Breast milk is easily digested by the preterm infant but may not have adequate iron content for the very premature infant. For full-term infants, human milk will supply easily absorbed iron.

Signs

Recognition of anemia begins with daily physical assessment and with special attention to pallor, jaundice, tachycardia, tachypnea, apnea, hepatosplenomegaly, and poor capillary refill. When the infant is anemic, the decreased hemoglobin concentration and the decreased number of red blood cells result in a diminished oxygen-carrying capacity of the blood.

Clinical management

Periodic screening of hemoglobin and hematocrit levels is necessary for growing premature infants. The complete blood count can be obtained to determine the presence of immature red blood cells (reticulocytes), which is an attempt by the bone marrow to correct the anemia. The normal hemoglobin and hematocrit levels at birth are as follows: hemoglobin—16 to 20 mg/dl; hematocrit—48% to 60%. Values may differ according to the source of the specimen (i.e., whether it is from a venous or arterial source or from a capillary source).

The decision to transfuse an infant is made if marked symptoms are present, indicating that the infant is unable to adapt to the anemia. Transfusion will raise the hematocrit level but may also depress the bone marrow's efforts to produce new red blood cells. Warmed blood in the form of packed red blood cells is slowly transfused through a peripheral IV site by means of a pump. Whenever possible, the risks of transfusion are considered and discussed with parents before transfusion.

In recent years, the human erythropoietin gene has been cloned. Recombinant human erythropoietin can be administered to certain infants to stimulate the bone marrow to produce red blood cells; its use has been shown to reduce the need for transfusion (Gallagher, Ehrenkranz, 1993).

Polycythemia

Neonatal **polycythemia** occurs when the central (venous or arterial) hematocrit level rises above 65%. Blood vis-

cosity increases, and circulation in smaller vessels becomes sluggish. Microemboli may form and travel to the CNS, gastrointestinal tract, and kidneys, causing cerebrovascular accidents, NEC, and renal vein thrombosis.

Risk

Term or postterm SGA infants are at highest risk for polycythemia as a result of increased natural erythropoietin levels in response to hypoxia. Maternal diabetes and maternal-to-fetal and twin-to-twin transfusions are associated with an increased incidence of polycythemia. Delaying cord clamping or holding the newly born infant below the level of the placenta allows transfer of extra blood into the newborn and are ways in which obstetric practice can contribute to polycythemia.

Signs

Infants with polycythemia look *plethoric* with a ruddy or purplish, cyanotic tinge to the skin. Respiratory distress, cardiac enlargement, and CHF may be present. Hypoglycemia commonly occurs because red blood cells consume glucose. Jitteriness, lethargy, or seizures are seen with neurologic involvement. If renal function is compromised, the infant will have oliguria. The increased red blood cell mass contributes to the bilirubin load, producing higher levels of hyperbilirubinemia and jaundice.

Clinical management

Treatment is recommended for infants with symptoms, but it is controversial for those who are symptom free. A partial exchange transfusion removes some of the cellular blood components, which are replaced with fluids, such as normal saline, 5% albumin, or Plasmanate. This will lower the hematocrit level to a targeted 50% to 55% and decrease viscosity. The procedure is usually performed through an umbilical venous catheter.

Thrombocytopenia

Thrombocytopenia is a platelet count below $100,000/mm^3$ and may occur in both ill and well newborns. Thrombocytopenia is the most common bleeding disorder of newborns. It can result from factors related to decreased production of platelets or increased destruction of platelets. Causes include maternal-fetal platelet incompatibilities (similar to red blood cell isoimmunization), perinatal infections, birth asphyxia, inherited disorders, administration of adult doses of aspirin during pregnancy, trapping of platelets in a giant hemangioma, and disseminated intravascular coagulation (DIC) (see Chapter 22).

Signs

Infants with thrombocytopenia will have *petechiae* (microhemorrhages into the skin) and increased bleeding time after heel sticks, injections, and venipunctures.

Clinical management

When a clotting disorder is suspected, confirm that vitamin K had been given after delivery, since a deficiency will cause similar symptoms. A platelet count and other laboratory tests of blood coagulation will be ordered to diagnose the defect in coagulation. Depending on the cause, transfusions of platelets and other blood factors may be needed (see Chapter 21). It is important to prevent injury of fragile tissues.

IMMUNOLOGIC DYSFUNCTION

Infections with organisms that would cause minimal damage later in life can cause extensive damage in a developing fetus or a newborn. The timing of the infection frequently makes the difference. Infection may be acquired during pregnancy by transplacental transmission, during birth by infected secretions, or postnatally by infected persons and objects in the environment (see Chapters 25 and 28). Some organisms are more prevalent during perinatal or neonatal life.

Bacterial Sepsis

Bacterial sepsis can occur within the first few days of life. Before the use of antibiotics, most infants with sepsis died from infection. Though there has been a decline in the mortality rate of infants since the introduction of antibiotics, bacterial sepsis continues to be a predominant cause of morbidity and mortality of neonates. Sites for bacterial infections include the blood, cerebrospinal fluid, lungs, and urine. The most common pathogenic organism in newborns is *group B b-hemolytic streptococcus* (GBS). In most cases, the infant acquires the organism from the mother by vertical transmission (see Chapter 25). GBS infection may be *early-onset,* occurring in the first week of life. Infants with early-onset diseases are severely ill; the mortality rate may reach 50%. Other organisms that cause early-onset sepsis in neonates are *Escherichia coli, Listeria monocytogenes,* and *Haemophilus influenzae.*

Late-onset disease affects infants more than 1 week old. The causative organisms are *nosocomial* (derived from the hospital environment) *Staphylococcus aureus, Staphylococcus epidermidis,* and *Pseudomonas,* plus those implicated in early-onset disease. The mortality rate in preterm infants approaches 20%, and CNS damage from meningitis is common.

Viral and Protozoal Infections

Viral and protozoal infections are transmitted transplacentally from maternal to fetal circulations during pregnancy or are acquired during passage through the birth canal. Congenital infections, known as TORCH—an acronym for *t*oxoplasmosis, *o*ther (syphilis, human immunodeficiency virus [HIV], hepatitis B), *r*ubella, *c*ytomegalovirus, and *h*erpes, are present at birth or shortly after. Hepatitis B virus, herpes, and HIV can be acquired during the birth process (Connor et al, 1994).

Postnatally acquired viral infections that affect neonates include influenza strains, adenovirus, coxsackievirus B, echoviruses, and respiratory syncytial virus (RSV). Cardiorespiratory and gastrointestinal symptoms are common. Infected persons, including health care personnel and family members, are the sources of infection.

Risk

Preterm infants are at high risk for sepsis because they do not have the passive immunity normally acquired later in gestation and they lack a mature immune system to respond to infection. Other risk factors for neonatal infection include prolonged rupture of membranes, maternal fever before delivery, chorioamnionitis, early asphyxia, and invasive procedures such as umbilical catheterization or endotracheal intubation. Prolonged hospitalization increases the risk for nosocomial infection.

Signs

The neonate with prenatally acquired viral disease is frequently growth retarded. Other neurologic manifestations of viral infection include cerebral calcifications and hydrocephalus. The eyes may be affected with cataracts, microphthalmia, and chorioretinitis. Infection of other organ systems produces pneumonitis, myocarditis, hepatitis, and thrombocytopenia. Involvement of these systems causes respiratory distress, cardiovascular instability, jaundice, hepatosplenomegaly, petechiae, and increased bleeding time.

Early signs of bacterial sepsis are subtle. Comments by mothers and nursing staff members that the infant "just doesn't seem to be right" should be heeded as characteristic signs of early illness. Fever, generally regarded as a common sign of infection, is *rare* in the neonate. Newborns more frequently have hypothermia, feeding intolerance, respiratory distress, apnea, bradycardia, hypotension, and cyanosis. Altered neurologic signs may be seen even if the infant does not have meningitis. Jaundice is associated with urinary tract infections and congenital viral infections. Skin pustules, discharge from the eyes, and a foul-smelling, moist umbilical cord with a reddened base are signs of local infections. Generalized sepsis may follow, however, because neonates are less able to keep these infections localized.

Clinical management

Prevention of perinatal sepsis involves measures that encourage women to seek prenatal care, appropriately timed rubella immunization, and education concerning transmission of diseases. Avoidance of hazardous behaviors such as unsafe sex, IV drug use, and ingestion of raw or undercooked meat reduces the risks.

Prevention of neonatal illness is best accomplished by identifying the infant who is at risk for sepsis, following

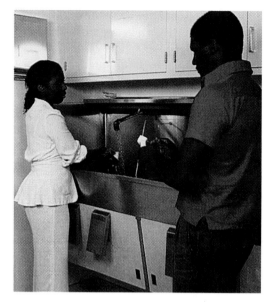

Figure 29-19 Before visitation, parents need to scrub arms and hands. (Courtesy Ross Laboratories, Columbus, Ohio.)

strict hand washing for all who come in contact with newborns, avoiding exposure to persons who are infectious, and educating parents (Figure 29-19).

Laboratory data are used to confirm the diagnosis of sepsis. The usual response of increased white blood cell count (leukocytosis) is replaced with a decreased count (leukopenia) in the ill infant. The white blood cell differential may reveal that more immature white blood cells are being released. Thrombocytopenia may occur. Blood and urine specimens are obtained for culture and sensitivity tests. Fluid from a lumbar puncture will also be evaluated for culture and sensitivity, examination of the cellular contents, and chemical analysis. Blood gas levels may reveal metabolic acidosis or hypoxemia. A urine specimen can detect the presence of bacterial antigens.

Laboratory data are helpful if intrauterine infection with the TORCH group is suspected. Levels of immunoglobulin M (IgM) over 20 mg/dl indicate that the fetal immune system has responded to an infection of some kind. Because there is a lag time between the time of infection and the production of IgM, elevated levels at birth indicate congenital infection. Identification of specific types of IgM confirm viral cause. Treatment of most viral diseases is symptomatic and consists of supportive care. Exceptions are the herpes simplex virus and HIV, for which specific therapy is available.

Therapies must be chosen carefully because side effects are common. Most side effects are related to differences in the ways neonates metabolize and excrete medications. If early-onset sepsis, pneumonia, or meningitis is suspected, therapy is started with broad-spectrum antibiotics. The results of the culture and sensitivity test are used to confirm the correct choice of antibiotic. Besides antimicrobial

| **Box 29-9** | **Clinical Manifestations of Neonatal Infections** |

GENERAL MANIFESTATIONS
Poor feeding
Lethargy
Irritability
Temperature instability
"Doesn't look right"

RESPIRATORY SYSTEM MANIFESTATIONS
Apnea or tachypnea
Grunting
Nasal flaring
Retractions

CARDIAC MANIFESTATIONS
Bradycardia or tachycardia
Hypotension
Diminished perfusion
Cyanosis

CENTRAL NERVOUS SYSTEM MANIFESTATIONS
Jittery
Hypotonia or hypertonia
High-pitched cry
Seizures

GASTROINTESTINAL SYSTEM MANIFESTATIONS
Feeding intolerance
Abdominal distention
Emesis

SKIN MANIFESTATIONS
Jaundice
Petechiae
Pustules

agents, infants will need supportive care, including assisted ventilation, during the time of illness.

Nursing responsibilities: immunologic dysfunction

Compliance with guidelines established by the Centers for Disease Control (CDC) for universal precautions is essential (see Chapter 25, Isolation Precautions). Policies and procedures developed by the hospital infection control department should address the following issues:
- Eye prophylaxis
- Skin and cord care
- Nursery staff
- Nursery design and environment
- Handwashing
- Staff dress code
- Isolation

- Visitors
- Employee health
- Epidemic control

Knowledge of the risk factors for sepsis is needed to identify infants who are at risk for developing infection. A complete physical assessment may reveal the multisystem effects of sepsis (Box 29-9). Frequent monitoring of vital signs, including BP determination, is necessary to assess cardiorespiratory stability. Electronic monitors provide continuous surveillance of heart rate, respiratory rate, BP, and oxygen saturation.

Maintenance of cardiorespiratory functions, blood volume, thermoregulation, fluid and electrolyte balance, and nutrition is essential if specific antibiotic therapy is to be effective. An awareness of the way neonates metabolize and excrete drugs is also essential for observing untoward effects. It is important to communicate with parents about the necessity of continuing therapy even after the infant improves clinically. Parents may carry an unusual burden of guilt if neonatal infection has resulted from maternal illness (see Nursing Care Plan).

Rarely do infected neonates need to be isolated. Although incubators isolate the infant from the environment, they do not separate the environment from the infant. Nursing measures to prevent nosocomial infection remain a high priority.

NEUROLOGIC DYSFUNCTION

Preservation of the CNS is the primary goal of neonatal therapy. Many factors, such as congenital disorders, injuries before, during, and after birth, drug effects, infectious agents, and the environment (which includes high-technology treatments), can affect neurologic functioning. Once a neurologic alteration is determined, the effect will usually continue throughout the infant's lifetime. Damage to sensitive, delicate neural pathways is difficult to repair. Therefore prevention is of the highest priority.

Parents of infants with neurologic alterations should be encouraged to participate in their infant's care, and a team effort is needed for support through the time of discharge. Often the best support will come from peer groups of parents of children with similar ongoing needs.

Intracranial Hemorrhage

Intracranial hemorrhage varies from a subarachnoid hemorrhage (which has a good prognosis) to subdural hemorrhage (which often has a poor outcome). *Periventricular/ intraventricular hemorrhage* (P/IVH) is the most common intracranial hemorrhage in neonates.

Risk

P/IVH occurs almost exclusively in small, preterm infants of less than 32 weeks' gestational age, primarily because cerebral blood flow is not effectively regulated. Treatments for other complications of prematurity often contribute to the pathogenesis of P/IVH. For example, after administration of hypertonic solutions (such as sodium bicarbonate for metabolic acidosis), the hypertonicity draws fluid into the blood, causing the intravascular volume to expand and increase cerebral flow. Infants with respiratory distress and hypercapnia are at risk because of the increase in cerebral blood flow that accompanies the rise in P_{CO_2}.

The origin of bleeding is the *subependymal germinal matrix,* where a rich but fragile capillary network is found. Rupture of vessels within this network causes bleeding close to the borders of the ventricular system into the periventricular tissue. The hemorrhage may extend into the ventricles, resulting in hydrocephalus when the flow of cerebrospinal fluid (CSF) is obstructed by clots. In the most severe form, bleeding extends from the germinal matrix into the cerebral parenchyma. A system of grading the P/IVH from least severe (grade I) to most severe (grade IV) was developed in 1978 by Papile et al and is still used today to describe the extent of the hemorrhage.

Signs

The signs of P/IVH may be dramatic if the infant's condition deteriorates rapidly or may be difficult to detect if it occurs over many hours. Therefore all infants at risk for IVH are carefully assessed clinically and with bedside ultrasound examinations. Infants with a rapid deterioration may have seizures, deepening coma, fixed pupils (not normally seen before 32 weeks of gestation), respiratory arrest, abnormal eye movements, and flaccidity over the course of a few minutes to hours. The hematocrit level may fall or may not rise after a transfusion. If there is obstruction to CSF flow, the anterior fontanelle will bulge. Alterations in temperature, fluid and electrolyte balance, BP, and glucose metabolism may also be seen. Only some of these signs will occur if the manifestation is more subtle than the dramatic form.

Clinical management

The prevention of P/IVH involves restricting environmental stimuli that may cause rapid changes in cerebral blood flow. Although cesarean delivery may help to preserve the normal cerebral circulation for the preterm infant, it is not the recommended mode of delivery unless there are other indications. Measures to maintain oxygenation can prevent P/IVH. Clustering of examinations and procedures, while allowing for rest, is advised, and any unnecessary stimuli should be avoided. Control of pain lessens agitation. Significant shifts in BP, administration of hypertonic solutions, and overventilation that could lead to pneumothorax should be avoided. Medications, such as Indomethacin, have been used with good success in an attempt to prevent the incidence of P/IVH in premature infants.

After P/IVH has been confirmed, the infant's condition will be followed closely by ultrasound examinations for evidence of ongoing bleeding or for signs of hydrocephalus. During the acute stage of hemorrhage, management involves maintenance of oxygenation, perfusion, temperature, and blood glucose level. If hydrocephalus develops, serial spinal taps to determine intracranial pressure or the placement of a ventriculoperitoneal shunt may be needed.

Seizures

Seizures are a common feature of a wide range of neonatal illnesses. Seizures are not a disease but a sign of a process causing a brain disturbance. Seizures may occur in sepsis, meningitis, drug withdrawal, hypoglycemia, hypocalcemia, fluid and electrolyte imbalances, perinatal asphyxia, and disorders of neurologic development. Chances for normal development depend on the cause and the effectiveness of treatment.

Risk

Seizures are associated with a variety of underlying problems (Box 29-10). The two most common processes that increase the risk for neonatal seizures are asphyxia and metabolic disturbances, such as hypoglycemia.

Signs

Neonatal seizure activity is subtle and easy to miss unless you observe very carefully. Although the classic grand mal seizure pattern is not seen in newborns, there are distinct varieties of seizures (Table 29-5). Jitteriness is frequently mistaken for seizures. The jittery infant has tremors and rapid movements of the extremities or fingers that can be stopped by flexing or holding the limbs. The jittery movements of the infant who is having a seizure cannot be stopped by holding the extremity. No other signs of seizures may occur. Although jitteriness can be normal, it may also be a sign of hypoglycemia or drug withdrawal.

Clinical management

An electroencephalogram (EEG) is obtained to document abnormal brain activity in the infant with seizures. Tests to discover the cause of the seizures are vital and

---

Box 29-10   Etiology of Neonatal Seizures

Perinatal asphyxia
Intracranial hemorrhage
Metabolic disturbances
 Hypoglycemia
 Hypocalcemia
 Hyponatremia
 Pyridoxine deficiency
Infection
 Bacterial meningitis
 Viral encephalopathy
 Congenital viral infection
Drug withdrawal
Genetic

Table **29-5**   **Neonatal Seizure Activity**

Appearance	Significance
SUBTLE	
Apnea (usually caused by an underlying problem)	Most frequent type and most common in preterm infant
Tonic horizontal deviation and/or jerking of the eyes (nystagmus); blinking, fluttering lids	
Drooling, sucking, and/or tongue thrusting	
Unusual movements of limbs (rowing, swimming, or pedaling)	
CLONIC	
Jerking activity	Full-term infant with hypoxic-ischemic encephalopathy
Multifocal: movement of one body part followed by another	Disturbances of the entire cerebrum
Focal: movement of one part	
TONIC	
Posturing similar to decerebrate posture in adults	Preterm infant with intraventricular hemorrhage
MYOCLONIC	
Single or multiple jerks of upper and lower extremities	Possible prediction of myoclonic spasms in early infancy

Data from Volpe JJ, Hill A: Neurologic disorders. In Avery G, ed: *Neonatology: pathophysiology of the newborn*, ed 3, Philadelphia, 1993, Lippincott.

include metabolic screens, appropriate cultures, cranial ultrasound and computerized axial tomography (CAT) scan.

Care for seizures involves treating the underlying cause. It is important to stop the seizure activity. An IV loading dose of phenobarbital is given over several minutes. Additional bolus doses may be necessary. The infant is given a maintenance dose when an adequate blood level of phenobarbital has been achieved. The dosage is adjusted to maintain a level (usually 15 to 30 g/ml) that will control the seizures, yet allow the newborn to behave normally.

T E S T *Yourself* **29-7**

Give the correct term from Table 29-5 for the following signs of neonatal seizure activity.
a. Periods of fluttering eyes, apnea, and bicycle movements of the legs
b. Rapid jerks of all extremities
c. Repetitive movements of one extremity
d. Movements of one body part followed by others

Hypoxic-Ischemic Encephalopathy

Hypoxic-ischemic encephalopathy (HIE) is a complication of hypoxemia and decreased cerebral perfusion that leads to ischemia. The combination of reduced arterial Po_2 and cerebral perfusion causes neurologic deficits of varying severity such as mental retardation, seizures, spasticity, and learning disorders. It is difficult to predict the extent of the deficits until cerebral edema, often seen after an asphyxial event, resolves. The immaturity of the newborn's brain makes this even more difficult.

Risk

Hypoxic-ischemic injury occurs in both preterm and term infants. Risk factors include perinatal asphyxia, abruptio placentae, prematurity, postmaturity, growth retardation, prolapsed cord, respiratory distress, and hypotension. Perinatal asphyxia has also been thought to be a cause of cerebral palsy. Recent studies, however, suggest that asphyxia, at or near the time of delivery, would have to be "nearly lethal" to cause cerebral palsy (ACOG, 1992).

Preterm infants with HIE are at risk for intraventricular hemorrhage followed by hydrocephalus, mental retardation, and motor deficits of the lower extremities. In contrast, the full-term infant is more likely to suffer edema and necrosis of the cerebral cortex and microcephaly as the cortex atrophies, which can be followed by motor deficits of the upper extremities, seizure disorders, mental retardation, and blindness (ACOG, 1992). Results of HIE are related to the site of injury. Cerebral palsy is more common in preterm infants. The prognosis depends on the extent of the insult.

Signs

Initially the infant with HIE will have low Apgar scores, decreased tone, and delay in the onset of spontaneous respirations. Most term infants demonstrate characteristic neurologic findings of seizures, altered level of consciousness, altered tone, altered activity, irregular respirations, apnea, poor or absent Moro reflex, abnormal cry, and poor suck.

Birth Injuries

Birth injuries involve trauma to the central or peripheral nervous systems, most commonly during the delivery process. Risk factors include macrosomia, dystocia, cephalopelvic disproportion, prematurity, abnormal presentation, instrumentation delivery, or prolonged or precipitous delivery. Injuries may involve the scalp (caput succedaneum, cephalhematoma), a skull fracture, the spinal cord, facial nerve palsy, or brachial plexus palsy.

Peripheral Nerve and Brachial Plexus Injuries

Facial nerve palsy occurs after a difficult forceps delivery or a prolonged labor during which the fetal face was compressed against the maternal sacrum. Injury to the brachial plexus results from excessive lateral traction on the neck. Brachial plexus injuries are often associated with shoulder dystocia, breech delivery, and prolonged labor or difficult delivery.

Signs

Manifestations of facial nerve palsy vary, depending upon the branch of the nerve that is involved. A complete injury results in the infant's inability to close the eye or open the mouth on the affected side. There is flattening of the nasolabial fold and absence of movement of the corner of the mouth on the involved side. There is a lack of movement on the affected side when the infant cries (Figure 29-20). Most facial nerve palsies improve spontaneously.

There are three types of brachial plexus palsy. Erb's palsy involves the arm muscles supplied by the C5-6 nerve roots. The arm is held in a characteristic "maitre d'" or "waiter's tip" posture (Figure 29-21). Klumpke paralysis involves the hand muscles supplied by the C7-T1 nerve roots. Erb-Duchenne paralysis involves the entire arm and hand from injury of the nerve roots from C5 to T1. Sequelae are common and include paralysis, loss of sensation, and poor bone growth.

Clinical management

Educating parents and preventing complications is the initial management for facial nerve palsy. Eye drops may be used to prevent corneal damage. Controversial therapies include electrical stimulation, massage, and physical therapy.

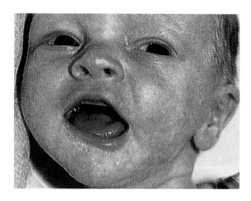

Figure 29-20   Facial nerve palsy. This infant incurred injury to the right facial nerve, resulting in loss of the nasolabial fold on the affected side and asymmetric movement of the mouth. The side of the mouth that appears to droop is the normal side. (From Zitelli BJ, Davis HW: *Atlas of pediatric physical diagnosis*, ed 3, St Louis, 1997, Mosby-Wolfe.)

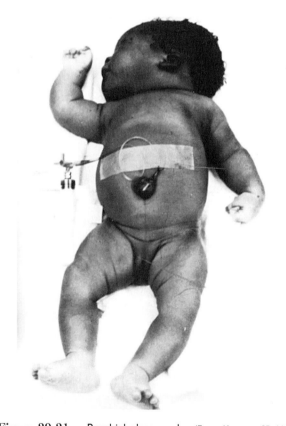

Figure 29-21   Brachial plexus palsy. (From Korones SB: *High-risk newborn infants: the basis for intensive nursing care*, ed 4, St Louis, 1986, Mosby.)

Initial management for brachial plexus therapy involves protecting the arm (i.e., by immobilization with splints) until the edema and pain subside. After edema resolves, gentle passive range of motion exercises can be performed. Ongoing physical therapy is needed.

Pain

Control of pain was not an issue in the NICU until recently. The belief that the neonatal nervous system was too immature to feel, transmit, and remember painful sensations, plus the fear of respiratory depression from analgesics and anesthetics, perpetuated this myth. Circumcisions, insertion of chest tubes, endotracheal intubation, and even PDA ligations were performed without any anesthesia or analgesia. It is now known that subjecting an infant to painful procedures without analgesia or anesthesia is inhumane.

It is not easy to assess pain in an infant. Most tools that have been developed to assess pain in children and adults depend on verbal communication. Physiologic and behavioral signs of pain have been identified by researchers, but the use of tools by nurses to quantify the pain that neonates experience is not yet standardized (Lawrence, 1993).

Research into neonatal and fetal physiology has helped find a rationale for relief of neonatal pain. The fetal nervous system is capable of transmitting painful experiences sometime between weeks 24 and 28 of gestation. The cerebral structures needed for memory are present by term. However, it has been noted that even in small infants, behavioral changes such as differences in sleep cycle and in the ability to regulate states persist beyond the immediate painful experience (Bell, 1994).

Signs

Neonates in pain exhibit changes in behavior, autonomic response, and metabolic response. Infants with pain cry differently than hungry, annoyed, or bored infants. They also have alterations in behavioral states and changes in tone and facial expressions. Physiologic changes during painful stimuli include lowered PO_2, elevated BP and heart rate, flushing, pallor, diaphoresis, and dilated pupils. Biochemical responses to pain in the infant include decreased insulin secretion and increased secretion of epinephrine, norepinephrine, and cortisol. Pain scales that specifically address neonatal signs have been developed but are not standardized (Bell, 1994).

Clinical management

Surgical procedures, including chest tube insertion and percutaneous central line insertion, cause pain. Neonates undergoing such procedures should receive medications for pain relief.

Neonatal pain may be alleviated with medications that act centrally or locally. Of those acting centrally, morphine and fentanyl are most commonly used for control of postoperative pain. Intraoperative anesthesia may be accomplished by general anesthetics. Lidocaine is used for local anesthesia during painful procedures. Drug Profile 29-4 reviews the use of medications to control pain. Behavioral and environmental interventions are useful during some painful procedures such as drawing blood by means of a

Box 29-4

DRUG PROFILE

Analgesics and Sedatives for the Neonate

Type and Dosage	Comments
ANALGESICS	
Narcotic	
Morphine 0.05-0.1 mg/kg/dose q2-4h prn IV, IM, or SC	Central nervous system and respiratory depressant; easily reversed with naloxone; slower onset but longer duration than fentanyl; may cause hypotension, ileus, urinary retention; withdrawal symptoms may occur
Meperidine (Demerol) 0.5-1.5 mg/kg/dose q4h prn IV, IM, SC, or PO	Same as morphine; less respiratory depression with therapeutic dose; less likely to induce sleep or sedation than morphine or fentanyl
Fentanyl (Sublimaze) 1-4 mcg/kg/dose q4-6h prn IV or SC Anesthesia: 5-50 mcg/kg/dose IV over 5-10 minutes	Rapid onset of action; decreases motor activity; does not increase intracranial pressure; easily reversed with naxolone; short duration of action; may cause hypotension, apnea, seizures, or rigidity if given too rapidly; withdrawal symptoms may occur
Local Anesthesia	
Lidocaine 0.5%-1.0% solution (to avoid systemic toxicity, volume should be <0.5 ml/kg of 1% lidocaine solution—5 mg/kg)	Local infiltration anesthesia for invasive procedures
SEDATIVES AND HYPNOTICS	
Barbiturate	
Phenobarbital Loading: 10-20 mg/kg IV to maximum of 40 mg/kg Maintenance: 3-5 mg/kg in 2 divided doses beginning 12 hr after last loading dose	Prolonged sedation possible once therapeutic levels achieved (20-25 µg/ml); depresses central nervous system—motor and respiratory; slow onset of action; little or no pain relief; not easily reversed; withdrawal symptoms may occur; incompatible with other drugs in solution
Benzodiazepine	
Diazepam (Valium) 0.02-0.3 mg/kg IV, IM q6-8h	Do not dilute injection; may displace bilirubin; respiratory depression; hypotension; may cause increased agitation; induces sleep; relaxes muscles; withdrawal symptoms may occur; no analgesic effect
Lorazepam 0.05-0.1 mg/kg/dose IV slowly	Respiratory depressant; has caused myoclonic jerks in premature infants
Midazolam 0.05-0.15 mg/kg slow IV or IM q2-4h	Respiratory depression and hypotension common when used with narcotics
OTHER	
Chloral hydrate 10-30 mg/kg/dose q6-8h prn PO to maximum daily dose of 50 mg/kg/day; PR	Gastric irritant—administer with or after feeding; paradoxic excitement may occur; not to be used for analgesia

Modified from Merenstein GB, Gardner SL: *Handbook of neonatal intensive care*, ed 3, St Louis, 1993, Mosby; data from Bell SG, Ellis LJ: *Neonatal Network* 6:27, 1987; Roberts RJ: *Drug therapy in infants*, Philadelphia, 1987, WB Saunders.

IM, Intramuscular; *IV,* intravenous; *PO,* orally; *PR,* by way of the rectum; *prn,* as required; *q,* every; *SC,* subcutaneous.

heel stick. Soothing the infant with rocking and offering a pacifier before puncture of the heel seems to decrease crying time and physiologic responses by distracting the infant or helping the infant to organize behavior. The use of a pacifier has been shown to be the most effective soothing intervention to reduce pain-induced stress (Campos, 1989, 1993). Improvements in NICU equipment designs and techniques can also help to make experiences less traumatic.

Stress. Control of stress is directly related to the reduction of noxious stimuli. The noise and bright lights of the NICU are not conducive to normal neurologic development. High levels of stress can contribute to the development of gastric ulcers and cause oxygen desaturation, apnea, bradycardia, jitteriness, and regurgitation. Even preterm infants exhibit specific behaviors that indicate high levels of stress (Box 29-11).

Box 29-11   **Signs of Stress in Preterm Infants**

MILD (EARLY)
Gaze aversion
Yawning
Hiccoughs
Grimacing, closing eyes
Slack jaw
Open mouth
Tongue thrusting
Bowel movements
Sneezing

MODERATE
Flushing
Mottling
Sighing
Regurgitation
Finger splaying
Extension of arms, legs
Jitteriness
Jerky movements
Limpness

SEVERE
Pallor
Cyanosis
Tachypnea
Bradypnea
Apnea
Decreased oxygen levels
Tachycardia
Bradycardia
Arrhythmias

Nursing Responsibilities

NEUROLOGIC DYSFUNCTION

ASSESSMENT

Several scales have been developed to assess neonatal pain. Nurses play a key role in assessing pain and providing comfort measures. An evaluation of facial expression, cry, breathing patterns, posture, and arousal state can determine the degree of pain being experienced by the neonate.

Assessment of the infant's ability to handle different types and levels of stress is possible through the use of the Assessment of Preterm Infant Behavior (APIB) (Als, 1982). The tool assesses the responses of the neonate's autonomic, motor, state, attentional-interactional, and regulatory systems to stimuli of increasing intensity.

NURSING DIAGNOSES

- Risk for injury related to seizures, sequela of illness, birth trauma
- Potential for delayed or altered neurodevelopment
- Parental guilt, regarding cause of infant illness
- Knowledge deficit, regarding care and stimulation of affected infant
- Pain and stress, related to procedures

EXPECTED OUTCOMES

- Exhibits normal neurologic responses and assumes normal growth rate.
- Experiences minimal pain and stress related to therapies.
- Parents participate in infant care, verbalize understanding of symptoms and treatment.
- Parents express anxiety or guilt feelings in discussion with caregiver.
- Parents demonstrate methods of consoling, stimulating, and interacting with infant.
- Parents verbalize where to find available support systems within family and community.

NURSING INTERVENTION

Stimulation

It was once assumed that the neonate lacked any perception of the environment; the neonate's ability to remember painful or pleasurable experiences was denied. Any signals recognized by mothers as purposeful responses to feelings and environmental changes were considered to be subjective. As a result of these beliefs, there was no plan for sensory stimulation. Fortunately, these assumptions are fading because of research into the newborn's capabilities (Burns et al, 1994).

Auditory stimuli should be soft and soothing and should mimic the intrauterine environment. Tapes of the maternal heartbeat, parents' voices, or soft music may be used. Visual stimulation is provided by dimming the lights and keeping the infant's eyes about 8 inches away from the source of stimulation. Because stimuli should be provided by people rather than by inanimate objects such as toys, social interaction is encouraged. Chronically ill neonates often have an aversion to any oral stimuli which, in turn, alters normal feeding behaviors. Providing oral stimulation with a pacifier during gavage feedings may allow a pleasurable association for objects placed in the mouth. Rocking and maintenance of the flexed position provides vestibular stimulation and security.

A new method of caring for preterm infants, **kangaroo care** (KC), promotes closeness between the infant and parent. Parents giving KC undress from the waist up. They provide skin-to-skin contact for their stable preterm infants by dressing them only in diapers and holding them upright and prone against their chests. Infants who are breast-feeding may even nurse in this position. Advocates of KC claim that infants cared for in this innovative way experience adequate oxygenation, more stable body temperature, and less apnea and crying (Gale et al, 1993). Parents find the skin-to-skin holding to be rewarding (Figure 29-22).

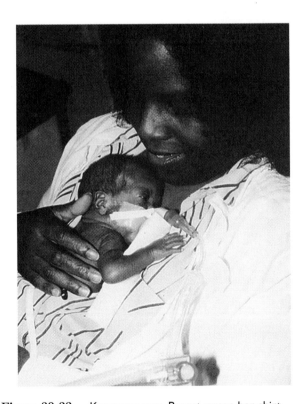

Figure 29-22   Kangaroo care. Parent wraps her shirt around the infant. The nurse will tape the ventilation tubing to the parent's outer garment at the shoulder area. (From Gale G et al: Skin-to-skin holding of the intubated premature infant, *Neonatal Network* 12(6):51, 1993.)

EVALUATION

- Upon going home, does the infant reflect appropriate interactions for the specific gestational or postconceptional age?
- Did the infant recover from stressful events with minimal, if any, adverse effects?
- Does the family, while participating in infant care, recognize the infant's signals of stress and thus adapt intensity of interaction?
- Have follow-up plans included supports for parents?

MUSCULOSKELETAL DYSFUNCTION

Musculoskeletal function is influenced by intrauterine forces (fetal position, uterine size and shape, and amount of amniotic fluid) and genetically determined conditions that affect muscle strength. The fetus must have a normal intrauterine environment to develop normally, thus the in utero position may influence muscular and skeletal development. No matter what the cause, abnormalities of

RESEARCH

PURPOSE OF STUDY

To explore the relationship between the developmental outcome and the behavior of very low birth weight infants (birth weight less than or equal to 1500 g) at high and low biologic risk.

REVIEW OF LITERATURE

Very low birth weight infants tend to be less socially responsive than full-term infants. They vocalize less and have less affective display. Mothers are less responsive to infant cues and also display less affectionate behaviors and fewer vocalizations.

FINDINGS AND IMPLICATIONS FOR STUDY

Low birth weight infants at higher biologic risk are less attentive and active through age 15 months than low birth weight infants at low biologic risk. These infants are also less adept in gross and fine motor skills through 24 months. The higher biologic risk infants are also found to have decreased attention spans and are less persistent in achieving goals.

Early developmental evaluation and intervention regarding play and appropriate stimulation must be instituted in order to improve the infant's attention span and facilitate cognitive and motor skills.

Oehler J et al: Behavioral characteristics of very low birth weight infants of varying biologic risk at 6, 15, and 24 months of age, *J Obstet Gynecol Neonatal Nurs* 25(3):233, 1996.

the musculoskeletal system can create significant distress for parents.

Musculoskeletal disorders include skeletal abnormalities and limb defects. Congenital hip dislocation, arthrogryposis (multiple congenital joint contractures), and osteogenesis imperfecta (connective tissue disorder with genetic etiology) are examples of skeletal dysplasias. Limb defects include clubfoot, syndactyly (fusion or webbing of digits), and polydactyly (duplication of digits). Torticollis is a tilting of the head and neck because of a defect of muscle or bone.

Nursing responsibilities

It is essential to use systematic observation to assess the musculoskeletal system. Begin with a head-to-toe visual inspection. Note posture, positioning, and any obvious anomalies. Spontaneous movements by the infant will indicate the equality of muscle tone. Passive range of motion will assess joint mobility.

Positioning. Since physical mobility is impaired by size and condition, skin integrity and positioning are crucial for the infant in the NICU. Clinical observations, electronic monitoring, and procedures are easier to accomplish when the infant is lying in the supine position with extremities extended. Maintenance of this position often requires restraint of the infant. The result is an infant who, although recovered from initial neonatal illness, is rigid (often to the extent that the position becomes arched), hard to cuddle or console, and restless. This does not happen if correct positioning is maintained.

Maintain the preterm infant in a position of *flexion* as much as possible. Keep in mind that this infant should really be in the weightlessness of the intrauterine world.

As gestation progresses, the infant naturally becomes more flexed because of lack of space. This helps develop tone in the flexor muscles. After term birth the normal infant's extensor tone develops gradually, and the two opposing forces become balanced. When preterm infants are forcibly placed in positions of extension, several alterations in normal growth and development appear. First, the scapulae are pulled together with the arms extended and abducted. Normal oral exploration is hampered when the growing infant's hands are not easily brought together and toward the mouth. Second, excessive extensor tone may develop in the lower portion of the legs, making it difficult to eventually walk on the entire sole of the foot.

Flexion can be maintained in the supine, side-lying, and prone positions through the use of soft rolls and stuffed animals (Figure 29-23, *A*). When lifting or holding an infant, bring the extremities toward the center of the body to encourage the flexed position (Figure 29-23, *B*). Education of parents of infants in the NICU should include instructions for proper positioning and its effects on development.

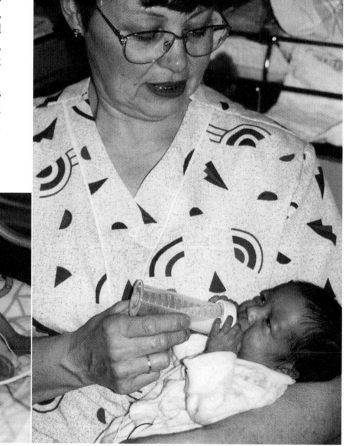

Figure 29-23 Positioning preterm infant to prevent deformity. **A,** Soft rolls minimize restlessness by providing boundaries. **B,** Swaddling brings extremities in, encourages hand-to-mouth activity, and maintains flexion. (Courtesy of Victoria Langer, RNC, MSN, NNP.)

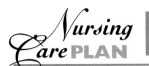

Nursing Care PLAN | *Premature Infant*

CASE

L. is a female AGA infant, 1785 g, 32 weeks' gestation, born to a 19-year-old G1 P1 mother by spontaneous vaginal delivery after 2 hours of ruptured membranes. *Maternal history:* Blood type O, Rh negative; rubella immune; rapid plasma reagin nonreactive; hepatitis B surface antigen negative. She had regular prenatal care and has no illnesses or history of familial disease; she does not smoke, abuse drugs, or drink alcohol. *Labor history:* Admitted in preterm labor, received terbutaline, then magnesium sulfate without stopping labor. Amniotic fluid clear on rupture of membranes. Neonatal team in attendance at birth. *Immediate neonatal care:* Infant cried spontaneously, weakly, with occasional grunting, nasal flaring, and mild intercostal retractions. Heart rate is 140 to 150 beats per minute. Tactile stimulation and free-flow oxygen were required to maintain adequate color and respiratory effort. Once stabilized, the infant was held briefly by the parents and transferred to the NICU.

Assessment

1. Review labor and delivery record.
2. Monitor vital signs, oxygen concentrations via pulse oximeter, blood gases, and response to treatments. Monitor for periods of apnea, signs of respiratory distress.
3. Observe for signs of hypoglycemia, hypocalcemia, hyperbilirubinemia, and complications related to immaturity (i.e., necrotizing enterocolitis) and therapies.
4. Monitor intake and output and weight loss/gain pattern.
5. Observe for nippling behaviors during oral feedings.
6. Determine parental response to crisis and their level of understanding of infant's status and procedures.

Nursing Diagnoses

1. Ineffective breathing patterns related to prematurity, grunting, retractions, and need for oxygen
2. Ineffective thermoregulation, hypothermia related to immaturity, lack of body fat, glucose balance
3. Risk for injury related to hypoxemia, hypoglycemia, and complications of prematurity
4. Risk for altered fluid and electrolyte balance, related to insensible water loss, IV therapy, phototherapy
5. Altered family processes related to situational crisis
6. Knowledge deficit, regarding infant status, management, procedures
7. Parental anxiety, Fear, Anticipatory Grieving, related to unknown outcome

Expected Outcomes

1. Exhibits unimpaired gas exchange evidenced by normal respiratory rate and pattern and pulse oximeter readings.
2. Maintains temperature in neutral thermal environment.
3. Maintains blood glucose greater than 45 mg/dl and serum calcium greater than 7 mg/dl. No evidence of necrotizing enterocolitis occurs. Bilirubin levels never exceed that which will cause injury.
4. Regains birth weight after loss of less than 10%; assumes expected growth rate. Demonstrates effective feeding patterns and retains oral feedings.
5. Parents express understanding of plan and procedures in therapy.
6. Parents demonstrate increasing confidence in infant care and exhibit attachment behaviors.

Nursing Interventions

1. Deliver warmed, humidified oxygen as prescribed. Maintain clear airway and pulmonary hygiene.
2. Adjust environmental temperature controls as needed, relate control to procedures and stressful events. Provide pain relief and stress reduction interventions.
3. Evaluate blood glucose levels via capillary samples. Give oral or parenteral glucose as needed.
4. Observe weight gain patterns; compare intake and output with weight. Provide gavage feeding, observe for nippling behaviors. Encourage mother to give feedings, to use breast pump, and to begin breast-feeding as soon as possible.
5. Explain all equipment and procedures. Help parents care for infant. Plan for discharge with appropriate referrals.
6. Describe infant behaviors and expected development. Demonstrate stimulation activities. Support attachment behaviors. Reinforce appropriate responses. Encourage parents to involve extended family.

Continued.

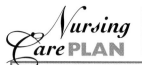

Nursing Care PLAN | *Premature Infant—cont'd*

Evaluation

1. Are vital signs within normal parameters? Is there any indication of risk of sudden infant death syndrome, bronchopulmonary dysplasia, or retinopathy of prematurity?
2. Can infant maintain temperature in an open crib? Are parents aware of protection from environmental temperature extremes?
3. Is growth following the newborn curve? Has infant regained birth weight?

4. What is the feeding pattern on discharge? Is the mother choosing to breast-feed and is she fully knowledgeable about breast-feeding?
5. Have all referrals been made? Do parents understand sequence of follow-up?
6. Do parents express relative confidence in assuming infant care?

Parents of children with musculoskeletal deformities need to know how long treatment will last and whether complete correction is possible. They must be shown how to remove and correctly reapply any corrective devices and to perform range of motion exercises.

TRANSPORT TO A REGIONAL CENTER

Improvement in the survival rate and the quality of survival of the high-risk and ill neonate are due partially to improvements in regionalization of care. Approximately 10% of all live births require specialized neonatal intensive care that can be provided at tertiary-level hospitals with NICUs or at secondary hospitals with neonatal special care units. Although high-risk neonates usually need to be transported from smaller to larger hospitals, personnel trained to perform resuscitation of the newborn and to provide support to stabilize the infant until a transport team arrives are essential in any obstetric unit. The AHA and the AAP are making a joint national effort to ensure that these personnel are available at every delivery.

Classification of the different levels of hospitals and efficient transport systems is established around the country. A well-equipped transport facility is important to the tiny neonate during the period when early extrauterine adjustment is taking place. Allowing the mother to give birth at a tertiary facility reduces the risks of delay involved in transport of a very ill infant.

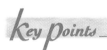

Key Points

- Neonatal nursing is a specialty that requires advanced knowledge and skills. Nurses need to develop supportive means of maintaining perspective.
- Stress in NICU nursing results from environmental noise, caring for many infants who may not survive or who survive with problems, and dealing with anxious, grieving parents.
- Understanding asphyxia will allow better, more rapid interventions in the immediate period after birth. Never wait for the Apgar score results to begin necessary interventions.
- Resuscitation is a team responsibility and may require two or three persons to be carried out correctly.
- RDS is a developmental problem that is now better controlled with exogenous surfactant administration.
- Heart defects are among the most common birth defects and usually require surgery for correction. The nurse's role is a supportive one, assessing status and maintaining life support.
- Because blood volume is so small, fluid and electrolyte balance is crucial.

- Premature infants need to grow at the fetal rate and thus require more calories per kilogram, although they have more difficulty in digesting feedings.
- Hypoglycemia may be as damaging as hypoxia and must be assessed and corrected promptly.
- Premature infants cannot regulate body temperature. A sign of maturity is the neonate's ability to sustain a temperature greater than 98° F—while wrapped—in an open crib.
- Preterm infants are vulnerable to anemia, hyperbilirubinemia, and sepsis.
- Stress and pain must be minimized. Analgesics are available for very small infants during procedures.
- Positioning prevents contractures and skin breakdown. The preterm infant preferably should be in a flexed position.
- Parents must be included in all plans, providing as much care as is comfortable for them. Education enables parents to assume total responsibility for the infant on the day of discharge from the NICU.

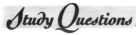

29-1. Select the terms that apply to the following statements:
  a. Blood shunted to more "valuable" organs from the periphery during perinatal asphyxia is the _____.
  b. _____ is accomplished by changes in position, percussion, and vibration of the chest wall.
  c. _____ consists of fibrin and sloughed cells, which further compromise gas exchange in the infant with RDS.
  d. A breathing pattern in a term or preterm infant in which respiration ceases for 15 to 20 seconds with pathophysiologic changes is _____.
  e. Process by which water is lost through the lungs (respiratory water loss) and the skin is _____.
  f. _____ causes a mechanical obstruction that allows air to reach the alveoli during inspiration but then traps it in the air sacs during expiration.
  g. _____ causes petechiae and increased bleeding time after heel sticks, injections, and venipunctures.
  h. _____ is caused by the interaction of normal bacterial contamination of the gut, plus formula feeding and ischemia in infants who have sustained ischemic injury to the intestines as a result of asphyxia or shock.
  i. _____ causes infants to look plethoric, with a ruddy or purplish, cyanotic tinge to the skin.
  j. _____ provides distending pressure to the alveoli to prevent atelectasis.
  k. _____ is a surface-active material instilled into the trachea of the neonate to reduce the surface tension.

29-2. You attend the delivery of a female infant, who is under a radiant warmer; she is dried and positioned, and bulb suction has been performed. Respiratory effort is good, heart rate is 130 beats per minute, mucous membranes are cyanotic, extremities are partially flexed, and she grimaced during suctioning. You identify signs of mild cardiorespiratory depression. The next step in resuscitation would be to:
  a. Provide a direct flow of oxygen over the infant's nose and mouth.
  b. Force the infant's thighs onto her abdomen to improve her muscle tone.
  c. Wait until the infant is 1-minute-old before intervening.
  d. Observe for the infant's improvement because this delay is caused by suctioning.

29-3. You have been providing a male infant with positive pressure ventilation with 100% oxygen for 30 seconds after birth. Heart rate is 70 beats per minute and respirations are gasping. A colleague has offered to assist you. What should be done next?
  a. Move the infant to the newborn ICU.
  b. Continue bag-and-mask ventilation while your colleague begins chest compressions.
  c. Administer sodium bicarbonate.
  d. Provide vigorous tactile stimulation.

29-4. You are caring for a growing and well preterm infant who is having periods of apnea and bradycardia during handling for feeding and for obtaining vital signs. Which nursing action is most appropriate?
  a. Assess the infant's ability to handle different types and levels of stress.
  b. Increase light on the incubator to facilitate observations of respirations and color.
  c. Use latches to close the incubator doors quietly rather than forcing them shut.
  d. Increase tactile and auditory stimuli to encourage spontaneous respirations.

29-5. Which of the following is not a cause of IWL?
  a. Single-walled incubator   c. Humidified air
  b. Phototherapy lamps   d. Radiant warmer

29-6. Which of the following is most likely to increase the risk for P/IVH in the preterm infant?
  a. Rapid infusion of hypertonic solutions
  b. Careful attention to respiratory status, especially P_{CO_2} level
  c. Clustering of treatment activities and procedures
  d. Sedation of infants requiring respiratory therapy

29-7. A female infant has a hematocrit level of 26%. She was born at 27 weeks' gestation and is now 5 weeks old. Which of the following assessment findings indicate that she is being compromised by her anemia?
  a. Demonstrates exaggerated reflexes and hyperirritability.
  b. Exhibits frequent episodes of apnea and desaturation.
  c. Regurgitates oral fluids within 5 minutes of feedings with occasional projectile vomiting.
  d. Skin and sclera appear yellow, and serum bilirubin is 10 g/dl.

Answer Key

References

AAP Provisional Committee for Quality Improvement and Subcommittee on Hyperbilirubinemia: Practice parameter: management of hyperbilirubinemia in the healthy term newborn, *Pediatrics* 94(4):558, 1994.

*Als H: Toward a synactive theory of development: promise for the assessment and support of infant individuality, *Infant Ment Health J* 3(4):229, 1982.

*Als H et al: Individualized behavioral and environmental care for the very low birth weight preterm infant at high risk for bronchopulmonary dysplasia: neonatal intensive care unit and developmental outcome, *Pediatrics* 78:1123, 1986.

American College of Obstetricians and Gynecologists: *Fetal and neonatal neurologic injury*, ACOG Technical Bulletin 163, January, 1992.

Anand KJS: Analgesia and sedation in ventilated neonates, *Neonatal Respiratory Diseases* 5(5):1, Ross Products Division, 1995, Abbott Laboratories.

Avery GB: *Neonatology: pathophysiology and management of the newborn*, ed 3, Philadelphia, 1993, JB Lippincott.

Bell SG: The national pain management guideline: implications for neonatal intensive care, *Neonat Netw* 13(3):9, 1994.

*Bellig L: A window on the neonate's brain, *Neonat Netw* 7(4):13, 1989.

Blackburn S: Hyperbilirubinemia and neonatal jaundice, *Neonat Netw* 14(7):15, 1995.

Bloom RS, Cropley CC: *Textbook of neonatal resuscitation*, Dallas, 1995, American Heart Association.

Burns K et al: Infant stimulation: modification of an intervention based on physiologic and behavioral cues, *J Obstet Gynecol Neonatal Nurs* 23(7):581, 1994.

*Campos RG: Soothing pain-elicited distress in infants with swaddling and pacifiers, *Child Dev* 60(4):781, 1989.

Campos RG: Soothing neonate's responses to a stressful procedure, *Neonat Netw* 12(6):93, 1993 (abstract).

Connor EM et al: Reduction of maternal-infant transmission of human immunodeficiency virus type I with zidovudine treatment, *N Engl J Med* 331(18):1173, 1994.

Darby MK, Loughead JL: Neonatal nutritional requirements and formula composition: a review, *J Obstet Gynecol Neonatal Nurs* 25(3):209, 1996.

Dodd V: Gestational age assessment, *Neonat Netw* 15(1):27, 1996.

*Farquhar JW: Children of diabetic women, *Arch Dis Child* 34:76, 1959.

Flyer DC, Lang P: Neonatal heart disease. In Avery GB, ed: *Neonatology: pathophysiology and management of the newborn*, Philadelphia, 1993, JB Lippincott.

Gale G et al: Skin-to-skin (Kangaroo) holding of the intubated premature infant, *Neonat Netw* 12(6):49, 1993.

Gallagher PG, Ehrenkranz RA: Erythropoietin therapy for anemia of prematurity, *Clin Perinatol* 29(1):169, 1993.

Gracey KM et al: Caring for the infant with retinopathy of prematurity undergoing cryotherapy, *Neonat Netw* 9(7):7, 1991.

Hicks M: A systematic approach to neonatal pathophysiology: understanding respiratory distress syndrome, *Neonat Netw* 14(1):29, 1995.

*Classic reference.

Hodges C, Vincent PA: Why do NICU nurses not refeed gastric residuals prior to feeding by gavage? *Neonat Netw* 12(8):37, 1993.

Kirsten D: Patent ductus arteriosus in the preterm infant, *Neonat Netw* 15(2):19, 1996.

Lawrence J et al: The development of a tool to assess neonatal pain, *Neonat Netw* 12(6):59, 1993.

Long WA, ed: *Fetal and neonatal cardiology*, Philadelphia, 1990, WB Saunders.

Ludington-Hoe SM et al: Kangaroo care: research results, and practice implications and guidelines, *Neonat Netw* 13(1):19, 1994.

*Maisels MI, Gifford KL: Normal serum bilirubin levels in the newborn and the influence of breastfeeding, *Pediatrics* 78(5):837, 1986.

Miller C: Nitric oxide therapy for persistent pulmonary hypertension of the newborn, *Neonat Netw* 14(8):9, 1995.

*Papile L et al: Incidence and evolution of subependymal and intraventricular hemorrhage: a study of infants with birth weights less than 1500 g, *J Pediatr* 92:529, 1978.

Parker LA: Necrotizing enterocolitis, *Neonat Netw* 14(6):17, 1995.

Paul KE: Recognition, stabilization, and early management of infants with critical congenital heart disease presenting in the first days of life, *Neonat Netw* 14(5):13, 1995.

Pickler RH, Terrell BV: Nonnutritive sucking and necrotizing enterocolitis, *Neonat Netw* 13(8):15, 1994.

Prevost RR: Comparing surfactant products, *Therapy Consultation* 10:909, 1991.

*Volpe JJ: Intraventricular hemorrhage and brain injury in the premature infant: neuropathology and pathogenesis, *Clin Perinatol* 16(2):387, 1989.

*Weibley TT et al: Gavage tube insertion in the premature infant, *MCN Am J Matern Child Nurs* 12:24, 1987.

Wong DL: *Whaley and Wong's essentials of pediatric nursing*, ed 5, St Louis, 1997, Mosby.

Young TE, Mangum OB: *NeoFax '95: a manual of drugs used in neonatal care*, ed 8, Columbus, Ohio, 1995, Ross Products Division, Abbott Laboratories.

 Student Resource Shelf

Beachy P, Deacon J, eds: *Core curriculum for neonatal intensive care nursing*, AWHONN, Philadelphia, 1993, WB Saunders.
A text written in outline format; includes study questions, extensive reference lists, and standards of care.

Hussey B: *Understanding my signal: help for parents of premature infants*, Palo Alto, Calif, VORT Corporation.
A pamphlet written for parents of premature infants from the infant's point of view; informs parents about behavioral cues.

Kenner C et al, eds: *Comprehensive neonatal nursing: a physiologic perspective*, Philadelphia, 1993, WB Saunders.
A complete textbook of neonatal nursing for the experienced NICU nurse.

Nugent J, ed: *Acute respiratory care of the neonate*, Petaluma, Calif, 1991, Neonatal Network.
The Neonatal Network provides the most comprehensive instruction for care of NICU infants. This is a soft-cover self-study guide for CE credits.

Seven

Maternal-Infant Nursing Issues

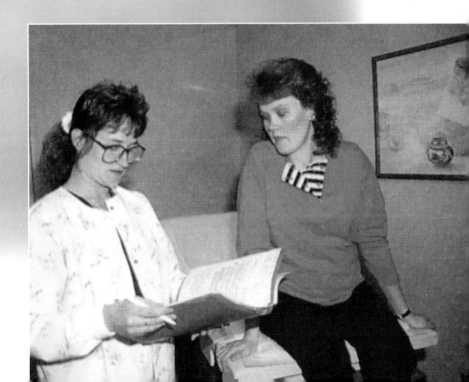

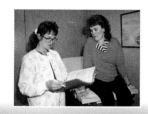

30

Legal *&* Ethical Issues *in* Maternal-Infant Nursing

ETHICAL DECISION MAKING

As a nurse, you must know the "right" thing to do. Rightness or wrongness can be applied to any nursing decision made or action taken. Many people, including your clients, the nursing staff, and your instructors, will evaluate your nursing care. Doing the right or best thing for each client is the objective of all nursing care.

The definition of the correct thing varies from person to person; it is not what an individual feels like doing. Rightness involves ethics and morality. Everyone uses personal standards to judge whether attitudes, behavior, actions, and decisions are good or bad. The profession of nursing also has standards of moral behavior that describe how a nurse should behave and act when practicing nursing. Nurses function within a code of ethics and a code of conduct and learn principles of ethics.

Much of what you have learned in maternal-infant nursing is based on the idea that pregnancy and childbearing are natural, normal, happy events. This, however, is not the case for all families. Because childbearing is a healthy process, nurses must orient care giving to the health of their clients and the prevention of disease. Because health during pregnancy is the responsibility of the pregnant woman or couple, the nurse's primary role is to offer information, support the healthy behaviors of the woman or couple, and encourage self-care. Self-care requires that women be motivated to be healthy and that they receive information that they can understand and use. This sharing of information involves the ethical principles of truth-telling, informed consent with minimal bias, and respect for the humanness of each client and family. Sharing knowledge requires that you have an adequate, up-to-date knowledge base and competence in nursing practice and especially in ethics and health care.

Ethics, Morals, and Values

There is an ethical dimension to every nursing situation. People interact best with other people when they act responsibly, respect one another, and care about each other. Self-respect and caring for oneself play an important role in this interaction. All of these behaviors are based on ethical principles: respect for human dignity, caring, and competence in professional practice.

Asking yourself what you should do in a situation and why you should do this are moral questions. An understanding of morals, ethics, and values can help you provide nursing care that is right for the client and performed the right way.

Morals are what a person should and ought to do; *moral* means relating to principles of right or wrong. Moral questions suggest that there are at least two answers available. Sometimes, several different options are possible—some helpful and some harmful—depending on the viewpoint. Even when a person refuses to decide, a choice has been made (to do nothing). **Ethics** is the branch of philosophy dealing with the reasons why we should or ought to do something. Each reason involves the ethical principle of **autonomy** (self-determination or choice by the client).

Values are the attitudes or belief that underlie how a person feels about some decision or toward someone else. Values are also attitudes or beliefs that are practiced as you interact with other people or that guide the decisions you make in life. You have many values; you grew up with them.

Personal values

As you were growing up, many people gave you advice and direction on the right or wrong thing to do or say. Parents and families are important sources for learning values. So, too, are religious groups, schoolmates, books, and television. Even your geographic neighborhood and your family's wealth were important influences on the values you now have.

Personal values that could influence the practice of maternal-infant nursing include ideas about life in general, procreation, sex, parenting, love, telling the truth, the Golden Rule, suffering, and pain. You will be asked to care for many women who share your personal values. You will also take care of women who do not share your values. The first step in analyzing a conflict is to remember that respect for people and their values does not mean you have to agree with them. Your professional judgment is also worthy of respect, though you must remember that it may be based on values with which the client disagrees.

Professional values

The nursing profession has its own standards of proper conduct (moral behavior) for nurses. These values or moral standards are stated in the American Nurses Association (ANA) *Code for Nurses with Interpretive Statements* (1986). The code says nurses should practice with respect for human dignity and should support client choice. Nurses should also practice in a competent and responsible manner (exercising accountability) and be **advocates** who protect clients from the "unethical, illegal, or immoral actions" of anyone else.

The nursing profession exports nurses to understand and practice safe care. Nurses should always balance safety with client preferences. The ANA code also states that nurses are morally obligated to provide care without discrimination. You may disagree with a choice a client or family has made, but you cannot *abandon* them. If a choice is appropriate or correct for a woman, you must care for her, at least until another nurse is available to provide care.

Personal and professional values sometimes conflict. Nurses are expected to overcome personal biases and provide respectful care to all clients. It is also wrong for you to impose your values on clients, especially without acknowledging or admitting it. When your most deeply held values are called into question, however, you may be supported in refusing to care for a client.

The Church Amendment was passed by the federal government in the wake of the early abortion controversy. This amendment allows health professionals who are morally opposed to abortion and other legal health care options to refuse to care for women who have selected options that are contrary to a nurse's deeply held personal and professional values (Rushton and Scanlon, 1995). However, your employer needs to know about your beliefs ahead of time so another health professional can be found to provide care.

When a dilemma occurs after employment, the nurse may not abandon the client but instead must go through a process of consultation with peers and supervisors and ultimately the bioethics committee of the institution. Being forced to act in a professional manner that is contrary to one's personal values will lead to *moral distress*. Over time, this distress leads to suffering and burnout. Newly practicing nurses are especially vulnerable to moral distress.

Moral Development as Moral Authority

Kohlberg (1984) spent many years studying how human beings develop intellectually and morally. Kohlberg's cross-cultural theory of moral development offers some insight into how individuals make moral choices (choices of right or wrong).

Kohlberg's first level of *preconventional* moral development has two stages. In the first stage, a person determines what the right thing is based on external authority—on whether a reward or punishment will result from the action. Young children function in this way. Adults functioning at this stage of moral development may decide that driving above the speed limit is wrong because they will get a ticket (punishment) if they are caught speeding. At the second stage in this level, people do good things for others so they can get something in return, or they act on the basis that what is right is what is fair. You can observe school-aged children and many adults involved in "what is fair."

Most adults in society function at the *conventional* level of moral development. At this level of Kohlberg's model, "right" is defined by individuals in positions of authority. For example, a staff nurse may decide to follow a physician's advice for a client because the nurse believes the physician is always right. The law becomes the moral authority for right or wrong; for example, a man might drive 55 miles an hour on the highway, not because he might get a ticket but because that is the law, and the law is right. This stage involves doing what is right because others expect it of you or of your role.

Nurses who place their moral authority in others (e.g., head nurse, physician, client, law, or hospital rules) often practice in an ethical manner. They also have fewer options for action because they believe that authority figures are always right. Even if they think another choice is better, these nurses will still follow the authority figure.

At these two levels of moral development, nurses may face conflict when others hold values and moral positions different from their own. They may favor the action that will avoid punishment or that agrees with the authority figure, even if the client disagrees.

The *postconventional* level of morality allows individuals to choose from ethical principles as guides for right and wrong, rather than choosing from other persons or because of fear of results. The major guide at this level is *utilitarianism*, the action or choice that will result in the greatest good for the greatest number of people (see Box 30-2). *Deontology* is also used as a guiding set of principles (see Box 30-1).

Systems of Ethical Thought

There are many different values, moral standards, and ethical principles in the world. Ethical principles are familiar ideas such as telling the truth, practicing the Golden Rule, doing good and not harm; for nursing, this means showing *respect for persons, client autonomy, quality and sanctity of life,* and *justice and mercy.*

Deontology

The ethical principle of respect for persons is based on the idea that persons should never be treated as objects or used for gain. Every human being, despite age, physical or mental condition, work status, or educational level, is worthy of respect. If a person is respected, his or her competency to make decisions is also respected. Thus the principle of client autonomy or self-determination is a critical idea. This is why **informed consent** is so critical in client care. It is linked to the idea of telling the truth to the client, or **veracity**, the obligation to tell the truth. If you respect a person's competence to handle information and critical issues, you will not cover up the truth.

Clients too young or too weak to speak for themselves need special protection in health care. When caring for newborns and children, special caution must be used in deciding what is in their best interest. Nurses expect parents to make decisions for their infant with the assumption that they will do what is best for their own child. There may be occasions, however, when this assumption is not true, and another person may be called in to represent the infant, such as a court-appointed guardian.

The second major idea in deontology is the obligation to do good rather than harm. The term **beneficence** refers to the obligation to do good, meaning the benefit of the treatment should outweigh the risks of harm to the client. **Nonmaleficence** is the obligation to do no harm. (Compare the use of these terms). The third major idea is that of **justice**, or equal treatment for individuals, with benefits and burdens shared equally in the society. This last principle is gradually being eroded by current cost containment policies in managed care. Box 30-1 lists the ethical principles found in deontology.

Utilitarianism

The utilitarianism system of ethical thought suggests that immediate or short-term pain or harm can be tolerated when greater harm is avoided. Immunization, medication to cure disease, and surgery all can hurt, but they can also save lives. Utilitarianism views these interventions as having *good ends,* and therefore being justified.

Utilitarianism is also defined as actions or decisions that promote the greatest happiness of usefulness for the greatest number of people. For example, several years ago, visiting hours for maternity wards reflected the same rules used in the rest of the hospital, meaning that any child under 15 could not visit the mother or new sibling and that fathers could only come for 2 to 3 hours a day. These hospital rules were established to avoid the potential for infections to be passed from children to already ill clients and to control traffic patterns and congestion in busy hospital corridors; these ends were considered the greatest good. Now, it is clear that the higher value is in sibling visitation, unrestricted visiting hours for fathers and grandparents, and rooming-in for family development so the utilitarian-based hospital rules were changed.

Concepts of justice may also be viewed as a part of utilitarianism. Box 30-2 lists the ethical principles of utilitarianism. These principles will underlie many of the ethical dilemmas the nurse might face. Questions may arise concerning the following issues:

Box 30-1 | **Ethical Principles of Deontology**

AUTONOMY OR SELF-DETERMINATION
The right and responsibility of a competent individual to make decisions about the "rightness" or "wrongness" of her or his own actions or beliefs.

RESPECT FOR PERSONS
Closely associated with the principle of autonomy and adherence to recognition of individualism; also includes a connection to the broader community or society. This principle recognizes the obligation or duty to others and to self in making decisions.

BENEFICENCE
The obligation to "do good."

NONMALEFICENCE
The obligation to "do no harm."

JUSTICE
The principle of equal or comparative treatment of individuals. Justice seeks to distribute benefits and burdens equally throughout society.

VERACITY
The obligation to tell the truth.

INFORMED CONSENT
An example of adherence to the principle of veracity.

From Lagana K, Dunderstadt K: *Ethical decision making for perinatal nurses,* White Plains, NY, 1995, March of Dimes Birth Defects Foundation.

- Are resources allocated justly? Is it *just* to use so much money and personnel time caring for an infant who cannot possibly survive? (See the case of Baby M and Baby K in Glover and Rushton, 1996).
- What is the value of life in itself versus the quality of life? When should the machines be turned off? What constitutes a living person? When is it futile (meaning no improvement is possible) to continue treatment? (Nelson and Nelson, 1992)
- Who decides what will be done, the partially educated client or the intensely educated physician? *Paternalism* versus *autonomy* continues to be an issue.

A third alternative to these either/or questions has been developed by Gilligan (1982), a feminist philosopher. She contrasts the *justice* perspective with the *care* perspective. In women's issues especially, a different voice is needed that reflects a different orientation—that of relationships and care approaches. Justice and rights are rule-bound and have more abstract solutions; the care perspective, on the other hand, considers the relationships, situations, and struggles of the persons involved in the ethical dilemma. When women are in conflict, they demonstrate that these moral

Box 30-2 | **Ethical Principles of Utilitarianism**

ALLOCATION OF RESOURCES VS COST EFFECTIVENESS
Relates to distribution of scarce health resources.

QUALITY OF LIFE VS SANCTITY OF LIFE
Addresses the question of preservation of life at all costs.

WITHHOLDING VS INITIATION
Addresses choices regarding the delivery of care to individuals in society.
Questions when care should be initiated, withheld, or withdrawn.

PATERNALISM VS AUTONOMY
Addresses the questions of who should make decisions about health care delivery to individuals.

From Lagana K, Dunderstadt K: *Ethical decision making for perinatal nurses,* White Plains, NY, 1995, March of Dimes Birth Defects Foundation.

conflicts are influenced by the need to intensify and maintain relationships. They are more cognizant of how the decisions will affect the whole family structure (McFadden, 1996). Table 30-1 identifies a guide to assessment of ideas about morality. Use this guide to identify sources of conflict when there is an unresolved moral issue.

Natural law

Some describe and use a third system of ethical thought to justify health care actions and decisions. *Natural law* evaluates the correctness of actions on the basis of what is natural or what is the natural purpose of human beings and body organs. For example, contraception is viewed as morally wrong by some religious traditions; the only purpose of sexual intercourse is to reproduce. Therefore any action or device used to interfere with procreation is viewed as wrong by these groups. Natural law may also be the basis for opposition to artificial insemination, in vitro fertilization, surrogate motherhood, and medicated childbirth.

For some, natural law would justify refusal of the use of any biomedical technology or care. However, this refusal is rarely interpreted as total opposition because nurses have the capacity to help these individuals recover from illness and maintain their health. When a person is dying, those who believe in natural law are willing to let nature take its course rather than prolong the dying by invasive treatments, surgery, and medications intended to cure. They would argue that care and comfort should be the only goals of medical and nursing care when a cure is no longer possible. For people with these beliefs, all health care can be seen as a violation of nature (Sachs, 1994; Rhodes, 1995).

Table 30-1	**Guide to Assessment of Ideas about Morality**
Care Perspective	**Justice Perspective**
Response in relationships	Rights in relationships
Sees others in their terms and context	Sees others as they would like to be seen
Interdependent in relationships	Independence and equality in relationships
Connection through response	Connection through roles, obligation
Goal of understanding	Goal of critique, analysis, objectivity
Interdependent, listens to others	Objective, fairness, equality within their own context

From Lyons NP: Listening to voices we have not heard. In Gilligan NP, Lyons NP, Hanmer TJ, eds: *Making connections*, Troy, NY, 1989, Emma Willard School.

Some health care providers turn the naturalistic fallacy into a technologic fallacy. For example, suppose an infant is dying, but technology is available to keep him alive in a handicapped condition, Some say the technology must be used at all costs. Others say that the technologic imperative is false: it may allow interns to be trained, but it uses persons for the needs of others rather than focusing on the client's well-being. The *technologic imperative* in certain cases may do more harm than good. It may cause suffering—iatrogenic illness—rather than relieve it. Therefore *merely having the machinery does not mean it should be used*. Sometimes there are other reasons for using technology, including making money for the hospital, giving interns practice, giving doctors medical triumphs, or making nurses feel good. But these do not offset the suffering of the client and the violation of the ethical norms of health care.

A person may justify, based on ethical principles, why a particular action of response is chosen. For example, when a premature infant is born with little hope of survival, health professionals often ask whether they should treat the infant or allow him to die. Often, this decision, although emotional and heart-wrenching, is reached on the basis of the quality of life the infant will have if life-sustaining treatment is begun. Other persons use the ethical principle of *sanctity of life*, or life at all costs, to justify any and all treatment, even though this treatment sometimes causes great harm to the ill neonate (as in the Baby K case). Thus a nurse must weigh the risks and benefits of treatment versus nontreatment and ethical and moral principles. Most decision making in health and illness requires balancing of principles and balancing of benefits with risks or harms.

Ethical pluralism

We live in a society that supports ethical pluralism—several systems of ethical justification for making the right decision or choice. We have discussed the value systems we hold and differing levels of moral development that explain how people make choices in life and in health care. Because of these different systems, it is easy to understand how, at times, intelligent, sensitive, and caring individuals may make decisions that seem contradictory.

Ethical decision making requires that time be taken to understand the choices available and to gather information to make sure all the ethical principles and values involved are understood. Ethical decision making does not imply that everyone agrees with choices that are made. At the least, however, all individuals involved should understand why the choice was made. In difficult situations, the hospital ethics committee must be called upon for guidance.

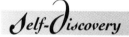
Self-Discovery

> Find out whether there is a hospital ethics committee in the setting where you have clinical practice. Discover which kinds of nursing ethical dilemmas have been brought to the committee for guidance. ~

PROCESS FOR ETHICAL DECISION MAKING

Ethical decision making is a complex process because it is based on *moral reasoning*, which means analyzing, weighing, justifying, choosing, and evaluating attitudes, behaviors, and actions. This process of critically examining the moral and ethical dimensions of nursing care takes into account personal and professional values, levels of moral development, and ethical theories used to justify choices of action. Because of the shift away from the belief that the health professional knows what is best for clients (*paternalism*) and the shift toward a client-defined health care goal (*client autonomy*), all individuals affected by the decision are included in the process of decision making. To make good decisions as a nurse, you must know and understand what you value, what you believe, and to what you are committed in nursing care.

Good decisions require time and the ability to listen carefully to the client. It is difficult to think critically in an emergency situation. Even when enough time is available, however, it is difficult to think critically about the options

| Box **30-3** | **Thompson and Thompson Bioethical Decision Model** |

STEP ONE

Review the situation to determine:
- Health problems
- Decisions needed
- Key individuals

STEP TWO

Gather additional information to:
- Clarify the situation
- Understand why that information is needed
- Understand legal constraints, if any

STEP THREE

Identify the ethical issues of concerns in the situation:
- Explore historical roots
- Explore current philosophic and religious positions
- Explore current societal views

STEP FOUR

Define personal and professional moral positions on the issues and concerns identified in Step Three, including:
- Review of personal constraints raised by issues
- Review of professional codes for guidance
- Identification of conflicting loyalties and obligations

STEP FIVE

Identify moral positions of key individuals involved

STEP SIX

Identify value conflicts, if any, and attempt to understand basis for conflict and possible resolution

STEP SEVEN

Determine who should make the needed decisions

STEP EIGHT

Identify the range of possible actions:
- Describe anticipated outcome for each action
- Include moral justification for each action
- Decide which actions fit criteria for decision making in this situation

STEP NINE

Decide on course of action and carry it out:
- Know reasons for choice of action
- Explain reasons to others
- Establish time frame for review of outcomes

STEP TEN

Evaluate the results of the decision and action:
- Did the expected outcomes occur?
- Is a new decision needed?
- Was the decision process complete?

Modified from Thompson JE, Thompson HO: *Bioethical decision making for nurses,* Norwalk Town, Conn, 1985, Appleton-Century-Crofts.

available for nursing care. You must be willing to ask questions and to gather information that will help you to understand as much about the client and her situation as possible. Listening carefully to the client's preferences and her reasons for making a decision is important. Listening to her and reflecting with her helps sort out the risks, benefits, costs, good results, or harm of each choice.

Good decision making also requires a person to identify whether personal values influence the information that is shared with a client about her condition, thereby possibly biasing her for or against an option. (Listen to explanations given to a client about decisions requiring informed consent. How often does the person doing the informing "forget" to include all facts on both sides of a decision?)

Understanding the client's sources of moral authority can also help in sorting through conflicts. Is the family's opinion paramount? The spouse's? If the client lacks the capacity to make a decision, whether because of age (infant), severe pain (difficult labor), or unconsciousness (anesthesia), others in her environment (parents, spouses, and physicians) will need to be involved so that appropriate decisions can be made.

The decision model in Box 30-3 can be used to analyze the ethical dimensions of maternal-infant nursing practice. It includes elements of decision theory, moral reasoning, applied ethics, and factors that might affect decision making in clinical practice. Use this model to analyze the ethical dimensions of your practice as a nurse. It works best when a group of individuals analyze the same case, but it can also be used by an individual.

Ethical Concerns in Maternal-Infant Nursing

We have focused on ethical decision making because many of the major concerns or issues in bioethics today can be found in maternal-infant nursing. Issues related to contraception or family planning, abortion, and genetics precede childbearing. Issues related to how, whom, and when to conceive are evident when considering conception. The issues surrounding unwanted pregnancy are ethical and moral ones. Because of the rise in world population and the strain on resources, the area of preventive care in childbearing assumes greater importance. Issues concerning the appropriate use of biomedical technology during pregnancy, labor, and birth and in the care of seriously ill neonates highlight the technologic imperative (Nelson and Nelson, 1992).

Biomedical technology has progressed rapidly in maternal-infant care in recent decades. The availability of cesarean births has saved many infants and women from death. However, it is now said that this procedure is used too often and may cause more harm than good for some women. Electronic fetal monitoring promised hope of saving infants in distress during labor, yet when used inappropriately, it can cause psychologic harm to the woman and her infant, as well as financial harm.

Many health care providers and parents believe they must save infants *because they can do it.* Many ethicists, professionals, and clients suggest otherwise, however. Technology is useful as an adjunct to clinical decision making, but it was never intended to replace it. The technologic imperative is a naturalistic fallacy.

In all aspects of family care during childbearing, you will be faced with the daily concerns of respect for human dignity, allocation of scarce resources, and ethical practice. These are the "ordinary ethics" for ordinary nursing practice. Many have suggested that the true measure of our morality as human beings is what we do *when no one else is looking.* Your code of ethics determines what you do from minute to minute in caring for childbearing families rather than what you do when a special situation occurs.

LEGAL ISSUES IN PERINATAL NURSING*

When you hear the words "high risk," you usually think of a client with complications of pregnancy. But this term takes on a new meaning when it refers to legal issues in perinatal nursing. Nurses working in this field face a high risk of lawsuit as compared with nurses in other specialty areas. Every year there is an increase in the number of nurses named as defendants in lawsuits. Now, more than ever, nurses must learn how to minimize their risk of being involved in a lawsuit. Only by investing time and effort to learn about legal issues can you effectively insulate yourself against becoming the defendant in a lawsuit. A **plaintiff** is the party who initiates a lawsuit and accuses another of wrongdoing. A **defendant** is the party against whom the lawsuit is filed and who is accused of wrongdoing.

By far, the best defense to any malpractice lawsuit is *prevention.* Avoidance of malpractice is no accident. It requires effort, and often, a commitment to change.

The first step in malpractice avoidance is to learn about the legal risks and pitfalls of malpractice. The next step is to use what is learned to make the necessary changes in daily practice. Although there is no guarantee that you will never be sued, you can adopt behaviors that will significantly reduce your chances of ending up in court.

*Mary Ann Shea, JD

Law is an unfamiliar area to most nurses. Before nurses can understand how to reduce their risk of being involved in litigation, they must understand the basic structure of the legal system.

Laws come in many variations. *Criminal law* involves the commission of a crime, such as murder, criminal assault, or manslaughter. Fortunately, nurses are not likely to be involved in these intentional wrongful acts that result in criminal prosecution. The penalty for being found guilty of a crime is usually incarceration or payment of a fine. The money paid for the fine does not go to the victim but to a governmental agency.

Civil law, on the other hand, is an area in which many nurses might be involved. Medical negligence or malpractice come under the category of *tort* or *personal injury law,* which is one type of civil law. The penalty when one is found liable in a civil case is usually payment of money damages to the person who was wronged.

Laws are derived from many sources. Some laws are actually written by legislators at both the state and federal levels. This type of law is also referred to as *statutory law.* *Case law* is determined by our judicial system and comes about when a court decides the outcome of a case. *Administative law* involves the regulation of agencies, such as the state board of nursing. These bodies are given legal authority to create regulations governing the actions of certain people.

Why So Many Lawsuits?

To avoid becoming a victim of the malpractice crisis, it is imperative that the mindset of those individuals filing the lawsuits be understood. To answer the question, "Why are there so many lawsuits?" three groups—the legal profession, the medical profession, and society—must be examined (Figure 30-1). Lawyers are quick to blame physicians and nurses for the increase in lawsuits, and physicians and nurses are just as quick to blame lawyers. Frequently *society's* impact is overlooked in the fingerpointing between physician's and lawyers. It is difficult, if not impossible, to avoid being sued without an understanding of what motivates people to file lawsuits. To better understand the propensity to file lawsuits, three categories must be explored:
1. Why are there lawsuits?
2. Why is there an increasing number of lawsuits against nurses?
3. Why is perinatal nursing considered a high-risk area for lawsuits?
These are complex issues that deserve careful attention.

Societal attitudes

The way members of society think affects their propensity to file lawsuits. Certain attitudes increase the likelihood of lawsuits.

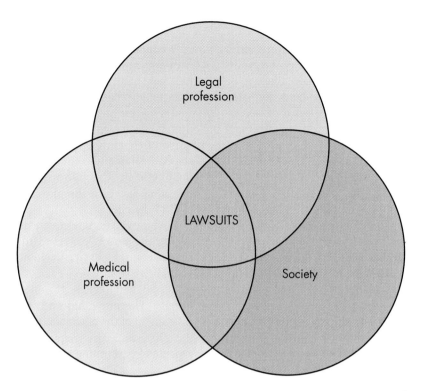

Figure 30-1 Relationship of lawsuits among society, the legal profession, and the medical profession.

Need to blame. When a person refuses to accept responsibility for his or her own actions, the result is the placing of blame on another person. For example, if a client who is 7 months pregnant exhibits signs of premature labor and is sent home with strict instructions to remain on bed rest, one would think that this same client would be willing to accept the consequences of not following medical instructions. Unfortunately, all too often the client who disregards medical advice by spending the day shopping at the mall instead of resting in bed files a lawsuit when her infant suffers as a result of being born prematurely.

Expectation of perfection. Clients often do not realize that medicine is not an exact science. They might think that everything can be cured by modern technology. The medical profession must take partial responsibility for conveying that attitude to the public.

The truth is that there generally are no guarantees that a proposed treatment regimen will produce the desired outcome. Clients who feel the medical system has wrongfully failed them are likely to pursue legal recourse. For example, a client who undergoes maternal serum alpha-fetoprotein testing during pregnancy must be told that a negative test result does *not* guarantee that the infant is free of genetic defects.

Lack of personalism. The sophisticated equipment in use today leads to advanced monitoring techniques that have substantially improved the quality of client care. Yet, the client's perception of the quality of care is often quite the opposite. Too often clients equate more equipment with less actual "hands-on" care. A client attached to a fetal monitor that continuously evaluates the status of the infant often feels she is better cared for by the nurse who comes in periodically and auscultates fetal heart tones. Clients who perceive that they receive good care often do not initiate lawsuits, even when faced with an untoward result.

Well-educated public. Clients are now better educated regarding their health care. They want and get more information about diagnosis, medications, and prognosis. By being more involved in their own health care, they also are aware of an adverse outcome when it occurs. Clients faced with a poor result will probably ask what went wrong, and they should be told by the proper person. Clients today are likely to be aware when they have been treated negligently. In fact, one of the worst things a health care provider can do when faced with a bad result is attempt to cover up the truth because a client who later learns he or she has been the victim of a deception is likely to take legal action. Remember that *angry clients are potential plaintiffs.*

Box **30-1**

CLINICAL DECISION

Describe a situation in which a client was unhappy about her treatment. How was it handled? Discuss improvements in interactions.

Why Increased Lawsuits Against Nurses?

Years ago, if a nurse was involved in a lawsuit, it was most likely as a witness, one who had knowledge of the events resulting in the lawsuit. Now, nurses are more likely to be involved in a different manner—as defendants. By being named as defendants, nurses are also accused of wrongdoing. There are several reasons why nurses' involvement in lawsuits has evolved in this manner.

Nursing as a profession

Nurses used to merely be physicians' "handmaidens" whose function was to follow orders. They had little independence or autonomy. Nurses did not make major decisions or perform independent assessments. Nursing, however, has changed. Nurses are now recognized as professionals, and nursing is well-recognized as a practice that is independent of the practice of medicine.

Along with this recognition of nurses as professionals came nurse accountability. Because nurses present themselves to the public as independent professionals, they also declare that they are responsible for their own actions. Today's nurse operates with autonomy and makes independent judgments regarding client care. Although this has enhanced overall client care, it has increased the nurse's risk of being named as a defendant in a lawsuit.

Nurses as "deep pockets"

The responsibility of the plaintiff's attorney is to find sufficient financial resources to compensate the plaintiff in whatever amount the jury determines is fair. It is often essential to include several defendants to ensure that enough compensation is available. In this situation, the nurse becomes another "pocket" to dip into to satisfy the judgment.

The nurse might also be named as a defendant in an attempt to hold the hospital liable by the doctrine of "respondent superior" ("let the master respond"). This theory holds that the employer is responsible for the negligent acts of its employee when the employee is acting within the scope of employment. By showing the nurse (employee) was negligent, the plaintiff can then access the hospital's "deep pocket."

Why is Perinatal Nursing a High-Risk Practice?

In nursing, there is a high risk of lawsuit attached to the perinatal specialty area. Whenever nurses practice in a specialty area that requires increased skill, training, and experience beyond that which is taught in nursing school, those nurses will be held to a higher standard of care. Perinatal nursing is one such highly specialized area; therefore perinatal nurses are held to a higher standard of care.

Nursing autonomy issues

Whenever nurses practice in a specialty area and operate with a great degree of autonomy, the chance for errors in judgment increases. Whenever judgmental errors occur, the chance for a charge of medical malpractice increases.

The nature of the practice of perinatal nursing requires that nurses act with autonomy much of the time. Perinatal nurses frequently monitor clients throughout the first stages of labor and communicate pertinent information to the physician. This information is often what determines the point at which the physician goes to the hospital to tend to the client.

If incorrect or inadequate information regarding the client's progress is conveyed to the physician, there is a chance that the physician will not get to the hospital soon enough. In a situation such as this, the nurse, not the physician, will likely be the one who is held liable for negligence. The nurse has an obligation to make a correct assessment of the client and to communicate the results to the physician. This requires that the nurse always be capable of performing a proper assessment.

Client issues

High expectation of outcome. Obstetric clients often do not perceive themselves as sick and are therefore completely unprepared for any bad result to their pregnancies. When a bad result does occur, it is devastating to the expectant parent. In such a situation, it is often impossible for the parent to accept that sometimes things like this "just happen." When this fact is combined with society's general tendency to attach blame, physicians and nurses often bear the brunt of the accusation of wrongdoing in the form of a lawsuit.

Defective infant survival rate. With recent advances in perinatal technology, infants who formerly would have died in utero or shortly after birth are now being saved. Unfortunately, many of these infants suffer severe medical consequences, such as mental retardation, cerebral palsy, seizure disorders, brain damage, developmental delays, and many other conditions that will be costly to monitor and treat for the infant's lifetime.

Historically, lawsuits for the wrongful death of an infant have not garnered large dollar awards, but lawsuits based on permanent brain damage, for example, will often result in multimillion dollar recoveries.

Long statute of limitations for minors. Lawsuits must be filed within a certain amount of time after the act which gave rise to the lawsuit occurred. These time limits are prescribed by law and are called **statutes of limitations.** The length of time one has to bring legal action differs, depending upon what type of lawsuit is being filed and the law of the particular state.

Statutes of limitations are usually shorter for adults than for minors. The statute of limitations for medical malpractice claims often will be 1 to 3 years for adults, depending on state law. The client must file the lawsuit within the specified number of years after the alleged act of negligence. The statute of limitations for minors, however, often does not begin to run until the minor has reached the age of majority. When dealing with minors, more specifically with newborns, the health care practitioner can actually be at risk of lawsuit for as long as *20 or more years* before the statute of limitations expires. These extended statutes of limitations for minors operate to the disadvantage of perinatal nurses.

Several potential plaintiffs. The obstetric staff treating a pregnant woman really has two clients—the mother and the fetus. Care must be directed toward the best interests of both. In the event that something goes wrong, one or both clients can suffer injury, giving rise to lawsuits initiated by either party. In addition, the husband or father can have his own basis for a lawsuit involving either his wife or child. In any event, for a single treatment regimen, there can be at least three parties ready to initiate a lawsuit in the event of an adverse outcome

Long involvement in treatment. A pregnant woman may receive medical care for an extended period during the 40 weeks of gestation. Medical treatment is usually ongoing, resulting in a relatively significant amount of treatment being given during any pregnancy. Statistically, as more treatment is given, the chances that something will be done incorrectly increase.

Sometimes the close relationship the pregnant woman develops with the physician and nurses during the prolonged treatment period can serve to buffer the tendency to sue, even if there is a bad result. Physicians and nurses who have good **rapport** with their clients and who establish caring relationships with them often escape lawsuits even when medical malpractice exists. Clients are much less likely to sue their friends, those people whom they perceive genuinely care about them.

Standards of Care

All professionals practicing in the medical field are held to certain standards when they administer care. These standards dictate what type of care is appropriate for a particular client. The **standards of care** for physicians are different from those for nurses. Likewise, the standards of care are different for registered nurses than for practical nurses.

Standards of care ensure that you will be "judged by the company you keep." Perinatal nurses will be expected to know and to do what other nurses practicing that specialty are expected to know and do.

Standards of care come from several sources, including laws, organizational standards, and institutional policies and procedures. They are interpreted by case law, enumerated by expert witnesses, and constantly in a state of change.

Laws

The most common type of laws influencing the nursing standards of care are nursing practice acts. These acts broadly define the scope of nursing practice within a particular state. Laws also dictate the requirements for nursing licensure. Because laws differ from state to state, it is important to be familiar with one's own state licensure laws and nursing practice act. A copy of your state's nursing practice act can be obtained from your state's board of nursing.

Organizational standards

Nursing specialty areas often have state or national organizations to which nurses can look for clarification of their roles. The Association of Women's Health, Obstetric, and Neonatal Nurses (AWHONN) has published standards of practice for nurses, defining what is expected of nurses practicing in perinatology (see Appendix 1B).

Perinatal nurses are expected to be capable of evaluating fetal monitor tracings and identifying certain patterns using specified terminology. Inappropriate terminology would be difficult, if not impossible, to defend in court. It is expected that nurses will maintain the highest level of skill and training throughout the time they practice nursing. As standards of care change and are updated, nurses are expected to be aware of the most current standards of care.

Institutional policies and procedures

Whether the nurse is employed in a hospital, clinic, or outpatient setting, the employing institution has policies and procedures to be followed. It is imperative that nurses be aware of all applicable policies and procedures. Policies and procedures can differ between institutions. It is not at all unusual to find differing policies and procedures within the same metropolitan area. Violation of an internal policy or procedure might be used against the nurse to establish a failure to abide by the applicable standard of care.

Choices when standards differ. Occasionally, a nurse encounters a situation in which the institution's policy seems to conflict with the law or an organizational standard differs from an internal policy. How does one decide in this situation which action to take? The safest way to resolve this conflict—and to avoid legal problems—is to follow the directive that is the *most* restrictive (Figure 30-2).

TEST *Yourself* 30-1 _____

When a problem occurs, how do you discover the correct standard of care?

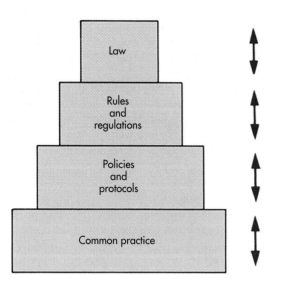

Figure 30-2 Relationship of law to rules, regulations, policies, and common practice. When questions arise, the most restrictive practice is the safest to follow.

Case law

When a case is decided in court, that decision sets a precedent for other courts addressing the same issue. How closely another court will follow an established precedent depends on how similar the issues are and where the original precedent was set. For example, a court in the Midwest is more likely to follow the precedent set by another court in the same region than one set on the West or East Coast.

When a court of similar jurisdiction has previously decided a case much like one in which you are involved, you can usually expect that your case will reach the same or a similar outcome. Case law lends an element of predictability to an otherwise unpredictable field. It is also sets a standard of care that is expected to be met in a similar situation in the future.

Expert witness testimony

Whenever a court case involves subject matter that is beyond the understanding of the average person, the court requires the use of an **expert witness**. The expert's role in a malpractice case is to clarify for the jury what the acceptable standard of care is for those accused of wrongdoing. After explaining to the jury what the reasonable and prudent nurse should have done in a particular situation, the expert is then asked if the nurse (defendant) abided by the acceptable standard of care.

To qualify as an **expert nurse witness**, the nurse must have expertise in the area that is the subject matter of the trial. The more highly credentialed the expert is shown to be, the more credible the expert's testimony will be to the jury. An expert nurse witness can only testify as to the standard of care for nurses, not to that for physicians.

Theories of Liability

Litigation may occur based on several different theories. Although the most common litigation is the allegation of negligence in the form of medical malpractice, causes of action can also be based on wrongful death, wrongful birth, and wrongful life.

Medical malpractice

Malpractice can be defined as "negligence by a professional that causes an injury." **Negligence** is the failure to act as a reasonable person would. The allegation of medical malpractice against a health care provider is difficult to prove in court. To satisfy the burden of proof "by a preponderance of the evidence," the plaintiff must establish that all four of the elements of a medical malpractice lawsuit exist:
- A *duty*
- A *breach of duty*
- An *injury*
- The *proximate causation* between the breach of duty and the injury

Duty to provide care. For health care professionals to successfully be charged with malpractice, it must be shown that they had a duty to provide care to the client. For a duty to arise, there must be a professional relationship with the client. If a client delivers an infant in a grocery store, she cannot sue the nurse at the hospital for malpractice because the nurse could not have had a legal duty to a client with whom the nurse did not have any relationship. Once the nurse-client relationship is established, however, the nurse has a duty to treat the client in accordance with acceptable standards of care.

Sometimes a nurse encounters a situation away from the clinical setting in which a delivery is imminent. A nurse who acts as a *good samaritan* enjoys some immunity from lawsuit. A good samaritan is a person who renders emergency assistance while off duty and without receiving compensation. Most states have some type of good samaritan legislation that makes it more difficult for the beneficiary of the treatment to sue the health care provider who acts as a good samaritan. However, the immunity from lawsuit is not absolute. Good samaritans can be sued for conduct that is grossly negligent, reckless, or blatantly outside of the scope of licensure. In all circumstances, the nurse must remain within the scope of nursing practice. For example, an off-duty nurse who encounters a situation in a supermarket in which delivery is imminent can assist in the delivery with minimal risk of being sued. But a nurse who decides to perform a cesarean section in the same situation will probably not be able to invoke the protection of good samaritan laws.

Although most states do not require a health care provider to act as a good samaritan, a few states do impose this legal duty to act. The legislative intent behind good samaritan laws is to encourage knowledgeable health care providers to assist in emergency situations by reducing the risk that they will be held liable for their actions.

Breach of duty. A breach of a nurse's duty is the failure to abide by or live up to the acceptable standard of care. The breach of the duty consists of *either* an act or an omission. The duty to a client can be breached by doing something that should not have been done or by not doing something that should have been done.

In a North Dakota case in which an infant was born with severe brain damage the court held that the nurse's failure to attach a client to a fetal monitor when it was ordered by the physician was a breach of the nurse's professional duty to the client. The jury in this case awarded $7,800,00 to the plaintiff.[1]

Injury or damages. The terms *injury* and *damages* are often used interchangeably in lawsuits. More exactly, however, the damages usually refer to the monetary value of the injury.

A client who does not sustain an injury as a result of an alleged negligent act does *not* have a malpractice case because one of the four necessary elements is missing. There must be an ascertainable injury for a lawsuit for malpractice to succeed.

Proximate causation. Proving proximate causation is probably the most difficult part of a malpractice action. The plaintiff must prove that the *breach* of the *duty* was the direct and *proximate cause* of the *injury* and that the injury was a foreseeable consequence of the breach of the duty (see Box 30-1).

Foreseeability means that the type of injury sustained must be the type of consequence that one would reasonably expect from a particular negligent act. For example, if a client is negligently over-medicated, it would be foreseeable that the client would require a longer hospital stay. But it is *not* foreseeable that the client would be injured by the collapse of a ceiling while continuing his hospital stay. The damage from the overmedication would *not* include the injuries sustained in the ceiling collapse.

On the other hand, if this same client developed a thrombosis as a direct result of the continued immobility from the treatment of the overmedication, that could become part of the suit for injury. The proximate causation is often the greatest challenge faced by the plaintiff's attorney. A lawsuit was brought in Louisiana alleging that the physician failed to arrive at the hospital in time. The client developed a concealed placental abruption that resulted in the death of the premature infant. The court held that although the obstetrician was negligent in his medical treatment of the woman in labor because his delay caused her needless suffering and anxiety, the evidence was insufficient to prove that the infant died as a result of his delay in arriving at the hospital. The court held that the signs of the abruption did not occur until after he was in attendance and could not have been detected earlier, even if he had been in attendance. The court awarded damages for pain and suffering the amount of $20,000, but no damages for the death of the infant were awarded. This case demonstrates how a negligent act can be present but may not be the proximate cause of the injury.[2]

Wrongful death

A pregnancy sometimes ends in tragedy, with the death of a viable infant. When a lawsuit for medical malpractice arises, it is the injured party who is the plaintiff. When the injury results in death, the survivors are the plaintiffs, and they file the lawsuit for the wrongful death of the person.

Wrongful death lawsuits usually allege that the death resulted from the negligence of the defendants. Often the death of the neonate cannot be prevented, and if the court makes such a finding, the lawsuit for wrongful death will be defeated. Such was the case in the Louisiana case where the jury concluded that the infant died as a result of placental abruption, not as a result of the physician's delay in arriving at the hospital.[3]

In some jurisdiction, for a wrongful death action to arise, there must have been a live birth. The issue in a Texas case revolved around whether or not the fetus had died in utero or just after birth. In this case, a fetus presented in footling breech position and was delivered to the shoulders, at which time the cervix clamped tightly around the fetus's neck and umbilical cord. The fetus's limbs were noted to be limp and cyanotic. When the infant was finally delivered, it was lifeless, and resuscitation attempts failed. The court held that no action for wrongful death could ensue.[4]

The courts are currently split on the issue of whether there must be a live birth, and some courts are allowing compensation on a wrongful death theory for the death of an unborn fetus if the fetus was viable at the time of delivery.[5]

Wrongful birth

Wrongful birth lawsuits arise when an "unwanted" child is born. These lawsuits sometimes arise in the context of failed sterilizations, but they also arise when a child is born with a defect that could have been discovered while options to terminate the pregnancy were still open. The premise behind a wrongful birth lawsuit is that the birth might have been prevented. A Virginia court awarded approximately $180,000 to a couple who gave birth to a child with Tay-Sachs disease after the father was mistakenly informed that he was not a carrier of the disease. The laboratory technician had apparently mislabeled his blood sample. The parents alleged that the erroneous test result prevented them from undergoing additional tests that would have confirmed Tay-Sachs early enough that they could have aborted the pregnancy.[6]

In another Tay-Sachs case, the allegation was that the physician failed to inform the parents of the risks of bearing a child with Tay-Sachs disease, so no tests were ever performed and their child was born with the disease.[7]

Wrongful birth actions are not limited to cases involving Tay-Sach but have also been filed by parents who gave birth to children with other defects, such as Down syndrome. Parents should be informed about available testing opportunities, such as amniocentesis, for the detection of possible fetal defects so that they can decide whether or not to avail themselves of these tests and the options they provide.

Wrongful life

Wrongful life is a relatively new cause of action that many states still do not recognize as compensable. In a lawsuit for wrongful life, it is the *child* who claims that he or she should not have been born. The courts in these cases have been reluctant to attach a damage award for the pain and suffering of having been born "defective" but have awarded damages to compensate for a child's care. This is an evolving area of law that can be expected to undergo dramatic changes in the next few years, as more courts must decide whether to recognize this doctrine.

Common Causes of Lawsuits

Who is responsible for what? It is sometimes difficult to determine with exactness where a physician's duty ends and a nurse's duty begins. Often the duties seem to overlap.

In an Illinois case, a breech presentation was not identified by the nurses throughout most of the labor, and once discovered, it was too late for the physician to perform a cesarean section. The infant suffered serious damage as a result of the difficult vaginal delivery. Both the physician and the nurses were sued, so the court held *both* parties responsible for failing to recognize the breech position and awarded $2,900,000 to the plaintiffs.[8]

Another case addressed the issue of whether or not a nurse could diagnose arrest of labor. The Louisiana court held that this diagnosis was the physician's responsibility. The nurse's responsibility was to report the observable facts to the physician.[9]

When differentiating between the nurse's responsibility and the physician's, *expert nurse witnesses*, not expert physician witnesses, must be called to determine the applicable standard of care for nurses. In a California case, the court held that a physician cannot testify as to an appropriate nursing standard of care.[10]

Frequently, when a physician is the defendant, the nurse will also be drawn into the lawsuit, and vice versa. Regardless of who is ultimately found to be responsible, both parties experience the trauma and disruption that accompany being subjected to a lawsuit. On a more positive note, it is clear that many lawsuits can be successfully defended by the nurses, the physician, or both.

Lawsuits against physicians

Lawsuits brought against physicians and nurses differ, reflecting the well-recognized differences between these professions and their responsibilities. Although there are many reasons for litigation, a likely allegation against a physician might be one of the following:

- Failure to diagnose a high-risk pregnancy
- Delay in performing a cesarean section
- Improper vaginal delivery or failure to perform a cesarean section
- Improper use of forceps
- Incidents surrounding inducing labor and the use of oxytocin
- Delay in arriving at the hospital
- Nonattendance at the delivery

Lawsuits against physicians occur much more frequently than those against nurses.

Lawsuits against nurses

Many of the bases for lawsuits against nurses do not arise out of issues unique to the perinatal specialty area. In fact, most of the liability issues facing perinatal nurses are very similar to those faced by nurses in other specialty areas. But for purposes of this chapter, these issues will be considered primarily in the context of the perinatal nurse.

Medications. Many lawsuits against nurses are the result of problems arising out of medication functions. Considering the amount of time nurses spend in various aspects of medication administration, this should come as no surprise. Allegations against nurses include (but are not limited to) improper client identification; wrong medication, dosage, route, or time; and failure to monitor for side effects. In the perinatal context, the administration of oxytocin is a factor in many of the lawsuits filed.

Nurses are often involved in the administration of oxytocin for the augmentation of labor. It is imperative that the nurses be aware of all nursing standards relating to the induction or augmentation of labor, including all AWHONN standards and hospital procedures. Nurses must also be aware of the signs and symptoms of any complications of oxytocin administration and must report any problems immediately (see Chapter 16).

Failure of client monitoring. Failure to assess the client and failure to recognize changes in the client's condition can lead to a charge of client abandonment. Nurses are expected to monitor their clients at appropriate time intervals that depend upon the client's condition.

Sometimes the physician's directive can be used to determine how often a client is to be monitored and for what. At other times, hospital policies and procedures dictate how often a particular aspect of client monitoring should be done. Without any specific directives, it is often up to nursing judgment.

Labor and delivery pose a unique monitoring challenge because there are two clients to monitor—the mother and the infant. The delivering mother must be adequately monitored to prevent any maternal complications during the antepartal period. Any substantial increases or decreases in the mother's blood pressure could affect the infant's welfare. The same is true for any other alterations of vital signs, such as elevated temperature or pulse. Any variation from the normal must be reported and corrected to prevent possible harm to the infant.

The fetus is the other client to be monitored, especially during labor. Many lawsuits have arisen as a result of problems related to fetal monitoring. In most institutions, electronic fetal monitoring has become the standard. Some institutions routinely monitor all labor and delivery situations. Whenever possible, it is prudent to use electronic fetal monitoring.

Lawsuits arising from problems regarding fetal monitoring can result in a variety of allegations against nurses. Allegations of wrongdoing often involve the failure to use a monitor when indicated, failure to continue monitoring, failure to correctly interpret the monitor strip, or failure to report nonreassuring or ominous fetal heart patterns (see Chapter 14).

Failure to use electronic fetal monitor when ordered or indicated. In North Dakota, a jury awarded a $7,800,000 judgment against a nurse who failed to place a client on a fetal monitor. The physicians had left standing orders that all of their clients were to be placed on monitors. The nurse mistakenly thought that all of the monitors were in use and thus did not attach the monitor until more than 1 hour after the client's arrival at the hospital. When finally applied, the fetal monitor indicated fetal distress and an emergency cesarean section was performed. The infant was severely brain damaged.[11]

Failure to leave monitor on. A nurse was found liable in a Nebraska case in which one of the allegations of negligence was that the fetal monitor was disconnected from a client about 12 hours before the client delivered an infant with cerebral palsy. The infant later died.[12]

Failure to correctly interpret fetal monitor tracings. In the previously referenced Nebraska case, the court also addressed the issue of whether it is the physician's or the nurse's responsibility to monitor and interpret fetal heart rate tracings. This case seems to say that the physician should be allowed to rely on a nurse's interpretation of fetal heart rate monitoring. Perinatal nurses are expected to be capable of interpreting fetal heart rate tracings and, according to AWHONN, they are expected to use appropriate and correct terminology when referring to the information on these tracings. Nurses have a tremendous responsibility to develop fetal monitor interpretation skills and to use them.

Failure to report abnormal fetal heart monitor results to the physician. A nurse should be able to recognize a nonreassuring fetal monitor tracing and then has an obligation to notify the physician to come to the hospital, according to the jury in a Washington case.[13] In another case in Virginia, the nurse was found liable when she did not notify the physician of trouble until almost a half hour after the problems were noticed on the fetal monitor tracing. The infant was born with severe neurologic deformities and the jury awarded the plaintiff $3,500,000; the Supreme Court of Virginia later affirmed the verdict.[14]

Failure to adequately assess the client. One of the most basic nursing responsibilities is that of client assessment. Every nurse, regardless of the area of practice, is expected by virtue of his or her licensure to be capable of performing a client assessment. The inability to do so is difficult, if not impossible, to defend in court. The nurse, after all, is the member of the health care team who is with the client constantly and is responsible for the minute-by-minute evaluation of the client's progress.

Nowhere is this more true than in labor and delivery, where monitoring the progress of the client's labor through delivery is the purpose of the unit's existence. The nurse must carefully and continuously assess the progress of both clients—mother and infant.

In addition to performing electronic fetal monitoring, the nurse is responsible for assessing the normal progress of labor by checking dilation, effacement, and contractions. The nurse must also be cognizant of changes that might indicate problems, such as alterations in vital signs. When the nurse is faced with premature rupture of the membranes, the client's temperature and white blood count must be monitored when assessing a client for infection.

Nurses in all specialty areas must maintain the highest level of assessment skills because these nurses often operate with a greater degree of autonomy than do nurses in other areas.

Failure to report client's changed conditions. Any abnormalities or changes in the patient's condition must be reported to the physician. The physician then has an obligation to the patient to provide the proper medical intervention.[15] In Ohio, a nurse's failure to report a client's elevated pulse, temperature, and white blood cell count to the physician was alleged to have denied the physician the opportunity to intervene sooner in the client's treatment, resulting in stillbirth from chorioamnionitis.[16]

When a nurse reports a client's changed condition to the physician and the nurse feels that the physician has not responded in a manner that is in the client's best interest, the nurse must *proceed up the chain of command,* according to the institution's policies and procedures, until proper medical care is given to the client. Usually the first step up the chain is to the nurse's supervisor. The nurse, as the client's advocate, is expected to take such action to protect the client.

TEST *Yourself* 30-2 _____

a. What is the nurse's responsibility when the client's condition changes?
b. You disagree intensely with how the woman's labor is being handled by the physician, and you fear malpractice. What is the best action for you to take?

Other causes of malpractice litigation

The kidnapping of infants from nurseries has increased over the years; consequently, most hospitals have taken steps to make their nurseries more secure. When a kidnapping does occur, a lawsuit frequently follows alleging that security was inadequate. Nurses sometimes wonder what their responsibility is in preventing newborn kidnapping. One obligation that can be imposed on nurses is to be alert on one's unit for suspicious persons or behavior and to question any unrecognized person claiming to be an employee. Any suspicious persons or incidents should be reported to security personnel (see Chapter 19).

Occasionally, lawsuits arise that seem to be based on facts that are almost too extraordinary to be believed. Yet some outrageous acts do occur and do result in lawsuits. For instance, in North Carolina, a nurse gave a sandwich to a client in labor, the client aspirated the food, and the infant suffered severe brain damage.[17] In yet another bizarre case, a nurse in New York was sued for injuries sustained when the nurse pushed a partially delivered infant back into the uterus.[18] In Michigan, a woman was told on admission to the hospital that her infant would not be born for hours because she was not dilated. Shortly thereafter, while she was returning to bed from the bathroom, she delivered the baby—onto the floor. The infant sustained a skull fracture and was mentally retarded.[19]

Consent

Treating a client without obtaining the proper consent can lead to a charge of assault or battery. These terms are often used together, but do have different meanings. **Assault** is the *threat* of an unauthorized touching of a client. **Battery** is the unauthorized touching of a client.

Informed consent

Informed consent is a well-recognized doctrine based on the client's right to autonomy. Clients have a right to decide what medical treatment they will have performed. To make an intelligent decision regarding medical treatment, clients have a right to sufficient information so the they can make an educated choice. Clients have a right to know that treatment is proposed, the expected outcome, the risks, and what alternative treatment is available.

Informed consent occurs most frequently when the client and the physician are discussing the proposed course of treatment. The physician should document informed consent in the medical record. The nurse is usually the one who obtains the client's signature on the consent form. Sometimes nurses are confused as to their proper role in this informed consent process, and understandably so. Nurses should realize that informed consent is not the same as the consent form. The consent form serves as written proof that informed consent took place.

The courts have generally held that it is the physician's duty to obtain informed consent. But the responsibility for obtaining the client's signature on the consent form can safely be delegated to the nurse, as long as the nurse follows the correct institutional policy and procedure for doing so.

The nurse should approach the client with the consent form and ask the client if the physician has explained the procedure and has answered all of the client's questions. If the client answers affirmatively, the nurse should then ask the client to read and sign the consent form for the hospital record. The nurse can then witness the client's signature. By doing so, the nurse is attesting to the fact that the client voluntarily signed the form.

If the client states that the physician has neither explained the procedure nor answered the client's questions, the nurse must realize that the client has not given informed consent. The nurse should *not* have the client sign the consent form but should instead notify the physician that the client still has questions. Having a client sign a consent form when the nurse knows that informed consent has not been given is substandard nursing practice and can result in the nurse being included with the physician in a lawsuit for assault and battery.

Implied consent

Sometimes a client is incapable of giving consent for treatments, such as in an emergency situation. No one would want to withhold lifesaving treatment from a client just because he or she was unconscious and could not give consent. The law presumes that if a person were capable of giving consent to lifesaving treatment, he or she would do so. This premise resulted in the doctrine of **implied consent**. In an emergency situation in which the client cannot consent to treatment, consent will be "implied-by-law," thereby protecting health care professionals from lawsuits for assault and battery.

Implied consent also applies to situations in which the client has not objected to a current course of treatment. This is often referred to as "implied-in-fact" consent. If you ask a labor and delivery client to hold our her arm so you can start an intravenous line and she does so, consent is implied.

Consent to treat a minor

A minor is defined in most states as a person who has not reached his or her eighteenth birthday. Once a person reaches the age of 18, he or she has legal capacity to consent for medical treatment. Nurses must check their own state's laws regarding minors, since they vary from state to state.

Treating a minor without the consent of the parent or guardian constitutes assault and battery. Some exceptions to this exist. First, in an emergency situation, the doctrine of implied consent covers any treatment given to save the minor's life. Parental consent is *not* necessary in an emergency situation. In fact, parents generally lack legal authority to refuse lifesaving treatment on behalf of their minor children, even if for religious reasons.

Second, an **emancipated minor** can consent to treatment. The definition of emancipation varies from state to state, but it usually includes minors who are married, have a child, are in the military, or are self-supporting. In most states, minors can also consent for pregnancy-related treatment.

When treating an emancipated minor, not only is parental notification and consent unnecessary, it might also lead to a charge of breach of confidentiality of privileged information.

TEST *Yourself* 30-3 _____

   a. What is the difference between informed and implied consent?
   b. What should you do if the client feels she still has unanswered questions and you have come to get a signature on the consent form?
   c. In a labor situation, give an example of assault as compared with an example of battery.

Right to refuse treatment

Generally speaking, competent adults have a right to refuse any medical treatment they do not want, even if it means they will die without it. Sometimes pregnant women wish to refuse treatment, even though the infant might suffer as a result of the mother's decision. This problem has led to an ethical dilemma. When is it appropriate to force unwanted treatment on the mother to benefit the infant?

This has not been an easy issue to resolve because someone's rights are violated regardless of which decision is made. The problem for the courts and for society is to make the determination of whose rights take precedence in a particular case.

Some courts have been known to order a mother to undergo a cesarean section in spite of religious opposition when there is a high likelihood that the infant will suffer damage or die during a vaginal delivery. However, other forms of treatment, particularly those which pose a greater risk to the mother, have not been imposed.

Another issue closely related to this one is whether a woman should be penalized for behavior that poses a risk to the fetus. The most prevalent example is that of substance abuse during pregnancy. How far can society go to protect the fetus? Some have advocated incarceration of pregnant drug abusers, though many others have spoken about the inappropriateness and ineffectiveness of such a directive. Again, the dilemma arises as we try to determine whose rights are superior and to what extent the other's rights can be violated.

There are no definitive answers to this conflict at this time, only more questions. Nurses should keep abreast of developments in this area.

Box 30-2
CLINICAL DECISION

Think of a clinical situation you have observed where there is potential for a lawsuit. Analyze the demeanor of the staff, the degree of informed consent, and the nursing responsibilities that may not have been met.

Abortion

Abortion is probably the most controversial issue any of us has faced in our lifetime. Those who favor abortion rights believe as passionately in their position as those who oppose abortion. So volatile is this controversy that violent attacks have occurred against employees at clinics that provide abortion services.

The nursing profession mirrors the societal conflict that exists concerning abortion. Many nurses consider themselves prochoice, whereas many others consider themselves prolife. Nurses on both sides of the issue are confronted with client care situations in which a woman is either having an abortion performed of is being treated for complications of an abortion. How will the nurse who morally opposes abortion deal with the above scenarios?

Nursing issues

Nurses cannot be forced to participate in procedures they find morally offensive. Nurses have a right to refuse to assist with abortions. However, a nurse cannot attempt to stop an abortion from being performed.[20]

The nurse also has a legal obligation to take care of a client who has undergone an abortion or who is being treated for complications of an abortion. To refuse care to a client in this situation is to make a character judgment upon which the provision of nursing care is based. Nurses are not allowed to do that. If a nurse refused to treat a client after an abortion and the client suffered because of the lack of nursing care, the nurse could be sued.

Minor requesting abortion

Several recent cases have addressed the issue of a minor's right to consent to abortion. Many states have attempted to pass laws limiting a minor's access to abortion without parental approval. The states differ tremendously on this issue, and the laws are in a constant state of change. Even when a law is passed, often an injunction is filed to block it before the law goes into effect. After this, the higher court either upholds the law or decides that it is unconstitutional.

This will be a difficult area for nurses to remain current in, but if a nurse is working in a setting where abortions are performed on minors, it is imperative that the nurse find a way to keep abreast of this constantly changing issue.

MALPRACTICE PREVENTION

The best defense to a malpractice action is *prevention*. However, malpractice prevention is no accident. It requires conscious attention to the two "Ds" of malpractice defense—demeanor and documentation.

Demeanor

The manner in which a nurse treats a client sets the stage for the likelihood of a lawsuit in the event of an adverse outcome. In malpractice prevention, nurses must never underestimate the power of rapport with the client.

Nursing care is delivered by human beings and consequently is subject to human error. When a negligent error results in an injury, the lawsuit climate is created. Whether the client takes the next step—going to the lawsuit—is likely to depend on the nurse's **demeanor** while treating the client. Simply put, given two identical poor client outcomes, the risk of a lawsuit might *not* be equal.

What determines whether an adverse outcome proceeds to a lawsuit? The nurse's rapport with the client. Remember this formula:

Adverse Outcome + *Uncaring Demeanor* = Lawsuit

Developing good rapport with clients is an important part of malpractice prevention. A lawsuit is often circumvented when the staff treats the client with warmth and caring.

Communication skills

The ability to develop good rapport with clients is dependent on the nurse's having good interpersonal communication skills. Listening is by far the most important communication skill. It is imperative that the nurse learn to listen to what the client says.

In a Kansas case, the jury found the nurse negligent when the client's husband's repeated requests to call the physician were ignored. The nurse told the husband that the client was dilated only 7 cm; therefore there was no need to notify the physician. The husband told the nurse that his wife had previously delivered an infant while dilated only 8 cm, but the nurse still ignored the request that the physician be called. The woman delivered only a few minutes later, with no physician in attendance.[21]

Besides listening to the client, the nurse must also be carefully attuned to the client's nonverbal communications. Communication is a two-way street. Information must be communicated from the nurse to the client in an understandable and appropriate manner. Be sure discharge instructions give the client enough information to adequately take care of herself and her infant after she goes home. Discharge instructions should be communicated orally *and* in writing.

The manner is which communication occurs between a nurse and a client has been at issue in court cases. In a Puerto Rican case, the court indicated that a reasonably prudent nurse would *not* make disparaging remarks to a client.[22]

Documentation

Once a lawsuit is filed, correct and complete documentation is by far the best defense. The client's medical record is a legal document and is admissible in court as evidence. It enjoys a privileged status in that it is presumed to be an accurate account of what transpired. This is because it was written at the time the alleged mistreatment occurred by someone with knowledge of the events and before litigation was initiated.

The **documentation** in the medical record must be able to stand on its own in proving that the standard of care was met. Omission of information from the medical record leads to the charge that the standard of care was violated. Unfortunately for the nurse, filling in the gaps in the medical record later—in court—will not suffice to prove that the standard of care was met. Spoken words have, at best, questionable credibility in a courtroom.

A case is only as good as the proof that is presented in court. Spoken words are often felt to be self-serving and therefore cannot prove the case. Why should a jury believe that you provided continuous nursing care when your documentation indicates otherwise? Given the opportunity, the jury will choose to believe what is documented in the medical record instead of the spoken words they hear in court. In addition, thorough documentation will help the nurse refresh his or her memory regarding the incident if a lawsuit is filed later. It often takes years for these cases to arise. If documentation is thorough and complete it will also be easier for you to later remember details of the incident.

Juries often assume that if something was not charted, it was not done. Nurses should give themselves credit for care they provided by thoroughly documenting it in the client's medical record.

Documentation format

The trend in recent years has been to move away from straight narrative charting and toward flow sheets. Sometimes nurses question whether these flow sheets are sufficient to defend them in a lawsuit. However, it is not the format but the completeness of the documentation that determines its adequacy. A complete and thorough flow sheet is better than an incomplete, vague narrative note, and a complete narrative note defends better than an incomplete flow sheet. The key is to provide all of the pertinent information about the client and the nursing care given. The format is secondary.

When using flow sheets, the nurse should be careful not to let the small spaces on the flow sheet discourage thorough reporting of information. If the flow sheet is not adequately telling the whole story, *it must be supplemented* with a narrative note. Nurses do not get into legal trouble by documenting too much—it is usually *too little documentation* that causes problems. A general documentation rule by which to live is, when in doubt as to how much to document, document *more* not *less.*

Documentation tips to stay out of court

1. *Write legibly.* An illegible entry cannot serve its intended purpose, which is to communicate information. If the jury cannot read it, it can not be relied on to provide a defense in court.
2. *Use ink.* The medical record is a legal document. When written, it is intended to be permanent. To ensure its permanency, always use ink. Using pencil is dangerous because anyone could erase the entry and replace it with something else.
3. *Never obliterate an entry.* If you make an error in the chart, follow your institution's policy for error correction, which usually entails drawing one line through the incorrect entry—so it can still be read—and inserting the correct information. An obliterated entry can be used by your opponent to imply that pertinent information has been removed from the record, and you might not be able to prove otherwise because no one can read what you obliterated.
4. *Fill in all blanks and lines.* A flow sheet should be completely filled in; otherwise someone else could come in later and fill in inaccurate information. In a narrative note, no lines should be left blank, despite a request by a co-worker that this be done so that he or she can fill it in later.
5. *Date and time entries.* Sometimes the time at which something happened is very important. If a nurse notifies a physician of a problem with a client, the nurse should document when the problems began, when the physician was notified, and when the physician arrived. Documenting this sequence can prove that the nurse acted properly and recorded his or her nursing assessment, as well as the physician notification and response.
6. *Document thought processes.* When faced with a situation where nursing judgment comes into play and decisions have to be made, document the process by

which the decision is reached. Doing so can ensure that the jury knows that the judgment made was the correct one in that situation. For example, you might have a physician's order to get the client "up in a chair twice a day for 15 minutes." You get her up, and after only 5 minutes, she complains of being lightheaded and nauseous and feels she will pass out. The appropriate nursing intervention is to return her to bed. If you only document "up in chair for 5 minutes,"it appears that you did not follow the physician's order. If, however, you document the details of your client's response to being up in the chair, it becomes clear that returning the client to bed was the correct decision.
7. *Be objective.* Document what you see and hear, not just conclusions. Do not document "client fell" unless you saw the client fall. Document your observations, such as "client found on floor."
8. *Describe behavior's, do not make personal judgments.* Do not document "client is hostile" or "client is drunk." Instead, describe the behaviors objectively, and leave the conclusion to the imagination of the reader. A record that describes a client who has "reddened eyes, staggering gait, slurred speech, and admits to consuming a case of beer" *informs* the reader, but it makes no personal judgment about the client's character.
9. *Never air grievances with personnel in the chart.* The chart is not a battleground for wars among the staff. Criticizing in the client's medical record the actions of the previous shift or the physician is inappropriate.
10. *Document the client's noncompliance with treatment.* In the event a client chooses to refuse to comply with medical advice, the client should not be able to sue the health care team for injuries brought on by his or her own noncompliance. Documenting the noncompliance in the medical record is imperative to defeat a lawsuit brought by the noncompliant client. If a client with threatened premature labor is sent home with strict instructions to stay in bed and the client admits to playing tennis, this admission should be documented. In the event this client's infant has problems, the defense will put the blame back on the woman in proving that the medical staff did not violate any standard of care.
11. *Document your assessment.* This proves that you attended to your client appropriately. If the client is attached to a fetal monitor, include this information in the medical record. If you do not document the results of your assessments, the jury might assume they were not done.
12. *Document your intervention.* When your assessment shows something abnormal about your client's condition, your duty is to address the problem. The chart must include what you did for the client at that point. For example, if a client complains of pain, and you

administer pain medication, that fact must be documented. If your client's blood pressure drops and you notify the physician, document that you did so. The record must reflect not only that problems were assessed but that the appropriate interventions were instituted.

13. *Document physician contact.* When a physician is notified, document the physician's name, the time the conversation took place, what the physician was told, and the physician's response. Many disputes erupt between nurses who claim they called the physician and physicians who allege they were never notified.

If you are involved in litigation, your documentation will be either your best friend or your worst enemy. Time spent documenting is time well spent in the prevention of a lawsuit.

Box **30-3**

CLINICAL DECISION

Do a chart review together with your classmates, analyzing labor documentation for the 13 documentation tips listed in this chapter.

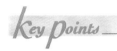

Key Points

- There may be no right or wrong answer in ethical dilemmas, and each person's perspective must be heard and valued.
- In this heterogeneous society, many cultures coexist side by side. The values of one group may conflict with the values of another, which results in laws that govern behavior.
- Law should be viewed both with respect and suspicion, and laws may be challenged.
- When laws and ethics clash, identify the dilemma, seek clarification, and work with others toward change.
- The professional standing of the perinatal nurse requires that standards of care are adhered to, demeanor is appropriate, and documentation is complete.
- There are ways to reduce the risk of lawsuits. Professional nurses strive to always ensure informed consent, client's rights, and full communication.

- If the nurse is unsure about whether to treat an infant, the best rule is to act.
- Decision making about fetal treatment when conflict is present may be based on four criteria: (1) How certain are the benefits to the client? (2) How great are the benefits? (3) How intrusive, coercive, or harmful will the treatment to the mother be? (4) Will anything be lost or gained by waiting until after birth?
- Decision making after birth must include the understanding that the statue of limitations might not expire for approximately 20 or more years after birth. In situations in which the physician is not following through on treatment in a high-risk case, the nurse has the responsibility to report this fact to an administrative officer and to document the report.

Study Questions

30-1. Select the terms that apply to the following statements:
   a. The level of skill and training expected of every nurse is the _____.
   b. The person bringing the lawsuit who claims to have been harmed is the _____.
   c. The failure to act as a reasonable person is _____.
   d. The nurse's best defense in court if sued is _____.
   e. The period of time in which one must file a lawsuit is the _____.
   f. The person who is sued is the _____.
   g. A person who testifies in court about the appropriate standard of care is an _____.
   h. The reasons why a decision should be made on a given course of action refers to _____.
   i. Attitudes or beliefs that guide how one interacts with others are called _____.

30-2. Which of the following are reasons why lawsuits are increasing?

    a. Clients often perceive a lack of professionalism in health care delivery.

    b. Members of society have a tendency to blame others rather than to take responsibility for their own actions.

    c. Clients may be misinformed about health care issues and what an adverse outcome is.

    d. There continues to be poor communication between physicians and clients.

30-3. Which of the following contributes to the increased risk of lawsuits against perinatal nurses?

    a. Perinatal nurses are more likely than other nurses to make mistakes.

    b. Obstetric clients are well aware that there might be complications of pregnancy and are prepared for them.

    c. Perinatal nurses are held to a higher standard of care and operate with more autonomy than do many other nurses.

    d. The statute of limitations for minors is brief, thereby limiting the amount of time to file a lawsuit.

30-4. Which of the following is *not* an element of informed consent?

    a. The client should be informed as to how long she will be hospitalized.

    b. The client should be told the nature of the procedure to be performed.

    c. The client should be told the risks of the procedure to be performed.

    d. The client should be told about alternative treatments that are available.

30-5. The nurse presents the consent form to the client for signature. The client states that she still has some questions about the proposed procedure. What should the nurse do?

    a. Ask the client to sign the form, and tell her that you will inform the physician immediately about her concerns.

    b. Delay having the client sign the form, and notify the physician that the client is requesting information.

    c. Notify the supervisor to come and explain the procedure to the client.

    d. Proceed with the preoperative medication orders so that the procedure is not delayed beyond its schedule time.

30-6. What four elements must be proven in order for a medical malpractice lawsuit to succeed?

    a. The duty, the breach, the injury, and the proximate causation

    b. The negligence, the proximate causation, the injury, and the neglect

    c. The duty, the intent, the injury, and the proximate causation

    d. The duty, the act, the omission, and the injury

Answer Key

30-1. *a*, Standard of care; *b*, plaintiff; *c*, negligence; *d*, documentation; *e*, statute of limitations; *f*, defendant; *g*, expert witness; *h*, ethics; *i*, values. 30-2: b. 30-3: c. 30-4: a. 30-5: a. 30-6: b.

Footnotes

[1]*Nelson v. Trinity Medical Center,* 419 N.W.2d 886 (1988).

[2]*Coleman v. Touro Infirmary of New Orleans,* 506 So.2d 571 (1987).

[3]*Coleman v. Touro Infirmary of New Orleans,* 506 So.2d 571 (1987).

[4]*Wheeler v. Yettie Kersting Memorial Hospital,* 761 S.W.2d 785 (1988), *The Regan Report on Nursing Law* 29(10):March, 1989.

[5]*Wallace v. Wallace,* 421 A.2d 134 (1980).

[6]*Naccash v. Burger,* 290 S.E.2d 825 (1982).

[7]*Goldberg v. Ruskin,* 471 N.E.2d 530 (1984).

[8]*Alvis v. Henderson Obstetrics, S.C.,* 592 N.E.2d 678 (1992), *The Regan Report on Nursing Law* 33(4):September, 1992.

[9]*Ewing v. Aubert,* 532 So.2d 876 (1988), *The Regan Report on Nursing Law* 29(8):June, 1989.

[10]*Alef v. Alta Bates Hospital,* 6 Cal.Rptr.2d 700 (1992), *The Regan Report on Nursing Law* 33(1):June, 1992.

[11]*Nelson v. Trinity Medical Center,* 419 N.W.2d 886 (1988).

[12]*Miles v. Box Butte County,* 489 N.W.2d 829 (1992), *The Regan Report on Nursing Law* 33(7):December, 1992.

[13]*Garcia v. Providence Medical Center,* 806 P.2d 766 (1991), *The Regan Report on Nursing Law* 32(12):May, 1991.

[14]*Fairfax Hospital System, Inc. v. McCarty,* 419 S.E.2d 621 (1992), *The Regan Report on Nursing Law* 33(6):November, 1992.

[15]*Guzeldere v. Wallin,* 593 N.E.2d 629 (1992), *The Regan Report on Nursing Law* 33(3):August, 1992.

[16]*Clancy v. Euclid General Hospital,* 584 N.E.2d 763 (1989), *The Regan Report on Nursing Law* 32(10):March, 1992.

[17]*Osborne v. Annie Penn Memorial Hospital,* 381 S.E.2d 794 (1989), *The Regan Report on Nursing Law* 30(5):October, 1989.

[18]*DeLeon v. Hospital of Albert Einstein College,* 566 N.Y.S.2d 213 (1991), *The Regan Report on Nursing Law* 31(11):April, 1991.

[19]*May v. William Beaumont Hospital,* 418 N.W.2d 497 (1989), *The Regan Report on Nursing Law* 31(1):June, 1990.

[20]*Collard v. Kentucky Board of Nursing,* 896 F.2d 179 (1990), *The Regan Report on Nursing Law* 30(11):April, 1990.

[21]*Hiatt v. Grace,* 523 P.2d 320 (1974).

[22]*DeLeon Lopez v. Corporacion Insular DeSeguros,* 931 F.2d 116 (1991), *The Regan Report on Nursing Law* 32(2):July, 1991.

References

American Nurses Association: *Protocols for women's primary care,* ANA Publication No. Ms-20, 1995.

Bernzweig EP: *The nurse's liability for malpractice: a programmed course,* ed 6, St Louis, 1996, Mosby.

Birkholz G: Malpractice data from the National Practitioner Data Bank, *Nurse Practitioner: American Journal of Primary Health Care* 20(3):32, 1995.

Calfee BE: Steering clear of trouble: litigation lessons . . . malpractice cases involving nurses, *Nursing* 24(1):64, 1994.

Fiesta J: Law for the nurse manager: failing to act like a professional, *Nursing Management* 25(7):15, 1994.

Fiesta J: *20 legal pitfalls for nurses to avoid,* Albany, NY 1994, Delmar Publishers.

Fiesta J: Law for the nurse manager: legal update, 1995—Part I, *Nursing Management* 27(5):22, 1996.

Glover JJ, Rushton CH: Introductions: from Baby Doe to Baby K: evolving challenges in pediatric ethics, *J Am Society of Law, Medicine, and Ethics,* 1997 (in press).

Hardy-Havens DM, Hannan C: Legislation to mandate maternal and newborn length of stay, *J Pediatr Health Care* 10(3):141, 1996.

McMullen P, Philipsen N: Legal issues. Fetal well-being III: strategies to diminish liability and improve patient care in all trimesters, *Nursing Connections* 8(1):50, 1995.

McRae MJ: Litigation, external fetal monitoring and the obstetric nurse, *J Obstet Gynecol Neonatal Nurs* 22(5):410, 1993.

Rhodes AM: Malpractice litigation, *MCN Am J Matern Child Nurs* 19(5):257, 1994.

Rhodes AM: Guardianship and the refusal of treatment, *MCN Am J Matern Child Nurs* 20(2):109, 1995.

Rhodes AM: Drug use during pregnancy, *MCN Am J Matern Child Nurs* 21(3):127, 1996.

Tammelleo AD: Fetal monitor delay: "proximate cause" issue, *The Regan Report on Nursing Law* 31(3):10, 1991.

Tammelleo AD: Nursing notes can be worth their weight in gold, *The Regan Report on Nursing Law* 33(8):3, 1992.

Ethical Issues

American Academy of Pediatrics Committee on Bioethics: Guidelines on forgoing life-sustaining medical treatment, *Pediatr Nurs* 20(5):517, 1994.

*American Nurses Association: *Code for nurses with interpretive statements,* Kansas City, Mo, 1986, ANA.

Bishop AH, Scudder JR: *The practical, moral, and personal sense of nursing: a phenomenological philosophy of practice,* Albany, NY 1990, State University of New York Press.

Cesar NS et al: Informed consent: an ethical dilemma, *Nursing Forum* 30(3):20, 1995.

Donahue M: Maternal-fetal health: Ethical issues, *AHWONNS Clin Issues Perinat Womens Health Nurs,* 4(4):561, 1993.

Doukas DJ et al: Compelled cesarean section: an ethical perspective, *Prim Care* 20(3):721, 1993.

Edgar A: Confidentiality and personal integrity, *Nursing Ethics* 1(2):86, 1994.

*Fry ST: Toward a theory of nursing ethics, *Advances in Nursing Science* 11(4):9, 1989.

Fry-Revere S: Anencephalic newborns: Legal and ethical comments regarding the matter of baby "K," *Pediatr Nurs* 20(3):283, 1994.

*Gilligan C: *In a different voice,* Cambridge, Mass, 1982, Harvard University Press.

*Gilligan C, Lyons NP, Hanmer TJ: *Making connections,* Troy, NY, 1989, Emma Willard School.

Harrison H: The principles for family-centered neonatal care, *Pediatrics* 92(5):643, 1993.

Heeg P: Ethics and the decision making process, *Contemp Nurse* 4(2):76, 1995.

*Classic reference.

Husted GL, Husted JH: *Ethical decision making in nursing,* St Louis, 1995, Mosby.

*Kohlberg L: *Essays on moral development,* vol 2, *The psychology of moral development,* New York, 1984, Harper & Row.

Lagana K, Dunderstadt K: *Ethical decision making for perinatal nurses,* White Plains, NY, 1995, March of Dimes Birth Defects Foundation.

Millette BE: Using Gilligan's framework to analyze nurse's stories of moral choices, *West J Nurs Res* 16(6):660, 1994.

Nelson LJ, Nelson RM: Ethics and the provision of futile, harmful, or burdensome treatment to children, *Crit Care Med* 20(3):427, 1992.

Online Database: BIOETHICSLINE, search through MEDLARS network.

Rose P: Best interests: a concept analysis and its implication for ethical decision making in nursing, *Nursing Ethics* 2(2):149, 1994.

Rushton CH: The baby K case: ethical challenges of preserving professional integrity, *Pediatr Nurs* 21(4):367, 1995.

Rushton CH, Hogue EE: Confronting unsafe practice: ethical and legal issues, *Pediatr Nurs* 19(3):284, 1993.

Rushton CH, Scanlon C: When values conflict with obligations: safeguards for nurses, *Pediatr Nurs* 21(3):260, 1995.

Sachs DA et al: Caring for the female Jehovah's Witness: balancing medicine, ethics and the first amendment, *Am J Obstet Gynecol* 170(2):452, 1994.

*Thompson JE, Thompson HO: *Bioethical decision making for nurses,* Norwalk Town, Conn, 1985, Appleton-Century-Crofts.

*Thompson JE, Thompson HO: Teaching ethics to nursing students, *Nurs Outlook* 37(2):84, 1989.

Tschudin V et al: Nursing ethics IV: theories and principles, *Nurs Standards* 9(2):51, 1994.

Viens DC: The moral reasoning of nurse practitioners, *J Am Acad Nurse Pract* 7(6):277, 1995.

 Student Resource Shelf

Fiesta J: Law for the nurse manager. Obstetrical liability update—Part I, *Nurs Manage* 26(7): 24, 1995.

Fiesta J: Law for the nurse manager. Obstetrical liability update—Part II, *Nurs Manage* 26(8):22, 1995.

Fiesta J: Law for the nurse manager. Obstetrical liability update—Part III, *Nurs Manage* 26(9):31, 1995.
   The author publishes updates at regular intervals, reviewing legal aspects for nursing practice.

Hogue EE: Managing your risk of legal liability, *Pediatr Nurs* 19(4):366, 1993.
   Outlines steps to reduce risk of liability.

McFadden EA: Moral development and reproductive health decision, *J Obstet Gynecol Nurs* 25(6):507, 1996.
   Reviews concepts of biomedical ethics, with the justice and care perspectives contrasted. Focuses on uniqueness of women's experiences.

Sorich MP, Letizia M: Nursing malpractice litigation: a personal journey, *MCN Am J Matern Child Nurs* 19(5):249, 1994.
   A personal experience that brings home the reality of being sued.

Glossary

A

abortion Termination of pregnancy when the fetus weighs less than 500 g or loss of pregnancy before 139 days (20 weeks from last menstrual period)

  complete Expulsion of all products of conception

  habitual Three or more consecutive spontaneous abortions

  incomplete Expulsion of some, but not all, products of conception

  induced Deliberate interruption of pregnancy for therapeutic or nontherapeutic reasons (elective termination)

  inevitable Progressive cervical dilation before week 20 without expulsion of fetus

  missed Embryo or fetus dies within the uterus but remains for 8 or more weeks

  spontaneous Termination of pregnancy without assistance (miscarriage)

abruptio placentae (premature separation) Separation of normally implanted placenta at 20 or more weeks of pregnancy, causing possible concealed or overt bleeding

acceleration of fetal heart rate Increase in fetal heart rate in response to fetal movement, contractions, or maternal medications

accoucheur Someone who assists in the delivery of an infant, such as an obstetrician or midwife

acinus (pl. acini) Smallest saccular division of a gland, occurring in grapelike clusters, as in the mammary gland

acrocyanosis Cyanotic or bluish discoloration of hands or feet of a newborn as a result of inadequate circulation or coldness

active phase *See* labor

afterbirth Products of conception (excluding the infant) expelled during delivery; includes placenta, membranes (sac), and umbilical cord; *syn.*, secundines

afterpains Discomfort caused by contraction of uterus after childbirth as it returns to its prepregnant condition, usually occurring in the multipara

allele Two copies of the same gene—one from father, one from mother; also called matching genes

alpha-fetoprotein (AFP) Protein produced by fetal yolk sac and liver, detectable by 7

weeks gestation, and used for determining and identifying certain birth defects and chromosomal anomalies; *see also* maternal serum alpha-fetoprotein (MSAFP)

amenorrhea Cessation or absence of menstruation

amniocentesis Removal of some amniotic fluid from the amniotic sac using a needle inserted through the abdominal wall of the mother; procedure to obtain fluid for detection of genetic diorders, fetal abnormalities, and fetal lung maturity

amnioinfusion Technique of infusing fluid into amniotic sac during labor via an intrauterine catheter

amnion Inner layer of fetal membranes or sac, that secretes amniotic fluid

amniotic fluid embolism Rare postpartum occurrence in which amniotic fluid enters the maternal circulation; the cells, debris, and fluid then form emboli, usually in the lungs

amniotomy Rupturing of amniotic sac by artificial means

androgens Hormones that help produce male secondary sex characteristics; anabolic agents produced in adrenal gland, testis, and ovary; *syn.*, male hormone

anencephaly Malformation of the cranium frequently associated with spina bifida; the cranial vault is absent; the cerebellum and basal ganglia sometimes are present

anorexia Severe loss of appetite

  a. nervosa Eating disorder based on fear of obesity and characterized by severe loss of appetite

anovulatory Associated with lack or absence of ovulation

anoxia (fetal) Severe oxygen deficiency caused by inadequate tissue perfusion; used interchangeably with, but not the same as, hypoxia

antenatal Prenatal, before birth

antepartal Occurring before labor and delivery

antibody Substance produced by the body for protection against the specific antigen that triggered its production

antigen Substance, usually of protein material, that triggers the production of antibodies and the immune response

Apgar score System of numeric evaluation of newborn status at 1 and 5 minutes of birth; based on newborn heart rate, respiration, muscle tone, reflexes, and color

apnea Absence or cessation of respirations

areola Pigmented area surrounding the nipple

arrest of descent Labor complication in which the fetus fails to descend through pelvic cavity, making medical intervention necessary for delivery of fetus

artifact Random marks on fetal heart rate tracing

asphyxia Insufficient oxygen and carbon dioxide exchange, generally resulting in respiratory failure

  birth or neonatal Insufficient exchange within 1 minute of birth

assisted birth Birth that involves use of medication, instrumentation, or surgery

asymptomatic bacteriuria More than $10^4/mm^3$ of bacteria in the urine; no symptoms

attitude Relationship of parts of fetus to each other; usual attitude is flexion (head flexed on chest, thighs folded on abdomen)

autonomic dysreflexia Abnormal response to stimulation that occurs in spinal injuries and results in severe muscle spasms and hypertension

autosome Any one of the 44 chromosomes (22 pairs) present in females and males; contain genes necessary for bodily function—except for sexual determination and function—which is contained in the remaining pair of two sex chromosomes (XY or XX)

B

ballottement Rebounding movement of fetus when uterus (or cervix) is tapped by an examiner; *syn.*, passive fetal movement

basal body temperature (BBT) Lowest usual temperature of the body taken before arising

baseline rate Rate of vital signs before stimulation; for fetal heart rate, before labor starts; during labor, rate between contractions

bilirubin   Yellowish-orange pigment resulting from breakdown of hemoglobin that can cause jaundice of the skin when bilirubin level rises above 5 mg/dl in the newborn

birth defect   Any alteration in fetal growth or development that takes place in utero and that may be evident at birth or later; *syn.*, congenital anomaly

blastocyst   State in early development when fluid accumulates in the morula, producing the inner cell mass at one side while its wall develops into the trophoblast

bradycardia   Fetal heart rate below 110 to 120 beats/min

Braxton Hicks contractions   Painless, intermittent contractions of uterus that occur throughout pregnancy and often are mistaken for early labor contractions

breech   Buttocks

> *breech presentation*   Delivery in which buttocks or feet of fetus appear first at the outlet

> *footling*   One or both feet of fetus appear first at the opening

> *frank*   Buttocks of fetus appear first at the opening

> *full or complete*   Buttocks and feet appear first

bulimia   Eating disorder characterized by episodes of self-induced vomiting after bouts of overeating

C

caput   Head

caput succedaneum   Swelling or edema on fetal scalp occurring in labor or delivery

cephalhematoma   Collection of blood on head of fetus between the bone and the periosteum as a result of trauma of labor and delivery, defined by the suture lines

cephalopelvic disproportion (CPD)   Fetus (fetal head) is too large to pass through bony ring of pelvic cavity; *syn.*, fetopelvic disproportion

cerclage procedure   Procedure for treatment of incompetent cervix; circling sutures

cesarean delivery or birth   Surgical removal of uterine contents through abdominal route after fetal viability testing

chorioamnionitis   Inflammation of amnion and chorion (fetal sac, bag of waters) surrounding fetus

chorion   Outermost membrane of developing fetus, that gives rise to fetal portion of placenta and extends to form the other layer of amniotic sac

chorionic gonadotropin   Hormone produced by the chorion and excreted in urine of the pregnant woman; its presence is a possible sign of pregnancy

chorionic villi   Fingerlike projections of the chorion that invade the decidua basalis and form fetal portion of placenta

chromosome   Units of DNA-containing hereditary material in each body cell; 23 are derived from each parent

cleavage   Process of early cell division by which the zygote divides into blastomeres

cleft lip   Congenital or genetic opening of upper lip extending from nares; may involve one or both nares

cleft palate   Congenital or genetic opening of roof of the mouth

colloid osmotic pressure (COP)   Pressure made up of various components of plasma that exerts influence over movement of fluid across all membranes; *syn.*, oncotic pressure

colonization   Presence of microorganisms on an epithelial surface

colostrum   Yellowish-white fluid expressed from breasts during pregnancy preceding development of milk; caloric and cathartic values of this substance are questioned

conception   Implantation of the blastocyst; not synonymous with fertilization

Coombs' test   Blood test to determine presence of antibodies

> *direct*   Determination of antibodies attached to blood cells, particularly maternal (anti-Rh) antibodies attached to fetal blood cells

> *indirect*   Determination of free-floating or unattached antibodies, particularly those (anti-Rh) in the maternal circulation (serum)

corpus luteum   Yellow body of material found in the site of the ruptured graafian follicle that persists for several months during pregnancy; secretes progesterone

cricoid pressure   Application of pressure to the cricoid cartilage at the critical time of tracheal intubation to prevent aspiration of gastric fluids

crowning   Appearance of the vertex, or head, at the external vaginal orifice

D

decidua   Enriched endometrial lining of pregnancy shed after pregnancy termination

> *d. basalis*   Portion of the endometrium underlying the embedded embryo from which maternal portion of placenta is formed

> *d. capsularis*   Outer portion of decidua surrounding the embryo

> *d. vera*   Remainder of endometrium not containing the embedded embryo

desquamation   Initial peeling of newborn's skin, particularly the wrist and ankle; occurs primarily in postmature infants

developmental crisis   Disruption of life caused by an event common to all in a particular age-group

diagnoses-related groups (DRGs)   System of determining the length of hospital stay to be covered by insurance; based on predefined medical diagnoses and treatments

dilation   Enlargement of an organ or orifice

> *of the cervix*   State of enlargement or opening of cervix to allow for passage of fetus

dilation and curettage (D&C)   Surgical procedure involving dilation of cervix and removal of uterine contents

dilation and evacuation (D&E)   Removal of uterine lining and contents by dilating cervix and evacuating contents by suctioning

discharge (vaginal)   Shedding of accumulated cells, mucus, or blood from the vagina

discoverable documents   Those created in the care of a client that can be subpoenaed by a court and used to present evidence in a lawsuit

disease (infectious)   Infections that produce physical complaints, signs, and symptoms

disseminated intravascular coagulation (DIC)   A bleeding or clotting malfunction that greatly complicates correction of hemorrhage

Down syndrome   Formerly known as mongolism; a congenital or genetic abnormality in which 47 chromosomes are present; *syn.*, trisomy 21 syndrome

dystocia   Difficult or abnormal labor

E

eclampsia   Abnormal reaction of the body to pregnancy, resulting in convulsions and possible coma; usually preceded by hypertension, albuminuria, and edema

ectopic pregnancy   Pregnancy that does not implant in the usual uterine sites

effacement   Thinning of cervix to allow for passage of fetus; in primigravidas, occurs before dilation, and in multigravidas, occurs with dilation

embryo   Conception up to week 10 after the last menstrual period or 8 weeks after fertilization

empowering   Carrying out nursing interventions in a manner in which family members acquire a sense of control over their own development course as a result of their efforts to meet their own needs

enabling   Creating opportunities for family members to become more competent and self-sustaining with respect to their abilities to mobilize their social networks to attain desired goals

endometriosis   Presence of endometrial tissue in the fallopian tube, peritoneum, or bladder, usually leading to infertility with signs of dysmenorrhea

endometritis   Inflammation of the endometrium

engagement Descent of fetus into pelvic canal until presenting part reaches the level of the ischial spines

engorgement Increase of blood and lymph in breast, causing tenderness, firmness, and discomfort before onset of lactation

epidural anesthesia Loss of sensation as a result of injection of local anesthetic drug into epidural space

episiotomy Surgical incision of perineum that enlarges the external vaginal opening to prevent laceration of vulva, perineum, and adjacent structures

erythema toxicum Newborn rash; characteristically blotchy rash seen initially with no pathogenic cause

erythroblastosis fetalis Hemolytic disorder of fetus or newborn in which maternal anti-Rh antibodies destroy fetal blood cells, causing jaundice and other effects

estrogenic hormone Hormone that produces female secondary sexual characteristics; *syn.,* female hormone

F

fertilization Process of penetration of secondary oocyte by spermatozoon; completed with fusion of male and female pronuclei; *syn.,* syngamy

fertilization age Age from fertilization of the ovum to birth

fetal Pertaining to the fetus

fetal death Death in utero after 20 weeks of gestation

fetus Offspring from the moment of conception until pregnancy is terminated or completed

fontanelle Space at the junction of three or more fetal and cranial bones, covered with a tough membrane

　anterior junction of sagittal, frontal, and coronal sutures, or anterior portion of skull; *syn.,* "soft spot," greater fontanelle

　posterior Junction of lambdoid and sagittal sutures; *syn.,* lesser fontanelle

foramen ovale Opening between the right and left atria of the heart in the fetus; closes after birth

fundus Upper portion of uterus

G

gap junction Cell-to-cell communication points that develop in uterine smooth muscle during last week of pregnancy to facilitate coordinating muscle contractions

gaze aversion Avoiding looking at another person's face—particularly seen as a compensation in the overstimulated newborn

gingivitis Inflammation of the gums

G6PD Glucose-6-phosphate dehydrogenase deficiency; inherited erythrocyte enzyme deficiency

gene Functional unit of heredity, situated on a chromosome in the cell nucleus

genotype Assortment of genes of an individual

gestation Length of time necessary for intrauterine growth and development of a fetus

gestational age Estimated age of fetus using the first day of last normal menstrual period, expressed in completed weeks

　preterm Born up to 37 completed weeks (259 days after last menstrual period)

　term Born between 38 and 41 completed weeks (260 to 287 days)

　postterm Born after 288 days or beginning of the week 42

graafian follicle Fluid-filled sac in ovary housing maturing ovum

gravid Pregnant

gravida Pregnant woman

　primigravida Woman pregnant for the first time

　multigravida Woman pregnant for the second time or more

　nulligravida Woman who has never been pregnant

H

half-life (t^{1}/$_{2}$) Measurable amount of time in which half of a drug dose is metabolized in the body

hemorrhage In obstetrics, loss of blood in excess of 500 ml

heterozygous Presence of different genes at same location on DNA chain

homozygous Presence of identical genes at same location on DNA chain

horizontal transmission Passing of infection from one person to another

host defense mechanisms Occur when all areas of the immune system function (*see* immunity)

hyaline membrane disease *See* idiopathic respiratory distress syndrome (RDS)

hydatidiform mole Grapelike, cystic masses of degenerated chorionic villi, usually benign

hydramnios "Water;" excessive amniotic fluid; *syn.,* polyhydramnios

hydrocephaly Abnormal accumulation of cerebrospinal fluid in the brain

hyperemesis gravidarum Excessive, severe vomiting during pregnancy

hypofibrinogenemia Reduced amounts of fibrinogen in blood

hypospadias Congenital or genetic defect in which the urethra of the male opens on underside of penis

hypoxemia Oxygen deficiency in blood

hypoxia Deficient amount of oxygen

I

icterus Jaundice

　icterus gravis neonatorum *See* erythroblastosis fetalis

idiopathic respiratory distress syndrome

Severe respiratory syndrome of the newborn or preterm infant resulting in the development of a hyaline membrane in the lungs; may be fatal; *syn.,* RDS, hyaline membrane disease

immunity Specific response to antigens whereby specific antibodies, which ordinarily combine only with the antigen when the body is again invaded, are formed

　active Inoculation with specific antigens to promote antibody formation

　passive Extrinsic antibodies transferred to fetus across placental membrane or to infant through milk or administered by intramuscular injection to infant, child, or adult; has a time-limited effectiveness

inertia (uterine) Inefficient, weak, or absent uterine contractions

　primary Occurring early in labor

　secondary Occurring after labor is established; *syn.,* uterine dysfunction

infant mortality rate Rate of death, per 1000 births of infants, from birth until the first birthday

inheritance pattern Scheme of inheritance of maternal or paternal genes by dominant, codominant, or recessive patterns

insemination Introduction of semen into vagina

　artificial Concentrated semen introduced into vagina by syringe

　heterologous Semen used is not from woman's partner—artificial insemination donor (AID)

　homologous Semen is from woman's partner—artificial insemination, homologous (AIH)

involution Return of pelvic organs and structures to their prepregnant state or condition

ischemia Reduction of blood supply to an area

J

jaundice Yellowish color of skin, sclera, mucous membrane, and excretions; *syn.,* icterus

K

kernicterus Excessive bilirubin deposits in the brain, causing neurologic changes and possibly permanent brain damage or death

L

labor Process by which muscular contractions of the myometrium cause dilation and effacement of cervix to allow full descent of fetus into vaginal canal and then though vaginal opening

　active phase Cervical dilation from 4 to 10 cm

　accelerated Cervical dilation from 4 to 7 cm

advanced Cervical dilation from 8 to 10 cm; also called transition phase

latent phase Early labor; cervical dilation from 0 to 3 cm

stages of labor
I:—Full cervical dilation and effacement
II:—Descent and delivery of infant
III:—Delivery of infant to delivery of placenta
IV:—Immediate recovery (optional stage)

lanugo Soft, fine, downy hair found on preterm and newborn infants

leukorrhea Excessive mucous discharge from genital tract; common in pregnancy; usually nonitchy and odorless

lightening Tilting or dropping of fetus forward and downward into the true pelvis; occurs 2 or 3 weeks before end of gestation in the primigravida or at beginning of labor in many multigravidas

linea nigra Darkening of the abdominal line between umbilicus and symphysis pubis during pregnancy caused by hormonal changes

lochia Uterine discharge after delivery that consists of the sloughing decidua, tissue, blood, and cells; lasts 2 or 3 weeks

low birth weight Weight at birth below tenth percentile for gestational age; a weight below 2500 g at birth

M

mastalgia Pain in the breast

mastitis Inflammation of the breast

maternal death Death of any woman from any cause while pregnant or within 42 days of termination of pregnancy; *syn.,* maternal mortality

direct Resulting from obstetric complications

indirect Resulting from previously existing problems and aggravated by effects of pregnancy

nonmaternal Accidental causes not related to pregnancy or its management

maternal mortality rate Total number of maternal deaths per 100,000 live births regardless of gestational age

maternal serum alpha-fetoprotein (MSAFP) Elevated serum levels of alpha-fetoprotein in maternal blood samples; *see also* alphafetoprotein (AFP)

melasma Darkened patches of skin on face or forehead caused by hormones of pregnancy; previously known as *chloasma*

menarche First menstrual flow

meningomyelocele Protrusion of the meninges and spinal cord through a defect in the spine

menopause Cessation of menses during middle age as part of the climacteric

menses *See* menstruation

menstruation Cyclic uterine discharge of blood, tissue, and cells as a result of hormonal changes in the body; *syn.,* menses

mentum Chin, used as landmark on fetal presenting part

milium (pl., milia) Tiny, white, or yellow beadlike sebaceous cysts found primarily on face of newborn

minimum effective concentration (MEC) Necessary level of a drug dissolved in the serum to cause a desired action

miscarriage Lay term for spontaneous abortion

mittelschmerz Lower abdominal pain generally associated with ovulation

molding Temporary changes in shape of head of newborn as it accommodates to birth canal during labor and delivery

mosaicism State of having two or more cell lines in a single person

multigravida Woman who has been pregnant more than once

multipara Woman who has delivered a viable fetus more than once

mutation Change in chromosomal integrity that may be passed to next generation

N

neonatal Referring to the newborn infant

neonatal death rate Number of deaths of live-born infants, per 1000 live births, from time of birth to beginning of day 28 of life

neonatal period From the hour of birth through 27 days, 23 hours, and 59 minutes of life

nephrotoxic Any substance or material that exerts a poisonous effect on kidneys

newborn infant Living infant during first 27 days, 23 hours and 59 minutes of its life

nidation Embedding of fertilized ovum into lining of uterus

nociception Initiation of pain signals, the cause of which is not always quickly determined

nondisjunction Failure of chromosomes at a pair to separate during meiosis, resulting in one cell containing the pair and the other cell having neither chromosome

nullipara Woman who has never delivered a viable infant

O

occiput Back of the head; occipital bone

oligohydramnios Abnormally small amount of amniotic fluid

ophthalmia neonatorum Acute, purulent conjunctivitis of eyes of newborn, usually caused by gonococcal infection

organogenesis Growth of tissues of the fetus into organs during first 12 weeks

osteoporosis Sequela of menopause, characterized by loss of calcium from bone tissue, leading to bone fragility

ototoxic Substance or material poisonous to ear

oxytocin Synthetic or natural substance that stimulates uterus to contract

ovulation Release of ovum from graafian follicle

ovum Female reproductive cell

P

papilledema Edema of optic nerve causing visual disturbances especially in preeclamptic or eclamptic clients

parity State of having given birth to an infant of 500 g or more, whether alive or stillborn; multiple births are considered one parous delivery

pelvimetry Clinical determination of pelvic size by internal or external measurements

perinatal death rate Rate of death of viable infants from week 20 in utero until end of neonatal period

pharmacokinetics Movement of drugs within biologic systems, as affected by uptake, distribution, biotransformation, and elimination

phenotype Way genetic inheritance is expressed overtly in an individual

phenylketonuria (PKU) Genetic disorder involving deficiency of the enzyme phenylalanine hydroxylase

phototherapy Treatment of hyperbilirubinemia by exposure to light

pica Craving for nonfood substances such as ice, starch, or clay

placenta previa Abnormally low implantation of placenta in the uterus

polyhydramnios Excessive amniotic fluid; *syn.,* hydramnios

position Relationship of a designated point on the presenting part of fetus to a designated point in maternal pelvis; divided into four quadrants

postpartum Period lasting 6 weeks after delivery

preeclampsia Abnormal bodily reaction to pregnancy characterized by edema, hypertension, and proteinuria; occurring after week 20 of pregnancy; often called toxemia

premature infant Infant born up through 37 completed weeks of gestation; *syn.,* preterm infant

presentation Relationship of long axis of fetus to long axis of mother; *syn.,* lie

presenting part Anatomic part of fetus closest to cervix and felt by examiner during vaginal or rectal examination; usually the head or buttocks

primigravida Woman pregnant for the first time

primipara Woman who has delivered for the first time a viable infant (older than 20 weeks' gestation)

prostaglandins Substances found in all body tissues that stimulate or inhibit smooth muscle activity

pruritus Itching

puerperium 42 days after birth, postpartal period

Q

quickening First active movements of fetus detectable by mother at approximately 16 to 18 weeks of gestation

R

respiratory distress syndrome (RDS) *See* idiopathic respiratory distress syndrome

respondeat superior "Let the master answer;" commonly interpreted in health care as: "Let the employer answer for the action of its employees"

resuscitation Restoration of breathing, life, or consciousness of one who is apparently dead and whose respirations have ceased

retrolental fibroplasia (RLF) Fibrous membrane that may occur behind the lens in eye as a result of high oxygen concentration administered to a preterm infant

risk-taking behaviors Persisting in a risky behavior, such as smoking, during pregnancy despite knowing of its potential harm

ruga Transverse fold of the vaginal mucous membrane

S

scotoma Blind spot in visual field

show Blood-tinged mucous discharge occurring during labor as the cervix dilates; *syn.,* bloody show

situational crisis Disruption in life caused by an event that occurs randomly and independently of normal life events; generally unexpected and may be unusual

socially high-risk condition Condition complicated by a variety of social problems, including substance abuse, homelessness, and economic, educational, or intellectual deprivation

spermatozoon Male reproductive cell; *syn.,* sperm

spinnbarkeit Changes in stretchability of cervical mucosa during ovulation

station Location of presenting part in relation to ischial spines of birth canal

statute of limitations Limited period of time, differing from state to state, between occurrence of an untoward incident and the filing of a lawsuit

stillborn Fetus of more than 20 weeks' gestation, born without life

striae gravidarum Reddened or bluish streaks in skin of breast, buttocks, or abdomen of pregnant woman, fades to silvery gray or brown scar tissue after birth

subinvolution Delay in return of pelvic organs and structures to their prepregnant state

substance abuse Use of substances that cause problems in an individual's personal, psychologic or social life

supine hypotensive syndrome Hypotension resulting from pressure of enlarged uterus on the vena cava, blocking venous return; *syn.* vena caval compression

suture
  of the fetal or infant skull Line of cartilage separating bony plates of skull
  of a wound Line approximating two aspects of a wound; may be stapled, clipped, or sewn together

syncope Fainting or lightheadedness; common in early pregnancy

T

tachycardia (fetal or newborn) Persistent heart rate greater than 160 beats/min

teratogen Agent or substance that alters fetal growth and development

term infant Live infant born after 38 to 42 weeks of gestation (from time of last menstrual period); *syn.,* full-term infant

thrombocytopenia Low blood platelet count

thrush White, patchy oral lesions of newborn caused by *Candida albicans*

tocolysis Use of medications to inhibit preterm uterine contractions to extend period of pregnancy when preterm labor is threatened

toxin Poisonous substance that may be part of a cell or tissue or may be excreted by the cell

toxoid Toxin treated so that its toxic properties are destroyed but is still capable of initiating the immune response and therefore of inducing immunity in the host

tracheoesophageal fistula Congenital or genetic disorder in which esophagus and trachea are connected or esophagus ends in a blind pouch and there is a lower connection in trachea to esophagus

Trichomonas vaginalis Protozoan infection of vagina; Skene's ducts and urinary tract also may be infected

trimester Approximately one third of gestational period calculated from the last menstrual period
  first First day of last normal menstrual period through 14 weeks' gestation
  second Weeks 15 through 28 of gestation
  third Weeks 29 through 41 of gestation and birth

U

ultrasonography Use of ultrasonic waves to obtain visual or telemetric measurements in diagnosing pregnancy and assessing gestational age and fetal condition or size

umbilical cord Life line between fetus and placenta through which nourishment and waste pass; contains two arteries and one vein surrounded by Wharton's jelly; *syn.,* funis

V

vacuum extraction Application of suction cap to fetal head to assist in delivery during the second stage of labor; *syn.,* ventouse

Valsalva's maneuver Bradycardia; increased intraabdominal pressure and reduced venous return caused by holding breath and keeping glottis closed while pushing during delivery

variability Degree of change in fetal heart rate within 1 minute

variable deceleration Fall in fetal heart rate in response to cord compression

vena caval syndrome (VCS) *See* supine hypotensive syndrome

vernix caseosa Cheeselike covering on fetus that protects skin from the drying and wrinkling properties of amniotic fluid

vertex Head
  vertex presentation Fetal position with the head against the inner cervix

vertical transmission Passage of infection from pregnant woman to fetus through placenta or to newborn through birth canal or breast milk

viability Capability of survival; more than 20 weeks' gestation

W

Wharton's jelly Gelatinous connective tissue surrounding umbilical vessels; gives support to umbilical cord

Z

zona Zone; belt or girdle

zygote Fertilized ovum ø

Appendix

Appendix 1A

Pregnant Patient's Bill of Rights

The Pregnant Patient has the right to participate in decisions involving her well-being and that of her unborn child, unless there is a clear-cut medical emergency that prevents her participation. In addition to the rights set forth in the American Hospital Association's "Patient's Bill of Rights," the Pregnant Patient, because she represents two patients rather than one, should be recognized as having the following additional rights[*]:

1. *The Pregnant Patient has the right*, before the administration of any drug or procedure, to be informed by the health care professional caring for her of any potential direct or indirect effects, risks, or hazards to herself or her unborn or newborn infant that may result from the use of a drug or procedure prescribed for or administered to her during pregnancy, labor, birth, or lactation.

2. *The Pregnant Patient has the right*, before the proposed therapy, to be informed not only of the benefits, risks, and hazards of the proposed therapy but also of any known alternative therapies, such as available childbirth education classes that could help prepare the Pregnant Patient physically and mentally to cope with the discomfort or stress of pregnancy and the experience of childbirth, thereby reducing or eliminating her need for drugs and obstetric intervention. She should be offered such information early in her pregnancy so that she may make a reasoned decision.

3. *The Pregnant Patient has the right*, before the administration of any drug, to be informed by the health care professional who is prescribing or administering the drug to her that any drug that she receives during pregnancy, labor, and birth, no matter how or when the drug is taken or administered, may adversely

affect her unborn infant, directly or indirectly, and that there is no drug or chemical that has been proven safe for an unborn child.

4. *The Pregnant Patient has the right* if cesarean birth is anticipated to be informed before the administration of any drug, and preferably before her hospitalization, that minimizing her and, in turn, her infant's intake of nonessential preoperative medicine will benefit her infant.

5. *The Pregnant Patient has the right*, before the administration of a drug or procedure, to be informed of the areas of uncertainty if there is *no* properly controlled follow-up research that has established the safety of the drug or procedure with regard to its direct or indirect effects on the physiologic, mental, and neurologic development of the child exposed, via the mother, to the drug or procedure during pregnancy, labor, birth, or lactation (this would apply to virtually all drugs and the vast majority of obstetric procedures).

6. *The Pregnant Patient has the right*, before the administration of any drug, to be informed of the brand and generic names of the drug so that she may advise the health care professional of any past adverse reaction to the drug.

7. *The Pregnant Patient has the right* to determine for herself, without pressure from her attendant, whether she will accept the risks inherent in the proposed therapy or refuse a drug or procedure.

8. *The Pregnant Patient has the right* to know the name and qualifications of the individual administering a medication or procedure to her during labor or birth.

9. *The Pregnant Patient has the right* to be informed, before the administration of any procedure, whether that procedure is being administered to her for her or her infant's benefit (medically indicated) or as an elective procedure (for convenience, teaching purposes, or research).

[*]From Haire DB: The pregnant patient's bill of rights, *J Nurse Midwifery* 20:29, 1975. (From Committee on Patient's Rights, Box 1900, New York, NY 10001.)

10. *The Pregnant Patient has the right* to be accompanied during the stress of labor and birth by someone she cares for and someone to whom she looks for emotional comfort and encouragement.

11. *The Pregnant Patient has the right* after appropriate medical consultation to choose a position for labor and birth that is the least stressful to her infant and to herself.

12. *The Obstetric Patient has the right* to have her infant cared for at her bedside if her infant is normal and to feed her infant according to her infant's needs rather than according to the hospital regimen.

13. *The Obstetric Patient has the right* to be informed in writing of the name of the person who actually delivered her infant and the professional qualifications of that person. This information should also be provided on the birth certificate.

14. *The Obstetric Patient has the right* to be informed if there is any known or indicated aspect of her or her infant's care or condition that may cause her or her infant later difficulty or problems.

15. *The Obstetric Patient has the right* to have her and her infant's hospital medical records complete, accurate, and legible and to have their records, including nurses' notes, retained by the hospital until the child reaches at least the age of majority or to have the records offered to her before they are destroyed.

16. *The Obstetric Patient has the right,* both during and after her hospital stay, to have access to her complete hospital medical records, including nurses' notes, and to receive a copy of her records upon payment of a reasonable fee and without incurring the expense of retaining an attorney.

It is the obstetric patient and her infant, not the health care professional, who must sustain any trauma or injury resulting from the use of a drug or obstetric procedure. The observation of the rights listed will not only permit the obstetric patient to participate in the decisions involving her and her infant's health care but also will help to protect the health care professional and the hospital against litigation arising from resentment or misunderstanding on the part of the mother.

Appendix 1B

AWHONN's Standards for the Nursing Care of Women and Newborns*

Standard I: Nursing Practice

Comprehensive nursing care for women and newborns focuses on helping individuals, families, and communities achieve their optimum health potential. This is best achieved within the framework of the nursing process.

The nurse is responsible for decisions and actions within the domain of nursing practice, which may include the following:

• Integration of the nursing process components of assessment, planning, implementation, and evaluation in all areas of nursing practice

• Individualization and prioritization of nursing care to meet the physical, psychologic, spiritual, and social needs of clients

• Collaboration with the individual, family, and other members of the health-care team; promotion of a safe

*From *NAACOG Standards for the nursing care of women and newborns,* ed 4, Washington, DC, 1991, Nurses Association of the American College of Obstetricians and Gynecologists. (NAACOG is currently known as Association of Women's Health, Obstetric, and Neonatal Nurses [AWHONN].)

and therapeutic environment for both the recipients and providers of nursing care

• Demonstration and validation of competence in nursing practice

• Acquisition of specialized knowledge and skills and additional formal education to provide specialized care

• Provision for complete and accurate documentation of care

The written or computerized client record is the documented means of communication among all members of the health-care team. It also promotes continuity of care and provides a mechanism for evaluating care. The record should contain accurate and complete recordings of the client's health history, physical examinations, and the nursing plan of care, including goals, interventions, health education, and evaluation of client and family responses. Additional documentation may include planned follow-up examinations and appropriate referrals. All information contained in the client record and related to the care of the client and family is confidential and should be released only according to institutional policy.

Note: To apply this universal standard to a specific area of gynecologic, obstetric, or neonatal nursing practice, refer directly to the specialty-specific nursing practice standards section.

Standard II: Health Education and Counseling

Health education for the individual, family, and community is an integral part of comprehensive nursing care. Such education encourages participation in, and shared responsibility for, health promotion, maintenance, and restoration.

Comprehensive health education includes the following:
- Identification of the needs and abilities of the learner
- Collaboration with the client and other health care providers in design, content, and follow-up of the educational plan
- Provision of accurate and current information
- Provision of information based on educationally sound principles of teaching and learning
- Recognition of client rights, responsibilities, and alternative choices
- Use of available educational resources to provide health education information to individuals and families in the community
- Documentation and evaluation of health education including client response

The nurse participates in or coordinates the health education and counseling process. It begins with the initial client contact or admission to the unit or service and is an ongoing, continuous process.

Note: To apply this universal standard to a specific area of gynecologic, obstetric, or neonatal nursing practice, refer directly to the specialty-specific nursing practice standards section.

Standard III: Policies, Procedures, and Protocols

Written policies, procedures, and protocols clarify the scope of nursing practice and delineate the qualifications of personnel authorized to provide care to women and newborns within the health-care setting.

The components of policies, procedures, and protocols are based on the following:
- Recognition of the organization's philosophy
- Recognition of the unit's philosophy
- Coordination with the overall mission of the organization
- Assessment of the practice setting and determination of types of services to be provided
- Incorporation of a multidisciplinary approach in their development
- Identification of specific areas of practice to be addressed
- Reflection of current practice, standards, and local regulations

- Anticipated use as references for health-care providers, orientation of new personnel and students, quality assurance activities, or guides for nursing actions in emergency situations

The development of policies, procedures, and protocols should include consideration of staff availability, skill, and licensure; the physical plant and equipment; effects on other departments; and fiscal impact. Policies, procedures, and protocols should be reviewed and revised at least on an annual basis or more frequently as science and technology changes.

Note: To apply this universal standard to a specific area of gynecologic, obstetric, or neonatal nursing practice, refer directly to the specialty-specific nursing practice standards section.

Standard IV: Professional Responsibility and Accountability

Comprehensive nursing care for women and newborns is provided by nurses who are clinically competent and accountable for professional actions and legal responsibilities inherent in the nursing role.

Responsibility and accountability for knowledge and competence in nursing practice for women and newborns includes the following:
- Awareness of changing practices and professional and ethical issues
- Knowledge and clinical skills gained through in-service education, professional continuing education, research data, and professional literature
- Implementation of newly acquired knowledge and skills
- Collaboration through networking and sharing with other professionals
- Participation in the development of standards and policies, procedures, and protocols
- Participation with professional committees within the institution
- Participation in periodic peer and self-evaluations
- Recognition of certification as one mechanism for the demonstration of special knowledge within a specialty area of practice

Legal accountability extends to these following areas:
- Nurse practice acts
- Parameters of professional practice established by professional organizations
- Institutional standards
- Legislative changes that affect practice
- Policies, procedures, and protocols within the practice environment

Standard V: Use of Nursing Personnel

Nursing care for women and newborns is conducted in practice settings that have qualified nursing staff in sufficient numbers to meet client-care needs.

Each practice setting should have sufficient nursing personnel to meet client-care requirements. Nursing staff who provide direct care to women and newborns should be supervised by registered nurses who are clinically proficient in the specialty area of practice. The client-care unit or service is managed by a professional nurse who is prepared educationally and clinically to assume a leadership position. In all practice settings the nurse may practice independently or collaboratively with other health care team members. It is essential that nurses know both the responsibilities and limitations of professional nursing practice specific to the practice setting.

Many variables are considered in determining both the number and type of nursing staff needed for a practice setting. Among these variables are those related to the client, practice, organization, and personnel. Client-related variables may include the following:
- Client demographics and acuity of clients' service
- Length of stay
- Educational needs
- Cultural factors and level of comprehension
- Communication barriers
- Discharge or home-care needs

Practice-related variables may include the following:
- Difference in educational and experiential level of nursing staff
- Nursing philosophy
- Type of nursing-care delivery system
- Use of assistive personnel
- Use of nurses in expanded roles
- Participation in teaching programs

Organizational variables may include the following:
- Scope of services provided
- Availability of support services
- Client volume
- Mission or philosophy of the organization
- Risk-management concerns
- Quality assurance programs
- Policies, procedures, and protocols
- Physical plant
- Marketing strategies
- Fiscal considerations

Personnel variables relate to the type and number of professional and nonprofessional staff and may include the following:
- Education, skill, and experience of the nursing leadership
- Educational preparation, skill, and experience of staff; types and mix of nursing staff
- Availability of qualified alternative staff to deal with emergencies or unanticipated volumes
- Distribution of staff (e.g, temporary reassignment, floating, on-call, cross-training, and supplemental staffing)
- Responsibilities for orientation, precepting, or students
- Turnover rates
- Clerical and technical support

Competency-based job descriptions should be available for each level of the nursing staff. Orientation for all personnel should include a general overview of the organization and specific information about the individual practice setting. Performance evaluations for all personnel should be conducted, documented, and discussed on a regular basis with input from the individual, colleagues, and supervisory staff.

Standard VI: Ethics

Ethical principles guide the process of decision making for nurses caring for women and newborns at all times and especially when personal or professional values conflict with those of the client, family, colleagues, or practice setting.

The nurse should have the opportunity to participate in the ethical decision-making process. To participate actively, nurses should be able to do the following:
- Clarify their own personal and professional values
- Recognize the difficulty in selecting a course of action that is morally and ethically acceptable to all parties
- Communicate openly and assertively
- Identify options
- Seek consultations

Nurses must carefully examine their own value systems because values influence the decision-making process. Opportunities should be provided in the practice setting for discussion of potential ethical issues. Each practice setting should have a framework for decision making regarding bioethical dilemmas. Ethical dilemmas generally arise when there is a conflict between loyalties, rights, duties, or values.

For nurses, most ethical dilemmas occur when there is a real or perceived requirement to act in a manner contrary to personal values or when care ordered to be provided does not seem compatible with the best interest of the client. Common areas of concern may include the following:
- Nursing autonomy and decision making
- Maternal interests versus fetal interests
- Issues of duty, obligation, and loyalty (e.g., employer to employee, professional to public, professional to professional)
- Clients' rights to resources, privacy, confidentiality, information, participation in decision making, and refusal of therapy
- The right to live or die
- Life cycle concerns, including contraception, sterilization, pregnancy termination, genetic manipulation, infanticide, sexuality, choices of lifestyle, and euthanasia
- Fetal or neonatal conditions incompatible with life
- Fetal tissue use
- Biomedical intervention

The bioethics literature can provide nurses with strategies to cope with or resolve decisions in situations when conflicts of values occur. For ethical decision-making frameworks to be applied to practice situations, working relationships must be established in which individuals may express their own points of view. All persons potentially affected by an ethical decision have the right to participate in the decision-making process.

Standard VII: Research

Nurses caring for women and newborns use research findings, conduct nursing research, and evaluate nursing practice to improve outcomes of care.

Knowledge of the research process and participation in scientific inquiry are necessary for the following:

- Participation in research according to ethical guidelines
- Use of research findings to provide appropriate and safe nursing care
- Use of research findings as a basis for validating standards of nursing care
- Evaluation of the relevance and application of research findings from nursing and related disciplines
- Validation of the effect of nursing practice on client outcomes

Standard VIII: Quality Assurance

Quality and appropriateness of client care are evaluated through a planned assessment program using specific, identified clinical indicators.

Each unit or service should have a written quality assurance plan that reflects a philosophy that is coordinated with the organization's mission and overall quality assurance program. Objectives of the unit-based or service-based quality assurance plan should include the following:

- Assurance of consistent quality client outcomes
- Identification and correction of potential nursing practice deficiencies
- Promotion of professional nursing practice based on appropriate nursing standards
- Education and participation of staff in quality assurance activities

The unit nurse manager is responsible for developing and implementing the unit-based quality assurance plan. The plan should include the following:

- Responsibilities of all personnel in the quality assurance process
- The scope of service provided
- Important aspects of care or service involving high-risk, high-volume, and problem-prone clients or activities
- Clinical indicators or measurable standards that affect the aspects of care and service that have been identified as important
- Specific criteria and thresholds for use in monitoring clinical indicators
- Methods for the collection and analysis of data, including reference to collection tools, sample size, time frame, and staff responsibility
- Determination of appropriate corrective action, when indicated, that will fall into one of three categories: educational, organizational, or behavioral change
- Follow-up assessment of identified problems
- Documentation of all aspects of the quality assurance program, including results
- A process for communication related to quality assurance activities within the total organization

Appendix 2A

Laboratory Values for Pregnant and Nonpregnant Women

Laboratory Values for Pregnant and Nonpregnant Women		
Values	**Nonpregnant**	**Pregnant (Second or Third Trimesters)**
HEMATOLOGIC		
Complete Blood Count (CBC)		
Hemoglobin, g/dl	12-16*	11-14*
Hematocrit, PCV, %	37-47	34-42
Red cell volume, ml	1600	1900
Plasma volume, ml	2400	3700

Continued.

Laboratory Values for Pregnant and Nonpregnant Women—cont'd

Values	Nonpregnant	Pregnant (Second or Third Trimesters)
Red blood cell count, million/mm$_3$	4.5-5[6]	3.75-4.5[6]
White blood cells, total per mm$_3$	4,500-10,000	5,000-16,000
Polymorphonuclear cells, %	54-62	60-85
Lymphocytes, %	38-46	15-40

Blood Coagulation and Fibrinolytic Activity[†]

Factors VII, VIII, IX, X		Increase in pregnancy, return to normal in early puerperium; Factor VIII increases during and immediately after delivery
Factors XI, XIII		Decrease in pregnancy
Prothrombin time (PT)	12-14 sec	Slight decrease in pregnancy
Partial thromboplastin time (PTT)	60-70 sec	Slight decrease in pregnancy and again during second and third stage of labor.
Activated (APTT)	30-40 sec	
Bleeding time	1-3 min (Duke) 2-4 min (Ivy)	No appreciable change
Coagulation time	6-10 min (Lee/White)	No appreciable change
Platelets	150,000 to 350,000/mm^3	No significant change until 3-5 days after birth, then marked increase; gradual return to normal
Fibrinolytic activity		Decreases in pregnancy, then abrupt return to normal
Fibrinogen	250 mg/dl	400 mg/dl

Mineral and Vitamin Concentrations

Serum iron, μg	75-150	65-120
Total iron-binding capacity, μg	250-450	300-500
Iron saturation, %	30-40	15-30
Folic acid (folate), μg/mL	5-20	Moderate decrease
Serum proteins		
Total g/dl	6.7-8.3	5.5-7.5
Blood glucose		
Fasting, mg/dl	70-80	65
2-hour postprandial, mg/dl	60-110	Less than 140 mg/dl after a 100 g carbohydrate meal

CARDIOVASCULAR

Blood pressure, mm Hg	110/70[‡]	105/60 (−5-10 systolic, 10-15 diastolic)
Mean arterial pressure (MAP)		< 90 in second trimester
Venous pressure, cm H$_2$O		
Femoral	9	24
Antecubital	8	8
Pulse, beats/min	70	80-90
Stroke volume, ml per beat	65	65-100 ml
Cardiac output, L/min	4.5	5.5-7.5
Circulation time (arm-tongue), sec	15-16	12-14
Blood volume, ml		
Whole blood	4000	5500-6000
Plasma	2400	3700
Red blood cells	4.0-5.0[6]/mm^3	3.75[6]-4.5[6]/mm^3
Blood Gases		
P$_{O_2}$	95-100 mm Hg	104-108 mm Hg
P$_{CO_2}$	35-45 mm Hg	27-32 mm Hg
pH	7.38	7.40-7.42
Bicarbonate	25±1.00 mEq/L	12-16 mEq/L

Continued.

Laboratory Values for Pregnant and Nonpregnant Women—cont'd

Values	Nonpregnant	Pregnant (Second or Third Trimesters)
HEPATIC		
Bilirubin total	Not more than 1 mg/dl	Unchanged
Serum cholesterol	110-300 mg/dl	Increases 60% from 16-32 weeks of pregnancy; remains at this level until after delivery
Thymol turbidity	0-4 units	Positive in 15%
Serum alkaline phosphatase	2-4.5 units (Bodansky)	Increases from week 12 of pregnancy to 6 weeks after delivery
Serum lactate dehydrogenase (LDH)		Unchanged
Serum glutamic-oxaloacetic transaminase (SGOT)		Unchanged
Serum globulin albumin	1.5-3.0 g/dl	Slight increase
A/G ratio		Decrease
Serum cholinesterase		Decrease
RENAL		
Renal plasma flow (RPF), ml/min	490-700	Increase by 25% to 612-875
Glomerular filtration rate (GFR)	105-132 ml/min	Increase by 50% to 160-198
Nonprotein nitrogen (NPN)	25-40 mg/dl	Decrease
Blood urea nitrogen (BUN)	13 ± 3 mg/dl	8.7 ± 1.5 mg/dl (decrease)
Creatinine clearance, mg/kg/24 h	85-120 ml/min	120-180 ml/min (increase)

Modified from Lowdermilk DL, Perry SE, Bobak IM: *Maternity and women's health care*, ed 6, St Louis, 1997, Mosby.

*At sea level. Permanent residents of higher levels (e.g., Denver) require higher levels of hemoglobin.

†Pregnancy represents a hypercoagulable state.

‡Average for a woman approximately 20 years of age; 30 years of age: 123/82; 40 years of age: 126/84.

Appendix **2B**

Laboratory Values for Infants

Laboratory Values for Infants

VALUE	RANGE	VALUE	RANGE
Red blood cells		Prothrombin time (PT)	
Newborn	4.0^6-6.0^6/mm^3	Newborn	<17 seconds
Infant (1-12 months)	2.7^6-5.4^6/mm^3	Hemoglobin (Hb)	
White blood count		1-3 days old	13.5-21.0 g/dl
Newborn	18,000/mm^3	2 months old	9.0-14.0 g/dl
Infant	6,000-17,500/mm^3	Hematocrit (Hct)	
Platelet count		Newborn	45% - 65%
Newborn	100,000-400,000/mm^3	Infant	28% - 42%
Partial thromboplastin time (PTT)	60-85 seconds nonactivated	Serum iron concentration	30-70 µg/g
	25-35 seconds activated	Total serum bilirubin	
		At birth	<2-5 mg/dl

Continued.

Laboratory Values for Infants—cont'd

VALUE	RANGE	VALUE	RANGE
Total serum bilirubin—cont'd		Creatine	
Up to 1 month	≤ 1 mg/dl	Newborn	0.3-1.0 mg/dl
Arterial blood gases		Infant	0.2-0.4 mg/dl
Partial pressure of oxygen (Po_2)	75-100 mm Hg	Serum glucose	50-100 mg/dl
Partial pressure of carbon dioxide (Pco_2)	27-40 mm Hg	Sweat test	Negative
		Albumin in meconium	Negative
pH		Urinalysis	
Newborn	7.27-7.47	Specific gravity	1.003-1.035
Infant	7.35-7.45	pH	5.0-7.0
Serum electrolytes		Protein	Negative
Sodium (Na^+)		Blood	Negative
Premature Infant	132-140 mmol/L	Sugar	Negative
Infant	139-146 mmol/L	Ketones	Negative
Potassium (K^+)		Cerebrospinal fluid (CSF)	
Infant	4.1-5.3 mEq/L	Specific gravity	1.007-1.009
Chlorine (Cl^-)	98-106 mmol/L	Glucose	60-80 mg/dl
Serum calcium		Protein	45-100 mg/dl
Premature infant	7-10 mg/dl	pH	7.33-7.42
Full-term infant	7.5-11 mg/dl		
Blood urea nitrogen (BUN)			
Newborn	8-18 mg/dl		
Infant	5-18 mg/dl		

Data from Betz CL, Sowden L: *Mosby's pediatric nursing reference*, ed 3, St Louis 1996, Mosby.

Appendix 3A

Drug Recommendations for Lactation

Drug Recommendations for Lactation

	Not Used*	Used with Caution†
Analgesics and narcotics	Heroin	Acetylsalicylic acid (aspirin)
	Cocaine	Methadone
	Crack	Propoxyphene ‡
	Phenylbutazone ‡	Indomethacin ‡
Anticoagulants	Phenindione	
	Dicumarol	Bishydroxycoumarin
	Ethyl biscoumacetate	Warfarin sodium (Coumadin)
Anticholinergics	Dicyclomine	Atropine ‡
		Scopolamine ‡

Continued.

Drug Recommendations for Lactation—cont'd

	Not Used*	Used with Caution†
Anticonvulsants	Ethosuximide ‡	Carbamazepine ‡ Clonazepam Mephobarbital Phenobarbital Phenytoin sodium ‡ (Dilantin) Pimidone
Antidepressants	Doxepin	All other antidepressants including: Amitriptyline, nortriptyline, amoxapine, bupropion, clomipramine, imipramine, desipramine, dothiepin, fluoxetine, impradole, maprotiline, opipramol, sertraline, trazodone
Antihistamines	Bromopheniramine ‡ Cimetidine ‡ (Ranitidine and nizatidine similar to cimetidine) Clemastine Diphenhydramine Tripelennamine	Chlorpheniramine
Antihypertensives/diuretics	Ethacrynic acid Reserpine Thiazide diuretics ‡	Acetazolamide ‡ Beta blockers ‡ Propranolol (Inderal)
Antimicrobials	Tetracyclines ‡ Sulfonamides Trimethoprim Metronidazole	
Chemotherapeutics	Antimetabolites/antineoplastics Radioactive elements for therapy or diagnostic purposes	
Hallucinogens	Lysergic acid diethylamide (LSD) Marijuana Phencyclidine hydrochloride (PCP)	
Laxatives and antidiarrheals	Bromides Loperamide ‡ Senna ‡	Cascara ‡ Mandelic acid Phenolphthalein
Oxytocics	Ergot alkaloids: Brocriptine Ergotamine Ergonovine	Methylergonovine
Psychotropics	Chlorpromazine and all propylamino phenothiazines Lithium carbonate	Flupenthixol Haloperidol Mesoridazine Perphenazine
Sedatives and hypnotics	Chlordiazepoxide Diazepam Florazepam Meprobamate Oxazepam	Alpraxolam Chloral hydrate Lorazepam Phenobarbital Temazepam
Respiratory Drugs	Prednisolone ‡	Prednisolone Theobromide Theophylline

Continued.

Drug Recommendations for Lactation—cont'd

	Not Used*	Used with Caution†
Stimulants	Amphetamines	Alcohol
		Caffeine
		Nicotine
Thyroid Drugs	Carbimizole	Levothyroxine
	Iodides	Liothyronine, Liotrix
	Methimazole	Thyroid
	Thiouracil	Thyroxine
	Tyropanoate	
Other Drugs or Foods	Clomid	All OTC medication
	Combined oral contraceptives	Carisoprodol
	Cyclosporine	Carrots (large amounts)
	Dihydrotachysterol	Fluoride tablets
	(DHT)	Mesalamine
	Estrogens	Metoclopramide
	Etretinate	Mexiletine
	L-dopa	Olsalazine
	Lovastatin	Penicillamine
	Misoprostol	Progestogen
		Vitamin D

*Adverse effects have been reported.
†High doses may cause adverse effects; benefits should outweigh risks.
‡Considered safe by American Academy of Pediatrics; other sources disagree.

Appendix 3B

Immunization during Pregnancy

Immunization during Pregnancy

	Risk from Disease			Indications for	
Pregnant Woman	Neonate	Immunizing Agent	Immunization during Pregnancy	Comments, Dose Schedule
LIVE VIRUS VACCINES					
Measles					
Significant morbidity, low mortality; not altered pregnancy	Significant increase in abortion rate; may cause malformations	Live-attenuated virus vaccine	Contraindicated (see immune globulins)	Vaccination of susceptible women should be part of postpartum care Single dose

Continued.

Immunization during Pregnancy—cont'd

Risk from Disease		Immunizing Agent	Indications for Immunization during Pregnancy	Comments, Dose Schedule
Pregnant Woman	Neonate			

Mumps

| Low morbidity and mortality; not altered by pregnancy | Probable increased rate of abortion in first trimester; questionable association of fibroelastosis in neonates | Live-attenuated virus vaccine | Contraindicated | Single dose |

Poliomyelitis

| No increased incidence in pregnancy but may be more severe if it occurs | Anoxic fetal damage reported; 50% mortality in neonatal disease | Live-attenuated virus (OPV) and inactivated virus (IPV) vaccine* Vaccine indicated for susceptible pregnant women traveling in endemic areas | Not routinely recommended for adults in United States, except persons at increased risk of exposure | *Primary:* Three doses of IPV at 4-8 wk intervals and fourth dose 6-12 mo later; two doses of OPV with 6-8 wk interval and third dose at least 6 wk later, customarily 8-12 mo later *Booster:* Every 5 years until 18 years of age for IPV |

Rubella

| Low morbidity and mortality; not altered by pregnancy | High rate of abortion and congenital rubella syndrome | Live-attenuated virus vaccine | Contraindicated | Vaccination of susceptible women in postpartum care Single dose |

Yellow fever

| Significant morbidity and mortality | Unknown | Live-attenuated virus vaccine | Contraindicated except if exposure unavoidable | Postponement of travel preferable to vaccination, if possible Single dose |

INACTIVATED VIRUS VACCINES

Influenza

| Possible increase in morbidity and mortality during epidemic of new antigenic strain | Possible increased abortion rate; no malformations confirmed | Inactivated type A and type B virus vaccines New types as developed | Usually recommended only for clients with serious underlying diseases | Criteria for vaccination of pregnant women same as for all adults Consult with public health authorities; recommendations change each year |

Rabies

| Near 100% fatality; not altered by pregnancy | Determined by maternal disease | Killed virus vaccine, or rabies immune globulin (RIG) | Indications for prophylaxis not altered by pregnancy; each case considered individually Postexposure for RIG | Public health authorities to be consulted for indications and dosage |

Continued.

Immunization during Pregnancy—cont'd

Risk from Disease		Immunizing Agent	Indications for Immunization during Pregnancy	Comments, Dose Schedule
Pregnant Woman	Neonate			

INACTIVATED BACTERIAL VACCINES

Cholera

Significant morbidity and mortality; more severe during third trimester	Increased risk of fetal death during third-trimester maternal illness	Killed bacterial vaccine	Only to meet international travel requirements	Vaccine is of low efficacy Two injections, 4-8 wk apart

Meningococcus

No increased risk during pregnancy	Unknown	Killed bacterial vaccine	Indications not altered by pregnancy; vaccination recommended only in unusual outbreak situations	Public health authorities to be consulted

Pneumococcus

No increased risk during pregnancy; no increase in severity of disease	Unknown	Polyvalent polysaccharide vaccine	Indications not altered by pregnancy; vaccine used only for high-risk individuals	In adults, one dose only

Typhoid

Significant morbidity and mortality; not altered by pregnancy	Unknown	Killed bacterial vaccine	Not recommended routinely except for travel to endemic areas	*Primary:* Two injections, 4 wk apart *Booster:* Single dose

TOXOIDS

Tetanus-diphtheria

Severe morbidity; tetanus mortality 60%; diphtheria mortality 10%; unaltered by pregnancy	Neonatal tetanus mortality 60%	Combined tetanus-diphtheria toxoids preferred: adult tetanus-diphtheria formulation	Lack of primary series, or no booster within past 10 yr	Updating of immune status should be part of antepartum care *Primary:* Two doses at 1-2 mo interval with third dose 6-12 mo later *Booster:* Single dose every 10 yr

Tetanus-Postexposure

Severe morbidity/ mortality	High neonatal mortality	Tetanus immune globulin (TIG)	Postexposure prophylaxis	Used with tetanus toxoid, 250 units in single dose TIG.

IMMUNE GLOBULINS: HYPERIMMUNE

Hepatitis B

Possible increased severity during third trimester	Possible increase in abortion rate and prematurity;	Hepatitis B immune globulin (HBIG)	Postexposure prophylaxis	Woman receives 0.06 ml/kg HBIG immediately and 1 mo later

Continued.

Immunization during Pregnancy—cont'd

Risk from Disease		Immunizing Agent	Indications for Immunization during Pregnancy	Comments, Dose Schedule
Pregnant Woman	Neonate			

IMMUNE GLOBULINS: HYPERIMMUNE

Hepatitis B—cont'd

| | neonatal hepatitis can occur if mother is a chronic carrier or is acutely infected | Recombinant DNA vaccine now available: Recombivax HB or Engerix B | | *Vaccine:* Three doses Infants of HBsAg-positive mothers receive 0.5 ml of HBIG within 12 hr of birth plus recombinant vaccine, which is repeated 1 and 6 mo later |

Varicella

| Possible increase in severe varicella pneumonia | Can cause congenital varicella; rarely causes congenital defects | Varicella-zoster immune globulin (VZIG) | Given to pregnant women with high risk of varicella pneumonia | Indicated only for newborns of mothers who developed varicella within 4 days before or 2 days after delivery; 1 vial/kg in one dose of VZIG, up to 5 vials |

IMMUNE GLOBULINS: POOLED

Hepatitis A

| Possible increased severity during third trimester | Possible transmission to neonate at delivery if mother is incubating the virus or is acutely ill | Pooled immune globulin (IG) | Postexposure prophylaxis | 0.02 ml/kg in one dose of IG should be given as soon as possible and within 2 wk of exposure; infants receive one dose of 0.5 ml as soon as possible after birth |

Measles

| Significant morbidity; low mortality; not altered by pregnancy | Significant increase in abortion rate; may cause malformations | Pooled immune globulin (IG) | Postexposure prophylaxis | Unclear if prevents abortion; must be given within 6 days of exposure 0.25 ml/kg in one dose of IG, up to 15 ml |

*IPV recommended for nonimmunized adults at increased risk.

IPV, Inactivated polio vaccine; *OPV,* oral polio vaccine.

Appendix 4A

Answers to "Test Yourself" Questions

Chapter 1

1-1. a. Insurance considerations control length of hospital stay and types of procedures that will be paid for, rather than client needs. May result in too early of discharge for the client's condition.

b. (1) Client may not have physically recovered enough to manage self-care.
(2) Client may not know how to feed or care for infant.
(3) Nursing assessment of potential complications in mother or newborn is incomplete.

Chapter 3

3-1. a. Seminiferous tubules
b. Leydig's cells
c. Epididymis
d. Seminal vesicles

3-2. a. Cells of fallopian tube
b. Fimbriae
c. Cilia
d. Ampulla
e. Myometrium
f. Cells of the cervix

3-3. a. Epithelial cells of acini
b. Ductules
c. Lactiferous sinuses
d. Tubercles of Montgomery

Chapter 4

4-1. a. **Menopause:** (1) Hot flashes—treat with relaxation techniques, layered clothing; (2) reduced vaginal secretions—treat with water soluble jelly, estrogen creams

b. **Postmenopause:** (1) Potential osteoporosis—exercise, brisk walking, increased calcium intake with vitamin D; (2) changes in CV health—dietary increase in fiber, reduction in fat, weight loss

4-2. a. Lung: Smoking, environmental pollution
b. Breast: Family history, benign breast disease, high dose ERT, late menopause, high fat and caffeine intake, smoking
c. Cervical: Frequent infections, herpes virus or papillomavirus, smoking, multiple partners
d. Endometrial: Family history, older age, early pregnancy and menopause
e. Colorectal: Family history, polyps, high fat–low fiber diet

4-3. a. Regular pap smears, mammograms, and rectal examinations with guaiac stool samples
b. No early detectable symptoms

Chapter 5

5-1. The symptothermal method has the best "perfect use" rating, with a 20% failure rate. Compared with use of no contraceptive method, there is a 70% failure rate (number of pregnancies within a period of 1 year of use).

5-2. a. She may have heavy menses or be at high risk for STDs. String irritates cervix when infection is present.
b. Ovum may become fertilized but may not implant.

5-3. Cost, frequency of clinic visits, stability of sexual relationship, number of partners, type of body structure and menses, age, spacing of children or avoiding pregnancy all together

Chapter 6

6-1. a. See Table 6-2. Drug abuse, smoking, drinking, exposure to noxious chemicals and high environmental temperatures, strenuous exercise, obese, underweight
b. Temperance in drug, alcohol, nicotine use; Change in lifestyle, reduction in excessive exercise; use of hot tub; use of tight underclothes for men

Chapter 7

7-1. a. 22,1
b. Crossing over
c. Because each oocyte enters a resting phase from puberty until its maturity (at ovulation), there is a period of "suspended time" in meiosis. During this time there is opportunity for damage to genetic material. In contrast, spermatocytes take only approximately 72 hours to mature.
d. Zygote

7-2. a. Testes determining factor
b. Trophoblast
c. Cushions fetus, thermal regulation, allows fetal movement, fetal swallowing, creates wedge against cervix thus protecting fetal head during labor

7-3. a. Mesoderm
   b. 13, 26; 27, 40 (term)
   c. There are not enough alveoli for gas exchange, plus lack of surfactant allows alveoli to collapse with each expiration.
7-4. a. Direct blood to developing brain, away from developing lungs, and to and from placenta
   b. Foramen ovale
   c. Ductus arteriosus
7-5. a. Dissipated to mother via the placenta
   b. Linked with development of birth defects, especially CNS defects
7-6. a. Black tarry substance consisting of bile pigments and fetal hair and cells. Found in fetal GI tract.
   b. Hypoxia, breech presentation
7-7. a. Has higher affinity for oxygen
   b. Vitamin K needs bacteria to be synthesized. Injection covers the initial period before oral feedings have established bacteria in the gut.
7-8. a. Fetal RBCs are larger and have a shorter life span than adult RBCs.
   b. Through placental passage of antibodies

Chapter 8

8-1. a. (1) *Acceptance:* Realizing fetus is actually present and incorporating it into one's life plans
   (2) *Fetal embodiment:* Personalizing infant, as different from oneself
   (3) *Separation:* Emotionally letting fetus be born, to be a separate person from oneself
   b. Imagery helps by forming a fantasy scenario. It is similar to visualization—thinking about oneself in a situation and rehearsing one's reactions.
8-2. a. Stability of relationship, financial security, timing of pregnancy
   b. Woman assists in struggle for relevance by involving partner in tasks related to pregnancy needs, discussing parenting questions, and sharing feelings.

Chapter 9

9-1. Because values reflect iron levels, inquire about current diet and pattern of menstrual flow when nonpregnant. Normal levels fall slightly during second and third trimesters.
9-2. Explain the increase in amount of blood to supply fetus and placenta also affect pressure in veins of legs.
   a. Similar to sitting for long periods, need to elevate legs or lie on side
   b. Need to sit up first before jumping up from a horizontal position
   c. Pressure expands walls of superficial veins of legs

9-3. a. Potential for infection because of pooled urine pockets related to stasis
   b. Could signal onset of mild diabetes
   c. Leads to fatigue, may indicate retention of excess fluid
9-4. (See Box 9-1) *Precautions:* Do not become short of breath, keep pulse below 140, do not exercise in supine position or get too warm, drink fluids, and eat carbohydrates
   Rationale: Blood diverted to skin and lungs from uterus and placenta. Fetus has no additional way to reduce heat.
9-5. a. Nägele's rule: March 6
   b. Method of nines: March 8
9-6. Breast fullness, beginning colostrum production, vaginal hyperemia, beginning abdominal enlargement

Chapter 10

10-1. a. Long boiling depletes vitamins
   b. Excessive sodium, above 4-5 g, will result in edema as a result of fluid retention and may affect blood pressure.
10-2. Rice plus legumes, soybeans, wheat, peanuts, sesame, milk, and vegetables listed in Table 10-6
10-3. a. Poor nutrition and fluid intake, alcohol, smoking
   b. She needs at least an amount that replaces the volume of milk
   c. 1-2 cups extra milk (provides extra protein mother needs)

Chapter 11

11-1. a. *Fetal well-being* refers to the appropriate growth for gestational age and to the normal form and function of the fetus.
   Fetal maturity refers to the status of pulmonary function, primarily whether the premature infant can sustain oxygen exchange.
   b. Age of fetus, maternal status
11-2. a. Ultrasonography can detect soft tissue position and some function. Bleeding may occur because of a wrong placement of the placenta so this test may help to diagnose any problem causing your bleeding.
   b. The tentative period includes the time from when tests for fetal well-being and maturity are being done and before results are final. The woman and her family must wait before continuing with prenatal bonding with the infant, usually while fighting fears about possible problems.
   c. Amniotic fluid leakage, bleeding, fetal death
11-3. a. *Reactive:* Two FHR accelerations within 10 minutes of > 15 bpm for > 15 seconds and occurring with fetal movements

Nonreactive: Lack of FHR accelerations matching the above criteria

b. *Fetal muscle tone:* Good criteria are one episode of flexion-extension of limbs, spine, or hand in 30 minutes
Movement: Three gross or rolling movements in 30 minutes
Breathing: 30-second episode of breathing within a 30-minute period
Amniotic fluid volume: One or more pockets of fluid of more than 2 cm

Chapter 12

12-1. Three of many examples requiring adaptation in the classes' content and timing include many more single working women, women beginning pregnancy in their late 30s, and shortened hospital stays requiring much better preparation for childbirth and parenting.

12-2. Educator must focus on teaching practical and realistic methods of coping with labor process and pain. She must remind couples that all the techniques taught in class are to be practiced and applied. She can emphasize the parents' own responsibility for managing pain by ensuring that they understand these techniques.

12-3. *Focused attention:* Gaze at selected photos, use visualization
Reduction of anxiety, fatigue, muscle tension: Encourage verbalization, massage, relaxation response
Controlled sensory input: Use of audio earphones and favorite music, hydrotherapy, effleurage

Chapter 13

13-1. a. LOA
b. Over lower left abdomen

Chapter 14

14-1. a. Rate limits for *tachycardia* above 160 for a 10-minute period or an elevation of 20 bpm above baseline for a 10-minute period
Rate limits for *bradycardia* below 110 bpm for a 10-minute period or a decrease from the normal baseline of 20 bpm for a 10-minute period
b. See Table 14-2 for etiologic factors for *tachycardia* and *bradycardia.*
c. *Tachycardia* indicates infection, response to drugs, or beginning hypoxia, thus is a warning sign of further trouble developing.
Bradycardia indicates increasing hypoxia and is ominous.

14-2. Reflected in the beat-to-beat or short term variability, which normally ranges from 3 to 10 beats above or below an imaginary line drawn as an average through the wavy line on the paper.

14-3. Determine type of nonreassuring pattern. Reposition client, and observe response. Notify second care person if first interventions do not improve pattern. If receiving oxytocin, turn off IV pump. Begin O_2 by face mask at 8 to 10 L/min. Check maternal blood pressure and pulse. Do not delay in getting a second opinion.

14-4. a. pH of 7.25
b. A damaged placental perfusion leads to build up of carbon dioxide, beginning respiratory acidosis. Without relief, further conversion from aerobic to anaerobic paths cause lactic acid to accumulate. A mixed respiratory and metabolic acidosis result, and pH falls as lactic acid builds up (see Figure 14-12).

14-5. Baseline variability increases above 25 bpm, variable decelerations that do not respond to position changes, decreased or absent variability not responding to stimulation, and bradycardia

Chapter 15

15-1. a. Joe could speak firmly to Ann by reminding her of learned responses to contraction, providing a cool washcloth and back pressure, and helping to support legs and changes in body position. A warm wet towel over the perineum or an ice compress over the clitoris during crowning may also help.
b. Calm her fears and build self-confidence, supervise and support the labor partner

15-2. a. See Box 15-1
b. *Phase 1:* Full dilation, internal rotation almost completed. *Phase 2:* To station 3, head rotating to AP or OP position. Phase 3: Station 4-5, head on perineum and extending labia just before birth.

15-3. a. There is dystocia because of position of presenting part.
b. Have woman sit up or use hands-and-knees position.

Chapter 16

16-1. a. A drug that is 80% protein bound will be more available during pregnancy because maternal hormones take up some of the usual binding sites, allowing a greater percent of free drug to go to receptor sites.
b. Mucous membranes are more vascular during pregnancy, and therefore drug absorption through these tissues will be more rapid.

16-2. a. Drugs of low molecular weight and lipid soluble drugs are transferred easily.
b. In late labor because of drug equilibrium, maternal and fetal drug levels will be almost

equal, especially if the maternal drug is via the intravenous route. Therefore newborns must be observed for delayed excretion of the maternal drug and for adverse effects resulting from a higher than usual dose in the newborn circulation.

16-3. a. 0.075 mL/min, 4.5 mL/hr

16-4. a. *For:* Comfort, fluid and nutritional balance, newborn normoglycemia
Against: Slowed stomach emptying always occurs during labor, potential for emesis, especially with anesthesia, potential for aspiration
a. Always position any vulnerable client with head and shoulders to the side, and slightly elevate the shoulders in a semi-Fowler's position. Observe closely during recovery.

Chapter 17

17-1. *WBC* Up to 18,000-20,000
Lochial color and amount: Bright red, moderate amount
Temperature (oral): 98-99° F
Appetite: Fair to very hungry
Fatigue level: Sleep and fatigued

Chapter 18

18-1. a. As circulation through the umbilical cord ceases, the newborn's systemic blood pressure rises causing blood flow through the ductus arteriosus to *reverse* its direction. As the former right-to-left shunt is reversed, the ductus arteriosus constricts, and by the end of the first day there is little blood flow through this structure.
Increased blood flow to the lungs, and therefore from the lungs, causes pressure on the foramen ovale, forcing the opening between the atria to close.
b. Respiration rate is irregular, and short periods of apnea are expected.
c. Grunting respirations on expiration indicate a difficulty expelling air. This abnormal finding is a warning sign of respiratory distress and must be evaluated at once.

18-2. a. The newborn responds to a drop in ambient temperature by chemical thermogenesis. Heat is produced by increasing the metabolic rate and metabolism of brown adipose tissue. Newborns do not shiver.
b. Factors that predispose a newborn to hypoglycemia include: maternal history of diabetes, intrapartal medications, and a newborn who is LGA or SGA or pre- or postmature. Findings in the newborn that indicate hypoglycemia include tremors, seizures, tachypnea, lethargy, and a serum blood glucose < 45 mg/dl.

18-3. a. To prevent retraction of the testicle into the abdominal cavity.
b. The pseudomenstruation is caused by the withdrawal of maternal hormones following birth.
c. Swollen genitalia would be an expected finding in newborns who had breech presentations and were delivered vaginally or by cesarean delivery following a lengthy labor that did not progress.

18-4. a. Equal, round, reactive to light
b. Skin tags or sinuses near the ears may be insignificant findings or may be associated with renal malformations.
c. Molding is the overlapping of the cranial bones during labor and delivery to accommodate the fetal head through the birth canal.

18-5. a. (1). General assessment; (2) evaluation of motor function, developmental reflexes, and cranial nerves; (3) behavioral assessment
Ortolani's test is performed to assess for a congenital hip dislocation.
b. The rooting reflex occurs when the newborn turns the head toward a stimulus. A breast-feeding mother can stimulate this reflex by stroking the infant's face with her nipple causing the infant to turn toward the stimulus and most likely to begin nursing.

Chapter 19

19-1. a. Test 30 minutes after birth and then every hour for 4 hours, then if stable, every 4 hours for the next 24 hours. A finding of 60 mg/dl glucose is within normal range; chart as such.
b. Check temperature, presence of tremors, acrocyanosis, high pitched cry, and respiratory distress. Note volume of feed already taken or taken in relation to time of birth.

19-2. Erythromycin ointment provides prophylaxis against gonorrhea and chlamydia if the ribbon of ointment is allowed to remain in the conjunctiva for at least 1 minute before excess is wiped off.

19-3. 448 calories in 24 hours; fluid and caloric needs achieved by taking in 22.4 ounces of formula/day.

Chapter 20

20-1. Support infant's head and neck with one hand, place face downward with head lower than trunk on your forearm, supported on your thigh. Deliver five back blows between shoulder blades, using heel of your hand.
Then sandwich between your two arms, flip infant to a chest-up position and deliver five chest thrusts midline, just below nipple line.
Then place infant on a flat surface. Assess for an open airway and dislodged foreign body in mouth.

Do not do a finger sweep of the mouth because this might push any object down further and worsen the situation.

If infant is still not breathing and no foreign object is seen, repeat series of back blows and chest thrusts one more time. If the infant is unconscious, begin CPR.

20-2. Infants who have altered immune systems, whether from HIV infection, malignancy, medications, chemotherapy, or radiation, will be on an individualized immunization schedule.

Chapter 21

21-1. a. An irritable uterus precedes preterm labor. Current interventions may extend pregnancy from 48 hours to several weeks.
b. See Boxes 21-1 and 21-2.

21-2. a. Expected changes are due to increased pressure on maternal organs. These include more edema in legs, potential for varicosities, increased potential for VCS, heartburn, constipation, and difficulty sleeping through the night.
b. Increased fiber, fluid, and protein to counteract constipation, and increased folic acid. Six small meals a day help facilitate digestion.
c. Loss of calcium from bones, muscle atrophy, depression, venous stasis, glucose intolerance, constipation, fatigue

21-3. a. Expected enlargement of uterus, although there is some growth of uterus.
No gestational sac in uterus.
b. Tube cannot stretch large enough to hold a pregnancy past 14 weeks

21-4. a. Bed rest. Wait and watch signs of progression. May be given an antiprostaglandin.
b. The doses differ markedly because, for induction, the fetal response to contractions must be considered. With the dose for abortion, there may be side effects of nausea and vomiting, which will receive treatment.

Chapter 22

22-1. a. Vascular: Generalized relaxation allowing increased blood volume without hypertension; fall in diastolic and rise in femoral venous pressure
b. Cardiac output: Increase of 50%
c. Heart rate at least 15 bpm faster

22-2. Needs earliest BP reading, prior history of hypertension, family history. MAP is 94.

22-3. a. *Gestational-transient* has onset during pregnancy without edema or proteinuria; resolves after birth.
Chronic hypertension has onset before pregnancy and may or may not have PIH signs superimposed. Chronic hypertension may show esca-

lating blood pressure to high readings, with accompanying signs of fatigue, headache, and dizziness.
Pregnancy induced hypertension, although process begins with implantation, has onset of symptoms after 20th week that include edema, proteinuria, and hypertension.
b. PIH signs include developing excess edema seen by weight gain >2 lb/week after 20 weeks. Early onset of proteinuria and edema are serious signs of vasoconstriction.

22-4. a. Avoid tight, constrictive knee-high stockings and long periods of standing. Use support hose, walk regularly, and sit with legs elevated on footstool.
b. Observe for relapse of symptoms. Follow preventive instructions for varicose veins.
c. Do not rub site; follow insulin protocol. Rotate sites; bruising may occur.

22-5. a. *Pulmonary edema:* SOB, rales, cough
Pulmonary embolism: SOB, sense of impending death, anxiety, chest pain, cough, cyanosis
b. Maintain high Fowler's position, begin nasal oxygen, notify physician at once.
Monitor vital signs; begin IV fluids.

Chapter 23

23-1. a. Beans, green leafy vegetables, dried fruits, eggs, enriched cereals, whole grains
b. Tea, coffee, milk, antacids, alcohol
c. Alcohol, antibiotics, anticonvulsants

23-2. a. Fatigue, hypervolemia of pregnancy, nausea, and vomiting
b. Avoid stress and fatigue, maintain prescribed drug intake
c. Lack of oxygen to fetus may occur, precipitate labor

23-3. 1. Migraine: c. 2. Muscle contraction: b. Traction-inflammatory: a.

23-4. a. Self-care includes adequate rest and avoiding excessive heat, sunlight, and infections.
b. Urinary infections
c. During recovery

23-5. The woman's body responses of vasoconstriction to protect her blood pressure will reduce perfusion to the "nonvital" organs, including the placenta.

Chapter 24

24-1. a. She may have weight loss, diarrhea, or susceptibility to infection. Fetal health is threatened, and fetal loss is common.
b. In third trimester
c. Careful drug regimen; observe for onset of fever or sore throat; report eye dryness. Keep pills safely away from children.

24-2. a. See Table 24-1: Lethargy, dry thick skin at elbows and knees, coarse hair, slowed mental capacity, anorexia, constipation
24-3. a. Fetal overproduction of insulin leading to LGA infant or, if severe, to intrauterine growth retardation
    b. Hyperinsulinism delays pulmonary maturation and depresses surfactant synthesis.

Chapter 25

25-1. a. *Toxoids:* From extracellular toxin that is treated to still induce antibodies in the immunized person
    Attenuated live virus: After a series of steps, a virus loses its virulence but retains ability to induce antibodies
    Killed bacteria: Actual bacteria cells or pieces that are inactive yet can induce antibodies
    b. Attenuated live virus may have a rare chance to cause subclinical illness.
25-2. a. Internal monitoring and scalp sampling puncture fetal skin integrity, and maternal HIV-positive blood covers infant, whether born by C-section or vaginally. An access puncture allows entry of virus, in addition to what may have crossed the placenta.
    b. Cleansing the skin removes the most accessible maternal blood and fluids from the skin before it is punctured or eye medication is instilled. What is the practice in your setting?
25-3. a. Use of nontreponemal antibody tests such as VDRL and RPR titers to observe for a rise in titer, indicating reinfection or poor response to treatment
    b. There is a window of 4 to 6 weeks in which these tests may be negative in spite of infection. A newborn may be symptom free at birth, yet its mother may be positive. HIV-positive women are treated for 3 weeks rather than 1 because of poor immunologic responses. Follow-up examinations with both is important.
25-5. a. The fetal risks for Jane at 14 weeks are improved from the first trimester. She may not become ill even though exposed (ask about prior immunization).
    b. Ann probably already has antibodies against toxoplasmosis so her risk is low. However, she should not change the litter box and should be tested for antibody titers. Anyone with HIV-positive status has a much higher risk of reactivated toxoplasmosis.
    c. There is rare transmission to the fetus but a high rate of transmission to the newborn.
25-6. a. Hepatitis B viral load is very high, increasing risk of infection if someone is exposed to blood and bodily fluids of an infected person.

    b. Because many of these diseases may not show clinical symptoms, just "guessing" who is infected is dangerous. Don't skip universal precautions.

Chapter 28

28-1. a. 44, 2, X, Y
    b. Codon
    c. A mutation alters protein synthesis by coding for a different, incorrect amino acid, which then changes the amount of protein produced or its function.
28-2. a. A recessive gene is expressed only if both copies of the gene are identical, whereas a dominant gene is expressed even if only one gene of the pair is affected.
    b. Consanguinity is mating between close relatives. It increases the chances for genetic diseases because the two parents share a greater number of abnormal genes than would two people who are not blood relatives.
28-3. a. 50%
    b. Because people with the AB genotype are typed as AB because neither A nor B is dominant over the other
    c. Because type 0 is recessive. To be expressed it must be inherited from both parents.
28-4. a. The infant may have an abnormality of protein, carbohydrate, or fat metabolism that will deprive him or her of some nutrients while allowing an excess of toxic metabolites to accumulate. This often results in developmental delays.
    b. Sickle cell hemoglobin causes the red blood cell to assume a cresentlike shape under certain conditions, such as hypoxia. The sickled cells are less flexible and occlude small blood vessels, causing ischemia.
28-5. a. The child has inherited two "color blind" sex-linked recessive genes from her parents.
    b. Females have a second, normal X chromosome that dominates over the abnormal recessive gene.
    c. Fragile X syndrome causes abnormal development in affected males; retinoblastoma on chromosome 13
28-6. The child is hypotonic with Brushfield's spots, epicanthal folds, a flat nasal bridge, and characteristic dermal creases. Cardiac defects are frequently found.
28-7. a. Genetics, environment, multifactorials
    b. Separate
    c. 21, Down
28-8. a. A factor or substance that causes congenital malformations in the developing fetus
    b. Timing of the exposure
    c. Lead, mercury, radiation, PCBs

28-9. a. Risk to fetus and mother, benefit to fetus and mother

  b. Certainly Accutane should be avoided by all women who are planning to become pregnant. However, many health care workers are advising all women of childbearing age to avoid Accutane therapy.

28-10. a. Drug therapy to replace missing enzymes, insertion of normal genes into target tissue, organ transplantation

  b. The nurse must provide accurate information about the genetic disease and options for continuing or terminating the pregnancy. The family should be supported during this process and in the future when decisions about future pregnancies will arise.

Chapter 29

29-1. a. Lack of pulmonary surfactant, atelectasis, hyaline membrane

  b. Allows oxygen exchange until infant able to produce sufficient surfactant

29-2. A=b, B=c, C=a

29-3. a. Cyanotic heart disease: Cyanosis, tachypnea, tachycardia
     Cyanotic defects: Diminished peripheral pulses

  b. Abnormal cardiac rhythm, abnormal heart sounds (murmurs)
     Acyanotic defects: Difficulty feeding

29-4. Fluid requirements: 150ml/kg/day
     Caloric requirements: 100-120 kcal/kg/day

29-5. a. 2. 5.0ml
  b. 12.5%

29-6. a. Conjugated bilirubin
  b. Facilitates biliary excretion of unconjugated

bilirubin; can prevent bilirubin toxicity

  c. Nursing interventions: Blindfold infant, check intake and output, feed extra fluids, touch and stroke infant for stimulation

29-7. a. Subtle seizure
  b. Myoclonic seizure
  c. Focal clonic seizure
  d. Multifocal seizure

Chapter 30

30-1. Find protocols and procedures for the unit. Sometimes these are outdated. Look up current journal articles. Check nursing professional standards and what other hospital units in your vicinity do. Check with the ethics committee of the hospital.

30-2. a. Report changes at once to physician. Take correct steps with nursing role; record changes and actions.

  b. Proceed up chain of command to obtain second opinion. Act as an ombudsman for client.

30-3. a. *Implied consent* is considered when a person is incapable of consenting to a life-saving procedure in an emergency. *Informed consent* is a result of a person who is alert and fully aware of the implications of the procedure or test *before* signing the consent.

  b. Find the physician or midwife to complete the explanation. Allow client to voice concerns. Wait to get signature.

  c. Threatening the client who won't cooperate versus actually forcing her to have a vaginal examination, for instance

Appendix 4B

Answers to Selected "Clinical Decisions"

Chapter 13

13-1.
Mary's labor graph indicates an arrest of descent.

13-2.
Reinforce support techniques with Jim. Give him simple comfort tasks to do. Give anticipatory guidance. Help Mary

talk about her feelings and anxiety. Stay with couple until they are more synchronized.

13-3.
Reassure that progress is good. Determine if analgesia is desired. Facilitate pain relief. Give anticipatory guidance. Allow time for ventilation of feelings. Reinforce comfort techniques.

Chapter 14

14-1.

Late decelerations are evident with indication of beginning bradycardia at the end of the strip. Notify physician, check temperature, reposition client, and begin oxygen by mask.

14-2.

Risk factors for this labor are extended ROM without well-established labor. She may show signs of intrauterine infection with fetal tachycardia. Chronic hypertension may affect placental integrity and give indication of late decelerations. She is also at risk for placental separation (see Chapter 21).

Chapter 15

15-1.

Note the positions of father and mother and nurse. What is wrong?

Chapter 16

16-1.

a. Pain behaviors
b. Nociception: Pain from visceral and somatic causes during transition
c. Pain description
d. Suffering expressed in her need for presence of significant other.

Chapter 17

17-1.

A temperature of 101.4°F 30 hours after birth indicates an infectious process somewhere. Assessment includes a systems overview for REEDA at wound sites, localized or generalized pain, malaise, I & O, dehydration, and Homan's sign. Notify physician after assessment.

Chapter 18

18-1.

Choose c. to report because unequal pulses indicate obstruction.

18-2.

May indicate onset of infection. Check vital signs of mother and infant. Closely observe, document intake and output, and notify pediatrician of findings.

18-3.

Ann has both a cephalhematoma and caput swelling. See Figure 18-19. Cephalhematoma may result in increased jaundice. In severe cases, a skull fracture may be present.

18-4.

a. A floppy infant indicates neurologic deficit, either temporary or permanent.

b. An asymmetric Moro response indicates that motor control, either peripherally or centrally, is affected. The infant should be evaluated for brachial palsy, central nerve damage, hypoxia, and hypoglycemia.

18-5.

The infant is approximately 40 to 41 weeks gestational age but is SGA by weight.

Chapter 19

19-1.

Counsel Mrs. Jones that there will be adequate milk if she nurses on demand, uses correct positioning, drinks adequate fluids, gets enough rest, and has a balanced diet. She can observe the infant's stools for soft consistency, the urine for its light color, and the skin turgor and weight gain to be assured that she is producing enough milk.

19-2.

The hematocrit and hemogobin are high. A high hematocrit will result in increased jaundice potential. The timing is related to the "dumping" of fetal RBC with their higher oxygen sensitivity; the liver recycling process becomes temporarily overloaded.

Chapter 20

20-1.

Talk in a normal voice. Tell the infant about the day's activities and his own feelings. Make a special time for father and son, perhaps giving the evening bath. Teach him games to play with the infant.

20-2.

Help her realize that Andy was preterm and thus initially less active in sucking. He will need coaxing and patience at feeding times. Her impatience is being reflected in the infant's frustration level. Feed him more often, carry him around in a body pack, talk with him, and share feeding times with partner.

Chapter 21

21-1.

Lisa needs evaluation of skin for flushing and an oral temperature. Vasodilation is an early reaction to magnesium sulfate. Monitor BP and pulse and uterine contractions. Expect to find a minimal decrease in BP and a gradual decrease in frequency of contractions.

21-2.

a. Findings are appropriate for gestational age for multiple pregnancy.
b. Review all ADL, nutrition, early monitoring requirements.

21-3.

a. Ann's immediate care includes assessment for signs of pain, bleeding, and hypovolemia. After decisions are made regarding treatment, she will need preparation for the procedures.

Chapter 22

22-1.

Urine output indicates oliguria. Because reflexes are still +2, you might consider that the dose is insufficient, but the respiratory rate of 10 breaths/min is a serious warning. Notify physician and arrange for magnesium sulfate levels to be drawn and sent to laboratory. Make frequent assessments of level of consciousness, BP, pulse, and reflexes.

22-2.

Observe all mucous membranes for oozing blood. Notify physician. Draw stat blood for PTT, PT times and platelets, hemoglobin and hematocrit. When monitoring, work quickly to avoid prolonged pressure on arm tissues.

Chapter 23

23-1.

Randi should be asked the number of times per day and week she uses an inhaler and for how long (dosage).

23-2.

Deborah should be asked the questions about headaches in Box 23-1.

Chapter 25

25-1.

a. Fetal heart indicates early decelerations with a partial late component.
b. Tachycardia is evident. Interventions must include more frequent temperature readings, IV fluids, and increased IV fluids. Antibiotics should have been started earlier. The physician should have checked the client frequently and evaluated fetal condition. Pediatrician should be notified of chorioamnionitis during late labor and should be present at the birth.

Chapter 26

26-1.

Their responses reflect denial, anger, and blaming as they grieve loss of their ideal pregnancy. The nurse may intervene by accepting these behaviors and using reflective responses, assisting the parents to work through these feelings.

Chapter 27

27-1.

Discuss what she really means by "a glass." Discuss alternatives of nonalcoholic wines. Does she also smoke or take any drugs? Discuss the fetal effects of alcohol consumption in each trimester—First: damage to organs during formation, second: increase of spontaneous abortion, third: interference with growth of fetus.

Chapter 29

29-1.

Notify the NICU team, heat radiant warmer, gather warm towels and blankets, resuscitation medications nearby, check all resuscitation equipment: (1) Bag with premature mask in working order, (2) laryngoscope with small straight blade, (3) endotracheal tubes of various sizes with stylets. Explain to mother and her support person(s) what to expect at the time of delivery.

29-2.

1. Correct answer
2. Despite spontaneous respiration, effort is ineffective to adequately ventilate.
3. These values are abnormal and require prompt intervention.

29-3.

Do not advance if the infant is vomiting, there are large gastric residuals, the abdomen is distended, or bowel sounds are absent.

Index